Procedures

Clinical
Procedures
for Medical
Assistants

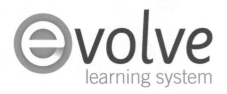 **evolve** learning system

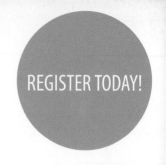 REGISTER TODAY!

To access your Student Resources, visit:

http://evolve.elsevier.com/Bonewit

Register today and gain access to:

- **Interactive Games and Activities**
  - Various activities that provide entertainment while learning important concepts related to the textbook material

- **Animations**
  - Helpful video clips that illustrate chapter concepts

- **Procedure Videos**
  - Videos that provide students with an invaluable learning tool by bringing the chapter procedures to life

ELSEVIER
SAUNDERS

Clinical Procedures for Medical Assistants

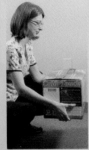
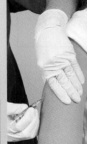

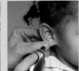
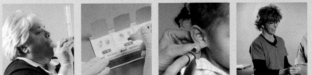

Eighth Edition

Kathy Bonewit-West, BS, MEd

Coordinator and Instructor
Medical Assistant Technology
Hocking College
Nelsonville, Ohio
Former Member, Curriculum Review Board
   of the American Association of Medical Assistants

ELSEVIER
SAUNDERS

ELSEVIER
SAUNDERS

3251 Riverport Lane
St. Louis, Missouri 63043

Executive Editor: Susan Cole
Developmental Editor: Jennifer Bertucci
Publishing Services Manager: Catherine Jackson
Senior Project Manager: Karen M. Rehwinkel
Design Direction: Teresa McBryan

Printed in China

Last digit is the print number: 9 8 7 6 5 4 3 2 1

Reviewers

Jen Gouge, MA, RT
Medical Assisting Coordinator
Peninsula College
Port Angeles, Washington

Carolyn Helms, BS, RMA
Medical Assisting Program Director
Atlanta Technical College
Atlanta, Georgia

Elizabeth Hoffman, MAEd, CMA (AAMA), CPT (ASPT)
Associate Dean of Health Sciences
Baker College of Clinton Township
Clinton Township, Michigan

Kathleen Hudson, BS, MS
Department Chair, Health Care Technology and
    Ambulatory Service
Program Director, Medical Assisting Program
Northern Essex Community College
Lawrence, Massachusetts

Pamela Jeffcoat, MA, CMA (AAMA)
Medical Assisting Program Director
Renton Technical College
Renton, Washington

Belinda King, MA, CMA (AAMA)
Instructor, Medical Assisting Program and Phlebotomy
Gaston College
Dallas, North Carolina

Darlene Kinney, MA, RD, CMA (AAMA)
Medical Assisting Program Director
University of Cincinnati, Clermont College
Batavia, Ohio

Wilsetta McClain, MBA, RMA, NCICS, NCPT, ABD
Phlebotomy Technician Program Department Chair
Baker College
Auburn Hills, Michigan

Christine Mills, MA
Medical Assisting Instructor
Rasmussen College
Ocala, Florida

Diane Morlock, BA, CMA (AAMA)
Medical Assisting Coordinator
Owens Community College
Toledo, Ohio

Lisa Nagle, CMA (AAMA), BS
Medical Assisting Program Director
Augusta Technical College
Augusta, Georgia

Emily Noel, BA
Medical Assisting Instructor
Kaplan University
Des Moines, Iowa

Sarah Olson, MHA, BS
Assistant Chair, School of Health Sciences
Kaplan University
Fort Lauderdale, Florida

Lauren Perlstein, RN, MSN
Medical Assisting Coordinator
Norwalk Community College
Norwalk, Connecticut

Julie Pepper, CMA (AAMA), BS
Medical Assisting Instructor
Chippewa Valley Technical College
Eau Claire, Wisconsin

Ruben Ramos, BS, NCPT, CHI
Medical Assisting Instructor
Southwest Career College, University of Texas El Paso
El Paso, Texas

Valentina Ramos, RN
Medical Assisting Instructor
Michael Berry Career Center
Dearborn, Michigan

Janet Roberts-Andersen, EdD, MT (ASCP)
Assistant Professor, Medical Assisting
Mercy College of Health Sciences
Des Moines, Iowa

Cheryl Steele, RMA
Medical Assisting Instructor
49er Regional Occupational Program
Auburn, California

Cathy Soto, PhD, MBA
Medical Assisting Technology Coordinator
El Paso Community College
El Paso, Texas

Deb Stockberger, MSN, RN
Medical Assisting Program Director
North Iowa Area Community College
Mason City, Iowa

Janice Vermiglio-Smith, RN, MS, PhD
Health Careers District Program Division Chair
Central Arizona College
Apache Junction, Arizona

Lori Warren, MA, RN, CPC, CPC-I, CCP, CLNC
Medical Department Co-Director
Medical Coding/Healthcare Reimbursement Program
    Director and Instructor
AAPC Approved PMCC Instructor
Spencerian College
Louisville, Kentucky

Helen Weeks, MA, BAS, RMA
Medical Assisting Program Director
Henry Ford Community College
Dearborn, Michigan

Dr. Barbara Worley, DPM, DS
Medical Assisting Program Manager
King's College
Charlotte, North Carolina

Shannon Ydoyaga, MS, BBA
Health Professions Program Administrator
Richland College
Dallas, Texas

Your laughter is contagious;
Your determination never swayed;
Your quest for knowledge is heart-warming;
Your generous spirit runs deep;
Your ability to overcome any obstacle is unmatched;
You are the medical assisting students of today and
the future of health care tomorrow.

Preface

Medical assistants, for many years an integral part of most physicians' staff, now fulfill an ever-expanding and varied role in the medical office, both clinically and administratively. With increased responsibilities has come a greater need for professional knowledge and skills. This text has been designed to meet that need.

The underlying principle of the text is to provide a format for the achievement of professional competency in clinical skills performed in the medical office and the understanding of their application to real-life or on-the-job situations. When professional competency is achieved in the classroom, less of a gap should exist between the academic world and the real world, and thus the transition from student to practicing medical assistant is more easily made.

Although I have emphasized the book's usefulness to students in medical assisting training programs, the practicing medical assistant will also find this text helpful as a learning and reference source. The organization of the text lends itself well to individualized instruction and convenient reference use.

NEW FEATURES IN THIS EDITION

In this eighth edition, the text has been expanded to encompass additional clinical procedures and the theory relating to each. This additional material will help students and instructors meet the demand for the increasing number and variety of clinical skills required of the practicing medical assistant by providing the most current and up-to-date procedures performed in the medical office. The reader will find that nearly every chapter incorporates new information to assist in the educational process.

Important Additions Include the Following:

- Expanded information on the Electronic Medical Record
- Current information on the OSHA Bloodborne Pathogens Standard
- Latex glove allergy information
- Automated blood pressure cuff information
- Theory and step-by-step procedure for proper body mechanics and wheelchair transfer of a patient
- Updated pediatric immunization schedule
- Comprehensive updated pharmacology drug table of medications commonly administered and prescribed in the medical office

- Prescriptions and the EMR
- The theory of the two-step tuberculin test
- New guidelines for interpreting tuberculin test results
- Tuberculosis blood test
- Theory and assistance required for mole removal
- The theory and step-by-step procedure for application of a computerized Holter monitor
- The theory and step-by-step procedure for measuring peak flow rate using a peak flow meter
- The theory of home oxygen therapy
- The new fecal immunochemical test and fecal DNA test for detecting occult blood in the stool
- New American Cancer Society recommendations for prostate screening
- Patient preparation for colonoscopy
- Bone density scan
- Expanded information on CLIA-waived testing kits and CLIA-waived automated analyzers
- Expanded information on quality control in the laboratory setting
- Laboratory documents and the EMR
- Red blood cell indices
- The PT/INR laboratory test and PT/INR home testing
- New ADA guidelines for interpreting blood glucose test results

STANDARD PEDAGOGICAL FEATURES IN THIS EDITION

Other very important features to the eighth edition are the inclusion of some valuable learning aids:

- **Resources on the Web** have been completely updated. These resources allow students to access websites containing additional information relating to the chapter.

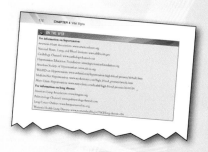

- The organizational format of this edition facilitates the learning process by providing students and educators with detailed objectives and an in-depth study of the most current and up-to-date clinical procedures performed in the medical office. Presented at the beginning of each chapter are **Learning Objectives** and their **related Procedures**, a **Chapter Outline**, and **Key Terms.** The learning objectives address the cognitive knowledge required to perform the procedures. Procedures coincide with the objectives to delineate the task or skill to be mastered by the student. (In the student Study Guide, the procedures are expanded into detailed performance objectives, including outcomes, and conditions and standards of acceptable performance.) The chapter outline provides a quick reference of the cognitive knowledge included in that chapter. The Key Terms list designates the terms that should be mastered for each chapter.

- The **knowledge** or **theory** that the student must acquire to perform each skill is presented in a clear and concise manner. **Numerous illustrations** accompany the theory section to aid the student in acquiring the knowledge relating to each skill.

- **Procedures** for each skill follow the theory section and are designed to help the student perform the skill with the level of competency required on the job. Each procedure is presented in an organized step-by-step format, with underlying principles and illustrations accompanying the techniques. A charting example follows each procedure to provide the student with a guide for charting his or her own procedure. Students should find it much easier to acquire competency in charting with these examples.

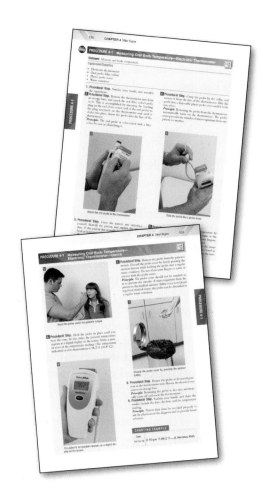

- The unique and memorable medical assistant biographical profiles (**Memories of Externship** and **Putting it All Into Practice**) help students "connect" with their future beyond the classroom. The MAs featured are real people sharing their fears, likes, hopes, and aspirations, providing a "real-world" feel to the book and an inspiration for the student.

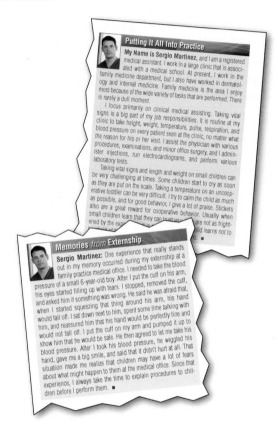

- **Patient Teaching** boxes emphasize this important aspect of the medical assistant's job and present it in context to make it more relevant, thereby making it more memorable.

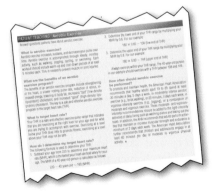

- **Case Studies** are designed to assist the student in responding to "real-life" situations that occur in the medical office. A practitioner's response is also given for each case study as a means of comparison for the student.

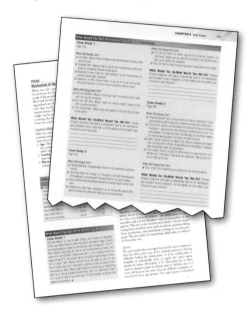

- Key Terms identified at the beginning of the chapter are defined at the end of the chapter in the **Terminology Review,** providing students with a valuable terminology overview for each chapter. Word parts (prefixes, suffixes, and combining forms) for the medical terms are also included in the Terminology Review sections of some chapters to help the student understand the meaning of the medical term through its word parts.

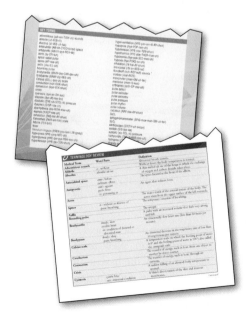

- A **Certification Review** of important points to know after each chapter helps the student to master the important elements covered in the medical assisting certification examination.

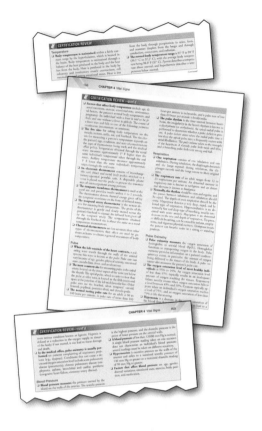

- Legal issues are important for medical assisting students to understand; it is damage control for the medical practice for which they will eventually work. **Medical Practice and the Law** boxes at the end of each chapter provide the student with current legal information pertaining to the chapter.

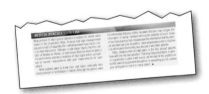

Continuing education is of utmost importance in such a rapidly changing profession. New techniques and developments in the field of medicine have a direct influence on the medical assisting profession. Continuing education helps the medical assistant maintain and improve existing skills and to learn new skills. The AAMA is a professional organization for medical assistants that is dedicated to continuing education. Information on the AAMA can be obtained by writing to:

American Association of Medical Assistants
20 N. Wacker Dr., No.1575
Chicago, IL 60606–2903
312-899-1500
www.aama-ntl.org

It is the author's hope that individuals who use this approach to medical assisting will view this text not as a stopping place but as a means of opening doors to new paths to be explored in the medical assisting profession.

EXTENSIVE SUPPLEMENTAL RESOURCES

Student DVDs

The most impressive feature of this book is the inclusion of clinical skills DVDs that present the skills outlined in the text. (An icon **see DVD** is placed next to the procedures in this text that are included on the DVD.) Students will have the invaluable opportunity to watch these procedures at home on their own DVD players or computers. This should greatly enhance the learning of these clinical skills and provide the medical assistant graduate with competence and confidence in performing clinical skills in the medical office.

Study Guide

The **Study Guide** that accompanies the textbook greatly enhances the learning value of the textbook. Included are extensive exercises for each chapter, practice for competency worksheets and performance evaluation checklists. Pretests, posttests, and apply your knowledge questions help better prepare students for chapter tests. Textbook and Study Guide assignment sheets are incorporated into the study guide for documenting completion of assignments and calculating points earned for each assignment. Laboratory assignment sheets allow the student to keep track of performance of procedures. New to this edition are video evaluation sheets that assess the student's knowledge of key points in the clinical skills presented on the DVDs accompanying the textbook. Also new to this edition are Practicum Activity worksheets that are completed at the student's practicum site. These worksheets assist the student in relating classroom knowledge to the "real-world" setting of the medical office.

Evolve Resources

The Evolve site (http://evolve.elsevier.com/Bonewit) includes all instructors' materials (for instructors only), content updates, weblinks, and a link to Clinical Medical Assisting Online.

The Evolve site offers many opportunities for students to apply the theory and skills learned throughout the textbook. Organized by chapter, the Evolve site includes several games (i.e., "Quiz Show" and "Road to Recovery") to provide entertainment while learning important concepts related to selected chapters, matching exercises, labeling exercises, identification exercises, and other helpful activities for the student.

Clinical Medical Assisting Online

Completely revised and up-to-date, Clinical Medical Assisting Online is a complete online course that can stand alone as a distance education course (when combined with an on-site lab component) or provide additional reinforcement to a traditional classroom course. It covers all key accredited clinical competencies in an exciting, interactive format.

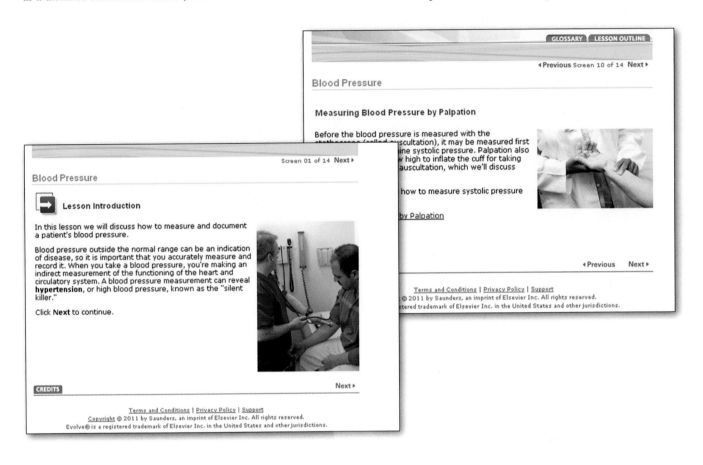

Acknowledgments

The completion of the eighth edition of this text permits the opportunity to relay appreciation to the medical assisting educators who so eagerly and enthusiastically use and enjoy this text. To them I am also indebted for their helpful assistance and suggestions for the eighth edition.

The following professionals served as invaluable consultants and reviewers and deserve special recognition and appreciation:

Sharlene K. Aasen, CMA.-C, Globe College, Oakdale, Minnesota.

Diana Bennett, RN, BSN, MAT, Indiana Vocational Technical College, Indianapolis, Indiana.

Julie A. Benson, AS, RMA, RPhbt, EKG, Medical Program Director, Platt College, Tulsa, Oklahoma.

Cathy Bierly, CMA, Athens Obstetrics and Gynecology, Athens, Ohio.

Lisa Breitbard, AA, LVN, Maric College of Medical Careers, San Diego, California.

Carol S. Champagne, RMA, CMA-C, ICEA, CCE, Clearwater Family Practice Clinic, Clearwater, Kansas; Chairperson, RMA, Continuing Education Committee; Certified Childbirth Education, Private Practice.

Gary A. Clarke, PhD, Assistant Professor of Biology, Roanoke College, Salem, Virginia.

Beverly G. Dugas, TN, Douglas College, New Westminster, British Columbia, Canada.

Amy Fought, CMA, Medical Assistant, Athens, Ohio.

Julie D. Franklin, MT(ASCP), MHE, Former Program Director, Medical Office Assisting, Chattanooga State Technical Community College, Chattanooga, Tennessee.

Cathy Goodwin, CMA-AC, Medical Assistant, San Diego, California.

Jeanne Howard, CMA, AAS, Medical Assisting Technology, El Paso Community College, El Paso, Texas.

Susan K. Ipacs, RN, MS, Associate Dean, School of Nursing, Hocking College, Nelsonville, Ohio.

Gail I. Jones, MS, MT(ASCP), Dettman-Connell School of Medical Technology, Fort Worth, Texas.

Jeannette Keiter, CMA, Athens Orthopedic Center, Athens, Ohio.

Richard W. Kocon, PhD, Laboratory Director, Damon Medical Laboratory, Inc., Needham Heights, Massachusetts.

Louis Komarmy, MD, Clinical Pathologist, Children's Hospital, San Francisco, California.

Albert B. Lowenfels, MD, Associate Director of Surgery, Westchester County Medical Center, Valhalla, New York.

Susan J. Matthews, RN, BSN, MEd, Watterson College, Louisville, Kentucky.

Sharon McCaughrin, CMA, Corporate Director of Education, Ross Medical Education Centers, Warren, Michigan.

Tracy Metcalf, CMA, Office Manager, Athens Bone and Joint Surgery, Athens, Ohio.

Deborah Montone, BS, RN, RMA, LLS-P, RCS, Dean of Academics, Hohokus School of Medical Sciences, Ramsey, New Jersey.

Sally A. Murdock, BSN, MS, RN, California Public Health Nursing Certification, Medical Assisting, San Diego Mesa College, San Diego, California.

Kathryn L. Murphy, RN, CMA, Medical Program Director, Department Chair, and Instructor, Springfield College, Springfield, Missouri.

Donna F. Otis, LPN, Medical Instructor, MAA Program, Metro Business College, Rolla, Missouri.

Raymond E. Phillips, MD, FACP, Senior Attending Physician, Phelps Memorial Hospital, North Tarrytown, New York.

Traci Powell, CMA, University Medical Associates, Athens, Ohio.

Vicki Prater, CMA, Concorde Career Institute, San Bernardino, California.

Linda Reed, Indiana Vocational Technical College, Indianapolis, Indiana.

Marjorie J. Reif, PA-C, CMA, Rochester Community College, Rochester, Minnesota.

Alan M. Rosich, Instructor of Radiologic Technology, Lorain County Community College, Elvira, Ohio.

Kimberly Rubesne, MA, Median School of Allied Health Careers, Pittsburgh, Pennsylvania.

Lynn G. Slack, CMA, ICM School of Business and Medical Careers, Pittsburgh, Pennsylvania.

Robin Snider-Flohr, MBA, RN, CMA, Jefferson Community College, Steubenville, Ohio.

Edward R. Stapleton, EMT-P, Assistant Clinical Professor and Director of Prehospital Care and Education, Department of Emergency Medicine, School of Medicine, University Hospital and Medical Center, State University of New York, Stony Brook, New York.

Rachel Stapleton, CMA, Neal J. Nesbitt, MD, Athens, Ohio.

Sandra E. Sterling, MT(ASCP), Boulder Valley Vocational-Technical School, Boulder, Colorado.

Marie Thomas, CLT(NCA), Berdan Institute, Totowa, New Jersey.

Joan K. Werner, PT, PhD, Director, Physical Therapy Program, University of Wisconsin, Madison, Wisconsin.

The photographs in the textbook were taken by Brian Blauser and Jack Foley, professional photographers. I am indebted to them for their careful precision and patience in taking and editing the photographs, thus greatly enhancing the learning value of this text.

A very special thanks to Marlene Donovan, Dawn Shingler, Kim Link, and Alisha Brown-Lewis for their dedication and hard work, not only on this edition, but also in the field of medical assisting education as a whole. They have contributed immensely to the recognition of medical assisting students and practitioners as valued members of the health care community.

I would like to gratefully acknowledge the following practicing medical assistants for contributing many hours to be photographed for demonstration of the clinical procedures in the text: Diana Arnold, Megan Baer, Dawn Bennett, Heather Bobo, Danielle Brown, Trudy Browning, Janet Canterbury, Theresa Cline, Marlyne Cooper, Hope Fauber, Dori Glover, Jennifer Hawk, Kevin Hickey, Cammie Lindner, Judy Markins, Korey McGrew, Natalie Morehead, Amber Nelson, Larry Nye, Traci Powell, Linda Proffitt, Latisha Sharpe, Michelle Shockey, Kara Van Dyke, Michelle Villers, and Huang Ying.

I would also like to acknowledge the following individuals who portrayed patients in the photographs in the text: Brian Adevc, David Arnold, Connie Arthur, Jessica Bennett, Kim Bingham, Pamela Bitting, Caitlin Brennan, David Brennan, Hollie Bonewit, LeAnn Brown, Phillip Carr, Chloe Cline, Angie Coffin, Chad Cron, Dawn Decaminada, Aja Fox, Markly Georges, Connie Hazlett, Gary Hazlett, Kyra Horn, Isabella Ipacs, Joey Ipacs, Susan Ipacs, Braylin Kemp, Charles Larimer, Pam Larimer, Christopher Mace, Mickey Midkiff, Deborah Murray, Delaney Murray, Michael Nkrumah, Heather Pike, Jan Six, Megan Skidmore, Colton Smith, Sydney Smith, Clinton Swart, Melanie Walker, Tristen West, and Lynn Witkowski.

I would like to extend my appreciation to the authors, publishers, and equipment companies who have granted me permission to use their illustrations.

The publication of the eighth edition was accomplished through the capable guidance of many talented individuals at Elsevier. Many thanks to Karen Rehwinkel for her outstanding production work. This edition could not have attained this level of excellence without the exceptional capabilities of Jennifer Bertucci, Developmental Editor. I want to relay a very special thank you to Michael Ledbetter, Publisher, for his dedication to quality medical assisting education and his encouragement in helping me achieve my very best in this edition.

With warm regard, I would like to recognize those very important individuals—the medical assisting students, graduates, and practicing medical assistants—who continually strive for excellence in meeting the demands and ever-increasing requirements of such a challenging profession. A quote by an unknown author really says it better: "Celebrate your talents, for they are what make you unique."

Kathy Bonewit-West, BS, MEd

Clinical Procedure Icons

The OSHA Bloodborne Pathogens Standard must be followed when performing many of the clinical procedures presented in this text. To assist the student in following the OSHA Standard, icons have been incorporated into the procedures. An illustration of each icon along with its description is outlined below.

HAND HYGIENE is an important medical aseptic practice and is crucial in preventing the transmission of pathogens in the medical office. The medical assistant should sanitize his or her hands frequently, using proper technique. When performing clinical procedures, the hands should always be sanitized before and after patient contact, before applying gloves and after removing gloves, and after contact with blood or other potentially infectious materials.

CLEAN DISPOSABLE GLOVES should be worn when it is reasonably anticipated that you will have hand contact with the following: blood and other potentially infectious materials, mucous membranes, nonintact skin, and contaminated articles or surfaces.

BIOHAZARD CONTAINERS are closable, leakproof, and suitably constructed to contain the contents during handling, storage, transport, or shipping. The containers must be labeled or color coded and closed before removal to prevent the contents from spilling.

APPROPRIATE PROTECTIVE CLOTHING such as gowns, aprons, and laboratory coats should be worn when gross contamination can reasonably be anticipated during performance of a task or procedure.

FACE SHIELDS OR MASKS IN COMBINATION WITH EYE-PROTECTION DEVICES must be worn whenever splashes, spray, spatter, or droplets of blood or other potentially infectious materials may be generated and pose a hazard through contact with your eyes, nose, or mouth.

Contents

1

The Medical Record

LEARNING OBJECTIVES

Components of the Medical Record
1. List and describe the functions served by the medical record.
2. Identify the information contained in each of the following medical office administrative documents: patient registration record NPP form, and correspondence.
3. Identify the information contained in each of the following medical office clinical documents: health history report, physical examination report, progress notes, medication record, consultation report, and home health care report.
4. State the purpose of a laboratory report and describe the information included in each of the following categories of laboratory reports: hematology, clinical chemistry, immunology, urinalysis, microbiology, parasitology, cytology, and histology.
5. List and describe the information included in each of the following diagnostic procedure documents: electrocardiogram report, Holter monitor report, sigmoidoscopy report, colonoscopy report, spirometry report, radiology report, and diagnostic imaging report.
6. State the purpose of each of the following therapeutic services: physical therapy, occupational therapy, and speech therapy.
7. Identify the information contained in each of the following hospital documents: history and physical report, operative report, discharge summary report, pathology report, and emergency department report.

Consent Documents
1. Identify the information contained in each of the following consent documents: consent to treatment form and release of medical information form.

Types of Medical Records
1. Explain the difference between a PPR and an EMR.
2. List the general functions of electronic medical record (EMR) software.
3. Explain the advantages and disadvantages of EMRs.
4. List the procedures performed by the physician and medical assistant using an EMR.

Medical Record Formats
1. Describe the organization of a source-oriented medical record and a problem-oriented medical record.
2. List and define the four subcategories included in the progress notes of a problem-oriented record (POR).

Health History
1. List and describe the seven parts of the health history.
2. List the guidelines that should be followed in recording the chief complaint.

PROCEDURES

Prepare a medical record for a new patient.

Obtain patient consent for treatment.
Assist a patient in completing a release of medical information form.
Release information according to a completed release of medical information form.

Identify the parts of a source-oriented medical record and a problem-oriented medical record.

Complete or assist the patient in completing a health history form.

1

Charting

1. List and describe the guidelines to follow to ensure accurate and concise charting.
2. List and describe the types of progress notes that are charted by the medical assistant.
3. List examples of subjective symptoms and objective symptoms.
4. List and describe common symptoms.

Chart the following:
- Procedures
- Administration of medication
- Specimen collection
- Laboratory tests
- Progress notes
- Instructions given to the patient

Obtain and record patient symptoms.

CHAPTER OUTLINE

Introduction to the Medical Record
Components of the Medical Record
Medical Office Administrative Documents
Patient Registration Record
NPP Acknowledgment Form
Correspondence
Medical Office Clinical Documents
Health History Report
Physical Examination Report
Progress Notes
Medication Record
Consultation Report
Home Health Care Report
Laboratory Documents
Hematology
Clinical Chemistry
Immunology
Urinalysis
Microbiology
Parasitology
Cytology
Histology
Diagnostic Procedure Documents
Electrocardiogram Report
Holter Monitor Report
Sigmoidoscopy Report
Colonoscopy Report
Spirometry Report
Radiology Report
Diagnostic Imaging Report

Therapeutic Service Documents
Physical Therapy
Occupational Therapy
Speech Therapy
Hospital Documents
History and Physical Report
Operative Report
Discharge Summary Report
Pathology Report
Emergency Department Report
Consent Documents
Consent to Treatment Form
Release of Medical Information Form
Types of Medical Records
Electronic Medical Record
Medical Record Formats
Source-Oriented Record
Problem-Oriented Record
Preparing a Medical Record for a New Patient
Medical Record Supplies
Taking a Health History
Components of the Health History
Charting in the Medical Record
Charting Guidelines
Charting Progress Notes
Charting Patient Symptoms
Other Activities that Need to Be Charted

KEY TERMS

attending physician
charting
consultation report
diagnosis (dye-ag-NOE-sis)
diagnostic procedure
discharge summary report
electronic medical record (EMR)
familial (fah-MIL-yul)

health history report
home health care
informed consent
inpatient
medical impressions
medical record
medical record format
objective symptom

paper-based patient record (PPR)
patient
physical examination
physical examination report
problem

prognosis (prog-NOE-sis)
reverse chronological order
SOAP
subjective symptom
symptom (SIMP-tum)

Introduction to the Medical Record

Medical records are a crucial part of a medical practice. A **medical record** is a written record of the important information regarding a patient, including the care of that individual and the progress of his or her condition. A **patient** is defined as an individual receiving medical care.

The patient's medical record serves many important functions. The physician uses the information in the medical record as a basis for decisions regarding the patient's care and treatment. The medical record documents the results of treatment and the patient's progress. The medical record provides an efficient and effective method by which information can be communicated to authorized personnel in the medical office.

The medical record also serves as a legal document. The law requires that a record be maintained to document the care and treatment being received by a patient. If something goes wrong, good documentation works to protect the physician and the medical staff legally. Incomplete records could be used as evidence in court to show that a patient did not receive the quality of care that meets generally accepted standards.

The medical assistant must always keep in mind that the information contained in a patient's medical record is strictly confidential and must not be read by or discussed with anyone except the physician or medical staff involved with the care of the patient (see *Highlight on the HIPAA Privacy Rule*).

COMPONENTS OF THE MEDICAL RECORD

A medical record consists of numerous documents. Each document in the medical record has a specific function or purpose. Most of these documents are preprinted forms that contain specific information entered by a physician or other health professionals. A large variety of forms are available; the type of form used is based on the specific requirements of each medical office.

Medical record documents can be classified into categories. Each of these categories is outlined in the box on page 6 along with the specific documents included in each.

It is important that the medical assistant be familiar with each type of document in the medical record. A description of the function or purpose of each type of medical record document follows (by category), along with the specific information that each contains.

MEDICAL OFFICE ADMINISTRATIVE DOCUMENTS

Administrative documents contain information necessary for the efficient (record-keeping) management of the medical office. Medical office administrative documents include the patient registration record and patient-related correspondence.

Patient Registration Record

The patient registration record (Figure 1-1) consists of demographic and billing information. All new patients must complete a patient registration record form. After the patient completes the registration record, the medical assistant enters the information into a computer. This allows the demographic and billing information to be used for numerous computerized functions, such as scheduling appointments, posting patient transactions, and processing patient statements and insurance claims. The original patient registration record is placed in the front of the patient's medical record.

Demographic Information

Demographic information required on a patient registration form includes the following:
- Full name
- Address
- Telephone number (home and work)
- Date of birth
- Gender
- Marital status
- Employer

Billing Information

Billing information is required to bill charges to the patient or an insurance company. Billing information required on a patient registration form includes the following:
- Name of responsible party (person responsible for the account)
- Social security number
- Address of responsible party
- Name of insured (policyholder)

Highlight on the HIPAA Privacy Rule

What Is the HIPAA Privacy Rule?

The acronym *HIPAA* stands for the *Health Insurance Portability and Accountability Act.* HIPAA is a federal law consisting of several components, one of which contains provisions to protect a patient's privacy, known as the HIPAA Privacy Rule.

The HIPAA Privacy Rule went into effect on April 14, 2003. The primary purpose of this rule is to provide patients with better control over the use and disclosure of their health information. All health care providers, health plans, and health care clearinghouses (e.g., billing services) that use, store, maintain, or transmit health information must comply with this rule.

What Is Included in the HIPAA Privacy Rule?

The HIPAA Privacy Rule is outlined here as it relates to the medical office:

1. The medical office must develop a written document known as a Notice of Privacy Practices (NPP). The NPP must explain to patients how their protected health information (PHI) will be used and protected by the medical office. *Protected health information* includes health information in any form (written, electronic, or oral) that contains patient-identifiable information (e.g., name, social security number, telephone number). The medical office must make a reasonable effort to provide an NPP to each patient and to obtain a signed acknowledgment from the patient that he or she has received an NPP.
2. A patient's written consent is not required for the use or disclosure of PHI for the following:
   - Medical treatment: *Examples:*
     (1) Patient referral to a specialist
     (2) Emergency care provided at a hospital
     (3) Tests on a patient performed by the laboratory
   - Payment: *Examples:*
     (1) Determination of eligibility for insurance benefits
     (2) Review of services provided for medical necessity
     (3) Utilization review activities
   - Health care operations: *Examples:*
     (1) Quality assessment activities
     (2) Contacting patients with information about care or treatment
     (3) Employee review activities
     (4) Training of health care students

3. Patients have the right to access their medical records and to request changes to the records if they believe them to be inaccurate.
4. To prevent unnecessary or inappropriate access to PHI, the medical office must make an effort to limit the use of, disclosure of, and requests for PHI to the minimum necessary to accomplish the intended purpose (e.g., a request from an insurance company for procedures performed on a patient). This requirement does not apply, however, to the use of PHI for the routine practice of medicine within the medical office.
5. Patients have a right to request an accounting of the transfer of their information for purposes other than treatment, payment, or health care operations.
6. Business associates to whom the medical office may disclose PHI must respect the HIPAA Privacy Rule. The medical office must execute a written agreement with each business associate to handle PHI in accordance with HIPAA. Business associates may include the following organizations and firms:
   - Medical laboratories
   - Transcription services
   - Law firms
   - Accounting firms
   - Software and hardware consultants
   - Billing services
7. The medical office must implement for all employees a basic training program on privacy and security of PHI.
8. The medical office is required to put in place appropriate administrative, physical, and technical security safeguards to protect the privacy of PHI from accidental use or disclosure or violation of the above-listed requirements.

What if a Medical Office Does *Not* Comply With the HIPAA Privacy Rule?

There are severe penalties if a medical office fails to comply with the HIPAA Privacy Rule, which can include civil and criminal penalties.

Where Can More Information on the HIPAA Privacy Rule Be Found?

The following websites contain current information on HIPAA:
   www.cms.hhs.gov/hipaa
   www.hhs.gov/ocr/privacy

- Insurance company
- Policy number and group number

NPP Acknowledgment Form

A Notice of Privacy Practices (NPP) is a written document that explains to patients how their protected health information will be used and protected by the medical office. The patient must sign a form acknowledging that he or she has received the NPP. The NPP form is then filed in the patient's chart.

Correspondence

Correspondence is an important part of the medical record. Correspondence regarding a patient may be received from various individuals or facilities, such as the patient's insurance company, the patient's attorney, and the patient himself or herself. Insurance correspondence includes such documents as a precertification authorization for a hospital admission and a request for additional information from the insurance company. Correspondence also includes copies of

PATIENT INFORMATION	CONFIDENTIAL		

File no. 10140
Date 11-21-12

(PLEASE PRINT)

Name: Carol (First) H (Middle) Jones (Last)   Birth date 1-20-68   Home phone 740-555-1248

Address 743 Evergreen Terrace   City Springfield   State OH   ZIP 12345

Check appropriate box: ☐ Minor ☐ Single ☒ Married ☐ Divorced ☐ Widowed ☐ Separated   Gender: ☐ Male ☒ Female

Employer Rockford, Inc.   Work phone 740-555-1234

Business address 1 Rockford Place   City Shelbyville   State OH   ZIP 21346

Spouse or parent's name John Jones   Employer Self-emp.   Work phone 740-555-8654

If patient is a student, name of school/college N/A   City ____ State ____

Whom may we thank for referring you? Henry Peterson, MD

Person to contact in case of emergency John Jones   Phone 740-555-1248

RESPONSIBLE PARTY

Name of person responsible for this account Carol Jones   Relationship to patient Self

Address 743 Evergreen Terrace   City Springfield   State OH   ZIP 12345   Home phone 740-555-1248

Employer Rockford, Inc.   Work phone 740-555-1234

Is this person currently a patient in our office? ☒ Yes   ☐ No

INSURANCE INFORMATION

Name of insured Carol Jones   Relationship to patient Self

Birth date 1-20-68   Social Security number 123-45-6789   Date employed 5-1-93

Name of employer Rockford, Inc.   Work phone 740-555-1234

Address of employer 1 Rockford Place   City Shelbyville   State OH   ZIP 21346

Insurance company Anthem BC/BS   Group number 51045

Insurance company address 521 Anthem Drive   City New Haberville   State OH   ZIP 21436

DO YOU HAVE ANY ADDITIONAL INSURANCE? ☐ YES ☒ NO   IF YES, COMPLETE THE FOLLOWING:

Name of insured ____   Relationship to patient ____

Birth date ____   Social Security number ____   Date employed ____

Name of employer ____   Work phone ____

Address of employer ____   City ____   State ____ ZIP ____

Insurance company ____   Group number ____

Insurance company address ____   City ____   State ____ ZIP ____

X *Carol Jones*

SIGNATURE OF PATIENT OR PARENT IF MINOR

Figure 1-1. Patient registration record. (Courtesy of and modified from Colwell Systems, Champaign, Ill.)

What Would You Do? What Would You *Not* Do?

Case Study 1

Moira Celeste, an account executive for a large insurance company, comes to the office complaining of insomnia and depression. Three months ago, her husband of 27 years left, and now they are legally separated. Since then, Moira has had a lot of trouble sleeping at night. She also feels lethargic during the day and hasn't been eating much. Moira says that she's been having some problems with alcohol. She wants to know of any community agencies that could help her with her problem but that would be sure to keep the information confidential. She has a very responsible job with her firm and does not want anyone to know about her alcohol problem. She also does not want any information about her problem put in her chart, and she especially does not want the physician to know about it because he is friends with many of her colleagues at work. ■

Categories of Medical Record Documents

Medical Office Administrative Documents
- Patient registration record
- NPP acknowledgment form
- Correspondence

Medical Office Clinical Documents
- Health history report
- Physical examination report
- Progress notes
- Medication record
- Consultation report
- Home health care report

Laboratory Documents
- Hematology report
- Clinical chemistry report

Laboratory Documents—cont'd
- Immunology report
- Urinalysis report
- Microbiology report
- Parasitology report
- Cytology report
- Histology report

Diagnostic Procedure Documents
- Electrocardiogram report
- Holter monitor report
- Sigmoidoscopy report
- Colonoscopy report
- Spirometry report
- Radiology report
- Diagnostic imaging report

Therapeutic Service Documents
- Physical therapy report
- Occupational therapy report
- Speech therapy report

Hospital Documents
- History and physical report
- Operative report
- Discharge summary report
- Pathology report
- Emergency department report

Consent Documents
- Consent to treatment form
- Release of medical information form

Putting It All Into Practice

My Name is Dawn Bennett, and I work for an orthopedic surgeon. I work in the front area of the office as an administrative supervisor in billing and collections.

Working in billing and collections is very challenging and sometimes stressful. It can even be embarrassing. We are a new practice, and when we opened, there was no collection system. When it came time to review our accounts, we realized that, like every other business, we needed a collection system. We immediately jumped in and took charge.

The primary physician at our office is from New York, and we were unfamiliar with his family members. One day he walked into our office with a very puzzled look. I asked him what was wrong. He replied, "You guys are doing a great job with our collection rate. I asked you to be stern, but thoughtful, when sending out patient collection letters, but did you have to send one to my mother-in-law?!" Needless to say, we fixed the error immediately. This incident prompted us to restructure our collection system, and we added a comment screen to our computer system on all of our patients' accounts. Going into a medical office that already has a system in place may be easier, but you can learn a lot more by setting up an office system yourself. ■

letters concerning the patient that are sent out of the office; examples are a copy of a letter referring the patient to a specialist and a copy of a collection letter sent to the patient.

MEDICAL OFFICE CLINICAL DOCUMENTS

Medical office clinical documents include a variety of records and reports that assist the physician in the care and treatment of the patient. Common medical office clinical documents are listed and described next.

Health History Report

A **health history report** is a collection of subjective data about the patient. Most of this information is obtained by having the patient complete a preprinted form that is then reviewed for completeness by the medical assistant. Some of the information included in the health history is obtained by the physician or medical assistant by interviewing the patient.

Along with the physical examination and laboratory and diagnostic tests, the health history is used for the following reasons: to determine the patient's general state of health, to arrive at a diagnosis and to prescribe treatment, and to document any change in a patient's illness after treatment has been instituted. The term **diagnosis** refers to the scientific method of determining and identifying a patient's condition.

A thorough history of personal health is obtained for each new patient, and subsequent office visits provide additional information regarding changes in the patient's condition or treatment. A complete discussion of the health history report is presented later in this chapter.

Physical Examination Report

A **physical examination** is an assessment of each part of the patient's body. The purpose of the physical examination is to provide objective data about the patient, which assists the physician in determining the patient's state of health. (The physical examination is described in detail in Chapter 5.)

The **physical examination report** is a summary of the physician's findings from the assessment of each part of the patient's body and includes the following:
- General appearance
- Head and neck
- Eyes

- Ears
- Nose
- Mouth and pharynx
- Arms and hands
- Chest and lungs
- Heart
- Breasts
- Abdomen
- Genitalia and rectum
- Legs and feet

Progress Notes

Progress notes involve updating the medical record with new information each time the patient visits or telephones the medical office. Progress notes serve to document the patient's health status from one visit to the next. It is important that the date and time be included with each progress note, along with the signature and credentials of the individual making the entry. A thorough discussion of charting progress notes is presented later in this chapter.

Medication Record

A medication record consists of detailed information related to a patient's medications. The record may include one or more of the following categories: prescription medications, over-the-counter (OTC) medications, and medications ad-

ministered at the medical office. Most medical offices use one form to record prescription and OTC medications and another form to record medications administered to the patient at the medical office.

Prescription and Over-the-Counter Medication Record Form

A medication record form for recording the patient's prescription and OTC medications includes the following:
- Patient's name and date of birth
- Drug allergies
- Date the patient began taking the medication
- Name of the medication
- Dosage
- Frequency of administration of the medication
- Route of administration
- Refills (prescription medications only)
- Date the patient stopped taking the medication

Medication Administration Record Form

A form for recording medications administered to the patient at the medical office (Figure 1-2) includes the following:
- Patient's name and date of birth
- Drug allergies
- Name of the medication
- Dosage administered
- Route of administration

MEDICATION ADMINISTRATION RECORD								
PATIENT NAME _Kristen Antle_				BIRTH DATE _1/9/84_				
ALLERGIES _Ø_								

SITE ABBREVIATIONS:

RD: Right deltoid   RDG: Right dorsogluteal   RVL: Right vastus lateralis
LD: Left deltoid   LDG: Left dorsogluteal   LVL: Left vastus lateralis

MEDICATION AND DOSAGE	ROUTE	DATE	MANUFACTURER	LOT#	EXP DATE	SITE	ADMIN BY
Rocephin 500 mg	IM	2/5/12	Roche	1053	10/5/13	RDG	D. Bennett, CMA (AAMA)
Depo-Provera 150 mg	IM	8/14/12	Pharmacia & Upjohn	68FUF	12/5/12	LDG	D. Bennett, CMA (AAMA)
Fluzone 0.5 ml	IM	11/4/12	Aventis Pasteur	OF1120	6/10/13	RD	D. Bennett, CMA (AAMA)
Depo-Provera 150 mg	IM	11/4/12	Pharmacia & Upjohn	87FUF	12/7/13	RDG	D. Bennett, CMA (AAMA)

Figure 1-2. Medication record.

- Injection site
- Date of administration
- Manufacturer, lot number, and expiration date of the medication
- Signature and credentials of the individual administering the medication

Consultation Report

A **consultation report** is a narrative report of a clinical opinion about a patient's condition by a practitioner other than the primary physician, known as a *consultant* (Figure 1-3). The consultant is usually a specialist in a certain field of medicine (e.g., cardiology, endocrinology, urology). The consultant's opinion of the patient's condition is based on a review of the patient's record and an examination of the patient. The consultation report must include the following:

- Documentation that the consultant reviewed the patient's health history
- Documentation that the consultant examined the patient
- A report of the consultant's impressions
- Any care or treatment provided by the consultant
- A report of the consultant's recommendations

Home Health Care Report

Home health care is the provision of medical and non-medical care in a patient's home or place of residence. The purpose of home health care is to minimize the effect of disease or disability by promoting, maintaining, and restoring the patient's health. There is a growing preference for home health care over equivalent health care options. Research shows that familiar surroundings contribute positively to a patient's emotional and physical well-being.

Home health care must be ordered by the patient's physician and is provided by skilled professionals. Home health care professionals include nurses, home health aides, dietitians, physical therapists, occupational therapists, speech therapists, and social workers. Examples of specialized services available through home health care include cardiac home care, intravenous (IV) therapy, respiratory therapy, pain management, diabetes management, rehabilitation, and maternal-child care. Home health care providers must periodically provide a summary report (Figure 1-4) to the patient's physician that includes the following:

- Observations and evaluations
- Type of care or service provided
- Instructions given to the patient on medications
- Safety measures recommended for the home
- Diet
- Activities permitted

LABORATORY DOCUMENTS

A laboratory report is a report of the analysis or examination of body specimens. Its purpose is to relay the results of laboratory tests to the physician to assist in diagnosing and treating disease. A thorough discussion of laboratory documents is presented in Chapter 15. The specific categories of laboratory tests follow.

Hematology

Laboratory analysis in hematology deals with the examination and analysis of blood for the detection of abnormalities and includes areas such as blood cell counts, cellular morphology, clotting ability of the blood, and identification of cell types.

Clinical Chemistry

Laboratory analysis in clinical chemistry involves detecting the presence of chemical substances and determining the amount of these substances in body fluids, excreta, and tissues (e.g., blood, urine, cerebrospinal fluid). The largest area in clinical chemistry is blood chemistry.

Immunology

Laboratory analysis in immunology deals with studying antigen-antibody reactions to assess the presence of a substance or to determine the presence of disease.

Urinalysis

Laboratory analysis in urinalysis involves the physical, chemical, and microscopic analysis of urine.

Microbiology

Laboratory analysis in microbiology deals with the identification of pathogens in specimens taken from the body (e.g., urine, blood, throat, sputum, wound, urethral, vaginal, cerebrospinal).

Parasitology

Laboratory analysis in parasitology deals with the detection of disease-producing human parasites or eggs in specimens taken from the body (e.g., stool, vaginal, blood).

Cytology

Laboratory analysis in cytology deals with the detection of abnormal cells.

Histology

Laboratory analysis in histology deals with the detection of diseased tissues.

DIAGNOSTIC PROCEDURE DOCUMENTS

A diagnostic procedure report consists of a narrative description and interpretation of a diagnostic procedure. A **diagnostic procedure** is a type of procedure performed to assist in the diagnosis, management, or treatment of a patient's condition. The procedure may be performed by a physician, the medical assistant, or a technician specially trained in the procedure. A physician is responsible for in-

HAROLD B. COOPER, M.D.
6000 MAIN STREET
VENTURA, CA 93003

June 15, 2012

John F. Millstone, M.D.
5302 Main Street
Ventura, CA 93003

Dear Dr. Millstone:

RE: Elaine J. Silverman

This 69-year-old woman was seen at your request. The patient was admitted to the hospital yesterday because of chills, fever, and abdominal and back pain.

REVIEW OF HEALTH HISTORY: The history has been reviewed. A prominent feature of the history is the presence of intermittent, severe, shaking chills for four days with associated left lower back pain, left lower quadrant abdominal pain, and fever to as high as 103 or 104 degrees. The patient has had hypertension for a number of years and has been managed quite well with Aldomet 250 mg twice a day.

PHYSICAL EXAMINATION: On examination her temperature at this time is 100.6 degrees. The pulse is 110 and regular. Blood pressure is 190/100. The patient has partial bilateral iridectomies, the result of previous cataract surgery. Otherwise, the head and neck are not remarkable. Lung fields are clear throughout. The heart reveals a regular tachycardia, and heart sounds are of good quality. No murmurs are heard, and there is no gallop rhythm present. The abdomen is soft. There is no spasm or guarding. A well-healed surgical scar is present in the right flank area. There is considerable tenderness in the left lower quadrant of the left mid abdomen, but as noted, there is no spasm or guarding present. Bowel sounds are present. Peristaltic rushes are noted, and the bowel sounds are slightly high pitched. The extremities are unremarkable.

IMPRESSIONS: I believe the patient has acute diverticulitis. She may have some irritation of the left ureter in view of the findings on the urinalysis. She appears to be responding to therapy at this time in that her temperature is coming down and there has been a slight reduction in the leukocytosis from yesterday.

RECOMMENDATIONS: I agree with the present program of therapy, and the only suggestion would be to possibly increase the dose of gentamicin to 60 mg q8h, rather than the 40 mg q8h that she is now receiving.

Thank you for asking me to see this patient in consultation.

Sincerely,

Harold B. Cooper

Harold B. Cooper, M.D.

mtf

Figure 1-3. Consultation report. (Modified from Diehl MO: Medical transcription: techniques and procedures, ed 6, St Louis, 2007, Saunders.)

Form 3514/2 (if 2-part set) or
Form 3514/3 (if 3-part set)

BRIGGS, Des Moines, IA 50306 (800) 247-2343
PRINTED IN U.S.A.

Home Health Agency — Visit Report

| Date of Visit | 11/21/12 | Start: 7 | Mileage | Finish: 9 |

Patient's Name: Clarence Castor

BP: (L): 160/82   (R): 160/82   T: 97.7

P: (A): 78   (R): 76   Wt.: 151   R: 18

Financial:		Med. A:		Med. B:
GH:	VA:		Pvt:	Other: Hospice
Area:			Diagnosis: Lung cancer	
Procedures:			Age: 74	

Pt. Instruction: Continue O₂ as needed

Comments/Observations: (Physical, mental, emotional, activity level, Environ., S/S, Treatments & Effects, Procedures, Med. Effects, Other)

Pt complaining of some difficulty breathing and swelling of his feet. Pt was given Proventil Atrovent neb tx

and started on oxygen at 2 liters per nasal cannula. Tx was discussed with Dr. Shay.

Plan: Monitor vitals every 2 hrs.

Supplies Used: O₂ @ 2 liters

Signature: D. Talley, RN

Next Visit: 11/22/12	RN √	PT	HHA	MSW	Other
Freq. of Visits: daily	√				
Travel Time:			Service Time:		

Supervisory Visit:

Form 3514 © BRIGGS, Des Moines, IA 50306 (800) 247-2343 PRINTED IN U.S.A.

Figure 1-4. Home health care report. (Form Number 3514. Courtesy Briggs, Des Moines.)

terpreting the results of the diagnostic procedure and completing the written report. Examples of diagnostic procedure reports follow.

Electrocardiogram Report

An electrocardiogram (ECG) report is a narrative description of a cardiologist's interpretation of an ECG, including the implications for the patient. The graphic tracing is usually included with the report.

Holter Monitor Report

A Holter monitor report is a narrative description of the interpretation of a 24-hour ambulatory ECG, including the evaluator's impressions. Portions of the graphic tracing are usually included with the report.

Sigmoidoscopy Report

A sigmoidoscopy report is a narrative description of the interpretation of a sigmoidoscopic examination, including the practitioner's impressions.

Colonoscopy Report

A colonoscopy report is a narrative description of a colonoscopic examination, including the practitioner's impressions.

Spirometry Report

A spirometry report is a narrative and graphic description of the interpretation of a patient's breathing capacity using a spirometer.

Radiology Report

A radiology report is a narrative description of a diagnostic or therapeutic radiologic procedure (Figure 1-5). A radiologist examines the radiograph and provides a written report, which includes a detailed interpretation of the radiograph and his or her impressions. The patient's physician receives a copy of the radiology report; the actual radiographic film or digital images are kept on file in the hospital's radiology department but are available for review by the patient's physician.

Diagnostic Imaging Report

A diagnostic imaging report is a narrative description of a diagnostic imaging procedure (Figure 1-6). The report includes a detailed interpretation of the diagnostic image, along with the practitioner's impressions. Examples of common diagnostic imaging procedures include ultrasonography, computed tomography (CT) scan, and magnetic resonance imaging (MRI). The diagnostic computer image is

COLLEGE HOSPITAL
4567 BROAD AVENUE
WOODLAND HILLS, MD 21532

RADIOLOGY REPORT

Examination Date:	June 14, 2012	Patient:	Rose Baker
Date Reported:	June 14, 2012	X-ray No.:	43200
Physician:	Harold B. Cooper, M.D.	Age:	19
Examination:	PA Chest, Abdomen	Hospital No.:	80-32-11

FINDINGS

PA CHEST: Upright PA view of chest shows the lung fields are clear, without evidence of an active process. Heart size is normal. There is no evidence of pneumoperitoneum.

IMPRESSION: NEGATIVE CHEST

ABDOMEN: Flat and upright views of the abdomen show a normal gas pattern without evidence of obstruction or ileus. There are no calcifications or abnormal masses noted.

IMPRESSION: NEGATIVE STUDY

RADIOLOGIST: *Marian B. Skinner*

Marian B. Skinner, MD

Figure 1-5. Radiology report. (Modified from Diehl MO: Medical transcription: techniques and procedures, ed 6, St Louis, 2007, Saunders.)

kept on file at the hospital but is available for review by the patient's physician.

THERAPEUTIC SERVICE DOCUMENTS

A therapeutic service report documents the assessments and treatments designed to restore a patient's ability to function. Examples of therapeutic services that the physician may order follow.

Physical Therapy

Physical therapy involves the use of therapeutic exercise, thermal modalities, cold, hydrotherapy, electrical stimulation, massage, and other physical agents to restore function and promote healing after an illness or injury. A physical therapist might help a football player with a knee injury to regain normal functioning of the knee or assist a patient recovering from a stroke to use his or her legs to walk again. Figure 1-7 shows an example of a physical therapy report.

Occupational Therapy

Occupational therapy helps a patient learn new skills to adapt to a physically, developmentally, emotionally, or mentally disabling condition. This enables the patient to perform activities of daily living and to achieve as much independence as possible. An occupational therapist might help an individual with a physical disability learn how to get dressed and how to prepare meals.

Speech Therapy

Speech therapy refers to treatment for the correction of a speech impairment resulting from birth, disease, injury, or previous medical treatment.

HOSPITAL DOCUMENTS

Hospital documents are prepared by the physician responsible for the care of a patient while at the hospital; this physician is known as the **attending physician.** The attending physician may be the patient's regular physician or a different physician. An example of the latter is a physician attending a patient at an urgent care center or in the emergency department of a hospital.

Hospital documents are dictated by the attending physician and transcribed at the hospital. The original document is filed in the patient's hospital medical record, and a copy is sent to the patient's regular physician. Hospital documents assist the patient's physician in reviewing the patient's hospital visit and in providing follow-up care.

DIAGNOSTIC IMAGING REPORT				
Mt. Carmel Hospital, Columbus, OH 43201				
DATE REQUESTED 6/6/2012	DATE TO BE DONE 6/10/2012	TODAY'S DATE 6/10/2012	DATE OF BIRTH 8/19/1949	
☐ WHEELCHAIR	☐ PORTABLE	☒ AMBULATORY	☐ CART	

PATIENT: Vera Ruth **INSURANCE:** Industrial

SEX F	ROOM NO. OP	RESPONSIBLE PERSON OR EMPLOYER J.B. Warren, Inc.	RADIOLOGIST Richard W. Adams, MD
CLINICAL INFORMATION AND PROVISIONAL DIAGNOSIS Back injury			ATTENDING PHYSICIAN Christopher Robb, MD
			NURSE

EXAMINATION REQUESTED (PINPOINT AREA OF CONCERN IF POSSIBLE)
CT LUMBAR SPINE

TECHNIQUE:

CT of the lumbar spine without contrast was performed from L-3 through S-1.

FINDINGS:

The L3-4 level appears satisfactory without evidence of osseous proliferation or disc protrusion.

At the L4-5 level there is some increased density at the disc level, which may be more prominent on the left. This is partially obscured due to facet artifact crossing obliquely.

There does appear to be some retention of epidural fat plane. This, however, may represent left-sided disc bulge or protrusion with the appropriate corresponding clinical appearance. Osseous variation at this level is not identified.

At the L5-S1 level, significant variation is not apparent.

IMPRESSION:

Variation at the L4-5 level on the left, which may represent annular disc bulge or perhaps protrusion on the left. However, confirmation with myelography and/or Ampaque enhanced computed tomography of the lumbar spine should be suggested prior to any surgical intervention.

Richard W. Adams, MD

Richard W. Adams, MD

Figure 1-6. Diagnostic imaging (CT scan) report.

History and Physical Report

The term **inpatient** refers to a patient who has been admitted to the hospital for at least one overnight stay. A health history must be obtained and a physical examination performed on all inpatients. There is one exception to this: If a patient history and physical examination are performed at the medical office within 1 week before admission, a copy of these documents may be used. In the event that a reliable health history cannot be obtained from the patient, it must be obtained from the person best able to relay the facts.

The history and physical report is a physician's narrative report of the patient's history and physical examination, along with the physician's medical impressions (Figure 1-8). The purpose of the history is to document the patient's current complaints and symptoms, whereas the purpose of the physical examination is to assess the patient's current health status. **Medical impressions,** or simply impressions, are conclusions drawn from an interpretation of data. In this case, the physician interprets the data from the health history and physical examination and draws conclusions as to the patient's state of health. Other terms for impressions include *provisional diagnosis* and *tentative diagnosis.*

Operative Report

An operative report (Figure 1-9) must be completed for all patients who have had a surgical procedure. This report describes the surgical procedure and must be completed and signed by the surgeon who performed the operation. The operative report must include the following:

- Patient identification information
- Date and location of the surgery
- Names of primary surgeon and assistants
- Preoperative diagnosis

PHYSICAL THERAPY EVALUATION

OBJECTIVE DATA TESTS AND SCALES PRINTED ON REVERSE.

DATE OF SERVICE 9 / 23 / 12

HOMEBOUND REASON: ❑ Needs assistance for all activities ❑ Residual weakness
❑ Requires assistance to ambulate ❑ Confusion, unable to go out of home alone
❑ Unable to safely leave home unassisted ❑ Severe SOB, SOB upon exertion
❑ Dependent upon adaptive device(s) ❑ Medical restrictions
❑ Other (specify)_____

SOC DATE 9 / 23 / 12

(If Initial Evaluation, complete Physical Therapy Care Plan)

PERTINENT BACKGROUND INFORMATION

OTHER DISCIPLINES PROVIDING CARE: ❑ SN ❑ OT ❑ ST ❑ MSW ❑ Aide

MEDICAL HISTORY

❑ Hypertension ❑ Cancer
❑ Cardiac ❑ Infection
❑ Diabetes ❑ Immunosuppressed
❑ Respiratory ❑ Open wound
❑ Osteoporosis ❑ Falls with injury
❑ Fractures ❑ Falls without injury
❑ Other (specify)_____

REASON FOR EVALUATION (Diagnosis/Problem)

Hx Ⓛ knee pain x 5 yrs; little relief c̄ PT
_____
_____
_____
_____
_____

LIVING SITUATION

☒ Capable ❑ Able ❑ Willing caregiver available
❑ Limited caregiver support (ability/willingness)
❑ No caregiver available
HOME SAFETY BARRIERS:
❑ Clutter ❑ Throw rugs ❑ Bath bench/equipment ❑ Needs grab bar
❑ Needs railings ❑ Steps (number/condition) _____
❑ Other (specify)_____
_____

PRIOR LEVEL OF FUNCTION

ADLs:
☒ Independent ❑ Needed assistance ❑ Unable
Equipment used: _____

IN-HOME MOBILITY (gait or wheelchair/scooter):
☒ Independent ❑ Needed assistance ❑ Unable
Equipment used: _____

COMMUNITY MOBILITY (gait or wheelchair/scooter):
❑ Independent ❑ Needed assistance ❑ Unable
Equipment used: _____

BEHAVIOR/MENTAL STATUS

☒ Alert ❑ Oriented ❑ Cooperative ❑ Confused ❑ Memory deficits
❑ Impaired judgement ❑ Other (specify)_____
_____

VITAL SIGNS/CURRENT STATUS

Blood Pressure:_____
Temperature: _____
Pulse:_____
Respirations:_____
O$_2$ saturation _____% (when ordered): ❑ at rest ❑ with activity
Skin: _____
Edema: _____
Vision: ____glasses_____
Sensation: _____
Communication: _____

PAIN

INTENSITY: 0 1 2 3 4 ⑤ 6 7 8 9 10
LOCATION: _____
AGGRAVATING FACTORS: _____
_____
_____
RELIEVING FACTORS: _____
_____
_____
BEST PAIN GETS: 2 **WORST PAIN GETS:** 8
ACCEPTABLE LEVEL OF PAIN: _____
CURRENT LEVEL OF PAIN: _____
IMPACT ON THERAPY POC? ❑ None ❑ (describe) _____
_____
_____

Communication: _____
Hearing: _____
Posture: _____
Endurance: _____

PATIENT NAME – Last, First, Middle Initial
Johnson, Thomas, J.

ID#

Form 3507P © BRIGGS, Des Moines, IA 50306 (800) 247-2343 www.BriggsCorp.com
305 PRINTED IN U.S.A.

PHYSICAL THERAPY EVALUATION
❑ Continued on Reverse

Figure 1-7. Physical therapy report. (Form Number 3507P. Courtesy Briggs, Des Moines.) *Continued*

PHYSICAL THERAPY EVALUATION (Cont'd.)

MUSCLE STRENGTH/FUNCTIONAL ROM EVAL

	AREA	STRENGTH Right	STRENGTH Left	ACTION	ROM Right	ROM Left
UPPER EXTREM.	Shoulder	5	5	Flex/Extend		5
		5	5	Abd./Add.		5
		5	5	Int. Rot./Ext. Rot.		5
	Elbow	5	5	Flex/Extend		5
	Forearm	5	5	Sup./Pron.		5
	Wrist	5	5	Flex/Extend		5
	Fingers	5	5	Flex/Extend		5
LOWER EXTREM.	Hip	5	2 (knee pain)	Flex/Extend	3	10% to 70%
		5	3	Abd./Add.		3
		5	3	Int. Rot./Ext. Rot.		4
	Knee	5	2+→3-	Flex/Extend		3
	Ankle	5	3	Plant./Dors.		4
	Foot	5	3	Inver./Ever.		4
SPINE	AREA	STRENGTH		ACTION	ROM	

FUNCTIONAL INDEPENDENCE/BALANCE EVAL

	TASKS	ASSIST SCORE	ASSISTIVE DEVICES/COMMENTS
BED MOBILITY	Roll/Turn	Not assessed	2° surgery
	Sit/Supine	2	Assist to Ⓛ LE
	Scoot/Bridge	2	Uses overhead trapeze
TRANSFERS	Sit/Stand	2	
	Bed/Wheelchair	2	
	Toilet	2	
	Floor	Not assessed	
	Auto	Not assessed	
BALANCE	Static Sitting	5	
	Dynamic Sitting	5	
	Static Standing	3	
	Dynamic Standing	3	
W/C SKILLS	Propulsion	N/A	
	Pressure Reliefs	N/A	
	Foot Rests	N/A	
	Locks	N/A	

MANUAL MUSCLE TEST (MMT) MUSCLE STRENGTH

GRADE	DESCRIPTION
5	Normal functional strength - against gravity - full resistance.
4	Good strength - against gravity with some resistance.
3	Fair strength - against gravity - no resistance - safety compromise.
2	Poor strength - unable to move against gravity.
1	Trace strength - slight muscle contraction - no motion.
0	Zero - no active muscle contraction.

FUNCTIONAL RANGE OF MOTION (ROM) SCALE

GRADE	DESCRIPTION	GRADE	DESCRIPTION
5	100% active functional motion.	2	25% active functional motion.
4	75% active functional motion.	1	Less than 25%.
3	50% active functional motion.		

FUNCTIONAL INDEPENDENCE SCALE (bed mobility, transfers, balance, W/C skills)

GRADE	DESCRIPTION
5	Independent - physically able and independent.
4	Verbal cue (VC) only needed.
3	Stand-by assist (SBA) - 100% patient/client effort.
2	Minimum assist (Min A) - 75% patient/client effort.
1	Maximum assist (Max A) - 25% - 50% patient/client effort.
0	Totally dependent - total care/support.

GAIT

ASSISTANCE: ☐ Independent ☐ SBA ☒ Min. assist ☐ Mod. assist ☐ Max. assist ☐ Unable

SURFACES: ☐ Level ☐ Uneven ☐ Stairs (number/condition)_____ **DISTANCE/TIME:**_____

WEIGHT BEARING STATUS: ☐ FWB ☐ WBAT ☒ PWB ☐ TDWB ☐ NWB

ASSISTIVE DEVICE(S): ☐ Cane ☐ Quad Cane ☐ Crutches ☐ Hemi Walker ☒ Walker ☐ Wheeled Walker

☐ Other (specify)_____

QUALITY/DEVIATIONS/POSTURES: _____

SUMMARY

Instruction provided: ☐ Safety ☐ Exercise ☐ Other (describe)_____

Equipment needed (describe) __Walker_____

☐ PT Evaluation only. No further indications for PT services.

☐ Orders for PT evaluation only. Needs additional PT services. See PT Care Plan for recommendations.

  ☐ Need to obtain orders.

☐ Orders for PT services with specific treatments, frequency and duration. See PT Care Plan/485.

DISCHARGE DISCUSSED WITH: ☒ Patient/Family

☐ Care Manager ☐ Physician ☐ Other (specify)_____

CARE COORDINATION: ☐ Physician ☐ SN ☐ PT ☐ OT ☐ ST ☐ MSW

☐ Aide ☐ Other (specify)_____

APPROXIMATE NEXT VISIT DATE_____/_____/_____

PLAN FOR NEXT VISIT_____

_____

PATIENT SIGNATURE (if applicable) *Thomas Johnson J.*_____

THERAPIST'S SIGNATURE/TITLE___*Michael Howe, MD*_____

DATE __9__/__23__/__12__ **TIME IN**_____ **TIME OUT**_____

Figure 1-7, cont'd. Physical therapy report. (Form Number 3507P. Courtesy Briggs, Des Moines.)

HISTORY AND PHYSICAL
ST. MERCY HOSPITAL

Patient Name: __Carol Jacobs__   Room #: __215__

Physician: __Charles Thomas, MD__   Hospital #: __5422__

Admission Date: __12/14/12__

CHIEF COMPLAINT: Chest pain

HISTORY OF PRESENT ILLNESS: Patient is an 85-year-old female complaining of chest pain. Patient was found to have abnormal cardiac enzymes in the Emergency Room consistent with acute myocardial infarction. Patient denied any pain radiating; however, she did complain of left-sided chest pain and lower back pain. Patient did not admit to any shortness of breath, nausea, or diaphoresis.

MEDICATIONS: Lasix, Darvocet-N 100, Lisinopril, Lopressor, Glynase, Relafen, Cytotec, and Micro K.

ALLERGIES: No drug allergies known.

PAST MEDICAL HISTORY: Significant for congestive heart failure, chronic obstructive pulmonary disease, diabetes mellitus type 2, coronary atherosclerosis, hypertension, and osteoporosis.

SOCIAL HISTORY: Not a drinker and not a smoker. Patient resides in a nursing home.

PHYSICAL EXAMINATION:

General: Patient is in acute distress. She is obese.
HEENT: She has 2 centimeters jugular venous distention. Pupils are equal and reactive to light and accommodation. No evidence of scleral or conjunctival icterus.
Chest: +2 bibasilar rales.
Heart: Regular rate and rhythm. +2/6 systolic ejection murmur in the left sternal border.
Abdomen: Soft, nontender, no splenomegaly and no hepatomegaly and positive bowel sounds.
Extremities: No evidence of edema or deep venous thrombosis.
Neurological: Cranial nerves II through XII grossly intact.

IMPRESSIONS: Congestive heart failure
Rule out myocardial infarction

Charles Thomas, MD

Charles Thomas, MD

Figure 1-8. Hospital history and physical examination report.

- Name of the surgical procedure
- Full description of the findings at surgery (normal and abnormal)
- Description of the technique and procedures used during surgery
- Ligatures and sutures used
- Numbers of packs, drains, and sponges used
- Description of any specimens removed
- Condition of the patient at the completion of surgery
- Postoperative diagnosis
- Instructions for follow-up care

Discharge Summary Report

The **discharge summary report** is a brief (usually one-page) summary of the significant events of a patient's hospitalization (Figure 1-10). The report must be completed and signed by the attending physician. The discharge summary report includes a concise account of the patient's illness, course of treatment, and response to treatment, as well as the condition of the patient at the time of discharge from the hospital. The purpose of this report is to document information needed by the patient's physician to provide for

OPERATIVE REPORT
ST. MARY'S HOSPITAL

Name: ___Natalie Boyer___

Hospital #: ___291734___   Room #: ___OP___

Surgeon: ___Paul Cain, M.D.___   Date of Surgery: ___1/6/12___

Assistants: ___N/A___   Anesthesia: ___General___

Anesthesiologist: ___John Adams, M.D.___

PRE-OP DIAGNOSIS: Abnormal Pap test with history of cervical carcinoma.

POST-OP DIAGNOSIS: Same and awaiting path report.

PROCEDURE: D&C, laser cone of the cervix.

The patient was taken to the operating room and placed in the lithotomy position; perineum and vagina were prepped, and moist sterile drape was used. Laser precautions all in place. Bimanual examination revealed a uterus enlarged with a second-degree uterine prolapse. The cervix was dilated. Uterus sounded to around 9 cm. The endocervical canal was dilated and D&C was performed with tissue recovered and submitted to Pathology. The cervix was stained with iodine, and the nonstaining area was identified. The laser was brought in, 50 watts of current were used to remove laser cone, and we submitted that to Pathology. We then vaporized beyond the margins of the cone, 3-4 mm to a depth of 4-5 mm. Hemostasis was adequate. We placed O Vicryl figure-of-eight sutures at the 3- and the 9-o'clock positions in the cervix, and then we put Monsel solution on the cervix. Hemostasis adequate. Sponge and needle counts correct times two. The patient tolerated the procedure well, and she returned to the recovery room in stable condition. She will be discharged home when awake and stable on Cipro 250 mg twice a day for a week, Darvocet-N 100, #20 as needed for pain. If she continues to have abnormal Pap tests, we will probably want to do a vaginal hysterectomy.

SURGEON: ___Paul Cain, MD___

Paul Cain, MD

Figure 1-9. Operative report.

the continuity of future care. It also is used to respond to authorized requests for information regarding the patient's hospitalization. The discharge summary report must include the following:
- Patient identification information
- Dates of hospitalization
- Reason for the hospitalization (provisional diagnosis)
- Brief health history
- Significant findings from examinations and tests
- Course of treatment
- Response to treatment
- Condition of the patient at discharge
- Discharge diagnosis (final diagnosis)
- Prognosis
- Discharge instructions
- Recommendations and arrangements for follow-up care

Pathology Report

A pathology report consists of a macroscopic (gross) and a microscopic description of tissue removed from a patient during surgery or a diagnostic procedure. The macroscopic description includes information about the size, shape, and appearance of the specimen as it appears to the naked eye. The report also includes a diagnosis of the patient's condition (Figure 1-11). A pathologist is required to examine the tissue specimen, complete the report, and sign it.

Emergency Department Report

The emergency department report is a record of the significant information obtained during an emergency department visit (Figure 1-12). The report is prepared and signed by the emergency department physician, and a copy is sent to the patient's family physician for the purpose of providing follow-up care. The emergency department report includes the following:
- Date of service
- Patient identification information
- Nature of the illness or injury
- Laboratory or diagnostic test results
- Procedures performed
- Treatment rendered
- Diagnosis

DISCHARGE SUMMARY

Brennan, Susan
97-32-11
June 18, 2012

ADMISSION DATE:　June 14, 2012　　　**DISCHARGE DATE:**　June 16, 2012

HISTORY OF PRESENT ILLNESS:
This 19-year-old female, nulligravida, was admitted to the hospital on June 14, 2012, with fever of 102°, left lower quadrant pain, vaginal discharge, constipation, and a tender left adnexal mass. Her past history and family history were unremarkable. Present pain had started two to three weeks prior to admission. Her periods were irregular, with latest period starting on May 30, 2012, and lasting for six days. She had taken contraceptive pills in the past but had stopped because she was not sexually active.

PHYSICAL EXAMINATION:
She appeared well developed and well nourished, and in mild distress. The only positive physical findings were limited to the abdomen and pelvis. Her abdomen was mildly distended, and it was tender, especially in the left lower quadrant. At pelvic examination, her cervix was tender on motion, and the uterus was of normal size, retroverted, and somewhat fixed. There was a tender cystic mass about 4-5 cm in the left adnexa. Rectal examination was negative.

PROVISIONAL DIAGNOSIS:
1. Probable pelvic inflammatory disease (PID).
2. Rule out ectopic pregnancy.

LABORATORY DATA ON ADMISSION:
Hgb 10.8, Hct 36.5, WBC 8,100 with 80 segs and 18 lymphs. Sedimentation rate 100 mm in one hour. Sickle cell prep+ (turned out to be a trait). Urinalysis normal. Electrolytes normal. SMA-12 normal. Chest x-ray negative, 2-hour UCG negative.

HOSPITAL COURSE AND TREATMENT:
Initially, she was given cephalothin 2 gm IV q6h, and kanamycin 0.5 gm IM bid. Over the next two days the patient's condition improved. Her pain decreased and her temperature came down to normal in the morning and spiked to 101° in the evening. Repeat CBC showed Hgb 9.8, Hct 33.5. The pregnancy test was negative. She was discharged on June 16, 2012 in good condition. She will be seen in the office in one week.

DISCHARGE DIAGNOSIS:
Pelvic inflammatory disease.

Harold B. Cooper, MD
Harold B. Cooper, MD

Figure 1-10. Discharge summary report. (Modified from Diehl MO: Medical transcription: techniques and procedures, ed 6, St Louis, 2007, Saunders.)

- Condition of the patient at discharge
- Instructions regarding follow-up care

CONSENT DOCUMENTS

Consent forms are legal documents required to perform certain procedures or to release information contained in the patient's medical record.

Consent to Treatment Form

Completion of a consent to treatment form (Procedure 1-1) is required for all surgical operations and nonroutine therapeutic and diagnostic procedures (e.g., sigmoidoscopy) performed in the medical office. The form must be signed by the patient or his or her legally authorized representative and must provide written evidence that the pa-

COLLEGE HOSPITAL
4567 BROAD AVENUE
WOODLAND HILLS, MD 21532

PATHOLOGY REPORT

Date:	June 20, 2012	Pathology No.:	430211
Patient:	Molly Ramsdale	Room No.:	1308
Physician:	Harold B. Cooper, M.D.		
Specimen Submitted:	Tumor, right axilla		

FINDINGS

GROSS DESCRIPTION: Specimen A consists of an oval mass of yellow fibroadipose tissue measuring 4 x 3 x 2 cm. On cut section, there are some small, soft, pliable areas of gray apparent lymph node alternating with adipose tissue. A frozen section consultation at time of surgery was delivered as NO EVIDENCE OF MALIGNANCY on frozen section, to await permanent section for final diagnosis. Majority of the specimen will be submitted for microscopic examination.

Specimen B consists of an oval mass of yellow soft tissue measuring 2.5 x 2.5 x 1.5 cm. On cut section, there is a thin rim of pink to tan-brown lymphatic tissue and the mid portion appears to be adipose tissue. A pathologic consultation at time of surgery was delivered as no suspicious areas noted and to await permanent sections for final diagnosis. The entire specimen will be submitted for microscopic examination.

MICROSCOPIC DESCRIPTION: Specimen A sections show fibroadipose tissue and nine fragments of lymph nodes. The lymph nodes show areas with prominent germinal centers and moderate sinus histiocytosis. There appears to be some increased vascularity and reactive endothelial cells seen. There is no evidence of malignancy.

Specimen B sections show adipose tissue and 5 lymph node fragments. These 5 portions of lymph nodes show reactive changes including sinus histiocytosis. There is no evidence of malignancy.

DIAGNOSIS: A & B: TUMOR, RIGHT AXILLA: SHOWING 14 LYMPH NODE FRAGMENTS WITH REACTIVE CHANGES AND NO EVIDENCE OF MALIGNANCY.

Stanley T. Nason, MD

Stanley T. Nason, MD

Figure 1-11. Pathology report. (Modified from Diehl MO: Medical transcription: techniques and procedures, ed 6, St Louis, 2007, Saunders.)

EMERGENCY DEPARTMENT REPORT
CAMDEN CLARK HOSPITAL

Name: __John Larimer__   DOB: __2/2/72__

ER Physician: __John Parsons, MD__   Date: __7/7/12__

ER Number: __07398__

Physician: __James Woods, MD__

NATURE OF ILLNESS/INJURY: This 40-year-old male presents to the Emergency Department complaining of a laceration of the sole of his right foot. Patient cut his foot on a rock 2 days ago and thinks he might have an infection now. Patient also complains of coughing over the past several days.

PHYSICAL EXAMINATION: Temperature 97.4, Pulse 76, Respirations 20, Blood Pressure 120/70. Patient is alert and oriented and is in no acute distress. ENT is normal. Lungs show diffuse rhonchi without crackles or wheezing. Heart has a regular rate and rhythm. Right great toe with marked tenderness with edema and erythema and heat.

DIAGNOSIS: Asthmatic Bronchitis
         Cellulitis, right foot first MTP

TREATMENT: PCMX scrub to right foot. Bacitracin dressing. Tetanus Diphtheria 0.5 cc IM. Biaxin 500 mg bid x 10 days. Guaifenesin with codeine 2 tsp q4h prn. Entex LA,1 bid prn. Debridement of skin flap.

PATIENT INSTRUCTIONS: Patient to follow up with family doctor in 7 days. Discussed bronchospasms with the patient.

James Woods, MD
James Woods, MD

Figure 1-12. Emergency department report.

---

tient agrees to the procedure or procedures listed on the form (Figure 1-13).

For the patient's consent to be valid, it must be informed consent. **Informed consent** means that the patient has received the following information before giving consent:
- The nature of the patient's condition
- The nature and purpose of the recommended procedure
- An explanation of risks involved with the procedure
- Alternative treatments or procedures available
- The likely outcome (**prognosis**) of the procedure
- The risks of declining or delaying the procedure

The explanation must be given in terms the patient can understand, and the patient should be given an opportunity to ask questions regarding the information.

The consent to treatment form should not be signed until the patient has been provided with all necessary information related to the procedure. The patient's signature must be witnessed; this is usually the responsibility of the medical assistant. *Witnessing a signature* means only that the medical assistant verified the patient's identity and watched the patient sign the form; it *does not* mean that the medical assistant is attesting to the accuracy of the information provided.

The consent to treatment form outlines the details of the discussion with the patient and includes the following information:
- The patient's full name
- Name of the procedure to be performed
- Name of the surgeon
- A statement indicating that the patient agrees to receive the procedure
- Acknowledgment that a disclosure of information has been made
- Acknowledgment that all questions were answered in a satisfactory manner
- A statement that no guarantee as to the outcome has been made
- Signature of the patient or his or her legal representative
- Signature of the witness

Release of Medical Information Form

As previously explained in the box entitled *Highlight on the HIPAA Privacy Rule,* a patient's written consent is not required for the use or disclosure of protected health information (PHI) for the purpose of medical treatment, payment, and health care operations (TPO). If a request

Figure 1-13. Consent to treatment form.

for protected health information is required for purposes that are not part of TPO, however, a detailed form must be completed, known as a *release of medical information form* (Figure 1-14). If a patient is moving to another state and wants to transfer his or her medical record to a new physician, a release of medical information form must be completed.

The release of medical information form must be signed by the patient authorizing the disclosure of his or her PHI (Procedure 1-2). If the patient is a minor, the form must be signed by the parent or legal guardian of the minor. The release of medical information form must stipulate the following:

- The patient's full name and address
- Name of the medical practice releasing the information
- Name of the individual or facility to receive the information
- Specific information to be released
- The purpose of or the need for the information
- Method of release of the information
- Signature of the patient or his or her legal representative
- Date that the consent was signed
- Expiration date of the consent form

Mailed or Faxed Requests for Release of Medical Information

Most medical offices require that the patient come to the office to sign the release of medical information form; however, this may not always be possible. An example is a patient who has moved away and is requesting the transfer of his or her medical records to a new physician. In this instance, a completed and signed release of medical information form may be mailed or faxed to the medical office. The procedure for processing this type of request is outlined at the end of Procedure 1-2.

TYPES OF MEDICAL RECORDS

Many medical offices rely on the use of paper medical records, known as **paper-based patient records (PPRs).** Although most of the medical record is paper based, some patient data are maintained on the computer; these include patient registration information and patient charges and payments. As technology advances, more and more offices are converting to an **electronic medical record (EMR)** for maintaining patient health information. With an electronic medical record, the entire record is stored in a database on

RELEASE OF MEDICAL INFORMATION

All information contained in the medical record is confidential, and the release of information is closely controlled. A properly completed and signed authorization form is required for the release of the following information.

PATIENT INFORMATION

Patient Name _____

Address _____ Social Security # _____

City _____ State _____ ZIP _____ Birth date _____/_____/_____

Phone (Home) _____ Work _____

RELEASE FROM:

Name _____

Address _____

City _____ State _____ ZIP_____

RELEASE TO:

Name _____

Address _____

City _____ State _____ ZIP_____

INFORMATION TO BE RELEASED:

1. GENERAL RELEASE:

____Entire Medical Record (excluding protected information)

____Hospital Records only (specify)_____

____Lab Results only (specify) _____

____X-ray Reports only (specify) _____

____Other Records (specify) _____

2. INFORMATION PROTECTED BY STATE/FEDERAL LAW:
If indicated below, I hereby authorize the disclosure and release of information regarding:

____Drug Abuse Diagnosis/Treatment

____Alcoholism Diagnosis/Treatment

____Mental Health Diagnosis/Treatment

____Sexually Transmitted Disease

PURPOSE/NEED FOR INFORMATION:

____Taking records to another doctor

____Moving

____Legal purposes

____Insurance purposes

____Worker's Compensation

____Other/Explain:_____

METHOD OF RELEASE:

____ U.S. Mail

____ Fax

____ Telephone

____ To Patient

PATIENT AUTHORIZATION TO RELEASE INFORMATION:

Authorization is valid for 60 days only from the date of my signature. I reserve the right to revoke this authorization at any time prior to 60 days (except for action that has already been taken) by notifying the medical office in writing.

I understand that my records are protected under HIPAA (Health Insurance Portability and Accountability Act) Standards for Privacy of Individually Identifiable Information (45 CFR Parts 160 and 164) unless otherwise permitted by federal law. Any information released or received shall not be further relayed to any other facility or person without my written authorization. I also understand that such information will not be given, sold, transferred, or in any way relayed to any other person or party not specified above without my further written authorization.

I hereby grant authorization to release the information listed above. I certify that this request has been made voluntarily and that the information given above is accurate to the best of my knowledge.

_____   _____

Signature of Patient/Legally Responsible Party   Date

_____   _____

Witness Signature   Date

OFFICE USE ONLY

Information indicated above released on _____
                                          Date

Explanation of information released: _____

_____

Signature and credentials of individual releasing information: _____

Figure 1-14. Release of medical information form.

PROCEDURE 1-1 sidebar label (vertical): **PROCEDURE 1-1**

PROCEDURE 1-1   Completion of a Consent to Treatment Form

Outcome Complete a consent to treatment form.

Equipment/Supplies

Consent to treatment form

1. **Procedural Step.** Type or print all required information on the consent to treatment form in the spaces provided (e.g., patient's full name, name of the procedure to be performed).
2. **Procedural Step.** Ensure that the physician has had a discussion to give the patient complete information about the procedure to be performed.
   Principle. For the patient's consent to be valid, it must be informed consent.
3. **Procedural Step.** Greet the patient and introduce yourself. Identify the patient by his or her full name and date of birth. Explain to the patient the purpose of the consent form.
4. **Procedural Step.** Give the consent form to the patient and ask him or her to read it. Ask the patient whether he or she has any questions.
5. **Procedural Step.** Ask the patient to sign the consent form. Witness the patient's signature by signing your name in the appropriate space on the form. Include today's date.
   Principle. Witnessing a signature means only that the medical assistant verified the identity of the patient and watched the patient sign the form; it does not mean that the medical assistant is attesting to the accuracy of the information provided.
6. **Procedural Step.** Provide the patient with a copy of the completed consent form for his or her files.
7. **Procedural Step.** File the original consent to treatment form in the patient's medical record.
   Principle. Maintaining the form provides legal documentation that the patient gave permission for treatment.

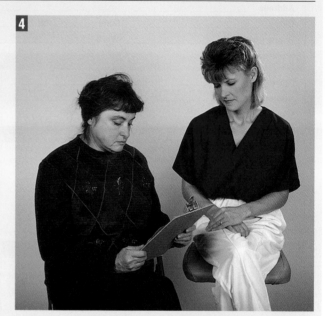

Ask the patient to read the consent form.

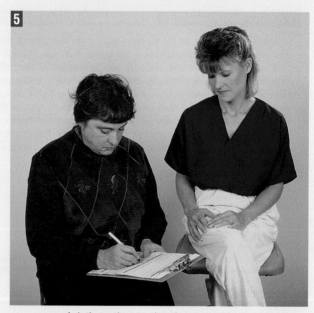

Ask the patient to sign the consent form.

PROCEDURE 1-2   Release of Medical Information

Outcome (1) Assist a patient in the completion of a release of medical information form. (2) Release medical information according to a completed release of medical information form.

Equipment/Supplies

Release of medical information form

1. **Procedural Step.** Greet the patient and introduce yourself. Identify the patient by his or her full name and date of birth. Explain the purpose of the release of medical information form. (**NOTE:** If you do not recognize the patient, ask him or her to provide photo identification such as a driver's license.)

2. **Procedural Step.** Provide the patient with a release of medical information form, and ask the patient to complete the form. Provide assistance if needed.
   Principle. Information from a patient's medical record can be released only on written authorization of the patient (except when permitted by law).

3. **Procedural Step.** Check to ensure that all information requested on the form has been completed by the patient.

4. **Procedural Step.** Ask the patient to sign the form. Witness the patient's signature by signing your name in the appropriate space on the form. Include today's date. If required by your medical office policy, ask the physician to initial the completed release of medical information form.
   Principle. For information to be released, the form must be signed by the patient authorizing the disclosure of medical information.

5. **Procedural Step.** Provide the patient with a copy of the release of medical information form for his or her files.

6. **Procedural Step.** Copy the information requested on the form. Release only the information requested. Include a copy of the completed release form with the medical information.

7. **Procedural Step.** Document what information is being released and the date of its release on the appropriate space on the release of information form. Sign the release of information form with your name and credentials verifying you were the individual releasing the information.

8. **Procedural Step.** File the original document and the release of medical information form in the patient's medical record.
   Principle. Maintaining the release form provides legal documentation that the patient gave permission for the release of his or her medical information.

9. **Procedural Step.** Send the medical information to the appropriate site according to your medical office policy.

Mailed or Faxed Requests for Release of Medical Information

These steps should be followed when a completed release of medical information form has been mailed or faxed to the medical office:

1. **Procedural Step.** Check the expiration date on the release of medical information form. If the authorization is outdated, a new release form needs to be completed.

2. **Procedural Step.** Verify the authenticity of the signature on the form. This can be accomplished by comparing the patient's signature on the form with the patient's signature in his or her medical record. If you have any doubt as to the authenticity of the signature, do not release the records.

3. **Procedural Step.** Copy the information requested on the form. Release only the information requested. Include a copy of the completed release form with the medical information.

4. **Procedural Step.** Document what information is being released and the date of its release. Sign the document with your name and credentials.

5. **Procedural Step.** File the original document and the release of medical information form in the patient's medical record.

6. **Procedural Step.** Send the medical information according to your medical office policy.

Witness the patient's signature.

PROCEDURE 1-2

the computer, including the health history report and physical examination report, progress notes, laboratory and diagnostic reports, and hospital reports. The electronic medical record is discussed in greater detail in the next section, whereas the remainder of this chapter focuses on the paper-based patient record.

Electronic Medical Record

The electronic medical record is a computerized record of the important health information regarding a patient, including the care of that individual and the progress of the patient's condition. Making the transition to an EMR is a major undertaking for a medical office. Medical offices are slowly moving toward the EMR. Approximately 25% of the medical offices in the United States have converted to an EMR and this percentage is expected to gradually increase over time. The biggest deterrent is the financial and time investment required for a medical office to make the conversion to the EMR.

EMR software allows for the creation, storage, organization, editing, and retrieval of medical records on a computer. The EMR software is usually linked to the practice management software. This allows the EMR to communicate with the practice management software and facilitates certain administrative tasks such as billing and insurance.

As was discussed at the beginning of this chapter, a medical record consists of numerous administrative and clinical documents. Each document in the medical record has a specific function. In a paper-based record (PPR), some of these documents consist of preprinted forms that contain specific information entered by a physician or other health care professional (e.g., patient registration form, health history form, medication record form, laboratory report form). With an EMR, the preprinted forms of a PPR are displayed on a computer screen and each form (known as a *template*) is filled out in much the same way as a paper form. A familiar example of an on-screen form is the form an individual completes when purchasing an item on the Internet; in this case, the form includes spaces (known as *fields*) for the individual to enter shipping and billing information.

Advantages of the Electronic Medical Record

The incorporation of an EMR in the medical office typically leads to better quality patient care through improved communication, faster access to data, and clearer and better documentation. These advantages are accomplished in the following ways:

Speed and Productivity: One of the principal advantages of an EMR is that the computer can retrieve requested documents from a patient's record very quickly (Figure 1-15). This avoids having to perform the much more time-consuming task of manually hunting through the record to locate this information. In addition, documents received from outside facilities, such as laboratory reports, can be stored very quickly in the EMR. EMRs do not need to be filed, as with a paper-based medical record. This saves considerable time and frees up the office space required to store paper records. Paper costs are also reduced and time is saved in not having to look for lost charts.

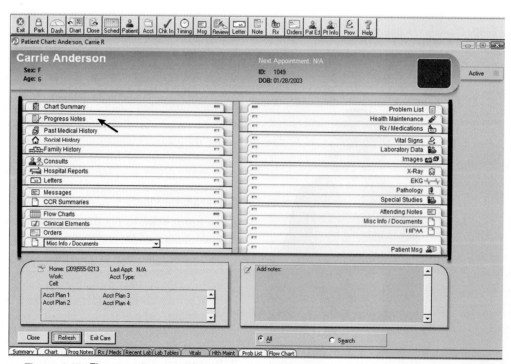

Figure 1-15. The computer can retrieve documents from a patient's EMR very quickly. (From Buck CJ: Electronic health record booster kit for the medical office, St Louis, 2009, Saunders. Screenshots used by permission of MCKESSON Corporation. All rights reserved. © MCKESSON Corporation 2008.)

Efficiency: EMR software facilitates the entry of data into the patient's medical record. To assist in entering data, EMR programs use point and click technology, such as check-boxes and drop-down lists. A familiar example of this is the drop-down list of states often used when an individual must indicate his or her state on an on-line address form. EMR programs also have the capability to print customized patient education instructions and handouts. For example, if a patient has been diagnosed with strep throat, patient education on strep throat can be printed and given to the patient. One of the principal advantages of an EMR is the ability to generate prescriptions, as described in detail in Chapter 11.

Accessibility: The EMR provides ready access to the patient's medical record. A patient's EMR is available at any EMR computer workstation, allowing more than one person to view the chart at the same time. The EMR is also readily accessible if a patient telephones the office. This avoids having to find the patient's record and call the patient back.

Disadvantages of the Electronic Medical Record

Disadvantages presented by the EMR in the medical office include the following:

Initial cost: An initial investment is required for the purchase of hardware and EMR software. Because computer access is required to use an EMR, the office must have a sufficient number of desktop computers, laptop computers, or tablet computers to accommodate the number of health care providers in the medical office. The combined expense of the hardware and software can easily fall into thousands of dollars. In addition, an office must periodically upgrade the EMR software, leading to further expense.

Time investment: It takes considerable time to learn an EMR program and use it with ease. Most software vendors provide on-site training of staff for a newly purchased program, as well as technical support when problems are encountered with the program. Even with all this assistance, however, learning an EMR program and using it with ease can take up to several months or longer.

Occupational tasks: Certain tasks must be performed before an EMR program becomes operational. To be effective, older records should be incorporated into a patient's EMR. This can be accomplished by manually scanning the records into a digital format using an input device known as a *scanner*. An application program known as an *optical character recognition (OCR)* program can also assist in this process. Once the record has been scanned into the computer, the OCR program converts typed text into text that can be manipulated by the computer. An OCR program can also convert a handwritten document into text, but it has a difficult time converting illegible handwriting into text.

Medical Assistants' Use of the EMR

EMR programs include an index that allows the medical assistant to access the various areas of information in the EMR program. The medical assistant must first select the patient who is being seen and enter information about the visit (Figure 1-16). Once the medical assistant begins working with the patient, there is a mechanism within the EMR program that is used to select an activity or topic. The selection may be made through a set of tabs on the screen or through a drop-down list. Selecting a tab such as *Medical History* moves the user to a screen containing information about the patient's medical history and allows the user to move to other screens with more specific information (see Figure 1-17). The EMR combines areas where data can be entered (e.g., blood pressure) and lists from which the user chooses an option (e.g., sitting, standing, lying).

Functions Performed by the Medical Assistant

The following functions are typically performed by the medical assistant using an EMR:
- Access the daily schedule.
- Select a patient.
- Enter the time that the patient has checked in.
- Enter the examination room number.
- Enter the patient's chief complaint (Figure 1-17).
- Enter or review the patient's history.
- Enter or review the patient's allergies.
- Enter or review the patient's current medications.
- Enter vital signs (Figure 1-18).
- Enter measurements such as height and weight.
- Enter results of tests, such as vision screening or hearing screening.
- Enter results of laboratory tests performed at the office (e.g., urinalysis, hemoglobin, strep testing).

Physicians' Use of the EMR

The physician enters data into the EMR about the physical examination, assessments, and plan for the patient. The physician can also review and update all information entered by the medical assistant. If the program is linked to

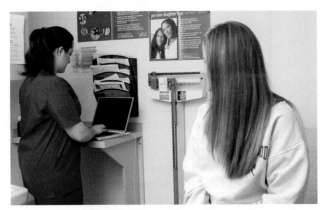

Figure 1-16. **Medical assistant taking patient symptoms using a computer and an electronic medical record program.**

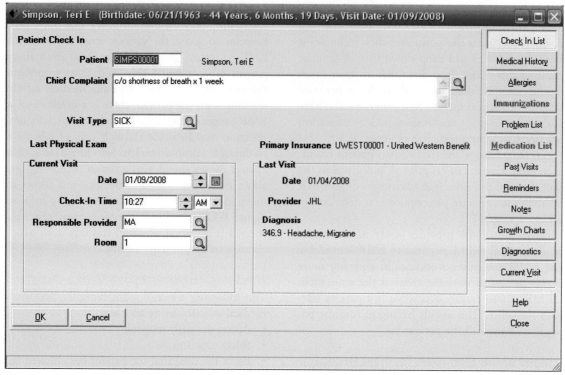

Figure 1-17. Electronic medical record screen. (Courtesy AltaPoint Data Systems, LLC, Midvale, Utah.)

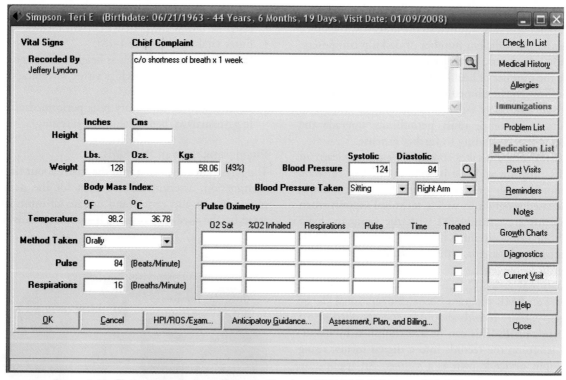

Figure 1-18. Electronic medical record screen. (Courtesy AltaPoint Data Systems, LLC, Midvale, Utah.)

the practice management software, the physician can specify the type of visit and the patient diagnosis. This assists in billing as part of the checkout procedure. The physician can also print a summary of the visit for the patient by selecting information from a list on the screen to include in the sum-

mary. Examples include physical examination findings, laboratory test results, vital signs, and treatment recommendations. The physician can also enter notes and reminders. Often there is a capacity to electronically send messages to other physicians or staff members within the system in a manner similar to e-mail. For example, the physician may send an electronic message to the medical assistant to schedule a patient for a particular test or to call in a prescription refill for a patient.

MEDICAL RECORD FORMATS

The way a medical record is organized is known as its *format*. The two main types of **medical record formats** are the *source-oriented record* and the *problem-oriented record*. Each of these formats is described.

Source-Oriented Record

The source-oriented format is used most often in the medical office for organizing a medical record. The documents in a source-oriented record are organized into sections based on the department, facility, or other source that generated the information (e.g., laboratory, hospital, consultant). Because documents from each source are filed together, it is easy to compare information from laboratory and diagnostic test results, assessments, and treatments.

Each section in a source-oriented record is separated from the other sections by a chart divider. Attached to each divider is a color-coded tab labeled with the title of its section (Figure 1-19). Within each of these sections, the documents are arranged according to date. Most offices use reverse chronological order to arrange the documents. **Reverse chronological order** means that the most recent document is placed on top or in front of the others, and thus the oldest document is on the bottom or at the end of that section.

What Would You Do? What Would You *Not* Do?

Case Study 2

Tessa Walsh, her husband, and two children are moving to another state. They will be leaving in 2 days. Tessa calls the office to have their medical records transferred to their new physician. Tessa's daughter has type 1 diabetes, so it is important that this be done as soon as possible. Tessa is quite annoyed to learn that she has to come in and sign a special form. She says that their medical records belong to them. Tessa says that the whole family has been coming there for the past 8 years and is well known by the physician and staff. She says that they have been good patients, have followed the physician's advice, and have always paid their bills on time. Tessa thinks that verbal permission should be enough. She's extremely busy packing and taking care of other moving details and doesn't have a minute to spare. ■

The titles that identify each section vary depending on the medical office's preference; however, typical examples include the following:

- History and physical
- Progress notes
- Medications
- Laboratory reports
- ECG
- X-ray reports
- Consultations
- Rehabilitation therapy
- Home health care
- Hospital reports
- Insurance
- Consents
- Correspondence
- Miscellaneous

Problem-Oriented Record

The documents in a problem-oriented record (POR), or problem-oriented medical record (POMR), are organized according to the patient's health problems. The advantage of using the POR is that each of the patient's problems can be defined and followed individually. The POR is developed in four stages:

1. Establishing a *database*
2. Compiling a *problem list*
3. Devising a *plan* of action for each problem
4. Following each problem with *progress notes*

Database

The first step in developing a POR is to establish a database. The database consists of a collection of subjective and objective data. These data include the health history report, the physical examination report, and results of baseline laboratory and diagnostic tests. The information in the database is used to identify and compile a problem list.

Problem List

The problem list is developed shortly after the database is completed and consists of a list of all of the patient's problems (Figure 1-20). A **problem** is defined as any patient condition that requires observation, diagnosis, management, or patient education. This includes not only medical problems but also psychological and social problems. The problem list is a crucial part of the POR and is always located in the front of the medical record.

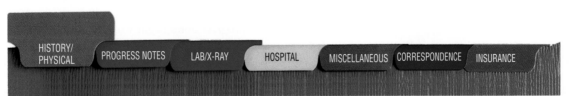

Figure 1-19. Chart dividers in a source-oriented record.

PATIENT RECORD								

Name ___ Morani, Betty

Number _____ **Blood Type:** A+

ALLERGIES/SENSITIVITY Codeine, Sulfa

Prob. No.	Date	PROBLEM DESCRIPTION	Date Resolved	Index	Prob. No.	Date	PROBLEM DESCRIPTION	Date Resolved	Index
1	10/05	Hypertension - essential		✓					
2	10/05	Diabetes mellitus (mild)		✓					
3	1/08	L. Retinopathy	see below						
4	4/2012	Atherosclerosis with cerebral vascular insuffic.							
5	4/2012	Hearing loss							
6	1/2012	HBP Non-compliance	2/12						
3	1/2012	Bilat. Grade II Retinopathy							

Prob. No.	CONTINUING MEDICATIONS	Start	Stop	Prob. No.	CONTINUING MEDICATIONS	Start	Stop
1	Sinoserp 1 mg. b.i.d.	10/05	10/09				
2	Orinase 0.5 gm. daily	10/05	10/09				
1	Hydrodiuril 50 mg. A.M.	10/05					
2	1500 cal. diet low Na hi K	2/2012					

Periodic Health Examination	Dates	1/04	4/06	2/08	1/10						

Figure 1-20. **POR** problem list. (Courtesy of and modified from Miller Communications, Norwalk, Conn.)

The problem list should be thought of as a table of contents for the record. Each problem in the list is numbered and titled. The problem title is stated as a diagnosis, a physiologic finding, a symptom, or an abnormal test result. All subsequent data (plans and progress notes) added to the medical record are cross-referenced to these numbered problems.

The problem list is modified as needed. If a new problem is identified, it is added to the list and dated accordingly. When a problem is resolved, it is marked as such, and the date is recorded.

Plan

After examining the problem list, the physician develops the third section of the POR. This involves devising a plan of action for further evaluation and treatment of each prob-

lem. Each plan begins with a heading that identifies the number of the problem, followed by the plan of action for the problem. This may include plans for laboratory and diagnostic tests, medical or surgical treatment, therapy, and patient education.

Progress Notes

The last stage in the development of the POR is the follow-up for each problem, or the progress notes (Figure 1-21). The progress notes begin with the number of the problem and include the following four categories:

1. *Subjective data:* Subjective data obtained from the patient
2. *Objective data:* Objective data obtained by observation, physical examination, and laboratory and diagnostic tests

PROBLEM ORIENTED - PROGRESS NOTES

Date	Time	Problem Number	FORMAT:	Problem Number and TITLE: S = Subjective O = Objective A = Assessment P = Plan			
11/15/12	9:30 AM	1	S:	Mother states that her child has had a runny nose and her throat has been			
				sore for 2 days.			
			O:	Vital signs: T 98.8 P 96 R 24			
				Weight: 42 lb.			
				General: alert and active. HEENT: sclera clear. TMs negative. Positive clear			
				rhinorrhea. Pharynx benign. Heart: regular without murmur.			
				Lungs: clear to auscultation and percussion. Abdomen: negative tenderness.			
				Positive bowel × 4. GU: negative. Neuro: good tone.			
			A:	Upper respiratory tract infection.			
			P:	1. A prescription for Rondec DM, 1/2 tsp q6h prn cough and congestion.			
				2. Instructed mother to contact office if child does not improve.			

NAME–Last	First	Middle	Attending Physician	Record No.	Room/Bed
Michaels	Jessica	L	Frank Edwards, MD	1	24

Form 653/2S © BRIGGS, Des Moines, IA 50306 (800) 247-2343 www.BriggsCorp.com
R404   PRINTED IN U.S.A.   **PROBLEM ORIENTED - PROGRESS NOTES**

Figure 1-21. POR SOAP progress notes. (Form Number 653/2S. Courtesy Briggs, Des Moines.)
Continued

PROBLEM ORIENTED - PROGRESS NOTES

Date	Time	Problem Number	FORMAT: Problem Number and TITLE: S = Subjective O = Objective A = Assessment P = Plan

NAME–Last	First	Middle	Attending Physician	Record No.	Room/Bed
Michaels	Jessica	L	Frank Edwards, MD	1	24

PROBLEM ORIENTED - PROGRESS NOTES

Figure 1-21, cont'd. POR SOAP progress notes. (Form Number 653/2S. Courtesy Briggs, Des Moines.)

3. *Assessment:* The physician's interpretation of the current condition based on analysis of the subjective and objective data

4. *Plan:* Proposed treatment for the patient

The acronym for this process is **SOAP,** and the writing of progress notes in this format is called *soaping.* Some physicians who use the source-oriented format have found it advantageous to record progress notes in SOAP format. This structured type of note increases the physician's ability to deal with each problem clearly and to analyze data in an orderly, systematic manner.

PREPARING A MEDICAL RECORD FOR A NEW PATIENT

When a patient comes to the medical office for his or her first visit, a medical record must be prepared for that patient (Procedure 1-3). The method used to prepare the record depends on the following criteria: the format used to organize the record, the filing system, and the type of storage equipment. Most medical offices use the source-oriented format to organize their medical records, the alphabetic filing system to arrange the records, and shelf filing units to store the medical records. Methods used to prepare a medical record are described in the following sections and are based on these criteria.

Medical Record Supplies

Certain supplies are required to prepare a medical record. These supplies are categorized and described next.

File Folders

A file folder is a protective cover made of a heavy material such as manila card stock. A file folder is used to hold medical record documents in an organized format. Flexible metal fasteners are typically used to hold documents in the folder. Folders are available with fasteners located on the top or left side of the folder.

Folders are available with tabs. A tab is a projection extending from a folder that is used to identify its contents.

PROCEDURE 1-3   Preparing a Medical Record

Outcome   Prepare a medical record.

The following procedure outlines the method for preparing a medical record for a new patient using the following organization: a source-oriented format stored in shelf files using a color-coded alphabetic filing system.

Equipment/Supplies

- Patient registration form
- Notice of Privacy Practices (NPP)
- NPP acknowledgment form
- File folder with a full cut side tab
- Metal fasteners
- Name labels

- Color-coded alphabetic bar labels
- Miscellaneous chart labels
- Set of chart dividers
- Blank preprinted forms
- Two-hole punch

1. **Procedural Step.** Greet the patient when he or she arrives at the medical office. Introduce yourself and identify the patient. Verify that the patient is a new patient.

2. **Procedural Step.** Ask the patient to do the following:
   a. Complete a patient registration form.
   b. Read a Notice of Privacy Practices (NPP).
   c. Sign an NPP acknowledgment form.

3. **Procedural Step.** When the patient returns the completed forms, check the patient registration form for accuracy, and make sure that you can read the patient's handwriting. If you have any questions regarding the information on the form, ask the patient for clarification. If required by the medical office policy, ask the patient for his or her insurance card and make a copy of it.
   Principle. A copy of the patient's insurance card is used for third-party billing.

4. **Procedural Step.** Enter into the computer the data on the completed registration record.

5. **Procedural Step.** Assemble supplies needed to prepare the medical record. Type the patient's full name on a name label while following these guidelines:
   a. Type the patient's name in transposed order as follows: last name, first name, middle name (or initial).
   b. Type the patient's name two or three typewritten spaces from the left edge of the label and one line down from the top of the label.
   c. Ensure that the patient's name is spelled correctly.
   Principle. Following these guidelines facilitates the accurate and efficient filing of the patient's medical record.

6. **Procedural Step.** Determine the first two letters of the patient's last name and select the appropriate alphabetic color-coded labels. Attach the color-coded labels to the (full cut) side tab. The labels should be

Continued

PROCEDURE 1-3   Preparing a Medical Record—cont'd

affixed to the folder using the label placement indentations on the tab.

Principle. Using the label placement indentations ensures that all labels on medical records are affixed at the same place.

7. Procedural Step. Affix the name label immediately above the first color-coded alphabetic label.

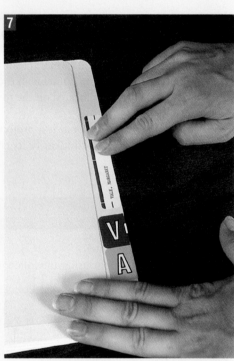

Affix the name label.

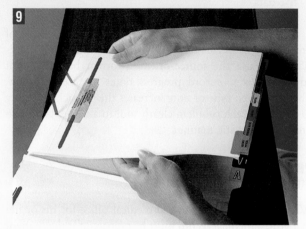

Insert the chart dividers into the metal fasteners.

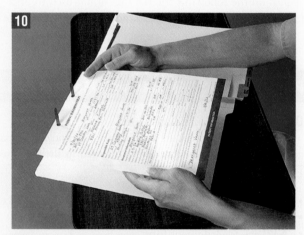

Place the patient registration form in the front of the medical record.

8. Procedural Step. Attach any additional chart labels, such as a year label and miscellaneous chart labels (e.g., allergy, insurance), to the folder according to the office policy.

9. Procedural Step. Insert the chart dividers onto the metal fasteners of the file folder.

10. Procedural Step. Place the original patient registration form in the front of the medical record. Place the signed NPP acknowledgment form and the copy of the patient's insurance card in the appropriate section of the record.

11. Procedural Step. Label preprinted forms to be placed in the record with required information such as the

patient's name and date. These forms typically include the medical history form, the physical examination form, progress note sheets, and a medication record form. If the forms are not prepunched, the medical assistant must use a two-hole punch to insert two holes into the top or side of the form.

12. Procedural Step. Insert each form under its proper chart divider. Refer to the box on page 33 for a list of chart divider subject titles and documents typically filed under each title.

13. Procedural Step. Check the medical record to ensure that it has been prepared properly.

The tab is located on either the side or the top of the folder. A folder with a tab extending across its entire side or top is called a *full cut tab.*

In the medical office, a file folder with a full cut side tab is typically used to prepare a new patient's chart. There are indentations at intervals along the full cut tab to indicate the placement of adhesive labels. This ensures that the labels

on all medical records are affixed at the same place on the file folders.

Folder Labels

Labels to identify the medical record are commercially available in rolls or continuous folded strips for typewriter use. Labels also are available on 8½ × 11-inch sheets for use with a computer and printer. The types of labels most commonly used in the medical office include name labels, alphabetic color-coded labels, color-coded year labels, and miscellaneous chart labels.

Chart Dividers

Chart dividers are used to identify each section of the medical record by subject (see Figure 1-19). Chart dividers consist of a heavy material such as manila card stock. Attached to each divider is a color-coded tab labeled with a subject title; the most frequently used subject titles are illustrated in the box below, along with the documents typically filed under each title.

TAKING A HEALTH HISTORY

The health history is a collection of subjective health data obtained by interviewing the patient and by having the patient complete a preprinted health history form that is then reviewed for completeness by the medical assistant. A thor-

---

Chart Divider Subject Titles and Documents Typically Filed Under Each Title

History and Physical
- Health history
- Physical examination report

Progress Notes
- Progress notes
- Medication record

Laboratory/X-ray
- Hematology report
- Clinical chemistry report
- Immunology report
- Urinalysis report
- Microbiology report
- Parasitology report
- Cytology report
- Histology report
- Electrocardiogram report

Laboratory/X-ray—cont'd
- Holter monitor report
- Sigmoidoscopy report
- Colonoscopy report
- Spirometry report
- Radiology report
- Diagnostic imaging report

Hospital
- History and physical report
- Operative report
- Pathology report
- Discharge summary report
- Emergency department report

Correspondence
- Consultation report
- Letter from patient

Correspondence—cont'd
- Letter from patient's attorney
- Referral letter

Insurance
- Copy of patient's insurance card
- Precertification authorization for hospital admission
- Request for additional information from insurance company

Miscellaneous
- Consent to treatment form
- Release of medical information form
- Home health care report
- Physical therapy report
- Occupational therapy report
- Speech therapy report

Memories *from* Externship

Dawn Bennett: During my externship as a medical assisting student, I was placed in a family practice clinic. I was very nervous my first day, wondering how in the world I would be able to remember everything I had learned in school. My first patients were an elderly couple. The wife was there for some test results for cancer. I looked at the results, and they were positive. After the physician relayed the results, the husband broke down. He had just lost his granddaughter to a heart attack and his son-in-law to a stroke. You could tell that he just could not bear losing his wife too.

One week later, the elderly man's wife was placed in a nursing home. He came into our office for an appointment. As I was working him up, he was telling me stories about himself and his wife when they were first married. He looked so sad. I sat with him for a few minutes after completing his workup and gave his stories my full attention. As I was leaving the room, a smile came across his face, and he thanked me for listening to him. I realized that working in a physician's office is more than just knowing what I learned in school. Compassion and showing patients you really do care about them are just as important. I felt good about myself that day. ■

What Would You Do? What Would You *Not* Do?

Case Study 3
Brett Oberlin is 21 years old and lives at home. He commutes to a local college and is a junior majoring in art education. His mother and father have come to the medical office and ask to see his medical record. The physician is attending a medical conference and will not return for another 4 days. Mr. and Mrs. Oberlin found some medications in Brett's room and looked them up on the Internet.

They found out that they are used to treat HIV infection. Brett would not talk to them about the medications and told them he is an adult and it is none of their business. Mr. and Mrs. Oberlin are very concerned about Brett. They also are worried about other members of the family being exposed to HIV. They say that because they are supporting him, they should be allowed to see his record. ■

ough history is taken for each new patient, and subsequent office visits (in the form of progress notes) provide information regarding changes in the patient's illness or treatment. A quiet, comfortable room that allows for privacy encourages the patient to communicate honestly and openly. Showing genuine interest in and concern for the patient reduces apprehension and facilitates the collection of data.

In an office with an EMR, the patient may complete a health history paper-and-pencil form, and the medical assistant then enters the data into the computer. An alternative is for the medical assistant to enter the information directly into the computer while asking the patient questions related to his or her health status. Although not yet in widespread use, computer-guided questionnaires are available for some patients to complete their own health histories. The medical office must provide a private area for the patient to complete the questionnaire, and the medical assistant must be available to answer questions.

Components of the Health History

The health history is taken before the physical examination is performed, providing the physician the opportunity to compare findings. The health history consists of seven parts or sections.

Identification Data

The identification data section is included at the beginning of the health history form to obtain basic demographic data on the patient (Figure 1-22, *A*). The patient completes the identification data section.

Chief Complaint

The chief complaint (CC) identifies the patient's reason for seeking care—that is, the symptom that is causing the patient the most trouble. The CC is used as a foundation for the more detailed information obtained for the present illness and review of systems sections of the health history. The medical assistant is usually responsible for obtaining the CC from the patient and recording it in the patient's chart. In most offices, this information is recorded on a preprinted, lined form (see Figure 1-22, *F*). Certain guidelines must be followed in obtaining and recording the CC, as follows:

- An open-ended question should be used to elicit the CC from the patient: What seems to be the problem? How can we help you today? What can we do for you today?
- The CC should be limited to one or two symptoms and should refer to a specific, rather than vague, symptom.
- The CC should be recorded concisely and briefly, using the patient's own words as much as possible.
- The duration of the symptom (onset) should be included in the CC.
- The medical assistant should avoid using names of diseases or diagnostic terms to record the CC.

Recording Chief Complaints

Following are correct and incorrect examples of recording chief complaints.

Correct Examples
- Burning during urination that has lasted for 2 days
- Pain in the shoulder that started 2 weeks ago
- Shortness of breath for the past month

Incorrect Examples
- Has not felt well for the past 2 weeks (This statement refers to a vague, rather than a specific, complaint.)
- Ear pain and fever (The duration of the symptoms is not listed.)
- Pain upon urination indicative of a urinary tract infection (Names of diseases should not be used to record the chief complaint; the duration of the symptom is not listed.)

Present Illness

The present illness (PI) is an expansion of the chief complaint and includes a full description of the patient's current illness from the time of its onset. The medical assistant is often responsible for completing this section of the health history, which is recorded on the same form as the chief complaint (see Figure 1-22, *F*). To complete this section of the health history, the medical assistant asks the patient questions to obtain a detailed description of the symptom causing the greatest problem. Much skill and practice in asking the proper questions are required to elicit detailed information. A general guide for obtaining further information on symptoms is presented in Procedure 1-4, and a more thorough study for analyzing a symptom is included in the *Study Guide for Students* (see Chapter 1).

Past History

The past medical history is a review of the patient's past medical status (see Figure 1-22, *B*). Obtaining information on past medical care assists the physician in providing optimal care for the current problem. Most medical offices ask the patient to complete this section of the health history through a checklist type of form. The medical assistant should assist the patient with this section as necessary by offering to answer any questions regarding the information required. The past history includes the following areas:
- Major illnesses
- Childhood diseases
- Unusual infections
- Accidents and injuries
- Hospitalizations and operations
- Previous medical tests
- Immunizations
- Allergies
- Current medications

Family History

The family history is a review of the health status of the patient's blood relatives (see Figure 1-22, *C*). This section of the health history focuses on diseases that tend to be familial. A **familial** disease is one that occurs in or affects blood relatives more frequently than would be expected by chance. Examples of familial diseases include hypertension, heart disease,

Text continued on p. 39.

PATIENT HEALTH HISTORY

A   **IDENTIFICATION DATA**   Please print the following information.

Today's date _____

Name _____   ____ Male ____ Female

Address _____   ____ Married ____ Separated ____ Divorced ____ Widowed ____ Single

_____   Date of Birth _____

Telephone _____   _____
         Home number   Work number

B   **PAST HISTORY**

Have you ever had the following: (Circle "no" or "yes", leave blank if uncertain)

Measles _____ no yes	Heart Disease _____ no yes	Diabetes _____ no yes	Hemorrhoids _____ no yes
Mumps _____ no yes	Arthritis _____ no yes	Cancer _____ no yes	Asthma _____ no yes
Chickenpox _____ no yes	Sexually Transmitted ____ no yes Disease	Polio _____ no yes	Allergies _____ no yes
Whooping Cough ___ no yes	Anemia _____ no yes	Glaucoma _____ no yes	Eczema _____ no yes
Scarlet Fever _____ no yes	Bladder Infections ___ no yes	Hernia _____ no yes	AIDS or HIV+ _____ no yes
Diphtheria _____ no yes	Epilepsy _____ no yes	Blood or Plasma ____ no yes Transfusions	Infectious Mono ____ no yes
Pneumonia _____ no yes	Migraine Headaches _ no yes	Back Trouble _____ no yes	Bronchitis _____ no yes
Rheumatic Fever ____ no yes	Tuberculosis _____ no yes	High Blood _____ no yes Pressure	Mitral Valve Prolapse no yes
Stroke _____ no yes	Ulcer _____ no yes	Thyroid Disease ____ no yes	Any other disease ___ no yes
Hepatitis _____ no yes	Kidney Disease _____ no yes	Bleeding Tendency _ no yes	Please list: _____ _____

MAJOR HOSPITALIZATIONS: If you have ever been hospitalized for any major medical illness or operation, write in your most recent hospitalizations below.

Hospitalizations	Year	Operation or illness	Name of hospital	City and state
1st Hospitalization				
2nd Hospitalization				
3rd Hospitalization				
4th Hospitalization				

TESTS AND IMMUNIZATIONS: Mark an X next to those that you have had.

Tests: Immunizations:

☐ TB Test   ☐ Electrocardiogram   ☐ Influenza

☐ Rectal/Hemoccult   ☐ Chest x-ray   ☐ Hepatitis B

☐ Sigmoidoscopy   ☐ Mammogram   ☐ Tetanus

☐ Colonoscopy   ☐ Pap Test   ☐ MMR

                                             ☐ Polio

ALLERGIES: List all allergies (foods, drugs, environment). ☐ None

_____

_____

_____

_____

CURRENT MEDICATIONS: List the following that you are currently taking: Prescription medications, over-the-counter (OTC) medications, vitamin supplements, and herbal supplements. ☐ None

Medication   Frequency

_____   _____

_____   _____

_____   _____

ACCIDENTS/ INJURIES: Describe all serious accidents, severe injuries, head injury, or fractures. Include the date each occurred. ☐ None

Accident/Injury: Date:

_____

_____

_____

_____

Figure 1-22. Health history form.   *Continued*

C FAMILY HISTORY

For each member of your family, follow the purple or blue line across the page and check boxes for:
1. His or her present state of health
2. Any illnesses he or she has had

	Good Health	Poor Health	Deceased	If deceased, write in age and cause of death.	Allergies or Asthma	Diabetes	Heart Disease	Stroke	Cancer	High Blood Pressure	Glaucoma	Arthritis	Ulcer	Kidney Disease	Mental Health Problems	Alcohol/Drug Abuse	Obesity	High Cholesterol	Thyroid Disease
Father:																			
Mother:																			
Brothers/Sisters:																			

D SOCIAL HISTORY

EDUCATION _____ High school _____ College _____ Postgraduate

Occupation _____ Years _____

Previous occupations _____ Years _____

_____ Years _____

Have you ever been exposed to any of the following in your environment?

☐ Excess dust (coal, lime, rock)　☐ Cleaning fluids/solvents　☐ Radiation　☐ Other toxic materials

☐ Sand　☐ Hair spray　☐ Insecticides

☐ Chemicals　☐ Smoke or auto exhaust fumes　☐ Paints

Please answer the following questions by placing an X in the box in front of the word Yes or No, except where you are asked for specific information. This information is obviously highly confidential and will be released to other health care professionals or insurance carriers ONLY with your consent.

DIET:

Do you eat a good breakfast? ☐ Yes ☐ No

Do you snack between meals (soft drinks, chips, candy bars)? ☐ Yes ☐ No

Do you eat fresh fruits and vegetables each day? ☐ Yes ☐ No

Do you eat whole grain breads and cereals? ☐ Yes ☐ No

Is your diet high in fat content? ☐ Yes ☐ No

Is your diet high in cholesterol content? ☐ Yes ☐ No

Is your diet high in salt content? ☐ Yes ☐ No

Are you allergic to any foods? ☐ Yes ☐ No

How many glasses of water do you drink each day? _____

How would you describe your overall eating habits? ☐ Excellent ☐ Good ☐ Fair ☐ Poor

PERSONAL HISTORY:

Do you find it hard to make decisions? ☐ Yes ☐ No

Do you find it hard to concentrate or remember? ☐ Yes ☐ No

Do you feel depressed? ☐ Yes ☐ No

Do you have difficulty relaxing? ☐ Yes ☐ No

Do you have a tendency to worry a lot? ☐ Yes ☐ No

Have you gained or lost much weight recently? ☐ Yes ☐ No

Do you lose your temper often? ☐ Yes ☐ No

Are you disturbed by any work or family problems? ☐ Yes ☐ No

Are you having sexual difficulties? ☐ Yes ☐ No

Have you ever considered committing suicide? ☐ Yes ☐ No

Have you ever desired or sought psychiatric help? ☐ Yes ☐ No

EXERCISE:

Do you exercise on a regular basis? ☐ Yes ☐ No

Does your job require strenuous, sustained physical work? ☐ Yes ☐ No

SLEEP PATTERNS:

Do you seem to feel exhausted or fatigued most of the time? ☐ Yes ☐ No

Do you have difficulty either falling asleep or staying asleep? ☐ Yes ☐ No

USE OF TOBACCO/ALCOHOL/CAFFEINE/DRUGS: Amt:

How much do you smoke per day? ☐ Cigarettes ___

☐ Don't smoke ☐ Cigars/pipes ___

Do you take two or more alcoholic drinks per day? ☐ Yes ☐ No

Do you drink six or more cups of coffee or tea per day? ☐ Yes ☐ No

Are you a regular user of sleeping pills, marijuana, tranquilizers, pain killers, etc? ☐ Yes ☐ No

Have you ever used heroin, cocaine, LSD, PCP, etc? ☐ Yes ☐ No

List any country outside the USA you have visited in the past six months. _____

When did you have your last physical examination? _____

Figure 1-22, cont'd. Health history form.

Patient's Name_____

E REVIEW OF SYSTEMS

HEAD AND NECK
_____ Frequent headaches
_____ Neck pain
_____ Neck lumps or swelling

EYES
_____ Wears glasses
_____ Blurry vision
_____ Eyesight worsening
_____ Sees double
_____ Sees halo
_____ Eye pain or itching
_____ Watery eyes
_____ Eye trouble

EARS
_____ Hearing difficulties
_____ Earaches
_____ Running ears
_____ Buzzing in ears
_____ Motion sickness

MOUTH
_____ Dental problems
_____ Swelling on gums or jaws
_____ Sore tongue
_____ Taste changes

NOSE AND THROAT
_____ Congested nose
_____ Running nose
_____ Sneezing spells
_____ Head colds
_____ Nosebleeds
_____ Sore throat
_____ Enlarged tonsils
_____ Hoarse voice

RESPIRATORY
_____ Wheezes or gasps
_____ Coughing spells
_____ Coughs up phlegm
_____ Coughed up blood
_____ Chest colds
_____ Excessive sweating,
      night sweats

CARDIOVASCULAR
_____ High blood pressure
_____ Racing heart
_____ Chest pains
_____ Dizzy spells
_____ Shortness of breath
_____ Shortness of breath at night
_____ More pillows to breathe
_____ Swollen feet or ankles
_____ Leg cramps
_____ Heart murmur

DIGESTIVE
_____ Heartburn
_____ Bloated stomach
_____ Belching
_____ Stomach pains
_____ Nausea
_____ Vomited blood
_____ Difficulty swallowing
_____ Constipation
_____ Loose bowels
_____ Black stools
_____ Grey stools
_____ Pain in rectum
_____ Rectal bleeding

URINARY
_____ Night frequency
_____ Day frequency
_____ Wets pants or bed
_____ Burning on urination
_____ Brown, black, or bloody urine
_____ Difficulty starting urine
_____ Urgency

MALE GENITAL
_____ Weak urine stream
_____ Prostate trouble
_____ Burning or discharge
_____ Lumps on testicles
_____ Painful testicles

FEMALE GENITAL
__/__/__ Last menstrual period
__/__/__ Last Pap test
_____ Postmenopausal or hysterectomy
_____ Noticed vaginal bleeding
_____ Abnormal LMP
_____ Heavy bleeding during periods
_____ Bleeding between periods
_____ Bleeding after intercourse
_____ Recent vaginal itching/discharge
_____ No monthly breast exam
_____ Lump or pain in breasts
_____ Complications with birth control

OBSTETRIC HISTORY
_____ Gravida
_____ Para
_____ Preterm
_____ Miscarriages
_____ Stillbirths
_____ Has had an abortion

MUSCULOSKELETAL
_____ Aching muscles
_____ Swollen joints
_____ Back or shoulder pains
_____ Painful feet
_____ Disability

SKIN
_____ Skin problems
_____ Itching or burning skin
_____ Bleeds easily
_____ Bruises easily

NEUROLOGICAL
_____ Faintness
_____ Numbness
_____ Convulsions
_____ Change in handwriting
_____ Trembles

F PROGRESS NOTES

Date	

Figure 1-22, cont'd. Health history form.

Common Symptoms

Symptom	Definition
Integumentary System	
Diaphoresis	Excessive perspiration.
Flushing	A red appearance to the skin, which generally affects the face and neck. A flushed appearance is commonly present with a fever.
Jaundice	A yellow appearance to the skin, first evident in the whites of the eyes.
Rash	An eruption on the skin.
Circulatory System	
Bradycardia	An abnormally slow pulse rate.
Dehydration	A decrease in the amount of water in the body. The patient has a flushed appearance, dry skin, and decreased output of urine.
Edema	The retention of fluid in the tissues, resulting in swelling. Skin over the area is tight. Edema is most easily observed in the extremities.
Tachycardia	An abnormally fast pulse rate.
Gastrointestinal System	
Anorexia	A loss of appetite and a lack of interest in food.
Constipation	A condition in which the stool becomes hard and dry, resulting in difficult passage from the rectum. The consistency of the stool, rather than the frequency of defecation, is used as a guide in determining the presence of constipation. (Frequency of bowel movements varies with the individual; some people have a bowel movement only every 2 to 3 days but are not constipated.) Other symptoms of constipation include headache, nausea, and general malaise.
Diarrhea	The passage of an increased number of loose, watery stools. The fecal material moves rapidly through the intestinal tract, resulting in decreased absorption by the body of water, electrolytes, and nutrients. Other symptoms usually associated with diarrhea are intestinal cramping and general weakness.
Flatulence	The presence of excessive gas in the stomach or intestines.
Nausea and vomiting	Nausea is a sensation of discomfort in the stomach with a feeling that vomiting may occur. Vomiting is the ejection of the stomach contents through the mouth, also known as *emesis*. The ejected content is known as *vomitus*.
Respiratory System	
Cough	An involuntary and forceful exhalation of air followed by a deep inhalation. A cough may be productive (meaning a discharge is produced) or nonproductive (no discharge is present).
Cyanosis	A bluish discoloration of the skin due to lack of oxygen.
Dyspnea	Labored or difficult breathing.
Epistaxis	Hemorrhaging from the nose (nosebleed).
Nervous System	
Chills	A feeling of coldness accompanied by shivering. Chills are generally present with a fever.
Convulsions	Involuntary contractions of the muscles.
Fever or pyrexia	A body temperature that is higher than normal.
Headache	A feeling of pain or aching in the head. It is a common symptom that accompanies many illnesses. Tension, fatigue, and eyestrain can result in a headache.
Malaise	A vague sense of body discomfort, weakness, and fatigue, often marking the onset of a disease and continuing through the course of the illness.
Pain	Irritation of pain receptors, resulting in a feeling of distress or suffering. Pain is an important indication that a part of the body is not working properly.
Pruritus	Severe itching.
Vertigo	A feeling of dizziness or light-headedness.

allergies, and diabetes mellitus. The patient usually completes this section of the health history and is asked to provide the following information about each blood relative:

- State of health
- Presence of any significant disease
- If deceased, cause of death

Social History

The social history section of the health history includes information on the patient's lifestyle, such as health habits and living environment (see Figure 1-22, *D*). The social history is important because the patient's lifestyle may have an impact on his or her condition and may influence the course of treatment chosen by the physician. The social history also provides the physician with information regarding the effect that the illness may have on the patient's daily living pattern. If it is necessary for the individual to make a major lifestyle adjustment (e.g., stop smoking, reduce working hours), the physician may recommend support services to assist in this transition. This section of the history is usually completed by the patient and includes the following areas:

- Education
- Occupation (past and present)
- Living environment
- Diet
- Personal history
- Exercise

Review of Systems

A review of systems (ROS) is a systematic review of each body system to detect any symptoms that have not yet been revealed. The importance of the ROS is that it assists in identifying symptoms that might otherwise remain undetected. The physician usually completes the ROS by asking a series of detailed and direct questions related to each body system; the results of this section of the health history assist the physician in a preliminary assessment of the type and extent of physical examination required. Figure 1-22, *E* shows an example of an ROS form.

CHARTING IN THE MEDICAL RECORD

Charting is the process of making written entries about a patient in the medical record and is performed by medical office personnel who are directly involved with the health care of the patient. The medical record is considered a legal document; the information must be charted as completely and accurately as possible. Developing good charting skills requires a thorough knowledge of charting guidelines combined with much repeated practice. To provide guidance in attaining this important skill, PPR charting guidelines are presented in this section, followed by examples of proper charting entries. With an EMR, the medical assistant enters charting information into a computer using free-text entry, drop-down lists, and check-boxes.

Charting Guidelines

To ensure accurate and concise charting, specific guidelines must be followed. These are listed and described as follows:

1. *Check the name on the chart before making an entry to ensure you have the correct chart.* If the medical assistant records in the wrong patient's chart by mistake, information such as a procedure that was performed on a patient may be excluded from the correct patient's record. As previously stated, from a legal standpoint, a procedure not documented was not performed.

2. *Use black ink to make entries in the patient's chart.* Black ink must be used to provide a permanent record. In addition, entries made in black ink are easier to reproduce when a record must be duplicated for insurance company purposes and patient referral.

3. *Write in legible handwriting.* For the medical record to be meaningful to others, the medical assistant must chart information legibly. If the medical assistant's cursive script is not legible, the information should be printed.

4. *Chart information accurately, using clear and concise phrases.*
   - The medical assistant should be brief but thorough and should avoid vagueness and duplication of information.
   - It is not necessary to include the patient's name in the entry because the entire medical record centers on one patient; it is assumed the information refers to that patient.
   - Each phrase should begin with a capital letter and end with a period.
   - Each new entry should begin on a separate line and be dated with the month, day, year, and time (either AM/PM or military time).
   - Standard abbreviations, medical terms, and symbols can be used to help save time and space. It is *crucial* that the medical assistant first check the office policy to determine the abbreviations, medical terms, and symbols that are commonly used in that office. Using commonly accepted terminology avoids confusing others who read the chart. A list of abbreviations and symbols commonly used in medical offices is presented in the box on pages 41 to 44.
   - *Spell correctly.* Correct spelling is essential for accuracy in charting. If you are in doubt about the spelling of a word, consult a dictionary.

5. *Chart immediately after performing a procedure.* When a procedure has been performed, it should be charted without delay. If a time lapse occurs between performing the procedure and charting it, the medical assistant may not remember certain aspects of the procedure, such as the results of the treatment or the patient's reaction. Procedures should never be charted in advance. The individual performing the procedure should be the one to chart it; in other words, never chart for someone else.

6. *Each charting entry should be signed by the person making it.* The signature should include the medical assistant's

first initial, full last name, and title (e.g., D. Bennett, CMA [AAMA]). The following title abbreviations are often used for medical assistants:

CMA (AAMA): certified medical assistant
RMA: registered medical assistant
MA: medical assistant
SMA: student medical assistant

7. *Never erase or obliterate an entry.* If an error is made in charting, the medical assistant must never erase or obliterate it. Should the physician or medical staff be involved in litigation, erased or obliterated entries tend to reduce credibility. If incorrect information is charted, the medical assistant should draw a single line through the incorrect information, permitting it to remain legible. The word *error* is then written above the incorrect data, including the date and the medical assistant's first initial, last name, and credentials. Some medical offices may request that the reason for the change also be recorded. The correct information is then inserted next to the error (Figure 1-23).

The medical assistant should always take the time to chart properly in the patient's medical record. Good charting helps coordinate efforts in the medical office and leads to high-quality health care.

Charting Progress Notes

After completion of the initial health history, a system is needed to update the medical record with new information each time the patient visits the medical office. Most offices use progress notes to fulfill this function. Progress notes document the patient's health status and the care and treatment being received by the patient in chronological order. Progress notes provide effective communication among medical office personnel and serve as a legal document.

The medical assistant is frequently responsible for charting progress notes in the medical record. They are usually charted on special preprinted lined sheets known as *progress note sheets.* These sheets have a column for the date and a column for charting information (see Figure 1-22, *F*). Types of progress notes that are often charted by the medical assistant are presented next, along with a charting example of each.

Charting Patient Symptoms

The medical assistant takes patient symptoms during office visits and telephone conversations. Information conveyed during a telephone conversation helps the medical assistant determine whether the patient needs to be seen and the immediacy of the situation.

A **symptom** is any change in the body or its functioning that indicates the presence of disease. Symptoms can be classified as subjective or objective. A **subjective symptom** is one that is felt by the patient and cannot be observed by another person. Pain, pruritus, vertigo, and nausea are examples of subjective symptoms. An **objective symptom** is one that can be observed by another person and by the patient. Rash, coughing, and cyanosis are objective symptoms. The medical assistant should have a thorough knowledge of common symptoms and should be able to recognize them. The box on page 38 lists and describes common symptoms.

Taking patient symptoms during an office visit consists of the following:

1. Obtaining a chief complaint (see earlier discussion)
2. Obtaining additional information about the chief complaint

If the patient complains of pain in the abdomen that has lasted for 2 days (chief complaint), additional information is needed to describe the pain, including its type, specific location, onset, intensity, precipitating factors, and duration. The procedure for taking patient symptoms during an office visit is outlined in Procedure 1-4. Additional skills and practice on taking patient symptoms are included in Chapter 1 of the *Study Guide* for students.

Other Activities That Need to Be Charted

Procedures

The medical assistant frequently charts procedures performed on the patient, including vital signs, weight and height, visual acuity, and ear irrigations. Procedures should be charted immediately after they are performed; from a legal standpoint, a procedure that is not documented was not performed. In general, the following information should be included: the date and time, the type of procedure, the outcome, and the patient reaction. The specific information to be charted is included with each procedure presented in this text.

CHARTING EXAMPLE	
Date	
6/30/12	9:15 a.m. Irrigated Ⓡ ear c̄ 200 ml of
	normal saline at 98.6° F. Mod amt of
	cerumen in returned solution. Pt states can
	hear better. ——— D. Bennett, CMA (AAMA)

Procedure.

	error 10/15/12 —— D. Bennett, CMA (AAMA)
10/15/12	9:30 a.m. Tubersol Mantoux test: 9mm induration. ———
	————————————— 12 ——— D. Bennett, CMA (AAMA)

Figure 1-23. Proper method for correcting an error in a patient's medical record.

Abbreviations and Symbols Commonly Used in the Medical Office

Abbreviations Used to Chart Symptoms and Procedures		Abbreviations Used to Chart Symptoms and Procedures—cont'd	
aa	of each	DTaP	diphtheria and tetanus toxoids and acellular pertussis vaccine
Ab	abortion	D&V	diarrhea and vomiting
abd	abdomen	DVA	distance visual acuity
abs	absent	ea	each
ac	before meals	ED	emergency department
ad lib	as desired	EDD	expected date of delivery
admin	administer	Fe	iron
AM or a.m.	before noon	flex sig	flexible sigmoidoscopy
amt	amount	freq	frequent
AP	apical pulse	F/U	follow-up
approx	approximately	Fx	fracture
appt	appointment	GYN	gynecology
ASA	acetylsalicylic acid (aspirin)	h or hr	hour
ASAP	as soon as possible	H/A	headache
BA	backache	HBP	high blood pressure
b/c	because	HC	head circumference
BC	birth control	Hep B	hepatitis B vaccine
bid	twice a day	Hg	mercury
BM	bowel movement	H_2O	water
BP	blood pressure	HR	heart rate
BPM	beats per minute	HRT	hormone replacement therapy
BS	blood sugar	hs	at bedtime
BSE	breast self-examination	ht	height
c̄	with	ID	intradermal
caps	capsules	IM	intramuscular
cath	catheter, catheterize	IPV	inactivated polio vaccine
CC	chief complaint	IV	intravenous
chemo	chemotherapy	lab	laboratory
CMA (AAMA)	certified medical assistant (American Association of Medical Assistants)	lac	laceration
c/o	complains of	lat	lateral
CS	cesarean section	lax	laxative
Cx	cervix	LB	lower back
d	day	LBP	lower back pain
/d	per day	liq	liquid
d/c	discontinue	LMP	last menstrual period
D&I	dry and intact	med, meds	medication, medications
dil	dilute	min	minute
disch	discharge	MMR	measles, mumps, and rubella
DNKA	did not keep appointment	mod	moderate
DOB	date of birth	N/A	not applicable
DOI	date of injury	NB	newborn
DRE	digital rectal examination	N/C	no complaints
DSD	dry, sterile dressing	neg	negative

Continued

Abbreviations and Symbols Commonly Used in the Medical Office—cont'd

Abbreviations Used to Chart Symptoms and Procedures—cont'd		Abbreviations Used to Chart Symptoms and Procedures—cont'd	
NH	nursing home	qod	every other day
NICU	newborn intensive care unit	QS	quantity sufficient
NKA	no known allergies	quad	quadriplegic
NKDA	no known drug allergies	R	respiration
NMP	normal menstrual period	RE	rectal examination
noct	nocturnal	reg	regular
NS	normal saline	rehab	rehabilitation
N&V	nausea and vomiting	RMA	registered medical assistant
NVA	near visual acuity	Rx	prescription
NVD	nausea, vomiting, and diarrhea	s̄	without
OB	obstetrics	SC or SQ	subcutaneous
occ	occasionally	S/E	side effects
oint	ointment	sec	second
op	operation	sigmoid	sigmoidoscopy
OR	operating room	sl	slight
OT	occupational therapy	sm	small
OTC	over-the-counter (nonprescription medication)	SOB	shortness of breath
OV	office visit	sol	solution
P	pulse	spec	specimen
Pap	Pap test	STAT	immediately
path	pathology	surg	surgery
pc	after meals	T	temperature
peds	pediatrics	tab, tabs	tablet, tablets
PEN	penicillin	temp	temperature
per	by or through	ther	therapy
pharm	pharmacy	tid	three times a day
PM or p.m.	afternoon	TLC	total lung capacity, tender loving care
PMS	premenstrual syndrome	TPR	temperature, pulse, and respiration
po or PO	by mouth	tr	trace
pos	positive	TSE	testicular self-examination
postop	postoperative (after surgery)	vag	vagina, vaginal
preop	preoperative (before surgery)	VE	vaginal examination
prep	preparation	vit	vitamin
prn	as needed	VO	verbal order
PT	physical therapy, prothrombin time	VS	vital signs
Pt or pt	patient	wk	week
qd	every day	WNL	within normal limits
qh	every hour	WO	written order
q(2,3,4)h	every (2,3,4) hours	w/o	without
qid	four times a day	wt	weight
qn	every night	W/U	workup
QNS	quantity not sufficient		

Abbreviations and Symbols Commonly Used in the Medical Office—cont'd

Abbreviations Used to Chart Body Parts and Locations

abd	abdomen
AD	right ear
AS	left ear
AU	in each ear, both ears
EENT	eye, ear, nose, and throat
GI	gastrointestinal
GU	genitourinary
Ⓛ or lt	left
ⓁⒶ	left arm
ⓁⓁ	left leg
LLQ	lower left quadrant
LRQ	lower right quadrant
LUQ	left upper quadrant
OD	right eye
OS	left eye
OU	in each eye, both eyes
Ⓡ or rt	right
ⓇⒶ	right arm
ⓇⓁ	right leg
RLQ	right lower quadrant
RUQ	right upper quadrant

Abbreviations Used to Chart Measurement

C	Celsius
cc	cubic centimeter
cm	centimeter
dL	deciliter
F	Fahrenheit
g	gram
kg	kilogram
L	liter
lb	pound
m	meter
mcg	microgram
mg	milligram
ml	milliliter
mm	millimeter
oz	ounce
pt	pint
qt	quart
ss	one half
T	tablespoon
tsp	teaspoon

Miscellaneous Abbreviations

Patient Examination

Dx	diagnosis
H/O	history of
H&P	history and physical
Hx	history
MHx	medical history
PE or Px	physical examination
prog	prognosis
Sx	symptoms
Tx	treatment

Conditions

BPH	benign prostatic hyperplasia
CA	cancer
CAD	coronary artery disease
CHF	congestive heart failure
COPD	chronic obstructive pulmonary disease
CRC	colorectal cancer
CVA	cerebrovascular accident
DM	diabetes mellitus
DVT	deep vein thrombosis
Fe def	iron deficiency
GC	gonorrhea
GDM	gestational diabetes mellitus
HTN	hypertension
IBS	irritable bowel syndrome
MI	myocardial infarction
MS	multiple sclerosis
OA	osteoarthritis
OM	otitis media
PID	pelvic inflammatory disease
RA	rheumatoid arthritis
RF	rheumatic fever
STD	sexually transmitted disease
TB	tuberculosis
URI	upper respiratory infection
USI	urinary stress incontinence
UTI	urinary tract infection

Diagnostic Procedures

CT, CAT	computed axial tomography
CXR	chest x-ray
ECG	electrocardiogram
Echo	echocardiogram

Continued

Abbreviations and Symbols Commonly Used in the Medical Office—cont'd

Miscellaneous Abbreviations—cont'd
Diagnostic Procedures—cont'd

EEG	electroencephalogram
FOBT	fecal occult blood test
IVP	intravenous pyelogram
LP	lumbar puncture
MRI	magnetic resonance imaging
NST	nonstress test
PFT	pulmonary function test
TRUS	transrectal ultrasound
US	ultrasound

Laboratory Tests

ABG	arterial blood gas
BG	blood glucose
Bx	biopsy
CBC	complete blood count
C&S	culture and sensitivity
diff	differential
ESR	erythrocyte sedimentation rate
FBG	fasting blood glucose
FBS	fasting blood sugar
GCT	glucose challenge test
GTT	glucose tolerance test
Hct	hematocrit
Hgb	hemoglobin
OGTT	oral glucose tolerance test
PET	positron emission tomography
PPBS	postprandial blood sugar
PSA	prostate-specific antigen
PT	prothrombin time
RBC	red blood cell

Miscellaneous Abbreviations—cont'd
Laboratory Tests—cont'd

RBS	random blood sugar
SG	specific gravity
trig	triglycerides
UA	urinalysis
U/C	urine culture
WBC	white blood cell

Symbols

∅	none, no
√	check
>	greater than
<	less than
↑	increase
↓	decrease
♀	female
♂	male
°	degree
@	at
×	times
$\bar{x}$	except
$\bar{p}$	after
#	number
1°	primary
2°	secondary
+	positive
−	negative
Ⓡ	rectal temperature
Ⓐ	axillary temperature
"	inches
'	feet

Administration of Medication

Charting medications administered to the patient is an important responsibility in the medical office. The recording should include the date and time, the name of the medication, the lot number (if required), the dosage given, the route of administration, the injection site used (for parenteral medication), and any significant observations or patient reactions.

CHARTING EXAMPLE	
Date	
6/30/12	10:15 a.m. Bicillin (Lot # T61420) 900,00 units IM, Ⓛ
	dorsogluteal. ———————— D. Bennett, CMA (AAMA)

Administration of medication.

Specimen Collection

Each time a specimen is collected from a patient, the medical assistant should chart the date and time of the collection, the type of specimen, and the area of the body from which the specimen was obtained. If the specimen is to be sent to an outside laboratory for testing, this information also should be charted, including the tests requested, the date the specimen was sent, and where it was sent. In this way, the physician would know that the specimen was collected and sent to the laboratory when test results are not back yet.

Diagnostic Procedures and Laboratory Tests

Diagnostic procedures and laboratory tests ordered for a patient should always be charted in the medical record. If the patient does not undergo the test, documented proof exists

PROCEDURE 1-4   Obtaining and Recording Patient Symptoms

Outcome Obtain and record patient symptoms.

Equipment/Supplies

- Medical record of the patient to be interviewed
- Black ink pen

1. **Procedural Step.** Assemble the equipment. Ensure that you have the correct patient's record and a black ink pen for charting patient symptoms.
   Principle. Black ink must be used to provide a permanent record.
2. **Procedural Step.** Go to the waiting room and ask the patient to come back.
3. **Procedural Step.** Escort the patient to a quiet, comfortable room, such as an examination room, that allows for privacy.
   Principle. Patient symptoms should be taken in a room that encourages communication.
4. **Procedural Step.** In a calm and friendly manner, greet the patient and introduce yourself. Identify the patient by his or her full name and date of birth.
   Principle. A warm introduction sets a positive tone for the remainder of the interview.
5. **Procedural Step.** Ask the patient to be seated. You should seat yourself so that you face the patient at a distance of 3 to 4 feet.
   Principle. This type of seating arrangement facilitates open communication.
6. **Procedural Step.** Use good communication skills to interact with the patient. These include the following:
   a. Use the patient's name of choice.
   b. Show genuine interest and concern for the patient.
   c. Maintain appropriate eye contact.
   d. Use terminology the patient can understand.
   e. Listen carefully and attentively to the patient.
   f. Pay attention to the patient's nonverbal messages.
   g. Avoid judgmental comments.
   h. Avoid rushing the patient.
7. **Procedural Step.** Locate the progress note sheet in the patient's medical record. Chart the date and time and the abbreviation for chief complaint (CC).
8. **Procedural Step.** Use an open-ended question to elicit the chief complaint, such as "What seems to be the problem?"
   Principle. An open-ended question allows the patient to verbalize freely.
9. **Procedural Step.** Chart the chief complaint while following the charting guidelines outlined on pages 39 to 40. In addition, these guidelines should be followed:
   a. Limit the chief complaint to one or two symptoms, and refer to a specific rather than a vague symptom.
   b. Chart the chief complaint concisely and briefly, using the patient's own words as much as possible.

   c. Include the duration of the symptom (onset) in the chief complaint.
   d. Avoid using names of diseases or diagnostic terms to record the chief complaint.
10. **Procedural Step.** Obtain additional information regarding the chief complaint using *what, when,* and *where* questions. While following proper charting guidelines, chart this information after the chief complaint.

What Questions:

- What exactly have you been experiencing?
- Does the symptom occur suddenly or gradually?
- Does anything make it worse?

Where Question:

- Where is the symptom located?

When Questions:

- When did the symptom first occur?
- How long does it last?
- Does anything cause it to occur?
   Principle. This information provides a complete description of the chief complaint.
11. **Procedural Step.** Thank the patient and proceed to the next step in the patient workup. (This usually includes measuring vital signs and height and weight and preparing the patient as needed for the physical examination [see Chapters 4 and 5].)
12. **Procedural Step.** Inform the patient that the physician will be with him or her soon.
13. **Procedural Step.** Place the patient's medical record where it can be reviewed by the physician (as designated by the medical office policy).
   Principle. The physician will want to review the patient's medical record before examining the patient.

CHARTING EXAMPLE	
Date	
6/30/12	3:15 p.m. CC: Intense pain in the Ⓛ ear for the
	past 2 days. Pt states pain is sharp and
	continuous. Pt noted sl yellow discharge
	from Ⓛ ear. Fever of 101° F began last night
	about 9 p.m. Took Tylenol 2 tabs at 8 a.m.
	———— D. Bennett, CMA (AAMA)

CHARTING EXAMPLE

Date	
6/30/12	1:30 p.m. Venous blood spec collected from Ⓡ
	arm. Sent to Ross Lab for CBC and diff on
	6/30/12 —————— D. Bennett, CMA (AAMA)
Date	
6/30/12	2:00 p.m. Throat spec collected. Sent to
	Ross Lab for C&S on 6/30/12 —————
	—————— D. Bennett, CMA (AAMA)

Specimen collection.

that the test was ordered. Charting diagnostic procedures and laboratory tests protects the physician legally and refreshes the physician's memory of the procedures and tests being run on the patient when results are not yet back from the testing facility. Information to include in the charting entry consists of the date and time, the type of procedure or test ordered, the scheduling date, and where it is being performed.

CHARTING EXAMPLE

Date	
6/30/12	10:15 a.m. Mammography scheduled for
	7/5/12 at Grant Hospital. —————
	—————— D. Bennett, CMA (AAMA)
Date	
6/30/12	11:30 a.m. Pt given lab request for GTT at
	Ross Lab. ————— D. Bennett, CMA (AAMA)

Diagnostic/laboratory tests.

Results of Laboratory Tests

It is usually unnecessary to chart results from laboratory reports returned from outside laboratories because the report itself is filed in the patient's record. In case of a STAT request or critical findings, the test results may be telephoned to the medical office, requiring the medical assistant to record the results on a report form. Careful recording is essential to avoid errors, which could affect the patient's diagnosis. Results of laboratory tests performed by the medical assistant in the office should be charted in the medical record and must include the date and time, name of the test, and test results.

Patient Instructions

It often is necessary to relay instructions to a patient regarding medical care (e.g., wound care, cast care, care of sutures). The medical assistant should chart this information, taking care to include the date and time and the type of instructions relayed to the patient. Many medical offices have printed instruction sheets that are given to the patient. The patient is asked to sign a form, which is filed in the patient's record, indicating that he or she has read and understands the instructions (Figure 1-24). The form also should be signed by the medical assistant, who functions as a signature witness. This protects the physician legally in the event that the patient fails to follow the instructions and causes further harm or damage to a body part.

Other areas that the medical assistant is responsible for charting in the medical record include missed or canceled appointments, telephone calls from patients, medication refills, and changes in medication or dosage by the physician.

CHARTING EXAMPLE

Date	
6/30/12	9:30 a.m. Instructions provided for BSE. Pt
	given a BSE educational brochure. —————
	—————— D. Bennett, CMA (AAMA)
Date	
6/30/12	10:00 a.m. Explained wound care. Written
	instructions provided. Signed copy in chart.
	To return in 2 days for suture removal. ———
	—————— D. Bennett, CMA (AAMA)
Date	
6/30/12	10:25 a.m. Provided instructions for applying
	a heating pad to the lower back. —————
	—————— D. Bennett, CMA (AAMA)

Patient instructions.

CHARTING EXAMPLE

Date	
6/30/12	8:00 a.m. FBS: 82 mg/dL.—————
	—————— D. Bennett, CMA (AAMA)
Date	
6/30/12	4:15 p.m. Quick Vue+ Mono Test: neg ———
	—————— D. Bennett, CMA (AAMA)

Laboratory test results.

CHARTING EXAMPLE

Date	
6/30/12	11:15 a.m. Phoned office. States that
	swelling in the Ⓡ ankle is almost gone.
	—————— D. Bennett, CMA (AAMA)
Date	
6/30/12	1:15 p.m. Missed appointment scheduled for
	6/30/12 at 1:00 p.m. ——— D. Bennett, CMA (AAMA)

Telephone call and missed appointment.

PATIENT INSTRUCTIONS FOR WOUND CARE

Name of patient: _____

Follow the instructions indicated below for care of your wound:

1. Use ice bag and elevate to reduce swelling and pain. Elevate higher than your heart.
2. You may take aspirin/Tylenol for pain.
3. Keep the dressing clean and dry.
4. Replace the dressing within _____ days.
5. Discard the dressing within _____ days.
6. Cleanse the wound daily as instructed.
7. Stitches should be removed in _____ days.
8. Despite the greatest of care, any wound can become infected. If your wound becomes red or swollen, shows pus or red streaks, or feels more sore instead of less sore, contact the physician **immediately.**

I have received and understand the above instructions:

Patient (or representative): _____

Relationship to patient: _____

Witness: _____   Time and date: _____

Figure 1-24. Instruction sheet for patients.

MEDICAL PRACTICE and the LAW

Documentation can be a deciding factor in a legal case. Everything you do for a patient should be documented in a factual manner in the medical record, or "chart." When a legal issue arises, often several years pass before it comes to trial. If you are involved, you will be asked detailed questions as to your actions on a particular day for a particular patient. Few people have accurate memories for that long. Juries give more credibility to documentation performed at the time of the action than to a memory of years ago. Ethically, you owe the patient thorough documentation to provide optimal continuity of care. Remember that all patient information is confidential.

Proper charting is a crucial skill for a medical assistant to master. Although proper documentation would not prevent a lawsuit, it might determine the outcome. Pay particular attention to the rules for consents and charting guidelines outlined in this chapter, and follow them to the letter. ■

---

evolve *Check out the Evolve site to access additional interactive activities.*

What Would You Do? What Would You *Not* Do? RESPONSES

Case Study 1
Page 5

What Did Dawn Do?

❏ Listened carefully to Mrs. Celeste and relayed concern through both verbal and nonverbal behavior.
❏ Reassured Mrs. Celeste that her information would be kept completely confidential. Explained to Mrs. Celeste that health care professionals are required by law to keep all patient information confidential.
❏ Told Mrs. Celeste how important it is to chart information that relates to her health. Explained that the physician must have accurate data to diagnose and treat her. Stressed that certain medications can be harmful to a patient if consumed with alcohol.
❏ Gave Mrs. Celeste information (including brochures) on community agencies that could help her. Explained that these agencies are required to maintain confidentiality and encouraged her to contact them.

What Did Dawn Not *Do?*

❏ Did not tell Mrs. Celeste to go to a different physician to ensure that her information remained private.
❏ Did not tell Mrs. Celeste that she needed to stop drinking before it affected her health.

What Would You Do/What Would You *Not* Do? Review Dawn's response and place a checkmark next to the information you included in your response. List the additional information you included in your response.

_____

_____

_____

_____

Continued

Case Study 2
Page 27

What Did Dawn Do?
- ❏ Reassured Tessa that she and her family have been good patients and apologized for the inconvenience.
- ❏ Told Tessa that it is against the law to transfer medical records without the patient's written authorization. Explained that the reason for the law is to safeguard a patient's privacy.
- ❏ Asked Tessa if she has a fax machine because the forms could be faxed to her for signing and then faxed back to the office. If not, explained that Tessa and her husband would need to come to the office to sign release forms.

What Did Dawn Not *Do?*
- ❏ Did not get defensive about Tessa being so annoyed.
- ❏ Did not send their medical records to the new physician without the signed release forms.

What Would You Do/What Would You *Not* Do? Review Dawn's response and place a checkmark next to the information you included in your response. List the additional information you included in your response.

_____

_____

_____

_____

Case Study 3
Page 33

What Did Dawn Do?
- ❏ Listened to and empathized with Mr. and Mrs. Oberlin's concerns.
- ❏ Told Mr. and Mrs. Oberlin that because Brett is of adult age, it would be against the law to let them see his medical record without his written authorization. Explained that the law is there to protect a patient's right to privacy, and just as it protects Brett's right, the law also protects their right, so that no one can obtain information from their medical records without their authorization.
- ❏ Suggested that they talk with Brett again regarding the situation.

What Did Dawn Not *Do?*
- ❏ Did not give them any information from Brett's medical record.

What Would You Do/What Would You *Not* Do? Review Dawn's response and place a checkmark next to the information you included in your response. List the additional information you included in your response.

_____

_____

_____

CERTIFICATION REVIEW

- ❏ **The patient registration record** must be completed by all new patients and consists of demographic and billing information.
- ❏ **The health history** (along with the physical examination and laboratory and diagnostic tests) is used to determine the patient's general state of health, to arrive at a diagnosis and prescribe treatment, and to observe any change in a patient's illness after treatment has been instituted.
- ❏ **The physical examination report** is a summary of the findings from the physician's assessment of each part of the patient's body.
- ❏ **The medication record** consists of detailed information relating to a patient's medications and includes one or more of the following categories: prescription medications, over-the-counter (OTC) medications, and medications administered at the medical office.
- ❏ **A consultation report** is a narrative report of a specialist's opinion about a patient's condition and is based on a review of the patient's medical record and an examination of the patient.
- ❏ **Home health care** provides medical and nonmedical care in a patient's home or place of residence to minimize the effect of disease or disability.
- ❏ **A laboratory report** is a report of the analysis or examination of body specimens. Its purpose is to relay the results of laboratory tests to the physician to assist him or her in diagnosing and treating disease.
- ❏ **A diagnostic procedure report** consists of a narrative description and interpretation of a diagnostic procedure and includes the following reports: electrocardiogram, Holter monitor, sigmoidoscopy, colonoscopy, spirometry, radiology, and diagnostic imaging.
- ❏ **A therapeutic service report** documents the assessments and treatment designed to restore a patient's ability to function, such as physical therapy, occupational therapy, and speech therapy.
- ❏ **Hospital documents** are prepared by the attending physician and include the history and physical examination of a hospitalized patient, operative report, discharge summary report, pathology report, and emergency department report.
- ❏ **A consent to treatment form** is required for all surgical operations and nonroutine diagnostic or therapeutic procedures performed in the medical office. The form must be signed by the patient and provides written evidence that the patient agreed to the procedure(s) listed on the form.

CERTIFICATION REVIEW—cont'd

❏ **A release of medical information form** is required to release information that is not part of medical treatment, payment, and health care operations.

❏ The **electronic medical record** is a computerized record of the important health information regarding a patient, including the care of that individual and the progress of the patient's condition. EMR software allows for the creation, storage, organization, editing, and retrieval of medical records on a computer. Advantages of an EMR include speed and productivity, efficiency, and accessibility; disadvantages include the initial cost, the time investment, and occupational tasks that need to be performed before an EMR program becomes operational.

❏ **A source-oriented medical record** is organized into sections based on the department, facility, or other source that generated the information. Each section of a source-oriented record is separated from the others by a chart divider labeled with the title of its respective section.

❏ **The documents in a problem-oriented record (POR)** are organized by the patient's specific health problems and include a database, a problem list, a plan of action for each problem, and progress notes. Progress notes for a POR include four categories: subjective data, objective data, assessment, and plan (SOAP).

❏ **A health history** consists of the following components: identification data, chief complaint, present illness, past history, family history, social history, and review of systems. A health history is taken for each new patient, and subsequent office visits (in the form of progress notes) provide information regarding changes in the patient's illness or treatment.

❏ **Charting** is the process of making written entries about a patient in the medical record. The medical record is a legal document, and the information must be charted as completely and accurately as possible, while following established charting guidelines.

❏ **Progress notes** update the medical record with new information each time the patient visits or telephones the medical office. Types of progress notes often charted by the medical assistant include patient symptoms, medical procedures, administration of medication, specimen collection, diagnostic procedures and laboratory tests ordered on a patient, results of laboratory tests, instructions given to the patient regarding medical care, missed or canceled appointments, telephone calls from patients, medication refills, and changes in medication or dosage by the physician.

TERMINOLOGY REVIEW

Medical Term	Word Parts	Definition
Attending physician		The physician responsible for the care of a hospitalized patient.
Charting		The process of making written entries about a patient in the medical record.
Consultation report		A narrative report of an opinion about a patient's condition by a practitioner other than the attending physician.
Diagnosis	*dia-:* through, complete *-gnosis:* knowledge	The scientific method of determining and identifying a patient's condition.
Diagnostic procedure	*dia-:* through, complete *gnos/o:* knowledge *-ic:* pertaining to	A procedure performed to assist in the diagnosis, management, or treatment of a patient's condition.
Discharge summary report		A brief summary of the significant events of a patient's hospitalization.
Electronic medical record (EMR)		A medical record that is stored on a computer.
Familial	*famil:* family *-al:* pertaining to	Occurring in or affecting members of a family more frequently than would be expected by chance.
Health history report		A collection of subjective data about a patient.
Home health care		The provision of medical and nonmedical care in a patient's home or place of residence.
Informed consent		Consent given by a patient for a medical procedure after he or she has been informed of the nature of his or her condition and the purpose of the procedure, and has been given an explanation of risks involved with the procedure, alternative treatments or procedures available, the likely outcome of the procedure, and the risks involved with declining or delaying the procedure.

Continued

TERMINOLOGY REVIEW—cont'd

Medical Term	Word Parts	Definition
Inpatient		A patient who has been admitted to a hospital for at least one overnight stay.
Medical impressions		Conclusions drawn by the physician from an interpretation of data. Other terms for impressions include *provisional diagnosis* and *tentative diagnosis.*
Medical record		A written record of important information regarding a patient, including the care of that individual and the progress of the patient's condition.
Medical record format		The way a medical record is organized. The two main types of medical record formats are the source-oriented record and the problem-oriented record.
Objective symptom		A symptom that can be observed by an examiner.
Paper-based patient record (PPR)		A medical record in paper form.
Patient		An individual receiving medical care.
Physical examination		An assessment of each part of the patient's body to obtain objective data about the patient that assists the physician in determining the patient's state of health.
Physical examination report		A report of the objective findings from the physician's assessment of each body system.
Problem		Any condition that requires further observation, diagnosis, management, or patient education.
Prognosis	*pro-:* before *-gnosis:* knowledge	The probable course and outcome of a disease and the prospects for a patient's recovery.
Reverse chronological order		Arranging documents with the most recent document on top or in the front, which means that the oldest document is on the bottom or at the back of a section or file.
SOAP format		A method of organization for recording progress notes. The SOAP format includes the following categories: subjective data, objective data, assessment, and plan.
Subjective symptom		A symptom that is felt by the patient but is not observable by an examiner.
Symptom		Any change in the body or its functioning that indicates the presence of disease.

ON THE WEB

For information on the medical record:

American Health Information Management Association: www.ahima.org

Privacy Rights Clearinghouse: www.privacyrights.org

Getting Medical Records: www.genetichealth.com

Electronic Medical Record: www.openclinical.org

For information on communication assistance:

Toll-Free Directory: inter800.com

U.S. Postal Service Zip Code Access: www.usps.com/zip4

United Parcel Service: www.ups.com

Federal Express: www.fedex.com

2

Medical Asepsis and the OSHA Standard

LEARNING OBJECTIVES	PROCEDURES
Microorganisms and Medical Asepsis	

Microorganisms and Medical Asepsis

1. Define a microorganism and give examples of types of microorganisms.
2. Explain the difference between a nonpathogen and a pathogen.
3. Define medical asepsis.
4. List the six basic requirements for growth and multiplication of microorganisms.
5. Outline the infection process and cycle, including the following:
   Give examples of the means of entry of microorganisms into the body.
   Give examples of the means of transmission of microorganisms from one person to another.
   Give examples of the means of exit of microorganisms from the body.
   List and explain the protective mechanisms the body uses to prevent the entrance of microorganisms.
6. Explain the difference between resident flora and transient flora.
7. State when each of the following is performed: handwashing, antiseptic handwashing, and alcohol-based hand rub.
8. Identify medical aseptic practices that should be followed in the medical office.
9. Explain how proper handwashing helps prevent the transmission of microorganisms.
10. List examples of when to wear clean disposable gloves.

Handwashing.

Applying an alcohol-based hand rub.

Application and removal of clean disposable gloves.

OSHA Bloodborne Pathogens Standard

1. Explain the purpose of OSHA.
2. Describe the purpose of the Needlestick Safety and Prevention Act.
3. List and describe the elements that must be included in the OSHA exposure control plan.
4. Explain the purpose of each of the following OSHA requirements: labeling requirements and sharps injury log.
5. Define and give examples of each of the following: engineering controls, work practice controls, personal protective equipment, and housekeeping procedures.
6. Identify the guidelines for use of personal protective equipment.

Adhere to the OSHA Bloodborne Pathogens Standard.

Regulated Medical Waste

1. List examples of medical waste and explain how to discard each type of waste.
2. Explain how to handle and dispose of regulated medical waste.

Prepare regulated waste for pickup by an infectious waste service.

Bloodborne Diseases

1. Describe postexposure prophylaxis for hepatitis B.
2. Explain the difference between acute and chronic hepatitis B.
3. Explain the possible effects and consequences of chronic hepatitis C.
4. List and describe the four stages of the AIDS infection cycle.
5. List and describe the AIDS-defining conditions.

KEY TERMS

aerobe (AIR-obe)
anaerobe (AN-er-obe)
antiseptic
asepsis (ay-SEP-sis)
cilia (SIL-ee-ya)
contaminated (kon-TAM-in-ated)
decontamination (DEE-kon-tam-in-AY-shun)
hand hygiene
infection
medical asepsis
microorganism (MYE-kroe-OR-gan-iz-um)
nonintact (NON-in-takt) skin
nonpathogen (non-PATH-oh-jen)

opportunistic (OP-pore-tune-IS-tik) infection
optimum (OP-tuh-mum) growth temperature
parenteral (pare-EN-ter-al)
pathogen (PATH-oh-jen)
perinatal (pare-ee-NAY-tul)
pH (PEE-AYCH)
postexposure prophylaxis (proe-fil-ACKS-is) (PEP)
regulated medical waste (RMW)
reservoir (REZ-er-vwar) host
resident flora (FLOE-ruh)
susceptible (sus-SEP-tih-bul)
transient (TRAN-zee-ent) flora

Introduction to Medical Asepsis and the OSHA Standard

Medical **asepsis** and **infection** control are crucial in preventing the spread of disease. The medical assistant should always practice good medical aseptic techniques to provide a safe and healthy environment in the medical office. The Occupational Safety and Health Administration (OSHA) Bloodborne Pathogens Standard is important for infection control. This standard is required by the federal government to reduce the exposure of health care employees to infectious diseases. This chapter presents a thorough discussion of medical asepsis, infection control, and the OSHA Bloodborne Pathogens Standard.

MICROORGANISMS AND MEDICAL ASEPSIS

Microorganisms are tiny living plants or animals that cannot be seen with the naked eye, but instead must be viewed with the aid of a microscope. Common types of microorganisms include bacteria, viruses, protozoa, fungi, and animal parasites. Most microorganisms are harmless and do not cause disease. They are termed **nonpathogens.** Other microorganisms, known as **pathogens,** are harmful to the body and can cause disease.

In the medical office, practices must be employed to reduce the number and hinder the transmission of pathogenic microorganisms. These practices are known as medical asepsis. **Medical asepsis** means that an object or area is clean and free from infection. Nonpathogens would still be present on a clean or medically aseptic substance or surface, but all the pathogens would have been eliminated.

Growth Requirements for Microorganisms

For microorganisms to survive, certain growth requirements must be present in the environment, as follows:

1. **Proper nutrition.** Microorganisms that use inorganic or nonliving substances as sources of food are known as *autotrophs.* Microorganisms that use organic or living substances for food are known as *heterotrophs.*
2. **Oxygen.** Most microorganisms need oxygen to grow and multiply and are termed **aerobes.** Other microor-

ganisms, known as **anaerobes,** grow best in the absence of oxygen.

3. **Temperature.** Each microorganism has a temperature at which it grows best, known as the **optimum growth temperature.** Most microorganisms grow best at 98.6° F (37° C), the human body temperature.
4. **Darkness.** Microorganisms grow best in darkness.
5. **Moisture.** Microorganisms need moisture for cell metabolism and to carry away wastes.
6. **pH.** Most microorganisms prefer a neutral pH. If the environment of the microorganisms becomes too acidic or too basic, they die.

If growth requirements are taken away from the environment of microorganisms, they are unable to survive. Eliminating these conditions is one way to reduce the growth and transmission of pathogens in the medical office.

Infection Process Cycle

For a pathogen to survive and produce disease, a continuous cycle must be followed; this is known as the *infection process cycle* (Figure 2-1). If the cycle is broken at any point, the pathogen dies. The medical assistant has a responsibility to help break this cycle in the medical office by practicing good techniques of medical asepsis. These techniques are discussed in the next section.

Protective Mechanisms of the Body

The body has protective mechanisms to help prevent the entrance of pathogens, and these help break the infection process cycle. Protective mechanisms of the body are as follows:

1. The skin is the body's most important defense mechanism; it serves as a protective barrier against the entrance of microorganisms.
2. The mucous membranes of the body, which line the nose and throat and respiratory, gastrointestinal, and genital tracts, help protect the body from invasion by microorganisms.
3. Mucus and cilia in the nose and respiratory tract fight off pathogens. Mucus traps the smaller microorganisms that enter the body, and the hairlike **cilia** constantly beat toward the outside to remove them from the body.
4. Coughing and sneezing help force pathogens from the body.
5. Tears and sweat are secretions that aid in the removal of pathogens from the body.

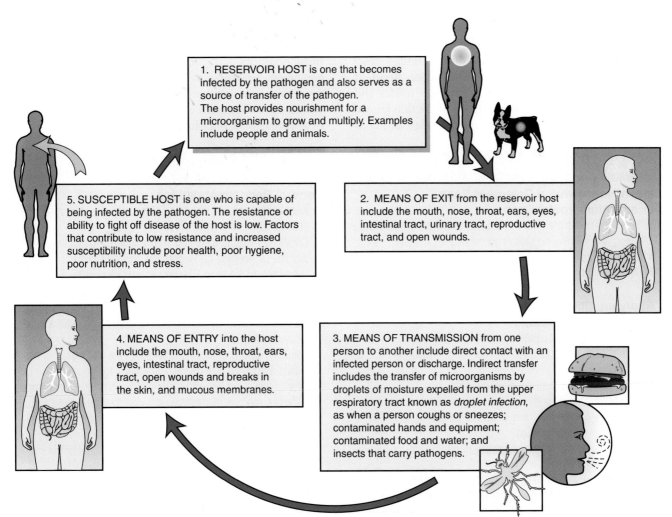

Figure 2-1. The infection process cycle.

6. Urine and vaginal secretions are acidic. Pathogens cannot grow in an acidic environment.

7. The stomach secretes hydrochloric acid, which helps in the process of digestion. This acidic environment discourages the growth of pathogens that enter the stomach.

Medical Asepsis in the Medical Office

Hand Hygiene

Hand hygiene refers to the process of cleansing or sanitizing the hands. Hand hygiene is considered the most important medical aseptic practice in the medical office for preventing the spread of infection. Specific techniques for sanitizing the hands in the medical office include the following:

- Handwashing with a detergent soap and water
- Handwashing with an antimicrobial soap and water
- Applying an alcohol-based hand rub

The Centers for Disease Control and Prevention (CDC) has issued new recommendations for hand hygiene in health care settings. The purpose of these guidelines is to promote improved hand hygiene practices and to reduce transmission of pathogenic microorganisms to patients and employees in health care settings. The CDC guidelines for hand hygiene as they apply to the medical office are outlined in Box 2-1. They are also discussed further in this section.

Resident and Transient Flora

Microorganisms on the hands are classified into the following categories: resident flora and transient flora. **Resident flora** (also known as *normal flora*) normally resides and grows in the epidermis and deeper layers of the skin known as the *dermis*. Resident flora is generally harmless and non-

Putting It All Into Practice

My Name is Jennifer Hawk, and I work for a large group of physicians in a multispecialty clinic. I work in both the front and back areas of the office. I really enjoy experiencing all of these areas of the office, and I definitely never get bored.

The most interesting experience I have had as a practicing medical assistant is seeing the impact that I make in patients' lives. They rely on you and look to you first for help in their health care situation. You are most often the first person they come into contact with in the office, and they look to you for understanding and empathy. Especially patients who come to your office on a regular basis see you as a kind of family member. They appreciate a familiar face and a smile. Most often, you are the individual giving patients instructions concerning testing they will be having done or medication they will be taking. Patients truly do count on your knowledge and assistance throughout their course of care. I was genuinely surprised at what an impact I could have on others. ∎

pathogenic. Because resident flora is attached to the deeper skin layers, it is difficult to remove from the skin.

Transient flora lives and grows on the superficial skin layers, or epidermis. It is picked up on the hands in the course of daily activities. In the medical office, this may include contact with an infected patient, contaminated equipment, or contaminated surfaces. Transient flora is often pathogenic, but because it is attached loosely to the skin, it can be removed easily with proper handwashing or by applying an alcohol-based hand rub.

BOX 2-1 CDC Guidelines for Hand Hygiene in Health Care Settings

Wash Hands with a Detergent Soap or an Antimicrobial Soap

- When the hands are visibly soiled with dirt or body fluids (e.g., blood, feces, urine, respiratory secretions)
- Before eating
- After using the restroom

Apply an Alcohol-Based Hand Rub (or Wash Hands)

- Before having direct patient contact
- After contact with a patient's intact skin (e.g., measuring pulse or blood pressure)
- Before applying and after removing gloves
- After contact with body fluids or excretions, mucous membranes, nonintact skin, and wound dressings as long as the hands are not visibly soiled
- When moving from a contaminated body site to a clean body site during patient care
- After contact with inanimate objects (e.g., medical equipment) when providing health care to a patient

General Recommendations

- Keep natural nail tips less than ¼ inch long. Avoid wearing artificial nails.
- Do not add soap to a partially empty liquid soap dispenser. The practice of "topping off" dispensers can lead to bacterial contamination of the soap. The correct procedure is either to dispose of an empty dispenser or to rinse an empty dispenser thoroughly and then refill it.
- Multiple-use cloth towels of the hanging or roll type are not recommended.
- Use hand lotions or creams to minimize the occurrence of dermatitis associated with frequent handwashing.
- Wear gloves if contact with blood or other potentially infectious materials, mucous membranes, and nonintact skin could occur.
- Change gloves during patient care if moving from a contaminated body site to a clean body site.
- Remove gloves after caring for a patient. Do not wear the same pair of gloves for the care of more than one patient.

Handwashing

Handwashing refers to washing the hands with a detergent soap and water. Detergent soap (commonly known as *plain soap*) contains agents that help break down and emulsify dirt and oil present on the skin. Soap is used to sanitize the hands through the physical removal of dirt and transient flora. It is important to use adequate friction during handwashing to ensure the removal of all transient flora. The CDC recommends that the hands be rubbed together for at least 15 seconds, making sure to cover all surfaces and to focus on the fingertips and fingernails. Procedure 2-1 outlines the handwashing procedure.

The CDC hand hygiene guidelines recommend that handwashing be performed when the hands are visibly soiled with dirt or body fluids, before eating, and after using the restroom (see Box 2-1). If the hands are not visibly soiled, the CDC recommends that an alcohol-based hand rub, rather than handwashing, be used to sanitize the hands. This is because repeated handwashing tends to dry out the hands, leading to irritation, chapping, and dermatitis.

Antiseptic Handwashing

Washing the hands with an antimicrobial soap is termed *antiseptic handwashing*. Antimicrobial soaps contain an **antiseptic,** which is an agent that functions to kill or inhibit the growth of microorganisms (Figure 2-2, *A*). Antiseptic handwashing sanitizes the hands through the mechanical scrubbing action and through the action of the antiseptic. Proper handwashing with an antimicrobial soap removes all soil and transient flora from the hands. Most antimicrobial soaps also deposit an antibacterial film on the skin that discourages bacterial growth. Antiseptic handwashing should be performed by the medical assistant before assisting with minor office surgery. Examples of antiseptics contained in antimicrobial soaps include triclosan, chlorhexidine, hexachlorophene, iodine, and chloroxylenol.

Alcohol-Based Hand Rubs

CDC guidelines recommend the use of an alcohol-based hand rub for sanitizing the hands when they are not visibly soiled (see Box 2-1). Alcohol-based hand rubs, also known as *hand sanitizers,* consist of 60% to 90% alcohol (ethanol or isopropanol) and come in the forms of gels, lotions, and foams (Figure 2-2, *B*). Studies have shown that hand rubs are more effective than traditional soap and water handwashing in removing transient flora and reducing bacterial counts on the hands. The advantages that alcohol-based hand rubs offer over traditional handwashing are as follows:

- Alcohol-based hand rubs are usually more accessible than sinks.
- They do not require rinsing; water or hand drying with a towel is not needed.
- Less time is required to perform hand hygiene. It takes 20 to 30 seconds to sanitize the hands with an alcohol-

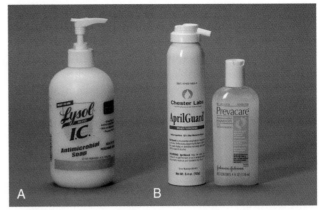

Figure 2-2. **A,** Antimicrobial soap. **B,** Alcohol-based hand rubs.

based hand rub compared with 1 to 2 minutes to perform proper handwashing.

- They are less damaging to the skin, resulting in less dryness and irritation. Most alcohol-based hand rubs contain emollients, which help prevent the skin of the hands from overdrying. As the alcohol dries, protective fats and oils remain on the hands.

Alcohol-based hand rubs have disadvantages. They are more expensive than plain soap. They also cause a brief stinging sensation if they are applied to broken skin, such as a cut or abrasion on the hand. Procedure 2-2 describes the proper steps for performing an alcohol-based hand rub.

Infection Control

In addition to hand hygiene, other good aseptic practices in the medical office include the following:

1. Follow the OSHA Bloodborne Pathogens Standard (presented in this chapter).
2. Keep the medical office free from dirt and dust, which can collect and carry microorganisms.
3. Ensure that the reception area and examining rooms are well ventilated. Stuffy rooms encourage microorganisms to settle on objects.
4. Keep the reception area and examining rooms bright and airy. Light discourages the growth of microorganisms.
5. Eliminate insects by the use of insecticides or window screens. Insects are a means of transmission of microorganisms.
6. Carefully dispose of wastes, such as urine, feces, and respiratory secretions; all wastes should be handled as though they contained pathogens.
7. Do not let soiled items touch clothing.
8. Avoid coughs and sneezes of patients. Moisture droplets expelled from the lungs with coughing and sneezing may contain pathogens.
9. Use discretion in the amount of jewelry worn; wear minimal jewelry or no jewelry at all. Microorganisms can become lodged in the grooves and crevices of jewelry and serve as a means of transmission of pathogens.
10. Teach patients aseptic practices to control the spread of infection at home.

PROCEDURE 2-1

Gloves

Gloves reduce hand contamination by 70% to 80%, reduce cross-contamination between patients, and protect patients and health care workers from infection. The CDC recommends that clean disposable gloves be worn when the medical assistant is likely to come in contact with any body substance, such as blood, urine, feces, mucous membranes, and nonintact skin. Clean disposable gloves should be worn when administering an injection, performing a venipunc-ture, or performing a urinalysis. Clean disposable gloves come in the following sizes: small, medium, large, and extra large, and sometimes extra small. Procedure 2-3 presents the proper method for applying and removing clean disposable gloves.

Sterile gloves are used to perform sterile procedures, such as a dressing change, or to assist the physician during minor office surgery, which is described in greater detail in Chapter 10.

---

see DVD **PROCEDURE 2-1   Handwashing**

Outcome Perform handwashing.

Equipment/Supplies

- Liquid soap
- Paper towels
- Waste container

---

1. **Procedural Step.** Remove your watch or push it up on the forearm so that the wrist is clear. Avoid wearing rings. If you wear rings, remove all except a plain wedding band and put them in a safe place.
   Principle. Microorganisms can lodge in the crevices and grooves of rings.
2. **Procedural Step.** Stand at the sink, making sure clothing does not touch the sink.
   Principle. The sink is considered contaminated, and if the uniform touches the sink, it may pick up microorganisms and transfer them.
3. **Procedural Step.** Turn on the faucets, using a paper towel.
   Principle. The faucets are considered contaminated because they harbor microorganisms.

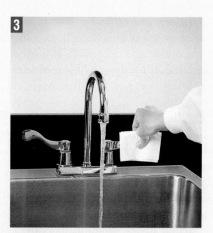

Turn on the faucets using a paper towel.

4. **Procedural Step.** Adjust the water temperature. The water should be warm to make the best suds.
   Principle. Water that is too hot or too cold tends to dry the skin, causing chapping and cracking and mak-

ing it easy for pathogens to enter the body or be transferred to patients.
5. **Procedural Step.** Discard the paper towel in the waste container.
   Principle. The paper towel is considered contaminated after touching the faucets.
6. **Procedural Step.** Wet the hands and forearms thoroughly with water. The hands should be held lower than the elbows at all times. Do not touch the inside of the sink because it is also contaminated.
   Principle. When you hold the hands lower than the elbows, bacteria and debris are carried away from the arms and body and into the sink.
7. **Procedural Step.** Apply soap to the hands. Apply 1 teaspoon of liquid soap (approximately the size of a nickel) to the palm of one hand.

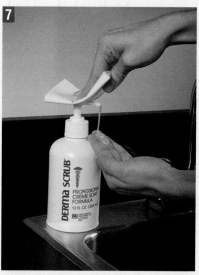

Apply soap to the hands.

PROCEDURE 2-1   Handwashing—cont'd

8. Procedural Step. Wash the palms and backs of the hands with 10 circular motions. Use friction along with the circular motions to wash the palm and back of each hand.

Principle. Friction helps to dislodge and remove microorganisms from the hands.

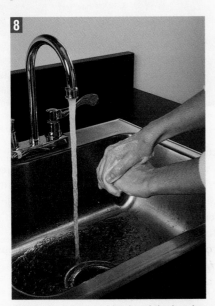

Wash the palms and backs of the hands.

9. Procedural Step. Wash the fingers with 10 circular motions while focusing on the fingertips and fingernails. Interlace the fingers and thumbs, and use friction and circular motions while rubbing the fingers back and forth.

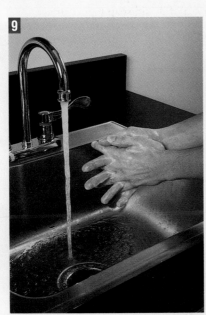

Interlace the fingers and thumbs, and use friction.

Principle. This kind of movement helps remove microorganisms and debris that have accumulated between the fingers.

10. Procedural Step. Rinse well, making sure to hold the hands lower than the elbows.

Principle. Running water helps to rinse away dirt and microorganisms.

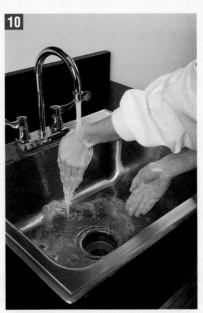

Rinse well, holding the hands lower than the elbows.

11. Procedural Step. Wash the wrists and forearms, using friction along with circular motions.

(**Note:** The hands are washed first because they are the most contaminated; microorganisms and dirt are washed away and do not spread to the wrists and forearms.)

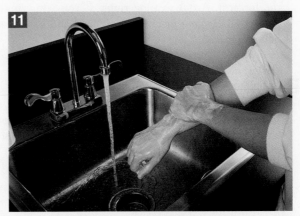

Wash wrists and forearms using friction.

Continued

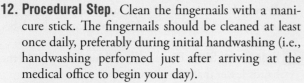

PROCEDURE 2-1   Handwashing—cont'd

12. Procedural Step. Clean the fingernails with a manicure stick. The fingernails should be cleaned at least once daily, preferably during initial handwashing (i.e., handwashing performed just after arriving at the medical office to begin your day).
Principle. Dirt and microorganisms collect underneath the fingernails.

13. Procedural Step. Rinse the arms and hands.
Principle. The running water rinses away the dirt and microorganisms.

14. Procedural Step. Repeat the handwashing procedure. For initial handwashing or when the hands come into contact with blood or other potentially infectious materials, the handwashing procedure should be repeated to ensure removal of all pathogens.

15. Procedural Step. Dry the hands gently and thoroughly, and discard the paper towel.
Principle. Gently drying the hands prevents them from becoming chapped. Microorganisms can lodge in the crevices of chapped hands. Ensure that the hands are dried completely, because wet skin also may cause chapping.

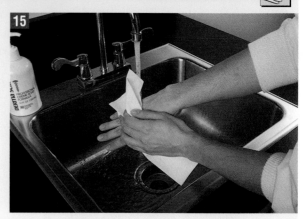

Dry the hands gently and thoroughly.

16. Procedural Step. Turn off the water, using a paper towel, and discard the paper towel in a waste container.
Principle. The faucet is considered contaminated, whereas the hands are medically aseptic or clean.

17. Procedural Step. Do not touch the sink with the bare hands.
Principle. The hands are now medically aseptic, and the sink is considered contaminated.

 ## PROCEDURE 2-2   Applying an Alcohol-Based Hand Rub

Outcome Apply an alcohol-based hand rub.

Equipment/Supplies

- Alcohol-based hand rub

1. Procedural Step. Inspect the hands to ensure that they are not visibly soiled. Hands that are visibly soiled must be washed with soap and water.
Principle. Alcohol-based hand rubs are not intended for the removal of visible soil.

2. Procedural Step. Remove your watch or push it up on the forearm. Avoid wearing rings. If you wear rings, remove all except a plain wedding band and put them in a safe place.
Principle. Microorganisms can lodge in the crevices and grooves of rings.

3. Procedural Step. Apply the alcohol-based hand rub to the palm of one hand as follows:
Gel or Lotion. Apply approximately 1 ml of the gel or lotion to the palm of one hand; this amount is approximately equal to the size of a dime.
Foam. Apply 3 grams of foam to the palm of one hand; this amount is approximately equal to the size of a walnut.

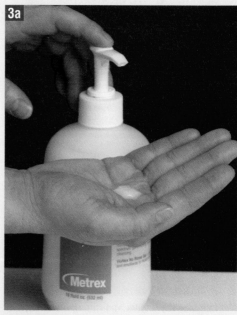

Apply lotion equal to the size of a dime.

PROCEDURE 2-2   Applying an Alcohol-Based Hand Rub—cont'd

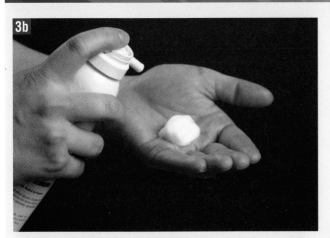

Apply foam equal to the size of a walnut.

Principle. Using more than the recommended amount results in a prolonged (and unnecessary) period of time for your hands to dry.

4. **Procedural Step.** Thoroughly spread the hand rub over all surfaces of both hands (and fingers) up to ½ inch above the wrist. Spread the hand rub around the fingertips and around and under your fingernails.

   Principle. Failure to cover all surfaces can leave areas of the hands contaminated. Microorganisms tend to collect around and underneath the fingernails.

5. **Procedural Step.** Rub the hands together until they are dry; this usually takes 10 to 30 seconds. Allow your hands to dry completely before touching anything. The hands are now medically aseptic.

   Note: After cleaning your hands 5 to 10 times with a hand rub, a buildup of emollients may occur on your hands. The emollients can be easily removed by washing your hands with soap and water.

   Principle. If you have applied a sufficient amount of hand rub, it should take at least 10 to 30 seconds for your hands to feel dry. Your hands will still feel a little wet at first. Let them dry completely before touching anything.

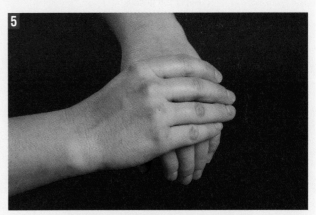

Rub the hands together until they are dry.

PROCEDURE 2-3   Application and Removal of Clean Disposable Gloves

Outcome Apply and remove clean disposable gloves.

Equipment/Supplies

• Clean disposable gloves

Applying Clean Disposable Gloves

No special technique is required when clean disposable gloves are applied. This is because the hands are clean and the gloves are clean; the medical assistant can touch any part of the gloves during application without contaminating them.

1. **Procedural Step.** Remove all rings, and sanitize your hands. Handwashing should be performed if the hands are visibly soiled. If this is not the case, use an alcohol-based hand rub to sanitize the hands. Ensure that your hands are completely dry.

   Principle. Rings may cause the gloves to tear. The warm, moist environment inside gloves provides ideal

growing conditions for the multiplication of transient microorganisms present on the hands. Sanitizing the hands removes these microorganisms and prevents the transmission of pathogens. Moisture encourages the growth of microorganisms.

2. **Procedural Step.** Choose the appropriate size of gloves; they should not be too small or too large. The gloves should fit snugly but not be too tight. Apply the gloves, and adjust them so they fit comfortably.

   Principle. If your gloves are too small, they may rip as you are applying them or may become uncomfortable to wear. If they are too large, you may find it difficult to perform your tasks.

PROCEDURE 2-3   Application and Removal of Clean Disposable Gloves—cont'd

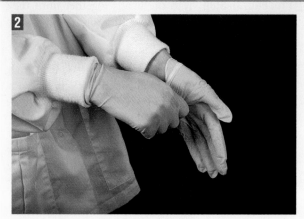

Apply the gloves.

3. Procedural Step. Inspect the gloves for tears. If a tear is present, a new pair of gloves must be applied.

Removing Clean Disposable Gloves

Gloves must be removed in a manner that protects the medical assistant from contaminating his or her clean hands with pathogens that may be present on the outsides of the gloves. This is accomplished by not allowing the bare hands to come in contact with the outsides of the gloves.

1. Procedural Step. Grasp the outside of the left glove 1 to 2 inches from the top with your gloved right hand. (**NOTE:** It does not matter which glove is removed first. You may start with the right glove if you prefer.)

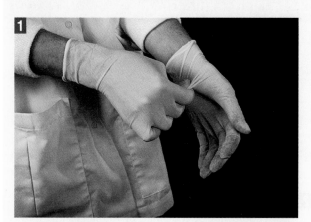

Grasp the glove 1 to 2 inches from the top of the glove.

2. Procedural Step. Slowly pull the left glove off the hand. It will turn inside out as it is removed from your hand.

3. Procedural Step. Pull the left glove free, and scrunch it into a ball with your gloved right hand.

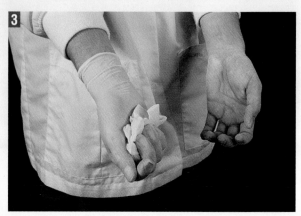

Scrunch the glove into a ball.

4. Procedural Step. Place the index and middle fingers of the left hand on the inside of the right glove. Do not allow your clean hand to touch the outside of the glove.

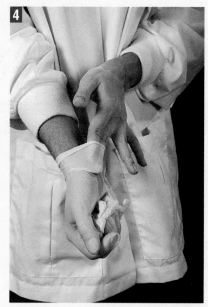

Place the index and middle fingers inside the glove.

5. Procedural Step. Pull the glove off the right hand. It will turn inside out as it is removed from your hand, enclosing the balled-up left glove. Discard both gloves in an appropriate container. If your gloves are visibly

PROCEDURE 2-3   Application and Removal of Clean Disposable Gloves—cont'd

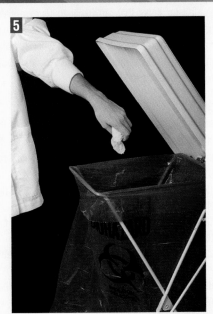

Discard both gloves in an appropriate container.

contaminated with blood or other potentially infectious materials, discard them in a biohazard waste container. Otherwise, they can be discarded in a regular waste container.

6. **Procedural Step.** Sanitize your hands to remove any microorganisms or other contaminants that may have come in contact with your hands during glove removal.

Highlight on Latex Glove Allergy

Latex Gloves

Since the establishment of the OSHA Bloodborne Pathogens Standard, there has been an increase in latex allergies among health care workers because of the expanded use of latex gloves. It has been shown that if an individual is repeatedly exposed to latex, the risk of latex allergy substantially increases. Individuals with other allergies or asthma are also at greater risk for developing a latex allergy. It is estimated that between 8% and 12% of health care workers are allergic to latex, whereas the prevalence of latex allergy in the general population is between 1% and 6%.

Latex gloves are made from natural rubber latex (NRL), which is a milky liquid extracted from rubber trees. Along with gloves, latex rubber is used to make many products used in the medical office. Examples of medical supplies that contain latex are stethoscopes, blood pressure cuffs, percussion hammers, syringes, rubber stoppers on medication vials, adhesive tape, tourniquets, and goggles. Examples of offices supplies made from latex include mouse pads, desktop and chair pads, rubber stamps, rubber bands, and erasers. Household products that contain latex include balloons, rubber balls, tires, hoses, pacifiers, carpeting, shoe soles, utility gloves, and condoms.

Cause of Latex Glove Allergy

The primary substance causing a latex glove allergy is a protein present within the latex that enters the body through direct contact or through inhalation. When latex gloves are donned by an allergic individual, the protein comes in direct contact with the skin. The protein is absorbed into the skin, which then triggers an allergic reaction. Cornstarch powder is sometimes applied to the inside of latex gloves to provide lubrication for easier application and removal of the gloves. The latex proteins adhere to the surface of the cornstarch particles and are released into the atmosphere when the gloves are applied or removed. These protein particles can then be inhaled by an allergic health care worker, leading to an allergic reaction. Other sources of an allergic reaction to latex gloves are chemicals that are added to the gloves during the manufacturing process. When gloves are applied, these chemicals enter the skin of an allergic individual and trigger a reaction.

Latex Glove Reactions

There are three types of adverse reactions caused by latex gloves, which are described below:

1. **Irritant contact dermatitis:** Irritant contact dermatitis is the most common reaction that occurs from latex gloves. It is not an allergic reaction, but rather is caused by irritation of the outer layers of the skin. In the medical office, this irritation is often due to frequent handwashing, along with irritation and rubbing from latex gloves and glove powder. Irritant contact dermatitis is characterized by dry, red, itchy, and cracked areas on the skin of the hands.

Highlight on Latex Glove Allergy—cont'd

2. **Allergic contact dermatitis:** Allergic contact dermatitis is an allergic reaction to the chemical additives used in the manufacturing process of gloves. It is characterized by a skin rash similar to poison ivy, with itchy, dry, red, crusted areas of skin that are cracked and blistered. Dermatitis occurs approximately 24 to 48 hours after direct contact with the gloves.

3. **Latex hypersensitivity reaction:** A hypersensitivity reaction is a more serious reaction that is caused by direct contact with or inhalation of the latex proteins. This type of reaction ranges from mild to severe. A mild reaction causes the following symptoms: redness of the skin, urticaria (hives), and itching. A more severe reaction causes sneezing, itchy red eyes, runny nose, and asthma symptoms (shortness of breath, coughing, and wheezing). Symptoms typically begin within minutes after contact with the latex. The most serious reaction to latex, although rare, is an anaphylactic reaction, which can be life threatening. Individuals with irritant contact dermatitis or allergic contact dermatitis have an increased risk of developing a latex hypersensitivity, because of breaks in the skin that allow easier entry of latex proteins into the body.

Treatment

There is no known treatment that will cure a latex allergy. Medications are available to reduce the symptoms of a latex allergy. The most effective approach is to avoid direct contact with latex and to avoid inhaling airborne powder from latex gloves. The most frequently used non-latex glove alternatives are nitrile gloves and vinyl gloves. In addition, the health care worker should wear a medical alert bracelet and should inform his or her employer and other staff members of the latex allergy.

NIOSH Recommendations

The National Institute for Occupational Safety and Health (NIOSH) has issued the following recommendations to help prevent the development of latex allergies in the workplace:

1. Use non-latex gloves for tasks that are not likely to involve contact with infectious materials (e.g., using non-latex gloves to perform an ear irrigation for the removal of cerumen). Because of their proven barrier protective capability, latex gloves are recommended for tasks that are likely to involve contact with infectious materials.

2. Appropriate barrier protection is necessary when handling infectious materials. If you choose latex gloves, use powder-free gloves with a reduced protein content.

3. Use appropriate work practices to reduce the chance of a reaction to latex:
   - After removing latex gloves, wash hands with a mild soap and dry thoroughly.

4. Use good housekeeping practices to remove latex-containing dust from the workplace:
   - Frequently clean areas contaminated with latex dust (e.g., upholstery, carpets, and ventilation ducts).
   - Frequently change ventilation filters and vacuum bags used in latex-contaminated areas.

5. Take advantage of any latex allergy education and training provided by your employer:
   - Become familiar with procedures for preventing latex allergy.
   - Learn to recognize the symptoms of latex allergy.

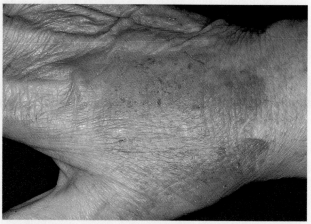

Latex glove allergy. (Goodman CC: Pathology: implications for the physical therapist, ed 3, St Louis, 2010, Saunders.)

Types of Gloves

There are two general types of gloves: latex and non-latex. Latex gloves are made from natural rubber latex (NRL), which is a milky liquid that is extracted from rubber trees. Non-latex gloves are made from synthetic rubber. Examples of non-latex gloves include nitrile, vinyl, and polychloroprene (Neoprene) gloves.

Natural rubber latex gloves have a number of advantages over non-latex gloves. Latex gloves are soft and elastic and therefore stretch to fit more comfortably, whereas some non-latex gloves (e.g., vinyl gloves) are stiffer and are not as comfortable to wear. Latex gloves are thin, which allows the health care worker better feel, dexterity, and grip, and they are lower in cost than most non-latex gloves. In addition, latex has been in use for more than 100 years and has proven barrier protective capability, whereas the barrier effectiveness of non-latex gloves is not as well established at this time. The primary disadvantage of latex gloves is that they can cause an allergic reaction in individuals with a hypersensitivity to latex (see *Highlight on Latex Glove Allergy*).

Glove Guidelines

The medical assistant should adhere to the following glove guidelines:

1. Keep fingernails trimmed short (less than ¼ inch long) to reduce the risk of tearing the gloves during application and use.

2. Wear the correct size glove. Gloves that are too small may rip as they are applied or may become uncomfort-

able to wear. Gloves that are too large may make it difficult to perform tasks.

3. Do not use oil-based hand lotions or creams because they can damage and deteriorate natural rubber latex gloves.

4. Do not store gloves in areas where there are extremes in temperatures (e.g., near a heater or air conditioner). These conditions can cause deterioration of the gloves.

OSHA BLOODBORNE PATHOGENS STANDARD

Purpose of the Standard

The federal government established OSHA (Occupational Safety and Health Administration) to assist employers in providing a safe and healthy working environment for their employees. To provide a safe working environment for health care workers, OSHA developed a comprehensive set of regulations known as the *OSHA Occupational Exposure to Bloodborne Pathogens Standard.*

These regulations went into effect in 1992 and are designed to reduce the risk to employees of exposure to infectious diseases.

The OSHA Bloodborne Pathogens Standard must be followed by any employee with occupational exposure to pathogens, regardless of the place of employment. In addition to medical assistants, employees with occupational exposure include physicians, nurses, dentists, dental hygienists, medical laboratory personnel, and emergency medical technicians. Employees who may have less obvious occupational exposure are correctional and law enforcement officers, firefighters, hospital laundry workers, morticians, and custodians.

Failure by employers to comply with the OSHA standard could result in a citation carrying a maximum penalty of $7000 for each violation and a maximum penalty of $70,000 for repeat violations.

Needlestick Safety and Prevention Act

Since the adoption of the OSHA Bloodborne Pathogens Standard, needlestick injuries among health care workers have continued to be a problem because of their high frequency of occurrence and the severity of the health effects associated with exposure to bloodborne pathogens. To address this problem, Congress passed the Needlestick Safety and Prevention Act (NSPA). The NSPA directed OSHA to revise the Bloodborne Pathogens Standard to incorporate stronger measures to reduce needlesticks and other sharps injuries among health care workers. In response to this mandate, the primary measure instituted by OSHA was to establish detailed requirements that employers identify and make use of safer medical devices. This revised OSHA Bloodborne Pathogens Standard went into effect in 2001 and is described in detail in this chapter.

OSHA Terminology

The following definitions help clarify terms related to the OSHA Bloodborne Pathogens Standard.

Occupational exposure *Occupational exposure* is reasonably anticipated skin, eye, mucous membrane, or parenteral contact with blood or other potentially infectious materials that may result from the performance of an employee's duties.

Parenteral *Parenteral* refers to the piercing of the skin barrier or mucous membranes, such as through needlesticks, human bites, cuts, and abrasions.

Blood *Blood* means human blood, human blood components, and products made from blood. Blood components include plasma, serum, platelets, and serosanguineous fluid (e.g., exudates from wounds). An example of a blood product is a medication derived from blood, such as immune globulins.

Bloodborne pathogens *Bloodborne pathogens* are pathogenic microorganisms in human blood that can cause disease in humans. Bloodborne pathogens include, but are not limited to, hepatitis B virus (HBV), hepatitis C virus (HCV), and human immunodeficiency virus (HIV).

Other potentially infectious materials *Other potentially infectious materials* (OPIM) include the following:
- Semen and vaginal secretions
- Cerebrospinal, synovial, pleural, pericardial, peritoneal, and amniotic fluids
- Any body fluid that is visibly contaminated with blood
- Any body fluid that has not been identified
- Saliva in dental procedures
- Any unfixed human tissue
- Any tissue culture, cells, or fluid known to be HIV infected

Contaminated *Contaminated* is defined as the presence or reasonably anticipated presence of blood or other potentially infected materials on an item or surface.

Decontamination *Decontamination* is the use of physical or chemical means to remove, inactivate, or destroy pathogens on a surface or item to the point where they are no longer capable of transmitting infectious particles, and the surface or item is rendered safe for handling, use, or disposal.

Nonintact skin *Nonintact skin* is skin that has a break in the surface. It includes, but is not limited to, skin with dermatitis, abrasions, cuts, burns, hangnails, chapping, and acne.

Exposure incident *Exposure incident* is defined as a specific eye, nose, mouth, or other mucous membrane, nonin-

---

What Would You Do? What Would You *Not* Do?

Case Study 1

Petra Meyer has come in for her annual gynecologic examination. She notices that alcohol-based hand rubs are being used in the medical office. Petra wants to know if they are as good as regular soap and water for washing hands. Petra says she likes to garden and wants to know if hand rubs are effective in removing ground-in soil from the hands. Petra also is curious to know why they are now being used so much in health care settings. ■

tact skin, or parenteral contact with blood or other potentially infectious materials that results from an employee's duties.

Components of the OSHA Standard

The OSHA Bloodborne Pathogens Standard is presented on the following pages as it pertains to the medical office and includes the following categories:

- Exposure control plan
- Safer medical devices
- Labeling requirements
- Communication of hazards to employees
- Record-keeping

Exposure Control Plan

The OSHA standard requires that the medical office develop an exposure control plan (ECP) (Figure 2-3). The ECP is a written document stipulating the protective measures that must be followed in that medical office to eliminate or minimize employee exposure to bloodborne pathogens and other potentially infectious materials. The ECP must be made available for review by all medical office staff. The ECP must include the following elements:

1. **An exposure determination.** The purpose of this section of the ECP is to identify employees who must receive training, protective equipment, hepatitis vaccination, and other protections required by the OSHA Bloodborne Pathogens Standard. The exposure determination must include (1) a list of all job classifications in which *all* employees are likely to have occupational exposure, such as physicians, medical assistants, and laboratory technicians, and (2) a list of job classifications in which only *some* employees have occupational exposure, such as custodians. For the second classification of jobs, the determi-

nation must include a list of tasks in which occupational exposure may occur, such as emptying the trash.

2. **The method of compliance.** The method of compliance section of the ECP must document the specific health and safety control measures that are taken in the medical office to eliminate or minimize the risk of occupational exposure. These measures are extremely important in reducing the risk of infectious disease for the medical assistant and are discussed in greater detail later in this section (see *Control Measures*).

3. **Postexposure evaluation and follow-up procedures.** Postexposure evaluation and follow-up must specify the procedures to follow in the event of an exposure incident in the medical office, including the method of documenting and investigating an exposure incident and the postexposure evaluation, medical treatment, and follow-up that would be made available to the employee. (Refer to the *OSHA Postexposure Evaluation and Follow-Up Procedures* box.)

OSHA requires employers to review and update their ECP at least annually to ensure that the plan remains current with the latest information on eliminating or reducing exposure to bloodborne pathogens. The ECP also must be updated whenever necessary to reflect new or modified tasks and procedures that affect occupational exposure.

Labeling Requirements

The OSHA Bloodborne Pathogens Standard requires that containers and appliances containing biohazardous materials be labeled with a *biohazard warning label*. The biohazard warning label must be fluorescent orange or orange-red and must contain the biohazard symbol and the word BIOHAZARD in a contrasting color (Figure 2-4, *A*).

A warning label must be attached to the following: (1) containers of regulated waste; (2) refrigerators and freezers used to store blood and other potentially infectious materials; and (3) containers and bags used to store, transport, or ship blood or other potentially infectious materials (Figure 2-4, *B*). Red bags or red containers may be substituted for biohazard warning labels. The labeling requirement is designed to alert employees to possible exposure, particularly in situations in which the nature of the material or contents is not readily identifiable as blood or other potentially infectious materials.

Communicating Hazards to Employees

According to the OSHA standard, employers must ensure that all medical office employees with risk of occupational exposure participate in a training program. This program must present the ECP for the medical office, while focusing on the measures that employees are to take for their safety. Training must be provided at the time an employee is initially assigned to tasks in which occupational exposure may occur and at least annually thereafter.

The employer must maintain records of the training sessions, which must include presentation dates, content of the sessions, names and qualifications of the trainers, and

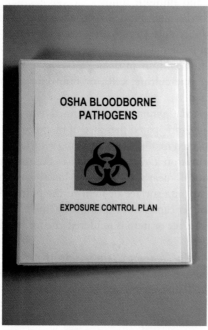

Figure 2-3. Example of an exposure control plan.

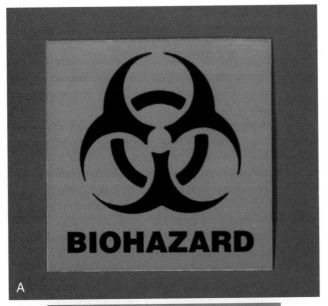

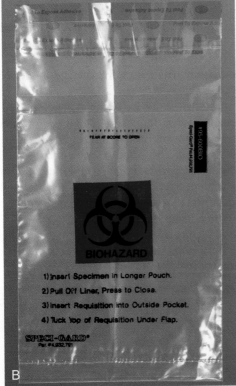

Figure 2-4. **A,** Biohazard warning label. **B,** Biohazard bag used to hold and transport blood or other potentially infectious materials.

OSHA Postexposure Evaluation and Follow-up Procedures

An exposure incident is a specific eye, nose, mouth, or other mucous membrane, nonintact skin, or parenteral contact with blood or other potentially infectious materials that results from an employee's duties. In the event of an exposure incident to blood-borne pathogens or other potentially infectious materials, OSHA requires the following steps to be performed:

1. Perform initial first aid measures immediately (e.g., wash a needlestick injury thoroughly with soap and water).
2. Document the route of exposure and the conditions and circumstances of the exposure incident. This includes such information as the engineering controls, the work practice controls, and personal protective equipment being used at the time of the incident.
3. Identify and document the source individual (unless the employer can establish that identification is not feasible or is prohibited by state or local law). A source individual is any person, living or dead, whose blood or OPIM may be a source of occupational exposure to the health care worker.
4. Obtain consent to test the source individual's blood. Test it as soon as possible to determine HBV, HCV, and HIV infectivity. The following guidelines apply to this requirement:
   - If consent is not obtained, the employer must document that legally required consent cannot be obtained.
   - If the source individual's consent is not required by law, the source individual's blood (if available) must be tested and the results documented.
   - If the source individual is already known to be infected with HBV, HCV, or HIV, testing does not need to be repeated.
5. Provide the exposed employee with the source individual's test results. Inform the employee of applicable laws and regulations concerning disclosure of the identity and infectious status of the source individual.
6. Obtain consent to test the employee's blood. Collect and test the blood of the employee as soon as possible for HBV, HCV, and HIV serologic status. If the employee does not give consent for HIV serologic testing, the baseline blood sample must be preserved for at least 90 days. If the employee elects to have the baseline sample tested during the 90-day waiting period, such testing must be done as soon as feasible.
7. When medically indicated, provide the employee with appropriate postexposure prophylaxis, as recommended by the U.S. Public Health Service.

names and job titles of employees who attended. These records must be maintained for 3 years from the date of the training session.

Record-Keeping

The OSHA Bloodborne Pathogens Standard requires that the following records be maintained:

1. **OSHA medical record.** The OSHA standard requires that the employer maintain an accurate OSHA record of every medical office employee at risk for occupational exposure. These records must be kept confidential except for review by OSHA officials and as required by law. The record must include the following: employee's name; social security number; hepatitis B vaccination status, including dates of vaccination; results of any postexposure examinations, medical testing, and follow-up procedures; and a written evaluation of any exposure incident along with a copy of the exposure incident report. The employer is required to maintain records for the duration of employment plus 30 years.

2. **Sharps injury log.** Employers with more than 10 employees at risk for occupational exposure are required to maintain a log of injuries from contaminated sharps. The log must be maintained in a way that protects the confidentiality of injured employees (e.g., removal of personal identification). The purpose of the log is to help employers and employees keep track of all needlestick injuries. This tracking helps in identifying problem areas that need attention and ineffective devices that need to be replaced. The sharps injury log must contain the following information:

- Type and brand of device involved in the injury
- Location of the incident (i.e., work area)
- Explanation of how the incident occurred

Control Measures

Specific health and safety control measures are required by OSHA to eliminate or minimize the risk of occupational exposure in the medical office. These measures are divided into six categories: engineering controls, work practice controls, personal protective equipment, housekeeping, hepatitis B vaccination, and universal precautions.

Engineering Controls

The medical office must use engineering controls to eliminate or minimize the risk of occupational exposure. *Engineering controls* include all control measures that isolate or remove health hazards from the workplace. Engineering controls must be examined and maintained or replaced as required to ensure their effectiveness. Examples of engineering controls include the following:

- Readily accessible handwashing facilities
- Safer medical devices
- Biohazard sharps containers and biohazard bags
- Autoclaves

Safer Medical Devices

Safer medical devices are one example of an engineering control. A *safer medical device* is a device that, based on reasonable judgment, would make an exposure incident involving a contaminated sharp less likely. *Reasonable judgment* refers to the judgment of the health care worker who would be using the device.

Safer medical devices include sharps with engineered sharps injury protection and needleless systems. A *sharp with engineered sharps injury protection (SESIP)* is a non-needle sharp or a needle device with a built-in safety feature used for procedures that involve the risk of sharps injury. Examples of SESIPs include safety-engineered syringes and phlebotomy devices (Figure 2-5).

A *needleless system* is a device that does not use a needle for (1) the administration of medication or other fluids, (2) the collection or withdrawal of body fluids after initial access to a vein or artery is established, or (3) any other procedure involving the potential for occupational exposure to bloodborne pathogens as a result of percutaneous injuries from contaminated sharps. An example of a needleless system is a jet injection syringe, which uses compressed air to administer an injection rather than a needle.

Employers are required to evaluate and implement commercially available safer medical devices and other engineering controls that eliminate occupational exposure to the lowest extent feasible. Input from employees involved in direct patient care must be taken into consideration in making this determination. This helps to ensure that the individuals who are using the devices have the opportunity for input. As part of the annual review of the exposure control plan, the following information must be documented: (1) safer medical devices that reflect changes in technology are being evaluated and implemented in the workplace, and (2) input was obtained from employees in selecting safer medical devices.

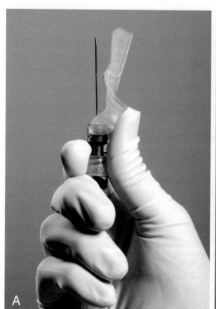
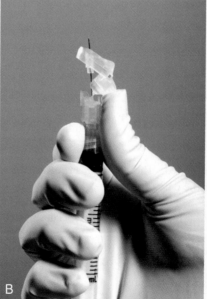
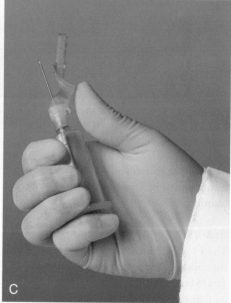

Figure 2-5. **A-B,** Safety-engineered syringes. **C,** Safety-engineered phlebotomy device.

Work Practice Controls

Work practice controls reduce the likelihood of exposure by altering the manner in which the technique is performed. It is important that the medical assistant consistently adhere to these safety rules, which include the following:

1. Perform all procedures involving blood or other potentially infectious materials in a manner that minimizes splashing, spraying, spattering, and generation of droplets of these substances.
2. Observe warning labels on biohazard containers and appliances. Bags or containers that bear a biohazard warning label or are color-coded red indicate that they hold blood or other potentially infectious materials. Refrigerators, freezers, and other appliances that contain hazardous materials also must bear a biohazard warning label.
3. Bandage cuts and other lesions on the hands before gloving.
4. Sanitize the hands after removing gloves, regardless of whether or not the gloves are visibly contaminated.
5. If your hands or other skin surfaces come in contact with blood or other potentially infectious materials, thoroughly wash the area as soon as possible with soap and water.
6. If your mucous membranes (e.g., eyes, mouth, nose) come in contact with blood or other potentially infectious materials, flush them with water as soon as possible.
7. Do not break or shear contaminated needles.
8. Do not remove, recap, or bend a contaminated needle except in unusual circumstances when no other alternative is possible, or when this is required by a specific medical procedure. Such actions must be performed by a method other than the traditional two-handed procedure. Needle removal can be accomplished with a one-handed technique using a sharps container with a well-designed unwinder. Recapping must be performed through the use of a one-handed technique; using a two-handed technique is strictly prohibited. The one-handed recapping technique involves holding the syringe in the dominant hand and picking up the needle with the cap, using a scooping motion. The cap is secured onto the needle by pushing it against a hard surface. (*Note:* Sterile needles may be recapped, such as after the withdrawal of medication from a vial or ampule.)
9. Immediately after use, place contaminated sharps in a puncture-resistant, leakproof container that is appropriately labeled or color-coded. *Contaminated sharps* are contaminated objects that can penetrate the skin, including (but not limited to) needles, lancets, scalpels, broken glass, and capillary tubes.
10. Do not eat, drink, smoke, apply cosmetics or lip balm, or handle contact lenses in areas where you may be exposed to blood or other potentially infectious materials.
11. Do not store food or drink in refrigerators, freezers, or cabinets or on shelves or countertops where blood or other potentially infectious materials are present.
12. Place blood specimens or other potentially infectious materials in containers that prevent leakage during collection, handling, processing, storage, transport, or shipping. Ensure that the containers are closed before they are stored, transported, or shipped, and are labeled or color-coded for easy identification.
13. Before any equipment that might be contaminated is serviced or shipped for repair or cleaning, such as a centrifuge, it must be inspected for blood or other potentially infectious materials. If such material is present, the equipment must be decontaminated. If it cannot be decontaminated, it must be appropriately labeled to indicate clearly the contamination site, to enable those coming into contact with the equipment to take appropriate precautions.
14. If you are exposed to blood or other potentially infectious materials, perform first aid measures immediately (e.g., wash a needlestick injury thoroughly with soap and water). After taking these measures, report the incident to your physician-employer as soon as possible so that postexposure procedures can be instituted. (See the box entitled *OSHA Postexposure Evaluation and Follow-Up Procedures.*) The most obvious exposure incident is a needlestick, but any eye, mouth, or other mucous membrane, nonintact skin, or parenteral contact with blood or other potentially infectious materials constitutes an exposure incident and should be reported.

Personal Protective Equipment

The OSHA standard specifies that personal protective equipment must be used in the medical office whenever occupational exposure remains after engineering and work practice controls are instituted. *Personal protective equipment* is clothing or equipment that protects an individual from contact with blood or other potentially infectious materials; examples include gloves, chin-length face shields, masks, protective eyewear, laboratory coats, and gowns. The type of protective equipment appropriate for a given task depends on the degree of exposure that is anticipated, as outlined here:

1. Wear gloves when it is reasonably anticipated that your hands will have contact with blood and other potentially infectious materials, mucous membranes, or nonintact skin; when performing vascular access procedures; and when handling or touching contaminated surfaces or items. Gloves cannot prevent a needlestick or other sharps injury, but they can prevent a pathogen from entering the body through a break in the skin, such as a cut, abrasion, burn, or rash.
2. Wear chin-length face shields or masks in combination with eye-protection devices whenever splashes, spray, spatter, or droplets of blood or other potentially infectious materials may be generated, posing a hazard through contact with the eyes, nose, or mouth (e.g., removing a stopper from a tube of blood, transferring serum from whole blood) (Figure 2-6).

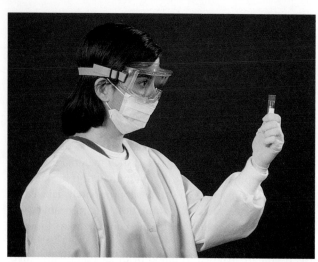

Figure 2-6. Jennifer wears a combination mask and eye-protection device and a laboratory coat to protect against splashes, spray, spatter, and droplets of blood.

3. Wear appropriate protective clothing, such as gowns, aprons, and laboratory coats, when gross contamination can reasonably be anticipated during performance of a task or procedure (e.g., laboratory testing procedure). The type of protective clothing needed depends on the task and degree of exposure anticipated.

Personal Protective Equipment Guidelines

Certain guidelines must be followed when using protective equipment:

1. Protective equipment must not allow blood or other potentially infectious materials to pass through or reach the skin, underlying garments (e.g., scrubs, street clothes, undergarments), eyes, mouth, or other mucous membranes under normal conditions of use and for the duration of time the protective equipment is used.
2. The employer must provide appropriate personal protective equipment at no cost to you. The employer is responsible for ensuring that the equipment is available in appropriate sizes, is readily accessible, and is used correctly. In addition, the employer must ensure that the equipment is cleaned, laundered, repaired, replaced, or disposed of as necessary to ensure its effectiveness.
3. Alternatives must be provided for employees who are allergic to latex gloves. Examples of alternatives include non-latex gloves and powderless gloves.
4. If gloves become contaminated, torn, or punctured, replace them as soon as practical.
5. All eye-protection devices must have solid side shields; chin-length face shields, goggles, and glasses with solid side shields are acceptable (Figure 2-7); standard prescription eyeglasses are unacceptable as eye protection.
6. If a garment is penetrated by blood or other potentially infectious materials, it must be removed as soon as pos-

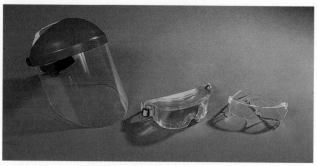

Figure 2-7. Examples of eye-protection devices. *Left,* Face shield; *center,* goggles; *right,* glasses with solid side shields.

sible and placed in an appropriately designated container for washing.

7. All personal protective equipment must be removed before leaving the medical office.
8. When protective equipment is removed, it must be placed in an appropriately designated area or container for storage, washing, decontamination, or disposal.
9. Utility gloves may be decontaminated and reused unless they are cracked, peeling, torn, punctured, or no longer provide barrier protection.
10. If you believe that using protective equipment would prevent proper delivery of health care or would pose an increased hazard to your safety or that of a coworker, in extenuating circumstances you may temporarily and briefly decline its use. After such an incident, the circumstances must be investigated to determine whether the situation could be prevented in the future.

Housekeeping

The OSHA standard requires that specific housekeeping procedures be followed to ensure that the work site is maintained in a clean and sanitary condition. The medical office must develop and implement a written schedule for cleaning and decontaminating each area where exposure occurs. The cleaning and decontamination method must be specified for each task and should be based on the type of surface

---

What Would You Do? What Would You *Not* Do?

Case Study 2

Tracy Smith is pregnant and is at the medical office to have her blood drawn for a prenatal profile. Tracy says she does not understand why gloves have to be worn when her blood is drawn. She says that it makes her feel like a leper, and she is absolutely sure that she doesn't have any diseases. Tracy says she has been reading information about the hepatitis B vaccine because she knows her baby will be given this vaccine soon after birth. She wants to know why it is recommended that an infant be immunized for hepatitis B. Tracy says that infants are not at risk for contracting hepatitis B because the way it is transmitted is mostly through sexual contact and illegal drug use. ∎

to be cleaned, the type of soil present, and the tasks or procedures being performed in that area. Housekeeping procedures include the following:

1. Clean and decontaminate equipment and work surfaces after completing procedures that involve blood or other potentially infectious materials. Cleaning is accomplished using a detergent soap, and decontamination is performed using an appropriate disinfectant (Figure 2-8).

2. Clean and decontaminate all equipment and work surfaces as soon as possible after exposure to blood or other potentially infectious materials. For decontamination of blood spills, OSHA recommends the use of a 10% solution of sodium hypochlorite (household bleach) in water ✕(1 part bleach to 10 parts water). ✕

3. Inspect and decontaminate all reusable receptacles, such as bins, pails, and cans, on a regular basis. If contamination is visible, the item must be cleaned and decontaminated as soon as possible.

4. Do not pick up broken, contaminated glassware with the hands, even if gloves are worn. Use mechanical means, such as a brush and dustpan, tongs, and forceps (Figure 2-9).

5. Protective coverings, such as plastic wrap and aluminum foil, may be used to cover work surfaces or equipment, but they must be removed or replaced if contamination occurs.

6. Handle contaminated laundry as little as possible and with appropriate personal protective equipment. Place all contaminated laundry in leakproof bags that are properly labeled or color-coded. Contaminated laundry must not be sorted or rinsed at the medical office.

7. If the outside of a biohazard container becomes contaminated, it must be placed in a second suitable container.

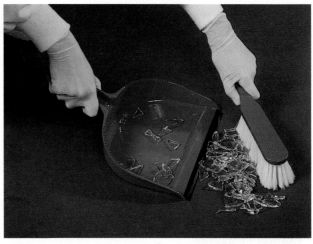

Figure 2-9. Use mechanical means to pick up broken contaminated glass.

8. Biohazard sharps containers (Figure 2-10) must be closable, puncture-resistant, and leakproof. They must bear a biohazard warning label and must be color-coded red to ensure identification of the contents as hazardous. To ensure effectiveness, the following guidelines must be observed:

   • Locate the sharps container as close as possible to the area of use to avoid the hazard of transporting a contaminated needle through the workplace.

   • Maintain sharps containers in an upright position to keep liquid and sharps inside.

   • Do not reach into the sharps container with your hand.

   • Replace sharps containers on a regular basis, and do not allow them to overfill. (It is recommended that sharps containers be replaced when they are three-quarters full.)

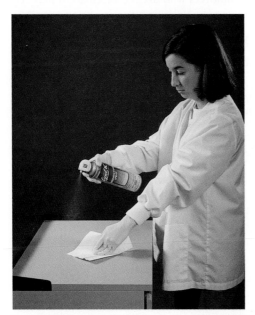

Figure 2-8. Clean and decontaminate work surfaces with an appropriate disinfectant after completing procedures involving blood and other potentially infectious materials.

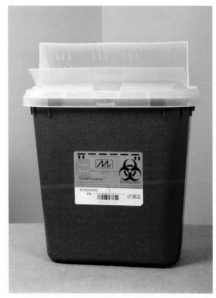

Figure 2-10. Biohazard sharps container.

Highlight on OSHA Bloodborne Pathogens Standard

General Information

The exposure control plan must be made available to OSHA on request.

OSHA inspectors are responsible for determining whether the medical office meets the Bloodborne Pathogens Standard. This is accomplished through careful review of the exposure control plan, interviews with the medical office employer and employees, and observation of work activities.

Feces, nasal secretions, saliva, sputum, sweat, tears, urine, and vomitus are not considered by OSHA to be potentially infectious materials unless they contain blood.

Control Measures

Employees must be trained in proper use of the following: engineering controls (including safer medical devices), work practice controls, and personal protective equipment.

General work clothes, such as scrubs, uniforms, pants, shirts, and blouses, are not intended to function as protection against a hazard and are not considered personal protective equipment.

Employees are not permitted to launder contaminated clothing at home; it is the employer's responsibility to have contaminated clothing laundered.

If an employee is allergic to standard latex gloves, the employer must provide a suitable non-latex alternative.

Needlestick Injuries

The CDC estimates that every year, 600,000 to 800,000 health care workers in the United States experience needlestick and other sharps injuries, and 1000 of these individuals contract serious infections as a result of these injuries. The CDC estimates that 62% to 88% of sharps injuries can be prevented by the use of safer medical devices.

A wide variety of commercially available safer medical devices has been developed to reduce the risk of needlestick and other sharps injuries.

Safer medical devices that eliminate exposure to the lowest extent feasible must be evaluated and implemented in the health care setting. Lack of injuries on the sharps injury log does *not* exempt the employer from this provision. ∎

Hepatitis B Vaccination

The OSHA standard requires employers to offer the hepatitis B vaccination series free of charge to all medical office personnel who have occupational exposure. The vaccination must be offered within 10 working days of initial assignment to a position with occupational exposure, unless the following factors exist: (1) the individual has previously received the

hepatitis B vaccination series, (2) antibody testing has revealed that the individual is immune to hepatitis B, or (3) the vaccine is contraindicated for medical reasons.

Medical office personnel who decline vaccination must sign a hepatitis B waiver form documenting refusal. This form must be filed in the employee's OSHA record (Figure 2-11). Employees who decline vaccination may request the

---

HEPATITIS B DECLINATION FORM

I understand that due to my occupational exposure to blood or other potentially infectious materials, I may be at risk of acquiring hepatitis B virus (HBV) infection. I have been given the opportunity to be vaccinated with hepatitis B vaccine at no charge to myself. However, I decline hepatitis B vaccination at this time. I understand that by declining this vaccine I continue to be at risk of acquiring hepatitis B, a serious disease. If in the future I continue to have occupational exposure to blood or to other potentially infectious materials and I want to be vaccinated with hepatitis B vaccine, I can receive the vaccination series at no charge to me.

_____

Employee Name (printed)

_____   _____

Employee Signature   Date

_____   _____

Witness Signature   Date

Figure 2-11. Hepatitis B declination form. This form must be signed by an employee with occupational exposure who declines hepatitis B vaccination.

vaccination later; the employer must then provide it, according to the aforementioned criteria.

Universal Precautions

Before the release of the OSHA standard, the CDC issued recommendations for health care workers known as the Universal Precautions. According to the concept of Universal Precautions, all human blood and certain human body fluids are treated as though they are known to be infectious for HIV, HBV, HCV, and other bloodborne pathogens. The OSHA standard states that the Universal Precautions must be observed; these precautions form the heart of the OSHA standard itself.

REGULATED MEDICAL WASTE

Medical waste is generated in the medical office through the diagnosis, treatment, and immunization of patients. Some of this waste poses a threat to health and safety and is known as **regulated medical waste (RMW)**. The OSHA Bloodborne Pathogens Standard defines RMW as follows:
- Any liquid or semiliquid blood or OPIM
- Items contaminated with blood or OPIM that would release these substances in a liquid or semiliquid state if compressed
- Items that are caked with dried blood or OPIM and are capable of releasing these materials during handling
- Contaminated sharps
- Pathologic and microbiologic wastes that contain blood or OPIM

Regulated medical waste must be discarded properly so as not to become a source of transfer of disease. According to the OSHA definition, a dressing saturated with blood is considered RMW and must be discarded in a biohazard bag. A bandage with a spot of blood on it is not considered RMW and can be discarded in a regular waste container. Box 2-2 gives the guidelines for discarding medical waste in the medical office.

BOX 2-2 Guidelines for Discarding Medical Waste in the Medical Office

Regular Waste Container

The following items that have been used for health care *are not* considered regulated medical waste and can be discarded in a covered waste container lined with a regular trash bag.
- Disposable drapes
- Disposable patient gowns
- Examining table paper
- Disposable clean or sterile gloves
- Gauze tinged with blood or other body fluids
- Disposable probe covers for thermometers
- Tongue depressors
- Tissues with respiratory secretions
- Disposable ear speculums
- Empty urine containers
- Urine testing strips
- Disposable diapers
- Feminine hygiene products

Biohazard Sharps Container

The following items are sharps. They *are* considered regulated medical waste and must be discarded in a biohazard sharps container.
- Hypodermic syringes and needles
- Venipuncture needles
- Lancets
- Razor blades
- Scalpel blades
- Suture needles
- Blood tubes
- Capillary pipets
- Microscope slides and coverslips
- Broken glassware

Biohazard Bag Waste Container

The following items *are* considered regulated medical waste. They are not sharps and can be discarded in a covered waste container lined with a biohazard bag.
- Any item saturated or dripping with blood or OPIM (e.g., dressings, gauze, cotton balls, paper towels, tissues that are saturated or dripping with blood)
- Any item caked with dried blood or OPIM, such as dressings and sutures
- Disposable clean or sterile gloves contaminated with blood or OPIM
- Disposable vaginal speculums and collection devices (e.g., swabs, spatulas, brushes)
- Tissue or fluid removed during minor office surgery
- Microbiologic waste, such as specimen cultures and collection devices
- Discarded live and attenuated vaccines

Sanitary Sewer

Disposal of small quantities of blood and other body fluids to the sanitary sewer is considered a safe method of disposing of these waste materials. The following fluids can be carefully poured down a utility sink, drain, or toilet. (*Note:* State regulations may dictate the maximum volume allowable for discharge of blood or body fluids into the sanitary sewer.)
- Blood
- Body excretions such as urine
- Body secretions such as sputum

Highlight on Hepatitis B Vaccine

The hepatitis B vaccine became available in 1982 and is 95% effective in providing immunity. The hepatitis B vaccine is administered intramuscularly in a series of three doses. The hepatitis B vaccine is well tolerated by most patients. The most common side effect is soreness at the injection site, including induration, erythema, and swelling. Occasionally, a low-grade fever, headache, and dizziness occur.

Approximately 5% of the population does not form antibodies to the hepatitis B vaccine. Because of this, the CDC recommends that an antibody titer test be performed on all health care workers between 1 and 2 months after the last dose of the hepatitis B vaccine. The titer test is performed to determine if the health care worker has developed protective antibodies to hepatitis B and has immunity to HBV infection. Health care workers who do not respond to the primary vaccination series, as indicated by a negative titer test, must be revaccinated with a second three-dose vaccination series and then have a repeat titer test. If the titer test is still negative, this means that the health care worker probably lacks immunity to HBV infection.

Current data show that vaccine-induced antibodies may decline over time, but the immune system memory that programs the body to produce these antibodies remains intact indefinitely. Because of this, an individual with declining antibodies is still protected against hepatitis B. At present, the CDC does not recommend a booster dose once an individual has received the initial (three-dose) vaccine series.

The hepatitis B vaccine is recommended for all infants and children, and for adolescents who are 18 years old or younger. It also is recommended for adults older than 18 years who are increased risk for developing hepatitis B. This population includes employees with occupational exposure (e.g., health care workers), hemodialysis patients, hemophiliacs, individuals with multiple sex partners, homosexually active men, injection drug users, individuals with HIV infection, household and sexual contacts of individuals infected with HBV, individuals with chronic liver or kidney disease, residents and staff in institutions for the developmentally disabled, and people who travel to countries where hepatitis B is common.

The number of individuals contracting hepatitis B has decreased sharply since the development of the hepatitis B vaccine. As more people become immune to hepatitis B through the immunization of infants, the goal of eliminating hepatitis B in the United States may be realized. ∎

Handling Regulated Medical Waste

Regulated medical waste must be handled carefully to prevent an exposure incident. The OSHA Bloodborne Pathogens Standard outlines specific actions to take when handling regulated medical waste, as follows:

1. Separate regulated waste from the general refuse at its point of origin. Disposable items containing regulated medical waste should be placed directly into biohazard containers and should not be mixed with the regular trash.
2. Ensure that biohazard containers are closable, leakproof, and suitably constructed to contain the contents during handling, storage, and transport. These containers include biohazard bags and sharps containers.
3. To prevent spillage or protrusion of the contents, close the lid of a sharps container before removing it from an examining room. Never open, empty, or clean a contaminated sharps container. If there is a chance of leakage from the sharps container, the medical assistant should place it in a second container that is closable, leakproof, and appropriately labeled or color-coded.
4. Securely close biohazard bags before removing them from an examining room. To provide additional protection, some medical offices double-bag by placing the primary bag inside a second biohazard bag.
5. Transport full biohazard containers to a secured area away from the general public, using personal protective equipment (e.g., gloves).

Disposal of Regulated Medical Waste

Each state is responsible for developing policies for disposal of regulated medical waste. To avoid noncompliance, it is important for the medical assistant to know and understand the specific regulated waste policies and guidelines set forth in his or her state. Regulated waste policies and guidelines for each state can be found at the following website: www.envcap.org/statetools/rmw/rmwlocator.html.

Most medical offices use a commercial medical waste service to dispose of regulated medical waste. This service is responsible for picking up and transporting the medical waste to a treatment facility for incineration to destroy pathogens and render them harmless. The waste can then be safely disposed of in a sanitary landfill. Regulated waste treatment facilities must be licensed and hold permits issued by the Environmental Protection Agency (EPA), allowing them to dispose of regulated medical waste.

A series of steps must be followed for preparing and storing regulated medical waste for pickup by the service. Although these steps may vary slightly from state to state, general measures required by most states include the following:

1. Place biohazard bags and sharps containers into a receptacle provided by the medical waste service. The receptacle is usually a cardboard box (Figure 2-12). The box should be securely sealed with packing tape, and a biohazard warning label must appear on two opposite sides of the box.

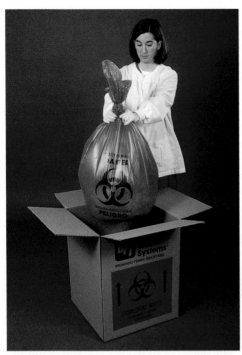

Figure 2-12. Jennifer places a biohazard bag inside a cardboard box in preparation for pickup by the medical waste service.

2. Store the biohazard boxes in a locked room inside the facility or in a locked collection container outside for pickup by the medical waste service. This step is aimed at preventing unauthorized access to items such as needles and syringes. The regulated waste storage area should be labeled with one of the following:
   • "Authorized Personnel Only" sign
   • International biohazard symbol
3. Many states require that a tracking record be completed when the waste is picked up by the medical waste service. This form includes such information as the type and quantity of waste (weighed in pounds) and where it is being sent. The form must be signed by a representative of the medical waste service and the medical office. After the waste has been destroyed at the regulated waste

---

What Would You Do? What Would You _Not_ Do?

Case Study 3

Giles Lee is 45 years old and is at the medical office. Twenty-five years ago, he was in a serious car accident and had to have a blood transfusion. He says that he donated blood for the first time 2 months ago. Last week he received a letter saying that his blood tested positive for hepatitis C and that he should see his physician. Giles says that he must have gotten hepatitis C from the blood transfusion he received when he was 20. He does not understand how that could have happened because the blood supply is tested for these types of diseases. Giles wants to know why he has not had any symptoms. He also wants to know if he can give hepatitis C to his wife and teenage children. ■

---

treatment facility, a record documenting its disposal is mailed to the medical office.

BLOODBORNE DISEASES

The biggest threats to health care workers from occupational exposure are HBV, HCV, and HIV. Hepatitis is much easier to transmit than HIV. After a needlestick exposure to blood infected with HBV, health care workers who are not immune to hepatitis B have a 6% to 30% chance of developing the disease. The risk of infection after a needlestick exposure to blood infected with HCV is approximately 2%. After a needlestick exposure to HIV-infected blood, a health care worker has a 0.3% chance of developing AIDS; he or she has a 0.1% chance of developing AIDS after a mucous membrane exposure of the eyes, nose, or mouth.

Hepatitis B

Hepatitis B is an infection of the liver caused by HBV. The most common means of transmitting hepatitis B in the health care setting are blood and blood components, such as serum and plasma.

Health care workers are most likely to contract hepatitis B through needlesticks and cuts with contaminated sharps. The virus also is spread in the health care setting, but less effectively, through blood splashes to the eyes, mouth, and nonintact skin and through body fluids such as semen and vaginal secretions.

The number of health care workers who contract hepatitis B in the workplace has declined dramatically since the development of the OHSA standard and the hepatitis B vaccine. Statistics show that in 1983 there were more than 10,000 health care workers who contracted hepatitis B in the workplace, but by 2001, that number had decreased to fewer than 400 health care workers. Preventive treatment is available for individuals exposed to hepatitis B who have not been vaccinated.

Postexposure Prophylaxis

Postexposure prophylaxis (PEP) refers to treatment administered to an individual after exposure to an infectious disease, to prevent the disease. PEP for unvaccinated individuals exposed to hepatitis B involves the administration of a passive and an active immunizing agent. It is important to administer both of these agents as soon as possible after an exposure incident—preferably within 24 hours, but no later than 7 days.

The passive immunizing agent provides temporary immunity to hepatitis B, giving the active agent a chance to take effect. The passive agent is hepatitis B immune globulin (HBIG), which contains antibodies that provide immunity to hepatitis B for 1 to 3 months.

The active immunizing agent in the hepatitis B vaccine (Figure 2-13) is produced from genetically altered yeast cells; brand names are Recombivax HB and Engerix-B. The

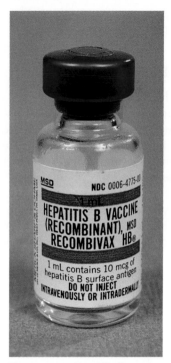

Figure 2-13. Hepatitis B vaccine.

hepatitis B vaccine is administered intramuscularly in a series of three doses. The second dose is given 1 month after the first dose, and the third dose is administered 6 months after the first dose (i.e., 0, 1 month, and 6 months). Mild side effects, such as soreness at the injection site, may occur, but serious reactions to the vaccine are extremely rare.

As previously discussed, the OSHA standard recommends that all health care workers receive the hepatitis B vaccine (an active immunizing agent) as a preventive measure against hepatitis B. After an exposure incident, a medical assistant who has previously been vaccinated probably would not require further treatment.

Acute Viral Hepatitis B

After a person becomes infected, the acute symptoms of hepatitis B usually last 1 to 4 weeks, but it can take 6 months for the patient to recover fully. Symptoms vary greatly in intensity from one individual to another and can range from mild to severe. Approximately one third of people who become infected are asymptomatic and unaware that they have the disease. Another one third have relatively mild flulike symptoms that often are mistaken for influenza or similar conditions. The remaining one third of infected patients have such severe symptoms that hospitalization may be required.

Initial symptoms, if present, occur approximately 12 weeks after exposure and include fatigue, headache, loss of appetite, nausea, vomiting, malaise, and muscle and joint pain. In patients with severe acute viral hepatitis, these symptoms progress to abdominal pain, dark urine, and clay-colored stools, followed several days later by jaundice. After the onset of jaundice, the liver enlarges and becomes

tender. A small percentage of patients (0.5% to 2% of those infected) develop fulminant hepatitis, which is almost always fatal. Fulminant hepatitis is characterized by a sudden onset of nausea and vomiting, chills, high fever, severe and early jaundice, convulsions, coma, and death as a result of hepatic failure, usually within 10 days of its onset.

There is no specific treatment or drug to treat the acute phase of hepatitis B. Supportive care is prescribed to help the patient's natural defenses overcome the disease. Supportive care includes restricted activity, rest, avoidance of alcohol, a well-balanced diet, adequate fluid intake, and precautionary measures to prevent spread of the disease.

Most patients (90%) are able to clear the virus from their bodies by producing antibodies that completely destroy the virus. These individuals recover fully and have lifelong immunity to hepatitis B and are not infectious to others.

Chronic Viral Hepatitis B

The remaining 10% of patients with acute viral hepatitis B remain infected and go on to develop chronic hepatitis B. These individuals produce antibodies to hepatitis B, but they are not sufficient to remove the virus from their body. Individuals with chronic hepatitis may or may not experience symptoms; nonetheless, they become carriers of hepatitis B and are capable of transmitting the disease to others. In addition, patients with chronic hepatitis face an increased risk of liver damage, which leaves them vulnerable to diseases such as cirrhosis of the liver and liver cancer. A significant number of these patients (25%) subsequently die from liver failure. In recent years, antiviral drugs have been developed to treat chronic hepatitis. They are effective in removing the virus from approximately 40% of patients infected with chronic hepatitis B.

Hepatitis C

Hepatitis C is an infection of the liver caused by HCV. Currently, no vaccine is available for the prevention of hepatitis C. In the medical office, the most likely means of contracting hepatitis C is through parenteral exposure to contaminated blood such as through needlesticks and other sharps injuries. The chance of contracting hepatitis C in the health care setting is much lower than that of contracting hepatitis B.

Memories *from* Externship

Jennifer Hawk: As a student, I was extremely nervous to go out on externship. I was so scared to think that I was actually going to be in a medical office setting and would have to put everything I had learned into practice. Would I remember everything? Would I do something wrong and hurt the patient? It was such an overwhelming feeling! But to my relief, I had a very good experience. The office staff was so friendly and helpful to me, and I surprised myself at how easily everything I had learned stayed with me. It was so exciting to see that I was actually functioning as a team member in the health care field. I could not have had better training. ■

Most individuals with acute hepatitis C have no symptoms; if symptoms do occur, they are mild and flulike. Approximately 55% to 85% of individuals with acute hepatitis C develop chronic hepatitis C. After 10 to 30 years, about 20% of these individuals develop serious liver disease, including cirrhosis of the liver and cancer of the liver. Ultimately, 1% to 5% of individuals with chronic hepatitis C die from liver failure (see the *Highlight on Viral Hepatitis*). Antiviral drugs have been developed to treat chronic hepatitis C and are effective in 40% of cases.

Other Forms of Viral Hepatitis

In addition to hepatitis B and C, three other strains that cause viral hepatitis have been identified: hepatitis A, D, and E. Among all strains of hepatitis, hepatitis B poses the greatest threat to health care workers and has already been discussed in detail. Hepatitis A occasionally has been transmitted to health care workers but is not considered a major occupational hazard. In all cases of viral hepatitis, the virus invades the liver and causes inflammation, resulting in simi-

---

Highlight on Viral Hepatitis

In 2007, there were an estimated 85,000 new cases of viral hepatitis in the United States. Approximately 51% of these infections were caused by the hepatitis B virus, 29% were caused by the hepatitis A virus, and 20% were caused by the hepatitis C virus.

Symptoms common to all types of hepatitis include fatigue, nausea, loss of appetite, abdominal pain, and jaundice.

Hepatitis A, B, and C are designated by the CDC as nationally notifiable diseases. When the physician diagnoses a case of hepatitis A, B, or C, a reportable disease form must be completed and filed with the local public health department.

In recent years, antiviral drugs have been developed to treat chronic forms of hepatitis B and C; however, not all infected individuals are candidates for treatment. These drugs, which must be taken for a prolonged time, are effective in removing the virus from approximately 40% of chronically infected patients.

Hepatitis B

The virus that causes hepatitis B is found in the blood and in certain body fluids (e.g., semen, vaginal secretions) of HBV-infected individuals. The most common means of transmission of hepatitis B is through sexual contact with an infected individual, by sharing needles for injection drug use with an infected individual, and perinatally from an infected mother to her infant during birth. Other modes of transmission include contact with blood or open sores of an infected individual and sharing of items such as razors or toothbrushes with an infected individual. Hepatitis B is not spread by sneezing, coughing, hugging, kissing, casual contact, breastfeeding, food, water, or sharing eating utensils or drinking glasses.

The highest rate of new hepatitis B infection occur in adults, particularly among males between 25 and 44 years of age. The greatest decline has occurred among children and adolescents as a result of routine hepatitis B immunization.

It is estimated that more than 1.25 million people in the United States are infected with chronic hepatitis B; this means that these individuals are carriers of hepatitis B and are capable of transmitting the disease to others. Many of these individuals do not know that they are carriers.

Every year, approximately 3000 Americans die as a result of the long-term consequences of chronic hepatitis B, such as cirrhosis and liver cancer.

Whether or not an HBV-infected individual goes on to develop chronic hepatitis B depends primarily on age. After infection with acute viral hepatitis B occurs, chronic infection develops in 90% of infants infected by their mothers at birth, 30% of children infected between ages 1 and 5 years, and 6% of individuals infected after age 5 years.

Hepatitis B can survive outside the body in a dried state for at least 1 week and still can be capable of causing infection. Examples of surfaces that could harbor dried blood or body fluids infected with HBV include contaminated worktables, equipment, and instruments.

Hepatitis C

Chronic hepatitis C is the most common chronic viral infection in the United States. Approximately 4 million Americans have been diagnosed with chronic hepatitis C, and each year it causes an estimated 12,000 deaths resulting from cirrhosis and liver cancer.

The most common means of transmission of hepatitis C is by sharing needles for injection drug use with an infected individual. Hepatitis C is not spread by casual contact, such as sneezing, coughing, hugging, sharing food or water, or sharing eating utensils or drinking glasses. It is rarely transmitted through sexual contact.

Individuals infected with hepatitis C should not share with other members of the household personal items that may have blood on them (e.g., toothbrushes, nail-grooming equipment, razors).

Chronic hepatitis C is known as "an epidemic that occurred in the past." Numerous individuals became infected with hepatitis C more than 30 years ago and are now being diagnosed with it. This is because the symptoms of chronic hepatitis C often do not appear until 10 to 30 years after infection, and many times the first symptoms come only with advanced liver disease. Chronic hepatitis C surpasses alcoholism as the leading cause of liver cirrhosis and liver transplantation in the United States.

Before 1992, a blood test to determine the presence of hepatitis C did not exist. Because of this, a significant number of people contracted hepatitis C from HCV-infected blood transfusions. The CDC encourages people who received blood transfusions before July 1992 to ask their physicians if they should be tested for hepatitis C.

Postexposure prophylaxis with immune globulin is not effective in preventing hepatitis C, and no vaccine exists yet to prevent hepatitis C. Vaccines for hepatitis C are difficult to develop because the virus mutates so frequently. The only way to control the disease is by preventing exposure to the hepatitis C virus. ■

lar symptoms. The medical assistant should have a general knowledge of each of the forms of viral hepatitis. Table 2-1 outlines the incubation period, means of transmission, characteristics, onset and symptoms, and prognosis for all strains of viral hepatitis.

Acquired Immune Deficiency Syndrome

Acquired immune deficiency syndrome (AIDS) is a chronic disorder of the immune system that eventually destroys the body's ability to fight off infection. AIDS is caused by a retrovirus known as *human immunodeficiency virus (HIV)*. The following description helps to clarify the difference between these two terms. The virus and the infection itself are known as *HIV*, whereas the term *AIDS* is used to refer to the last stage of HIV infection. Simply put, the terms *HIV infection* and *AIDS* refer to different stages of the same disease.

When HIV gains entrance into the body, it begins to attack and destroy certain white blood cells known as *CD4$^+$ T cells*, which are involved in protecting the body against viral, fungal, and protozoal infections. As more and more CD4$^+$ T cells are destroyed, the immune system is gradually weakened. After a period of time, which may last 10 years or longer, the body's immune system becomes so ravaged by the attack that it succumbs to the diseases associated with AIDS.

AIDS is characterized by the presence of severe and life-threatening opportunistic infections and unusual cancers that rarely affect individuals with healthy immune systems. An **opportunistic infection** is an infection that results from a defective immune system that cannot defend itself from pathogens normally found in the environment. Opportunistic infections are extremely difficult to treat because the infection tends to recur quickly after a course of therapy is completed.

Stages of AIDS

The AIDS infection cycle has four stages; however, all stages may not be experienced by every infected individual. These four stages are described next.

Stage 1: Acute HIV Infection

An individual infected with HIV may first experience a transient flulike illness known as *acute HIV infection*, which occurs 1 to 4 weeks after exposure. Many people do not develop any symptoms, however, when they first become infected with HIV. If they do occur, symptoms of acute HIV infection include fever, sweats, fatigue, loss of appetite, diarrhea, pharyngitis, myalgia, arthralgia, and adenopathy. These symptoms usually disappear within 1 week to 1 month and are often mistaken for symptoms of another viral infection.

Stage 2: Asymptomatic Period

After the early symptoms subside (if they occur at all), the infected individual normally experiences a long incubation period, lasting months to years depending on the individ-

ual. During this time, the individual is asymptomatic and looks and feels completely well. Because of this, the individual may not realize the HIV infection is present. The only evidence of HIV infection during this stage is production by the body of antibodies to HIV that are detectable by blood tests. These HIV antibodies are unable to destroy the virus; however, they are used as a basis for the test procedure to indicate that the HIV infection is present. Because of the length of time required by the body to develop HIV antibodies, however, these tests may fail to detect HIV for 3 to 6 months after an individual has been infected. Although an infected person may appear perfectly healthy, the virus is very active during this stage in destroying CD4$^+$ T cells, a process that gradually weakens the immune system. Because HIV may be transmitted with or without symptoms, it is during this asymptomatic period that the danger of accidental transmission is greatest.

Stage 3: Symptomatic Period

Before the development of full-blown AIDS, many HIV-infected individuals experience a series of lesser symptoms caused by a weakened immune system. One of the first such symptoms experienced by many people infected with HIV is lymph nodes that remain enlarged for longer than 3 months. Other symptoms often experienced months to years before the onset of AIDS include progressive generalized lymphadenopathy, lack of energy, unexplained weight loss, recurrent fevers and sweats, diarrhea, persistent or frequent yeast infections (oral or vaginal), and persistent skin rashes or flaky skin. Some people develop frequent and severe herpes infections that cause mouth, genital, or anal sores or a painful nerve disease known as *shingles*.

Stage 4: AIDS

AIDS is the last stage of the infection cycle that began with HIV infection. As previously described, full-blown AIDS is characterized by the presence of opportunistic infections and unusual cancers known as *AIDS-defining conditions*. They do not usually occur, or produce only mild illness, in individuals with healthy immune systems. A severe and rare type of pneumonia caused by the organism *Pneumocystis jirovecii* is frequently associated with AIDS patients, as is Kaposi sarcoma, a rare type of cancer. Box 2-3 describes these and other AIDS-defining conditions. AIDS is also known to damage the nervous system, which eventually results in varying degrees of dementia and other symptoms. As HIV infection progresses, the individual becomes overwhelmed by infection and cancer. The body is unable to fight back because of a severely damaged immune system, and the patient eventually dies from AIDS-defining conditions.

Transmission of AIDS

Research has shown that HIV is not transmitted through casual contact or even extensive contact, such as occurs among family members of AIDS patients. In the general population, HIV is spread primarily through sexual contact

Table 2-1 Forms of Viral Hepatitis

	Hepatitis A (HAV)	Hepatitis B (HBV)	Hepatitis C (HCV)	Hepatitis D (HDV)	Hepatitis E (HEV)
Incubation period	2-6 wk	6 wk to 6 mo	2 wk to 6 mo	2 wk to 5 mo	3-6 wk
Means of transmission	Caused by a virus found in the feces of HAV-infected individuals. Transmitted almost exclusively by the fecal-oral route through practices of poor hygiene; also transmitted by the consumption of food and water contaminated with human feces	Caused by a virus found in the blood and certain body fluids of HBV-infected individuals. Transmitted by exposure to contaminated semen and vaginal secretions through personal contact, especially sexual contact; parenteral exposure to contaminated blood and blood components, such as through injecting drugs using contaminated needles and accidental needlestick injuries by health care workers; perinatally from an infected mother to her infant during birth	Caused by a virus found in the blood of HCV-infected individuals. Parenteral exposure to contaminated blood or blood components, primarily from injecting drugs using contaminated needles. It is possible to transmit HCV during intercourse, but it is uncommon	Same as hepatitis B	Fecal-oral route through practices of poor hygiene; consumption of food and water contaminated with feces
Characteristics	Usually occurs in children and young adults, especially in environments of poor sanitation and overcrowding; often a mild disease with symptoms similar to the flu and lasting 1-2 wk; there is a vaccine available to prevent hepatitis A	Symptoms usually last 1-4 wk, but it may be 6 mo before the individual fully recovers; there is a vaccine available to prevent hepatitis B	At risk are individuals who received a blood transfusion before 1992; currently a vaccine does not exist for hepatitis C	Affects only those already infected with hepatitis B; a person who has received the hepatitis B vaccine also is protected from hepatitis D	Rare in the United States; generally seen in developing countries; usually occurs in epidemics rather than as sporadic cases
Symptoms	Symptoms include fever, malaise, fatigue, anorexia, nausea, vomiting, and abdominal discomfort, followed in some people by dark urine, clay-colored stools, and mild jaundice	Symptoms include fatigue, headache, loss of appetite, nausea, vomiting, malaise, and muscle and joint pain, followed in some people by dark urine, clay-colored stools, abdominal pain, and jaundice	Symptoms are similar to those of hepatitis B	Occurs as a coinfection or superinfection with hepatitis B and intensifies the symptoms of hepatitis B	Symptoms are similar to those of hepatitis B
Prognosis	Most people recover fully within 6-10 wk and become immune to the virus; rarely fatal; chronic hepatitis does not develop; carrier states do not develop	Most people recover fully and become immune to this disease; some people (10%) go on to develop chronic hepatitis and may develop cirrhosis and liver cancer; these people also are carriers of hepatitis B. Eventually 25% of people with chronic hepatitis B die from liver failure	Approximately 55%-85% of people infected with hepatitis C are unable to clear the virus from their body and develop chronic hepatitis, which may lead to liver damage, such as cirrhosis and liver cancer. These people are also carriers of hepatitis C. Eventually 1% to 5% of people with chronic hepatitis C die from liver failure	Frequently leads to chronic hepatitis; high fatality rate (30% of chronic hepatitis patients)	Does not progress to chronic hepatitis; hepatitis E is particularly dangerous if contracted by pregnant women (10%-20% fatality rate in these individuals)

Highlight on AIDS

Prevalence

AIDS was first reported in the United States in 1981, but most likely it existed here and in other parts of the world for many years before that. Since 1981, more than 1 million cases of AIDS have been reported in the United States, and every year approximately 40,000 people in the United States are newly infected with HIV. Since 1981, there have been an estimated 550,000 deaths from AIDS in the United States.

Currently, almost 75% of those individuals newly diagnosed with HIV are adolescent and adult males, and the largest proportions of these are men who have sex with men, followed by individuals infected through high-risk heterosexual contact. Individuals between the ages of 25 and 44 account for the largest proportion of newly diagnosed HIV cases.

Transmission

HIV is spread primarily through sexual contact with an infected individual and by sharing drug injection needles with infected individuals. Scientific evidence shows that HIV is not spread through casual, everyday contact. There is no evidence that HIV is spread by sharing facilities or equipment, such as telephones, computers, food utensils, bedding, doorknobs, and bathrooms. Because HIV is not passed through the air, it is not spread through coughing and sneezing. HIV also is not spread through tears or sweat, or by shaking hands, hugging, or donating blood.

Most individuals infected with HIV show no symptoms and may not develop full-blown AIDS for 10 years or longer. After infection with HIV, the individual is infected for life.

Women can transmit HIV to their fetuses during pregnancy or birth. Approximately one quarter to one third of pregnant women infected with HIV who are not being treated with antiretroviral drugs pass the infection to their infants. HIV also can be spread to infants through the breast milk of mothers infected with the virus. Because of this, the CDC recommends that testing for HIV be included in the routine panel of prenatal screening tests for all pregnant women, and that separate written consent is not required. The CDC further recommends that the patient should be notified that HIV testing will be performed, unless the patient declines the test (known as opt-out screening). The CDC recommends that repeat HIV screening be performed in the third trimester in areas that have elevated rates of HIV infection among pregnant women.

Worldwide, more than 700,000 infants are infected with HIV each year. If antiretroviral drugs are taken during pregnancy and the infant is delivered by cesarean section, the chance of transmitting HIV to the infant is reduced significantly. In developing countries, such as sub-Saharan Africa, women seldom know their HIV status, and treatment is often unavailable.

HIV Testing

The CDC recommends HIV screening for patients in all health care settings after the patient is notified that the testing will be performed, and separate written consent is not required. HIV screening should be performed unless the patient declines (known as opt-out screening). The CDC further recommends that individuals at high risk for HIV infection undergo HIV screening at least annually.

The enzyme immune assay (EIA) test and the enzyme-linked immunosorbent assay (ELISA) test are used as screening tests for the presence of HIV. Newer rapid HIV testing kits are also commercially available; brand names include Uni-Gold Recombigen HIV (Trinity Biotech, County Wicklow, Ireland), Clearview HIV (Inverness Medical, Princeton, NJ), and OraQuick Rapid HIV test (OraSure Technologies, Bethlehem, PA). Because of the possibility of a false-positive result, a second screening test is always performed if a blood specimen tests positive. If the second test also is positive, a more specific test, such as the Western blot test, is performed to confirm the test results. An individual who tests positive for HIV is seropositive.

A negative HIV test is not conclusive for the absence of HIV infection. If an individual has recently been infected with HIV, the antibodies may not have had time to develop. It generally takes 2 to 12 weeks (but possibly as long as 6 months for the HIV antibodies to appear in the blood.

CDC Definition of AIDS

As scientists have learned more about the disease, the CDC's definition of AIDS has changed several times since the beginning of the AIDS epidemic. The current AIDS definition includes the presence of one or both of the following conditions:

1. HIV positive and a CD4$^+$ T cell count below 200 cells/μL (normal CD4$^+$ T cell count for a healthy individual ranges from 500 to 1500 cells/μL)
2. Presence of one or more AIDS-defining conditions

Treatment

There is no known cure for AIDS; there is no vaccine to prevent it. Powerful antiviral drugs have been developed that slow the reproduction of the virus and reduce the viral load in the body. In many patients, these drugs have dramatically delayed HIV from progressing to full-blown AIDS, thereby allowing them to live longer. These drugs can have serious side effects, and they do not prevent the spread of the disease to someone else. Numerous drugs also are available to treat the opportunistic infections and cancers that occur with AIDS. ■

BOX 2-3 AIDS-Defining Conditions

Neoplasms
Kaposi Sarcoma
Malignant Neoplasm

Kaposi sarcoma is the most common neoplasm occurring in AIDS patients. It is an aggressive tumor that involves multiple body organs, but it generally occurs initially on the skin. It is characterized by multiple dark-red or purplish blotches on the skin. The areas of the body most commonly affected are the trunk, arms, head, and neck. Diagnosis of Kaposi sarcoma is made by tissue biopsy. Other body sites commonly affected by this neoplasm are the lymph nodes, the lungs, and the gastrointestinal tract. Kaposi sarcoma is rarely the primary cause of death but does further weaken the AIDS patient, who may die eventually as a result of opportunistic infections.

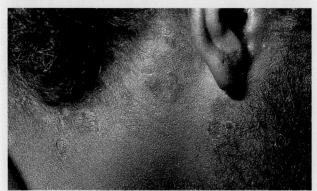

Kaposi sarcoma. (Forbes CD: Color atlas and text of clinical medicine, ed 3, St Louis, 2003, Mosby.)

Opportunistic Infections
Pneumocystis jirovecii *Pneumonia*
Protozoa

Pneumocystis jirovecii pneumonia (PCP) is the most common opportunistic infection causing death in individuals with AIDS. This protozoan lung infection previously was considered rare and in most instances not fatal. PCP occurs at least once in more than 65% of AIDS patients, and 25% of patients initially infected experience a recurrence. PCP is characterized by moderate to severe difficulty in breathing, fever, and a nonproductive cough in the early stages and a productive cough in the later stages of the disease. Death occurs in 30% of PCP-infected patients and is generally caused by acute respiratory failure.

Cytomegalovirus Infection
Virus

Cytomegalovirus is a virus that belongs to the herpes virus group and that rarely causes disease in healthy adults. Most AIDS patients have active cytomegalovirus infection. The most common signs of its presence in AIDS patients are spots on the retinas, which may lead to blindness. This virus also causes pneumonia, esophagitis, and colitis. Specific symptoms include fever, profound fatigue, muscle and joint aches, night sweats, impaired vision, cough, dyspnea, abdominal pain, and diarrhea.

Opportunistic Infections—cont'd
Herpes Simplex 1 and 2
Virus

Herpes simplex 1 is spread by contact with oral secretions, and herpes simplex 2 is spread by contact with genital secretions. Herpes simplex causes painful vesicular lesions, usually of the nasopharynx, oral cavity, skin, and genital tract. This virus tends to have periods of latency followed by reactivation of symptoms. In AIDS patients, herpes simplex is apt to cause cervical lymphadenopathy and proctitis.

Mycobacterial Infections
Bacteria

Mycobacterial infections are among the most frequent opportunistic infections in AIDS patients. One strain (*Mycobacterium avium* complex) causes fever, fatigue, weight loss, diarrhea, and malabsorption. Another strain *(Mycobacterium tuberculosis)* causes pulmonary tuberculosis, which is not considered an opportunistic infection. In AIDS patients, tuberculosis is characterized by a productive, purulent cough, fever, dyspnea, fatigue, weight loss, and wasting. The AIDS epidemic seems to be causing a resurgence of tuberculosis in the United States. Because tuberculosis is more contagious than most AIDS-defining conditions, it seems to be spreading beyond AIDS patients and into the general population.

Candidiasis
Yeastlike Fungus

Candida albicans is a fungus that inhabits the oropharynx, large intestine, and skin, causing no harm in individuals with healthy immune systems. Infection with *C. albicans* is often one of the first

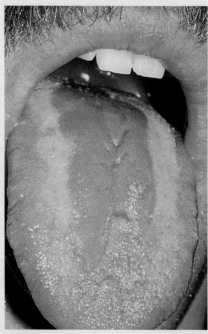

Candida. (Christensen BL: Adult health nursing, ed 5, St Louis, 2006, Mosby.)

Continued

BOX 2-3 AIDS-Defining Conditions—cont'd

signs of a weakened immune system in HIV-infected individuals. It is characterized by a white, patchy growth on the mouth, throat, or esophagus (thrush). AIDS patients develop an extremely severe case of candidiasis that makes eating and swallowing difficult and painful. In female AIDS patients, this organism causes severe vaginitis.

Cryptosporidiosis
Protozoa
In AIDS patients, this condition usually causes profuse, watery diarrhea along with anorexia, vomiting, fatigue, malaise, and fever. This condition may become chronic, resulting in dehydration and electrolyte imbalance, which lead to weight loss and eventual death.

Toxoplasmosis
Protozoa
Toxoplasmosis is one of the most common causes of encephalitis in AIDS patients, resulting in the following symptoms: headache, altered mental state, visual disturbances, cranial nerve palsy, and motor disorders. Toxoplasmosis also may result in infections of the heart, lungs, skin, stomach, abdomen, and testes.

Cryptococcosis
Fungus
Cryptococcosis is a common cause of meningitis in AIDS patients and includes chronic symptoms of low-grade fever, malaise, and headaches. Other symptoms manifested after these initial symptoms include photophobia, stiff neck, nausea, vomiting, and seizures.

---

with an infected person and by sharing drug injection needles with someone who is infected. Untreated HIV-infected women also can transmit the virus to their infants during pregnancy and birth and through their breast milk.

Because HIV is not easily transmitted, the risk to health care workers is low. Since reporting began in 1985, the CDC has received reports of 57 documented cases and 138 possible cases of HIV infection from occupational exposure to health care workers (as of December 2001). Despite the low risk of infection, however, the serious nature of HIV infection warrants the use of the OSHA Blood-borne Pathogens Standard by all health care workers. Because most HIV carriers are asymptomatic and may be unaware of their infection, precautions minimizing the risk of exposure to blood and body fluids should be taken with all patients at all times. These precautions also are recommended as a means of protection against other bloodborne pathogens, such as hepatitis B, hepatitis C, and syphilis.

⊝**volve** *Check out the Evolve site to access additional interactive activities.*

PATIENT TEACHING Acquired Immune Deficiency Syndrome

Teach patients the ways in which AIDS is transmitted.
- Having unprotected sex (vaginal, anal, or oral) with someone who is infected with HIV. The virus is most commonly found in semen, blood, and vaginal secretions.
- Sharing needles for injection drug use with someone who is infected with HIV. This occurs as follows: If an HIV-infected individual uses a needle to pierce his or her skin, there will be a tiny amount of blood left on the needle. If another person uses the same needle, the person will be injecting the HIV-infected blood into his or her body.
- Transmitting in utero. A pregnant woman with HIV can pass it on to her fetus. Infants born with HIV usually develop AIDS by 2 years of age.
- Receiving a blood transfusion or blood products (before 1985) from someone infected with HIV. (In 1985, blood banks began screening blood for AIDS, so this is largely a problem of blood received before then.)
- There is a greater risk of contracting AIDS if a patient already has another sexually transmitted disease, such as chlamydia, gonorrhea, syphilis, herpes, or bacterial vaginosis.

Teach patients how to prevent AIDS.
- Know your sexual partners and their sexual history and drug use.
- Use a latex condom during sexual intercourse to minimize the risk of infection. HIV cannot pass through the latex if the condom

does not break and is used properly. If a lubricant is used with the condom, it should be water based, such as K-Y jelly, because an oil-based lubricant such as petroleum jelly could break down the latex.
- Avoid sexual practices that involve the exchange of body fluids, such as semen or vaginal secretions.
- If you think that you could have HIV, never let your blood, semen, or vaginal fluid enter another person's body.
- Do not share needles for injectable drug use.

Teach patients to recognize the symptoms of AIDS.
- Unexplained fatigue
- Weight loss of 10 to 15 lb in less than 2 months, but without dieting
- Unexplained fever, chills, and sweating at night for longer than 2 weeks
- Unexplained swollen glands for longer than 1 month
- Unexplained diarrhea or bloody stools for longer than 2 weeks
- Unexplained persistent dry cough, shortness of breath, or difficulty in breathing
- White patches on the tongue or mouth that cannot be scraped off
Explain to patients that these symptoms also could be signs of other diseases. If they have any of these symptoms, however, they should consider having an HIV test. The earlier the infection is detected, the earlier treatment can begin that may delay the onset of other symptoms. ■

MEDICAL PRACTICE and the LAW

There are three behaviors that are crucial in protecting yourself from a lawsuit:

1. Establish a rapport. If patients believe that you truly care about them and have their best interests at heart, they rarely sue, even if you make a mistake.
2. Follow all procedures according to your procedures manual. If you do everything right and the patient has an adverse outcome, you will not likely be found liable.
3. Document everything you do objectively. Lawsuits often come to court years after the incident, and nobody's memory is as good as written documentation. Document only the facts, not your opinion. Document the patient's reactions to treatments.

Ethics and Law

Ethics is the highest standard of behavior and is loosely based on the Golden Rule. No law can force you to behave ethically, but most major professions, including the American Association of Medical Assistants (AAMA), have a written code of ethics. Ethics uses words such as *should* and *may*. If you are angry with someone, ethically, you should not yell at him or her. This is not against the law, but it is unethical.

Law is the lowest standard of behavior and is enforced by federal, state, and local law enforcement personnel. Laws use words such as *must* and *shall*. If you are angry with someone, legally, you must not hit him or her. This behavior is illegal, and you could be charged with assault and battery.

Regarding medical asepsis and infection control, you have a duty and a responsibility to protect yourself, your coworkers, and, most important, your patients. Follow specific guidelines established by OSHA and the CDC to prevent the transmission of pathogens. ■

What Would You Do? What Would You *Not* Do? RESPONSES

Case Study 1
Page 63

What Did Jennifer Do?

❏ Told Petra that the hand sanitizers (alcohol-based hand rubs) are as good as, if not better than, soap and water for removing germs from the hands.
❏ Stressed to Petra that hand sanitizers are not designed to remove soil from the hands and that she should wash her hands with soap and water when they are visibly soiled.
❏ Explained that the Centers for Disease Control and Prevention now recommends that hand sanitizers be used in health care settings to help prevent the spread of disease.

What Did Jennifer Not *Do?*

❏ Did not tell Petra that she should switch from soap and water to hand sanitizers.

What Would You Do/What Would You *Not* Do? Review Jennifer's response and place a checkmark next to the information you included in your response. List additional information you included in your response.

_____
_____
_____
_____

Case Study 2
Page 68

What Did Jennifer Do?

❏ Explained to Tracy that a federal agency known as the Occupational Safety and Health Administration (OSHA) requires that gloves be worn when drawing a patient's blood in the office. Told her that the office could be fined if they were not worn.

❏ Told Tracy that having her infant immunized for hepatitis B is an investment in her child's future. Explained that her child could come into contact with the virus anytime in his or her life. Stressed that if a young child becomes infected with hepatitis B, the child has a higher risk of developing chronic hepatitis, which can cause serious liver problems later in life.
❏ Gave Tracy a brochure on hepatitis B to take home.

What Did Jennifer Not *Do?*

❏ Did not discourage Tracy from having her baby immunized for hepatitis B.

What Would You Do/What Would You *Not* Do? Review Jennifer's response and place a checkmark next to the information you included in your response. List additional information you included in your response.

_____
_____
_____
_____

Case Study 3
Page 73

What Did Jennifer Do?

❏ Explained to Giles that the blood supply was not tested for hepatitis C until 1992 because a test to detect the presence of hepatitis C was not developed until then.
❏ Told Giles that it is possible for someone to have hepatitis C and not exhibit any symptoms.
❏ Told Giles that he should ask the physician his question about giving hepatitis C to others.

Continued

What Would You Do? What Would You *Not* Do? RESPONSES—cont'd

What Did Jennifer Not *Do?*

❑ Did not automatically assume that Giles had hepatitis C because he had not yet been seen by the physician. It would be up to the physician to make a diagnosis of hepatitis C.

❑ Did not tell Giles about the serious complications of hepatitis C. If Giles is diagnosed with hepatitis C, it would be the physician's responsibility to relay this information.

What Would You Do/What Would You *Not* Do? Review Jennifer's response and place a checkmark next to the information you included in your response. List additional information you included in your response.

_____

_____

_____

_____

CERTIFICATION REVIEW

❑ **Microorganisms** are tiny living plants or animals that cannot be seen with the naked eye; examples include bacteria, viruses, protozoa, fungi, and animal parasites. Microorganisms that do not cause disease are nonpathogens. Microorganisms that are harmful to the body and can cause disease are pathogens.

❑ **Medical asepsis** refers to practices that are employed to reduce the number and hinder the transmission of pathogenic microorganisms. Nonpathogens would still be present, but all the pathogens would have been removed.

❑ **Microorganisms** that use inorganic substances as sources of food are autotrophs; microorganisms that use organic substances for food are heterotrophs. Aerobes are microorganisms that need oxygen to grow and multiply, and anaerobes are microorganisms that grow best in the absence of oxygen.

❑ **The body has protective mechanisms** to help prevent the invasion of pathogens, which include the following: the skin and mucous membranes, mucus and cilia in the nose and respiratory tract, coughing and sneezing, tears and sweat, urine and vaginal secretions, and hydrochloric acid secreted by the stomach.

❑ **Hand hygiene** refers to the process of cleaning or sanitizing the hands and is the most important medical aseptic practice for preventing the spread of infection. *Handwashing* refers to washing the hands with a detergent soap; *antiseptic handwashing* refers to washing the hands with an antimicrobial soap. The CDC now recommends that an alcohol-based hand rub should be used to sanitize the hands when they are not visibly soiled.

❑ **Resident flora,** also known as *normal flora,* normally resides and grows in the epidermis and dermis. Resident flora is generally harmless and nonpathogenic. Transient flora lives and grows on the superficial skin layers and is picked up in the course of daily activities. Transient flora is often pathogenic but can be removed easily by handwashing or by applying an alcohol-based hand rub.

❑ **OSHA** was established by the federal government to assist employers in providing a safe and healthy working environment for their employees. The OSHA standard must be followed by any employee with occupational exposure, regardless of the place of employment.

❑ **Occupational exposure** is defined as reasonably anticipated skin, eye, mucous membrane, or parenteral contact with bloodborne pathogens or other potentially infectious materials that may result from the performance of an employee's duties. Bloodborne pathogens are pathogenic microorganisms in human blood that can cause disease in humans. An exposure incident is a specific eye, mouth, or other mucous membrane, nonintact skin, or parenteral contact with blood or other potentially infectious materials that results from an employee's duties.

❑ **The OSHA standard** requires that the medical office develop a written exposure control plan designed to eliminate or minimize employees' exposure to bloodborne pathogens and other potentially infectious materials. The ECP must be reviewed and updated annually to ensure that it remains current with the latest information on eliminating or reducing exposure to bloodborne pathogens.

❑ **Engineering controls** include all measures that isolate or remove health hazards from the workplace; examples include safer medical devices and biohazard containers. A safer medical device is a device that, based on reasonable judgment, would make an exposure incident involving a contaminated sharp less likely (e.g., sharps with engineered sharps injury protection, needleless systems).

❑ **Work practice controls** reduce the likelihood of exposure by altering the manner in which a technique is performed and include such practices as bandaging cuts before gloving; sanitizing hands as soon as possible after removing gloves; immediately placing contaminated sharps in a biohazard sharps container; and not eating, drinking, or smoking in areas where you may be exposed to blood or other potentially infectious materials. If exposed to blood or OPIM, perform first-aid measures immediately and then report the incident to the physician so that PEP can be instituted.

CERTIFICATION REVIEW—cont'd

❏ **Personal protective equipment** is clothing or equipment that protects an individual from contact with blood or other potentially infectious materials; examples include gloves, chin-length face shields, masks, protective eyewear, laboratory coats, and gowns. The type of protective equipment appropriate for a given task depends on the degree of exposure that is anticipated.

❏ **Regulated medical waste** is waste that may pose a substantial threat to health and safety if exposed to the public. RMW must be properly handled and contained in the medical office so as not to become a source of transfer of disease. Regulated medical waste must be disposed of in accordance with all applicable state laws.

❏ **The biggest threats to health care workers** from occupational exposure are hepatitis B, hepatitis C, and HIV. Hepatitis is an infection of the liver. The most common means of transmission of hepatitis in the health care setting are blood and blood products through needlesticks and cuts with contaminated sharps.

❏ **AIDS** is a disorder of the immune system that eventually destroys the body's ability to fight infection. AIDS is characterized by the presence of severe and life-threatening opportunistic infections and unusual cancers. AIDS is caused by HIV, which is transmitted through contaminated body fluids, particularly blood and semen.

TERMINOLOGY REVIEW

Medical Term	Word Parts	Definition
Aerobe	*aer/o:* air	A microorganism that needs oxygen to live and grow.
Anaerobe	*an-:* without *aer/o:* air	A microorganism that grows best in the absence of oxygen.
Antiseptic	*anti-:* against *septic:* infection	An agent that inhibits the growth of or kills microorganisms.
Asepsis	*a-:* without *sepsis:* infection	Free from infection or pathogens; the actions practiced to make and maintain an area or object free from infection or pathogens.
Cilia		Slender, hairlike projections that constantly beat toward the outside to remove microorganisms from the body.
Contaminate		To soil or to make impure. An aseptic object is contaminated when it touches something that is not clean.
Decontamination		The use of physical or chemical means to remove, inactivate, or destroy pathogens on a surface or item to the point where they are no longer capable of transmitting infectious particles; the surface or item is rendered safe for handling, use, or disposal.
Hand hygiene		The process of cleansing or sanitizing the hands.
Infection		The condition in which the body, or part of it, is invaded by a pathogen.
Medical asepsis	*a-:* without *sepsis:* infection	Practices that are employed to reduce the number and hinder the transmission of pathogens.
Microorganism	*micro-:* small *organism:* organism	A microscopic plant or animal.
Nonintact skin	*non-:* not	Skin that has a break in the surface. It includes, but is not limited to, abrasions, cuts, hangnails, paper cuts, and burns.
Nonpathogen	*non-:* not *path/o:* disease *-gen:* producing	A microorganism that does not normally produce disease.
Opportunistic infection		An infection that results from a defective immune system that cannot defend the body from pathogens normally found in the environment.
Optimum growth temperature		The temperature at which an organism grows best.
Parenteral	*para-:* apart from *enter/o:* intestine *-al:* pertaining to	Taken into the body through piercing of the skin barrier or mucous membranes, such as through needlesticks, human bites, cuts, and abrasions.

Continued

TERMINOLOGY REVIEW—cont'd

Medical Term	Word Parts	Definition
Pathogen	*path/o:* disease *-gen:* producing	A disease-producing microorganism.
Perinatal	*peri-:* surrounding *natal:* pertaining to birth	Relating to the period shortly before and after birth.
pH		The degree to which a solution is acidic or basic.
Postexposure prophylaxis (PEP)	*post-:* after *pro:* before *phylaxis:* prevention of disease	Treatment administered to an individual after exposure to an infectious disease to prevent the disease.
Regulated medical waste (RMW)		Medical waste that poses a threat to health and safety.
Reservoir host		The organism that becomes infected by a pathogen and serves as a source of transfer of the pathogen to others.
Resident flora		Harmless, nonpathogenic microorganisms that normally reside on the skin and usually do not cause disease. Also known as *normal flora.*
Susceptible		Easily affected; lacking resistance.
Transient flora		Microorganisms that reside on the superficial skin layers and are picked up in the course of daily activities. They are often pathogenic but can be removed easily from the skin by sanitizing the hands.

ON THE WEB

For information on federal regulations and recommendations for infection control:

Occupational Safety and Health Administration (OSHA): www.osha.gov

Centers for Disease Control and Prevention (CDC): www.cdc.gov

National Institute for Occupational Safety and Health (NIOSH): www.cdc.gov/niosh

CDC Recommendations for Hand Hygiene in the Healthcare Setting: www.cdc.gov/handhygiene

Food and Drug Administration (FDA): www.fda.gov

Environmental Protection Agency: www.epa.gov

Association for the Advancement of Medical Instrumentation (AAMI): www.aami.org

Division of Healthcare Quality Promotion (DHQP): www.cdc.gov/ncidod/dhqp

Epidemiology Program Office: www.cdc.gov/epo

Morbidity and Mortality Weekly Report: www.cdc.gov/mmwr

For information on hepatitis:

CDC National Center for Infectious Diseases: www.cdc.gov/hepatitis

Hepatitis Foundation International: www.hepfi.org

Hepatitis B Foundation: www.hepb.org

National Institute of Allergy and Infectious Diseases: www.niaid.nih.gov

HealthTalk: www.healthtalk.com

ON THE WEB—cont'd

For information on AIDS:

CDC National Center for Infectious Diseases: www.cdc.gov/ncidod/diseases

AIDS Education Global Information System: www.aegis.com

AIDS Information: www.aidsinfo.nih.gov

The Body—AIDS and HIV Information Resource: www.thebody.com

About AIDS: aids.about.com

HIV Positive.Com: www.hivpositive.com

Mayo Clinic: www.mayoclinic.com

3

Sterilization and Disinfection

LEARNING OBJECTIVES	PROCEDURES
Hazard Communication Standard	
1. Explain the purpose of the Hazard Communication Standard.	Read and interpret an MSDS.
2. List and describe the information that must be included on the label of a hazardous chemical.	
3. List and describe the information that must be included in a material safety data sheet (MSDS).	
Sanitization	
1. State the purpose of sanitization.	Sanitize instruments.
2. State the advantages of using an ultrasonic cleaner to clean instruments.	
3. List and describe the guidelines that should be followed when sanitizing instruments.	
Disinfection	
1. State the uses of the three levels of disinfection: high, intermediate, and low.	Chemically disinfect articles.
2. Explain the differences among the following: critical item, semicritical item, and noncritical item.	
3. List and describe the guidelines for disinfecting articles.	
4. List and describe the primary use of disinfectants in the medical office.	
Sterilization	
1. Explain how the autoclave functions to sterilize articles.	Wrap articles to be autoclaved.
2. List the components of a sterilization monitoring program.	Sterilize articles in the autoclave.
3. List and describe types of sterilization indicators.	Maintain the autoclave.
4. Identify the advantages and disadvantages of each of the following types of wraps: sterilization paper, sterilization pouches, and muslin.	
5. List the guidelines that should be followed when the autoclave is loaded.	
6. Identify the sterilization times for each of the following categories: unwrapped articles, wrapped articles, liquids, and large wrapped packs.	
7. Describe the method for storing wrapped articles.	
8. Describe the daily, weekly, and monthly maintenance of the autoclave.	
Other Sterilization Methods	
1. State the primary use of each of the following types of sterilization methods: dry heat, ethylene oxide gas, chemicals, and radiation.	

KEY TERMS

antiseptic (an-tih-SEP-tik)
autoclave (AU-toe-klave)
contaminate (kon-TAM-in-ate)
critical item
decontamination (DEE-kon-tam-in-AY-shun)
detergent
disinfectant (dis-in-FEK-tant)
hazardous chemical
incubate (IN-kyoo-bate)

load
material safety data sheet (MSDS)
noncritical item
sanitization (san-ih-tih-ZAY-shun)
semicritical item
spore
sterilization (stare-ill-ih-ZAY-shun)
thermolabile (ther-moe-LAH-bul)

Introduction to Sterilization and Disinfection

The air and all objects around us contain microorganisms. The medical assistant is responsible for helping to reduce and eliminate microorganisms to prevent the spread of disease. This can be accomplished by practicing good techniques of medical and surgical asepsis (see Chapters 2 and 10).

Physical and chemical agents are used to destroy microorganisms in the medical office. The agent selected depends on the intended use of the article. Articles that penetrate sterile tissue or the vascular system, such as surgical instruments, must be sterilized. Articles that come in contact with the skin, such as stethoscopes, blood pressure cuffs, and percussion hammers, should be disinfected.

Sanitization, disinfection, and sterilization involve hazardous chemicals. It is essential for the medical assistant to know the precautions that are required when working with hazardous chemicals.

DEFINITIONS OF TERMS

Terms that aid in understanding this chapter are listed and defined here.

Sanitization Sanitization is a process that removes organic material and reduces the number of microorganisms to a safe level as determined by public health requirements. Sanitization removes all organic material, such as blood, body fluids, and tissue, from an article. For articles that are used in examinations, treatments, and office surgery to be properly sterilized or disinfected, they must first be sanitized.

Decontamination Decontamination refers to the use of physical or chemical means to remove or destroy pathogens on an item so that it is no longer capable of transmitting disease; this makes the item safe to handle.

Detergent A detergent is an agent that cleanses by emulsifying dirt and oil.

Disinfectant A disinfectant is an agent used to destroy pathogenic microorganisms; however, it does not kill the resistant bacterial spores. Disinfectants are generally applied to inanimate objects.

Spore A spore is a hard, thick-walled capsule that some bacteria form by losing moisture and condensing their contents to contain only the essential parts of the protoplasm of the cell. Spores represent a resting and protective stage of the bacterial cell and are more resistant to drying, sunlight, heat, and disinfectants than is the vegetative form of the bacterium. Favorable conditions cause the spore to germinate into a vegetative bacterium again that is capable of reproducing. Two examples of species of bacteria that form spores are *Clostridium botulinum*, which causes botulism, and *Clostridium tetani*, which causes tetanus.

Sterilization Sterilization is the process of destroying all forms of microbial life, including bacterial spores. An object that is *sterile* is free of all living microorganisms and spores. There can be no relative degrees of sterility—an object is either sterile or not sterile. The device most commonly used to sterilize articles in the medical office is the autoclave.

HAZARD COMMUNICATION STANDARD

The Hazard Communication Standard (HCS) is a requirement of the Occupational Safety and Health Administration (OSHA). The purpose of the HCS is to ensure that employees are informed of the hazards associated with chemicals in their workplaces. Chemicals can be in the form of a liquid, a solid, or a gas. A **hazardous chemical** is any chemical that presents a threat to the health and safety of an individual coming into contact with it. Hazardous chemicals are those that are corrosive, toxic, irritating, carcinogenic, flammable, or reactive.

The HCS is based on the concept that employees have a right to know about the hazardous chemicals in their workplace and the precautions to take to protect themselves when working with hazardous chemicals. In the medical office, sanitization, disinfection, and sterilization procedures involve the use of hazardous chemicals; the medical assistant must have a thorough knowledge of the HCS.

The HCS consists of the following components:
- Development of a hazard communication program
- Inventory of hazardous chemicals
- Labeling requirements
- Material safety data sheet requirements
- Employee information and training

Hazard Communication Program

As part of the HCS, employers are required to develop a hazard communication program. The hazard communication program consists of a written plan that describes what the facility is doing to meet the requirements of the HCS. The information in the plan must be made available and communicated to all employees who work with hazardous chemicals.

Inventory of Hazardous Chemicals

The employer must develop and maintain a list of hazardous chemicals that are used and stored in the workplace. This list must include the name of the chemical, the name of the manufacturer, the hazardous ingredients, and the health and safety ratings of the chemical. The list must be updated as new chemicals are introduced into the workplace. In the medical office, hazardous chemicals often include the following:
- Products used for sanitization, disinfection, and sterilization (e.g., chemical disinfectants, autoclave cleaners)
- Chemicals used for laboratory testing (e.g., laboratory testing reagents, developing solutions, controls)
- Pharmaceutical products such as local anesthetics (e.g., lidocaine [Xylocaine])

- Front office products (e.g., toner for copying machine and laser printer)
- Cleaning products (e.g., drain cleaner)

Labeling of Hazardous Chemicals

The HCS requires that each container of a hazardous chemical be labeled by the manufacturer with a warning to alert the user that the chemical is dangerous (Figure 3-1). This label must include the possible hazards of the chemical and the steps that can be taken to protect against those risks. Hazard warnings can use words, pictures, or symbols to provide the user with an understanding of the physical and health hazards of the chemical. If a label falls off a product or is damaged or obscured, a replacement label must be applied. If a chemical is transferred to a new container, a label with all the required information must be attached to the new container.

Container Label Requirements

The HCS requires that manufacturers label the containers of hazardous chemicals they produce with specific information. This information allows the user of the chemical to tell at a glance the hazards of using the chemical and the basic steps to take to protect oneself. Information required by the HCS includes the following:

1. **Name of the chemical.** The name of the chemical must be clearly indicated on the label.
2. **Manufacturer information.** The name, address, and emergency phone number of the company that manufactures the chemical must be stated on the label.
3. **Physical hazards of the chemical.** Physical hazards that must be stated include the potential of the chemical to catch fire, explode, or react with other chemicals or materials.
4. **Health hazards of the chemical.** Health hazards include the potential of the chemical to cause irritation to tissue, cancer, a sensitivity reaction, or a toxic or corrosive reaction.
5. **Safety precautions.** The protective clothing, equipment, and procedures that are recommended when working with the chemical must be stated on the label. Examples include gloves, protective eyewear, and working with the chemical in a well-ventilated area.
6. **Storing, handling, and disposal of the chemical.** Information on how the chemical should be stored, handled, and disposed of must be stated on the label.

Material Safety Data Sheets

A **material safety data sheet (MSDS)** provides more detailed information than the container label regarding the chemical, its hazards, and measures to take to prevent injury and illness when handling the chemical (Figure 3-2). The HCS requires that a current MSDS be kept on file for each hazardous chemical used or stored in the workplace. MSDSs must be readily accessible to employees and provided to them on request. It is important that the medical assistant review the MSDS before working with a hazardous chemical.

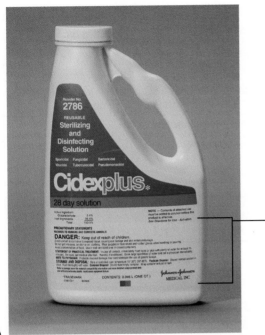

PRECAUTIONARY STATEMENTS
HAZARDS TO HUMANS AND DOMESTIC ANIMALS
DANGER: Keep out of reach of children.
Direct contact is corrosive to exposed tissue, causing eye damage and skin irritation/damage. Do not get into eyes, on skin, or on clothing. Wear goggles or face shield and rubber gloves when handling or pouring. Avoid contamination of food. Use in well-ventilated area in closed containers.
STATEMENT OF PRACTICAL TREATMENT: In case of contact, immediately flush eyes or skin with plenty of water for at least 15 minutes. For eyes, get medical attention. Harmful if swallowed. Drink large quantities of water and call a physician immediately.
NOTE TO PHYSICIAN: Probable mucosal damage may contraindicate the use of gastric lavage.
STORAGE AND DISPOSAL: Store at controlled room temperature 15°-30°C (59°-86°F).
Disposal: Discard residual solution in drain. Flush thoroughly with water.
Container disposal: Do not reuse empty container. Wrap container and put in trash.
Refer to package insert for material compatibility information and more detailed usage/product data.
Use with polycarbonate plastic could cause equipment failure.

*TRADEMARK   CONTENTS: 0.946 L (ONE QT.)
2786 C2-1   830006

A   B

Figure 3-1. **A,** Hazardous chemical container label. **B,** The label must indicate the possible hazards of the chemical.

Companies that manufacture and distribute hazardous chemicals must provide an MSDS with every product. A hazardous chemical should never be used unless an MSDS is available. In the event of an accidental exposure, information on the MSDS must be readily available as a reference for emergency treatment. If an MSDS is missing, it must be replaced. This can be accomplished by contacting the supplier or the manufacturer of that chemical for a replacement or by going to the manufacturer's website; most manufacturers post their MSDSs on their websites for easy access.

An MSDS does not have to be kept on file for a hazardous chemical that is used in the workplace in the same way that a household consumer would use it. For example, correction fluids, such as Wite-Out and Liquid Paper, contain a hazardous chemical. If the medical assistant uses it in the same way, however, that a household consumer would use it (i.e., to correct errors on a document), an MSDS does not need to be kept on file. If household bleach (sodium hypochlorite) is used to decontaminate blood spills in the medical office, an MSDS would need to be kept on file because the bleach is not being used in the same way that a household consumer would use it.

What Would You Do? What Would You *Not* Do?

Case Study 1

Elba Cordera has brought her daughter Maria in for a well-baby visit. Maria is 9 months old and is just starting to crawl. Mrs. Cordera is taking precautions to baby-proof her house to protect Maria from accidents. Mrs. Cordera wants to know how to tell whether a cleaning product is poisonous. She also wants to know what she should do if Maria gets into a cleaning product and spills it on herself or swallows it. ■

Material Safety Data Sheet Requirements

The HCS requires that manufacturers of hazardous chemicals include the following information on the MSDS (see Figure 3-2):

1. **Identification.** This section provides information used to identify the chemical and must include the chemical's generic name and its brand name; the name, address, and emergency phone number of the manufacturer; and the date the MSDS was prepared.

2. **Composition of ingredients.** This section provides a list of the ingredients in the hazardous chemical and exposure limits of each chemical.

3. **Physical and chemical properties.** Physical and chemical properties of the chemical must be listed in this section; these include the following:
   - Appearance and odor
   - Boiling point
   - Vapor pressure
   - Solubility in water
   - Evaporation rate
   - Specific gravity
   - Vapor density
   - pH level
   - Melting point
   - Freezing point
   - Odor threshold

4. **Fire and explosion data.** Some hazardous chemicals may cause a fire or explosion if used improperly. This section indicates under what circumstances this may occur and what to do if it does occur, including recommended extinguishing agents.

5. **Reactivity data.** Some chemicals react when combined with other chemicals or materials. The reactivity data list the substances and conditions that the chemical should

MATERIAL SAFETY DATA SHEET **(MSDS)**		
Date of Issue: 4/28/04		Date of Revision: 8/8/10

SECTION 1   IDENTIFICATION

GENERIC NAME: Glutaraldehyde	**INFORMATION TELEPHONE NUMBER:** 1 (800) 733-8690
BRAND NAME: Aldecide	**EMERGENCY TELEPHONE NUMBER:**
MANUFACTURER'S NAME: Brennan Corporation	1 (800) 331-0766
MFG. ADDRESS: P.O. Box 93	
CITY: Camden **STATE:** NJ **ZIP:** 08106	

SECTION 2   COMPOSITION OF INGREDIENTS

CAS NUMBER	CHEMICAL NAME OF INGREDIENTS	PERCENT	PEL	TLV
111-30-8	Glutaraldehyde	2.5	0.2 ppm	0.2 ppm
7732-18-5	Water	97.4	None	None
7632-00-0	Sodium Nitrite	<1	None	None

SECTION 3   PHYSICAL AND CHEMICAL PROPERTIES

BOILING POINT: 212° F	**SPECIFIC GRAVITY (H$_2$O = 1):** 1.004
VAPOR PRESSURE (mm Hg): 0.20 at 20° C	**VAPOR DENSITY (AIR = 1):** 1.1
ODOR: Sharp odor	**pH:** 7.5-8.5
SOLUBILITY IN WATER: Complete (100%)	**MELTING POINT:** n/a
APPEARANCE: Bluish-green liquid	**FREEZING POINT:** 32° F
EVAPORATION RATE: 0.98 (Water = 1)	**ODOR THRESHOLD:** 0.04 ppm

SECTION 4   FIRE AND EXPLOSION HAZARD DATA

FLASH POINT: Not flammable (aqueous solution)	**NFPA Rating:**
FLAMMABILITY LIMITS: **LEL:** n/a	**Health: 2**
EXTINGUISHING MEDIA: n/a (aqueous solution)	**Flammability: 0**
SPECIAL FIRE FIGHTING PROCEDURES: n/a	**Reactivity: 0**
UNUSUAL FIRE/EXPL HAZARDS: None	

SECTION 5   REACTIVITY DATA

STABILITY: Stable under recommended storage conditions.
CONDITIONS TO AVOID: Avoid direct sunlight and temperatures above 104° F (40° C).
INCOMPATIBILITY (MATERIAL TO AVOID): Strong acids and alkalines will neutralize active ingredient.
HAZARDOUS DECOMPOSITION BY-PRODUCTS: None
HAZARDOUS POLYMERIZATION: Will not occur

Figure 3-2. Material safety data sheet (MSDS).

be kept away from to prevent a dangerous reaction. This information helps in determining where and how to store the chemical.

6. **Health hazard data.** This section is one of the most important areas for health care workers and includes the following information:
   - Route of entry, which indicates how the chemical can enter the body, including skin contact, eye contact, inhalation, and ingestion
   - Signs and symptoms of overexposure (e.g., burning eyes, nausea, dizziness, difficulty in breathing)
   - Medical conditions that are aggravated by exposure to the chemical (e.g., asthma, dermatitis)
   - Acute and chronic health hazards that could result from overexposure (e.g., skin irritation, eye damage, lung damage)

This section also indicates whether the hazardous chemical has been identified as a potential carcinogen by the

MATERIAL SAFETY DATA SHEET   PAGE 2

SECTION 6   HEALTH HAZARD DATA

ROUTE OF ENTRY: SKIN: yes   EYES: yes   INHALATION: yes   INGESTION: yes

SIGNS AND SYMPTOMS OF OVEREXPOSURE:

SKIN: Moderate irritation. May aggravate existing dermatitis.

EYES: Serious eye irritant. May cause irreversible damage, which could permanently impair vision.

INHALATION: Vapors may be severely irritating and cause stinging sensations in the eyes, nose, throat, and lungs. May aggravate pre-existing asthma.

INGESTION: May cause irritation or chemical burns of the mouth, throat, esophagus, and stomach. May cause vomiting, diarrhea, epigastric distress, headache, dizziness, faintness, mental confusion, and general systemic illness.

CARCINOGENICITY DATA: NTP: No   AIRC: No   OSHA: No

SECTION 7   EMERGENCY FIRST AID PROCEDURES

SKIN: Wash skin with soap and water for 15 minutes. If skin redness or irritation persists, seek medical attention. Remove contaminated clothing and wash before reuse.

EYES: Immediately flush with water for 15 minutes. Seek medical attention.

INHALATION: Remove to fresh air. If irritation persists, seek medical attention.

INGESTION: Do not induce vomiting. Seek medical attention immediately. Call a physician or Poison Control Center.

SECTION 8   PRECAUTIONS FOR SAFE HANDLING AND USE

SPILL PROCEDURES: Ventilate area, wear protective gloves and eye gear. Wipe with sponge, mop, or towel. Flush with large quantities of water. Collect liquid and discard it.

WASTE DISPOSAL METHOD: Container must be triple rinsed and disposed of in accordance with federal, state, and/or local regulations. Used solution should be flushed thoroughly with water into sewage disposal system in accordance with federal, state, and/or local regulations.

PRECAUTIONS IN HANDLING AND STORAGE: Store in a cool, dry place (59-86° F) away from direct sunlight or sources of intense heat. Keep container tightly closed when not in use.

SECTION 9   CONTROL MEASURES

VENTILATION: Ensure adequate ventilation to maintain recommended exposed limit.

RESPIRATORY PROTECTION: None normally required for routine use.

SKIN PROTECTION: Wear chemical-resistant protective gloves. Butyl rubber, nitrile rubber, polyethylene, or double-gloved latex.

EYE PROTECTION: Safety goggles or safety glasses

WORK/HYGIENE PRACTICES: Prompt rinsing of hands after contact. Handle in accordance with good personal hygiene and safety practices. These practices include avoiding unnecessary exposure.

Figure 3-2, cont'd. Material safety data sheet (MSDS).

National Toxicology Program (NTP), the International Agency for Research on Cancer (IARC), and OSHA.

7. **Emergency first-aid procedures.** This section identifies the first-aid measures to take if exposed to the chemical (e.g., in case of eye contact, immediately flush eyes with water for 15 minutes).

8. **Precautions for safe handling and use.** This section tells what to do for a spill or leak, the method of disposal of the chemical, and how to handle and store the chemical.

9. **Control measures.** This section lists engineering controls, work practice controls, and personal protective equipment that should be used to protect oneself from the hazardous chemical. Examples of these measures include using chemical-resistant gloves and eye protection and working in a well-ventilated area.

Employee Information and Training

The HCS requires that employees be provided with information and training regarding hazardous chemicals in the workplace. The training session must be offered at the time of an employee's initial assignment to a work area where hazardous chemicals are present, and whenever a new chemical hazard is introduced into the work area. The train-

Putting It All Into Practice

My Name is Kara VanDyke, and I work for two physicians in a family practice medical office. As a medical assistant, one of the situations you deal with on an almost daily basis is drug representatives who come to the office to promote their products. Their job is anything but easy. The waiting and the frequent rejections would make most people think twice before applying for the job.

One winter day, I am sure I made one drug representative really think twice about his career choice. As the representative stopped at our office, he, being a polite young man, let a patient enter the building first with wet, snow-covered feet. Trying to make a good impression with a new suit and dress shoes, he soon found himself doing a "Spanish fandango" while trying to maintain his balance and eventually crashed to the floor.

I thought I would help by mopping up the snow-tracked floor. What I did not know was the mop had wax on it. Needless to say, when he returned with the requested drug samples, we were not able to keep him from falling a second time! ■

ing program must be an ongoing activity, and each training session must be documented. The HCS requires that the following information be relayed to employees who work with hazardous chemicals:

1. Requirements making up the HCS.
2. Physical and health hazards associated with exposure to chemicals in the workplace.
3. Measures employees can take to protect themselves from injury or illness from hazardous chemicals.
4. Emergency procedures to carry out in the event of exposure to a hazardous chemical or a chemical spill.
5. The meaning of the information on container labels and how to use that information.
6. The meaning of the information on the MSDS and how to use that information.
7. The location of the following: hazard communication program plan, list of hazardous chemicals in the workplace, and MSDS for each chemical in the workplace.

SANITIZATION

Sanitization involves a series of steps designed to remove organic material from an article and to reduce to a safe level the number of microorganisms on the article (Procedure 3-1). Organic material on an article may result in incomplete sterilization or disinfection. This is because the organic material acts as a physical barrier preventing the physical or chemical agent from reaching the surface of the article to kill microorganisms.

Sanitizing Instruments

Items most frequently sanitized in the medical office are medical and surgical instruments. This section focuses on the theory and procedure for sanitizing instruments. The

general steps in the sanitization procedure of instruments are as follows:

1. *Rinse* the instruments to prevent organic material from drying on the instruments.
2. *Decontaminate* the instruments with a chemical disinfectant to remove pathogenic microorganisms, making the instrument safe to handle.
3. *Clean* the instruments to remove all organic matter.
4. *Thoroughly rinse* the instruments to remove all detergent residue.
5. *Dry* the instruments to prevent stains on the instruments.
6. *Check the instruments* for defects and working condition.
7. *Lubricate* hinged instruments to make the instruments function well and last longer.

Cleaning Instruments

Two methods can be used to perform the cleaning step (step 3 in the preceding list) of the sanitization procedure: the manual method and the ultrasound method.

Manual Method

The manual method is used most often in the medical office. It involves the manual cleaning of instruments using a cleaning solution and a brush. Manual cleaning is recommended for delicate instruments because vibrations that occur with the ultrasound method may damage these instruments.

Ultrasound Method

The ultrasound method uses a machine known as an *ultrasonic cleaner* (Figure 3-3). The ultrasound method offers a safety advantage in that instruments do not have to be handled during the cleaning process. This decreases the incidence of an accidental puncture or cut from a sharp instrument. An ultrasonic cleaner works by converting sound waves into mechanical energy, which creates small bubbles all over the instruments. When the bubbles burst, vibrations occur that loosen and remove debris from the instru-

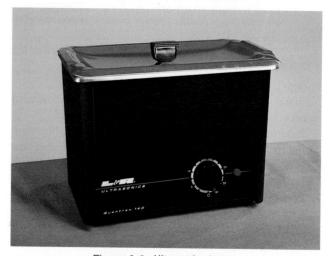

Figure 3-3. Ultrasonic cleaner.

ments. Ultrasonic cleaners are especially good at removing debris from hard-to-reach areas, such as box locks of hemostats and screw locks of scissors.

Before the instruments are placed in the ultrasonic cleaner, they should be separated according to the type of metal (e.g., stainless-steel, aluminum, brass). Instruments made of dissimilar metals should not be cleaned together in the ultrasonic cleaner. When different metals are in close contact, the ions from one metal can flow to another. This may result in a permanent blue-black stain on an instrument, which can be removed only by having the instrument refinished.

Guidelines for Sanitizing Instruments

The following guidelines should be followed when sanitizing surgical instruments:

1. **Wear gloves during the sanitization process.** While following the OSHA Bloodborne Pathogens Standard, the medical assistant should wear disposable gloves during the entire sanitization procedure. This protects the medical assistant from bloodborne pathogens and other potentially infectious materials. The medical assistant should be especially careful when working with hazardous chemicals and when handling sharp instruments. Heavy-duty utility gloves should be worn over the disposable gloves to provide protection from the irritating effects of chemical agents and accidental punctures or cuts from sharp instruments.

2. **Handle instruments carefully.** Instruments are expensive and delicate, yet durable. They can last for many years if handled and maintained properly. Dropping an instrument on the floor or throwing an instrument into a basin may damage it. Instruments should never be piled in a heap because they become entangled and may be damaged when separated. Keep sharp instruments separate from other instruments to prevent damaging or dulling the cutting edge. Also, keep delicate instruments separate to protect them from damage.

3. **Follow instructions on labels of chemical agents.** Before using a chemical agent such as a chemical disinfectant, an instrument cleaner, or an autoclave cleaner, review the product's MSDS, and carefully read the label on the container. Check the label to determine the use, mixing, and storage of the chemical agent. Read and observe precautions listed on the label regarding personal safety, such as the use of gloves and eye protection. Also, check the expiration date on the label of the chemical agent. Chemicals have a tendency to lose their potency over time and should not be used past the expiration date.

4. **Use a proper cleaning agent.** A low-sudsing detergent with a neutral pH should be used to clean the instruments. Commercially available instrument cleaners meet these criteria (Figure 3-4). These cleaners usually come in a concentrated liquid or powder form and must be diluted with water before use. Never substitute any other type of detergent, such as dishwasher detergent or

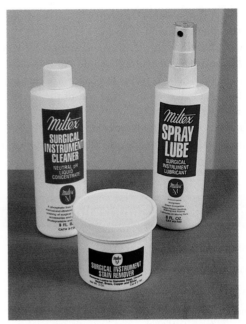

Figure 3-4. Commercially available surgical instrument cleaners. *Left*, Instrument cleaner; *center*, stain remover; *right*, spray lubricant.

laundry detergent; these detergents may not be low-sudsing or may not have the proper pH for sanitizing instruments. If a detergent with an alkaline pH is used and is not completely rinsed off, it could leave a residue on the instrument. This could result in an orange-brown stain on the instrument that resembles rust. Using an acid detergent also can cause staining and permanent corrosion.

5. **Use proper cleaning devices.** Proper cleaning devices should be used for the manual cleaning of surgical instruments. A stiff nylon brush should be used to clean the surface of the instrument. A stainless-steel wire brush can be used to clean grooves, crevices, or serrations. A stain on an instrument often can be removed by using a commercial instrument stain remover (see Figure 3-4). Never use steel wool or other abrasives to remove stains because damage to the instrument could occur.

6. **Carefully inspect each instrument for defects and proper working condition.** After cleaning, rinsing, and drying the instrument, it is important to check it for defects and proper working condition as follows:
   - The blades of an instrument should be straight and not bent.
   - The tips of an instrument should approximate tightly and evenly when the instrument is closed.
   - An instrument with a box lock (e.g., hemostatic forceps, needle holders) should move freely but must not be too loose. The pin that holds the box lock together should be flush against the instrument.
   - An instrument with a spring handle (e.g., thumb and tissue forceps) should have sufficient tension to grasp objects tightly.

- The cutting edge of a sharp instrument should be smooth and devoid of nicks.
- Scissors should cut cleanly and smoothly. To test for this, the medical assistant should cut into a thin piece of gauze. The scissors are in proper working condition if they cut all the way to the end of the blade without catching on the gauze.
7. **Lubricate hinged instruments.** Lubricate box locks, screw locks, scissor blades, and any other moving part of

each instrument. The lubricant makes the instrument function better and last longer. Use a lubricant that can be penetrated by steam, such as a commercial spray lubricant or a lubricant bath (see Figure 3-4). Lubricate after performing the final rinse (and drying of the instrument); otherwise, the lubricant would be rinsed off the instrument. Never use industrial oils or silicon sprays. These substances are not steam penetrable and can build up on the instrument, affecting its working condition.

 see DVD

PROCEDURE 3-1   Sanitization of Instruments

Outcome Sanitize instruments.

Equipment/Supplies

- Sink
- Disposable gloves
- Heavy-duty utility gloves
- Contaminated instruments
- EPA-approved chemical disinfectant and MSDS
- Disinfectant container
- Cleaning solution and MSDS

- Basin
- Stiff nylon brush
- Stainless-steel wire brush
- Paper towels
- Cloth towel
- Instrument lubricant

1. **Procedural Step.** Review the MSDS for the hazardous chemicals you will be using in the sanitization process.
   Principle. The MSDS provides information regarding the chemical, its hazards, and measures to take to prevent injury and illness when handling the disinfectant.
2. **Procedural Step.** Apply disposable gloves. Transport the contaminated instruments to the cleaning area as soon as possible after use. The instruments should be carried in a covered basin from the examining room to the cleaning area.
   Principle. Disposable gloves act as a barrier to protect the medical assistant from infectious materials. Transporting contaminated instruments in a covered basin promotes infection control.
3. **Procedural Step.** Apply heavy-duty utility gloves over the disposable gloves.
   Principle. Utility gloves help protect the hands from the irritating effects of chemical solutions.
4. **Procedural Step.** Separate sharp instruments and delicate instruments from other instruments.
   Principle. Separating sharp instruments from others prevents damage to or dulling of the cutting edge of these instruments. Delicate instruments should be separated to protect them from damage.
5. **Procedural Step.** Immediately rinse the instruments thoroughly under warm, not hot, running water (approximately 110° F [44° C]) to remove organic material, such as blood, body fluids, tissue, and other debris.
   Principle. Rinsing the instruments as soon as possible prevents organic material from drying on the instru-

ments, making it difficult to remove later. Hot water may cause coagulation of organic material, making it more difficult to remove.

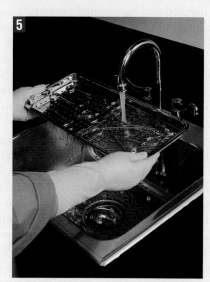

Rinse instruments under warm water to remove organic matter.

6. **Procedural Step.** Decontaminate the instruments by disinfecting them in an EPA-approved chemical disinfectant as follows:
   a. Select the proper chemical disinfectant; check the expiration date on the container label.

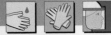

PROCEDURE 3-1   Sanitization of Instruments—cont'd

b. Observe all personal safety precautions listed on the label of the disinfectant (e.g., wearing safety goggles).

c. Follow the manufacturer's directions on the label for proper mixing and use of the disinfectant.

d. Label the plastic or stainless steel disinfecting container with the name of the disinfectant and the date when the disinfectant is no longer effective and must be discarded (reuse life).

e. Pour the disinfectant into the labeled container and immerse the articles into the disinfectant. Ensure the articles are completely submerged in the disinfectant.

f. Cover the container that holds the chemical disinfectant.

g. Disinfect the articles for 10 minutes.

Principle. Decontaminating the instruments removes pathogenic microorganisms from them, making them safe to handle. A disinfectant past its expiration date loses its potency and should not be used. An EPA-approved disinfectant has been determined by the U.S. Environmental Protection Agency to be effective when used as directed, without causing an unreasonable risk to the public or the environment. The container must be kept covered to prevent the escape of toxic fumes and to prevent evaporation of the disinfectant, which could change its potency.

7. **Procedural Step.** Clean the instruments. The instruments can be cleaned using the manual method or the ultrasound method as follows:

Manual Method for Cleaning Instruments

a. Obtain the instrument cleaning solution; check its expiration date.

b. Observe all personal safety precautions listed on the label of the cleaning agent.

c. Follow the directions on the manufacturer's label for proper mixing and use of the cleaning agent. The detergent may need to be diluted with water.

d. Remove the articles from the chemical disinfectant and place them in the basin containing the cleaning solution.

e. Use a stiff nylon brush to clean the surface of each instrument. Scrub all parts of the instrument thoroughly. Brush delicate instruments carefully to prevent damaging them.

f. Use a stainless-steel wire brush to clean grooves, crevices, or serrations where contaminants such as blood and tissue may collect.

g. If there is a stain on the instrument, attempt to remove it using a damp cloth or sponge to which a commercial stain remover has been applied.

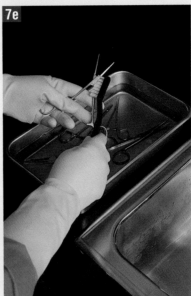

Clean the surface of the instrument with a stiff nylon brush.

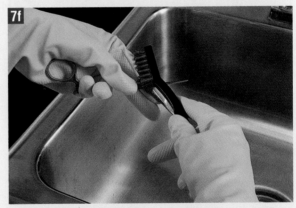

Clean grooves, crevices, or serrations with a wire brush.

h. Scrub each instrument until it is visibly clean and free from organic material and stains.

Principle. A cleaning agent past its expiration date loses its potency and should not be used. Taking appropriate precautions with cleaning agents prevents harm to the medical assistant from hazardous chemicals. All organic material must be removed from the instruments to ensure complete sterilization in the autoclave.

Ultrasound Method for Cleaning Instruments

a. Using a cleaning agent recommended by the manufacturer, prepare the cleaning solution in the ultrasonic cleaner. Observe all personal safety precautions listed on the label.

Continued

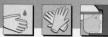

PROCEDURE 3-1   Sanitization of Instruments—cont'd

b. Remove the articles from the chemical disinfectant, and separate instruments made of dissimilar metals, such as stainless steel, aluminum, and bronze.

c. Place the instruments in the ultrasonic cleaner with hinged instruments in an open position.

d. Ensure that sharp instruments do not touch other instruments.

e. Ensure that all instruments are fully submerged in the cleaning solution.

f. Place the lid on the ultrasonic cleaner.

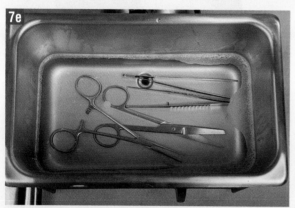

Completely submerge instruments in the cleaning solution.

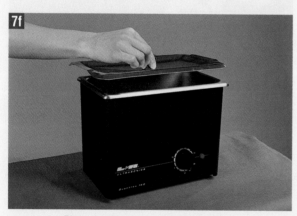

Place the lid on the ultrasonic cleaner.

g. Turn on the ultrasonic cleaner, and clean the instruments for the length of time recommended by the manufacturer.

h. After completion of the cleaning cycle, remove the instruments from the machine.

Principle. Taking appropriate precautions with chemical agents prevents harm to the medical assistant from hazardous chemicals. Mixing dissimilar metals together could result in permanent stains on the instruments. Instruments must be completely submerged with hinged instruments in an open position so the solution can reach all parts of the instrument.

8. Procedural Step. Rinse each instrument thoroughly with warm, not hot, water (110° F [44° C]) for at least 20 to 30 seconds to remove all traces of the detergent. Open and close hinged instruments while rinsing to ensure the solution is completely rinsed out of every part of the instrument.

Principle. Detergent residue left on the instrument could cause stains, which could build up and interfere with proper functioning of the instrument. Using warm water helps to remove the cleaning solution and facilitates the drying process.

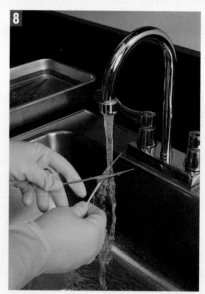

Rinse thoroughly with warm water.

9. Procedural Step. Dry each instrument with a paper towel, and place the instrument on a cloth towel for additional air drying.

Principle. If the instrument is not completely dry, stains may occur on the instrument.

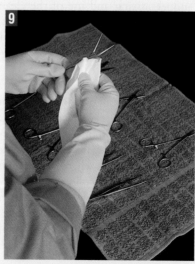

Dry the instrument with a paper towel.

PROCEDURE 3-1

PROCEDURE 3-1   Sanitization of Instruments—cont'd

10. **Procedural Step.** Check each instrument for defects and proper working condition. Scissors should cut all the way to the end of a thin piece of gauze without catching. If defects are noted, or the instrument is not working properly, it must be discarded or sent to the manufacturer for repair.

Principle. Instruments that have defects or are not in proper working condition are unsafe to use on a patient during a medical or surgical procedure.

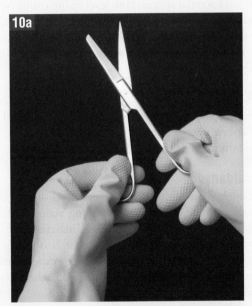

Check the instrument for defects and proper working order.

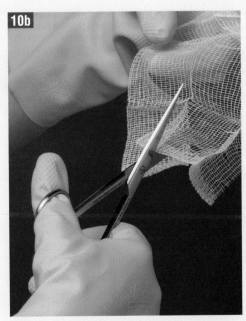

Scissors should cut through gauze without catching.

11. **Procedural Step.** Lubricate hinged instruments using a steam-penetrable lubricant as follows:
   a. Apply the lubricant to a hinged instrument in its open position.
   b. Open and close the instrument after applying the lubricant so it reaches all parts of the hinged area.
   c. Place the instrument back on the towel and allow it to drain. Rinsing or wiping is unnecessary.

Principle. Lubricating an instrument makes it function better and last longer.

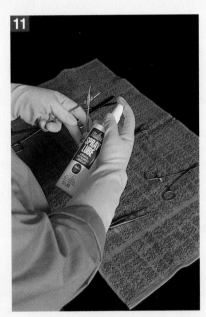

Lubricate hinged instruments.

12. **Procedural Step.** Dispose of the cleaning solution according to the manufacturer's instructions. Remove both sets of gloves, and sanitize your hands.

13. **Procedural Step.** Wrap the instruments and sterilize them in the autoclave according to the medical office policy.

PROCEDURE 3-1

DISINFECTION

Disinfection is the process of destroying pathogenic microorganisms, but it does not kill bacterial spores. Disinfection is accomplished in the medical office through the use of liquid chemical agents that are applied to inanimate objects (Procedure 3-2). Chemical disinfection has been discussed with respect to its role in the sanitization process to decontaminate surgical instruments and make them safe to handle. This section discusses the use of chemical disinfection to disinfect semicritical and noncritical items so they can be used for patient care.

Levels of Disinfection

Based on killing action, disinfection can be classified according to three levels.

High-Level Disinfection

High-level disinfection is a process that destroys all microorganisms with the exception of bacterial spores. High-level disinfection is used to disinfect semicritical items. A **semicritical item** is an item that comes in contact with nonintact skin or intact mucous membranes, such as a flexible fiberoptic sigmoidoscope. A frequently used high-level disinfectant is 2% glutaraldehyde (e.g., Cidex, MetriCide). A newer high-level disinfectant that is growing in popularity is Cidex OPA (ortho-phthalaldehyde). Cidex OPA does not contain glutaraldehyde, which means it is less toxic and is safer to handle.

Intermediate-Level Disinfection

Intermediate-level disinfection is a process that inactivates tubercle bacilli (the causative agents of tuberculosis), all vegetative bacteria, most viruses, and most fungi, but it does not kill bacterial spores. Intermediate-level disinfection is used to disinfect noncritical items. **Noncritical items** are items that come in contact with intact skin but not with mucous membranes, including stethoscopes, blood pressure cuffs, tuning forks, percussion hammers, and crutches. A common intermediate-level disinfectant is isopropyl alcohol, which is frequently used in the form of alcohol wipes.

Low-Level Disinfection

Low-level disinfection is a process that kills most bacteria, some viruses, and some fungi, but it cannot be relied on to kill resistant microorganisms, such as tubercle bacilli, and it cannot kill bacterial spores. Low-level disinfectants typically are used to disinfect surfaces such as examining tables, laboratory countertops, and walls. Low-level disinfectants used in the medical office include sodium hypochlorite (household bleach) and phenolics.

Types of Disinfectants

The disinfectants used most frequently in the medical office are described next. Table 3-1 lists these disinfectants, along with common names and uses for each.

Glutaraldehyde

Glutaraldehyde is often used as a high-level disinfectant in the medical office. It has a rapid killing action and is not inactivated by the presence of organic material. Because it does not corrode lenses, metal, or rubber, it is the agent of choice for semicritical items that cannot be exposed to heat, such as flexible fiberoptic sigmoidoscopes. Brand names for glutaraldehyde include Cidex and MetriCide.

Glutaraldehyde is highly toxic and can cause harm to the body if not handled properly. When working with glutaraldehyde, the medical assistant must work in an area that is well ventilated. Utility gloves and safety goggles must be

Table 3-1 Disinfectants Used in the Medical Office		
Disinfectant	**Common Names**	**Use in the Medical Office**
Glutaraldehyde	Cidex MetriCide ProCide Omnicide Wavicide	Disinfection of flexible fiberoptic sigmoidoscopes.
Alcohol	Isopropyl alcohol	Disinfection of stethoscopes, blood pressure cuffs, tuning forks, and percussion hammers; isopropyl alcohol wipes are used to disinfect rubber stoppers of multiple-dose medication vials.
Chlorine and chlorine compounds	Sodium hypochlorite (household bleach)	Recommended by OSHA for decontamination of blood spills.
Phenolics	Carbolic acid Hydroxybenzene Phenic acid Phenyl hydroxide Phenylic acid	Disinfection of walls, furniture, floors, and laboratory work surfaces.
Quaternary ammonium compounds	Benzalkonium chloride	Disinfection of walls, furniture, floors, and laboratory work surfaces.

worn to protect oneself from the irritating effects of this chemical (Figure 3-5). If the hands or any other part of the body comes in contact with glutaraldehyde, the area should be rinsed thoroughly under running water.

Alcohol

Alcohol is frequently used as a disinfectant in the medical office. The two most common types are *ethyl alcohol* and *isopropyl alcohol.* The disinfecting action of alcohol is increased by the presence of water; a 70% solution of alcohol is recommended. Stronger concentrations (95% to 100%) are not as effective. A disadvantage of alcohol is that it tends to dissolve the cement from around the lenses of instruments.

Ethyl alcohol and isopropyl alcohol provide intermediate- to low-level disinfection and can be used to disinfect stethoscopes, blood pressure cuffs, and percussion hammers. Isopropyl alcohol wipes are used to disinfect small surfaces such as the diaphragm of a stethoscope and rubber stoppers on multiple-dose medication vials.

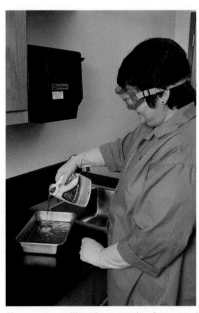

Figure 3-5. Kara wears utility gloves and safety goggles to protect herself from the irritating effects of glutaraldehyde.

Chlorine and Chlorine Compounds

Chlorine and chlorine compounds are some of the oldest and most used disinfectants. Their most important use is in the chlorination of water. In the medical office, chlorine is used in the form of hypochlorites, such as liquid sodium hypochlorite (household bleach). A 10% solution of household bleach in water inactivates tuberculosis bacteria, hepatitis B and C viruses, human immunodeficiency virus, and many bacteria in 10 minutes at room temperature. Because of this, household bleach is recommended by OSHA for the decontamination of blood spills. A disadvantage of this disinfectant is that it can irritate skin and mucous membranes and is highly corrosive to metal.

Phenolics

Phenolics are used mainly to disinfect walls, furniture, floors, and laboratory work surfaces. This disinfectant is a corrosive poison and tends to be irritating to the eyes and skin. For this reason, eye and skin protective devices should be worn when working with phenolics in the pure form. Many derivatives of phenolics are commonly used and are usually nonirritating, including Lysol and hexachlorophene.

Quaternary Ammonium Compounds

The quaternary ammonium compounds are sometimes used in the medical office for the disinfection of noncritical surfaces, such as floors, furniture, and walls.

Guidelines for Disinfection

Certain guidelines should be followed when disinfecting articles with a chemical agent.

Sanitize Articles Before Disinfecting Them

The article to be disinfected must first be thoroughly sanitized. As previously described, sanitization includes the following steps: initial rinse, decontamination with a chemical disinfectant, cleaning, rinsing, drying, and checking for working order. It is important to remove all organic matter from the article before it is disinfected. If organic

---

What Would You Do? What Would You *Not* Do?

Case Study 2
Alecia Scout brings in her 2-year-old son, Benjamin, for a preschool physical examination. Benjamin is very unhappy and is crying loudly. Mrs. Scout says that Benjamin is upset because she wouldn't let him play with the toys in the waiting room. She is afraid that he will catch a disease from a sick child who has played with the toys. Mrs. Scout is visibly annoyed and says that medical offices should not keep toys in the waiting room because they might spread disease and cause problems for parents who do not want their children to play with the toys. ■

Memories *from* Externship

Kara VanDyke: During my externship experience, I was placed in a pediatrician's office. I wanted to go to a pediatric site because I love being around children. One day I was in the examining room with my patient, a 4-year-old boy who was there with his mother. It was standard procedure at this office to take every patient's temperature. I started getting out our electronic thermometer to take his temperature when I noticed he looked a little frightened. He was looking at the thermometer funny, and he said, "Can you do it in my ear?" I said I was sorry but we didn't have that kind of thermometer. I told him I could do it under his arm or under his tongue. His mom looked at him, and he said, "But I want it in my ear." He finally agreed to let me do it under his arm. When I was finished taking his temperature, he smiled and said, "You're the nicest doctor!" ■

material is still present on the article after it is sanitized, this prevents the chemical disinfectant from reaching the surface of the article to kill microorganisms. In addition, with some disinfectants, organic material can absorb the chemical disinfectant and inactivate it. The article should be thoroughly rinsed of the detergent after cleaning because detergent residue may interfere with the disinfecting process. The article must be completely dry before placing it in the disinfectant, because water dilutes the chemical and decreases its effectiveness.

Observe Safety Precautions

The medical assistant should carefully read the MSDS and the container label before using a chemical disinfectant. All safety precautions should be followed when using the chemical to protect against illness or injury from a hazardous chemical.

Properly Prepare and Use the Disinfectant

Products vary substantially among manufacturers; it is important that the manufacturer's directions on preparation, dilution, and use of the chemical disinfectant be followed carefully. The disinfectant should be prepared exactly as indicated on the container label. Some disinfectants are used at their full strength, whereas others require dilution. Some disinfectants (e.g., glutaraldehyde) require the addition of an activator before they can be used. Properly preparing the disinfectant ensures the destruction of microorganisms. A disinfectant must be applied for a certain length of time to kill microorganisms. The medical assistant must be sure to disinfect for the length of time indicated on the container label.

Properly Store the Disinfectant

Chemical disinfectants should be closed tightly and stored properly under the storage conditions recommended by the manufacturer. Chemical disinfectants lose their potency over time; the medical assistant should strictly adhere to the manufacturer's recommendations for the disinfectant's shelf life, use life, and reuse life. Each of these terms is defined next as it relates to chemical disinfectants.

Shelf life Shelf life is the length of time a chemical disinfectant may be stored before use and still retain its effectiveness. The shelf life is indicated by an expiration date on the container. The expiration date should always be checked before using the chemical. Outdated disinfectants should not be used.

Use life Some disinfectants must be combined with another chemical, or activated, before they are used. Use life is the period of time a disinfecting solution is effective after it has been activated. Cidex Plus (Johnson & Johnson) is effective for 28 days after activation. At the end of this time, any chemical remaining in the container must be discarded. When a chemical disinfectant is activated, the date on which it will expire should be written on the label of the container.

Reuse life Reuse life is the period of time that a disinfecting solution being used and reused remains active. For example, Cidex Plus can be reused for 28 days to disinfect articles after it has been poured into a disinfecting container. At the end of this time, the disinfectant must be discarded. The name of the disinfectant and the date when the disinfectant must be discarded should be written on an adhesive label and affixed to the container into which the disinfectant will be poured.

PROCEDURE 3-2   Chemical Disinfection of Articles

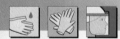

Outcome Chemically disinfect articles.

Equipment/Supplies

- Sink
- Disposable gloves
- Heavy-duty utility gloves
- Contaminated articles

- EPA-approved chemical disinfectant and MSDS
- Disinfectant container
- Paper towels

1. **Procedural Step.** Sanitize the articles by performing procedural steps 1 through 10 in Procedure 3-1.
2. **Procedural Step.** Review the MSDS for the EPA-approved chemical disinfectant that you will be using.
   Principle. The MSDS provides information regarding the chemical disinfectant, its hazards, and measures to take to prevent injury and illness when handling the disinfectant.
3. **Procedural Step.** Check the expiration date of the chemical disinfectant.
   Principle. A disinfectant past its expiration date loses its potency and should not be used.

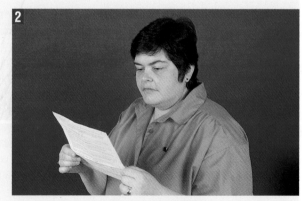

Review the MSDS.

PROCEDURE 3-2   Chemical Disinfection of Articles—cont'd

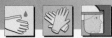

4. Procedural Step. Observe all personal safety precautions listed on the label. Follow the directions on the manufacturer's label for proper mixing, use, and reuse of the disinfectant. The disinfectant may need to be diluted with distilled water. Label the disinfecting container with the name of the disinfectant and its reuse life expiration date.

Principle. Taking appropriate precautions with chemical agents prevents harm to the medical assistant from hazardous chemicals. When a disinfectant that is being used and reused reaches its expiration date, it is no longer effective and must be discarded.

5. Procedural Step. Immerse the articles in the chemical disinfectant. Ensure that the articles are completely submerged in the disinfectant.

Principle. The articles must be completely submerged to allow the disinfectant to reach all parts of the instrument.

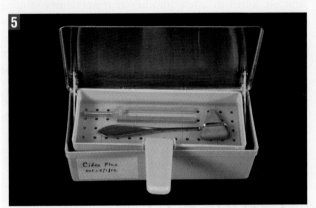

Completely immerse the articles in the disinfectant.

6. Procedural Step. Cover the container that holds the chemical disinfectant.

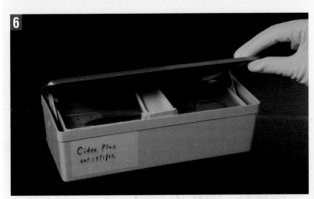

Cover the disinfectant container.

Principle. The container must be kept covered to prevent the escape of toxic fumes and to prevent evaporation of the disinfectant, which could change its potency.

7. Procedural Step. Disinfect the articles for the proper length of time as indicated on the label of the container.

Principle. Proper time requirements must be followed to ensure complete destruction of all microorganisms.

8. Procedural Step. Remove the articles from the disinfectant, and rinse them thoroughly. Dry the articles with paper towels. Dispose of the disinfectant according to the manufacturer's instructions.

Principle. All traces of the chemical disinfectant must be removed to prevent irritation to the patient's tissues. The disinfectant must be disposed of properly to prevent harm to the environment.

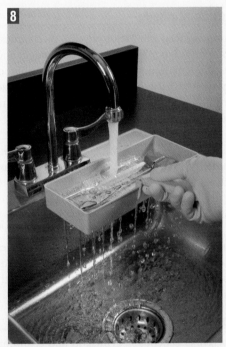

Rinse articles thoroughly to remove the disinfectant.

9. Procedural Step. Remove both sets of gloves, and sanitize your hands.

10. Procedural Step. Store the articles according to the medical office policy.

PROCEDURE 3-2

STERILIZATION

Sterilization is the process of destroying all forms of microbial life, including bacterial spores. An item that is sterile is free of all living microorganisms and spores. Sterilization must be used to process all critical items. A **critical item** is an item that comes in contact with sterile tissue or the vascular system.

As previously described, a semicritical item (one that comes in contact with nonintact skin or with intact mucous membranes) can be chemically disinfected using a high-level disinfectant. Most offices prefer instead to sterilize semicritical items in the autoclave (e.g., vaginal specula, nasal specula). The autoclave provides a convenient, efficient, safe, and inexpensive method for destroying microorganisms. Chemical disinfectants not only are more expensive to use, but also are more hazardous and create problems regarding their proper disposal. The exception is any semicritical item that is heat sensitive. Flexible fiberoptic sigmoidoscopes would be damaged by the heat of an autoclave and must be chemically disinfected.

Sterilization Methods

Sterilization involves the use of physical or chemical methods. Each method of sterilization has advantages and disadvantages. The method used to achieve sterility depends primarily on the nature of the item to be sterilized. The most common physical and chemical sterilization methods include the following:

Physical Methods	Chemical Methods
Steam under pressure (autoclave)	Ethylene oxide gas
Hot air (dry heat oven)	Cold sterilization (chemical agents)
Radiation	

The most common method for sterilizing articles in the medical office is steam under pressure using an autoclave. The autoclave is discussed in detail in this chapter; the other methods of sterilization are briefly described.

Autoclave

The autoclave is dependable, efficient, and economical and can be used to sterilize items that are not harmed by moisture or high temperature. Refer to the box *Items Sterilized in the Autoclave* for a list of heat-resistant items that can be sterilized in the autoclave.

An **autoclave** consists of an outer jacket surrounding an inner sterilizing chamber. Under pressure, distilled water is converted to steam, which fills the inner sterilizing chamber. The pressure plays no direct part in killing microorganisms; rather, it functions to attain a higher temperature than could be reached by the steam from boiling water (212° F [100° C]). The cooler, drier air already in the chamber is forced out through the air exhaust valve.

It is important that all the air in the chamber be replaced by steam. When air is present, the temperature in the autoclave is reduced, and a temperature that is adequate for sterilization is not reached. When all the air has been removed, the air exhaust valve seals off the inner chamber, and the temperature in the autoclave begins to increase.

During the sterilization process, the steam penetrates the materials in the sterilizing chamber. The materials are cooler, so the steam condenses into moisture on them, giving up its heat. This heat serves to kill all microorganisms and their spores.

The autoclave is usually operated at approximately 15 pounds of pressure per square inch (psi) at a temperature of 250° F (121° C). Vegetative forms of most microorganisms are killed in a few minutes at temperatures ranging from 130° F to 150° F (54° C to 65° C), but certain bacterial spores can withstand a temperature of 240° F (115° C) for longer than 3 hours. No organism, however, can survive direct exposure to saturated steam at 250° F (121° C) for 15 minutes or longer.

The sterilization process using the autoclave is discussed in this section (with the exception of sanitization, which was already presented). The sterilization process consists of the following components:
- Monitoring program
- Sanitizing articles
- Wrapping articles
- Operating the autoclave (autoclave cycle)
- Handling and storing packs
- Maintaining the autoclave

Monitoring Program

To ensure that instruments and supplies are sterile when used, the Centers for Disease Control and Prevention (CDC) recommends that the medical office establish and maintain a monitoring program of the sterilization process. The monitoring program should consist of the following:
1. Written policies and procedures for each step of the sterilization process.
2. Sterilization indicators to ensure that minimum sterilizing conditions have been achieved.
3. Records for each cycle maintained in an autoclave log (Figure 3-6).

The information that should be recorded for each autoclave cycle includes the following:
- Date and time of the cycle
- Description of the load
- Exposure time
- Exposure temperature
- Results of the sterilization indicator
- Initials of the operator

Items Sterilized in the Autoclave

Surgical instruments	Brushes
Medical instruments	Dressings
Minor office surgery trays	Glassware
Liquids	Reusable syringes

AUTOCLAVE LOG						
Date/Time	Description of the Load	Cycle Time (min)	Temperature (°F)	Indicator* (+/–)	Initials	Comments
7/25/12 4:00 PM	Surgical instruments	20	250	—	KV	
7/26/12 3:00 PM	MOS tray setups	30	250	—	KV	

*Indicator Interpretation:
Positive (+): Spores not killed indicating sterilization conditions have not been met.
Negative (–): Spores killed indicating sterilization conditions have been met.

MAINTENANCE: (Indicate date, vendor name, service, etc.)

Figure 3-6. Example of an autoclave log.

Some autoclaves have recorders that automatically print out a portion of this information at the end of the cycle (Figure 3-7).

Sterilization Indicators

Materials that are being sterilized must be exposed to steam at a sufficient temperature and for a proper length of time. Sterilization indicators are available to determine the effectiveness of the procedure and to check against improper wrapping of articles, improper loading of the autoclave, and faulty operation of the autoclave.

An article is not considered sterile unless the steam has penetrated to its center; most sterilization indicators are placed in the center of the pack. The medical assistant should carefully read the instructions that come with the sterilization indicators. The most reliable indicators check for the attainment of the proper temperature and indicate the duration of the temperature.

If an indicator does not change properly, a problem may be present in the sterilization technique or in the working condition of the autoclave. The manufacturer's guidelines

for proper sterilization techniques should be reviewed, and the articles should be resterilized while following these guidelines. If the indicator still does not change properly, the autoclave is in need of repair and should not be used until it has been serviced.

What Would You Do? What Would You Not Do?

Case Study 3

Cassie Augusta is in the examining room and is being prepared for the removal of a sebaceous cyst. Cassie is concerned about the instruments that the physician will be using to perform the procedure. She wants to know if they are "safe." Cassie says that her friend Mackenzie got a tattoo several years ago and developed hepatitis 3 weeks later. Mackenzie thinks she got hepatitis from the instruments that were used for her tattoo procedure. Cassie wants to know if it is possible for an instrument to give someone hepatitis. She says she heard that hepatitis can cause liver cancer and wants to know if this is true. Cassie also wants to know if there is a vaccine to prevent hepatitis. ■

```
READY

BEGIN

SET  TEMP:      270 F        Temperature
SET  TIME:      015  ←────── Time
RUN #           011  ←────── Cycle number

DATE    7/25/12

HEAT UP
DEG       PSI       MIN
066       00.0      000
066       00.0      002
074       00.0      004  ──┐ Heat-up
164       00.0      006    │ phase
219       04.1      008    │
234       09.4      010    │
261       22.6      012  ──┘

STERILIZE
DEG       PSI       MIN
272       30.2      000
272       30.7      001
273       31.3      002
274       31.0      003
273       30.7      004
273       30.4      005
273       30.1      006
272       30.0      007  ──┐ Sterilization
272       30.1      008    │ phase
272       30.4      009    │
272       30.4      010    │
272       30.7      011    │
273       31.0      012    │
273       30.8      013    │
274       31.0      014    │
273       30.7      015  ──┘

VENT
COMPLETE
```

Figure 3-7. Example of a printout of an autoclave cycle.

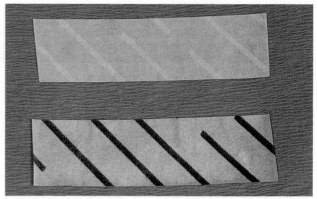

Figure 3-8. Autoclave tape. *Top,* Autoclave tape as it appears before the sterilization process. *Bottom,* Diagonal lines appear on the tape during autoclaving and indicate that the wrapped article has been autoclaved.

Sterilization Strips. Sterilization strips are commercially prepared paper or plastic strips that contain a thermolabile dye and that change color when exposed to steam under pressure for a certain length of time (Figure 3-9). Most sterilization strips are designed to change color after being exposed to a temperature of 250° F (121° C) for 15 minutes. The indicator strip should be placed in the center of the wrapped pack, with the end containing the dye placed in an area of the pack considered to be the hardest for steam to penetrate.

Biologic Indicators

Biologic indicators are the best means available for determining the effectiveness of the sterilization procedure. The CDC recommends that medical office personnel use a biologic indicator to monitor all autoclaves at least once a week.

A biologic indicator is a preparation of living bacterial spores. Biologic indicators are commercially available in the form of dry spore strips in small glassine envelopes. Biologic monitoring of an autoclave requires the use of a preparation of spores of *Geobacillus stearothermophilus,* which is a microorganism whose spores are particularly resistant to moist heat and are not harmful to humans.

Sterilization indicators should be stored in a cool, dry area. Excessive heat or moisture can damage the indicator. The most common sterilization indicators are chemical indicators and biologic indicators, which are described next.

Chemical Indicators

Chemical indicators are impregnated with a **thermolabile** dye that changes color when exposed to the sterilization process. If the chemical reaction of the indicator does not show the expected results, the item may not be sterile and must be resterilized. Chemical indicators include autoclave tape and sterilization strips.

Autoclave Tape. Autoclave tape contains a chemical that changes color if it has been exposed to steam. The tape is available in a variety of colors, can be written on, and is useful for closing and identifying the wrapped article (Figure 3-8). Autoclave tape has some limitations as an indicator. Because it is placed on the outside of the pack, it cannot ensure that steam has penetrated to the center of the pack. It also does not ensure that the item has been sterilized; it merely indicates that an article has been in the autoclave and that a high temperature has been attained.

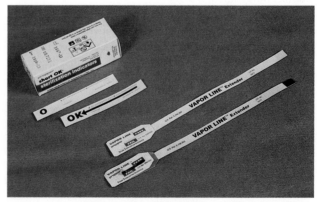

Figure 3-9. Sterilization strips. Sterilization strips contain a thermolabile dye and change color when exposed to steam under pressure for a certain length of time.

Each biologic testing unit includes two spore tests that are sterilized and one spore control that is not sterilized (Figure 3-10). The biologic indicator is placed in the center of two wrapped articles. The articles are placed in areas of the autoclave that are the least accessible to steam penetration, such as on the bottom tray of the autoclave, near the front of the autoclave, and in the back of the autoclave.

After the indicators have been exposed to sterilization conditions, they must be processed before the results can be obtained. The two methods for processing results are the in-house method and the mail-in method.

In-House Method. The in-house method involves processing and interpreting the results at the medical office. After sterilization, the processed spores are incubated for 24 to 48 hours. If sterilization conditions have been met, the color or condition of the processed spores is different from those of the control, and the spore test is interpreted as negative. If sterilization conditions have not been met, the processed spores and the unprocessed control display the same color or condition, and the spore test is interpreted as positive.

Mail-In Method. With this method, the processed bacterial spores and the (unprocessed) control are mailed to a processing laboratory. The test is performed by the laboratory, and the results are returned to the medical office.

If spores are not killed in routine spore tests, the autoclave should be checked immediately for proper use and function, and the spore test should be repeated. If the spore test remains positive, the autoclave should not be used until it is serviced.

Wrapping Articles

Articles to be sterilized in the autoclave first must be thoroughly sanitized (see Procedure 3-1). Next, the articles are prepared for autoclaving by wrapping them. The purpose of wrapping articles is to protect them from recontamination during handling and storage. Articles that are wrapped and handled correctly remain sterile after autoclaving until the package seal is broken.

The wrapping material should be made of a substance that is not affected by the sterilization process and should allow steam to penetrate while preventing contaminants, such as dust, insects, and microorganisms, from entering during handling and storage. It should not tear or puncture easily and should allow the sterilized package to be opened without contamination of the contents. A wrapper should not be used if it is torn or has a hole. Examples of wrapping materials used for autoclaving are sterilization paper, sterilization pouches, and muslin.

Sterilization Paper

Sterilization paper is a disposable and inexpensive wrapping material. It consists of square sheets of paper of different sizes (Figure 3-11). The most common sizes (in inches) are 12 × 12, 15 × 15, 18 × 18, 24 × 24, 30 × 30, and 36 × 36. Articles must be wrapped in such a way that they do not become contaminated when the pack is opened. The proper method for wrapping instruments using sterilization paper is outlined in Procedure 3-3. This method of wrapping can be used for all types of instruments and supplies.

The disadvantage of sterilization paper is that it is difficult to spread open for removal of the contents. It has a "memory" and tends to flip back easily, so it may not open flat to provide a sterile field. (*Memory* is the ability of a material to retain a specific shape or configuration.) Because sterilization paper is opaque, it is impossible to view the contents of a pack before opening it.

Sterilization Pouches

Sterilization pouches typically consist of a combination of paper and plastic; paper makes up one side of the pouch, and a plastic film makes up the other side (Figure 3-12). Sterilization pouches are available in different sizes; the most common sizes (in inches) are 3 × 9, 5 × 10, and 7 × 12.

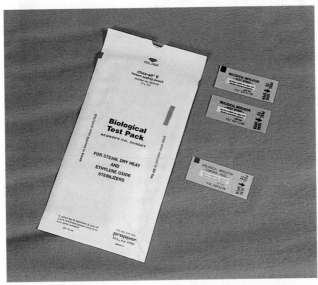

Figure 3-10. Biologic indicator. A biologic indicator includes two spore tests that are sterilized *(top right)* and one spore control that is not sterilized *(bottom right)*.

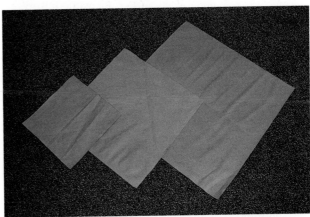

Figure 3-11. Sterilization paper wraps. Sterilization paper consists of square sheets of paper that are available in different sizes.

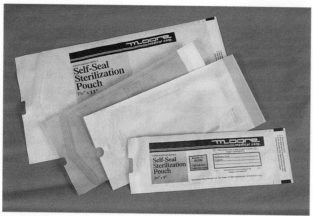

Figure 3-12. Sterilization pouches. Sterilization pouches consist of a combination of paper and plastic and are available in different sizes.

Most pouches have a peel-apart seal on one end that is used later to open the pouch for removal of the sterile item. The other end of the pouch is open and is used to insert the item into the pouch. When the article has been inserted, this end is sealed with heat or adhesive tape. The proper method for wrapping an instrument by using a pouch is outlined in Procedure 3-4.

Sterilization pouches provide good visibility of the contents on the plastic side. Most manufacturers include a sterilization indicator on the outside of the pouch. After removing a pouch from the autoclave, the medical assistant should check the indicator for proper color change. If the indicator does not change to the appropriate color (as specified by the manufacturer), the contents of the pouch must be resterilized.

Muslin

Muslin is a reusable woven fabric that is available in different sizes. Muslin is flexible and easy to handle and is considered the most economical sterilization wrap because it can be reused. Because of its durability, muslin is frequently used to wrap large packs, such as tray setups for minor office surgery. Muslin is "memory free," so it lies flat when opened. A pack wrapped in muslin may be opened on a table so that the wrapper becomes a sterile field. The procedure for wrapping an article with muslin is the same as that for sterilization paper (see Procedure 3-3).

 PROCEDURE 3-3   Wrapping Instruments Using Paper or Muslin

Outcome Wrap an instrument for autoclaving.

Equipment/Supplies

- Sanitized instrument
- Appropriate-sized wrapping material (sterilization paper or muslin)

- Sterilization indicator strip
- Autoclave tape
- Permanent marker

1. **Procedural Step.** Sanitize your hands.
2. **Procedural Step.** Assemble the equipment. Select the appropriate-sized wrapping material for the instrument being wrapped. Check the expiration date on the sterilization indicator box. If the sterilization strips are outdated, do not use them.
   Principle. Instruments are wrapped so they are protected from recontamination after they have been sterilized. Outdated strip indicators may not provide accurate test results.
3. **Procedural Step.** Place the wrapping material on a clean, flat surface. Turn the wrap in a diagonal position to your body so that it resembles a diamond shape.
4. **Procedural Step.** Place the instrument in the center of the wrapping material with the longest part of the instrument pointing toward the two side corners. If the instrument has a movable joint, place it on the wrap in a slightly open position. If necessary, a gauze square can be used to hold the instrument in an open position.

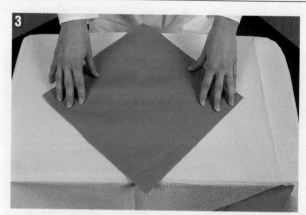

Turn the wrap in a diagonal position.

Principle. Instruments with movable joints must be in an open position to allow steam to reach all parts of the instrument. If the instrument is in a closed position, heat exposure could cause the instrument to crack at its weakest part, such as the lock area.

PROCEDURE 3-3   Wrapping Instruments Using Paper or Muslin—cont'd

5. Procedural Step. Place a sterilization indicator in the center of the pack next to the instrument.
Principle. Sterilization indicators assess the effectiveness of the sterilization process.

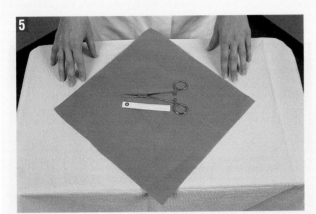

Place a sterilization indicator in the center of the pack next to the instrument.

6. Procedural Step. Fold the wrapping material up from the bottom, and double-back a small corner, creating a flap. This flap will later be used to open the sterile pack without contaminating the instrument.

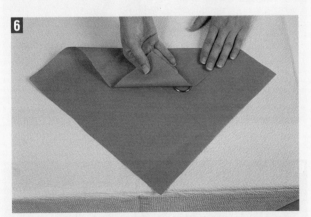

Fold the wrapping material up from the bottom, and double-back a small corner.

7. Procedural Step. Fold over one edge of the wrapping material, and double-back the corner.

8. Procedural Step. Fold over the other edge of the wrapping material, and double-back the corner.

9. Procedural Step. Fold the pack up from the bottom, pull the top flap down, and secure it with autoclave tape. Ensure that the pack is firm enough for handling but loose enough to permit proper circulation of steam.
Principle. Instruments must be wrapped properly to permit full penetration of steam and to prevent contaminating them when the wrap is opened. Using

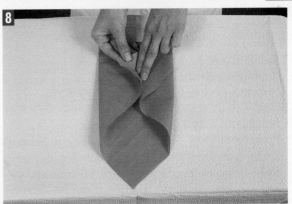

Fold over the other edge of the wrapping material, and double-back the corner.

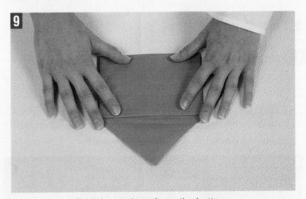

Fold the pack up from the bottom.

autoclave tape indicates that the pack has been through the autoclave cycle and prevents mix-ups with packs that have not been processed.

10. Procedural Step. Label the pack according to its contents. Mark the pack with the date of sterilization and your initials.
Principle. Dating the pack ensures that the most recently sterilized packs are stored in back of previously sterilized packs.

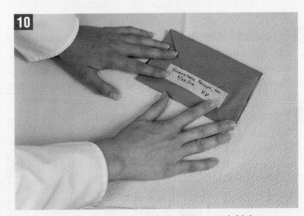

Label and date the pack. Include your initials.

PROCEDURE 3-3

PROCEDURE 3-4   Wrapping Instruments Using a Pouch

Outcome Wrap an instrument for autoclaving.

Equipment/Supplies

- Sanitized instrument
- Appropriate-sized sterilization pouch
- Permanent marker

1. **Procedural Step.** Sanitize your hands.
2. **Procedural Step.** Assemble the equipment. Select the appropriate-sized sterilization pouch for the instrument being wrapped. For hinged instruments, use a bag wide enough so the instrument can be placed in a slightly open position inside the bag.
   Principle. Instruments are wrapped so they are protected from recontamination after they have been sterilized.
3. **Procedural Step.** Place the sterilization pouch on a clean, flat surface.
4. **Procedural Step.** Label the pack according to its contents. Mark the pack with the date of sterilization and your initials.
   Principle. Dating the pack ensures that the most recently sterilized packs are stored in back of previously sterilized packs.

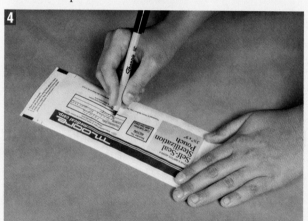

Label and date the pack. Include your initials.

5. **Procedural Step.** Insert the instrument to be sterilized into the unsealed, open end of the pouch. If the instrument has a movable joint, place it in the pouch in a slightly open position. If necessary, a gauze square can be used to hold the instrument in an open position.
6. **Procedural Step.** Seal the open end of the pouch as follows:
   Adhesive Closure. Peel off the paper strip located above the perforation to expose the adhesive. Fold along the perforation and press firmly to seal the paper to the plastic. Ensure that the seal is secure by running your fingers back and forth on both sides of the pouch over the entire sealing area.

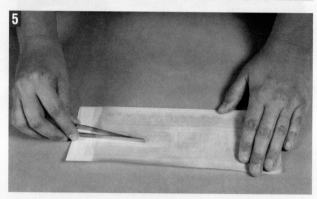

Insert the instrument into the pouch.

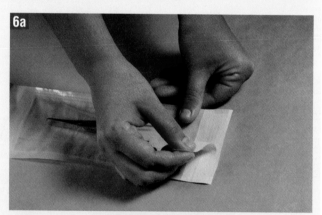

Peel off the paper strip.

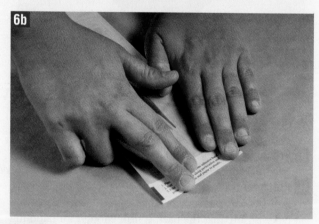

Press firmly to seal the pack.

   Heat Closure. Seal the pouch using a heat-sealing device.
7. **Procedural Step.** Sterilize the pack in the autoclave.

Operating the Autoclave

The autoclave must be operated according to the manufacturer's instructions. The medical assistant should read the operating manual carefully before running the autoclave for the first time. Thereafter, the manual should be kept in an accessible location so that it is available if needed as a reference. Procedure 3-5 outlines a general procedure for sterilizing articles in the autoclave.

The steps involved in achieving sterilization using an autoclave are known as the *autoclave cycle.* Accomplishment of each step varies based on whether the autoclave is operated manually or automatically. Figure 3-13 illustrates the autoclave cycle for manual and automatic autoclave operation.

Guidelines for Autoclave Operation

Location of the Autoclave

The autoclave must be placed on a level surface to ensure that the chamber fills correctly. The front of the autoclave should be near the front of the support surface so that water can be easily drained from the drain tube into a container when the autoclave is being flushed.

Filling the Water Reservoir

Distilled water is used to fill the water reservoir of the autoclave. Normal tap water contains minerals, such as chlorine, which have corrosive effects on the stainless-steel chamber of the autoclave. In addition, using tap water may cause a mineral buildup that can block the air exhaust valve. This causes air pockets, which prevent the temperature from

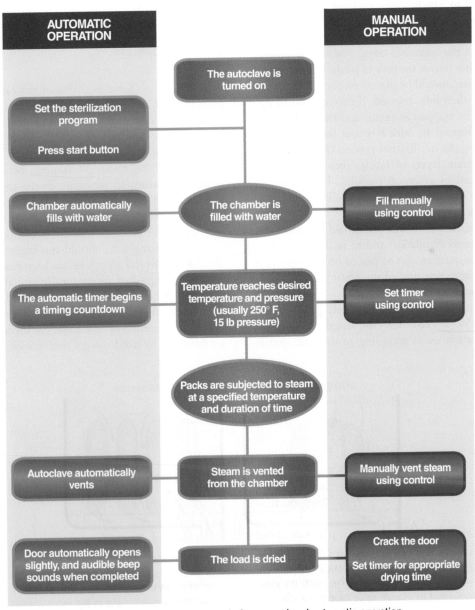

Figure 3-13. The autoclave cycle for manual and automatic operation.

increasing in the autoclave. The water reservoir is filled to the proper level as indicated in the operating manual. An autoclave malfunction may occur if the reservoir is overfilled, or if there is not enough water in the reservoir.

Loading the Autoclave

For an item to attain sterility, steam must penetrate every fiber and reach every surface of the item at a required temperature and for a specified time. To accomplish this, all packs must be positioned in the chamber to allow free circulation and penetration of steam. The following guidelines should be followed when loading the autoclave:

1. Small packs are best because steam penetrates them more easily; it takes longer for steam to reach the center of a large pack to ensure sterilization. A pack should be no larger than 12 × 12 × 20 inches.

2. To allow for proper steam penetration, the packs should be packed as loosely as possible inside the autoclave, with approximately 1 to 3 inches between small packs and 2 to 4 inches between large packs. Packs should not be allowed to touch surrounding walls, and at least 1 inch should separate the autoclave trays. Placing the articles too close together retards the flow of steam (Figure 3-14).

3. Jars and glassware should be placed on their sides in the autoclave with their lids removed. If they are placed upright, air may be trapped in them, and they would not be sterilized. Trapped air must flow out and be replaced by steam during the sterilization process (Figure 3-15).

4. Packs that contain layers of fabric, such as dressings, should be placed in a vertical position. Because steam flows from top to bottom, this method allows the steam to penetrate the layers of fabric.

5. Sterilization pouches should be positioned on their sides to maximize steam circulation and to facilitate the drying process. Pouches can also be placed on the autoclave tray with the paper side up and the plastic side down.

Timing the Load

The autoclave is operated at approximately 15 psi with a temperature of 250° F (121° C). The length of time required for sterilization varies according to the item that is

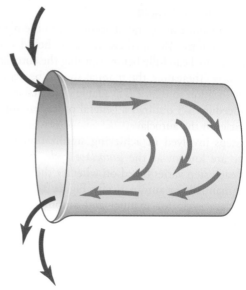

Figure 3-15. Jars and glassware should be placed on their sides in the autoclave with their lids removed. (Courtesy AMSCO/American Sterilizer Company, Erie, Pa.)

being sterilized (Table 3-2). Steam can easily reach the surfaces of hard, nonporous items such as unwrapped instruments (e.g., vaginal specula) to kill microorganisms; these items require approximately 15 minutes of sterilization time. A large minor office surgery pack requires a longer sterilization time, about 30 minutes, because more time is needed for steam to penetrate to the center of the pack. Rubber goods may be damaged, however, by exposure to excessive heat. To prevent this, the medical assistant should sterilize rubber items for only the prescribed length of time.

The sterilizing time should not begin until the desired temperature in the autoclave has been reached. Timing the load is accomplished automatically or manually. Autoclaves with automatic operation begin timing the load automatically when the desired temperature has been reached. With the manual method of operation, the medical assistant must set the timer by hand using a timing control on the front of

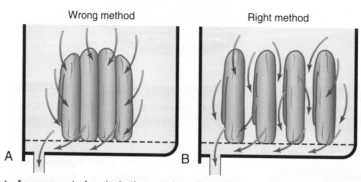

Figure 3-14. Arrangement of packs in the autoclave. **A,** Improper arrangement of packs in the autoclave. This arrangement prevents adequate penetration of steam, resulting in failure to sterilize the portions in the center of the mass. **B,** Proper arrangement of packs in the autoclave. The packs are separated from each other, and steam can now permeate each pack quickly and in the much shorter period of exposure needed. (Courtesy of and modified from AMSCO/American Sterilizer Company, Erie, Pa.)

Table 3-2 Minimum Sterilizing Times

Items (Manual Operation)*	Program (Automatic Operation)†	Time (Min at 250° F [121° C])
Unwrapped nonsurgical instruments	Unwrapped	15
Open glass or metal canisters		
Nonsurgical rubber tubing		
Wrapped instruments	Wrapped	20
Fabric or muslin		
Wrapped trays of loose instruments		
Rubber tubing		
Minor office surgery tray setup (wrapped)	Packs	30
Liquids or gels	Liquids	30

*Manual operation: The sterilizing time is selected on the basis of the items being sterilized, as indicated in this column. The sterilizing time is set by using the manual timing control when the autoclave has reached a temperature of 250° F (121° C).

†Automatic operation: The sterilization program selected from this column is based on the item being autoclaved. This program is selected by pressing the appropriate program button on the front of the autoclave (i.e., unwrapped, wrapped, packs, liquids). The autoclave automatically begins the proper timing countdown when it reaches 250° F (121° C).

the autoclave. The medical assistant should not set the timer until the temperature gauge reaches the desired temperature. The articles in the load are not considered sterile unless they have been subjected to steam for the proper length of time at the proper temperature.

Drying the Load

The sterilized articles are moist and must be allowed to dry before they are removed from the autoclave. Microorganisms can move quickly through the moisture on a wet wrap and onto the sterile article inside, resulting in contamination.

When the load has been subjected to steam for the proper length of time and temperature, the chamber must be vented of steam. Venting the chamber permits the pressure in the autoclave to decrease to zero and the chamber to cool, making it safe for the door to be opened. Most autoclaves are designed to vent automatically, which eliminates having to vent them manually.

The door of the autoclave should be opened approximately ½ inch but no more than 1 inch. Opening the door more than 1 inch causes cold air from the outside to rush into the autoclave, resulting in condensation of water on the packs. Cracking the door allows the moisture on the articles to change from a liquid to a vapor and to escape through the crack. The residual heat in the inner chamber also helps to dry the articles. The load should be allowed to dry for 15 to 60 minutes, depending on the type of autoclave and the load. Loads that contain large packs require a longer drying time than loads with smaller packs. The medical assistant should follow the manufacturer's recommendations for proper drying times of various loads.

Handling and Storing Packs

Sterilized wrapped articles should be handled carefully and as little as possible. If a wrapped article is crushed, compressed, or dropped, the sterility of the contents cannot be assumed, and the pack must be resterilized. This is known as *event-related sterility*, meaning that a sterile pack is con-

sidered sterile indefinitely, unless an event occurs that interferes with the sterility of the article.

Sterilized packs should be stored in clean, dry areas that are free from dust, insects, and other sources of contamination. Wrapped articles should be stored with the most recently sterilized articles placed in the back. The medical assistant should thoroughly check each sterilized pack at least twice: before storing it and before using it. If the pack is torn or opened, or if it is wet, it is no longer sterile and must be rewrapped and resterilized.

Maintaining the Autoclave

For the autoclave to work efficiently, it must be maintained properly. The operating manual that accompanies the autoclave provides specific information for the care and maintenance of that type of autoclave.

Safety precautions should be followed when performing maintenance procedures. Before proceeding with preventive maintenance, the autoclave must be cool, the pressure gauge at zero, and the power cord disconnected from the wall socket. Autoclave maintenance is performed on a daily, weekly, and monthly basis as follows:

Daily Maintenance

1. Wipe the outside of the autoclave with a damp cloth and a mild detergent.
2. Wipe the interior of the autoclave and the trays with a damp cloth.
3. Clean the rubber gasket on the door of the autoclave with a damp cloth.
4. Inspect the rubber door gasket for damage that could prevent a good seal.

Weekly Maintenance

1. Wash the inside of the chamber and the trays with a commercial autoclave cleaner according to the manufacturer's instructions, while observing all personal safety

precautions. This usually involves the following steps: The water reservoir must be drained first. A soft cloth or a soft brush should be used to clean the chamber. Do not use steel wool, a steel brush, or other abrasive agents because they can damage the chamber. When the chamber is clean, it should be rinsed thoroughly with distilled water. The chamber must be dried thoroughly and the door left open overnight.

2. Wash the metal shelves with an autoclave cleaner, and rinse them thoroughly with distilled water.

Monthly Maintenance

1. Flush the system to remove any buildup of residue, which could cause corrosion of the chamber lines. Carefully follow the manufacturer's directions in the instruction manual to perform this procedure.
2. Check the air trap jet to ensure it is functioning properly. The air trap jet prevents air pockets from occurring in the chamber, to ensure adequate sterilization.
3. Check the safety valve to ensure it is functioning properly. The safety valve releases pressure in the chamber if it gets too high.

Other Sterilization Methods

In addition to the autoclave, other methods can be used to sterilize articles. These methods are not generally used in the medical office and are discussed only briefly in this chapter.

Dry Heat Oven

Dry heat ovens are used to sterilize articles that cannot be penetrated by steam or may be damaged by it. Dry heat is less corrosive than moist heat for instruments with sharp edges; it does not dull their sharp edges. Oil, petroleum jelly, and powder cannot be penetrated by steam and must be sterilized in a dry heat oven. Moist heat sterilization tends to erode the ground-glass surfaces of reusable syringes, whereas dry heat does not.

Dry heat ovens operate similarly to ordinary cooking ovens. A longer exposure period is needed with dry heat because microorganisms and spores are more resistant to dry heat than to moist heat and because dry heat penetrates more slowly and unevenly than moist heat. The most commonly used temperature for dry heat sterilization is 320° F

(160° C) for 1 to 2 hours, depending on the article being sterilized. The recommended wrapping material for dry heat sterilization is aluminum foil because it is a good conductor of heat, and it protects against recontamination during handling and storage. Dry heat sterilization indicators are available to determine the effectiveness of the sterilization process.

Ethylene Oxide Gas Sterilization

Ethylene oxide is a colorless gas that is toxic and flammable. It is used to sterilize heat-sensitive items that cannot be sterilized in an autoclave. After items are sterilized with this gas, they must be aerated to remove the toxic residue of the ethylene oxide.

Ethylene oxide sterilization is a more complex and expensive process than steam sterilization. It frequently is used in the medical manufacturing industry for producing prepackaged, presterilized disposable items, such as syringes, sutures, catheters, and surgical packs.

Cold Sterilization

Cold sterilization involves the use of a chemical agent for an extended length of time. Only chemicals that are designated *sterilants* by the U.S. Environmental Protection Agency (EPA) can be used for sterilizing articles. If a chemical agent holds this status, the word *sterilant* is printed on the front of the container.

The item to be sterilized must be completely submerged in the chemical for a long time (6 to 24 hours depending on the manufacturer's instructions). Prolonged immersion of instruments can damage them. In addition, each time an instrument is added to the instrument container, the clock must be restarted for the entire amount of time. For these reasons, and because this method involves the use of a hazardous chemical, cold sterilization should be used only when an autoclave, gas, or a dry heat oven is not indicated or is unavailable.

Radiation

Radiation uses high-energy ionizing radiation to sterilize articles. Medical manufacturers use radiation to sterilize prepackaged surgical equipment and instruments that cannot be sterilized by heat or chemicals.

 PROCEDURE 3-5   Sterilizing Articles in the Autoclave

Outcome Sterilize a load of contaminated articles in the autoclave.

Equipment/Supplies

- Autoclave and instruction manual
- Distilled water
- Wrapped articles
- Heat-resistant gloves

PROCEDURE 3-5   Sterilizing Articles in the Autoclave—cont'd

1. Procedural Step. Assemble the equipment.

2. Procedural Step. Check the level of water in the autoclave and add distilled water, if needed.

Principle. Water contained in the water reservoir of the autoclave is converted to steam during the sterilization process. Distilled water is used to prevent corrosion of the stainless-steel chamber of the autoclave.

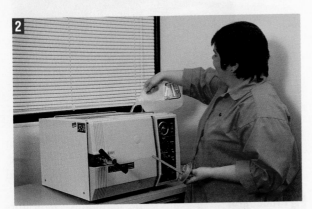

If needed, add distilled water to the autoclave.

3. Procedural Step. Properly load the autoclave while following these guidelines:

a. Do not overload the chamber. Small packs should be placed 1 to 3 inches apart, and large packs should be placed 2 to 4 inches apart. The packs should not touch the chamber walls.

b. Ensure that at least 1 inch separates the autoclave trays.

c. Place jars and glassware on their sides.

d. Place dressings in a vertical position.

e. When sterilizing dressings and hard goods together, place dressings on the top shelf and hard goods on the lower shelf.

f. When using sterilization pouches, set the pouches on their sides to maximize steam circulation and to facilitate drying.

Principle. The autoclave must be loaded properly to ensure adequate steam penetration of all articles.

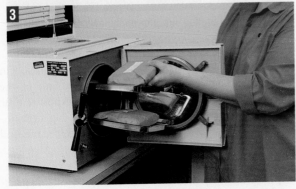

Properly load the autoclave.

4. Procedural Step. Operate the autoclave according to the procedure described in the instruction manual. A general procedure for the manual and the automatic methods of operation follows.

Manually Operated Autoclave

a. Determine the sterilizing time for the types of articles being autoclaved (see Table 3-2).

b. Turn on the autoclave.

c. Fill the chamber with water using the appropriate control.

d. Securely close and latch the door of the autoclave.

e. Set the timing control when the temperature gauge reaches the desired temperature (usually 250° F [121° C]). At the end of the steam exposure time, an indicator light usually comes on, or a beeper sounds.

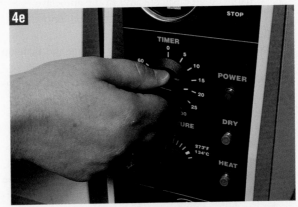

Set the timing control.

f. If the autoclave does not vent automatically, use the appropriate control to release steam from the chamber.

g. Dry the load by cracking open the door approximately ½ inch but no more than 1 inch. Set the drying time using the timing control. The drying time varies between 15 and 60 minutes, depending on the autoclave and the type of load.

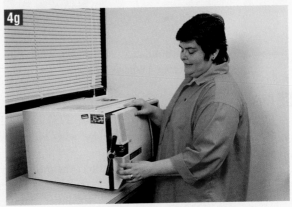

Crack the door to dry the load.

Continued

PROCEDURE 3-5   Sterilizing Articles in the Autoclave—cont'd

Principle. To ensure sterilization, the load should not be timed until the proper temperature has been reached. The sterility of wrapped packs cannot be ensured unless the wrapped articles are allowed to dry fully. Microorganisms can move through the moisture on a wet wrap and contaminate the sterile article inside.

Automatically Operated Autoclave

a. Securely close and latch the door of the autoclave.
b. Turn on the autoclave.
c. Determine the sterilization program according to what is being autoclaved (see Table 3-2). Press the appropriate program button on the front of the autoclave to select the program. Press the start button.
d. Indicators on the front of the autoclave tell you what is happening (automatically) in the autoclave:
Filling Indicator. Lights up when the chamber is filling with water
Sterilizing Indicator. Lights up during the heat-up and sterilization phases of the cycle
Temperature Display. Digital display of the temperature in the autoclave
Time Display. Digital countdown of the time remaining in the sterilization program
Drying Indicator. Lights up during the drying phase of the cycle
Complete or Ready Indicator. Illuminates when the autoclave has completed the cycle and sterilized articles can be removed from the autoclave

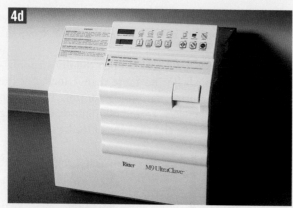

Automatic autoclave buttons and indicators.

5. **Procedural Step.** Turn off the autoclave. Wearing heat-resistant gloves, remove the load. Do not touch the inner chamber of the autoclave with your bare hands.
Principle. Heat-resistant gloves protect the medical assistant's hands when the warm packs from the chamber of the autoclave are being removed. The inner chamber of the autoclave is hot and could burn bare skin.

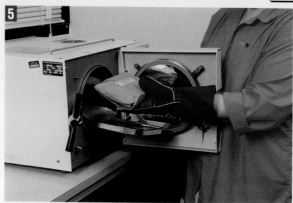

Remove the load with heat-resistant gloves.

6. Procedural Step. Inspect the packs as you take them out of the autoclave. If the packs show any damage, such as holes or tears, the articles should be rewrapped and resterilized.
7. **Procedural Step.** Check the sterilization indicators located on the outside of the pack to ensure the proper response has occurred.
Principle. Autoclave tape indicates only that the article has been through the autoclave cycle; it does not ensure that sterilization has taken place. Sterilization is confirmed when the pack is opened for use and the sterilization strip indicator in the center of the pack is checked for its proper response.

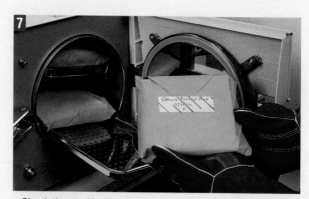

Check the sterilization indicator on the outside of the pack.

8. Procedural Step. Record monitoring information in the autoclave log. Include the date and time of the cycle, a description of the load, and the exposure time and temperature. If a biologic indicator has been included in the load, process it according to the medical office policy, and record results on the autoclave log.
9. Procedural Step. Store the packs in a clean, dust-proof area with the most recently sterilized packs placed behind previously sterilized packs.

PROCEDURE 3-5 Sterilizing Articles in the Autoclave—cont'd

10. **Procedural Step.** Maintain appropriate daily care of the autoclave, while following the manufacturer's recommendations. Daily care of the autoclave includes the following:

a. Wipe the outside of the autoclave with a damp cloth and a mild detergent.

b. Wipe the interior of the autoclave and the trays with a damp cloth.

c. Clean the rubber gasket located on the door of the autoclave with a damp cloth.

d. Inspect the rubber door gasket for damage that could prevent a good seal.

Principle. For the autoclave to work efficiently, it must be properly maintained.

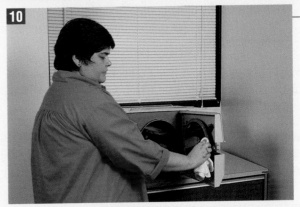

Clean the rubber gasket with a damp cloth.

evolve *Check out the Evolve site to access additional interactive activities.*

MEDICAL PRACTICE *and the* LAW

If not performed properly, sterilization and disinfection can adversely affect patients, which can make the medical assistant and other office personnel liable for resultant injuries. Meticulous care must be taken to ensure that all procedures are performed correctly and completely.

Sterilization and disinfection procedures include the use of hazardous chemicals. These chemicals must be stored, used, and disposed of in specific ways mandated by law. The autoclave can be a dangerous machine if it is not used correctly, and it could harm others with hot steam. If you use the autoclave without proper instruction, you could be liable for injuries or accidents resulting from misuse.

Whenever you are dealing with contaminated articles, you have a duty to protect yourself, other employees, patients, and other articles from cross-contamination. ■

What Would You Do? What Would You *Not* Do? RESPONSES

Case Study 1
Page 89

What Did Kara Do?

❑ Complimented Mrs. Cordera for her concern and efforts to baby-proof her home.

❑ Gave Mrs. Cordera a patient information brochure on baby-proofing the home.

❑ Told Mrs. Cordera that she should assume that all cleaning products are poisonous. Got out a disinfectant container and showed Mrs. Cordera the information on the label that tells what to do in case of an accidental poisoning.

❑ Gave the National Poison Control hotline number (1-800-222-1222) to Mrs. Cordera and told her that was the fastest way to obtain information on what to do in case of an accidental poisoning. Told her to keep this number by her phone.

What Did Kara Not Do?

❑ Did not take Mrs. Cordera's question lightly.

What Would You Do/What Would You *Not* Do? Review Kara's response and place a checkmark next to the information you included in your response. List additional information you included in your response.

_____

_____

_____

Case Study 2
Page 99

What Did Kara Do?

❑ Explained to Mrs. Scout that toys are in the waiting room for children to play with to make their visit more comfortable and less stressful.

❑ Reassured Mrs. Scout that the medical office personnel do everything they can to prevent the spread of germs in the office and that the toys are sanitized every day.

Continued

What Would You Do? What Would You *Not* Do?   RESPONSES—cont'd

❏ Relayed to Mrs. Scout that only toys that can be sanitized are kept in the medical office.

❏ Told Mrs. Scout that her concern would be brought up at the weekly office meeting.

What Did Kara Not Do?

❏ Did not get defensive because Mrs. Scout was just being concerned about her child's health.

What Would You Do/What Would You *Not* Do? Review Kara's response and place a checkmark next to the information you included in your response. List additional information you included in your response.

_____

_____

_____

_____

Case Study 3
Page 103

What Did Kara Do?

❏ Told Cassie through verbal and nonverbal behavior that her concern was valid.

❏ Told Cassie that hepatitis can be transmitted through dirty instruments.

❏ Reassured Cassie that all instruments are sterilized in the autoclave, which has special indicators to ensure all germs have been killed.

❏ Gave Cassie a patient information brochure on hepatitis. Told her that individuals with chronic hepatitis can develop liver cancer and that the best way to avoid hepatitis is through measures and behaviors recommended for prevention.

❏ Told Cassie that a vaccine is available to prevent hepatitis B, but not hepatitis C.

What Did Kara Not Do?

❏ Did not dismiss her concern about dirty instruments as unimportant.

❏ Did not overly alarm her about the consequences of chronic hepatitis.

What Would You Do/What Would You *Not* Do? Review Kara's response and place a checkmark next to the information you included in your response. List additional information you included in your response.

_____

_____

_____

_____

CERTIFICATION REVIEW

❏ **The Hazard Communication Standard (HCS)** is required by OSHA for any facility that uses or stores hazardous chemicals. Its purpose is to ensure that employees are informed of the hazards associated with chemicals in their workplaces and the precautions to take to protect themselves when working with hazardous chemicals.

❏ **A hazardous chemical** is any chemical that presents a threat to the health and safety of an individual coming into contact with it.

❏ **A hazard communication program** must be developed by employers who use and store hazardous chemicals in their workplace; it describes what their facility is doing to meet the requirements of the HCS.

❏ **A hazardous chemical** must contain a label that includes the name of the chemical, manufacturer information, physical and health hazards of the chemical, safety precautions, and storing and handling information.

❏ **A material safety data sheet (MSDS)** provides information regarding the chemical, its hazards, and measures to take to prevent injury and illness when handling the chemical. An MSDS must be kept on file for each hazardous chemical used or stored in the workplace.

❏ **The HCS requires** that employees be provided with information and training regarding hazardous chemicals in the workplace. The training program must be offered at the time of an employee's initial assignment to a work area where hazardous chemicals are present and whenever a new chemical hazard is introduced into the workplace.

❏ **Sanitization** is a process that removes organic material from an article and lowers the number of microorganisms to a safe level. The items most frequently sanitized in the medical office are medical and surgical instruments.

❏ **Instruments can be cleaned** manually or by using an ultrasonic cleaner. The manual method uses a brush, instrument cleaner, and friction to clean instruments. An ultrasonic cleaner uses a cleaning solution and sound waves to clean the instruments. To prevent the formation of a permanent stain, items made of dissimilar metals should not be cleaned together.

❏ **Disinfection** is the process of destroying pathogenic microorganisms; it does not kill bacterial spores. Disinfectants consist of chemical agents that are applied to inanimate objects. The disinfectants used most often in the medical office are glutaraldehyde, alcohol, sodium hypochlorite (household bleach), phenolics, and quaternary ammonium compounds.

❑ **Disinfection can be classified** into the following levels: high, intermediate, and low. High-level disinfection is used to disinfect semicritical items that are heat sensitive, such as flexible fiberoptic sigmoidoscopes. Intermediate-level disinfection is used for noncritical items, such as stethoscopes and blood pressure cuffs. Low-level disinfection is used to disinfect surfaces such as examining tables, countertops, and walls.

❑ **Sterilization** is the process of destroying all forms of microbial life, including bacterial spores. Sterilization must be used for critical items. Critical items are items that come in contact with sterile tissue or the vascular system.

❑ **The autoclave** is used most often in the medical office for sterilization. The autoclave is usually operated at approximately 15 pounds of pressure per square inch at a temperature of 2508° F (1218° C).

❑ **To ensure that instruments and supplies are sterile** when used, a monitoring program should be established in the medical office. This program should include reviewing sterilization policies and procedures, checking the use of sterilization indicators, and maintaining records for each autoclave cycle.

❑ **Sterilization indicators** determine the effectiveness of the sterilization process and include chemical indicators and biologic indicators. Chemical indicators use a thermolabile dye that changes color when exposed to the sterilization process. Biologic indicators are the best

indicators available for determining the effectiveness of the sterilization procedure. They consist of a preparation of heat-resistant living bacterial spores.

❑ **The purpose of wrapping articles** for autoclaving is to protect them from recontamination during handling and storage. Examples of wraps commonly used include sterilization paper, sterilization pouches, and muslin.

❑ **The autoclave cycle** refers to the steps involved in achieving sterilization with an autoclave. The autoclave must be loaded properly so that steam can easily penetrate the contents of the load. The length of time for sterilization varies according to the item that is being sterilized. The sterilizing time should not begin until the desired temperature in the autoclave has been reached. To prevent recontamination, articles must be completely dry before they are removed from the autoclave. Sterilized wrapped articles should be handled carefully and as little as possible. They should be stored in a clean, dustproof area. The autoclave should be properly maintained while following a daily, weekly, and monthly schedule.

❑ **Event-related sterility** means that a sterile pack is considered sterile indefinitely unless an event occurs that interferes with the sterility of the article. If a pack is torn or opened, or if it is wet, it is no longer sterile and must be rewrapped and resterilized.

❑ **Other methods that can be used to sterilize articles** include dry heat, ethylene oxide gas, chemical agents, and radiation. Ethylene oxide and radiation are used by the medical manufacturing industry for producing prepackaged and presterilized disposable items.

TERMINOLOGY REVIEW

Antiseptic A substance that kills disease-producing microorganisms but not their spores. An antiseptic is usually applied to living tissue.

Autoclave An apparatus for the sterilization of materials, using steam under pressure.

Contaminate To soil, stain, or pollute; to make impure.

Critical item An item that comes in contact with sterile tissue or the vascular system.

Decontamination The use of physical or chemical means to remove or destroy pathogens on an item so that it is no longer capable of transmitting disease; this makes the item safe to handle.

Detergent An agent that cleanses by emulsifying dirt and oil.

Disinfectant An agent used to destroy pathogenic microorganisms but not their spores. Disinfectants are usually applied to inanimate objects.

Hazardous chemical Any chemical that presents a threat to the health and safety of an individual coming into contact with it.

Incubate To provide proper conditions for growth and development.

Load The articles that are being sterilized.

Material safety data sheet (MSDS) A sheet that provides information regarding a chemical, its hazards, and measures to take to prevent injury and illness when handling the chemical.

Noncritical item An item that comes into contact with intact skin, but not with mucous membranes.

Sanitization A process to remove organic matter from an article and to reduce the number of microorganisms to a safe level as determined by public health requirements.

Semicritical item An item that comes into contact with nonintact skin or intact mucous membranes.

Spore A hard, thick-walled capsule formed by some bacteria that contains only the essential parts of the protoplasm of the bacterial cell.

Sterilization The process of destroying all forms of microbial life, including bacterial spores.

Thermolabile Easily affected or changed by heat.

ON THE WEB

For information on infection control in the health care setting:

Centers for Disease Control and Prevention: www.cdc.gov

Environmental Protection Agency: www.epa.gov

National Institute of Environmental Health Sciences: www.niehs.nih.gov

National Institute for Occupational Safety and Health: www.cdc.gov/niosh

Infection Control Today: www.infectioncontroltoday.com

Association for Professionals in Infection Control and Epidemiology: www.apic.com

To locate a material safety data sheet:

MSDS-Search: www.msdssearch.com

HazCom: www.hazard.com/msds

4

Vital Signs

LEARNING OBJECTIVES	**PROCEDURES**

Temperature

1. Define a vital sign.
2. Explain the reasons for taking vital signs.
3. Explain how body temperature is maintained.
4. List examples of how heat is produced in the body.
5. List examples of how heat is lost from the body.
6. State the normal body temperature range and the average body temperature.
7. List and explain factors that can cause variation in the body temperature.
8. List and describe the three stages of a fever.
9. List the sites for taking body temperature, and explain why these sites are used.
10. List and describe the guidelines for using a tympanic membrane thermometer and a temporal artery thermometer.

Measure oral body temperature.
Measure axillary body temperature.
Measure rectal body temperature.
Measure aural body temperature.
Measure temporal artery body temperature.

Pulse

1. Explain the mechanism of pulse.
2. List and explain the factors that affect the pulse rate.
3. Identify a specific use for each of the eight pulse sites.
4. State the normal range of pulse rate for each age group.
5. Explain the difference between pulse rhythm and pulse volume.

Measure radial pulse.
Measure apical pulse.

Respiration

1. Explain the purpose of respiration.
2. State what occurs during inhalation and exhalation.
3. State the normal respiratory rate for each age group.
4. List and explain the factors that affect the respiratory rate.
5. Explain the difference between rhythm and depth of respiration.
6. Describe the character of each of the following abnormal breath sounds: crackles, rhonchi, wheezes, and pleural friction rub.

Measure respiration.

Pulse Oximetry

1. Explain the purpose of pulse oximetry.
2. State the normal oxygen saturation level of a healthy individual.
3. List and describe the functions of the controls, indicators, and displays on a pulse oximeter.
4. Describe the difference between a reusable and a disposable oximeter probe.
5. List and describe factors that may interfere with an accurate pulse oximetry reading.

Perform pulse oximetry.

Blood Pressure
1. Define blood pressure.
2. State the normal range of blood pressure for an adult.
3. List and describe factors that affect the blood pressure.
4. Identify the different parts of a stethoscope and a sphygmomanometer.
5. Identify the Korotkoff sounds.
6. State the advantages and disadvantages of an automated oscillometric blood pressure device.
7. Explain how to prevent errors in blood pressure measurement.

Measure blood pressure.
Determine systolic pressure by palpation.

CHAPTER OUTLINE

Introduction to Vital Signs
Temperature
  Regulation of Body Temperature
  Body Temperature Range
  Assessment of Body Temperature
Pulse
  Mechanism of the Pulse
  Assessment of Pulse

Respiration
  Mechanism of Respiration
  Assessment of Respiration
Pulse Oximetry
  Assessment of Oxygen Saturation
Blood Pressure
  Mechanism of Blood Pressure
  Assessment of Manual Blood Pressure

KEY TERMS

adventitious (ad-ven-TISH-us) sounds
afebrile (uh-FEB-ril)
alveolus (al-VEE-uh-lus)
antecubital (AN-tih-CYOO-bi-tul) space
antipyretic (AN-tih-pye-REH-tik)
aorta (ay-OR-tuh)
apical-radial pulse
apnea (AP-nee-uh)
axilla (aks-ILL-uh)
bounding pulse
bradycardia (BRAY-dee-CAR-dee-uh)
bradypnea (BRAY-dip-NEE-uh)
Celsius (SELL-see-us) scale
conduction (kon-DUK-shun)
convection (kon-VEK-shun)
crisis
cyanosis (sye-an-OH-sus)
diastole (dye-AS-toe-lee)
diastolic (DYE-uh-STOL-ik) pressure
dyspnea (DISP-nee-uh)
dysrhythmia (dis-RITH-mee-uh)
eupnea (YOOP-nee-uh)
exhalation (EKS-hal-AY-shun)
Fahrenheit (FAIR-en-hite) scale
febrile (FEH-bril)
fever
frenulum linguae (FREN-yoo-lum LIN-gway)
hyperpnea (HYE-perp-NEE-uh)
hyperpyrexia (HYE-per-pye-REK-see-uh)
hypertension (HYE-per-TEN-shun)

hyperventilation (HYE-per-ven-til-AY-shun)
hypopnea (hye-POP-nee-uh)
hypotension (HYE-poe-TEN-shun)
hypothermia (HYE-poe-THER-mee-uh)
hypoxemia (hye-pok-SEE-mee-uh)
hypoxia (hye-POKS-ee-uh)
inhalation (IN-hal-AY-shun)
intercostal (IN-ter-KOS-tul)
Korotkoff (kuh-ROT-kof) sounds
malaise (mal-AYZE)
manometer (man-OM-uh-ter)
meniscus (men-IS-kus)
orthopnea (orth-OP-nee-uh)
pulse deficit
pulse oximeter
pulse oximetry
pulse pressure
pulse rhythm
pulse volume
radiation (RAY-dee-AY-shun)
SaO_2
sphygmomanometer (SFIG-moe-man-OM-uh-ter)
SpO_2
stethoscope (STETH-uh-skope)
systole (SIS-toe-lee)
systolic (sis-TOL-ik) pressure
tachycardia (TAK-ih-KAR-dee-uh)
tachypnea (TAK-ip-NEE-uh)
thready pulse

Introduction to Vital Signs

Vital signs are objective guideposts that provide data to determine a person's state of health. Vital signs include temperature, pulse, respiration (collectively called TPR), and blood pressure (BP). Another indicator of a patient's health status is pulse oximetry. Although some physicians order this measurement routinely on all patients as part of the patient workup, most physicians order this vital sign only when the patient complains of respiratory problems (e.g., shortness of breath).

The normal ranges of the vital signs are finely adjusted, and any deviation from normal may indicate disease. During the course of an illness, variations in the vital signs may occur. The medical assistant should be alert to any significant changes and report them to the physician because they indicate a change in the patient's condition. When patients visit the medical office, vital signs are routinely checked to establish each patient's usual state of health and to establish baseline measurements against which future measurements can be compared. The medical assistant should have a thorough knowledge of the vital signs and should attain proficiency in taking them to ensure accurate findings.

General guidelines that the medical assistant should follow when measuring the vital signs are as follows:

1. Be familiar with the normal ranges for all vital signs. Keep in mind that normal ranges vary based on the different age groups (infant, child, adult, elder).
2. Make sure that all equipment for measuring vital signs is in proper working condition to ensure accurate findings.
3. Eliminate or minimize factors that affect the vital signs, such as exercise, food and beverage consumption, smoking, and emotional state.
4. Use an organized approach when measuring the vital signs. If all of the vital signs are ordered, they are usually measured starting with temperature, followed by pulse, respiration, blood pressure, and pulse oximetry.

TEMPERATURE

Regulation of Body Temperature

Body temperature is maintained within a fairly constant range by the hypothalamus, which is located in the brain. The hypothalamus functions as the body's thermostat. It normally allows the body temperature to vary by only about 1° to 2° Fahrenheit (F) throughout the day.

Body temperature is maintained through a balance of the heat produced in the body and the heat lost from the body (Figure 4-1). A constant temperature range must be maintained for the body to function properly. When minor changes in the temperature of the body occur, the hypothalamus senses this and makes adjustments as necessary to ensure that the body temperature stays within a normal and safe range. If an individual is playing tennis on a hot day,

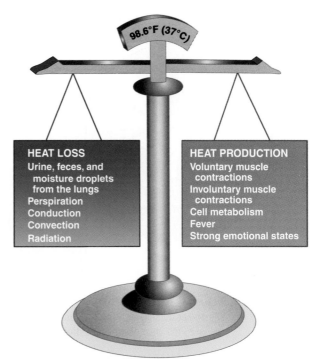

Figure 4-1. Body temperature represents a balance between the heat produced in the body and the heat lost from the body.

the body's heat-cooling mechanism is activated to remove excess heat from the body through perspiration.

Heat Production

Most of the heat produced in the body is through voluntary and involuntary muscle contractions. Voluntary muscle contractions involve the muscles over which a person has control, for example, the moving of legs or arms. Involuntary muscle contractions involve the muscles over which a person has no control; examples are physiologic processes such as digestion, the beating of the heart, and shivering.

Body heat also is produced by cell metabolism. Heat is produced when nutrients are broken down in the cells. Fever and strong emotional states also can increase heat production in the body.

Heat Loss

Heat is lost from the body through the urine and feces and in water vapor from the lungs. Perspiration also contributes to heat loss. Perspiration is the excretion of moisture through the pores of the skin. When the moisture evaporates, heat is released and the body is cooled.

Radiation, conduction, and convection all cause loss of heat from the body. **Radiation** is the transfer of heat in the form of waves; body heat is continually radiating into cooler surroundings. **Conduction** is the transfer of heat from one object to another by direct contact; heat can be transferred by conduction from the body to a cooler object it touches. **Convection** is the transfer of heat through air currents; cool air currents can cause the body to lose heat. These processes are illustrated in Figure 4-2.

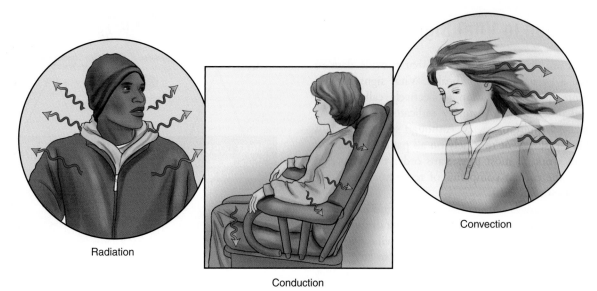

Radiation

Conduction

Convection

Figure 4-2. Heat loss from the body. With **radiation,** the body gives off heat in the form of waves to the cooler outside air. With **conduction,** the chair becomes warm as heat is transferred from the individual to the chair. With **convection,** air currents move heat away from the body.

Body Temperature Range

The purposes of measuring body temperature are to establish the patient's baseline temperature and to monitor an abnormally high or low body temperature. The normal body temperature range is 97° F to 99° F (36.1° C to 37.2° C), the average temperature being 98.6° F (37° C). Body temperature is usually recorded using the Fahrenheit system of measurement. Table 4-1 lists comparable **Fahrenheit** and **Celsius** temperatures and explains how to convert temperatures from one scale to the other.

Alterations in Body Temperature

A body temperature greater than 100.4° F (38° C) indicates a **fever,** or *pyrexia.* If the body temperature falls between 99° F (37.2° C) and 100.4° F (38° C), this is called a *low-grade fever.* When an individual has a fever, the heat the body is producing is greater than the heat the body is losing. A temperature reading greater than 105.8° F (41° C) is known as **hyperpyrexia.** Hyperpyrexia is a serious condition, and a temperature greater than 109.4° F (43° C) is generally fatal.

A body temperature less than 97° F (36.1° C) is classified as subnormal, or **hypothermia.** This means that the heat the body is losing is greater than the heat it is producing. A person usually cannot survive with a temperature less than 93.2° F (34° C). Terms used to describe alterations in body temperature are illustrated in Figure 4-3.

Variations in Body Temperature

During the day-to-day activities of an individual, normal fluctuations occur in the body temperature. The body temperature rarely stays the same throughout the course of a day. The medical assistant should take the following

Table 4-1 Equivalent Fahrenheit and Celsius Temperatures	
Fahrenheit	**Celsius**
93.2	34
95	35
96.8	36
97.7	36.5
98.6	37
99.5	37.5
100.4	38
101.3	38.5
102.2	39
104	40
105.8	41
107.6	42
109.4	43
111.2	44

Temperature Conversion

1. Celsius to Fahrenheit: To convert Celsius to Fahrenheit, multiply by $\frac{9}{5}$ and add 32:

$$°F = (°C \times \tfrac{9}{5}) + 32$$

2. Fahrenheit to Celsius: To convert Fahrenheit to Celsius, subtract 32 and multiply by $\frac{5}{9}$:

$$°C \times (°F - 32) \times \tfrac{5}{9}$$

points into consideration when evaluating a patient's temperature.

1. **Age.** Infants and young children normally have a higher body temperature than adults because their thermoregulatory system is not yet fully established. Elderly individuals usually have a lower body temperature owing to

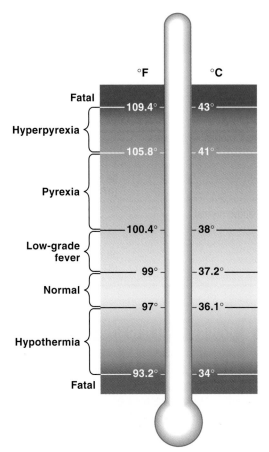

Figure 4-3. Terms that describe alterations in body temperature (adult oral temperature).

factors such as loss of subcutaneous fat, lack of exercise, and loss of thermoregulatory control. Table 4-2 shows the normal ranges of body temperature according to age group.

2. **Diurnal variations.** During sleep, body metabolism slows down, as do muscle contractions. The body's temperature is lowest in the morning before metabolism and muscle contractions begin increasing.

3. **Emotional states.** Strong emotions, such as crying and extreme anger, can increase the body temperature. This is important to consider when working with young chil-

dren, who frequently cry during examination procedures or when they are ill.

4. **Environment.** Cold weather tends to decrease the body temperature, whereas hot weather increases it.

5. **Exercise.** Vigorous physical exercise causes an increase in voluntary muscle contractions, which elevates the body temperature.

6. **Patient's normal body temperature.** Some patients normally run a low or high temperature. The medical assistant should review the patient's past vital sign recordings.

7. **Pregnancy.** Cell metabolism increases during pregnancy, and this elevates body temperature.

Fever

Fever, or pyrexia, denotes that a patient's temperature has increased to greater than 100.4° F (38° C). An individual who has a fever is said to be **febrile;** one who does not have a fever is **afebrile.**

Fever is a common symptom of illness, particularly inflammation and infection. When there is an infection in the body, the invading pathogen functions as a *pyrogen,* which is any substance that produces fever. Pyrogens reset the hypothalamus, causing the body temperature to increase to above normal. Fever is not an illness itself, but rather a sign that the body may have an infection. Most fevers are self-limited, that is, the body temperature returns to normal after the disease process is complete.

Stages of a Fever

A fever can be divided into the following three stages:

1. The *onset* is when the temperature first begins to increase. This increase may be slow or sudden, the patient often experiences coldness and chills, and the pulse and respiratory rate increase.

2. During the *course of a fever,* the temperature rises and falls in one of the following three fever patterns: continuous, intermittent, or remittent. Fever patterns are described and illustrated in Table 4-3. During this stage, the patient has an increased pulse and respiratory rate and feels warm to the touch. The patient also may experience one or more of the following: flushed appearance, increased thirst, loss of appetite, headache, and malaise. **Malaise** refers to a vague sense of body discomfort, weakness, and fatigue.

3. During the *subsiding stage,* the temperature returns to normal. It can return to normal gradually or suddenly (known as a **crisis**). As the body temperature is returning to normal, the patient usually perspires and may become dehydrated.

Assessment of Body Temperature

Assessment Sites

There are five sites for measuring body temperature: mouth, **axilla,** rectum, ear, and forehead. The locations in which temperatures are taken should have an abundant blood sup-

Table 4-2 Variations in Body Temperature by Age			
Age	**Site**	**Average Temperature**	
Newborn	Axillary	97° F-100° F	36.1° C-37.8° C
1 yr	Oral	99.7° F	37.6° C
5 yr	Oral	98.6° F	37° C
Adult	Oral	98.6° F	37° C
	Rectal	99.6° F	37.5° C
	Axillary	97.6° F	36.4° C
	Aural	98.6° F	37° C
Elderly (over 70 yr)	Oral	96.8° F	36° C

Table 4-3 Fever Patterns

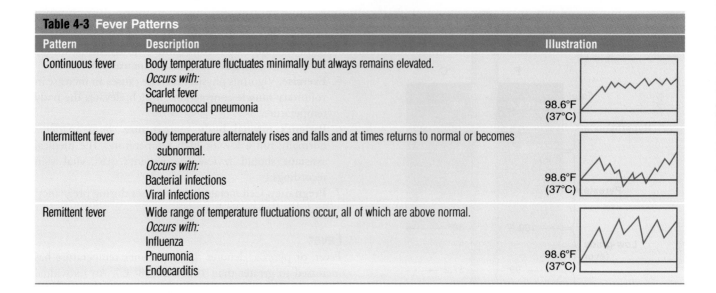

Pattern	Description	Illustration
Continuous fever	Body temperature fluctuates minimally but always remains elevated. *Occurs with:* Scarlet fever Pneumococcal pneumonia	98.6°F (37°C)
Intermittent fever	Body temperature alternately rises and falls and at times returns to normal or becomes subnormal. *Occurs with:* Bacterial infections Viral infections	98.6°F (37°C)
Remittent fever	Wide range of temperature fluctuations occur, all of which are above normal. *Occurs with:* Influenza Pneumonia Endocarditis	98.6°F (37°C)

Highlight on Fever

Although most fevers indicate an infection, not all do. Noninfectious causes of fever include heatstroke, drug hypersensitivity, neoplasms, and central nervous system damage.

A fever usually is not harmful if it remains less than 102° F (38.9° C). Research suggests that fever may serve as a defense mechanism to destroy pathogens that are unable to survive above the normal body temperature range.

The level of the fever is not related to the seriousness of the infection. A patient with a temperature of 104° F (40° C) may not be any sicker than a patient with a temperature of 102° F (38.9° C).

In children, fever often is one of the first signs of illness and has a tendency to become highly elevated. In contrast, in elderly patients, fever may be elevated to only 1° F to 2° F above normal, even with a severe infection.

During a fever, the body's basal metabolism increases by 7% for each degree of temperature elevation. Heart and respiratory rates also increase to meet this metabolic demand.

Chills during a fever result when the hypothalamus has been reset at a higher temperature. In an attempt to reach this temperature, involuntary muscle contractions (chills) occur, which produce heat, causing the temperature of the body to increase. After the higher temperature has been reached, the chills subside, and the individual then feels warm.

Increased perspiration during a fever occurs when the hypothalamus has been reset at a lower temperature, for example, after taking an **antipyretic** or after the cause of the fever has been removed. To cool the body and reach this lower temperature, the body perspires, often profusely; profuse perspiration is known as *diaphoresis.* ■

Putting It All Into Practice

My Name is Sergio Martinez, and I am a registered medical assistant. I work in a large clinic that is associated with a medical school. At present, I work in the family medicine department, but I also have worked in dermatology and internal medicine. Family medicine is the area I enjoy most because of the wide variety of tasks that are performed. There is rarely a dull moment.

I focus primarily on clinical medical assisting. Taking vital signs is a big part of my job responsibilities. It is routine at my clinic to take height, weight, temperature, pulse, respiration, and blood pressure on every patient seen at the clinic, no matter what the reason for his or her visit. I assist the physician with various procedures, examinations, and minor office surgery, and I administer injections, run electrocardiograms, and perform various laboratory tests.

Taking vital signs and length and weight on small children can be very challenging at times. Some children start to cry as soon as they are put on the scale. Taking a temperature on an uncooperative toddler can be very difficult. I try to calm the child as much as possible, and for good behavior, I give a lot of praise. Stickers also are a great reward for cooperative behavior. Usually when small children learn that they can trust you, they are not as frightened by the experience. It is rewarding when a child learns not to be afraid of being evaluated for routine vital signs. ■

ply so that the temperature of the entire body is obtained, not the temperature of only a part of the body. In addition, the site must be as closed as possible to prevent air currents from interfering with the temperature reading. The site chosen for measuring a patient's temperature depends on the patient's age, condition, and state of consciousness; the type of thermometer available; and the medical office policy.

Oral Temperature

The oral method is a convenient and one of the most common means for measuring body temperature. When the medical assistant records a temperature, the physician assumes it has been taken through the oral route, unless it is otherwise noted. There is a rich blood supply under the tongue in the area on either side of the **frenulum linguae.**

The thermometer should be placed in this area to receive the most accurate reading. The patient must keep the mouth closed during the procedure to provide a closed space for the thermometer.

Axillary Temperature

Axillary temperature is recommended as a site for measuring temperature in toddlers and preschoolers. The axillary site also should be used for mouth-breathing patients and for patients with oral inflammation or who have had oral surgery.

The temperature obtained through the axillary method measures approximately 1° F lower than the same person's temperature taken through the oral route (see Table 4-2). The medical assistant should make a notation to tell the physician that the temperature was taken through the axillary route.

Rectal Temperature

The rectal temperature provides an extremely accurate measurement of body temperature because few factors can alter the results. The rectum is highly vascular and, of the five sites, provides the most closed cavity. The temperature obtained through the rectal route measures approximately 1° F higher than the same person's temperature taken through the oral route (see Table 4-2). The medical assistant should make a notation on the patient's chart if the temperature has been taken rectally.

The rectal method is generally used for infants and young children, unconscious patients, and mouth-breathing patients, and when greater accuracy in body temperature is desired. The rectal site should not be used with newborns because of the danger of rectal trauma.

Aural Temperature

The aural (ear) site is used with the tympanic membrane thermometer. The ear provides a closed cavity that is easily accessible. Tympanic membrane thermometers provide instantaneous results, are easy to use, and are comfortable for the patient. They make it easier to measure the temperature of children younger than 6 years, uncooperative patients, and patients who are unable to have their temperatures taken orally.

Forehead Temperature

The temporal artery is a major artery of the head that runs laterally across the forehead and down the side of the neck. In the area of the forehead, it is located approximately 2 mm below the surface of the skin. Because the temporal artery is located so close to the skin surface and is easily accessible, the forehead provides an ideal site for obtaining a body temperature measurement. In addition, the temporal artery has a constant steady flow of blood, which assists in providing an accurate measurement of the patient's body temperature.

The forehead site can be used to measure body temperature using a temporal artery thermometer in individuals of all ages (newborns, infants, children, adults, elderly). The results compare in accuracy with other methods used to measure body temperature. The temperature obtained through the forehead site is about the same as a rectal temperature measurement. The temporal artery reading measures approximately 1° higher than oral body temperature and 2° higher than axillary temperature on the Fahrenheit scale.

Types of Thermometers

The four types of thermometers available for measuring body temperature are electronic thermometers, tympanic membrane thermometers, temporal artery thermometers, and chemical thermometers. Mercury glass thermometers are no longer used in the medical office because they break easily and release mercury. Mercury is a chemical that is dangerous to the human body because it can cause damage to the nervous system. If mercury is released into the environment, it can be harmful to wildlife. Many cities have banned the sale or use of mercury because of its potential hazards.

Electronic Thermometer

An electronic thermometer is often used in the medical office to measure body temperature. Electronic thermometers are portable and measure oral, axillary, and rectal temperatures ranging from 84° F to 108° F (28.9° C to 42.2° C).

An electronic thermometer measures body temperature in a brief time, which varies between 4 and 20 seconds, depending on the brand of thermometer used. The temperature results are digitally displayed on an LCD screen. An electronic thermometer consists of interchangeable oral and rectal probes attached to a battery-operated portable unit (Figure 4-4). The probes are color-coded for ease in identifying them. The oral probe is color-coded with blue on its collar and is used to take oral and axillary temperatures; the rectal probe is color-coded with red on its collar and is used to take rectal temperatures only.

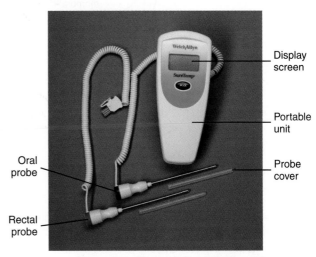

Figure 4-4. Electronic thermometer.

A disposable plastic cover is placed over the probe to prevent the transmission of microorganisms among patients. Depending on the method of taking the temperature, the probe may be inserted into the mouth, axilla, or rectum and is left in place until an audible tone is emitted from the thermometer. When the tone sounds, the patient's temperature in degrees Fahrenheit is displayed on the screen. The medical assistant ejects the plastic probe cover into a regular waste container.

The casing, probes, and attached cords of the electronic thermometer should be periodically cleaned with a soft cloth slightly dampened with a solution of warm water and a disinfectant cleaner.

Procedures 4-1, 4-2, and 4-3 outline the methods for measuring oral, axillary, and rectal temperatures using an electronic thermometer.

Tympanic Membrane Thermometer

The tympanic membrane thermometer is used at the aural site. The tympanic membrane thermometer functions by detecting thermal energy that is naturally radiated from the body. As with the rest of the body, the tympanic membrane gives off heat waves known as *infrared waves*. The tympanic thermometer functions like a camera by taking a "picture" of these infrared waves, which are considered a documented indicator of body temperature (Figure 4-5). The thermometer calculates the body temperature from the energy generated by the waves and converts it to an oral or rectal equivalent.

The tympanic membrane thermometer is battery operated and consists of a small handheld device with a sensor probe (Figure 4-6). To operate the thermometer, the probe

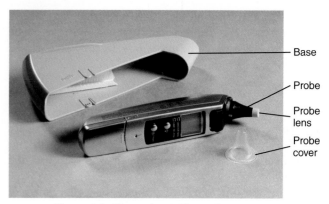

Figure 4-6. Tympanic membrane thermometer.

Base
Probe
Probe lens
Probe cover

is covered with a disposable soft plastic cover and is placed in the outer third of the external ear canal. An activation button is depressed momentarily, and the results are displayed in 1 to 2 seconds on a digital screen. The probe cover is ejected into a regular waste container. The procedure for taking aural body temperature using a tympanic membrane thermometer is presented in Procedure 4-4.

Temporal Artery Thermometer

Measuring temperature using a temporal artery thermometer is the newest method for assessing body temperature. A temporal artery thermometer is an electronic device consisting of a probe attached to a portable unit (Figure 4-7).

To perform the procedure, a scan button is continually depressed while the probe is gently and slowly moved across the patient's forehead. During this process, the probe sensor scans the forehead for the infrared heat given off by the temporal artery. The probe sensor captures the highest temperature or *peak temperature* in the area being scanned. The peak temperature represents the temperature given off by the temporal artery, or body temperature.

Along with measuring the peak temperature, the probe sensor automatically measures the *ambient temperature*, which is the surrounding air temperature. This is done because there is a small heat loss from the forehead that occurs

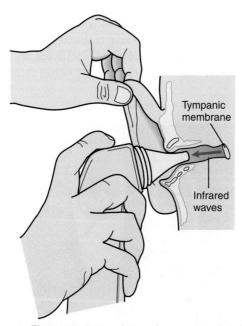

Figure 4-5. The tympanic membrane thermometer functions by detecting thermal energy that is naturally radiated from the tympanic membrane.

Tympanic membrane

Infrared waves

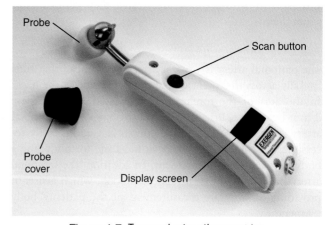

Probe

Scan button

Probe cover

Display screen

Figure 4-7. Temporal artery thermometer.

Guidelines for Using a Tympanic Membrane Thermometer

The following guidelines help ensure accurate aural temperature measurement with a tympanic membrane thermometer.

1. **Determine whether a tympanic thermometer can be used to measure the patient's temperature.** The tympanic thermometer should not be used on a patient with inflammation of the external ear canal (e.g., otitis externa) or when the ear contains a discharge such as blood or pus. The presence of otitis media and tympanostomy tubes does not significantly affect the temperature reading; a normal amount of cerumen also has no effect. An excessive buildup of cerumen that occludes the ear canal can result in a falsely low temperature reading.

2. **Determine whether external factors are present that may influence the temperature reading.** If any of these factors are present, remove the individual from the situation and wait 20 minutes before taking the temperature. External factors are present in an individual who has been lying on one ear or the other, who has had the ears covered (e.g., hat, ear muffs), who has been exposed to very hot or very cold temperatures, or who has been recently swimming or bathing. If an individual wears hearing aids, remove the hearing device from one ear and wait 20 minutes before taking temperature in that ear.

3. **Select the temperature measurement system desired.** The temperature of a tympanic membrane thermometer can be displayed in degrees Fahrenheit or degrees Celsius. Follow the manufacturer's instructions to change from one measurement to the other.

4. **Place the probe properly in the patient's ear.** The most important factor in obtaining an accurate temperature is proper placement of the probe in the patient's ear, which is outlined as follows.
   - **Straighten the ear canal.** The ear canal has an S shape that obstructs the view of the tympanic membrane. To obtain an accurate temperature measurement, the ear canal must be straightened before inserting the probe. This allows the probe sensor to obtain a clear picture of the tympanic membrane. In adults and children older than 3 years of age, the canal is straightened by gently pulling the ear auricle upward and backward. In children younger than 3 years of age, the canal is straightened by pulling the ear pinna downward and backward.
   - **Seal the opening of the ear.** The probe must be inserted tightly enough to seal the opening of the ear without causing patient discomfort. If the probe does not seal the ear canal, cooler external air can cause the thermometer to register a lower temperature.
   - **Correctly position the probe.** Position the tip of the probe toward the opposite temple (approximately midway between the opposite ear and the eyebrow). This allows the sensor to obtain the best possible picture of the tympanic membrane. If the tip is positioned incorrectly, it may be aimed at the ear canal, which results in a falsely low reading.

5. **Verify the accuracy of the temperature reading, if needed.** If you need to take the patient's temperature again, you can use the other ear. There are slight but insignificant differences between temperature readings in the right ear and those in the left ear. Before using the same ear, however, you must wait 2 minutes to allow the aural temperature to stabilize.

6. **Check the probe lens before taking the temperature.** The end of the probe is covered with a lens that is transparent to heat waves. To ensure an accurate temperature measurement, it is extremely important to keep this lens clean, dry, and intact. To protect the lens, always store the thermometer in its storage base when transporting or storing the thermometer. Before taking a temperature, always check to ensure that the lens is shiny and clear. Fingerprints, cerumen, and dust reduce the transparency of the lens, resulting in falsely low temperature readings. If the lens is dirty, it must be cleaned before taking the patient's temperature. If the lens is damaged, the thermometer cannot be used and must be repaired.

7. **Respond appropriately to digital messages.** A message to alert the user is displayed in the digital screen under the following circumstances:
   - An attempt is made to take a temperature without changing the cover after the last temperature.
   - An attempt is made to take a temperature with no probe cover in place.
   - The ambient (surrounding) temperature is not within the operating range for the thermometer 50° F (10° C) to 104° F (40° C).
   - The battery is low.
   - The thermometer is in need of repair.

8. **Care for the tympanic thermometer properly.**
   - **Probe lens.** Dust and other minute particles of environmental debris can build up on the probe lens during normal use. The lens should be cleaned as a part of routine maintenance or when it becomes dirty. If the thermometer is placed in the ear without a probe cover, immediately remove the probe and clean the lens. To clean the lens, gently wipe its surface with an antiseptic wipe and immediately wipe it dry with a cotton swab. After cleaning, allow at least 5 minutes before taking a temperature.
   - **Thermometer casing.** Clean the casing of the thermometer periodically by wiping it dry with a soft cloth slightly moistened with alcohol. Never submerge the thermometer in water or a cleaning solution. Do not use an abrasive cleaner on the casing, as this could damage the casing.

9. **Store the thermometer properly.** The thermometer must be stored in its storage base to protect the lens from damage and dirt. Store the thermometer in a clean, dry area within a temperature range of 50° F (10° C) to 104° F (40° C). Keep the thermometer away from temperature extremes, which could damage the thermometer.

as a result of cooling by ambient temperature. The thermometer's computer determines and automatically corrects for any effect from ambient temperature. An accurate body temperature reading is digitally displayed on the screen on the thermometer. The procedure for measuring temperature using a temporal artery thermometer is presented in Procedure 4-5.

Earlobe Temperature Measurement

Sweating of the forehead can cause an inaccurate temporal artery temperature reading. This is because perspiration causes the skin of the forehead to cool, resulting in a falsely low temperature reading. Sweating of the forehead occurs when a patient's fever breaks. It also occurs when a patient's skin is clammy; in this instance, forehead sweating may be present but not readily visible. To avoid this problem, the temperature of the neck area located just behind the earlobe also must be measured.

The area behind the earlobe is less affected by sweating than the forehead. During sweating, the blood vessels behind the earlobe dilate, resulting in a constant, steady flow of blood, which provides an accurate measurement of body temperature. After scanning the forehead, the medical assistant must place the probe of the thermometer in the soft depression of the neck just below the mastoid process of the ear. If the patient's forehead has cooled from sweating, the earlobe temperature automatically registers as the peak temperature, thereby overriding the forehead temperature.

The area behind the earlobe does not normally provide an accurate body temperature measurement and supersedes the forehead measurement only when the patient is in a diaphoretic state. Additional guidelines for temporal artery temperature measurement are presented in Box 4-1.

BOX 4-1 Temporal Artery Thermometer Guidelines

Guidelines

1. The operating environmental temperature for a temporal artery thermometer is 60° F to 104° F (15.5° C to 40° C).
2. Do not take temperature over scar tissue, open sores, or abrasions.
3. Ensure that the side of the head to be measured is exposed to the environment. Anything covering the area to be measured (e.g., hair, hat, wig, bandages) traps body heat, resulting in a falsely high reading.
4. A falsely low temporal artery reading can result from the following:
   - A dirty probe lens
   - Sweating of the forehead (in this instance, the earlobe measurement becomes the overriding temperature reading)
   - Scanning the forehead too quickly
   - Not keeping the button depressed while scanning the forehead and the area behind the earlobe

---

Care and Maintenance

The temporal artery thermometer should be stored in a clean, dry area. The thermometer must be protected from extremes in temperature, direct sunlight, and dust. The casing of the thermometer should be cleaned periodically with a soft cloth moistened with a solution of warm water and a disinfectant cleaner; never splash water on or immerse the unit in water because this could damage the internal components of the thermometer.

To obtain an accurate measurement, the probe lens must be clean and shiny. Dust and other minute particles of environmental debris can build up on the probe lens during normal use, preventing the probe sensor from getting an accurate "view" of the heat emitted by the temporal artery and resulting in a falsely low reading. The lens should be cleaned if it becomes dirty and as a part of routine maintenance. The lens is cleaned by gently wiping its surface with an antiseptic wipe and immediately wiping it dry with a cotton-tipped applicator stick.

Chemical Thermometers

Chemical thermometers contain chemicals that are heat sensitive and include disposable chemical single-use thermometers and temperature-sensitive strips. They are used most often by patients at home to measure body temperature. Although chemical thermometers are less accurate than other types of thermometers, they assist in providing a general assessment of body temperature. Because of their chemical makeup, they should be stored in a cool area, preferably colder than 86° F (30° C), and should not be exposed to direct sunlight because heat may cause the thermometer to register a higher temperature. Each type of chemical thermometer is described here.

Disposable Chemical Single-Use Thermometers

The disposable chemical single-use thermometer has small chemical dots at one end that respond to body heat by changing color (Figure 4-8, *A, B*). Each thermometer comes in its own wrapper. The protective wrapper must be peeled back to expose the handle of the thermometer. The thermometer is removed from the wrapper by pulling on the handle, taking care not to touch the dotted area. The thermometer is inserted under the tongue and is left in place for the duration of time recommended by the manufacturer (generally 60 seconds). After removal of the thermometer, the dots are observed for a change in color. The thermometer is read by noting the highest reading among the dots that have changed color (Figure 4-8, *C*). The thermometer is discarded after use.

Temperature-Sensitive Strips

A temperature-sensitive strip consists of a reusable plastic strip that contains heat-sensitive liquid crystals designed to measure body temperature. The plastic strip is pressed onto the forehead and is held in place until the colors stop changing, generally for 15 seconds. The results are read by observing the color change and noting the corresponding temperature indicated on the strip (Figure 4-9).

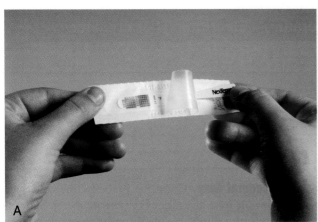
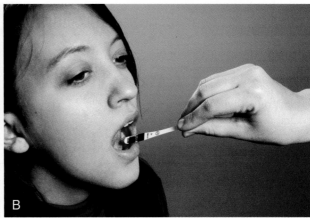

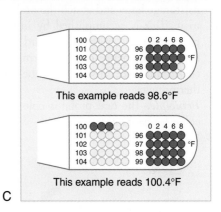

This example reads 98.6°F

This example reads 100.4°F

C

Figure 4-8. Disposable chemical single-use thermometers. **A,** The thermometer is removed from the wrapper by pulling on the handle. **B,** The thermometer is inserted under the tongue and is left in place for 60 seconds. **C,** The thermometer is read by noting the highest reading among the dots that have changed color.

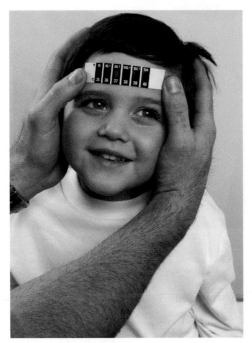

Figure 4-9. Temperature-sensitive strip. The plastic strip is pressed onto the forehead and is held in place until the color stops changing (generally for 15 seconds). The results are read by observing the color and noting the corresponding temperature indicated on the strip.

PROCEDURE 4-1   Measuring Oral Body Temperature—Electronic Thermometer

Outcome Measure oral body temperature.

Equipment/Supplies

- Electronic thermometer
- Oral probe (blue collar)
- Plastic probe cover
- Waste container

1. Procedural Step. Sanitize your hands, and assemble the equipment.

2. Procedural Step. Remove the thermometer unit from its storage base, and attach the oral (blue collar) probe to it. This is accomplished by inserting the latching plug (at the end of the coiled cord of the oral probe) to the plug receptacle on the thermometer unit until it clicks into place. Insert the probe into the face of the thermometer.

Principle. The oral probe is color-coded with a blue collar for ease in identifying it.

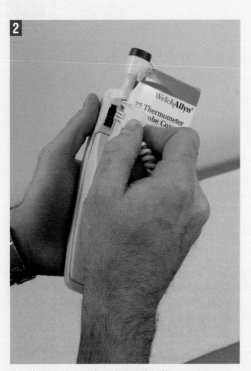

Attach the oral probe to the thermometer.

3. Procedural Step. Greet the patient and introduce yourself. Identify the patient and explain the procedure. If the patient has recently ingested hot or cold food or beverages or has been smoking, you must wait 15 to 30 minutes before taking the temperature.

Principle. Ingestion of hot or cold food or beverages and smoking change the temperature of the mouth, which could result in an inaccurate reading.

4. Procedural Step. Grasp the probe by the collar, and remove it from the face of the thermometer. Slide the probe into a disposable plastic probe cover until it locks into place.

Principle. Removing the probe from the thermometer automatically turns on the thermometer. The probe cover prevents the transfer of microorganisms from one patient to another.

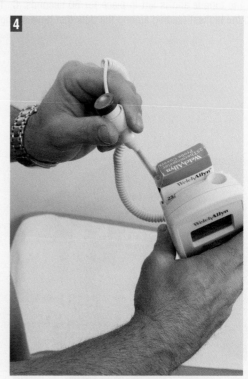

Slide the probe into a probe cover.

5. Procedural Step. Take the patient's temperature by inserting the probe under the patient's tongue in the pocket located on either side of the frenulum linguae. Instruct the patient to keep the mouth closed.

Principle. There is a good blood supply in the tissue under the tongue. The mouth must be kept closed to prevent cooler air from entering and affecting the temperature reading.

PROCEDURE 4-1   Measuring Oral Body Temperature—Electronic Thermometer—cont'd

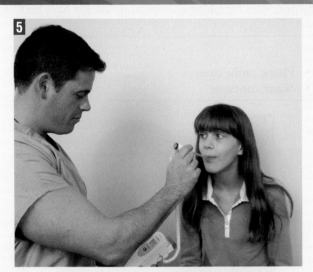

5

Insert the probe under the patient's tongue.

6. Procedural Step. Hold the probe in place until you hear the tone. At that time, the patient's temperature appears as a digital display on the screen. Make a mental note of the temperature reading. (The temperature indicated on this thermometer is 98.2° F [36.8° C]).

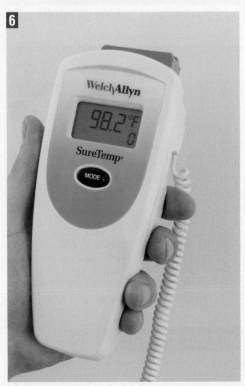

6

WelchAllyn

98.2°F
C

SureTemp®

MODE

The patient's temperature appears as a digital display on the screen.

7. Procedural Step. Remove the probe from the patient's mouth. Discard the probe cover by firmly pressing the ejection button while holding the probe over a regular waste container. Do not allow your fingers to come in contact with the probe cover.
Principle. The probe cover should not be touched so as to prevent the transfer of microorganisms from the patient to the medical assistant. Saliva is not considered regulated medical waste; the probe can be discarded in a regular waste container.

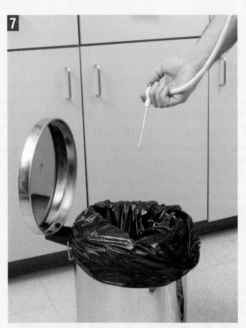

7

Discard the probe cover by pressing the ejection button.

8. Procedural Step. Return the probe to its stored position in the thermometer unit. Return the thermometer unit to its storage base.
Principle. Returning the probe to the unit automatically turns off and resets the thermometer.

9. Procedural Step. Sanitize your hands, and chart the results. Include the date, the time, and the temperature reading.
Principle. Patient data must be recorded properly to aid the physician in the diagnosis and to provide future reference.

CHARTING EXAMPLE

Date	
10/15/12	2:15 p.m. T: 98.2° F.____S. Martinez, RMA

PROCEDURE 4-1

PROCEDURE 4-2   Measuring Axillary Body Temperature—Electronic Thermometer

Outcome Measure axillary body temperature. *Note:* Many of the principles for taking a temperature already have been stated and are not included in this procedure.

Equipment/Supplies

- Electronic thermometer
- Oral probe (blue collar)
- Plastic probe cover
- Waste container

1. **Procedural Step.** Sanitize your hands, and assemble the equipment.
2. **Procedural Step.** Remove the thermometer unit from its storage base, and attach the oral (blue collar) probe to it. This is accomplished by inserting the latching plug (on the end of the coiled cord of the oral probe) to the plug receptacle on the thermometer unit until it locks into place. Insert the probe into the face of the thermometer.
3. **Procedural Step.** Greet the patient and introduce yourself. Identify the patient and explain the procedure.
4. **Procedural Step.** Remove clothing from the patient's shoulder and arm. Ensure that the axilla is dry. If it is wet, pat it dry with a paper towel or a gauze pad.
   Principle. Clothing removal provides optimal exposure of the axilla for proper placement of the thermometer. Rubbing the axilla causes an increase in the temperature in that area owing to friction, resulting in an inaccurate temperature reading.
5. **Procedural Step.** Grasp the probe by the collar, and remove it from the face of the thermometer. Slide the probe into a disposable probe cover until it locks into place.
6. **Procedural Step.** Take the patient's temperature by placing the probe in the center of the patient's axilla. Instruct the patient to hold the arm close to the body. Hold the arm in place for small children and other patients who cannot maintain the position themselves.
   Principle. Interference from outside air currents is reduced when the arm is held in the proper position.
7. **Procedural Step.** Hold the probe in place until you hear the tone. At that time, the patient's temperature appears as a digital display on the screen. Make a mental note of the temperature reading.
8. **Procedural Step.** Remove the probe from the patient's axilla. Discard the probe cover by firmly pressing the ejection button while holding the probe over a regular waste container. Do not allow your fingers to come in contact with the probe cover.
9. **Procedural Step.** Return the probe to its stored position in the thermometer unit. Return the thermometer unit to its storage base.
10. **Procedural Step.** Sanitize your hands, and chart the results. Include the date, the time, and the axillary temperature reading. The symbol Ⓐ must be charted next to the temperature reading to tell the physician that an axillary reading was taken.

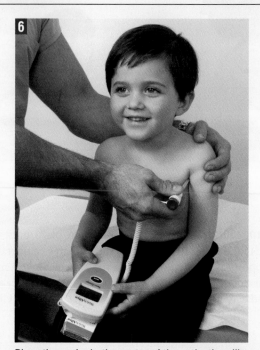

Place the probe in the center of the patient's axilla.

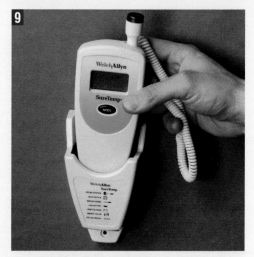

Return the thermometer to its base.

CHARTING EXAMPLE

Date	
10/15/12	9:30 a.m. T: 97.4° F Ⓐ S. Martinez, RMA

PROCEDURE 4-3   Measuring Rectal Body Temperature—Electronic Thermometer

Outcome   Measure rectal body temperature.

Equipment/Supplies

- Electronic thermometer
- Rectal probe (red collar)
- Plastic probe cover
- Lubricant

- Disposable gloves
- Tissues
- Waste container

1. **Procedural Step.** Sanitize your hands, and assemble the equipment.
2. **Procedural Step.** Remove the thermometer unit from its storage base. Attach the rectal (red collar) probe to it. This is accomplished by inserting the latching plug (on the end of the coiled cord of the rectal probe) to the plug receptacle on the thermometer unit. Insert the probe into the face of the thermometer.
   Principle. The rectal probe is color-coded with a red collar for ease in identifying it.
3. **Procedural Step.** Greet the patient and introduce yourself. Identify the patient and explain the procedure. If a patient is a child or an adult, provide him or her with a patient gown. Instruct the patient to remove enough clothing to provide access to the anal area and to put on the gown with the opening in the back. If the patient is an infant, ask the parent to remove his or her diaper.
   Principle. It is important to explain what you will be doing, because body temperature may be higher in a fearful or apprehensive patient. The patient gown provides the patient with modesty and comfort.
4. **Procedural Step.** Apply gloves. Position the patient. ***Adults and children:*** Position the patient in the Sims position, and drape the patient to expose only the anal area. ***Infants:*** Position the infant on his or her abdomen.
   Principle. Gloves protect the medical assistant from microorganisms in the anal area and feces. Correct positioning allows clear viewing of the anal opening and provides for proper insertion of the thermometer. Draping reduces patient embarrassment and provides warmth.
5. **Procedural Step.** Grasp the probe by the collar, and remove it from the face of the thermometer. Slide the probe into a disposable plastic probe cover until it locks into place. Apply a lubricant to the tip of the probe cover up to a level of 1 inch.
   Principle. A lubricated thermometer can be inserted more easily and does not irritate the delicate rectal mucosa.

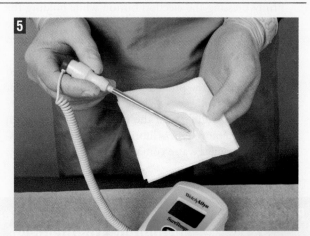

Apply a lubricant to the tip of the probe cover.

6. **Procedural Step.** Instruct the patient to lie still. Separate the buttocks to expose the anal opening, and gently insert the thermometer probe approximately 1 inch into the rectum of an adult, ⅝ inch in children, and ½ inch in infants. Do not force insertion of the probe. Hold the probe in place until the temperature registers.
   Principle. The probe must be inserted correctly to prevent injury to the tissue of the anal opening. The probe should be held in place to prevent damage to the rectal mucosa.

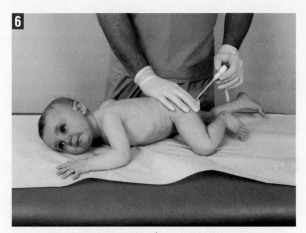

Gently insert the probe ½ inch into the rectum.

Continued

PROCEDURE 4-3

PROCEDURE 4-3   Measuring Rectal Body Temperature—Electronic Thermometer—cont'd

7. Procedural Step. Hold the probe in place until you hear the tone. At that time, the patient's temperature appears as a digital display on the screen. Make a mental note of the temperature reading.

8. Procedural Step. Gently remove the probe from the rectum in the same direction as it was inserted. Avoid touching the probe cover. Discard the probe cover by firmly pressing the ejection button while holding the probe over a regular waste container. Return the probe to its stored position in the thermometer unit. Return the thermometer unit to its storage base.

Principle. Fecal material is not considered regulated medical waste; the probe can be discarded in a regular waste container.

9. Procedural Step. Wipe the patient's anal area with tissues to remove excess lubricant. Dispose of the tissues in a regular waste container.

Principle. Wiping the anal area makes the patient more comfortable.

10. Procedural Step. Remove gloves, and sanitize your hands. Chart the results. Include the date, the time, and the rectal temperature reading. The symbol Ⓡ must be charted next to the temperature reading to tell the physician that a rectal reading was taken.

CHARTING EXAMPLE	
Date	
10/15/12	11:15 a.m. T: 99.8° F Ⓡ —————
	————— S. Martinez, RMA

PROCEDURE 4-4   Measuring Aural Body Temperature—Tympanic Membrane Thermometer

Outcome Measure aural body temperature.

Equipment/Supplies

- Tympanic membrane thermometer
- Probe cover
- Waste container

1. Procedural Step. Sanitize your hands, and assemble the equipment.

Principle. Your hands should be clean and free from contamination.

2. Procedural Step. Greet the patient and introduce yourself. Identify the patient and explain the procedure.

Principle. It is important to explain what you will be doing, because body temperature may be higher in a fearful or apprehensive patient.

3. Procedural Step. Remove the thermometer from its storage base. Ensure that the probe lens is clean and intact.

Principle. A dirty or damaged probe lens could result in a falsely low temperature reading.

4. Procedural Step. Attach a cover on the probe by pressing the probe tip straight down into the cover box. You will be able to see and feel the cover snap securely into place on the probe. This procedure automatically turns on the thermometer.

Principle. The probe cover protects the lens and provides infection control. The cover must be seated securely on the probe to activate the thermometer.

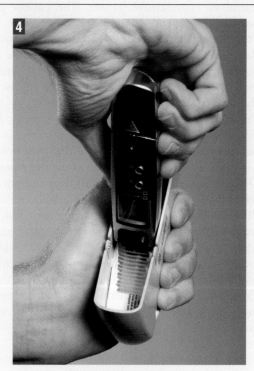

Place a cover on the probe.

PROCEDURE 4-4   Measuring Aural Body Temperature—Tympanic Membrane Thermometer—cont'd

5. Procedural Step. Pull the probe straight up from the cover box. Look at the digital display to see if the thermometer is ready to use.

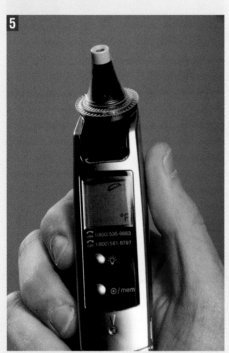

When the thermometer is ready, it displays the word READY.

6. Procedural Step. Hold the thermometer in your dominant hand. If you are right-handed, you should take the temperature in the patient's right ear. If you are left-handed, take the temperature in the patient's left ear.
Principle. Taking the temperature with the dominant hand assists in the proper placement of the probe in the patient's ear.

7. Procedural Step. Straighten the patient's external ear canal with your nondominant hand, as follows:
Adults and Children Older Than 3 Years Old. Gently pull the ear auricle upward and backward.
Children Younger Than 3 Years Old. Gently pull the ear pinna downward and backward.
Principle. Straightening the ear canal allows the probe sensor to obtain a clear picture of the tympanic membrane, resulting in an accurate temperature measurement.

8. Procedural Step. Insert the probe into the patient's ear canal tightly enough to seal the opening, but without causing patient discomfort. Point the tip of the probe toward the opposite temple (approximately midway between the opposite ear and eyebrow).
Principle. Sealing the ear canal prevents cooler external air from entering the ear, which could result in a

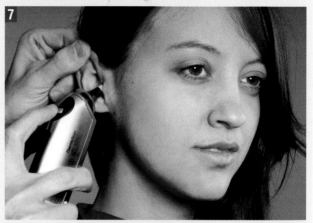

Straighten the canal of adults and children older than 3 years by pulling the ear auricle upward and backward.

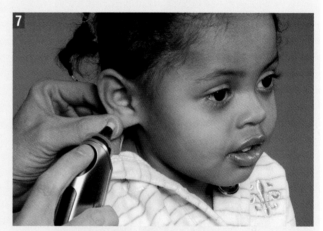

Straighten the canal of children younger than 3 years by pulling the ear auricle downward and backward.

falsely low reading. Correct positioning of the probe optimizes the sensor's view of the tympanic membrane, leading to an accurate temperature reading.

9. Procedural Step. Ask the patient to remain still. Hold the thermometer steady, and depress the activation button. Depending on the brand of the thermometer, perform one of the following:
a. Hold the button down for one full second, and then release it, or
b. Hold down the button down until an audible tone is heard.
Principle. The thermometer cannot take a temperature unless the activation button is depressed for 1 full second. When the button is depressed, the infrared sensor in the probe scans the thermal energy radiated by the tympanic membrane.

10. Procedural Step. Remove the thermometer from the ear canal. Turn the digital display of the thermometer toward you, and read the temperature. Make a mental note of the temperature reading. If the temperature

Continued

PROCEDURE 4-4   Measuring Aural Body Temperature—Tympanic Membrane Thermometer—cont'd

seems to be too low, repeat the procedure to ensure that you have used the proper technique. The temperature indicated on this thermometer is 99.8° F (37.7° C). The temperature remains on the display screen for 30 to 60 seconds or until another cover is inserted on the probe (whichever occurs first).

Principle. The temperature remains on the display screen until another cover is inserted on the probe. Improper technique can result in a falsely low temperature reading.

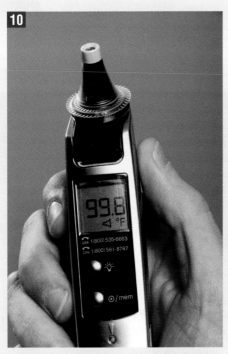

Read the temperature on the digital display.

11. **Procedural Step.** Dispose of the probe cover by ejecting it into a regular waste container.

12. Procedural Step. Replace the thermometer in its storage base.

Principle. The thermometer should be stored in its base to protect the probe lens from damage and dirt.

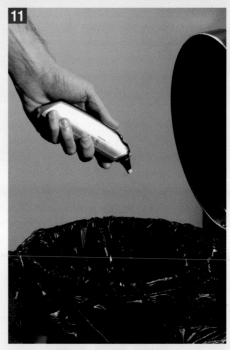

Dispose of the probe cover.

13. Procedural Step. Sanitize your hands.

14. Procedural Step. Chart the results. Include the date, the time, the aural temperature reading, and which ear was used to take the temperature (AD: right ear; AS: left ear). When these abbreviations are used, the physician knows that the temperature was taken through the aural route.

CHARTING EXAMPLE	
Date	
10/15/12	3:00 p.m. T: 99.8° F, AD ———————— ———————— S. Martinez, RMA

PROCEDURE 4-5   Measuring Temporal Artery Body Temperature

Outcome Measure temporal artery body temperature.

Equipment/Supplies

- Temporal artery thermometer
- Probe cover
- Antiseptic wipe
- Waste container

1. **Procedural Step.** Sanitize your hands, and assemble the equipment.
2. **Procedural Step.** Greet the patient and introduce yourself. Identify the patient and explain the procedure.
3. **Procedural Step.** Examine the probe lens of the temporal artery thermometer to ensure that the lens is clean and intact.
   Principle. A dirty or damaged probe lens could result in a falsely low temperature reading.
4. **Procedural Step.** Place a disposable cover over the probe. If the thermometer does not use disposable covers, clean the probe with an antiseptic wipe, and allow it to dry.
   Principle. Applying a probe cover or cleaning the probe with an antiseptic wipe provides infection control.

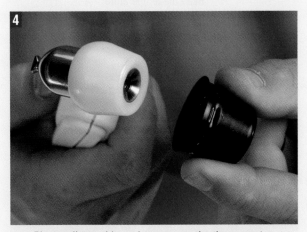

Place a disposable probe cover on the thermometer.

5. **Procedural Step.** Select an appropriate site; the right or left side of the forehead can be used. The site selected should be fully exposed to the environment.
   Principle. The temporal artery is located in the center of each side of the forehead, approximately 2 mm below the surface of the skin.
6. **Procedural Step.** Prepare the patient by brushing away any hair that is covering the side of the forehead to be scanned and the area behind the earlobe on the same side.
   Principle. Hair covering the area to be measured traps body heat, resulting in a falsely high temperature reading.

7. **Procedural Step.** Hold the thermometer in your dominant hand with your thumb on the scan button.
8. **Procedural Step.** Gently position the probe of the thermometer on the center of the patient's forehead, midway between the eyebrow and the hairline.

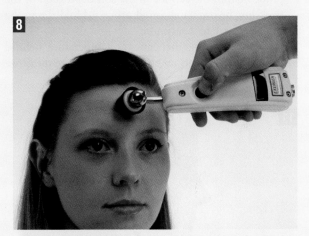

Position the probe on the center of the patient's forehead.

9. **Procedural Step.** Depress the scan button, and keep it depressed for the entire measurement.
   Principle. Not keeping the scan button depressed can result in a falsely low temperature reading.
10. **Procedural Step.** Slowly and gently slide the probe straight across the forehead, midway between the eyebrow and the upper hairline. Continue until the hairline

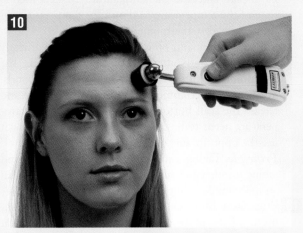

Slowly slide the probe straight across the patient's forehead.

Continued

PROCEDURE 4-5   Measuring Temporal Artery Body Temperature—cont'd

is reached. Keep the scan button depressed and the probe flush (flat) against the forehead. During this time, a beeping sound occurs and a red light blinks to indicate that a measurement is taking place. Rapid beeping and blinking indicate a rise to a higher temperature. Slow beeping indicates that the thermometer is still scanning but is not finding a higher temperature.

Principle. The thermometer continually scans for the peak temperature as long as the scan button is depressed. The probe must be held flat against the forehead to ensure accurate scanning of the temporal artery.

11. Procedural Step. Keeping the button depressed, lift the probe from the forehead, and gently place the probe behind the earlobe in the soft depression of the neck just below the mastoid process. Hold the probe in place for 1 to 2 seconds.

Principle. Taking the patient's temperature behind the earlobe prevents an error in temperature measurement in the event that the patient is sweating.

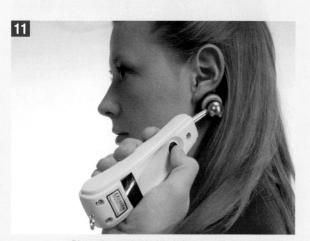

Place the probe behind the ear lobe.

12. Procedural Step. Release the scan button on the digital display, and read the temperature. Make a mental note of the temperature reading (The temperature indicated on this thermometer is 99.1° F [37.3° C]). The reading remains on the display for approximately 15 to 30 seconds after the button is released. The thermometer shuts off automatically after 30 seconds. To turn the thermometer off immediately, press and release the scan button quickly. If the patient's temperature needs to be taken again, wait 60 seconds, or use the opposite side of the forehead.

Principle. Taking a measurement cools the skin, and taking another measurement too soon may result in an inaccurate reading.

13. Procedural Step. Dispose of the probe cover by pushing it off the probe with your thumb and ejecting it into a regular waste container. Wipe the probe with an antiseptic wipe, and allow it to dry.

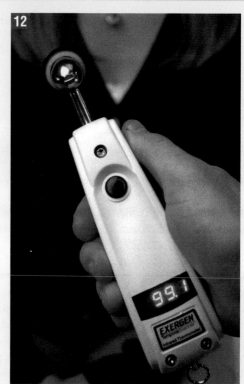

Read the temperature.

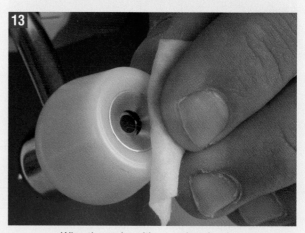

Wipe the probe with an antiseptic wipe.

14. Procedural Step. Sanitize your hands, and chart the results. Include the date, the time, and the temperature reading. The symbol (TA) must be charted next to the temperature reading to tell the physician that a temporal artery reading was taken. Store the thermometer in a clean, dry area.

CHARTING EXAMPLE

Date	
10/15/12	9:15 a.m. T: 99.1° F (TA) ——————
	—————————————— S. Martinez, RMA

PULSE

Mechanism of the Pulse

When the left ventricle of the heart contracts, blood is forced from the heart into the **aorta,** which is the major trunk of the arterial system of the body. The aorta is already filled with blood and must expand to accept the blood being pushed out of the left ventricle. This creates a pulsating wave that travels from the aorta through the walls of the arterial system. This wave, known as the *pulse,* can be felt as a light tap by an examiner. The pulse rate is measured by counting the number of "taps," or beats per minute. The heart rate can be determined by taking the pulse rate.

Factors Affecting Pulse Rate

Pulse rate can vary depending on many factors. The medical assistant should take each of the following into consideration when measuring pulse:

1. **Age.** The pulse varies inversely with age. As age increases, the pulse rate gradually decreases. Table 4-4 lists the pulse rates of various age groups.
2. **Gender.** Women tend to have a slightly faster pulse rate than men.
3. **Physical activity.** Physical activity, such as jogging and swimming, increases the pulse rate temporarily.

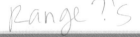

Table 4-4 Pulse Rates of Various Age Groups		
Age Group	**Pulse Range (beats/min)**	**Average Pulse (beats/min)**
Infant (birth to 1 yr)	120-160	140
Toddler (1-3 yr)	90-140	115
Preschool child (3-6 yr)	80-110	95
School-age child (6-12 yr)	75-105	90
Adolescent (12-18 yr)	60-100	80
Adult (after 18th yr)	60-100	80
Adult (after 60th yr)	67-80	74
Well-trained athletes	40-60	50

What Would You Do? What Would You *Not* Do?

Case Study 1

Marcela Mason comes in with Olivia, her 5-year-old daughter. Olivia has had a fever and sore throat for the past 2 days. Olivia's aural temperature is taken in her left ear, and it measures 103.3°F. Mrs. Mason says that she has an ear thermometer at home, but when she took Olivia's temperature with it, the readings were always below 97°F. She knew that could not be right because Olivia felt so warm. Mrs. Mason would like to be able to use her ear thermometer, but she thinks that it might be broken because of the low readings. Mrs. Mason says that she is thinking of switching back to a mercury glass thermometer, but she has heard that it isn't a good idea to use this type of thermometer anymore and wants to know why. ■

Memories *from* Externship

Sergio Martinez: One experience that really stands out in my memory occurred during my externship at a family practice medical office. I needed to take the blood pressure of a small 6-year-old boy. After I put the cuff on his arm, his eyes started filling up with tears. I stopped, removed the cuff, and asked him if something was wrong. He said he was afraid that, when I started squeezing that thing around his arm, his hand would fall off. I sat down next to him, spent some time talking with him, and reassured him that his hand would be perfectly fine and would not fall off. I put the cuff on my arm and pumped it up to show him that he would be safe. He then agreed to let me take his blood pressure. After I took his blood pressure, he wiggled his hand, gave me a big smile, and said that it didn't hurt at all. That situation made me realize that children may have a lot of fears about what might happen to them at the medical office. Since that experience, I always take the time to explain procedures to children before I perform them. ■

4. **Emotional states.** Strong emotional states, such as anxiety, fear, excitement, and anger, temporarily increase the pulse rate.
5. **Metabolism.** Increased body metabolism, such as occurs during pregnancy, increases the pulse rate.
6. **Fever.** Fever increases the pulse rate.
7. **Medications.** Medications may alter the pulse rate. For example, digitalis decreases the pulse rate, and epinephrine increases it.

Pulse Sites

The pulse is felt most strongly when a superficial artery is held against a firm tissue, such as bone. The locations of sites used for measuring the pulse are shown in Figure 4-10 and are described next.

Radial

The most common site for measuring the pulse is the radial artery, which is located in a groove on the inner aspect of the wrist just below the thumb. The radial pulse is easily accessible and can be measured with no discomfort to the patient. This site is also used by individuals at home monitoring their own heart rates, such as athletes, patients taking heart medication, and individuals starting an exercise program. The procedure for measuring radial pulse is outlined in Procedure 4-6.

Apical

The apical pulse has a stronger beat and is easier to measure than the other pulse sites. If the medical assistant is having difficulty feeling the radial pulse, or if the radial pulse is irregular or abnormally slow or rapid, the apical pulse should be taken (Procedure 4-7). This pulse site is often used to measure pulse in infants and in children up to 3 years old because the other sites are difficult to palpate accurately in these age groups. The apical pulse is measured

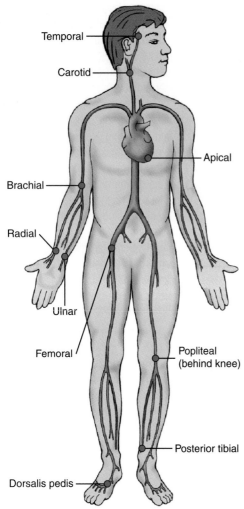

Figure 4-10. Pulse sites.

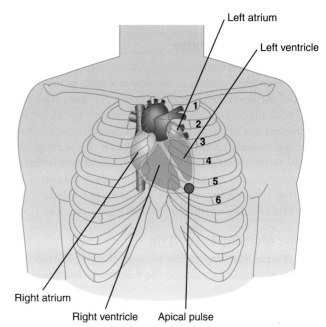

Figure 4-11. The apical pulse is found over the apex of the heart, which is located in the fifth intercostal space at the junction of the left midclavicular line.

using a stethoscope. The chest piece of the stethoscope is placed lightly over the apex of the heart, which is located in the fifth **intercostal** (between the ribs) space at the junction of the left midclavicular line (Figure 4-11).

Brachial

The brachial pulse is in the **antecubital space,** which is the space located at the front of the elbow. This site is used to take blood pressure, to measure pulse in infants during cardiac arrest, and to assess the status of the circulation to the lower arm.

Ulnar

The ulnar pulse is located on the ulnar (little finger) side of the wrist. It is used to assess the status of circulation to the hand.

Temporal

The temporal pulse is located in front of the ear and just above eye level. This site is used to measure pulse when the radial pulse is inaccessible. It is also an easy access site to assess pulse in children.

Carotid

The carotid pulse is located on the anterior side of the neck, slightly to one side of the midline, and is the best site to find a pulse quickly. This site is used to measure pulse in children and adults during cardiac arrest. The carotid site also is commonly used by individuals to monitor pulse during exercise.

Femoral

The femoral pulse is in the middle of the groin. This site is used to measure pulse in infants and children and in adults during cardiac arrest, and to assess the status of circulation to the lower leg.

Popliteal

The popliteal pulse is at the back of the knee and is detected most easily when the knee is slightly flexed. This site is used to measure blood pressure when the brachial pulse is inaccessible and to assess the status of circulation to the lower leg.

Posterior Tibial

The posterior tibial pulse is located on the inner aspect of the ankle just posterior to the ankle bone. This site is used to assess the status of circulation to the foot.

Dorsalis Pedis

The dorsalis pedis pulse is located on the upper surface of the foot, between the first and second metatarsal bones. This site is used to assess the status of circulation to the foot.

Assessment of Pulse

The purpose of measuring pulse is to establish the patient's baseline pulse rate and to assess the pulse rate after special procedures, medications, or disease processes that affect heart functioning. Pulse is measured using palpation at all of the pulse sites except the apical site.

Pulse is palpated by applying moderate pressure with the sensitive pads located on the tips of the three middle fingers. The pulse should not be taken with the thumb because the thumb has a pulse of its own. This could result in measurement of the medical assistant's pulse rather than the patient's pulse. Excessive pressure should not be applied when measuring pulse because this could obliterate, or close off, the pulse. It may not be possible to detect the pulse if too little pressure is applied, however. An accurate assessment of pulse includes determinations of the pulse rate, the pulse rhythm, and the pulse volume.

Pulse Rate

The pulse rate is the number of heart pulsations or heartbeats that occur in 1 minute; therefore, pulse rate is measured in beats per minute. Normal pulse rates vary widely in the various age groups, as shown in Table 4-4. For a healthy adult, the normal resting pulse rate ranges from 60 to 100 beats per minute, with the average falling between 70 and 80 beats per minute.

An abnormally fast heart rate of more than 100 beats per minute is known as **tachycardia.** Tachycardia may indicate disease states such as hemorrhaging or heart disease. Tachycardia usually occurs when an individual is involved in vigorous physical exercise or is experiencing strong emotional states.

Bradycardia is an abnormally slow heart rate—less than 60 beats per minute. A pulse rate of less than 60 beats per minute may occur normally during sleep. Trained athletes often have low pulse rates. If a patient exhibits tachycardia or bradycardia during radial pulse measurement, the apical pulse should also be measured.

Pulse Rhythm and Volume

In addition to measuring the pulse rate, the medical assistant should determine the rhythm and volume of the pulse. The **pulse rhythm** denotes the time interval between heartbeats; a normal rhythm has the same time interval between beats. Any irregularity in the heart's rhythm is known as a **dysrhythmia** (also termed *arrhythmia*) and is characterized by unequal or irregular intervals between the heartbeats. If a dysrhythmia is present, the physician may order one or

---

PATIENT TEACHING   Aerobic Exercise

Answer questions patients have about aerobic exercise.

What is aerobic exercise?
Aerobic exercise increases, sustains, and decreases your pulse over time. Aerobic exercise is accomplished through steady, nonstop activity, such as walking, jogging, cycling, or swimming. Each workout should include warm-up and cool-down periods of at least 5 minutes each. This is needed to prevent muscle or joint injuries.

What are the benefits of an aerobic exercise program?
The benefits of an aerobic exercise program include strengthening of the heart, a slower resting pulse rate, reduction of stress, increased energy, lowering of body fat, decreased "bad" (low-density lipoprotein) cholesterol, and increased "good" (high-density lipoprotein) cholesterol. The key to a safe and effective aerobic exercise program is the target heart rate (THR).

What is target heart rate?
Your THR is a safe and effective exercise pulse range that indicates that you are exercising at the right level for your age and for what you are trying to accomplish with exercise. Exercising at a level below your THR does little to promote fitness; exercising at a level above your THR may not be safe.

How do I determine my target heart rate?
The following formula is used to determine your THR:
1. Subtract your age from 220 to determine your maximum heart rate (MHR), which is the fastest your heart can beat safely for your age. The MHR of a 40-year-old person is calculated as follows:

$$220 - 40 \text{ years old} = 180 \text{ (MHR)}$$

2. Determine the lower end of your THR range by multiplying your MHR by 0.6. For our example:

$$180 \times 0.60 = 108 \text{ (low end of THR)}$$

3. Determine the upper end of your THR range by multiplying your MHR by 0.8. For our example:

$$180 \times 0.80 = 144 \text{ (upper end of THR)}$$

Always exercise within your THR range. The 40-year-old person in our example should exercise with a THR between 108 and 144.

How often should aerobic exercise be performed?
To promote and maintain health, the American Heart Association recommends that healthy adults aged 18 to 65 spend at least 30 minutes a day, 5 days a week, in moderately intense aerobic exercise (e.g., brisk walking), or 20 minutes, 3 days each week, in vigorous-intensity exercise (e.g., jogging), or a combination of moderate and vigorous exercise. These moderate- and vigorous-intensity recommendations should be added to the light-intensity activities of daily living such as washing dishes and taking out the trash. In addition, the AHA recommends that adults perform activities that maintain or increase muscular strength and endurance a minimum of 2 days each week. The American Heart Association further recommends that children and adolescents engage in at least 60 minutes per day of moderate to vigorous physical activity. ■

more of the following: an apical-radial pulse, an electrocardiogram, or Holter monitoring.

An **apical-radial pulse** is performed to determine whether a pulse deficit is present. Taking an apical-radial pulse involves measuring the apical pulse at the same time as the radial pulse for a duration of 1 full minute. A **pulse deficit** exists when the radial pulse rate is less than the apical pulse rate. If one medical assistant measures an apical pulse rate of 88 beats per minute, and another medical assistant simultaneously measures a radial pulse rate of 76 beats per minute, this results in a pulse deficit of 12 beats. A pulse deficit means that not all of the heartbeats are reaching the peripheral arteries. A pulse deficit is caused by an inefficient contraction of the heart that is not strong enough to transmit a pulse wave to the peripheral pulse site. A pulse deficit frequently occurs with atrial fibrillation, which is a type of dysrhythmia.

The **pulse volume** refers to the strength of the heartbeat. The amount of blood pumped into the aorta by each contraction of the left ventricle should remain constant, making the pulse feel strong and full. If the blood volume decreases, the pulse feels weak and may be difficult to detect. This type of pulse is usually accompanied by a fast heart rate and is described as a **thready pulse.** An increase in the blood volume results in a pulse that feels extremely strong and full, known as a **bounding pulse.**

Any abnormalities in the rhythm or volume of the pulse should be recorded accurately in the patient's chart by the medical assistant. A pulse that has a normal rhythm and volume is recorded as being regular and strong.

RESPIRATION
Mechanism of Respiration

The purpose of respiration is to provide for the exchange of oxygen and carbon dioxide between the atmosphere and the blood. Oxygen is taken into the body to be used for vital body processes, and carbon dioxide is given off as a waste product.

Each respiration is divided into two phases: **inhalation** and **exhalation** (Figure 4-12). During inhalation, or inspiration, the diaphragm descends and the lungs expand, causing air containing oxygen to move from the atmosphere into the lungs. Exhalation, or expiration, involves the removal of carbon dioxide from the body. The diaphragm ascends, and the lungs return to their original state

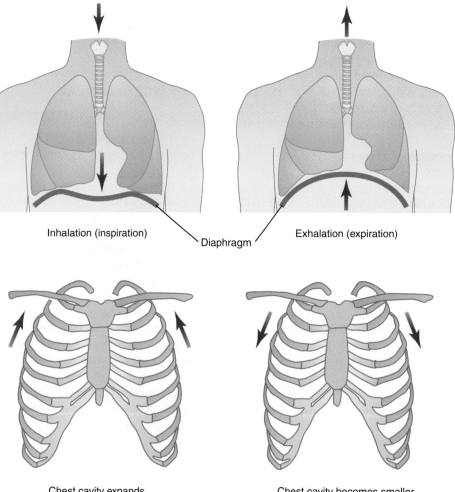

Inhalation (inspiration)   Diaphragm   Exhalation (expiration)

Chest cavity expands   Chest cavity becomes smaller

Figure 4-12. Inhalation and exhalation.

so that air containing carbon dioxide is expelled. One complete respiration is composed of one inhalation and one exhalation.

Respiration can be classified as *external* or *internal.* External respiration involves the exchange of oxygen and carbon dioxide between the **alveolus** (thin-walled sacs) of the lungs and the blood (Figure 4-13). The blood, located in small capillaries, comes in contact with the alveoli, picks up oxygen, and carries it to the cells of the body. At this point, the oxygen is given off to the cells, and carbon dioxide is picked up by the blood to be transported as a waste product to the lungs. The exchange of oxygen and carbon dioxide between the body cells and the blood is known as *internal respiration.*

Control of Respiration

The medulla oblongata, located in the brain, is the control center for involuntary respiration. A buildup of carbon dioxide in the blood sends a message to the medulla, which triggers respiration to occur automatically.

To a certain extent, respiration is also under voluntary control. An individual can control respiration during activities such as singing, laughing, talking, eating, and crying. Voluntary respiration is ultimately under the control of the medulla oblongata. The breath can be held for only a certain length of time, after which carbon dioxide begins to

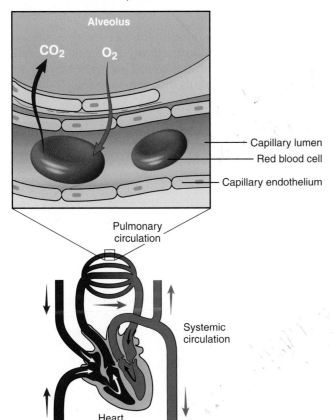

External Respiration

Alveolus

CO_2 O_2

Capillary lumen
Red blood cell

Capillary endothelium

Pulmonary circulation

Systemic circulation

Heart

Figure 4-13. Exchange of oxygen and carbon dioxide between the alveoli of the lungs and the blood.

Case Study 2

Alex Jacoby is 18 years old and a senior in high school. He comes to the office complaining of severe pain in his left shoulder. Alex is an outstanding competitive swimmer and is currently ranked first in the state in the 100-yard butterfly. Alex has a big meet coming up and must do well because he has a chance of getting an athletic scholarship to the University of Florida. He says he thinks he can take 2 seconds off his best time at this meet and he doesn't want anything to interfere with that. Alex wants the physician to do whatever he can to make his shoulder better and thinks that a steroid injection and OxyContin might be the answer. His vital signs are as follows: temperature 98.5° F, pulse 48 beats/min, respirations 12 breaths/min, and blood pressure 108/68 mm Hg. Alex asks why his pulse is so slow and wants to know if there is any medication that he can take to make it faster. ■

build up in the body, resulting in a stimulus to the medulla that causes respiration to occur involuntarily. Small children may voluntarily hold their breath during a temper tantrum. A parent who does not understand the principles of respiration may be concerned that the child would cease to breathe. The medical assistant should be able to explain that involuntary respiration would eventually occur and the child would resume breathing.

Assessment of Respiration

Because an individual can control his or her respiration, the medical assistant should measure respirations without the patient's knowledge. Patients may change their respiratory rate unintentionally if they are aware that they are being measured. An ideal time to measure respiration is after the pulse is taken. Procedure 4-6 outlines the procedures for taking pulse and respiration in one continuous procedure.

Respiratory Rate

The respiratory rate of a normal healthy adult ranges from 12 to 20 respirations per minute. With most adults, there is a ratio of one respiration for every four pulse beats. If the respiratory rate is 18, the pulse rate would be approximately 72 beats per minute. An abnormal increase in the respiratory rate of more than 20 respirations per minute is referred to as **tachypnea.** An abnormal decrease in the respiratory rate of less than 12 respirations per minute is known as **bradypnea.** When measuring the respiratory rate, the medical assistant should take into consideration the following factors:

1. **Age.** As age increases, the respiratory rate decreases. The respiratory rate of a child would be expected to be faster than that of an adult. Table 4-5 provides a chart of the respiratory rates for various age groups.
2. **Physical activity.** Physical activity increases the respiratory rate temporarily.
3. **Emotional states.** Strong emotional states temporarily increase the respiratory rate.

Table 4-5 Respiratory Rates of Various Age Groups

	Average Respiratory Range, breaths/min	Respiratory Average, breaths/min
Infant (birth to 1 yr)	30-40	35
Toddler (1-3 yr)	23-35	30
Preschool child (3-6 yr)	20-30	25
School-age child (6-12 yr)	18-26	22
Adolescent (12-18 yr)	12-20	16
Adult (after 18th yr)	12-20	16

4. **Fever.** A patient with a fever has an increased respiratory rate. One way that heat is lost from the body is through the lungs; a fever causes an increased respiratory rate as the body tries to rid itself of excess heat.

5. **Medications.** Certain medications increase the respiratory rate, and others decrease it. If the medical assistant is unsure of what effect a particular drug may have on the respiratory rate, he or she should consult a drug reference, such as the *Physician's Desk Reference* (PDR).

Rhythm and Depth of Respiration

The *rhythm* and *depth* should be noted when measuring respiration. Normally, the rhythm should be even and regular, and the pauses between inhalation and exhalation should be equal. The depth of respiration indicates the amount of air that is inhaled or exhaled during the process of breathing. Respiratory depth is generally described as normal, deep, or shallow and is determined by observing the amount of movement of the chest. For normal respirations, the depth of each respiration in a resting state is approximately the same. Deep respirations are those in which a large volume of air is inhaled and exhaled, whereas shallow respirations involve the exchange of a small volume of air. Normal respiration is referred to as **eupnea.** The rate is approximately 12 to 20 respirations per minute, the rhythm is even and regular, and the depth is normal.

Hyperpnea is an abnormal increase in the rate and depth of respirations. A patient with hyperpnea exhibits a very deep, rapid, and labored respiration. Hyperpnea occurs normally with exercise and abnormally with pain and fever. It also can occur with any condition in which the supply of oxygen is inadequate, such as heart disease and lung disease.

Hyperventilation is an abnormally fast and deep type of breathing that is usually associated with acute anxiety conditions, such as panic attacks. An individual who is hyperventilating is "overbreathing," which usually causes dizziness and weakness.

Hypopnea is a condition in which a patient's respiration exhibits an abnormal decrease in rate and depth. The depth is approximately half that of normal respiration. Hypopnea often occurs in individuals with sleep disorders.

PATIENT TEACHING   Chronic Obstructive Pulmonary Disease

Answer questions that patients have about chronic obstructive pulmonary disease (COPD).

What is COPD?
COPD is a chronic airway obstruction that results from emphysema or chronic bronchitis or a combination of these conditions. COPD is a chronic, debilitating, irreversible, and sometimes fatal disease.

How many people have COPD?
More than 12 million Americans have been diagnosed with COPD; however, it is estimated that an additional 12 million Americans have the disease but remain undiagnosed. COPD is the fourth leading cause of death in the United States behind heart disease, cancer, and stroke. Although COPD is much more common in men than in women, the greatest increase in death rates is occurring in women.

What causes COPD?
Cigarette smoking over a period of many years is the leading cause of COPD. Other causes include air pollution and occupational exposure to irritating inhalants, such as noxious dusts, fumes, and vapors.

What types of tests might the physician order?
Respiratory tests to diagnose COPD include various types of pulmonary function tests. Examples of pulmonary function tests are spirometry, lung volumes, diffusion capacity, arterial blood gas studies, pulse oximetry, and cardiopulmonary exercise tests.

What treatment might the physician prescribe?
Treatment is focused on improving breathing difficulties and may include bronchodilator drug therapy, breathing exercises, and oxygen therapy.

1. Encourage patients with COPD to comply with the therapy prescribed by the physician.
2. Provide the patient with information about smoking, emphysema, and chronic bronchitis. Educational materials are available from the American Lung Association, the American Heart Association, and the American Cancer Society.

Table 4-6 Abnormal Breath Sounds

Type	Cause	Character
Crackles* (rales)	Air moving through airways that contain fluid	Dry or wet intermittent sounds that vary in pitch (this sound can be duplicated by rubbing hair together next to ear)
Rhonchi*	Thick secretions, tumors, or spasms that partially obstruct air flow through large upper airways	Deep, low-pitched, rumbling sound more audible during expiration
Wheezes	Severely narrowed airways caused by partial obstruction in smaller bronchi and bronchioles; common symptom of asthma	Continuous, high-pitched, whistling musical sounds heard during inspiration and expiration
Pleural friction rub*	Inflamed pleurae rubbing together	High, grating sound similar to rubbing leather pieces together, heard on inspiration and expiration

*Audible only through a stethoscope.

Color of the Patient

The patient's color should be observed while the respiration is being measured. A reduction in the oxygen supply to the tissues (**hypoxia**) results in a condition known as **cyanosis,** which causes a bluish discoloration of the skin and mucous membranes. Cyanosis is first observed in the nail beds and lips because in these areas the blood vessels lie close to the surface of the skin. Cyanosis typically occurs in patients with advanced emphysema and in patients during cardiac arrest.

Apnea is a temporary absence of respirations. Some individuals experience apnea during sleep; this condition is known as *sleep apnea*. Apnea can be a serious condition if the individual's breathing ceases for more than 4 to 6 minutes because brain damage or death could occur.

Respiratory Abnormalities

A patient who is having difficulty breathing or shortness of breath has a condition known as **dyspnea.** Dyspnea may occur normally during vigorous physical exertion and abnormally in patients with asthma and emphysema. A patient with dyspnea may find it easier to breathe while in a sitting or standing position. This state is called **orthopnea** and occurs with disorders of the heart and lungs, such as asthma, emphysema, pneumonia, and congestive heart failure.

Breath Sounds

Breath sounds are caused by air moving through the respiratory tract. Normal breath sounds are quiet and barely audible. Abnormal breath sounds are referred to as **adventitious sounds** and generally signify the presence of a respiratory disorder. The causes and characters of abnormal breath sounds are presented in Table 4-6.

PULSE OXIMETRY

Pulse oximetry is a painless and noninvasive procedure used to measure the oxygen saturation of hemoglobin in arterial blood. Hemoglobin is a complex compound found in red blood cells that functions in transporting oxygen in the body. Pulse oximetry provides the physician with information on a patient's cardiorespiratory status, in particular,

the amount of oxygen being delivered to the tissues of the body. The procedure for performing pulse oximetry is presented in Procedure 4-8.

A **pulse oximeter** is the device used to measure and display the oxygen saturation of the blood. It is a computerized device that consists of a two-sided, cliplike probe connected by a cable to a monitor (Figure 4-14). A pulse oximeter also measures the patient's pulse rate in beats per minute. A constant-pitched audible beep is emitted with each pulse beat.

Assessment of Oxygen Saturation

Mechanism of Action

The probe of the pulse oximeter must be attached to a peripheral pulsating capillary bed, such as the tip of a finger. One side of the probe contains a **light-emitting diode (LED)** that transmits infrared light and red light through the patient's tissues to a light detector located on the other side of the probe, known as the *photodetector* (Figure 4-15).

Hemoglobin that is bright red in color has a high oxygen content *(oxygen-rich)* and absorbs more of the infrared light emitted by the LED. Hemoglobin that is dark red in color is low in oxygen *(oxygen-poor)* and absorbs more of the red light. The computer of the oximeter compares and calculates the light transmitted from the oxygen-rich hemoglobin and

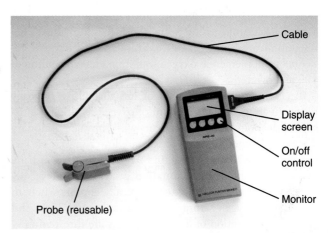

Figure 4-14. Pulse oximeter.

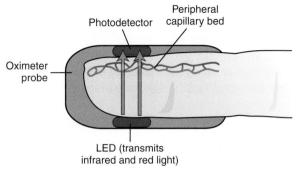

Figure 4-15. The probe of the pulse oximeter is attached to a peripheral capillary bed in the fingertip. The LED transmits light through the capillary bed to a light detector (photodetector) located on the other side of the probe to measure the oxygen saturation of hemoglobin.

the oxygen-poor hemoglobin and, from this ratio, is able to determine the oxygen saturation of the patient's hemoglobin. This measurement is converted to a percentage and is displayed as a digital readout on the screen of the monitor. Because the pulse oximeter measures the oxygen saturation of peripheral capillaries, the abbreviation **SpO$_2$** *(saturation of peripheral oxygen)* is used to record the reading.

A more complete but invasive measurement of oxygen saturation is arterial blood gas analysis, which requires drawing a blood specimen from an artery. The abbreviation for this type of arterial oxygen saturation measurement is **SaO$_2$** *(saturation of arterial oxygen).*

Interpretation of Results

The pulse oximetry reading represents the percentage of hemoglobin that is saturated (filled) with oxygen. Each molecule of hemoglobin can carry four oxygen molecules. If 100 molecules of hemoglobin were fully saturated with oxygen, they would be carrying 400 molecules of oxygen, and the oxygen saturation reading would be 100%. If these same 100 molecules of hemoglobin were carrying only 360 molecules of oxygen, however, the oxygen saturation reading would be 90%. The more hemoglobin that is saturated with oxygen, the higher the oxygen saturation of the blood.

The oxygen saturation level of most healthy individuals is 95% to 99%. Because the air we breathe is only 21% saturated with oxygen, it is unusual for an individual's hemoglobin to be fully or 100% saturated with oxygen. Patients on supplemental oxygen sometimes have a reading of 100%, however.

An oxygen saturation level of less than 95% typically results in an inadequate amount of oxygen reaching the tissues of the body, although patients with chronic pulmonary disease are sometimes able to tolerate lower saturation levels. Respiratory failure, resulting in tissue damage, usually occurs when the oxygen saturation decreases to a level between 85% and 90%. Cyanosis typically appears when an individual's oxygen saturation reaches a level of 75%, and an oxygen saturation of less than 70% is life threatening.

A decrease in the oxygen saturation of the blood (less than 95%) is known as **hypoxemia.** Hypoxemia can lead to

a more serious condition known as hypoxia. **Hypoxia** is defined as a reduction in the oxygen supply to the tissues of the body, and if not treated, it can lead to tissue damage and death. The first symptoms of hypoxia include headache, mental confusion, nausea, dizziness, shortness of breath, and tachycardia. The tissues most sensitive to hypoxia are the brain, heart, pulmonary vessels, and liver.

Purpose of Pulse Oximetry

In the medical office, pulse oximetry is often performed on patients complaining of respiratory problems (e.g., dyspnea). A decreased pulse oximetry reading (along with further testing and the patient's clinical signs and symptoms) assists the physician in proper diagnosis and treatment, which may include drug therapy and oxygen therapy.

Conditions that can cause a decreased SpO$_2$ value (hypoxemia) include the following:
- Acute pulmonary disease (e.g., pneumonia)
- Chronic pulmonary disease (e.g., emphysema, asthma, bronchitis)
- Cardiac problems (e.g., congestive heart failure, coronary artery disease)

In addition to assisting the physician in diagnosing a patient's condition, pulse oximetry is used to assess the following:
- Effectiveness of oxygen therapy
- Patient's tolerance to activity
- Effectiveness of treatment (e.g., bronchodilators)
- Patient's tolerance to analgesia and sedation

In the medical office, pulse oximetry is most often used as a "spot-check" measurement, in other words, as a single measurement of oxygen saturation. Occasionally, pulse oximetry may be used for the short-term *continuous monitoring* of a patient in the office for the following: to monitor a patient experiencing an asthmatic attack or to monitor a sedated patient during minor office surgery.

Components of the Pulse Oximeter

Most medical offices use a handheld pulse oximeter (see Figure 4-14), which is portable, lightweight, and battery operated. This is in contrast to a stand-alone oximeter, which is more apt to be used in a hospital setting for the continuous bedside monitoring of a patient's oxygen saturation level. A pulse oximeter not only measures oxygen saturation, it also measures the pulse rate in beats per minute. The two main parts of the pulse oximeter—the monitor and the probe—are described in detail next.

Monitor

The monitor contains controls, indicators, and displays (Figure 4-16). These may vary slightly depending on the brand of oximeter. Those that are found on most handheld pulse oximeters include the following:
1. **On/off control.** Turns the oximeter on and off.
2. **SpO$_2$% display.** A digital display of the patient's oxygen saturation expressed as a percent. This number is updated with each pulse beat.

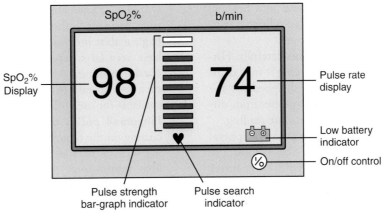

SpO₂%

SpO₂%
Display

98   74

Pulse rate
display

Low battery
indicator

On/off control

Pulse strength
bar-graph indicator

Pulse search
indicator

Figure 4-16. Pulse oximeter monitor: controls, indicators, and displays.

3. **Pulse rate display.** This display indicates the patient's pulse rate in beats per minute. This number is updated with each pulse beat. Most oximeters emit a constant-pitched audible beep with each pulse beat.

4. **Pulse strength bar-graph indicator.** This indicator provides a visual display of the patient's pulse strength at the probe placement site. The pulse strength indicator consists of a segmented display of bars. The pulse strength indicator "sweeps" with each pulse beat, and the stronger the pulse, the more segments that light up on the bar graph.

5. **Pulse search indicator.** This indicator lights up when the oximeter is searching for the patient's pulse.

6. **Adjustable volume control.** This control is used to adjust the beep that sounds with each pulse beat. In most oximeters, the settings are high, low, and off.

7. **Low battery indicator.** This indicator is used to warn that the battery is getting low. The indicator lights up and the monitor sounds an alarm when approximately 30 minutes of battery use remains.

8. **Alarm messages.** Alarm messages indicate a problem or condition that may affect the reading. Alarm messages must not be ignored and must be corrected before continuing.

When the pulse oximeter is turned on, it automatically performs a power-on self-test (POST), which takes approximately 3 to 5 seconds. During the POST, the oximeter checks its internal systems to ensure they are functioning properly. If the oximeter detects a problem, an alarm sounds and the monitor displays an error code. If this occurs, the medical assistant should refer to the troubleshooting section of the user's manual for interpretation of the error code and the necessary action that should be taken.

When the POST is completed, the oximeter begins searching for a pulse. During this time, the pulse search indicator lights up. It takes several seconds for the oximeter to locate a pulse and to calculate and display the SpO₂ reading. If the oximeter is unable to detect a pulse, or if the pulse is too weak to provide the data needed to calculate oxygen saturation, the oximeter is unable to make a measurement. In this case, an alarm sounds and the oximeter may automatically shut off. If this occurs, the medical as-

sistant should reposition the probe or move the probe to another finger and perform the procedure again.

Probe

The probe of the pulse oximeter may be reusable or disposable (Figure 4-17). Most offices use reusable clip-on probes. Reusable probes are convenient to use and easy to apply, but they are more susceptible to inaccurate readings owing to patient movement. Reusable probes must be cleaned and disinfected after each use. Disposable probes are expensive to use and are generally employed for the long-term moni-

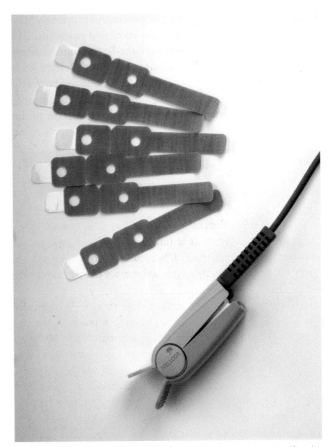

Figure 4-17. Disposable *(top)* and reusable *(bottom)* probes for the pulse oximeter.

toring of a patient's oxygen saturation level in a hospital setting. Disposable probes are made of an adhesive bandage–like material and are discarded after use.

It is important to handle reusable probes carefully. Hitting a probe against a hard object or dropping it may damage it. It is important to use the probe designed for the pulse oximeter that is being used. Mixing probes from different manufacturers can result in an inaccurate reading.

The probe must be attached to the patient at a peripheral site that is highly vascular and where the skin is thin. The most common site to apply a probe is the tip of a finger (Figure 4-18); other acceptable sites include the toe and earlobe. A specially designed probe is available for application to the earlobe; it is smaller than a finger probe and has a curved ear attachment to hold it in place.

A cable connects the probe to the monitor. The probe may be permanently attached to the cable, or it may be a separate device that requires connection to the cable. The pulse oximeter monitor should never be lifted or carried by the cable because this could damage the cable connections or could cause the cable to disconnect from the monitor and possibly drop on the floor or fall on the patient.

Factors Affecting Pulse Oximetry

Although pulse oximetry is an easy procedure to perform, the medical assistant must be aware of certain factors that may interfere with an accurate reading. These factors are listed, along with guidelines for correcting or preventing them.

1. **Incorrect positioning of the probe.** As previously discussed, the oximeter probe consists of two parts: an LED and a photodetector. Because light is transmitted from the LED through the tissues to the photodetector, it is important that these two components be aligned directly opposite to each other during the measurement. In most cases, this automatically occurs when the clip-on probe

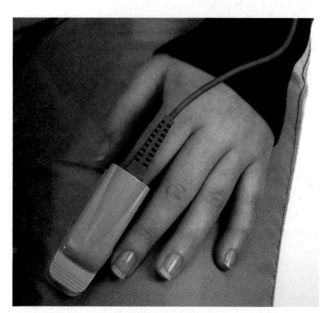

Figure 4-18. Applying a probe to the tip of a finger.

is applied. Proper alignment of the probe may be impossible, however, with patients who have very small fingers (e.g., a thin individual, a child) or with patients who have very large fingers (e.g., an obese individual). To obtain an accurate reading, another site must be used, such as the earlobe. In addition, pediatric probes are available for use with thin patients or children.

2. **Fingernail polish or artificial nails.** A dark, opaque coating on the fingernail may result in a falsely low reading. This is because the coating interferes with proper light transmission through the finger. The darker the coating, the more likely that the SpO_2 reading will be affected. Blue, black, and green fingernail polishes tend to cause the most problems. If the patient is wearing fingernail polish, it should be removed with acetone or fingernail polish remover. If the patient has artificial fingernails, another site should be used to take the measurement, such as the earlobe or the toe. Oil, dirt, and grime on the fingertip can also interfere with proper light transmission. If the patient's fingertip is dirty, cleanse the site with soap and water and allow it to dry. Areas with bruises, burns, stains, or tattoos should be avoided as a probe placement site. Darkly pigmented skin and jaundice do not usually affect the ability of the oximeter to obtain an accurate reading.

3. **Poor peripheral blood flow.** A pulse oximeter works best when there is a good strong pulse in the finger to which the probe is applied. Poor peripheral blood flow may cause the pulse to be so weak that the oximeter cannot obtain a reading. Conditions resulting in poor blood flow include peripheral vascular disease, vasoconstrictor medications, severe hypotension, and hypothermia. In these situations, the medical assistant should try using the earlobe because it is less affected by decreased blood flow. Sometimes patients with cold fingers (but who are not hypothermic) may have enough constriction of the peripheral capillaries that it interferes with obtaining a reading. To solve this problem, the medical assistant should ask the patient to warm his or her fingers by rubbing the hands together. The probe should never be attached to the finger of an arm to which an automatic blood pressure cuff is applied because blood flow to the finger would be cut off when the cuff inflates, resulting in loss of the pulse signal.

4. **Ambient (surrounding) light.** Ambient light shining directly on the probe, such as bright fluorescent light, direct sunlight, or an overhead examination light, may result in an inaccurate reading. This is because some of the ambient light may be picked up by the probe's photodetector and alter the reading. This problem can be corrected by one of the following: turning off the light, moving the patient's hand away from the light source, or covering the probe with an opaque material such as a washcloth.

5. **Patient movement.** Patient movement is a common cause of an inaccurate reading. Motion affects the ability of the light to travel from the LED to the photodetector

and prevents the probe from picking up the pulse signal. To avoid this problem, it is important that the medical assistant instruct the patient to remain still during the procedure. Occasionally, patient movement cannot be eliminated, such as when the patient has tremors of the hands. In these instances, the oxygen saturation level should be measured at a site that is less affected by motion, such as the toe or the earlobe.

Pulse Oximeter Care and Maintenance

The pulse oximeter monitor and cable should be cleaned periodically using a cloth slightly dampened with a solution of warm water and a disinfectant cleaner. The medical as-

sistant should make sure that the cloth is not too wet to prevent the solution from running into the monitor, which could damage the internal components. The probe should be cleaned periodically with a soft cloth moistened with warm water and a disinfectant cleaner. Cleaning the probe removes dirt and grime that could interfere with proper light transmission, leading to an inaccurate reading. The probe also should be disinfected after each use by wiping it thoroughly with an antiseptic wipe and allowing it to dry. The probe should never be soaked or immersed in a liquid solution because this would damage it. The probe is heat-sensitive and cannot be autoclaved. The pulse oximeter should be stored at room temperature in a dry environment.

 PROCEDURE 4-6 Measuring Pulse and Respiration

Outcome Measure pulse and respiration.

Equipment/Supplies

• Watch with a second hand

1. Procedural Step. Sanitize your hands. Greet the patient and introduce yourself. Identify the patient and explain the procedure. Observe the patient for any signs that might affect the pulse or respiratory rate.
Principle. Pulse rate can vary according to the factors listed on page 139.

2. Procedural Step. Have the patient sit down. Position the patient's arm in a comfortable position. The forearm should be slightly flexed to relax the muscles and tendons over the pulse site.
Principle. Relaxed muscles and tendons over the pulse site make it easier to palpate the pulse.

3. Procedural Step. Place your three middle fingertips over the radial pulse site. Never use your thumb to take a pulse. The radial pulse is located in a groove on the inner aspect of the wrist just below the thumb.
Principle. The thumb has a pulse of its own; using the thumb results in measurement of the medical assistant's pulse and not the patient's pulse.

4. Procedural Step. Apply moderate, gentle pressure directly over the site until you feel the pulse. If you cannot feel the pulse, this may be caused by:

a. Incorrect location of the radial pulse: Move your fingers to a slightly different location in the groove of the wrist until you feel the pulse.

b. Applying too much pressure or not enough pressure: Vary the depth of your hold until you can feel the pulse.
Principle. A normal pulse can be felt with moderate pressure. The pulse cannot be felt if not enough pressure is applied, whereas too much pressure applied to the radial artery closes it off, and no pulse is felt.

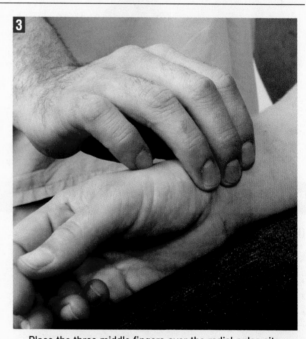

Place the three middle fingers over the radial pulse site.

5. Procedural Step. Count the pulse for 30 seconds and make a mental note of this number. Note the rhythm and volume of the pulse. If abnormalities occur in the rhythm or volume, count the pulse for 1 full minute.
Principle. A longer time ensures an accurate assessment of abnormalities.

6. Procedural Step. After taking the pulse, continue to hold three fingers on the patient's wrist with the same amount of pressure, and measure the respirations. This

Continued

PROCEDURE 4-6

PROCEDURE 4-6　Measuring Pulse and Respiration—cont'd

5

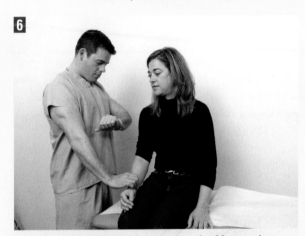

Count the pulse for 30 seconds.

6

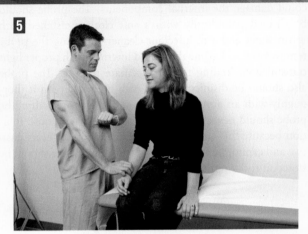

Count the number of respirations for 30 seconds.

helps to ensure that the patient is unaware that respirations are being monitored.

Principle. If the patient is aware that respiration is being measured, the breathing may change.

7. **Procedural Step.** Observe the rise and fall of the patient's chest as the patient inhales and exhales.

Principle. One complete respiration includes one inhalation and one exhalation.

8. **Procedural Step.** Count the number of respirations for 30 seconds and make a mental note of this number; note the rhythm and depth of the respirations. Also observe the patient's color. If abnormalities occur in rhythm or depth, count the respiratory rate for 1 full minute.

9. **Procedural Step.** Sanitize your hands, and chart the results. If you counted the pulse and respirations for 30 seconds, multiply each of the numbers counted by 2. This will give you the pulse rate and respiratory rate for 1 full minute. Include the date; the time; the pulse rate, rhythm, and volume; and the respiratory rate, rhythm, and depth.

CHARTING EXAMPLE

Date	
10/15/12	2:30 p.m. P: 74. Reg and strong. R: 18.
	Even and reg.————————S. Martinez, RMA

PROCEDURE 4-7　Measuring Apical Pulse

Outcome Measure apical pulse.

Equipment/Supplies

- Watch with a second hand
- Stethoscope
- Antiseptic wipe

1. **Procedural Step.** Sanitize your hands. Greet the patient and introduce yourself. Identify the patient and explain the procedure. Observe the patient for any signs that might increase or decrease the pulse rate.

2. **Procedural Step.** Assemble the equipment. If the stethoscope's chest piece consists of a diaphragm and a bell, rotate the chest piece to the bell position. Clean the earpieces and chest piece of the stethoscope with an antiseptic wipe.

Principle. The bell position allows better auscultation of heart sounds. Cleaning the earpieces helps prevent the transmission of microorganisms.

3. **Procedural Step.** Ask the patient to unbutton or remove his or her shirt. Have the patient sit or lie down (supine).

Principle. A sitting or supine position allows access to the apex of the heart.

4. **Procedural Step.** Warm the chest piece of the stethoscope with your hands. Insert the earpieces of the stethoscope into your ears, with the earpieces directed slightly forward, and place the chest piece over the apex of the patient's heart. The apex of the heart is located in the fifth intercostal space at the junction of the left midclavicular line.

PROCEDURE 4-7   Measuring Apical Pulse—cont'd

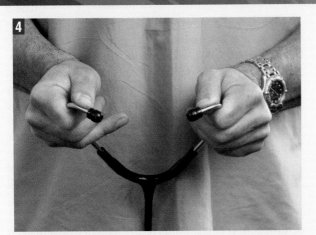

Insert the earpieces into your ears with the earpieces directed slightly forward.

Principle. Warming the chest piece reduces the discomfort of having a cold object placed on the chest. In addition, a cold chest piece could startle the patient, resulting in an increase in pulse rate. The earpieces should be directed forward to follow the direction of the ear canal, which facilitates hearing.

5. Procedural Step. Listen for the heartbeat, and count the number of beats for 30 seconds (and multiply by 2) if the rhythm and volume are normal or if the apical pulse is being taken on an infant or child. If abnormalities occur in the rhythm or volume, count the pulse for 1 full minute. You will hear a "lubb-dupp" sound through the stethoscope. This sound is the closing of the heart's valves. Each "lubb-dupp" is counted as one beat.

6. Procedural Step. Sanitize your hands, and chart the results. Include the date, the time, and the apical pulse rate, rhythm, and volume.

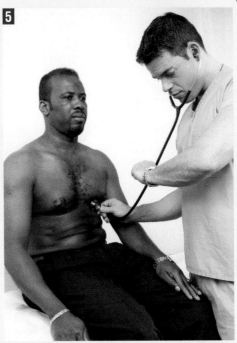

Count the number of beats for 30 seconds, and multiply by 2.

7. Procedural Step. Clean the earpieces and the chest piece of the stethoscope with an antiseptic wipe.

CHARTING EXAMPLE

Date	
10/15/12	10:15 a.m. AP: 68. Reg and strong. _____ _____ S. Martinez, RMA

PROCEDURE 4-8   Performing Pulse Oximetry

Outcome Perform pulse oximetry.

Equipment/Supplies

- Handheld pulse oximeter
- Reusable finger probe
- Antiseptic wipe

1. Procedural Step. Sanitize your hands.

2. Procedural Step. Assemble the equipment. Handle the probe carefully, and perform the following:
  a. Carefully inspect the probe to ensure it opens and closes smoothly. Inspect the probe windows (LED and photodetector) to ensure they are clean and free of lint.
  b. Disinfect the probe windows and surrounding platforms with an antiseptic wipe, and allow them to dry.
  c. If necessary, connect the probe to the cable.

PROCEDURE 4-8   Performing Pulse Oximetry—cont'd

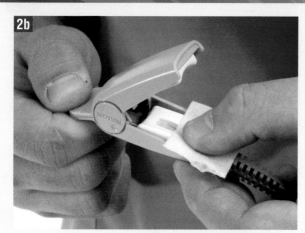

Disinfect the probe with an antiseptic wipe.

d. Connect the cable to the monitor by plugging it into the port on the monitor. Do not lift or carry the monitor by the cable.

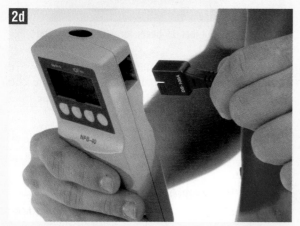

Connect the cable to the monitor by plugging it into the port on the monitor.

Principle. Misuse or improper handling of the probe could damage it. Dirt or lint on the probe windows could interfere with proper light transmission, leading to an inaccurate reading. Cross-contamination between patients is prevented by disinfecting the probe. Lifting the monitor by the cable could damage the cable connections.

3. **Procedural Step.** Greet the patient and introduce yourself. Identify the patient and explain the procedure. Explain to the patient that the clip-on probe does not hurt and feels similar to a clothespin attached to the finger. If the patient seems fearful, place the probe on your own finger first to reassure the patient that it is not painful.

4. **Procedural Step.** Seat the patient comfortably in a chair with the lower arm firmly supported and the palm facing down.

Principle. Supporting the lower arm helps prevent patient movement during the procedure.

5. **Procedural Step.** Select an appropriate finger to apply the probe. Use the tip of the patient's index, middle, or ring finger. If the patient's fingers are very small or very large, and the probe cannot seem to be aligned properly, use the earlobe to take the measurement. If the patient exhibits tremors of the hands, use the earlobe to obtain the reading.

Principle. The probe must be applied to a peripheral site with thin skin that is highly vascular. Very small or very large fingers may not allow for proper positioning of the probe on the finger.

6. **Procedural Step.** Observe the patient's fingernail. If the patient is wearing dark fingernail polish, ask him or her to remove it with acetone or nail polish remover. If the patient is wearing artificial nails, choose another probe site, such as the toe or earlobe.

Principle. An opaque coating on the fingernail may interfere with proper light transmission through the finger, leading to an inaccurate reading.

7. **Procedural Step.** Check to ensure that the patient's fingertip is clean. If it is dirty, cleanse the site with soap and water, and allow it to dry. Ensure that the patient's finger is not cold. If it is cold, ask the patient to rub his or her hands together.

Principle. Oils, dirt, or grime on the finger can interfere with proper light transmission through the finger, leading to an inaccurate reading. Sometimes patients with cold fingers may have enough constriction of the capillaries that it interferes with obtaining a reading.

8. **Procedural Step.** Ensure that ambient light does not interfere with the measurement. Position the probe securely on the fingertip as follows:

a. Ensure that the probe window is fully covered by placing the finger over the LED window, with the fleshy tip of the finger covering the window. The tip of the finger should touch the end of the probe stop.

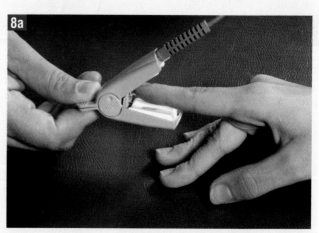

Position the probe securely on the fingertip.

PROCEDURE 4-8 Performing Pulse Oximetry—cont'd

b. Ensure that the light-emitting diode and the photodetector are aligned opposite to each other.

c. Allow the cable to lay across the back of the hand and parallel to the arm of the patient.

Principle. Ambient light can be picked up by the probe and alter the reading. Proper alignment of the LED and photodetector is necessary for an accurate reading.

9. **Procedural Step.** Instruct the patient to remain still and to breathe normally. Turn on the oximeter by pressing the on/off control. Wait while the oximeter goes through its power-on self-test (POST). If the monitor fails the POST, refer to the troubleshooting section of the user manual for interpretation of the error code and the necessary action that should be taken.

Principle. Patient movement may lead to an inaccurate reading. The monitor automatically conducts a POST to ensure that it is functioning properly.

10. **Procedural Step.** Allow several seconds for the pulse oximeter to detect the pulse and calculate the oxygen saturation of the blood. Ensure that the pulse strength indicator fluctuates with each pulsation and that the pulse signal is strong. If the oximeter sounds an alarm indicating that it was unable to locate a pulse, reposition the probe on the patient's finger or move the probe to another finger, and perform the procedure again.

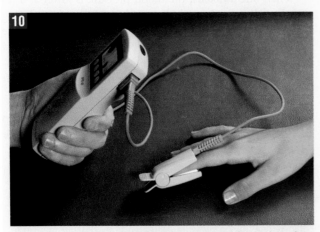

Allow several seconds for the pulse oximeter to detect the pulse.

Principle. The reading takes several seconds to display. The pulse strength indicator provides a quick assessment of pulse quality. If the oximeter is unable to locate a pulse, it will be unable to obtain a reading.

11. **Procedural Step.** Leave the probe in place until the oximeter displays a reading. Read the oxygen saturation value and pulse rate, and make a mental note of these readings. On this pulse oximeter, the oxygen saturation reading is 100% and the pulse rate is 75. If the SpO$_2$ reading is less than 95%, reposition the probe on the finger, and perform the procedure again.

Principle. A low SpO$_2$ reading may be caused by improper positioning of the probe on the finger.

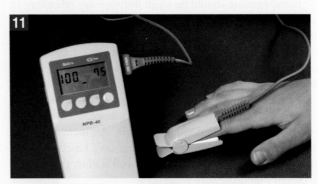

Read the oxygen saturation value and pulse rate.

12. **Procedural Step.** Remove the probe from the patient's finger, and turn off the oximeter.

13. **Procedural Step.** Sanitize your hands, and chart the results. Include the date, the time, the SpO$_2$ reading, and the pulse rate.

14. **Procedural Step.** Disconnect the cable from the monitor. Disinfect the probe with an antiseptic wipe. Properly store the monitor in a clean, dry area.

CHARTING EXAMPLE

Date	
10/15/12	2:30 p.m. SpO$_2$: 100%. P: 75. ————
	———————— S. Martinez, RMA

BLOOD PRESSURE
Mechanism of Blood Pressure

Blood pressure (BP) is a measurement of the pressure or force exerted by the blood on the walls of the arteries in which it is contained. Each time the ventricles contract, blood is pushed out of the heart and into the aorta and pulmonary aorta, exerting pressure on the walls of the arter-

ies. This phase in the cardiac cycle is known as **systole,** and it represents the highest point of blood pressure in the body, or the **systolic pressure.** The phase of the cardiac cycle in which the heart relaxes between contractions is referred to as **diastole.** The **diastolic pressure** (recorded during diastole) is lower because the heart is relaxed. Contraction and relaxation of the heart result in two different pressures—systolic and diastolic.

Interpretation of Blood Pressure

Blood pressure measurement is expressed as a fraction. The numerator is the systolic pressure, and the denominator is the diastolic pressure. The standard unit for measuring blood pressure is millimeters of mercury (mm Hg). A blood pressure reading of 110/70 mm Hg means that there was enough force to raise a column of mercury 110 mm during systole and 70 mm during diastole.

Based on guidelines from the National Heart, Lung, and Blood Institute (NHLBI), a blood pressure reading of less than 120/80 mm Hg is classified as normal, whereas a blood pressure reading of 120/80 is classified as *prehypertension*. These guidelines were issued as a result of scientific studies showing that the risk of heart disease begins at a blood pressure reading lower than previously thought. The NHLBI guidelines are outlined in Table 4-7.

Blood pressure should be taken during every office visit to allow the physician to compare the patient's readings over time. This is a good preventive measure in guarding against serious illness. A single blood pressure reading taken on one occasion does not characterize an individual's blood pressure accurately. Several readings, taken on different occasions, provide a good index of an individual's baseline blood pressure.

Blood pressure readings always should be interpreted using a patient's baseline blood pressure. An increase or decrease of 20 to 30 mm Hg in a patient's baseline blood pressure is significant, even if it is still within the normal accepted blood pressure range.

The most common condition that causes an abnormal blood pressure reading is **hypertension.** Hypertension, or high blood pressure, results from excessive pressure on the walls of the arteries. Hypertension is determined by a sustained systolic blood pressure reading of 140 mm Hg or greater, or a sustained diastolic reading of 90 mm Hg or greater. See Table 4-7 for the NHLBI classifications for hypertension. **Hypotension,** or low blood pressure, results from reduced pressure on the arterial walls. Hypotension is determined by a blood pressure reading of less than 95/60 mm Hg.

Pulse Pressure

The difference between systolic and diastolic pressures is the **pulse pressure.** It is determined by subtracting the smaller number from the larger. If the blood pressure is 110/70 mm Hg, the pulse pressure would be 40 mm Hg. A pulse pressure between 30 and 50 mm Hg is considered to be within normal range.

Factors Affecting Blood Pressure

Blood pressure does not remain at a constant value. Numerous factors may affect it throughout the course of the day. An understanding of these factors helps to ensure an accurate interpretation of blood pressure readings.

1. **Age.** Age is an important consideration when determining whether a patient's blood pressure is normal. As age increases, the blood pressure gradually increases: A 6-year-old child may have a normal reading of 90/60 mm Hg, whereas a young, healthy adult may have a blood pressure reading of 116/76 mm Hg, and it would not be unusual for a 60-year-old man to have a reading of 130/90 mm Hg. As an individual gets older, there is a loss of elasticity in the walls of the blood vessels, causing this increase in pressure to occur. Table 4-8 is a chart of the average optimal blood pressure readings for various age groups.
2. **Gender.** After puberty, women usually have a lower blood pressure than men of the same age. After menopause, women usually have a higher blood pressure than men of the same age.
3. **Diurnal variations.** Fluctuations in an individual's blood pressure are normal during the course of a day. When one awakens, the blood pressure is lower as a result of decreased metabolism and physical activity during sleep. As metabolism and activity increase during the day, the blood pressure rises.
4. **Emotional states.** Strong emotional states, such as anger, fear, and excitement, increase the blood pressure. If

Table 4-7	Classification of Blood Pressure for Adults Age 18 and Older			
Blood Pressure Classifications	**Systolic Blood Pressure, mm Hg**		**Diastolic Blood Pressure, mm Hg**	
Normal	Less than 120	*and*	Less than 80	
Prehypertension*	120-139	*or*	80-89	
Hypertension*				
Stage 1	140-159	*or*	90-99	
Stage 2	160 or higher	*or*	100 or higher	

From National Heart, Lung, and Blood Institute: Seventh report of the Joint National Committee on Detection, Evaluation, and Treatment of High Blood Pressure. Bethesda, Md: NIH Publication No. 03-5231, May, 2003, U.S. Department of Health and Human Services.
*Based on the average of two or more properly measured, seated blood pressure readings taken at each of two or more visits.

What Would You Do? What Would You *Not* Do?

Case Study 3

Tyrone Jackson, 45 years old, is at the medical office to have his blood pressure checked. Three months ago, Tyrone started taking a diuretic and an antihypertensive prescribed by the physician to reduce his blood pressure. The last recording in his chart indicates that Tyrone's blood pressure decreased from 180/112 mm Hg to 126/84 mm Hg; however, his blood pressure at this visit is 158/98 mm Hg. Tyrone says that he has not been very good at taking his medication lately. He says it is really hard to remember to take all those pills every day. He also says that he felt just fine before being put on blood pressure pills, but when he started taking them, he felt awful. He had to urinate more often; when he got up fast, he felt dizzy; and he had some problems with headaches. Tyrone says that he decided to cut back on his pills to see if these problems got better, and sure enough, they went away altogether. Tyrone wants to know if there's anything he can do to lower his blood pressure other than taking pills. ■

Table 4-8 Average Optimal Blood Pressure for Age	
Age	**Blood Pressure, mm Hg**
Newborn (6.6 lb)	40 (mean)
1 mo	85/54
1 yr	95/65
6 yr*	105/65
10-13 yr*	110/65
14-17 yr*	120/75
Adult	Less than 120/80

From National High Blood Pressure Education Program (NHBPEP); National Heart, Lung, and Blood Institute; National Institutes of Health: The seventh report of the Joint National Committees on Detection, Evaluation, and Treatment of High Blood Pressure, JAMA 239:2560, 2003.
*In children and adolescents, hypertension is defined as blood pressure that is, on repeated measurement, at the 95th percentile or greater adjusted for age, height, and gender (NHBPEP, 1997).

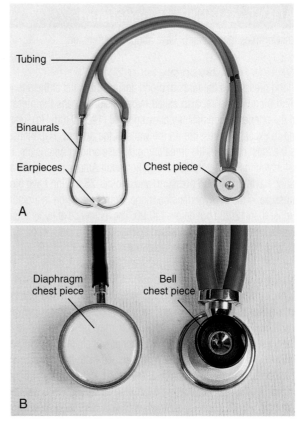

Figure 4-19. **A,** The parts of a stethoscope. **B,** Types of chest pieces.

the medical assistant observes such a reaction, an attempt should be made to calm the patient before taking his or her blood pressure.

5. **Exercise.** Physical activity temporarily increases the blood pressure. To ensure an accurate reading, a patient who has been involved in physical activity should be given an opportunity to rest for 20 to 30 minutes before blood pressure is measured.

6. **Body position.** The blood pressure of a patient who is in a lying or standing position is usually different from that measured when the patient is sitting. For example, the diastolic pressure of an individual in a sitting position is higher than his or her diastolic pressure in a lying position. A notation should be made on the patient's chart if the reading was obtained in any position other than sitting, by using the following abbreviations: *L* (lying) and *St* (standing).

7. **Medications.** Many medications may increase or decrease the blood pressure. Because of this factor, it is important to record in the patient chart all prescription and over-the-counter medications that the patient is taking.

8. **Other factors.** Other factors that may increase the blood pressure include pain, a recent meal, caffeine, smoking, and bladder distention.

Assessment of Manual Blood Pressure

The equipment needed to measure manual blood pressure includes a stethoscope and a sphygmomanometer. The **stethoscope** amplifies sounds produced by the body and allows the medical assistant to hear them.

Stethoscope

The most common type of stethoscope used in the medical office is the acoustic stethoscope. It consists of four parts: earpieces, sidepieces known as *binaurals,* plastic or rubber tubing, and a chest piece (Figure 4-19, *A*).

Stethoscope Chest Piece

There are two types of chest pieces: a *diaphragm,* which is a large, flat disc, and a bell, which has a bowl-shaped appearance (Figure 4-19, *B*). The chest piece of a stethoscope consists of a diaphragm and a bell, or just a diaphragm. If a chest piece consists of a diaphragm and a bell, the medical assistant must ensure that the desired piece is rotated into position before use. Failure to do so would not allow the medical assistant to hear sound through the earpieces.

The diaphragm chest piece is more useful for hearing high-pitched sounds, such as lung and bowel sounds, whereas the bell chest piece is more useful for hearing low-pitched sounds, such as those produced by the heart and vascular system. Before using a stethoscope, the medical assistant should ensure that it is in proper working condition.

Sphygmomanometers

The **sphygmomanometer** is an instrument that measures the pressure of blood within an artery. It consists of a **manometer,** an inner inflatable bladder surrounded by a covering known as the *cuff,* and a pressure bulb with a control valve to inflate and deflate the inner bladder. The manometer contains a scale for registering the pressure of the air in the bladder.

Two types of sphygmomanometers are used—aneroid and mercury. The *aneroid sphygmomanometer* is lightweight

PATIENT TEACHING Hypertension

Answer questions patients have about hypertension.

What is high blood pressure?

Blood pressure is the force of blood against the walls of the arteries. High blood pressure, also called hypertension, means the pressure in the arteries is consistently above normal (140/90 mm Hg), resulting in excessive pressure on the walls of the arteries. Hypertension is the most common life-threatening disease among Americans. It is estimated that approximately 74 million adult Americans, age 20 and older, have high blood pressure, and another 25 million have blood pressure in the prehypertension range. Prehypertension is a reading higher than 120/80 but below 140/90. The incidence of hypertension in the United States has increased dramatically as a result of an aging population and an increased incidence of obesity.

What are the symptoms of high blood pressure?

Approximately 20% of individuals who have high blood pressure are unaware of it because there are few or no symptoms and, as a result, an individual with hypertension may go undiagnosed for many years. If symptoms do occur, they may include one or more of the following: headaches, dizziness, flushed face, fatigue, epistaxis (nosebleed), excessive perspiration, heart palpitations, frequent urination, and leg claudication (cramping in the legs with walking). The only way to know for sure whether you have high blood pressure is to have it checked regularly.

What causes high blood pressure?

In 90% to 95% of cases, the precise cause of high blood pressure is unknown. This type of hypertension is known as *essential* or *primary hypertension.* Certain factors seem to increase the risk of developing essential hypertension, however; these include the following:

Uncontrollable Risk Factors
- **Heredity.** A family history of high blood pressure increases an individual's risk of developing high blood pressure.
- **Ethnicity.** Research has shown that more black than white Americans develop high blood pressure.
- **Age.** Blood pressure normally increases as one grows older. High blood pressure occurs most often in individuals over the age of 35. Men tend to develop high blood pressure most often between the ages of 35 and 55, whereas women are more likely to develop it after menopause.

Controllable Risk Factors
- **Obesity.** Individuals with a BMI (body mass index) of 30 or higher are more likely to develop high blood pressure.
- **Sodium intake.** Sodium, found in salt and processed, canned, and most snack foods, does not cause high blood pressure; however, it can aggravate high blood pressure. Most Americans consume more sodium than they need. The current recommendation is to consume less than 2.4 g (2400 mg) of sodium per day. This is equivalent to 6 g (about 1 teaspoon) of salt.

- **Lack of physical exercise.** A sedentary lifestyle makes it easier to gain weight and increases the chance of developing high blood pressure.
- **Chronic stress.** Research indicates that people who are under continuous stress tend to develop more heart and circulatory problems than people who are not under stress.
- **Smoking.** Smoking tobacco constricts blood vessels, causing an increase in blood pressure.
- **Alcohol consumption.** Heavy and regular alcohol consumption can increase blood pressure.

The remaining 5% to 10% of individuals with hypertension have *secondary hypertension.* This means that high blood pressure can be linked to a known cause, which includes chronic kidney disease, adrenal and thyroid diseases, narrowing of the aorta, steroid therapy, oral contraceptives, and preeclampsia associated with pregnancy.

What can happen if high blood pressure is not treated?

If high blood pressure is not brought under control, it can cause severe damage to vital organs, such as the heart, brain, kidneys, and eyes. This damage can result in a heart attack or heart failure, stroke, kidney damage, or damaged vision. Early detection and treatment of high blood pressure can prevent these complications. High blood pressure is often discovered during a routine medical examination or (less commonly) when an individual experiences one of the complications of hypertension caused by damage to a vital organ.

Can high blood pressure be cured?

Essential hypertension cannot be cured, but many treatments are used to bring it under control. These include lifestyle modifications, such as weight reduction, a healthy diet rich in fruits and vegetables and low in saturated fat, limitation of salt intake, regular aerobic exercise, cessation of smoking, limitation or elimination of alcohol consumption, and stress management. If lifestyle modifications alone are not enough, medications are available for reducing blood pressure, allowing the patient to lead a normal, healthy, active life.

How long will I undergo treatment?

Treatment for essential hypertension is usually lifelong. Even if you feel fine, you'll probably have to continue treatment for the rest of your life to maintain your blood pressure in a healthy range. If you discontinue your diet and lifestyle changes or stop taking your medication, your blood pressure will increase again.

- Encourage patients with hypertension to adhere to the treatment prescribed by the physician. Help patients remember to take their medication by telling them to associate their medication schedule with a daily routine, such as brushing their teeth or with meals.
- Provide the patient with educational materials about high blood pressure, available from sources such as the American Heart Association.

and portable, but the *mercury sphygmomanometer* is more accurate.

Aneroid Sphygmomanometer

The aneroid sphygmomanometer (Figure 4-20) has a manometer gauge with a round scale. The scale is calibrated in millimeters, with a needle that points to the calibrations (Figure 4-21). To ensure an accurate reading, the needle must be positioned initially at zero. The manometer must be placed in the correct position for proper viewing. The medical assistant should be no farther than 3 feet from the scale on the gauge of the manometer, and the manometer should be placed so that it can be viewed directly. At least

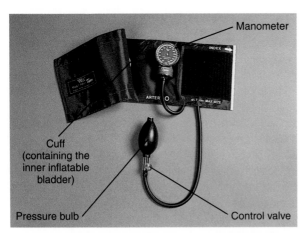

Figure 4-20. The parts of an aneroid sphygmomanometer.

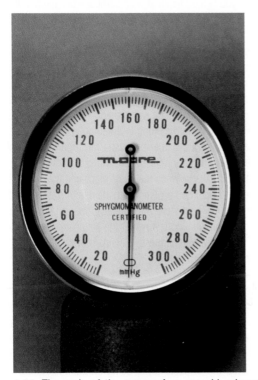

Figure 4-21. The scale of the gauge of an aneroid sphygmomanometer.

once a year, an aneroid sphygmomanometer should be recalibrated to ensure its accuracy.

Mercury Sphygmomanometer

The mercury sphygmomanometer (Figure 4-22) has a vertical tube calibrated in millimeters that is filled with mercury. Although more accurate than the aneroid sphygmomanometer, use of the mercury sphygmomanometer is being discouraged because mercury is a hazardous chemical that can be dangerous to humans and the environment.

If a mercury manometer is used to measure blood pressure, it must be placed in the correct position for proper viewing. The medical assistant should be no farther than 3 feet from the scale of the manometer. A portable mercury manometer should be placed on a flat surface so the mercury column is in a vertical position. The wall model mercury manometer is mounted securely on a wall, placing the mercury column in a vertical position.

The following guidelines must be followed when measuring blood pressure with a mercury sphygmomanometer. Before the blood pressure reading is obtained, the mercury must be even with the zero level at the base of the calibrated tube. Pressure created by inflation of the inner bladder causes the mercury to rise in the tube. The top portion of the mercury column, the **meniscus,** curves slightly upward. The blood pressure should be read at the top of the meniscus, with the eye at the same level as the meniscus of the mercury column.

Cuff Sizes

Blood pressure cuffs come in a variety of sizes and are measured in centimeters (cm) (Figure 4-23). The size of a cuff refers to its inner inflatable bladder, rather than its cloth cover. Table 4-9 lists the types of cuffs available and the size of the inner bladder of each cuff.

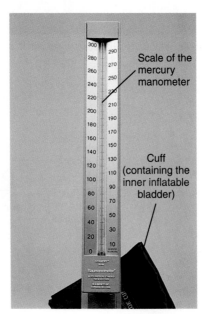

Figure 4-22. The parts of a mercury sphygmomanometer.

For accurate blood pressure measurement, the inner bladder of the cuff should encircle at least 80% (but not more than 100%) of the arm circumference and should be wide enough to cover two thirds of the distance from the axilla to the antecubital space (Figure 4-24). Child cuffs often must be used for adults with thin arms. The adult cuff is used for the average-sized adult arm, and the thigh cuff is used for taking blood pressure from the thigh or for adults with large arms. If the cuff is too small, the reading may be falsely high, as it would be, for example, when an adult cuff is used on a patient with a large arm. If the cuff is too large, the reading may be falsely low, as it would be when an adult

Table 4-9 Types of Blood Pressure Cuffs			
Cuff	Bladder Length, cm	Bladder Width, cm	Acceptable Circumference, cm
Child arm	21	8	16-21
Small adult arm	24	10	22-26
Adult arm	30	13	27-34
Large adult arm	38	16	35-44
Adult thigh	42	20	45-52

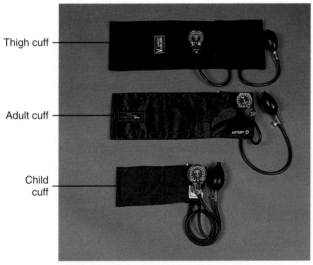

Figure 4-23. Blood pressure cuffs: child, adult, and thigh.

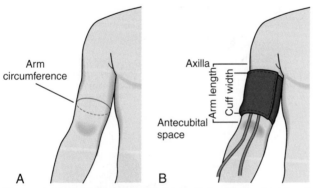

Figure 4-24. Determination of proper cuff size. **A,** The bladder of the cuff should be long enough to encircle 80% of the arm. **B,** The cuff should be wide enough to cover two thirds of the distance from the axilla to the antecubital space.

Highlight on Stethoscopes

The stethoscope was first introduced in the 1800s by a French physician named René Laennec. This early stethoscope consisted of a simple wooden tube with a bell-shaped opening at one end.

The selection of a stethoscope is an individual decision. One hears sounds differently when using different stethoscopes. The primary consideration in choosing a stethoscope should be that it is well made and fits well in your ears. Stethoscopes are available from uniform shops and medical supply companies.

The usual length of tubing on a stethoscope is 12 to 16 inches (30 to 40 cm), but you may prefer the longer 22-inch tubing. An argument against long tubing is that it transmits sound less efficiently. Research has shown, however, that 6 to 8 additional inches of tubing do not significantly alter the transmission of most sounds.

The stethoscope should have metal binaurals. The binaurals should allow you to angle the earpieces firmly to follow the direction of your ear canal. Binaurals that are too tight are uncomfortable and binaurals that are too loose do not allow you to hear as well as you should.

The earpieces should fit comfortably and snugly in the ear canal. If you can understand what someone is saying in the same room, they are too loose, which would interfere with effective auscultation. Some stethoscopes come with removable ear tips in different sizes. This offers the advantage of selecting an ear tip that fits your ear canal. Flexible ear tips of soft rubber are usually more comfortable than nonflexible tips of hard rubber or plastic.

The chest piece should be a key factor in the selection of a stethoscope. A stethoscope with a diaphragm and a bell offers the greatest versatility for listening to different types of sounds. Many stethoscopes have a rubber or plastic rim around the diaphragm and bell to avoid chilling the patient with a cold chest piece and to decrease air leaks between the chest piece and the patient.

The most common problem with the use of stethoscopes is air leaking. Air leaks interfere with effective sound transmission and allow environmental noise to enter the stethoscope. Air leaks may result from a cracked earpiece, a cracked or chipped chest piece, or a break in the tubing.

Stethoscopes must be cared for properly to ensure proper functioning and to prevent the transmission of disease in the medical office. The earpieces should be removed and cleaned regularly with a cotton-tipped applicator moistened with alcohol to remove cerumen. The chest piece should be cleaned with an antiseptic wipe to remove dirt, dust, lint, and oils. The tubing should be cleaned with a paper towel using an antimicrobial soap and water. Alcohol should not be used to clean the tubing because it can dry out the tubing and cause it to crack over time. ∎

cuff is used on a patient with a thin arm. The cuff should fit snugly and should be applied so that the center of the inflatable bag is directly over the brachial artery to allow for complete compression of the artery. The cuff has an interlocking, self-sticking substance (Velcro) that facilitates closing and fastening the cuff in place temporarily.

In obese patients with an arm circumference greater than 50 cm (20 inches), it may not be possible to fit even an adult thigh cuff around the patient's arm. In this situation, the American Heart Association (AHA) states that the patient's blood pressure can be measured using the forearm and radial artery; however, the AHA further states that this method may

Prevention of Errors in Blood Pressure Measurement

The following guidelines should be followed to prevent errors in blood pressure measurement:

1. **Instruct the patient** not to consume caffeine, use tobacco, or exercise for 30 minutes before blood pressure measurement.

2. **The patient should be comfortably seated** in a quiet room for at least 5 minutes before blood pressure is taken. Patient anxiety and apprehension can cause a spasm of the brachial artery, which can increase the blood pressure reading by as much as 30 to 50 mm Hg. This is known as the "white coat effect," which refers to the white lab coat worn by the physician. It tends to occur more frequently in older adults and young children.

3. **Always use the proper cuff size.** If the cuff is too small, it may come loose as the cuff is inflated, or the reading may be falsely high. If the cuff is too large, the reading may be falsely low. The inner inflatable bladder of the cuff should encircle at least 80% (but no more than 100%) of the patient's arm and should cover two thirds of the distance from the axilla to the antecubital space.

4. **Never take blood pressure over clothing.** Clothing interferes with the ability to hear Korotkoff sounds; this could result in an inaccurate blood pressure reading. Roll up the patient's sleeve approximately 5 inches above the elbow. If the sleeve is too tight after being rolled up, remove the arm from the sleeve. A tight sleeve causes partial compression of the brachial artery, resulting in an inaccurate reading.

5. **Position the patient properly.** The patient should be seated in a chair with the legs uncrossed and the back and arm supported. Crossing the legs can increase the systolic reading by 2 to 8 mm Hg. If the back is not supported (such as when a patient is seated on an examining table), the diastolic reading can be increased by as much as 6 mm Hg. Position the arm at heart level, and ensure that it is well supported with the palm facing upward. If the arm is above heart level, the blood pressure reading may be falsely low. If the arm is not supported or is placed below heart level, the blood pressure reading may be falsely high.

6. **Avoid extraneous sounds from the cuff.** Position the cuff approximately 1 to 2 inches above the bend in the elbow. The cuff should be up far enough to prevent the stethoscope from touching it; otherwise, extraneous sounds, which could interfere with an accurate measurement, may be picked up.

7. **Compress the brachial artery completely.** Center the inner bladder of the cuff directly over the artery to be compressed. Most cuffs are labeled with arrows indicating the center of the bladder for the right and left arms. Centering the inner bladder allows for complete compression of the brachial artery.

8. **Apply equal pressure over the brachial artery.** The cuff should be applied so that it fits smoothly and snugly around the patient's arm. This prevents bulging or slipping and permits application of an equal pressure over the brachial artery. A loose-fitting cuff can cause a falsely high reading.

9. **Instruct the patient to relax as much as possible and to not talk during the procedure.** Patient anxiety and apprehension can increase the blood pressure reading. Talking interferes with the medical assistant's ability to hear the Korotkoff sounds.

10. **Position the earpieces so that you can hear the sounds clearly.** Place the earpieces of the stethoscope in your ears with the earpieces directed slightly forward. This allows the earpieces to follow the direction of the ear canal, which facilitates hearing.

11. **Avoid extraneous sounds from the tubing.** Make sure the tubing of the stethoscope hangs freely and is not permitted to rub against any object. If the stethoscope tubing rubs against an object, extraneous sounds may be picked up, and this could interfere with an accurate measurement.

12. **Position the chest piece properly.** Palpate the brachial pulse to provide good positioning of the chest piece over the brachial artery. Place the chest piece firmly, but gently, over the brachial artery to assist in transmitting clear and audible sounds. Do not allow the chest piece to touch the cuff, to prevent extraneous sounds from being picked up, which could interfere with an accurate measurement.

13. **Release the pressure at a moderate steady rate.** Release the pressure in the cuff at a rate of 2 to 3 mm Hg/sec to ensure an accurate blood pressure measurement. Releasing the pressure too slowly is uncomfortable for the patient and could cause a falsely high diastolic reading. Releasing the pressure too quickly could cause a falsely low systolic reading.

14. **Avoid venous congestion.** If you need to take the blood pressure in the same arm again, wait 1 to 2 minutes to allow blood trapped in the veins (venous congestion) to be released. Venous congestion can result in a falsely high systolic reading and a falsely low diastolic reading.

15. **Measure and record the blood pressure in both arms during the initial blood pressure assessment of a new patient.** There may normally be a difference of 5 to 10 mm Hg between the two arms. During return visits, the blood pressure should be measured in the arm with the higher initial reading.

result in a falsely high systolic reading. When using this method, an appropriate sized cuff should be positioned midway between the elbow and the wrist, with the center of the bladder positioned over the radial pulse. The medical assistant should then place the diaphragm of the stethoscope over the radial pulse and should measure the patient's blood pressure using the same technique presented in Procedure 4-9.

Korotkoff Sounds

Korotkoff sounds are used to determine systolic and diastolic blood pressure readings. When the bladder of the cuff is inflated, the brachial artery is compressed so that no audible sounds are heard through the stethoscope. As the cuff is deflated, at a rate of 2 to 3 mm Hg per second, the sounds become audible until the blood flows freely, at which point the sounds can no longer be heard (Table 4-10). The medical assistant should practice listening to these sounds and should be able to identify the various phases.

Procedure 4-9 outlines the procedure for taking blood pressure using an aneroid sphygmomanometer. Procedure 4-10 outlines the procedure for determining systolic pressure by palpation.

Automated Oscillometric Blood Pressure Device

Automated oscillometric devices (Figure 4-25) are being used in some medical offices to measure blood pressure. They are becoming especially popular for use in home monitoring of blood pressure by patients with high blood pressure. It is important to use an automated device that has undergone a formal clinical validation process to assess its accuracy. A current list of clinically validated automated blood pressure devices can be found at the following websites: British Hypertension Society: www.bhsoc.org; and the Association for the Advancement of Medical Instrumentation: www.aami.org.

An automated oscillometric device uses an electronic sensor to measures oscillations from the wall of the brachial artery as the cuff gradually deflates. An oscillation is a back-and-forth movement that occurs in the brachial artery as the pulse wave travels through it. The point of maximum oscillation corresponds to the mean arterial pressure, which is an overall index of an individual's blood pressure. A computer in the device then uses this information to calculate the systolic blood pressure and the diastolic blood pressure. Results are then displayed on a screen. The automated blood pressure procedure takes approximately 30 seconds to complete from start to finish.

The medical assistant must make sure to follow the manufacturer's instructions for the particular brand and model of automated device used; these instructions are outlined in the user manual that accompanies the device. Many of the principles for the accurate measurement of blood pressure using an automated device are the same as those for

Table 4-10	Korotkoff Sounds	
Phase	**Description**	**Illustration**
	Inflation of cuff compresses and closes off brachial artery so that no blood flows through the artery.	

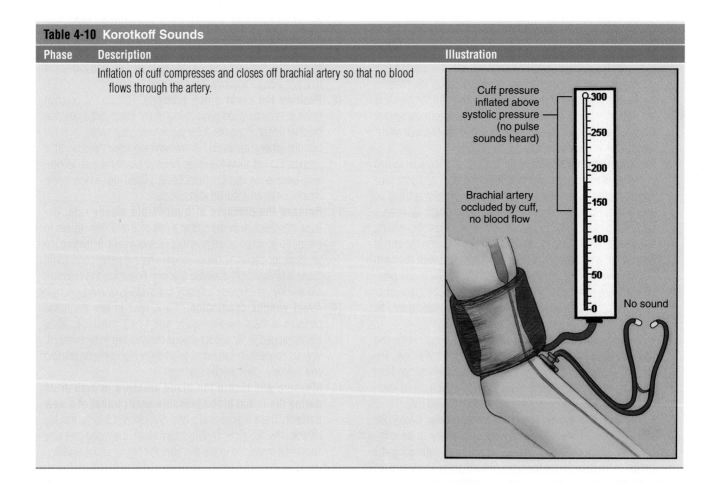

Table 4-10 Korotkoff Sounds—cont'd

Phase	Description	Illustration
Phase I	First faint but clear tapping sound is heard, and it gradually increases in intensity. First tapping sound is the systolic pressure.	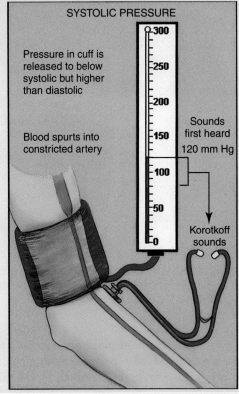
Phase II	As cuff continues to deflate, sounds have murmuring or swishing quality.	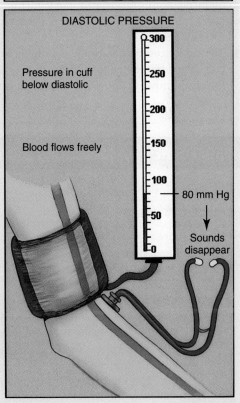
Phase III	With further deflation, sounds become crisper and increase in intensity.	
Phase IV	Sounds become muffled and have soft, blowing quality.	
Phase V	Sounds disappear. This is recorded as the diastolic pressure.	

SYSTOLIC PRESSURE

Pressure in cuff is released to below systolic but higher than diastolic

Blood spurts into constricted artery

Sounds first heard 120 mm Hg

Korotkoff sounds

DIASTOLIC PRESSURE

Pressure in cuff below diastolic

Blood flows freely

80 mm Hg

Sounds disappear

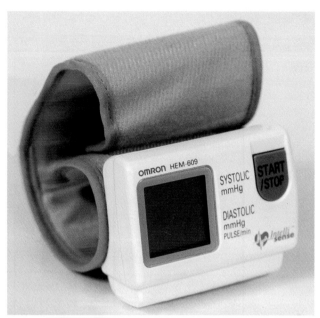

Figure 4-25. Automated oscillometric blood pressure device. (Robinson DS: Essentials of dental assisting, ed 4, St Louis, 2007, Saunders.)

manual measurement of blood pressure (refer to *Prevention of Errors in Blood Pressure Measurement*). The device should be calibrated periodically according to the manufacturer's recommendations. Automated oscillometric devices offer certain advantages and disadvantages, described as follows:

Advantages
1. The device can automatically determine how much the cuff should be inflated to reach a pressure that is approximately 30 mm Hg above the systolic pressure.

2. The cuff does not have to be manually inflated and deflated because this function is performed automatically by the device.
3. The patient's brachial artery does not need to be located, and the bladder of the cuff does not need to be centered over the brachial artery.
4. A stethoscope and user listening skills are not required to obtain the reading because the electronic sensor in the automated device measures oscillations from the wall of the brachial artery to obtain the reading.
5. Automated devices are less susceptible to external environmental noise than are manual devices.
6. The blood pressure measurement is easy to read because the systolic and diastolic readings are shown on a digital display screen.
7. The device allows multiple blood pressure measurements to be taken.
8. Most automated devices come equipped with an internal memory for storing multiple blood pressure measurements.

Disadvantages
1. There are certain factors that can cause an automated device to fail to obtain a reading. These include patient movement, muscle tremors, preeclampsia, dysrhythmias (such as atrial fibrillation), and a very weak pulse. If any of these conditions are present, an alternative method of blood pressure measurement should be used.
2. Because the device relies on brachial artery oscillations to obtain a reading, stiff arteries (especially in older patients) can interfere with obtaining an accurate reading.
3. Automated oscillometric devices are expensive.

PROCEDURE 4-9   Measuring Blood Pressure

Outcome Measure blood pressure.

Equipment/Supplies

- Stethoscope
- Sphygmomanometer
- Antiseptic wipe

1. Procedural Step. Sanitize your hands, and assemble the equipment. If the chest piece consists of a diaphragm and a bell, rotate it to the diaphragm position. Clean the earpieces and chest piece of the stethoscope with the antiseptic wipe.
Principle. The chest piece must be rotated to the proper position for sound to be heard through the earpieces.

2. Procedural Step. Greet the patient and introduce yourself. Identify the patient and explain the procedure. Explain to the patient that measuring blood

pressure may normally cause a little numbing and tingling in the arm when the cuff is inflated. While explaining the procedure, observe the patient for signs that might influence the reading, such as anger, fear, pain, and recent physical activity. If it is not possible to reduce or eliminate these influences, list them in the patient's chart. Determine how high to pump the cuff by checking the patient's chart for previously measured systolic readings, or determine the patient's systolic pressure by palpation (see Procedure 4-10).

PROCEDURE 4-9   Measuring Blood Pressure—cont'd

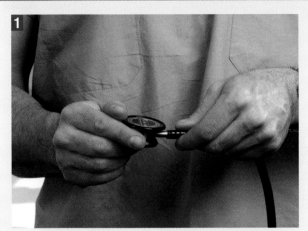

Rotate the chest piece to the diaphragm position.

3. **Procedural Step.** Have the patient sit quietly in a comfortable position in a chair with the legs uncrossed and the back supported. The patient should relax in a sitting position for at least 5 minutes before measuring his or her blood pressure. Roll up the patient's sleeve approximately 5 inches above the elbow. If the sleeve does not roll up or is too tight after being rolled up, remove the arm from the sleeve. The arm should be positioned at heart level and well supported, with the palm facing up.

Principle. Patient anxiety can cause a significant increase in blood pressure. Clothing interferes with the ability to hear Korotkoff sounds, which could result in an inaccurate blood pressure reading. A tight sleeve causes partial compression of the brachial artery, resulting in an inaccurate reading. The position of the arm allows easy access to the brachial artery. Placing the arm above heart level may cause the reading to be falsely low. Not supporting the arm or placing it below heart level may cause the reading to be falsely high.

4. **Procedural Step.** Select the proper cuff size. The inner inflatable bladder of the cuff should be long enough to encircle at least 80% (but no more than 100%) of the patient's arm and wide enough to cover two thirds of the distance from the axilla to the antecubital space.

Principle. The appropriate-size cuff must be used to ensure an accurate measurement. If the cuff is too small, it may come loose as the cuff is inflated, or the reading may be falsely high. If the cuff is too large, the reading may be falsely low.

5. **Procedural Step.** Locate the brachial pulse with the fingertips. The brachial pulse is located near the center of the antecubital space but slightly toward the little finger–side of the arm. Center the inner bladder over the brachial pulse site. (*Note:* Place the cuff on the

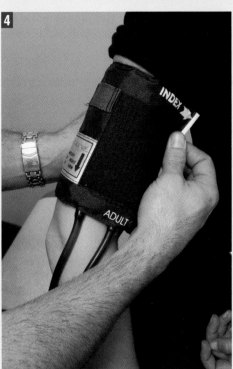

The inner bladder should encircle at least 80% of the patient's arm.

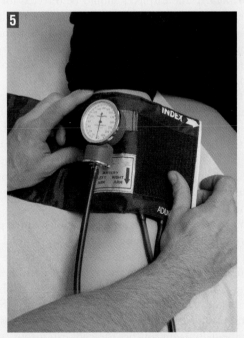

Center the inner bladder over the brachial pulse site.

patient's arm so that the lower edge of the cuff is approximately 1 to 2 inches above the bend in the elbow. Most cuffs are labeled with right and left arrows indicating the center of the bladder. The right arrow should be placed over the brachial pulse site when you

Continued

PROCEDURE 4-9

PROCEDURE 4-9   Measuring Blood Pressure—cont'd

are using the right arm, and the left arrow should be placed over the brachial pulse site when you are using the left arm.)

Principle. The cuff should be placed high enough to prevent the stethoscope from touching it; otherwise, extraneous sounds, which could interfere with an accurate measurement, may be picked up. Centering the inner bladder over the pulse site allows complete compression of the brachial artery.

6. **Procedural Step.** Wrap the cuff smoothly and snugly around the patient's arm, and secure the end of it.
   Principle. Applying the cuff properly prevents it from bulging or slipping. This technique permits application of an equal pressure over the brachial artery.

7. **Procedural Step.** Position the manometer for direct viewing and at a distance of no more than 3 feet.
   Principle. The medical assistant may have trouble seeing the scale on the manometer if it is placed more than 3 feet away.

8. **Procedural Step.** Instruct the patient not to talk or move. Place the earpieces of the stethoscope in your ears, with the earpieces directed slightly forward. During the blood pressure measurement, the tubing of the stethoscope should hang freely and should not be permitted to rub against any object.
   Principle. The earpieces should be directed forward, permitting them to follow the direction of the ear canal, which facilitates hearing. If the stethoscope tubing rubs against an object, extraneous sounds may be picked up; this would interfere with an accurate measurement.

9. **Procedural Step.** Making sure the arm is well extended, locate the brachial pulse again, and place the diaphragm of the stethoscope over the brachial pulse site. The diaphragm should be positioned to make a tight seal against the patient's skin. Enough pressure should be exerted to leave a temporary ring on the patient's skin when the disc is removed. Do not allow the chest piece to touch the cuff.
   Principle. A well-extended arm allows easier palpation of the brachial pulse. Locating the brachial pulse again is necessary for proper positioning of the chest piece over the brachial artery. Proper positioning of the diaphragm and good contact of the diaphragm with the skin help transmit clear and audible Korotkoff sounds through the earpieces of the stethoscope. If the diaphragm touches the cuff, extraneous sounds may be picked up; this would interfere with an accurate measurement.

10. **Procedural Step.** Close the valve on the bulb by turning the thumbscrew clockwise (to the right) with the thumb and forefinger of your dominant hand until it feels tight but can still be loosened with the thumb

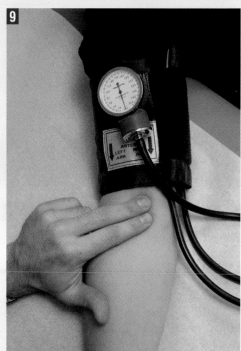

Locate the brachial pulse again before placing the diaphragm over the site.

and forefinger of one hand when you need to deflate the cuff. Pump air into the cuff as rapidly as possible to at least 30 mm Hg above the previously measured or palpated systolic pressure.

Principle. Inflation of the cuff compresses and closes off the brachial artery so that no blood flows through the artery. If the patient has had the blood pressure measured previously at the medical office, the recorded systolic pressure can be used to determine how

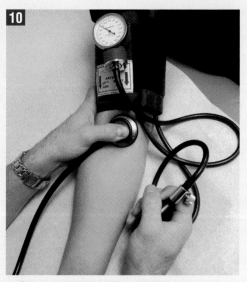

Pump air into the cuff as rapidly as possible.

PROCEDURE 4-9   Measuring Blood Pressure—cont'd

high to inflate the cuff. Preliminary determination of the systolic pressure by palpation allows the medical assistant to estimate how high to inflate the cuff.

11. Procedural Step. Release the pressure at a moderately steady rate of 2 to 3 mm Hg/sec by slowly turning the thumbscrew counterclockwise (to the left) with the thumb and forefinger. This opens the valve and allows the air in the cuff to escape slowly. Listen for the first clear tapping sound (phase I of the Korotkoff sounds). This represents the systolic pressure. Note this point on the scale of the manometer.

Principle. Releasing the pressure too slowly is uncomfortable for the patient and could cause a falsely high diastolic reading. Releasing the pressure too quickly could cause a falsely low systolic reading and a falsely high diastolic reading. The systolic pressure is the point at which the blood first begins to spurt through

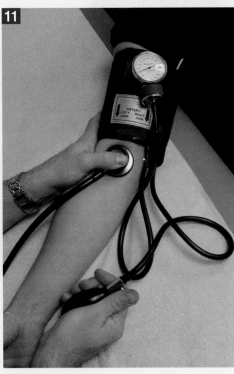

Release the pressure at a moderately steady rate.

the artery as the cuff pressure begins to decrease; it represents the pressure that occurs on the walls of the arteries during systole.

12. Procedural Step. Continue to deflate the cuff while listening to the Korotkoff sounds. Listen for the onset of the muffled sound that occurs during phase IV. Continue to deflate the cuff, and note the point on the scale at which the sound ceases (phase V). Continue to steadily deflate the cuff for another 10 mm Hg to ensure that there are no more sounds.

Principle. Phase V marks the diastolic pressure (which represents the pressure that occurs on the walls of the arteries during diastole); the cuff pressure is reduced, and blood is flowing freely through the brachial artery.

13. Procedural Step. Quickly and completely deflate the cuff to zero. If you could not obtain an accurate blood pressure reading, wait 1 to 2 minutes before taking another measurement on the same arm. Remove the earpieces of the stethoscope from your ears, and carefully remove the cuff from the patient's arm.

Principle. Venous congestion results when blood pressure is taken, which alters a second reading if it is taken too soon on the same arm.

14. Procedural Step. Sanitize your hands, and chart the results. Include the date, the time, and the blood pressure reading. Blood pressure is recorded using even numbers. Make a notation in the patient's chart if the lying or standing position was used to take blood pressure. Abbreviations that can be used are *L* (lying) and *St* (standing).

15. Procedural Step. Clean the earpieces and the chest piece of the stethoscope with an antiseptic wipe, and replace the equipment properly.

CHARTING EXAMPLE	
Date	
10/20/12	2:30 p.m. BP: 106/74.__ S. Martinez, RMA

PROCEDURE 4-10 Determining Systolic Pressure by Palpation

Outcome Determine systolic pressure by palpation.

Equipment/Supplies

*   Sphygmomanometer

1. **Procedural Step.** Sanitize your hands, and assemble the equipment.
2. **Procedural Step.** Locate the brachial pulse with the fingertips. Place the cuff on the patient's arm so that the inner bladder is centered over the brachial pulse site.
3. **Procedural Step.** Wrap the cuff smoothly and snugly around the patient's arm, and secure the end of it.
4. **Procedural Step.** Position the manometer for direct viewing and at a distance of no more than 3 feet.
5. **Procedural Step.** Locate the radial pulse with your fingertips.
6. **Procedural Step.** Close the valve on the bulb, and pump air into the cuff until the pulsation ceases.
7. **Procedural Step.** Release the valve at a moderate rate of 2 to 3 mm Hg per heartbeat while palpating the artery with your fingertips.
8. **Procedural Step.** Record the point at which the pulsation reappears as the palpated systolic pressure.
9. **Procedural Step.** Deflate the cuff completely, and wait 15 to 30 seconds before checking the blood pressure.

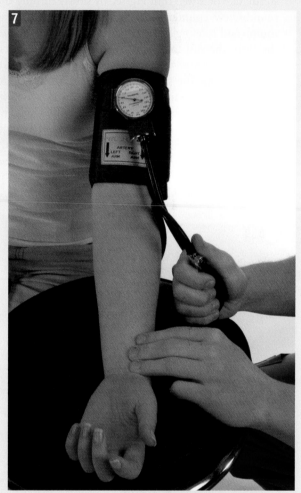

Release the valve while palpating the radial artery.

*e*volve *Check out the Evolve site to access additional interactive activities.*

MEDICAL PRACTICE *and the* LAW

Measurement of vital signs is standard procedure for almost every patient in the physician's office. Because vital sign measurements are performed so frequently, the medical assistant may tend to minimize their importance. Changes in vital signs may be the first indicator of disease or illness, so meticulous attention must be paid to the performance and documentation of vital signs and to comparison of current measurements with past measurements for each patient.

Most patients want to know their vital signs, especially their blood pressure or temperature if febrile. Although the patient owns the information that you collect, be aware that you may not give this information to family members without the patient's consent. Some offices have a policy that indicates specific information that the medical assistant can give the patient; some physicians prefer to disclose this information themselves and discuss it with their patients.

Often, measurement of vital signs is the first contact patients have with the medical assistant. The most important factor in determining whether a patient will sue is not the skill of the practitioner, but the level of rapport with the patient. In everything you do, convey your caring and concern to every patient. ∎

What Would You Do? What Would You *Not* Do? RESPONSES

Case Study 1
Page 139

What Did Sergio Do?
- ☐ Told Mrs. Mason that sometimes ear thermometers can be a little tricky to use.
- ☐ Showed Mrs. Mason how to use the ear thermometer and let her practice by taking Olivia's temperature.
- ☐ Explained how to care for and maintain the ear thermometer to prevent inaccurate readings.
- ☐ Explained to Mrs. Mason that the use of mercury is being discouraged because it can be toxic to humans and animals.

What Did Sergio Not *Do?*
- ☐ Did not ask Mrs. Mason if she had read the directions that came with her ear thermometer.
- ☐ Did not tell Mrs. Mason that she should switch back to the mercury thermometer.
- ☐ Did not ask Mrs. Mason why she waited so long to bring Olivia to the office.

What Would You Do/What Would You *Not* Do? Review Sergio's response and place a checkmark next to the information you included in your response. List the additional information you included in your response.

_____

_____

_____

_____

Case Study 2
Page 143

What Did Sergio Do?
- ☐ Recognized and congratulated Alex on his swimming achievements.
- ☐ Told Alex that it is normal for his pulse to be that slow because of his athletic training and it shows that he is in good shape.
- ☐ Assured Alex that the physician will do everything he can to help Alex.
- ☐ Stressed to Alex how important it is to follow the physician's advice so that his shoulder heals as soon as possible.

What Did Sergio Not *Do?*
- ☐ Did not comment on Alex's request for a steroid injection or OxyContin. Made sure to chart the information so that the physician could handle the situation.
- ☐ Did not criticize Alex for putting a swim meet before his health.

What Would You Do/What Would You *Not* Do? Review Sergio's response and place a checkmark next to the information you included in your response. List the additional information you included in your response.

_____

_____

_____

_____

Case Study 3
Page 148

What Did Sergio Do?
- ☐ Empathized with Tyrone about having to take so many pills. Suggested that he get a daily pill container to help him remember.
- ☐ Stressed to Tyrone the importance of taking his blood pressure medication. Explained to him that high blood pressure is a "silent disease." He may feel fine, but damage to his body organs can still be taking place if he does not take his pills.
- ☐ Gave Tyrone a brochure about high blood pressure and went over the long-term effects of hypertension and lifestyle changes that could help lower blood pressure.
- ☐ Encouraged Tyrone to call the office when he experiences side effects from medications because the physician may be able to do something to help.

What Did Sergio Not *Do?*
- ☐ Did not tell him it was all right to discontinue his medication.

What Would You Do/What Would You *Not* Do? Review Sergio's response and place a checkmark next to the information you included in your response. List the additional information you included in your response.

_____

_____

_____

_____

CERTIFICATION REVIEW

Temperature
- ☐ **Body temperature is maintained** within a fairly constant range by the hypothalamus, which is located in the brain. Body temperature is maintained through a balance of the heat produced in the body and the heat lost from the body. Heat is produced in the body by voluntary and involuntary muscle contractions, cell metabolism, and strong emotional states. Heat is lost from the body through perspiration; in urine, feces, and moisture droplets from the lungs; and through conduction, convection, and radiation.
- ☐ **The normal body temperature range** is 97° F to 99° F (36.1° C to 37.2° C), with the average body temperature being 98.6° F (37° C). *Pyrexia* describes a temperature above normal, and hypothermia describes a temperature below normal.

Continued

CERTIFICATION REVIEW—cont'd

❑ **Factors that affect body temperature** include age, diurnal variations, exercise, emotional state, environmental factors, the patient's normal body temperature, and pregnancy. An individual with a fever is said to be *febrile,* and one without a fever is *afebrile.* The course of a fever rises and falls in one of the following patterns: continuous, intermittent, or remittent.

❑ **The five sites** for taking body temperature are the mouth, rectum, axilla, ear, and forehead. The site chosen for measuring a patient's temperature depends on the patient's age, condition, and state of consciousness; the type of thermometer being used; and the medical office policy. Temperature obtained through the rectal route measures approximately 1° F higher than the same individual's temperature taken through the oral route. Axillary temperature measures approximately 1° F lower than the same individual's temperature taken through the oral route.

❑ **An electronic thermometer** consists of interchangeable oral (blue) and rectal (red) probes attached to a battery-operated portable unit. A disposable plastic cover is placed over the probe to prevent the transmission of microorganisms among patients.

❑ **The tympanic membrane thermometer** is used at the aural site and provides results within 1 to 2 seconds. The thermometer detects thermal energy given off by the tympanic membrane in the form of infrared waves.

❑ **The temporal artery thermometer** is the newest device for assessing body temperature. The probe of the thermometer is gently and slowly moved across the patient's forehead to capture the infrared heat given off by the temporal artery. The temperature obtained through the forehead site is about the same as a rectal temperature measurement.

❑ **Chemical thermometers** are less accurate than other types of thermometers; they often are used by patients at home to obtain a general assessment of body temperature.

Pulse

❑ **When the left ventricle of the heart contracts,** a pulsating wave travels through the walls of the arterial system; this wave is known as the *pulse.* Pulse rate can vary because of age, gender, physical activity, emotional state, metabolism, fever, and medications.

❑ **The most common site** for measuring pulse is the radial artery, located on the inner aspect of the wrist just below the thumb. The apical pulse, which is easier to hear than the pulse at other sites, is located in the fifth intercostal space at the junction of the left midclavicular line. Other pulse sites are the brachial, ulnar, temporal, carotid, femoral, popliteal, posterior tibial, and dorsalis pedis.

❑ **The normal resting pulse rate** for an adult is 60 to 100 beats per minute. A pulse rate of more than 100 beats per minute is tachycardia, and a pulse rate of less than 60 beats per minute is bradycardia.

❑ **The pulse rhythm** is the time interval between heartbeats. An irregularity in the heart's rhythm is known as a *dysrhythmia* (or *arrhythmia*). An apical-radial pulse is performed to determine whether a pulse deficit is present. A pulse deficit exists when the radial pulse rate is less than the apical pulse rate; it frequently occurs with atrial fibrillation. The *pulse volume* refers to the strength of the heartbeat. A thready pulse feels weak and thin, and a bounding pulse feels very strong and full.

Respiration

❑ **One respiration** consists of one inhalation and one exhalation. During inhalation, the diaphragm descends and the lungs expand; during exhalation, the diaphragm ascends and the lungs return to their original state.

❑ **The respiratory rate** of an adult ranges from 12 to 20 respirations per minute. An abnormal increase in respiratory rate is known as *tachypnea,* and an abnormal decrease is known as *bradypnea.*

❑ **Normally, the rhythm** should be even and regular, and the pauses between inhalation and exhalation should be equal. The depth of each respiration should be the same. Hyperpnea denotes a very deep, rapid, and labored type of respiration. Hyperventilation is an abnormally fast and deep type of breathing, usually associated with acute anxiety. Hypopnea is an abnormal decrease in the rate and depth of respiration. Dyspnea, or difficult breathing, can be caused by asthma, emphysema, and vigorous physical exertion. *Orthopnea* means the patient can breathe easier in a sitting or standing position.

Pulse Oximetry

❑ **Pulse oximetry measures** the oxygen saturation of hemoglobin in arterial blood (SpO_2). Hemoglobin functions in transporting oxygen in the body. Pulse oximetry provides information on a patient's cardiorespiratory status, in particular, the amount of oxygen being delivered to the tissues of the body. A pulse oximeter also measures the patient's pulse rate.

❑ **The oxygen saturation level of most healthy individuals** is 95% to 99%. An oxygen saturation level of less than 95% typically results in an inadequate amount of oxygen reaching the tissues. Respiratory failure usually occurs when oxygen saturation falls to a level between 85% and 90%. Cyanosis typically appears when an individual's oxygen saturation reaches a level of 75%, and an oxygen saturation of less than 70% is life threatening.

❑ **Hypoxemia** is a decrease in the oxygen saturation of the blood (less than 95%). Hypoxemia can lead to a

CERTIFICATION REVIEW—cont'd

more serious condition known as *hypoxia*. Hypoxia is defined as a reduction in the oxygen supply to tissues of the body; if not treated, it can lead to tissue damage and death.

❑ **In the medical office, pulse oximetry is usually performed** on patients complaining of respiratory problems (e.g., dyspnea). Conditions that can cause a decreased oxygen saturation level include acute pulmonary disease (pneumonia), chronic pulmonary disease (emphysema, asthma, bronchitis) and cardiac problems (congestive heart failure, coronary artery disease).

Blood Pressure

❑ **Blood pressure measures** the pressure exerted by the blood on the walls of the arteries. The systolic pressure is the highest pressure, and the diastolic pressure is the point of lesser pressure on the arterial walls.

❑ **A blood pressure** of less than 120/80 mm Hg is normal. A single blood pressure reading taken on one occasion does not characterize an individual's blood pressure; several readings must be taken on different occasions.

❑ **Hypertension** is excessive pressure on the walls of the arteries and refers to a sustained systolic pressure of 140 mm Hg or greater or a sustained diastolic reading of 90 mm Hg or greater.

❑ **Factors that affect blood pressure** are age, gender, diurnal variations, emotional state, exercise, body position, and medication.

TERMINOLOGY REVIEW

Medical Term	Word Parts	Definition
Adventitious sounds		Abnormal breath sounds.
Afebrile	*a-:* without	Without fever; the body temperature is normal.
Alveolus	*alveol/o:* air sac	A thin-walled air sac of the lungs in which the exchange of oxygen and carbon dioxide takes place.
Antecubital space	*ante-:* before *cubitum:* elbow	The space located at the front of the elbow.
Antipyretic	*anti-:* against *pyr/o:* fever *-ic:* pertaining to	An agent that reduces fever.
Aorta		The major trunk of the arterial system of the body. The aorta arises from the upper surface of the left ventricle.
Apnea	*a-:* without or absence of *-pnea:* breathing	The temporary cessation of breathing.
Axilla		The armpit.
Bounding pulse		A pulse with an increased volume that feels very strong and full.
Bradycardia	*brady-:* slow *cardi/o:* heart *-ia:* condition of diseased or abnormal state	An abnormally slow heart rate (less than 60 beats per minute).
Bradypnea	*brady-:* slow *-pnea:* breathing	An abnormal decrease in the respiratory rate of less than 10 respirations per minute.
Celsius scale		A temperature scale on which the freezing point of water is 0° and the boiling point of water is 100°; also called the *centigrade scale.*
Conduction		The transfer of energy, such as heat, from one object to another by direct contact.
Convection		The transfer of energy, such as heat, through air currents.
Crisis		A sudden falling of an elevated body temperature to normal.
Cyanosis	*cyan/o:* blue *-osis:* abnormal condition	A bluish discoloration of the skin and mucous membranes.

Continued

☟ TERMINOLOGY REVIEW—cont'd

Medical Term	Word Parts	Definition
Diastole		The phase in the cardiac cycle in which the heart relaxes between contractions.
Diastolic pressure		The point of lesser pressure on the arterial wall, which is recorded during diastole.
Dyspnea	*dys-:* difficult, painful, abnormal *-pnea:* breathing	Shortness of breath or difficulty in breathing.
Dysrhythmia	*dys-:* difficult, painful, abnormal *rhythm:* rhythm *-ia:* condition of diseased or abnormal state	An irregular rhythm; also termed *arrhythmia.*
Eupnea	*eu-:* normal, good *-pnea:* breathing	Normal respiration. The rate is 16 to 20 respirations per minute, the rhythm is even and regular, and the depth is normal.
Exhalation	*-ex:* outside, outward	The act of breathing out.
Fahrenheit scale		A temperature scale on which the freezing point of water is 32° and the boiling point of water is 212°.
Febrile		Pertaining to fever.
Fever		A body temperature that is above normal; synonym for *pyrexia.*
Frenulum linguae		The midline fold that connects the undersurface of the tongue with the floor of the mouth.
Hyperpnea	*hyper-:* above, excessive *-pnea:* breathing	An abnormal increase in the rate and depth of respiration.
Hyperpyrexia	*hyper-:* above, excessive *pyr/o:* fever *-ia:* condition of diseased or abnormal state	An extremely high fever.
Hypertension	*hyper-:* above, excessive *tension:* pressure	High blood pressure.
Hyperventilation	*hyper-:* above, excessive	An abnormally fast and deep type of breathing, usually associated with acute anxiety conditions.
Hypopnea	*hypo-:* below, deficient *-pnea:* breathing	An abnormal decrease in the rate and depth of respiration.
Hypotension	*hypo-:* below, deficient *tension:* pressure	Low blood pressure.
Hypothermia	*hypo-:* below, deficient *therm/o:* heat *-ia:* condition of diseased or abnormal state	A body temperature that is below normal.
Hypoxemia	*hypo-:* below, deficient *ox/i:* oxygen *-emia:* blood condition	A decrease in the oxygen saturation of the blood. Hypoxemia may lead to hypoxia.
Hypoxia	*hypo-:* below, deficient *ox/i:* oxygen *-ia:* condition of diseased or abnormal state	A reduction in the oxygen supply to the tissues of the body.
Inhalation	*in-:* in, into	The act of breathing in.

↻ TERMINOLOGY REVIEW—cont'd

Medical Term	Word Parts	Definition
Intercostal	*inter-:* between *cost/o:* rib *-al:* pertaining to	Between the ribs.
Korotkoff sounds		Sounds heard during the measurement of blood pressure that are used to determine the systolic and diastolic blood pressure readings.
Malaise	*-mal:* bad	A vague sense of body discomfort, weakness, and fatigue that often marks the onset of a disease and continues through the course of the illness.
Manometer	*-meter:* instrument used to measure	An instrument for measuring pressure.
Meniscus		The curved surface on a column of liquid in a tube.
Orthopnea	*orth/o:* straight *-pnea:* breathing	The condition in which breathing is easier when an individual is in a sitting or standing position.
Pulse oximeter	*ox/i:* oxygen *-meter:* instrument used to measure	A computerized device consisting of a probe and a monitor used to measure the oxygen saturation of arterial blood.
Pulse oximetry	*ox/i:* oxygen *-metry:* measurement	The use of a pulse oximeter to measure the oxygen saturation of arterial blood.
Pulse pressure		The difference between the systolic and diastolic pressures.
Pulse rhythm		The time interval between heartbeats.
Pulse volume		The strength of the heartbeat.
Radiation		The transfer of energy, such as heat, in the form of waves.
SaO_2 (saturation of arterial oxygen)		Abbreviation for the percentage of hemoglobin that is saturated with oxygen in arterial blood.
Sphygmomanometer	*sphygm/o:* pulse *-meter:* instrument used to measure	An instrument for measuring arterial blood pressure.
SpO_2 (saturation of peripheral oxygen)		Abbreviation for the percentage of hemoglobin that is saturated with oxygen in arterial blood as measured by a pulse oximeter.
Stethoscope	*steth/o:* chest *-scope:* to view, to examine	An instrument used for amplifying and hearing sounds produced by the body.
Systole		The phase in the cardiac cycle in which the ventricles contract, sending blood out of the heart and into the aorta and pulmonary aorta.
Systolic pressure		The point of maximum pressure on the arterial walls, which is recorded during systole.
Tachycardia	*tachy-:* fast, rapid *cardi/o:* heart *-ia:* condition of diseased or abnormal state	An abnormally fast heart rate (more than 100 beats per minute).
Tachypnea	*tachy-:* fast *-pnea:* breathing	An abnormal increase in the respiratory rate of more than 20 respirations per minute.
Thready pulse		A pulse with a decreased volume that feels weak and thin.

ON THE WEB

For information on hypertension:

American Heart Association: www.americanheart.org

National Heart, Lung, and Blood Institute: www.nhlbi.nih.gov

Cardiology Channel: www.cardiologychannel.com

Hypertension Education Foundation: www.hypertensionfoundation.org

American Society of Hypertension: www.ash-us.org

WebMD on Hypertension: www.webmd.com/hypertension-high-blood-pressure/default.htm

MedicineNet Hypertension: www.medicinenet.com/high_blood_pressure/article.htm

Mayo Clinic Hypertension: www.mayoclinic.com/health/high-blood-pressure/ds00100

For information on lung disease:

American Lung Association: www.lungusa.org

Pulmonology Channel: www.pulmonologychannel.com

Lung Cancer Online: www.lungcanceronline.org

Women's Health-Lung Disease: www.womenshealth.gov/FAQ/lung-disease.cfm

5

The Physical Examination

LEARNING OBJECTIVES	PROCEDURES
Preparation for the Physical Examination 1. Identify the three components of a complete patient examination. 2. List the guidelines that should be followed in preparing the examining room. 3. Identify equipment and instruments used during the physical examination.	Prepare the examining room. Operate and care for equipment and instruments used during the physical examination, according to the manufacturers' instructions. Prepare a patient for a physical examination.
Measuring Weight and Height 1. Explain the purpose of measuring weight and height. 2. List the guidelines that should be followed when measuring weight and height.	Measure weight and height.
Body Mechanics 1. Explain the importance of using proper body mechanics. 2. State the basic principles related to proper body mechanics that should be followed.	Demonstrate proper body mechanics when standing, sitting, and lifting an object.

Positioning and Draping
1. Explain the purposes of positioning and draping.
2. List one use of each patient position.
	Position and drape a patient in each of the following positions:
	    Sitting
	    Supine
	    Prone
	    Dorsal recumbent
	    Lithotomy
	    Sims
	    Knee-chest
	    Fowler's

Wheelchair Transfer 1. Explain the purpose of a wheelchair. 2. Describe the purpose of a transfer belt.	Transfer a patient from a wheelchair to the examining table and back again.
Assessment of the Patient 1. List and define the four techniques of examining the patient. 2. State an example of the use of each examination technique during the physical examination of a patient.	
Assisting the Physician 1. Describe the responsibilities of the medical assistant during the physical examination.	Assist the physician during the physical examination of a patient.

KEY TERMS

audiometer (aw-dee-OM-eh-ter)
auscultation (os-kul-TAY-shun)
bariatrics (BAR-ee-AT-riks)
body mechanics
clinical diagnosis
diagnosis
differential (diff-er-EN-shul) diagnosis
inspection
mensuration (men-soo-RAY-shun)

ophthalmoscope (off-THAL-meh-skope)
otoscope (AH-toe-skope)
palpation (pal-PAY-shun)
percussion (per-KUSH-un)
percussion hammer
prognosis
speculum (SPEK-yoo-lum)
symptom

Introduction to the Physical Examination

A complete patient examination consists of three parts: the *health history,* the *physical examination* of each body system, and *laboratory and diagnostic tests.* The physician uses the results to determine the patient's general state of health, to arrive at a diagnosis and prescribe treatment, and to observe any change in a patient's illness after treatment has been instituted.

An important and frequent responsibility of the medical assistant is to assist with a physical examination. Because health-promotion and disease-prevention activities have become an important focus of health care, individuals are becoming more aware of the need for a yearly physical examination to detect early signs of illness and to prevent serious health problems. Also, a physical examination may be a prerequisite for employment, participation in sports, attendance at summer camp, and admission to school. The physical examination is explained in detail in this chapter. Taking the health history, collecting specimens, and performing laboratory and diagnostic tests are discussed in other chapters.

DEFINITIONS OF TERMS

The medical assistant should know and understand the following terms related to the patient examination:

Final diagnosis. Often simply called the *diagnosis,* this term refers to the scientific method of determining and identifying a patient's condition through evaluation of the health history, the physical examination, laboratory tests, and diagnostic procedures. A final diagnosis is crucial because it provides a logical basis for treatment and prognosis.

Clinical diagnosis. The clinical diagnosis is an intermediate step in the determination of a final diagnosis. The clinical diagnosis of a patient's condition is obtained through evaluation of the health history and the physical examination without the benefit of laboratory or diagnostic tests. Laboratory and diagnostic imaging facilities provide a space to specify the clinical diagnosis on their request forms; this information assists the facility in correlating data from their test results with the physician's needs. When the physician has analyzed the test results, a final diagnosis can often be established.

Differential diagnosis. Two or more diseases may have similar symptoms. The differential diagnosis involves determining which of these diseases is producing the patient's symptoms so that a final diagnosis can be established. For example, streptococcal sore throat and pharyngitis have similar symptoms. A differential diagnosis is made by obtaining a throat specimen and performing a strep test.

Prognosis. The prognosis consists of the probable course and outcome of a patient's condition and the patient's prospects for recovery.

Risk factor. A risk factor is a physical or behavioral condition that increases the probability that an individual will develop a particular condition; examples are genetic factors, habits, environmental conditions, and physiologic

Highlight on Health Screening

The chance of developing certain diseases is greater at different ages. Periodic health screening is recommended for the detection and early treatment of disease.

Test or Procedure	Gender	Recommended Frequency (for individuals of average risk)
Beginning at Age 20 Years		
Blood pressure	M and F	Every year
Cholesterol levels	M and F	Every 5 years
Blood glucose level	M and F	Every 3-5 years
Breast self-examination	F	Every month
Beginning at the Age Specified		
Clinical breast examination (by a physician)	F	Every 3 years between the ages of 20 and 39 and then every year beginning at age 40
Pap test and pelvic examination	F	Begin within 3 years of the onset of vaginal intercourse or at age 21, whichever comes first, then every 1 to 2 years
Testicular self-examination	M	Every month beginning at age 15
Fecal occult blood test	M and F	Every year starting at age 50
Colonoscopy	M and F	Every 10 years beginning at age 50
Prostate cancer screening	M	Should be offered by a health provider every year beginning at age 50 to men with a life expectancy of at least 10 years
Mammography	F	Every year beginning at age 40
Electrocardiogram	M and F	One baseline recording starting at age 40

conditions. The presence of a risk factor for a certain disease does not mean that the disease will develop; it means only that a person's chances of developing that disease are greater than those of a person without the risk factor. For example, cigarette smoking is a risk factor for developing lung cancer and heart disease. A person who smokes has a higher risk of developing lung cancer than a person who does not or who has stopped smoking.

Acute illness. An acute illness is characterized by symptoms that have a rapid onset, are usually severe and intense, and subside after a relatively short time. In some cases, the acute episode progresses into a chronic illness. Examples of acute illness include colds, influenza, strep throat, and pneumonia.

Chronic illness. A chronic illness is characterized by symptoms that persist for longer than 3 months and show little change over a long time. Examples of chronic illness include diabetes mellitus, hypertension, and emphysema.

Therapeutic procedure. A therapeutic procedure is performed to treat a patient's condition with the goal of eliminating it or promoting as much recovery as possible. Examples of therapeutic procedures include administration of medication, ear and eye irrigations, and application of heat and cold.

Laboratory testing. Laboratory testing involves the analysis and study of specimens obtained from patients to assist in diagnosing and treating disease. Examples of laboratory testing include the hemoglobin test, glucose test, urinalysis, and strep testing.

Diagnostic procedure. A diagnostic procedure is a procedure performed to assist in the diagnosis of a patient's condition; examples include electrocardiography, colonoscopy, and mammography.

PREPARATION OF THE EXAMINING ROOM

Proper preparation of the examining room provides a comfortable and healthy environment for the patient and facilitates the physical examination. The following guidelines should be followed in preparing the examining room:

1. Ensure that the examining room is free of clutter and well lit.
2. Check the examining rooms daily to ensure there are ample supplies. Restock supplies that are getting low.
3. Empty waste receptacles frequently.
4. Replace biohazard containers as necessary. When removing biohazard containers from the examining room (see Chapter 2), follow the OSHA Bloodborne Pathogens Standard.
5. Make sure the room is well ventilated, and install an air freshener to eliminate odors.
6. Maintain room temperatures that are comfortable not only for a fully clothed individual, but also for an individual who has disrobed.
7. Clean and disinfect examining tables, countertops, and faucets daily.
8. Remove dust and dirt from furniture and towel dispensers.

9. Change the examining table paper after each patient by unrolling a fresh length. Check to ensure there is an ample supply of gowns and drapes ready for use.

10. Ensure that the examining room door is closed during the examination because patient privacy is paramount.

11. Properly clean and prepare equipment, instruments, and supplies that are used for patient examinations so that they are ready for use by the physician. Table 5-1 lists the equipment and supplies, along with their uses, that may be employed during a physical examination.

12. Check equipment and instruments regularly to verify that they are in proper working condition. This protects the patient from harm caused by faulty equipment.

13. Have equipment and supplies ready for the examination and arranged for easy access by the physician. Equipment and supplies needed for the physical examination vary according to the type of examination and the physician's preference (Figure 5-1).

14. Know how to operate and care for each piece of equipment and each instrument. The manufacturer provides an operating manual, which should be read carefully and thoroughly and kept available for reference.

PREPARATION OF THE PATIENT

It is the medical assistant's responsibility to prepare the patient for the physical examination. After greeting and escorting the patient to the examining room, the medical assistant should identify the patient by asking the patient to state his or her full name and date of birth. This information should be compared with the demographic data indicated in the patient's chart. The patient should *not* be asked whether he or she is a certain patient. For example, the patient should not be asked: "Are you Mary Williams?" The patient may not hear the medical assistant correctly or may not be paying attention and may answer in the affirmative even if he or she is not that patient. Proper identification is essential to avoid mistaking one patient for another. If the medical assistant performs a procedure on the wrong patient by mistake, he or she could be held liable. The medical

Table 5-1 Equipment and Supplies for the Physical Examination	
Item	**Description and Purpose**
Patient examination gown	Gown made of disposable paper or cloth that provides patient modesty, comfort, and warmth.
Drape	A length of disposable paper or cloth to cover a patient or parts of a patient to provide comfort and warmth and reduce exposure.
Sphygmomanometer	Instrument used to measure blood pressure.
Stethoscope	Instrument used to auscultate body sounds, such as blood pressure and lung and bowel sounds.
Thermometer	Instrument used to measure body temperature.
Upright balance scale	Device used to measure weight and height.
Otoscope	Lighted instrument with lens, used to examine external ear canal and tympanic membrane.
Tuning fork	Small metal instrument consisting of stem and two prongs, used to test hearing acuity.
Ophthalmoscope	Lighted instrument with lens, used for examining interior of eye.
Tongue depressor	Flat wooden blade used to depress patient's tongue during examination of mouth and pharynx.
Antiseptic wipe	Disposable pad saturated with antiseptic, such as alcohol, that is used to cleanse skin.
Tape measure	Flexible device calibrated in inches on one side and centimeters on the other side, used to measure patient (e.g., diameter of limb, head circumference).
Percussion hammer	Instrument with rubber head, used for testing neurologic reflexes.
Speculum	Instrument for opening body orifice or cavity for viewing (e.g., ear speculum, nasal speculum, vaginal speculum).
Disposable gloves	Gloves, usually latex, that are worn only once to provide protection from bloodborne pathogens and other potentially infectious materials.
Lubricant	Agent that is applied to physician's gloved hand or to speculum that reduces friction between parts to make insertion easier.
Specimen container	Container in which body specimen is placed for transport to laboratory (after it has been labeled).
Tissues	Used for wiping body secretions.
Cotton-tipped applicator	Small piece of cotton wrapped around the end of a slender wooden stick, used for collection of specimen from the body.
Overhead examination light	Light mounted on flexible movable stand to focus light on area for good visibility.
Basin	Container in which used instruments are deposited.
Biohazard container	Specially made container used for receiving items that contain infectious waste.
Waste receptacle	Container for used disposable articles that do not contain infectious waste.

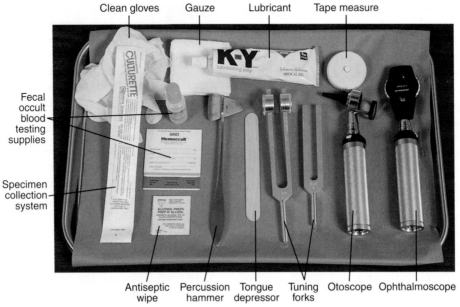

Figure 5-1. Common instruments and supplies used during the physical examination.

Highlight on Patient Teaching

The purpose of patient teaching is to help the patient develop habits, attitudes, and skills that enable the individual to maintain and improve his or her own health.

Fact: Patients who are active, informed participants in their health care are more apt to follow the physician's instructions than patients who are passive recipients of medical services.

Action: Provide patients with information on health care. Every patient interaction is an opportunity for teaching.

Fact: Adult learners are goal oriented and performance centered. They need and want information that would assist them in managing and improving their health.

Action: Review the information that you provide to patients, and determine whether it is nice to know or necessary to know. Select subject matter that is practical and useful and relates directly to the patient's needs.

Fact: The more information that is presented, the more the patient is likely to forget. Approximately one half of information presented to the patient is forgotten in the first 5 minutes after giving it.

Action: When teaching, use the following pointers to help patients learn and retain information:
- Keep it short and be specific.
- Speak in terms the patient can understand.
- Focus on "how," rather than "why."
- Repeat and reinforce important information.
- Give practical examples, and provide ample time for patient practice.

- Ask for feedback from the patient to determine whether he or she understands the information.
- Provide the patient with written information.

Fact: Each individual has a distinct style of learning and learns best when using his or her preferred learning style. The three main learning styles are reading, listening, and doing. People often use more than one style for learning.

Action: Use a variety of teaching strategies to engage the various learning styles of patients. Examples of teaching strategies include explanations, printed handouts, audiovisual aids, demonstrations, and discussions.

Fact: Only two thirds of patients comply with health care instructions prescribed by the physician. Factors that influence compliance include the patient's adaptation to illness, motivation to change, physical capability, and support systems.

Action: The following help increase patient compliance with prescribed treatment:
- Address the patient by his or her name of choice. (Keep in mind that many patients object to being called by their first name by strangers.)
- Encourage the patient to take an active role in personal health care.
- Help the patient set goals and objectives for change.
- Encourage care and support from family members.
- Make the patient aware of outside resources.
- Give positive reinforcement when the patient makes healthy changes.

assistant then takes vital signs and measures the weight and height of the patient. The results of these procedures are charted in the patient's medical record.

The medical assistant can reduce a patient's apprehension and embarrassment by addressing the patient by his or her name of choice, by adopting a friendly and supportive attitude, and by speaking clearly, distinctly, and slowly. The medical assistant should explain the purpose of the examination and offer to answer any questions. This also facilitates the physical examination of the patient.

The patient should be asked whether he or she needs to void before the examination. An empty bladder makes the examination easier and is more comfortable for the patient. If a urine specimen is needed, the patient is asked to void.

Instructions on disrobing for the examination should be specific so that the patient understands what items of clothing to remove and where to place the clothing. The disrobing area should be comfortable and should provide privacy. It is helpful to have a place for the patient to sit to make it easier to remove clothing and shoes. The area also should be equipped with hooks for hanging clothing. Instructions for putting on the examination gown and for locating the gown opening reduce patient confusion. If the medical assistant senses that the patient will have trouble undressing, assistance should be offered. Elderly and disabled patients sometimes have difficulty removing clothing.

The medical assistant is responsible for making the patient's medical record available for review by the physician. The medical office has a designated location where the record is placed, such as a small shelf mounted on the wall next to the outside of the examining room door or in a chart holder mounted on the outside of the examining room door. The medical assistant should ensure that the medical record is placed so that patient-identifiable information is not visible. This is required by the Health Insurance Portability and Accountability Act (HIPAA) Privacy Rule to protect a patient's health information.

The physical examination is performed with the patient positioned on an examining table, which is specially constructed to facilitate the examination. For safety, it is ad-

Putting It All Into Practice

My Name is Hope Fauber, and I am a certified medical assistant. I work in a medical clinic with a family medicine department of 10 physicians and 10 residents and interns. My duties cover a broad spectrum, from pediatrics to geriatrics, and include prenatal care, allergy injections, minor office surgery, electrocardiograms, colposcopies, immunizations, and wound care.

At our clinic, many of the patients are elderly. I occasionally come across geriatric patients who are not very cooperative and are "set in their ways." One 90-year-old woman, in particular, had a reputation in the office for being cantankerous and difficult to work with. One day, when the physician ordered laboratory work on her, I prepared to draw blood from her tiny, frail body, praying that everything would go smoothly. As I helped her up after a successful "stick," she, of all people, reached to give me a hug and said to me, "I like you. That didn't even hurt!" She continued to hold my hand and talk to me as I walked her out of the office. This turned out to be the last time I would see her because she moved out of town, but not out of my heart, leaving a lasting impression on my life. ■

visable to help the patient onto and off of the examining table.

MEASURING WEIGHT AND HEIGHT

The medical assistant routinely measures the weight and height of many types of patients. The process of measuring the patient is **mensuration.** A change in weight may be significant in the diagnosis of a patient's condition and in prescribing the course of treatment. Underweight and over-

What Would You Do? What Would You *Not* Do?

Case Study 2

Karen Steiner drops her 17-year-old daughter, Mikayla, off at the medical office for her sports physical examination. Mikayla is captain of the varsity cheerleading squad and is getting ready to start her senior year in high school. Mikayla's vital signs are normal, and she measures 5 feet 6 inches tall and weighs 105 pounds. With some reluctance, Mikayla admits that she's been having problems with heartburn, and she's pretty sure she knows what's causing it. She says that she has to keep her weight down for cheerleading, and after eating dinner with her family, she makes herself vomit to get rid of the food in her stomach. Mikayla is not too concerned about doing this because a lot of the popular girls at school are doing the same thing. She says it's the easy way to stay slim, and she would like to lose another 10 pounds before football season starts. Mikayla wants some prescription drug samples to help with the heartburn because the over-the-counter pills that she's been taking are not working anymore. She does not want her parents to know about any of this because she's afraid that they would not understand and might make her drop out of cheerleading. ■

What Would You Do? What Would You *Not* Do?

Case Study 1

Abbey Auden, 35 years old, is at the medical office. Her husband got a backyard trampoline for their two school-age children, and she decided to try it out. Abbey landed wrong on the trampoline and hurt her back and neck. For the past 5 days, she has been having headaches and back pain. Abbey refuses to have her weight taken because she has gained weight over the past several years and does not want to know how much she's gained. She does not understand why weight has to be taken at an office visit in the first place. Abbey says that many times when she should go to the doctor, she doesn't, just to avoid being weighed. She says she would not even be here now except that her husband insisted that she come. ■

weight patients who follow a diet therapy program should be weighed at regular intervals to determine their progress. Prenatal patients are weighed during each prenatal visit to assist in the assessment of fetal development and of the mother's health. Procedure 5-1 describes how to measure height and weight.

An adult's weight usually is measured during each office visit; an adult's height is typically measured only during the first visit or when a complete physical examination of the patient is requested. Children are weighed and their height (or length) is measured during each office visit to observe their pattern of growth and to calculate medication dosage.

The patient's height is used to interpret body weight (see the box *Highlight on Interpreting Body Weight*). Weight and height are compared against a standardized chart that serves as a general guide to determine whether the patient's weight falls within normal limits (Figure 5-2).

Highlight on Cultural Diversity

Culture consists of the values, beliefs, and practices of a particular group of people. Culture is deeply rooted and is passed on from one generation to the next through communication. It includes areas such as religion, dietary practices, family lines of authority, family life patterns, beliefs, and health practices.

As the demographics of the United States continue to change, the medical assistant is faced with the challenge of providing care to an increasing number of cultural groups. It is important for the medical assistant to learn as much as possible about the cultural values of patients coming to the medical office. This is known as *cultural awareness* and can be accomplished by carefully observing and listening to patients to acquire knowledge of their cultural values.

Cultural sensitivity is respect and appreciation for cultural diversity, whereas *cultural competence* is understanding and using the cultural background of a patient to assist with the resolution of a problem. Because health practices are part of a patient's culture, changing them may have a negative impact on the patient. Whenever possible, the medical assistant should incorporate factors from a patient's cultural background into his or her health care.

Guidelines for Achieving Cultural Competence

The following guidelines help the medical assistant in developing cultural awareness and sensitivity and in achieving cultural competence:

1. **Respect the patient's values, beliefs, and practices.** Even if you do not agree with them, it is important to respect the patient's right to hold these values and to not dismiss them as strange or odd. Cultural values play an important role in a patient's lifestyle. Patients from some cultures believe that losing blood depletes the body's strength and provides a route for the soul to leave the body. If a blood specimen is needed, these patients may become highly distressed or refuse to have their blood drawn. Members of some cultural groups believe that illness results when the body's natural balance or harmony is disturbed. To restore the balance, alternative forms of medicine, such as herbal remedies and aromatherapy, are used.

2. **Refrain from cultural stereotypes.** Not all people of a cultural group have the same beliefs, practices, and values. Assuming that all members of a cultural group are alike is known as *stereotyping* and should be avoided. Just as one would never assume that all people in the United States like hamburgers and baseball, every individual must be approached according to his or her specific beliefs and practices.

3. **Always address patients by their last names (and Mr., Mrs., Miss, Ms.) unless they give you permission to use other names.** In many cultures, using a first name to address anyone other than family or friends is considered disrespectful. Most older people in the United States dislike being called by their first name and feel it shows a lack of respect.

4. **Speak slowly and clearly.** Communicating with a patient may be difficult if the patient has a limited knowledge of English. With these patients, you should speak slowly and clearly in a normal tone and volume of voice. Speaking loudly does not help the patient understand any better and may be offensive to the patient.

5. **Show respect for cultural lines of authority.** In many cultures, respect is given based on age and gender. In certain cultures, elders are considered the holders of the culture's wisdom and are highly respected. In other cultures, youth is valued over age. In certain cultures, the male dominates, and women have very little status. Because of this, a female patient from this type of culture may not be permitted to give her own health history or to answer questions. In addition, a male patient from this culture may not accept instructions from a female medical assistant.

6. **Use appropriate eye contact.** In most cultures, direct eye contact is important and generally shows that the other is attentive and listening. It conveys self-confidence, openness, interest, and honesty, whereas the lack of eye contact may be interpreted as secretiveness, shyness, guilt, or lack of interest. Other cultures consider eye contact impolite or an invasion of privacy; these patients show respect by avoiding direct eye contact.

7. **Be aware of cultural responses to illness.** The conditions under which an individual assumes the role of a (sick) patient and the way he or she performs in that role vary with culture. Individuals of some cultures resist the sick role and blame sickness on external forces as a means of punishment. These individuals may deny their illness and fail to provide much information when the medical assistant takes their symptoms. In other cultures, individuals take an optimistic view of the outcome of health care and, because of this, are more likely to elicit information and to follow the physician's instructions.

8. **Learn to appreciate the richness of diversity as an asset, rather than a hindrance, to communication and effective interaction with patients.**

PATIENT TEACHING Health Promotion and Disease Prevention

Teach patients the essentials of health promotion and disease prevention. Help patients become aware of the following patterns of behavior that promote and support health:

- Keeping up to date with immunizations
- Eating nutritiously from the food pyramid
- Exercising regularly
- Maintaining normal weight
- Managing stress
- Maintaining high self-esteem
- Avoiding tobacco and drugs

- Using alcohol wisely
- Understanding how the environment affects health and taking appropriate action to improve it
- Knowing the facts about cardiovascular disease, cancer, infections, sexually transmitted diseases, and accidents, and using this knowledge to protect against them
- Understanding the changes that occur through the natural processes of aging
- Developing a sense of responsibility for health by taking an active role in establishing and maintaining a healthy lifestyle

---

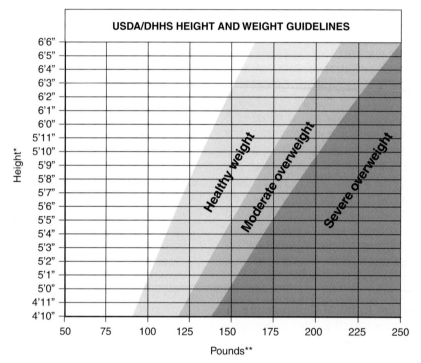

* Without shoes.
**Without clothes. The higher weights apply to people with more muscle and bone, such as many men.

Figure 5-2. U.S. Department of Agriculture (USDA)/Department of Health and Human Services (DHHS) height and weight guidelines. (From Report of the Dietary Guidelines Advisory Committee on the dietary guidelines for Americans, Washington, DC, 1995, U.S. Department of Health and Human Services.)

Guidelines for Measuring Weight and Height

When using an upright balance scale to measure weight and height, use the following guidelines.

Weight

1. **Locate the scale to provide privacy for the patient.** Place the scale on a hard, level surface in a private location. Many patients are self-conscious about having their weight measured and prefer that it be done in privacy. Do not make

weight-sensitive comments during the procedure. This is especially important for patients with weight control problems such as obesity and eating disorders.

2. **Balance the scale before measuring weight.** If the scale is not balanced, the weight measurement will be inaccurate. The scale is balanced when the upper and lower weights are on zero and the indicator point comes to a rest at the center of the balance area.

Guidelines for Measuring Weight and Height—cont'd

3. **Assist the patient.** Assist the patient onto and off of the scale platform. The scale platform moves slightly and may cause the patient to become unsteady.
4. **Obtain an accurate weight.** Always ask the patient to remove his or her shoes. Measure weight with the patient in normal clothing. Ask the patient to remove heavy outer clothing, such as a sweater or a jacket.
5. **Interpret the calibration markings accurately.** The lower calibration bar is divided into 50-lb increments (Figure 5-3, *A*). The upper calibration bar is divided into pounds and quarter pounds. The longer calibration lines indicate pound increments, and the shorter calibration lines indicate quarter-pound and half-pound increments (Figure 5-3, *B*).
6. **Determine the patient's weight correctly.** Add the measurement on the lower scale to the measurement on the upper scale. The result should be rounded to the nearest quarter pound. Occasionally, the patient's weight may need to be converted to kilograms, which is the metric unit of measurement for weight. This may be required when determining medication dos-

age. The following formulas are used to convert weight and height measurements from one system to another.

Weight Conversion
Pounds to Kilograms. Divide the number of pounds by 2.2:

$$136 \text{ lb} \div 2.2 = 61.8 \text{ kg}$$

Kilograms to Pounds. Multiply the number of kilograms by 2.2:

$$75 \text{ kg} \times 2.2 = 165 \text{ lb}$$

Height Conversion
Inches to Centimeters. Multiply the number of inches by 2.5:

$$64 \text{ inches} \times 2.5 = 160 \text{ cm}$$

Centimeters to Inches. Divide the number of centimeters by 2.5:

$$185 \text{ cm} \div 2.5 = 74 \text{ inches (or 6 feet 2 inches)}$$

Height
1. **Provide for the patient's safety.** Follow the proper procedure when measuring the patient's height. An error in technique could result in injury. If a patient is placed on the scale in a forward position, the measuring bar could fall into the patient's face when he or she steps off of the scale, causing a facial injury.
2. **Determine the calibration markings accurately.** Depending on the brand of scale, the calibration markings are divided into inches or feet and inches. (Figure 5-4 is an example of a scale divided into feet and inches.) The calibration rod also is calibrated into centimeters, which is the metric unit of mea-

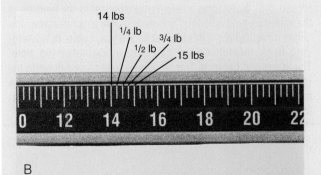

Figure 5-3. Calibration markings for measuring weight on an upright balance scale. **A,** The upper calibration bar is divided into pounds and quarter pounds. **B,** The longer calibration lines indicate pound increments, and the shorter calibration lines indicate quarter-pound and half-pound increments.

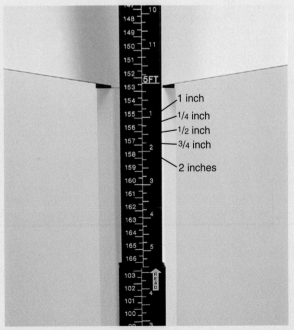

Figure 5-4. Calibration markings for measuring height on an upright balance scale.

Continued

Guidelines for Measuring Weight and Height—cont'd

surement for height. This unit of measurement is not typically used to measure height in the United States.

3. **Read the measurement correctly.** The height measurement is read from the top of the bar down and should be read to the nearest quarter inch. For most patients, you can read the height measurement at the junction of the stationary calibration rod and the movable calibration rod (Figure 5-5, *A*). If the patient's height is less than the top value of the stationary calibration rod, however, you must read the measurement from the bottom of the bar up directly on the stationary rod. For example, on most scales the highest calibration on the stationary rod is 50 inches; patients with a height of 50 inches or less would have their height read directly from the stationary rod (Figure 5-5, *B*).

4. **Record the height measurement correctly.** Record the height measurement in feet and inches. If the scale is calibrated in inches, convert the reading to feet and inches by dividing the number of inches by 12. A height measurement of 60 inches is recorded as 5 feet (60 inches ÷ 12 = 5). If the patient's height measurement is 64 inches, the results would be recorded as 5 feet, 4 inches.

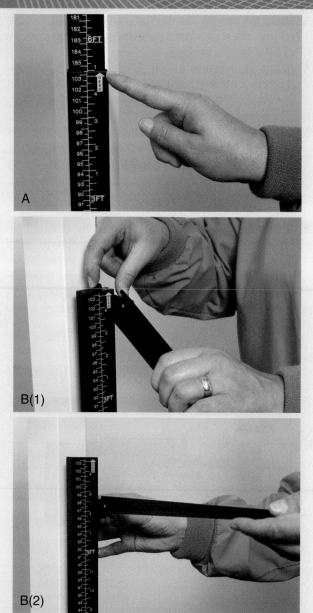

Figure 5-5. **A,** Reading a height measurement at the junction of the stationary calibration rod and the movable calibration rod. The height measurement in this illustration is 6 feet, 1 inch. **B(1),** Reading a height measurement on the stationary calibration rod. **Note:** The measuring bar must first be released and moved down to the stationary bar to measure the patient's height. **B(2),** Reading the height at the junction of the bar and the rod. The height measurement in this illustration is 3 feet, 2 inches.

Highlight on Interpreting Body Weight

The two common methods to interpret body weight are weight in relation to standard tables and calculation of the body mass index (BMI).

Height and Weight Tables

One way to interpret body weight is through the use of standardized height and weight tables. In 1959, the Metropolitan Life Insurance Company (MET) issued a set of tables indicating desirable height and weight ranges for men and women. In 1983, MET issued revised tables for men and women that showed height and weight ranges higher than those in the 1959 table. Many health experts believe that the desirable weight ranges of the revised tables are too high and do not represent healthy body weight.

In 1995, the U.S. Department of Agriculture (USDA) and the Department of Health and Human Services (DHHS) issued a set of weight guidelines (see Figure 5-2) that are lower than those of the MET tables. The USDA/DHHS guidelines do not distinguish between weights of men and women and must be interpreted by each individual as follows. Women usually have smaller bones and less muscle than men, so they should use the lower end of the range. Men and large-boned, muscular women should use the higher end of the weight range to find their healthy body weights.

Body Mass Index

Another method for interpreting body weight is the BMI. The BMI expresses the correlation of an individual's weight to his or her height. Except for trained athletes, the BMI strongly correlates with total body fat content in adults. This provides an indication of the risk of developing chronic health conditions associated with obesity. Many health experts believe that the BMI is a more accurate standard for interpreting body weight than are height and weight tables.

Method for Calculating BMI

a. Use the following website to have your BMI calculated automatically:
www.cdc.gov/nccdphp/dnpa/bmi

b. Use the following steps to calculate your BMI:
1. Multiply your weight in pounds (without clothes or shoes) by 703. For an individual who weighs 135 lb:

$$135 \times 703 = 94,905$$

2. Divide this number by your height in inches. If this individual is 66 inches tall:

$$94,905 \div 66 = 1438$$

3. Divide this amount again by your height in inches, and round off to the nearest whole number:

$$1438 \div 66 = 21.79, \text{ or } 22$$

The BMI of this individual is 22.

Interpretation of the BMI

In June 1998, the National Heart, Lung, and Blood Institute (NHLBI), a federal health agency, issued a set of guidelines for the classification of body weight in adults. One of these guidelines relates to interpretation of the BMI, as outlined here.

BMI	Interpretation
Below 18.5	Underweight
18.5-24.9	Healthy weight
25-29.9	Overweight
30-34.9	Obesity (I)
35.0-39.9	Obesity (II)
40 or more	Extreme obesity (III)

The NHLBI recommends that the BMI be determined in all adults. People of normal weight should have their BMI reassessed every 2 years.

Adult Obesity

The incidence of obesity in the United States has increased markedly, and obesity is now one of the most common problems encountered by primary care physicians. Approximately 66% of adults in the United States are either overweight or obese. That means that nearly two out of every three Americans are overweight or obese. Obesity is associated with premature death and, after smoking, is the second leading cause of preventable death in the United States today. Approximately 300,000 deaths in the United States each year are associated with obesity.

It has been determined that as the BMI increases to greater than 25, there is an increased risk of developing certain diseases associated with overweight and obesity, including the following:
- Hypertension
- Cardiovascular disease
- Dyslipidemia (high blood cholesterol levels, high blood triglyceride levels, or both)
- Type 2 diabetes
- Colon cancer
- Gallbladder disease
- Breast and endometrial cancers
- Sleep apnea and respiratory problems
- Osteoarthritis

Obesity is considered a chronic condition that requires a multiple treatment approach, including a behavioral therapy program, a low-calorie diet, and a suitable aerobic exercise program. Primary care physicians often manage individuals with mild and moderate obesity, but morbidly obese patients are usually referred to a bariatric specialist. **Bariatrics** is the branch of medicine that deals with the treatment and control of obesity and diseases associated with obesity. ■

PROCEDURE 5-1   Measuring Weight and Height

Outcome Measure weight and height.

Equipment Supplies

• Upright balance scale
• Paper towel

Weight

1. **Procedural Step.** Sanitize your hands.
2. **Procedural Step.** Check the scale to ensure it is balanced as follows:
   a. Make sure the upper and lower weights are on zero. When the weights are on zero, they are all the way to the left of the calibration bars.

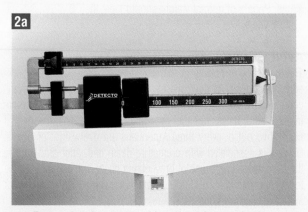

Ensure that the upper and lower weights are on zero.

   b. Look at the indicator point. If the scale is balanced, the indicator point is resting in the center of the balance area.
   c. If the indicator point rests below the center, adjust the screw on the balance knob by turning it clockwise (to the right) until the indicator point rests in the center of the balance area.

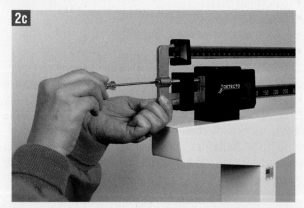

Correct the balance by adjusting the screw on the balance knob.

   d. If the indicator point rests above the center, adjust the screw on the balance knob by turning it counterclockwise (to the left) until the indicator point rests in the center of the balance area.

Principle. If the scale is not balanced, the weight measurement will be inaccurate.

3. **Procedural Step.** Greet the patient and introduce yourself.
4. **Procedural Step.** Identify the patient and explain to the patient that you will be measuring his or her height and weight.
5. **Procedural Step.** Instruct the patient to remove shoes and outer clothing such as a jacket or sweater. A good medical aseptic practice is to place a paper towel on the platform of the scale to protect the patient's feet.
   Principle. Removing heavy clothing and shoes allows a more accurate measurement of the patient's weight.
6. **Procedural Step.** Assist the patient onto the scale, and instruct the patient not to move.
   Principle. It is not possible to balance the scale if the patient is moving.
7. **Procedural Step.** Balance the scale as follows:
   a. Move the lower weight to the notched groove that does not cause the indicator point to drop to the bottom of the calibration area. Ensure that the lower weight is seated firmly in its groove.
   b. Slide the upper weight slowly along its calibration bar by tapping it gently until the indicator point comes to rest at the center of the balance area.
   Principle. Not seating the lower weight firmly in its groove results in an inaccurate reading.

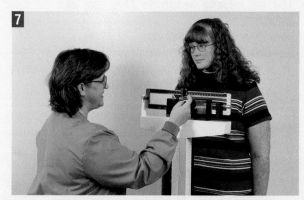

Slide the upper weight by tapping it gently.

8. **Procedural Step.** Read the results to the nearest quarter pound by adding the measurement on the lower scale to the measurement on the upper scale. Jot down this value or make a mental note of it.
9. **Procedural Step.** Ask the patient to step off of the scale platform. Provide assistance if needed.

PROCEDURE 5-1   Measuring Weight and Height—cont'd

Height

1. Procedural Step. Slide the movable calibration rod upward until the measuring bar is well above the patient's apparent height. Open the measuring bar to its horizontal position.

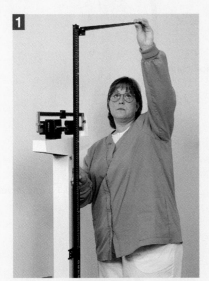

Slide the bar upward until it is well above the patient's height.

2. Procedural Step. Instruct the patient to step onto the scale platform with his or her back to the scale. Provide assistance if needed. Instruct the patient to stand erect and to look straight ahead.

Principle. Looking straight ahead helps the patient to stand erect and balanced, which ensures an accurate measurement.

3. Procedural Step. Carefully lower the measuring bar (keeping it horizontal) until it rests gently on top of the patient's head with the hair compressed. The measuring bar should form a 90-degree angle with the calibration rod.

Principle. The measuring bar must be at a 90-degree angle to ensure an accurate height measurement.

4. Procedural Step. Keeping the measuring bar in a horizontal position, instruct the patient to step down and put on his or her shoes. Hold the bar in a horizontal position until the patient has stepped off the scale.

5. Procedural Step. Read the height measurement from the top down to the nearest quarter-inch marking at the junction of the stationary calibration rod and the movable calibration rod. (*Note:* If the patient's height is less than the top value of the stationary rod, read the measurement from the bottom up directly on the stationary calibration rod.) Jot down this value or make a mental note of it.

6. Procedural Step. Return the measuring bar to its vertical (resting) position, and slide the movable calibration rod to its lowest position. Return the weights to zero.

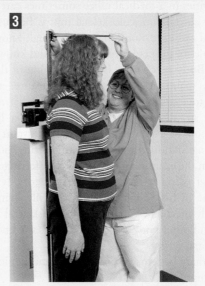

Lower the bar until it rests on top of the patient's head.

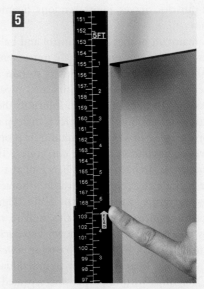

Read the measurement to the nearest quarter-inch marking.

7. Procedural Step. Sanitize your hands, and chart the results. Include the date and time and the patient's weight and height measurements. The weight should be charted in pounds to the nearest quarter pound, and the height should be charted in feet and inches to the nearest quarter inch.

CHARTING EXAMPLE	
Date	
11/5/12	10:15 a.m. Wt: 155 lbs. Ht: 5' 6¼"
	H. Fauber, CMA (AAMA)

BODY MECHANICS

Daily activities in a medical office sometimes carry the risk of acute or chronic musculoskeletal injury. Because of this, the medical assistant should have a thorough knowledge of the principles of proper body mechanics and know when to use them. **Body mechanics** is the utilization of the correct muscles to maintain proper balance, posture, and body alignment to accomplish a task safely and efficiently without undue strain on muscles or joints. Proper body mechanics should be used when the medical assistant performs the following: standing, walking, sitting, lifting, positioning a patient on the examining table, and transferring a patient. The medical assistant should also use proper body mechanics at home in his or her activities of daily living. Using proper body mechanics prevents musculoskeletal strains to the back and other body structures such as the knees, neck, shoulders, and wrists.

The primary benefits of proper body mechanics include the following:

1. Allows an individual to conserve energy, which makes it easier to perform a task
2. Protects the body from injury by reducing stress and strain on muscles, nerves, joints, tendons, ligaments, and soft tissues
3. Helps to maintain proper body control and balance
4. Promotes effective, efficient, and safe movement

Studies show that health care workers sustain a significantly higher incidence of back injuries as compared with other professions. To help prevent an injury to the back, a primary focus of proper body mechanics is to keep the natural curves of the spine or vertebral column in proper alignment. The vertebral column has four curvatures. These curvatures increase the strength and resilience of the vertebral column and include the cervical curvature, thoracic curvature, lumbar curvature, and sacral curvature (Figure 5-6). The vertebral column extends from the skull to the pelvis and consists of a series of bones known as *vertebrae*. The vertebrae are separated by shock-absorbing *intervertebral discs* (see Figure 5-6). These discs allow an individual to bend and twist. Over time, with improper and repeated bending and twisting (especially while carrying an object), the discs can deteriorate, which causes them to narrow, to harden, and even to crack and tear. This condition is known as *degenerative disc disease*. With degenerative disc disease, the discs lose their shock-absorbing ability and cause the patient to experience localized pain and stiffness in the area of disc deterioration. In addition, once a disc is weakened, it can bulge out or rupture; this is known as a herniated disc.

Principles

There are some basic principles related to proper body mechanics that should be followed:

1. Movements should be smooth and coordinated rather than jerky.
2. Keeping the body in good physical condition through exercising, stretching, and weight training helps to prevent musculoskeletal injury.

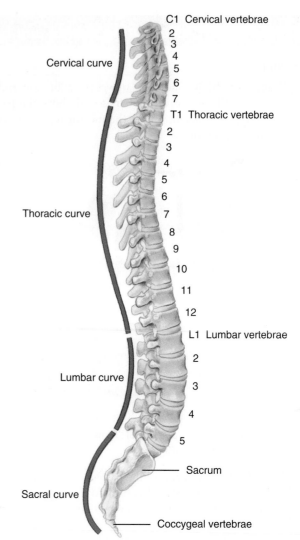

Figure 5-6. Vertebral column. (From Applegate EJ: The anatomy and physiology learning system, ed 3, St Louis, 2006, Saunders.)

3. To avoid straining the back, do not reach for something that is farther than 14 to 18 inches away.
4. Work at a comfortable height that avoids having to bend the neck or back forward to perform the task. People are usually most comfortable working at a height that falls between the waist and elbow levels.
5. If possible, push, pull, or slide an object rather than lift it. This conserves energy and places less strain on the back.
6. Lighter items should be stored on higher shelves or cabinets, and heavier items should be stored at or below waist level.
7. When an object from an overhead shelf or cabinet needs to be retrieved, use a step stool or chair to come up to the level of the object. Reaching for a stored overhead item can produce strain on the back.
8. When lifting an object or transferring a patient, the large muscles of the arms and legs should be used as much as possible and the back muscles as little as possible. The more muscle groups that are used, the more evenly the weight is distributed over the medical assistant's body, which puts less strain on the back.

9. When transferring a patient, encourage the patient to assist as much as possible.

10. If a patient becomes dizzy or faint or starts to fall, do not try to hold the patient in an upright position. Instead, balance yourself with your legs apart to form a wide base of support, and gently and gradually lower the patient to a chair or to the floor.

11. Always ask for assistance if you don't think you can lift a heavy object or transfer a patient.

Application of Body Mechanics

The medical assistant should practice proper body mechanics when standing, sitting, lifting an object, positioning a patient on the examining table, and transferring a patient from a wheelchair to an examining table and back again, as outlined on the following pages.

Standing

It is important to maintain good posture by positioning the body in the correct standing position as outlined below. This provides the medical assistant with good balance and stability and reduces strain on the back by keeping the vertebral column at its natural alignment.

1. Wear comfortable low-heeled shoes that provide good support.

2. Hold the head erect at the midline of the body, the back as straight as possible with the pelvis tucked inward, the chest forward with the shoulders back, and the abdomen drawn in and kept flat. This helps to maintain appropriate alignment of the vertebral column (Figure 5-7).

3. The knees should be slightly flexed with the feet pointing forward and parallel to each other about 3 inches apart.

This provides a broad base of support and improves balance.

4. The arms should be positioned comfortably at the side, and the weight of the body should be evenly distributed over both feet.

Sitting

The medical assistant should use proper body mechanics when in a sitting position (Figure 5-8), as outlined below.

1. Sit in a chair with a firm back.

2. Sit firmly with the back and buttocks supported against the back of the chair; avoid slumping. The body weight should be evenly distributed over the buttocks and thighs.

3. Use a small pillow or a rolled towel to support the lower back.

4. The feet should be flat on the floor, and the knees should be level with the hips.

5. If you need to sit for a prolonged period of time, use a footstool to raise one knee to reduce strain on the back.

6. Take frequent stretch breaks.

Lifting

The following steps outline the procedure for lifting an object while using proper body mechanics:

1. First determine the weight of the object to determine if you can safely lift it. Pushing the object with one foot can help you determine if you can lift it without assistance. Never lift anything heavier than you can easily manage.

2. Stand in front of the object and balance yourself with the feet about 6 to 8 inches apart, toes pointed outward, and

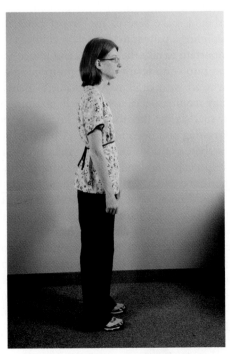

Figure 5-7. Proper standing position.

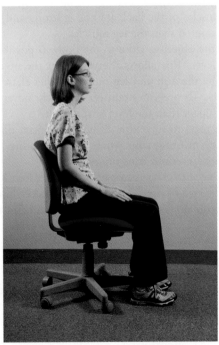

Figure 5-8. Proper sitting position.

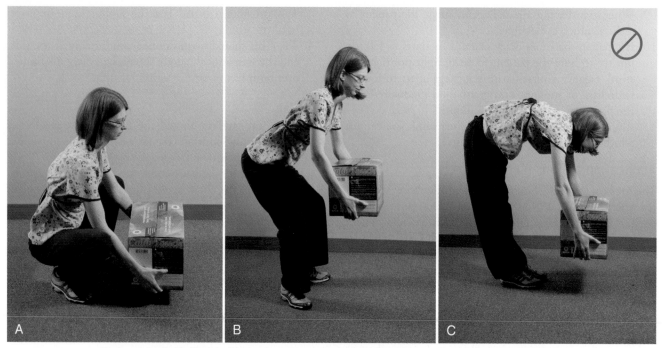

Figure 5-9. **A,** To lift the object, always bend the body at the knees and hips. **B,** Lift with the leg muscles, while keeping the back straight. **C,** Never bend from the waist.

one foot slightly forward to provide a wide base of support. Tighten the stomach and gluteal muscles in preparation for lifting the object.

3. To lift the object, always bend the body at the knees and hips (Figure 5-9, *A*). This helps to maintain your center of gravity and allows the strong muscles of the legs to do the lifting. Never bend from the waist (Figure 5-9, *C*).

4. Grasp the object firmly with both hands.

5. Keeping the back straight, lift the object smoothly with the leg muscles, not the back muscles (Figure 5-9, *B*). The muscles of the back are not as strong and are more easily injured than the leg muscles.

6. Hold the object as close to the body as possible and at waist level. This allows the weight of the object to be lifted by the arm and leg muscles rather than the back muscles. To prevent strain on the back, never lift anything higher than the level of the chest.

7. If you need to turn after lifting the object, don't twist. Turn by pivoting your whole body. Twisting the spine can cause a serious back injury.

8. If you need to carry the object to another location, make sure the area of transport is dry and free of clutter.

9. Lower the object slowly, making sure to bend from the knees to allow the leg muscles to do the work.

POSITIONING AND DRAPING

Correct positioning of the patient facilitates the examination by permitting better access to the part being examined or treated. The basic positions used in the medical office are sitting, supine, prone, dorsal recumbent, lithotomy, Sims, knee-chest, and Fowler's.

The position used depends on the type of examination or procedure to be performed. More than one position may be used to examine the same body part during the physical examination. The sitting and supine positions are both used to examine the chest. It is important to know the correct position for each examination or treatment. When positioning a patient, the medical assistant should explain the position to the patient and assist the patient in attaining it. The medical assistant should make sure to use proper body mechanics when positioning a patient to avoid musculoskeletal injuries.

It is important to take the patient's endurance and degree of wellness into consideration when positioning a patient. Patients who are weak or ill may be unable to assume a position or may require special assistance in attaining it. Some positions, such as the lithotomy and knee-chest positions, are embarrassing and uncomfortable. A patient should not be kept in these positions any longer than necessary. Some patients (especially the elderly) become dizzy after a time in certain positions, such as the knee-chest position. These patients should be allowed to rest before they get off the examining table. The medical assistant also should assist patients off the examining table to prevent falls.

The patient is draped during positioning to provide for modesty, comfort, and warmth. Only the part to be examined should be exposed. Patient gowns and drapes used in the medical office are usually made of paper but also may be made of cloth. Procedures 5-2 through 5-9 present proper positioning and draping of the patient.

PROCEDURE 5-2   Sitting Position

Outcome Position and drape a patient in the sitting position. The sitting position is used to examine the head, neck, chest, and upper extremities and to measure vital signs.

Equipment/Supplies

- Examining table
- Disposable patient gown
- Disposable patient drape

1. **Procedural Step.** Sanitize your hands. Greet the patient and introduce yourself.
2. **Procedural Step.** Identify the patient and explain the type of examination or procedure that will be performed.
3. **Procedural Step.** Provide the patient with a patient gown. Instruct the patient to remove clothing as appropriate for the type of examination being performed and to put on the patient gown with the opening in front. The disrobing facility should provide privacy, a place to sit, and a place to hang clothing.
4. **Procedural Step.** Pull out the footrest of the examining table, and assist the patient into a sitting position. The patient's buttocks and thighs should be firmly supported on the edge of the table.
5. **Procedural Step.** Place a drape over the patient's thighs and legs to provide warmth and modesty.
6. **Procedural Step.** After completion of the examination, assist the patient down from the table. Return the footrest to its normal position. Instruct the patient to get dressed. Discard the gown and drape in a waste container.

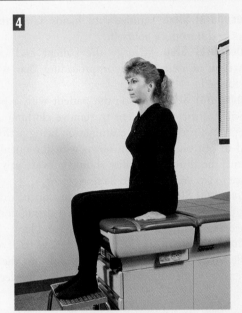

Sitting position.

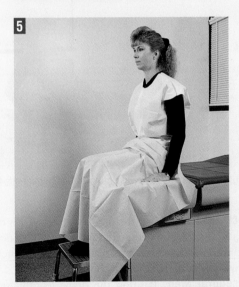

Place the drape over the patient's thighs and legs.

PROCEDURE 5-2

PROCEDURE 5-3   Supine Position

Outcome Position and drape a patient in the supine position. The supine position is used to examine the head, chest, abdomen, and extremities.

Equipment/Supplies

- Examining table
- Disposable patient gown
- Disposable patient drape

1. **Procedural Step.** Sanitize your hands. Greet the patient and introduce yourself.
2. **Procedural Step.** Identify the patient and explain the type of examination or procedure that will be performed.
3. **Procedural Step.** Provide the patient with a patient gown. Instruct the patient to remove clothing as appropriate for the type of examination being performed and to put on the patient gown with the opening in front. The disrobing facility should provide privacy, a place to sit, and a place to hang clothing.
4. **Procedural Step.** Pull out the footrest of the examining table, and assist the patient into a sitting position. Place a drape over the patient's thighs and legs.
5. **Procedural Step.** Ask the patient to move back on the table. As the patient is doing this, pull out the table extension while supporting the patient's lower legs.

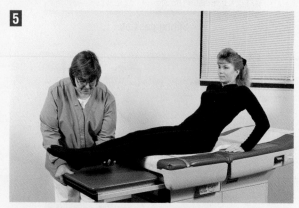

Pull out the table extension while supporting the patient's legs.

6. **Procedural Step.** Ask the patient to lie on his or her back with the legs together. Provide assistance if needed. The patient's arms may be placed above the head or alongside the body.
7. **Procedural Step.** Position the drape lengthwise over the patient to provide warmth and modesty. As the

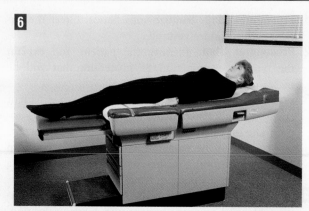

Position the patient on the back with the legs together.

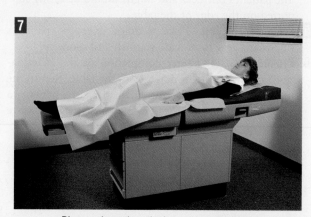

Place a drape lengthwise over the patient.

physician examines the patient, move the drape according to the body parts being examined.

8. **Procedural Step.** After completion of the examination, assist the patient into a sitting position. Slide the table extension back into place while supporting the patient's lower legs.
9. **Procedural Step.** Assist the patient down from the table. Instruct the patient to get dressed. Return the footrest to its normal position. Discard the gown and drape in a waste container.

PROCEDURE 5-4   Prone Position

Outcome Position and drape a patient in the prone position. The prone position is used to examine the back and to assess extension of the hip joint.

Equipment/Supplies

- Examining table
- Disposable patient gown
- Disposable patient drape

1. **Procedural Step.** Sanitize your hands. Greet the patient and introduce yourself.
2. **Procedural Step.** Identify the patient and explain the type of examination or procedure that will be performed.
3. **Procedural Step.** Provide the patient with a patient gown. Instruct the patient to remove clothing as appropriate for the type of examination being performed and to put on the patient gown with the opening in back. The disrobing facility should provide privacy, a place to sit, and a place to hang clothing.
4. **Procedural Step.** Pull out the footrest of the examining table, and assist the patient into a sitting position. Place a drape over the patient's thighs and legs.
5. **Procedural Step.** Ask the patient to move back on the table. As the patient is doing this, pull out the table extension while supporting the patient's lower legs.
6. **Procedural Step.** Ask the patient to lie on his or her back. Provide assistance if needed. Position the drape lengthwise over the patient.
7. **Procedural Step.** Ask the patient to turn onto his or her stomach by rolling toward you. Provide assistance for this step by helping him or her turn and adjusting the drape to provide modesty.
   Principle. This step prevents the patient from accidentally rolling off the table.
8. **Procedural Step.** Position the patient with the legs together and the head turned to one side. The arms can be placed above the head or alongside the body.
9. **Procedural Step.** Adjust the drape as needed so that it is positioned lengthwise over the patient to provide warmth and modesty. As the physician examines the patient, move the drape according to the body parts being examined.
10. **Procedural Step.** After completion of the examination, ask the patient to turn back over by rolling toward you. Assist the patient into a supine position and

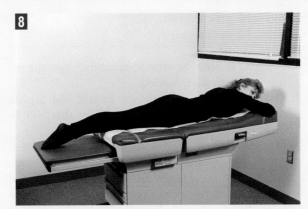

Position the patient's legs together with the head turned to one side.

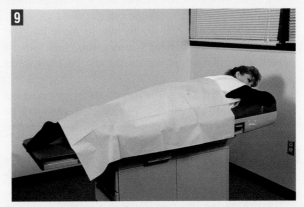

Place a drape lengthwise over the patient.

then into a sitting position. Slide the table extension back into place while supporting the patient's lower legs.
11. **Procedural Step.** Assist the patient down from the table. Return the footrest to its normal position. Instruct the patient to get dressed. Discard the gown and drape in a waste container.

PROCEDURE 5-5   Dorsal Recumbent Position

Outcome Position and drape a patient in the dorsal recumbent position. The dorsal recumbent position is used to perform vaginal and rectal examinations; to insert a urinary catheter; and to examine the head, neck, chest, and extremities of patients who have difficulty maintaining the supine position. The supine position is an uncomfortable position for patients with respiratory problems, back injury, or lower back pain. Bending the legs (rather than lying flat) is more comfortable for these patients and is easier to maintain.

Equipment/Supplies

- Examining table
- Disposable patient gown
- Disposable patient drape

1. **Procedural Step.** Sanitize your hands. Greet the patient and introduce yourself.
2. **Procedural Step.** Identify the patient and explain the type of examination or procedure that will be performed.
3. **Procedural Step.** Provide the patient with a patient gown. Instruct the patient to remove clothing as appropriate for the type of examination being performed and to put on the patient gown with the opening in front. The disrobing facility should provide privacy, a place to sit, and a place to hang clothing.
4. **Procedural Step.** Pull out the footrest of the examining table, and assist the patient into a sitting position. Place a drape over the patient's thighs and legs.
5. **Procedural Step.** Ask the patient to move back on the table. As the patient is doing this, pull out the table extension while supporting the patient's lower legs.
6. **Procedural Step.** Ask the patient to lie on his or her back. Provide assistance if needed. The arms can be placed above the head or alongside the body. Position the drape diagonally over the patient.
7. **Procedural Step.** Ask the patient to bend the knees and place each foot at the edge of the examining table with the soles of the feet flat on the table. Provide assistance during this step. Push in the table extension and the footrest.
8. **Procedural Step.** Adjust the drape as needed to provide the patient with warmth and modesty. The drape should be positioned diagonally, with one corner over the patient's chest; the opposite corner falls between the patient's legs and completely covers the pubic area.
9. **Procedural Step.** When the physician is ready to examine the genital area, the center corner of the drape is folded back over the abdomen.
10. **Procedural Step.** After completion of the examination, pull out the footrest and the table extension.

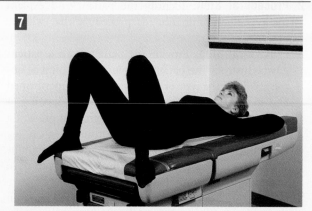

Ask the patient to bend the knees and place each foot at the edge of the examining table.

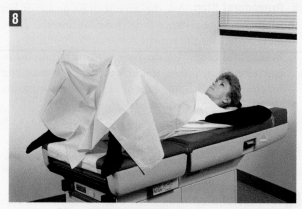

Place a drape diagonally over the patient.

Assist the patient into a supine position and then into a sitting position. Slide the table extension back into place while supporting the patient's lower legs.

11. **Procedural Step.** Assist the patient down from the table. Return the footrest to its normal position. Instruct the patient to get dressed. Discard the gown and drape in a waste container.

PROCEDURE 5-6   Lithotomy Position

Outcome Position and drape a patient in the lithotomy position. The lithotomy position is used for vaginal, pelvic, and rectal examinations. The lithotomy position is the same as the dorsal recumbent position except that the patient's feet are placed in stirrups. The lithotomy position provides maximal exposure to the genital area and facilitates insertion of a vaginal speculum. Because this is an uncomfortable position for the patient to maintain, the patient should not be put into this position until just before the examination.

Equipment/Supplies

- Examining table
- Disposable patient gown
- Disposable patient drape

1. **Procedural Step.** Sanitize your hands. Greet the patient and introduce yourself.
2. **Procedural Step.** Identify the patient and explain the type of examination or procedure that will be performed.
3. **Procedural Step.** Provide the patient with a patient gown. Instruct the patient to remove clothing as appropriate for the type of examination being performed and to put on the patient gown with the opening in front. If the patient is wearing socks, tell her that she may keep them on during the procedure. The disrobing facility should provide privacy, a place to sit, and a place to hang clothing.
   Principle. Socks help to keep the patient's feet warm after they are placed in the metal stirrups.
4. **Procedural Step.** Some medical offices use disposable stirrup covers. If this is the case, apply a cover to each stirrup. Pull out the footrest of the examining table, and assist the patient into a sitting position. Place a drape over the patient's thighs and legs.
   Principle. Stirrup covers provide a soft, warm, nonslip surface for the patient's feet.
5. **Procedural Step.** When the physician is ready to examine the patient, ask the patient to move back on the table. As the patient is doing this, pull out the table extension while supporting the patient's lower legs.
6. **Procedural Step.** Ask the patient to lie on the back. Provide assistance if needed. The arms can be placed above the head or alongside the body.
7. **Procedural Step.** Position the drape over the patient to provide warmth and modesty. The drape should be positioned diagonally with one corner over the patient's chest and the opposite corner between the patient's feet.
8. **Procedural Step.** Pull out the stirrups and position them at an angle. Position the stirrups so that they are level with the examining table and pulled out approximately 1 foot from the edge of the table. Check to make sure the stirrups are not too far apart or too close together. Lock the stirrups into place.
   Principle. If the stirrups are too far apart, it is uncomfortable for the patient. If the stirrups are too close

together, the patient will be unable to move her buttocks to the edge of the table as needed for the examination.

9. **Procedural Step.** Ask the patient to bend the knees and place each foot, one at a time, into a stirrup. Provide assistance during this step. Push in the table extension and the footrest.
10. **Procedural Step.** Instruct the patient to slide the buttocks all the way down to the edge of the examining table and to let her legs fall apart as far as is comfortable.

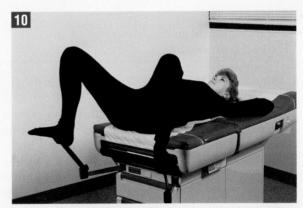

Ask the patient to slide the buttocks to the edge of the table and to rotate the thighs outward.

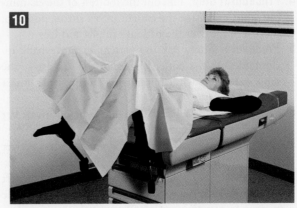

Position the drape diagonally.

Continued

PROCEDURE 5-6 Lithotomy Position—cont'd

11. **Procedural Step.** Reposition the drape as needed so that one corner is over the patient's chest and the opposite corner falls between the patient's legs and completely covers the perineal area. When the physician is ready to examine the genital area, the center corner of the drape is pulled up and folded back over the knees.

12. **Procedural Step.** After completion of the examination, pull out the footrest and table extension. Ask the patient to slide the buttocks back from the end of the table. Lift the patient's legs out of the stirrups at the same time, and place them on the table extension (supine position). Remove the stirrup covers and discard them in a waste container. Return the stirrups to their normal position. Assist the patient into a sitting position. Slide the table extension back into place while supporting the patient's lower legs.
    Principle. Lifting both the patient's legs out of the stirrups at the same time avoids strain on the back and abdominal muscles.

13. **Procedural Step.** Assist the patient down from the table. Return the footrest to its normal position. Instruct the patient to get dressed. Discard the gown and drape in a waste container.

PROCEDURE 5-7 Sims Position

Outcome Position and drape a patient in the Sims position. Sims position, also known as the *left lateral position,* is used to examine the vagina and rectum, to measure rectal temperature, to perform a flexible sigmoidoscopy, and to administer an enema.

Equipment/Supplies

- Examining table
- Disposable patient gown
- Disposable patient drape

1. **Procedural Step.** Sanitize your hands. Greet the patient and introduce yourself.
2. **Procedural Step.** Identify the patient and explain the type of examination or procedure that will be performed.
3. **Procedural Step.** Provide the patient with a patient gown. Instruct the patient to remove clothing from the waist down and to put on the patient gown with the opening in back. The disrobing facility should provide privacy, a place to sit, and a place to hang clothing.
4. **Procedural Step.** Pull out the footrest of the examining table, and assist the patient into a sitting position. Place a drape over the patient's thighs and legs.
5. **Procedural Step.** Ask the patient to move back on the table. As the patient is doing this, pull out the table extension while supporting the patient's lower legs.
6. **Procedural Step.** Ask the patient to lie on his or her back. Provide assistance if needed.
7. **Procedural Step.** Position the drape lengthwise over the patient to provide warmth and modesty.
8. **Procedural Step.** Ask the patient to turn onto the left side. Provide assistance during this step to prevent the patient from accidentally rolling off the table and to

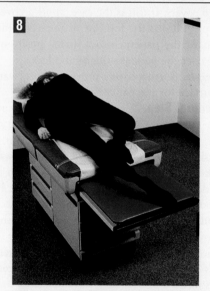

The right leg is flexed sharply, and the left leg is flexed slightly.

adjust the drape to provide modesty. The patient's left arm should be positioned behind the body and the right arm forward with the elbow bent. Assist the patient in flexing the legs. The right leg is flexed sharply, and the left leg is flexed slightly.

PROCEDURE 5-7　Sims Position—cont'd

9. **Procedural Step.** Adjust the drape as needed. When the physician is ready to examine the patient, a small portion of the drape is folded back to expose the anal area.

10. **Procedural Step.** After completion of the examination, assist the patient into a supine position and into a sitting position. Slide the table extension back into place while supporting the patient's lower legs.

11. **Procedural Step.** Assist the patient down from the table. Return the footrest to its normal position. Instruct the patient to get dressed. Discard the gown and drape in a waste container.

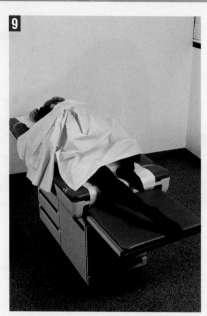

Adjust the drape as needed.

PROCEDURE 5-8　Knee-Chest Position

Outcome Position and drape a patient in the knee-chest position. The knee-chest position is used to examine the rectum and to perform a proctoscopic examination because it provides maximal exposure to the rectal area. This is a difficult position to maintain; the patient should not be put into this position until just before the examination.

Equipment/Supplies

- Examining table
- Disposable patient gown
- Disposable patient drape
- Pillow

1. **Procedural Step.** Sanitize your hands. Greet the patient and introduce yourself.

2. **Procedural Step.** Identify the patient and explain the type of examination or procedure that will be performed.

3. **Procedural Step.** Provide the patient with a patient gown. Instruct the patient to remove clothing from the waist down and to put on the gown with the opening in back. The disrobing facility should provide privacy, a place to sit, and a place to hang clothing.

4. **Procedural Step.** Pull out the footrest of the examining table, and assist the patient into a sitting position. Place a drape over the patient's thighs and legs.

5. **Procedural Step.** Ask the patient to move back on the table. As the patient is doing this, pull out the table extension while supporting the patient's lower legs.

6. **Procedural Step.** Assist the patient into the supine position and then into the prone position, making sure to have the patient roll toward you. Position the drape diagonally over the patient to provide warmth and modesty.

7. **Procedural Step.** Ask the patient to bend the arms at the elbows and rest them alongside the head. Ask the patient to elevate the buttocks while keeping the back straight. The patient's head should be turned to one side, and the weight of the body should be supported by the chest. A pillow under the chest can give additional support and aid in relaxation. The knees and lower legs are separated approximately 12 inches.

8. **Procedural Step.** Adjust the drape diagonally as needed with one corner over the patient's back and the opposite corner over the buttocks and falling between the patient's legs. When the physician is ready to ex-

Continued

PROCEDURE 5-8   Knee-Chest Position—cont'd

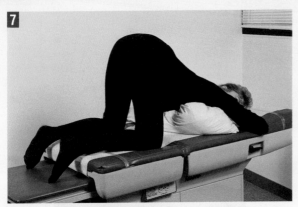

The buttocks are elevated, and the head is turned to one side.

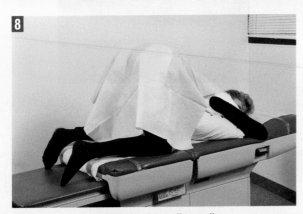

Position the drape diagonally.

amine the patient, a small portion of the drape is folded back to expose the anal area.

9. **Procedural Step.** After completion of the examination, assist the patient into a prone position and then into a supine position. Allow the patient to rest in the supine position before he or she sits up.
   Principle. Patients (especially elderly ones) frequently become dizzy after being in the knee-chest position and should be allowed to rest before they sit up.

10. **Procedural Step.** Assist the patient into a sitting position. Slide the table extension back into place while supporting the patient's lower legs.

11. **Procedural Step.** Assist the patient down from the table. Return the footrest to its normal position. Instruct the patient to get dressed. Discard the gown and drape in a waste container.

PROCEDURE 5-9   Fowler's Position

Outcome Position and drape a patient in Fowler's position. Fowler's position is used to examine the upper body of patients with cardiovascular and respiratory problems, such as congestive heart failure, emphysema, and asthma. These patients find it easier to breathe in this position than in a sitting or supine position. This position also is used to draw blood from patients who are likely to faint.

Equipment/Supplies

- Examining table
- Disposable patient gown
- Disposable patient drape

1. **Procedural Step.** Sanitize your hands. Greet the patient and introduce yourself.
2. **Procedural Step.** Identify the patient and explain the type of examination or procedure that will be performed.
3. **Procedural Step.** Provide the patient with a patient gown. Instruct the patient to remove clothing as appropriate for the type of examination being performed and to put on the patient gown with the opening in

front. The disrobing facility should provide privacy, a place to sit, and a place to hang clothing.
4. **Procedural Step.** Position the head of the table as follows:
   a. For the semi-Fowler's position, the table should be positioned at a 45-degree angle.
   b. For the full Fowler's position, the table should be positioned at a 90-degree angle.

PROCEDURE 5-9   Fowler's Position—cont'd

5. **Procedural Step.** Pull out the footrest of the examining table, and assist the patient into a sitting position. Place a drape over the patient's thighs and legs.

6. **Procedural Step.** Pull out the table extension while supporting the patient's lower legs. Ask the patient to lean back against the table head. Provide assistance during this step.

7. **Procedural Step.** Position the drape lengthwise over the patient to provide warmth and modesty. As the physician examines the patient, move the drape according to the body parts being examined.

8. **Procedural Step.** After completion of the examination, assist the patient into a sitting position. Slide the table extension back into place while supporting the patient's lower legs.

9. **Procedural Step.** Assist the patient down from the table. Instruct the patient to get dressed. Return the head of the table and the footrest to their normal positions. Discard the gown and drape in a waste container.

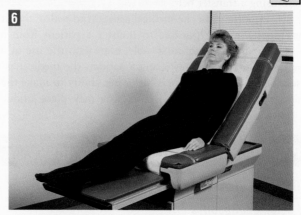

Ask the patient to lean back against the table head.

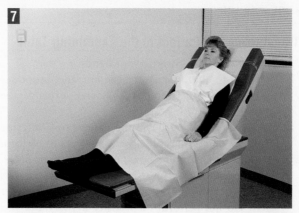

Position the table at a 45-degree angle for the semi-Fowler's position.

WHEELCHAIR TRANSFER

A wheelchair is a chair mounted on wheels designed to make mobility easier for individuals who cannot walk or who are having difficulty walking because of illness or disability. Although some patients who come to the medical office in a wheelchair are able to transfer themselves from a wheelchair to an examining table, others may need assistance. The medical assistant plays an important role in the safe and efficient transfer of a patient from a wheelchair to an examining table and back again.

The Occupational Safety and Health Administration (OSHA) recommends that assistive devices be used whenever possible to transfer patients. A transfer belt (also known as a gait belt) is a safety device that is approximately 1½ to 2 inches wide and 48 or 60 inches long and is made of a durable fiber such as canvas, nylon, or leather (Figure 5-10). It can be used to assist in the safe transfer of a patient from a wheelchair to an examining table and back again. The transfer belt is wrapped around the patient's waist over his or her clothing and is securely fastened. The belt pro-

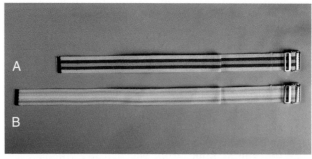

Figure 5-10. Transfer belts. **A**, Transfer belt that is 48 inches in length. **B**, Transfer belt that is 60 inches in length.

vides the medical assistant with a secure grip for holding onto the patient and controlling the patient's movement. This makes the transfer more comfortable for the patient by not having to grasp the patient around the rib cage or under the axillae to make the transfer. Using a transfer belt also reduces the chance of the medical assistant hurting his or her musculoskeletal system while transferring a patient.

Procedure 5-10 outlines the procedure for transferring a patient from a wheelchair to an examining table and back again using a transfer belt.

It is important for the medical assistant to realize that it may not always be possible to transfer a patient from a wheelchair to the examining table, even with the use of a transfer belt. Before transferring a patient, the medical assistant should carefully assess his or her ability to make the transfer. There are certain factors that may place undue strain on the medical assistant's musculoskeletal system. These factors include patients who are overweight or patients who have conditions that limit their mobility (e.g., leg paralysis), making it impossible for the patient to assist with the transfer. If factors exist that might cause strain to the medical assistant's musculoskeletal system, the medical assistant should ask for assistance or notify the physician that it is not possible to transfer the patient to the examining table.

PROCEDURE 5-10   Wheelchair Transfer

Outcome Transfer a patient from a wheelchair to the examining table and from an examining table to a wheelchair.

Equipment/Supplies

- Examining table
- Transfer belt

Transferring the Patient to the Examining Table

1. **Procedural Step.** Sanitize your hands.
2. **Procedural Step.** Greet the patient and introduce yourself. Identify the patient and explain the procedure.
3. **Procedural Step.** Evaluate the patient to determine his or her mental and physical capabilities to perform the transfer. Determine how heavy the patient is and if he or she is able to assist in the transfer. Assess whether or not you are able to perform the transfer safely. Do not perform the transfer if you think you may incur a musculoskeletal injury.
4. **Procedural Step.** Wrap the transfer belt snugly around the patient's waist over the patient's clothing with the buckle in front. Securely fasten the belt by threading it through the teeth of the buckle. Put the belt through the other two openings to lock it. The belt should be snug with just enough space between the belt and the patient's clothing to allow your fingers to be inserted comfortably between the belt and the patient's waist.
   Principle. Placing the transfer belt over the patient's clothing prevents abrasions to the patient's skin. The belt must be snug to prevent it from sliding upward on the patient's body.
5. **Procedural Step.** With the patient's stronger side next to the examining table, position the wheelchair at a 45-degree angle to the end of the examining table.
6. **Procedural Step.** If the examining table is height-adjustable, lower it to the same height as the wheelchair or slightly lower. If it is not height-adjustable, pull out the footrest of the examining table.
7. **Procedural Step.** Lock the brakes of the wheelchair and fold back the wheelchair footrests.
   Principle. The wheels must be locked to prevent the chair from moving during the transfer. The wheelchair

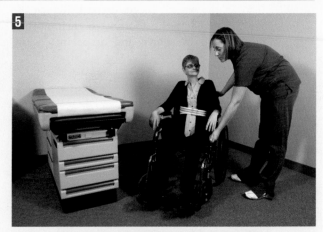

Position the wheelchair at a 45-degree angle.

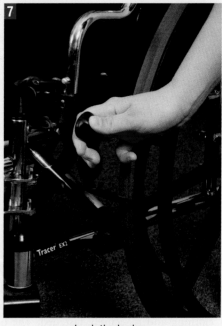

Lock the brakes.

PROCEDURE 5-10 Wheelchair Transfer—cont'd

footrests must be out of the way to provide an unobstructed path for making the transfer.

8. **Procedural Step.** Inform the patient of what he or she will be required to do during the transfer. During the transfer, clearly state in a step-by-step manner what the patient should do. Encourage the patient to help as much as possible during the transfer by using the muscles of his or her arms and legs.

9. **Procedural Step.** Make sure the patient's feet are positioned flat on the floor.
   Principle. Making sure the patient's feet are flat on the floor provides the patient with balance and stability when he or she stands.

10. **Procedural Step.** Stand in front of the patient with the feet apart about 6 to 8 inches, the toes pointed outward, one foot slightly forward, and the knees bent.
    Principle. This position conserves energy and provides a wide base of support for the transfer.

11. **Procedural Step.** Ask the patient to place his or her hands on the armrests of the wheelchair and to lean forward.

12. **Procedural Step.** Grasp the transfer belt on either side of the patient's waist using an underhand grasp.
    Principle. The transfer belt provides a secure handle for holding onto the patient and controlling the patient's movement.

13. **Procedural Step.** Tighten your abdominal gluteal muscles in preparation for the transfer. Ask the patient

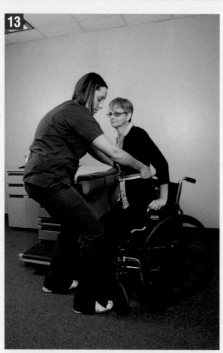

Assist the patient to a standing position.

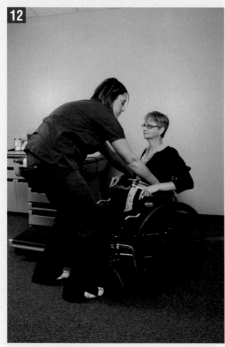

Grasp the transfer belt on either side of the patient's waist.

to push off the armrests and into a standing position on the count of 3. At the same time, straighten your knees and assist the patient to a standing position by pulling upward on the transfer belt, making sure to keep your back straight.
Principle. The patient pushing upward with his or her arm and leg muscles provides an additional lifting force and reduces the chance of straining your back muscles. Lifting the patient using your knees and the transfer belt allows the strong muscles of the legs and arms to do the lifting rather than the back muscles.

14. **Procedural Step.** Pivot the patient toward the examining table. Position the patient's buttocks and backs of the knees toward the examining table. Instruct the patient to step onto the footrest (backward) one foot at a time.
    Principle. Pivoting prevents twisting of the spine, which can result in a serious back injury.

15. **Procedural Step.** Gradually lower the patient into a sitting position on the examining table. Make sure the patient's buttocks and thighs are firmly supported on the table. Remove the transfer belt.

16. **Procedural Step.** Unlock the wheelchair and move it out of the way of the examining table. Push in the footrest of the examining table.

17. **Procedural Step.** Stay with the patient to prevent falls.

Continued

PROCEDURE 5-10

PROCEDURE 5-10   Wheelchair Transfer—cont'd

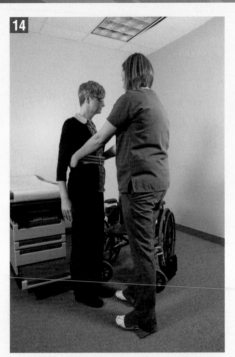

Position the patient toward the table.

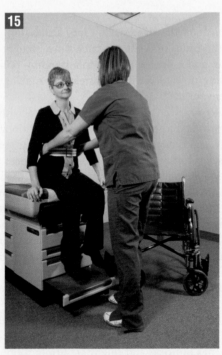

Gradually lower the patient onto the table.

Transferring the Patient to the Wheelchair

1. **Procedural Step.** Wrap the transfer belt snugly around the patient's waist and securely fasten it.
2. **Procedural Step.** Position the wheelchair at a 45-degree angle to the end of the examining table.

3. **Procedural Step.** If the examining table is height-adjustable, lower it to the same height as the wheelchair or slightly lower. If it is not height-adjustable, pull out the footrest of the examining table.
4. **Procedural Step.** Lock the wheelchair into place and fold back the footrests.
5. **Procedural Step.** Inform the patient of what he or she will be required to do during the transfer.
6. **Procedural Step.** Stand in front of the patient with the feet apart about 6 to 8 inches, the toes pointed outward, one foot slightly forward, and the knees bent.
7. **Procedural Step.** Ask the patient to place his or her arms on your shoulders. To prevent a neck injury, do not allow the patient to place his or her arms around your neck.

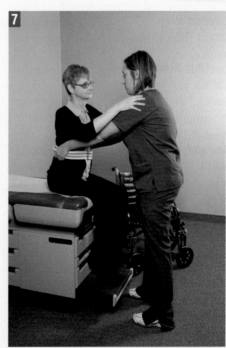

Ask the patient to put his or her arms on your shoulders.

8. **Procedural Step.** Grasp the transfer belt on either side of the patient's waist using an underhand grasp.
9. **Procedural Step.** Ask the patient to push to a standing position using his or her thigh and leg muscles on the count of 3. At the same time, straighten your knees and assist the patient to a standing position by pulling upward on the transfer belt.
10. **Procedural Step.** Instruct the patient to step down from the footrest, one foot at a time.

PROCEDURE 5-10   Wheelchair Transfer—cont'd

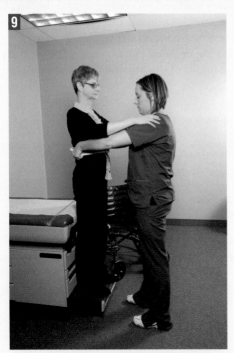

Assist the patient to a standing position.

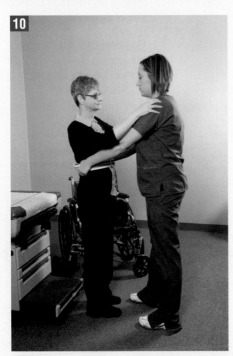

Instruct the patient to step down from the footrest.

11. **Procedural Step.** Pivot the patient toward the wheelchair. Position the backs of the patient's legs against the seat of the wheelchair.

12. **Procedural Step.** Bend at your knees and gradually lower the patient into a sitting position in the wheelchair with the patient's buttocks at the back of the chair. Remove the transfer belt and make sure the patient is comfortable.

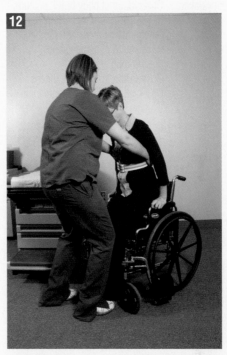

Gradually lower the patient into the wheelchair.

13. **Procedural Step.** Reposition the wheelchair footrests and place the patient's feet in the footrests. Unlock the wheelchair.

14. **Procedural Step.** Push in the footrest of the examining table.

ASSESSMENT OF THE PATIENT

The extent of patient assessment during the physical examination depends on the purpose of the examination and the patient's condition. A complete physical examination involves a thorough assessment of all body systems. Table 5-2 outlines the specific assessments included in a complete physical examination. The physician uses an organized and systematic approach in performing a physical examination, starting with the patient's head and proceeding toward the feet. Using this type of approach facilitates the examination process and requires the fewest position changes by the patient.

With a paper-based patient record (PPR), the physician notes the results of the physical examination in the patient's

Table 5-2 Physician Assessment During the Physical Examination

Body Structure	Assessment	Normal Findings	Abnormal Findings
General appearance	Observation of body build, posture, gait	Good posture and balance	Poor posture or balance
		Steady gait	Unsteady, irregular, or staggering gait
	Determination of weight and height	Weight within ideal range	Patient is overweight or underweight
	Observation of hygiene and grooming	Good hygiene and grooming	Poor hygiene and grooming
	Observation for signs of illness	No signs of illness	Obvious signs of illness
	Observation of attitude, emotional state, mood	Patient speaks clearly and is cooperative	Patient is uncooperative, withdrawn, incoherent, negative, or hostile
Skin	Inspection of skin for color, vascularity, lesions	Smooth, supple, free of blemishes	Blisters, wounds, lesions, rashes, swelling
		No unusual color	Unusual skin color (e.g., flushing, cyanosis, jaundice, pallor)
	Palpation of temperature, moisture, turgor, texture	Warm to touch	Rough, dry, flaky skin
			Poor skin turgor
Head and neck	Inspection of size, shape, contour of head	Round head with prominences in front and back	Head is asymmetric or of unusual size
	Inspection of hair and scalp	Hair is resilient, evenly distributed, and not excessively dry or oily	Loss of hair
			Scaliness or dryness of scalp
			Presence of lice or other parasites
	Palpation of head and neck	No lumps, swelling, tenderness, or lesions of head or neck	Lumps, swelling, tenderness, or lesions of head or neck
Eyes	Evaluation of visual acuity and color vision	Good visual ability with or without glasses or contact lenses	Poor visual acuity or blindness
		Appropriate color perception	Color blindness
	Evaluation of visual field	No visual field loss	Gaps in field of vision
	Inspection of eyelids and eyeballs	Eyes are bright	Dull or glossy eyes
	Inspection of conjunctiva	Pink mucous membranes	Inflamed mucous membranes
			Excessive tearing
			Drainage from eyes
	Inspection of eye movements	Eyes move equally in all directions	Drooping eyelids
			Uncoordinated eye movements
	Tests for pupillary reaction using penlight	Pupils are black, equal in size, react appropriately to light	Dilated, constricted, or unequal pupils
	Inspection of internal eye structures using ophthalmoscope	Reddish-pink retina, even caliber, intact retinal blood vessels	Cloudy lens or narrowed blood vessels
Ears	Test for hearing using tuning fork or audiometer	Good hearing ability	Limited hearing or deafness
	Inspection of size, shape, symmetry of ears	Ears are symmetric and proportionate to head	Ears are asymmetric and not proportionate to the head
	Inspection of external ear canal and tympanic membrane using an otoscope	Cerumen is soft and easily removed	Lesions, redness, or swelling of external ear canal
		No drainage or discomfort	Drainage from ear
		Skin of ear canal is intact, pink, warm, and slightly moist	Pain when ear is moved
			Impacted cerumen
		Tympanic membrane is pearly gray and semitransparent	Tympanic membrane is red, bulging, or perforated

Table 5-2 Physician Assessment During the Physical Examination—cont'd

Body Structure	Assessment	Normal Findings	Abnormal Findings
Nose	Inspection of size, shape, symmetry of nose	Nose is symmetric, straight, not tender	Nose is asymmetric, deformed, flaring, or tender
	Inspection of nostrils using nasal speculum	Septum is intact and midline Nasal mucosa is moist and pink	Deviation or perforation of septum Redness, swelling, polyps, or discharge Nostrils are obstructed
	Test for sense of smell	Correct or very few incorrect responses to odors	Absent, decreased, exaggerated, or unequal responses to test substances
Mouth and pharynx	Inspection of lips for contour, color, texture	Pink, moist, soft, smooth lips	Pallor, cyanosis, blisters, swelling, cracking, excessive dryness of lips
	Inspection of mucosa	Pink, moist mucous membranes	Pale or dry mucosa with ulcers or abrasions
	Inspection of gums and palate	Smooth, pink, moist, firm gums Hard palate is firm and white Soft palate is pink and cushiony	Gums are red, bleeding, swollen, tender, spongy, or receding
	Inspection of teeth	Smooth, white enamel; regularly spaced teeth or well-fitting dentures	Missing or loose teeth, dental caries, poor-fitting dentures
	Inspection of tongue	Moist, pink, slightly rough-surfaced tongue	Tongue is dry, furry, smooth, red, or ulcerated
	Inspection of pharynx	Pink and smooth pharynx Tonsils are pink and normal in size Gag reflex is present	Pharynx is red, swollen, or ulcerated Tonsils are red or swollen Absent gag reflex
Arms and hands	Inspection of hands and arms for general appearance	Firm, strong muscles	Muscle weakness, lack of control or coordination
		Normal range of motion in joints	Restricted range of motion
	Palpation of arm muscles	Good muscle control and coordination	
	Palpation for tenderness or lumps	No tenderness or lumps	Tenderness or lumps in hands or arms
	Inspection of fingernails	Colorless nail plate with a convex curve Smooth nail texture	Indentation, infection, brittleness, thickening, or angulation of nails Cyanosis or pallor of nails
Chest and lungs	Inspection of size and shape of chest	Chest is symmetric	Abnormal chest contour
	Assessment of respiratory rate, rhythm, depth	Normal respiratory rate, rhythm, depth	Labored, slow, rapid, or irregular respirations
	Percussion of chest		
	Auscultation of breath sounds	Normal breath sounds	Flat or dull lung sounds Noisy breath sounds
		No cough	Productive or nonproductive cough
	Palpation of ribs	No tenderness of ribs	Tenderness of ribs
Heart	Auscultation of heart sounds	Normal heart sounds	Irregular heartbeats or murmur
	Auscultation of apical pulse, rate, rhythm, volume	Regular, strong heartbeats	Rates slower or more rapid than normal
	Palpation of peripheral pulses	Palpable peripheral pulses	Weak or absent peripheral pulses
	Auscultation of blood pressure	Blood pressure within normal range for age	Low or high blood pressure
	Assessment of peripheral vascular perfusion	Skin is pink, resilient, moist Immediate return of color to nail beds	Cyanosis, pallor, edema Poor capillary filling in nail beds
	Electrocardiogram to assess heart function	Normal heart function	Abnormal electrocardiogram
Breasts	Inspection of size, symmetry, contour	Breasts are round, smooth, symmetric	Retraction, dimpling, redness, or swelling of breasts
	Inspection of nipple	Nipples are round and equal in size, similar in color, appear soft and smooth Areola is round and pink	Bleeding, cracking, discharge, or inversion of nipples
	Palpation of breasts and axillary lymph nodes	No lumps in or tenderness of breasts or axillary lymph nodes	Lumps in or tenderness of breasts or axillary lymph nodes

Continued

Table 5-2 Physician Assessment During the Physical Examination—cont'd

Body Structure	Assessment	Normal Findings	Abnormal Findings
Abdomen	Inspection of contour, symmetry, skin condition, integrity	Symmetric contour Unblemished skin Soft abdomen	Asymmetric contour Rash or other skin lesions Abdominal distention
	Auscultation of bowel sounds	Active bowel sounds	Increased, diminished, or absent bowel sounds
	Percussion to assess underlying organs Palpation of underlying organs, tenderness, lumps	Normal position and size of liver and spleen	Tenderness or lumps Enlarged liver or spleen
Genitalia and rectum	**Male** Inspection of penis and urethra Inspection of scrotum and palpation of testes	Penis is smooth Testicles are smooth, firm, and movable within scrotal sac Scrotum is symmetric	Ulceration or discharge from penis Lumps or tenderness of scrotum, testes, or prostate gland
	Palpation of rectum and prostate gland Stool specimen to test for occult blood	Increased pigmentation in anal area Good anal sphincter tone Absence of occult blood in stool	Enlarged prostate gland Hemorrhoids or relaxed anal sphincter Occult blood in stool
	Female Inspection of external genitalia	External genitalia are smooth and without lesions	Ulceration or redness or swelling of external genitalia
	Inspection of vagina and cervix using vaginal speculum Specimen collection from vagina and cervix for Pap test	Vaginal mucosa is pink and moist Cervix is pink and smooth Pap test is normal	Lacerations, tenderness, redness, or discharge from vagina or cervix Pap test is abnormal
	Bimanual pelvic examination	No tenderness or lumps in uterus and ovaries	Tenderness in or lumps of uterus and ovaries
	Palpation of rectum Stool specimen to test for occult blood	Good anal sphincter tone Increased pigmentation in anal area	Hemorrhoids or relaxed anal sphincter Occult blood in stool
Legs and feet	Inspection of legs for general appearance and palpation of legs	Firm, strong muscles Normal range of motion in joints	Muscle weakness, lack of control or coordination Restricted range of motion Tenderness or lumps Limp or foot dragging during walking
	Inspection of toenails	Smooth nail texture	Indentation, infection, brittleness, thickening, or angulation of nails
Neurologic	Determination of mental status and level of consciousness	Alert and responds appropriately Oriented to person, place, and time	Responds inappropriately Disoriented
	Determination of sense of pain and touch	Normal responses to pain and touch	Diminished or absent response to stimuli
	Use of percussion hammer to test reflexes	Normal reflexes	Abnormal or absent reflexes

Memories *from* Externship

Hope Fauber: During my externship at a student health center at a 4-year college, I was responsible for working up patients for gynecologic examinations. The two-piece drapes had the top opening in the front and the bottom opening in the back. After explaining this to an Asian student who spoke very little English, I noticed that she had the openings opposite of what I had explained. I explained again, with words and gestures, that she needed to reverse the openings. To my surprise, she stood up, turned around in a circle, and sat down! ∎

medical record. Figure 5-11 is an example of a preprinted form for this purpose. With an electronic medical record (EMR), the physician uses free-text entry, drop-down lists, and check-boxes to record findings on the screen of a computer monitor. The EMR program uses this information to generate the physical examination report. This means that by the end of the examination, the physical examination report is complete, and the physician does not need to dictate his or her findings at a later time. This alleviates the need for transcribing the physician's dictation into a written report.

PHYSICAL EXAMINATION

INSTRUCTIONS:
(WNL) Within Normal Limits
(POS) Positive findings (X) Omitted

1. GENERAL

a. Posture _____
b. Gait _____
c. Speech _____
d. Appearance _____
e. Emotion _____

2. HEAD

a. Hair _____
b. Masses _____
c. Shape _____
d. Bruits _____
e. Tenderness _____
f. Sinus _____
g. Articulations _____

3. EYES

a. Lids R ___ L ___   f. Pupils R ___ L ___
b. Sclera R ___ L ___   g. Fundi R ___ L ___
c. Conjunctiva R ___ L ___   h. Light R ___ L ___
d. Muscles R ___ L ___   i. Bruits R ___ L ___
e. Cornea R ___ L ___
j. Accommodation R ___ L ___

4. EARS

a. Pinna R ___ L ___
b. Canal R ___ L ___
c. Drum R ___ L ___
d. Weber _____
e. Rinne _____

5. NOSE

a. Septum _____
b. Mucosa R ___ L ___
c. Obstruction _____

6. MOUTH/THROAT

a. Lips _____   f. Teeth _____
b. Breath _____   g. Dentures _____
c. Tongue _____   h. Caries _____
d. Pharynx _____   i. Larynx _____
e. Tonsils _____   j. Floor _____

7. NECK

a. Thyroid _____   d. Nodes R ___ L ___
b. Trachea _____   e. Bruits R ___ L ___
c. Veins _____   f. Carotid R ___ L ___

8. LUNGS

a. Chest _____   e. Bruits _____
b. Symmetry _____   f. Sounds _____
c. Diaphragm _____   g. Fremitus _____
d. Rubs _____

9. HEART

a. PMI _____   e. Rub _____
b. Rate _____   f. Murmur _____
c. Rhythm _____   g. Palpation _____
d. Thrill _____

10. BREASTS

a. Nodes R ___ L ___
b. Nipple R ___ L ___
c. Areolae R ___ L ___
d. Symmetry _____
e. Discharge _____

11. ABDOMEN

a. Sounds _____   e. Hernia R ___ L ___
b. Masses _____   f. Bruits R ___ L ___
c. Tenderness _____   g. Femoral R ___ L ___
d. Organs _____   h. Ing. nodes R ___ L ___

12. MUSCULOSKELETAL

a. Cervical _____
b. Thoracic _____
c. Lumbar _____
d. Sacral _____
e. Pelvic _____
f. Rib cage _____

13. FEMALE GENITALS

a. Labia _____   e. Cervix _____
b. Bartholin _____   f. Uterus _____
   gland _____   g. Adnexa _____
c. Urethra _____   R ___ L ___
d. Vagina _____   h. Pap smear
                        done _____

14. MALE GENITALS

a. Penis _____   e. Scars _____
b. Scrotum _____   f. Meatus _____
c. Testicles _____   g. Epididymis _____
d. Discharge _____

15. RECTAL

a. Masses _____   f. Fissure _____
b. Anus _____   g. Hemorrhoids _____
c. Sphincter _____   h. Sigmoid _____
d. Prostate _____   _____cm.
e. Pilonidal _____   i. Mucosa _____
                     j. Other _____

16. SKIN

a. Scars _____
b. Marks _____
c. Texture _____
d. Sweat _____
e. Color _____
f. Ulcers _____

17. NEUROLOGICAL

	Strength*	Reflex**
a. Biceps	R ___ L ___	R ___ L ___
b. Triceps	R ___ L ___	R ___ L ___
c. Knee	R ___ L ___	R ___ L ___
d. Ankle	R ___ L ___	R ___ L ___

e. Romberg _____   i. Coordination _____
f. Babinsky _____   j. Tremor _____
g. Cranial N _____   k. Vibratory _____
h. Sensory _____

*When testing strength use grades:
  Weak (W); Normal (N); Strong (S)

**When testing reflexes use:
  Absent (A); Present (P); Brisk (B)

18. EXTREMITIES

a. Range of Motion
   Shoulder _____   Knee _____
   Elbow _____   Ankle _____
   Wrist _____   Hand _____
   Hip _____   Foot _____
            Phalanges _____

b. General   UR _____ UL _____ LR _____ LL _____
c. Muscular   UR _____ UL _____ LR _____ LL _____
d. Bruits   UR _____ UL _____ LR _____ LL _____
e. Edema   UR _____ UL _____ LR _____ LL _____
f. Varicosities   UR _____ UL _____ LR _____ LL _____

Signature _____

Figure 5-11. A preprinted form for recording the results of the physical examination.

Patients who exhibit symptoms of illness usually require only select portions of the physical examination. A patient who comes to the medical office with symptoms of bronchitis usually does not require a complete physical examination; rather, the physician examines the body system that is most likely to be associated with the symptoms. Four assessment techniques are used to obtain information during the physical examination: inspection, palpation, percussion, and auscultation.

Inspection

Inspection involves observation of the patient for any signs of disease, and of the four assessment techniques, it is the one most frequently used. Good lighting, either natural or artificial, is important for effective observation. The patient's color, speech, deformities, skin condition (e.g., rashes, scars, warts), body contour and symmetry, orientation to the surroundings, body movements, and anxiety level are assessed through inspection. The medical assistant should develop a high level of detailed observational skills to assist the physician in assessing physical characteristics.

Palpation

Palpation is the examination of the body using the sense of touch (Figure 5-12). The physician uses palpation to determine the placement and size of organs; the presence of lumps; and the existence of pain, swelling, or tenderness. Examining the breasts and taking the pulse are performed by palpation. Palpation often helps verify data obtained by inspection. The patient's verbal and facial expressions also are observed during palpation to assist in the detection of abnormalities.

The two types of palpation—light and deep—are categorized by the amount of pressure applied. *Light palpation* of

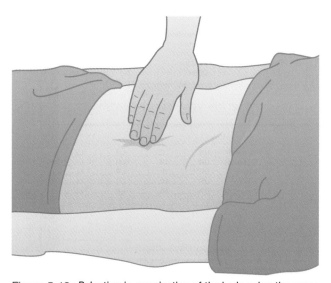

Figure 5-12. Palpation is examination of the body using the sense of touch.

structures is performed to determine areas of tenderness. The fingertips are placed on the part to be examined and are gently depressed approximately one half inch. *Deep palpation* is used to examine the condition of organs such as those in the abdomen. Two hands are used for deep palpation. One hand is used to support the body from below, and the other hand is used to press over the area to be palpated. Deep palpation is used by the physician to perform a bimanual pelvic examination.

Percussion

Percussion involves tapping the patient with the fingers and listening to the sounds produced to determine the size, density, and locations of organs. This technique is often used to examine the lungs and abdomen.

The fingertips are used to produce a sound vibration similar to that of tapping a drumstick on a drum. The nondominant hand is placed directly on the area to be assessed, with the fingers slightly separated. The dominant hand is used to strike the joint of the middle finger placed on the patient to produce the sound vibration (Figure 5-13). Structures that are dense, such as the liver, spleen, and heart, produce a dull sound. Empty or air-filled structures, such as the lungs, produce a hollow sound. Any condition that changes the density of an organ or tissue, such as fluid in the lungs, would change the quality of the sound.

Auscultation

Auscultation is an examination technique that involves listening with a stethoscope to the sounds produced within the body. This technique is used to listen to the heart and lungs or to measure blood pressure. Environmental noise interferes with effective auscultation of body sounds and should be minimized. The diaphragm of the stethoscope chest piece is used to assess high-pitched sounds, such as lung and bowel sounds; the bell of the stethoscope chest piece is used to assess low-pitched sounds, such as those produced by the heart and vascular system. The chest piece should be cleaned with an antiseptic wipe and warmed with the hands before being placed on the patient.

ASSISTING THE PHYSICIAN

During the patient assessment, the medical assistant should assist the physician as required. This includes helping the patient change positions for the physician's examination of

What Would You Do? What Would You *Not* Do?

Case Study 3

Ben-Yi Sun has brought his father, Chang-Yi Sun, to the medical office. Chang-Yi Sun is 76 years old and lives with Ben-Yi and his family. Because there is a large Asian population in the community, the medical office personnel have learned two things about the Asian culture: (1) They are brought up to respect elders, and elders are always considered first, and (2) Asians have a great respect for

harmony. If they do not understand something, they may not admit it to avoid disrupting harmony. Ben-Yi Sun speaks very good English, but his father understands only a few words of English. Chang-Yi Sun has been diagnosed with hypertension, and he needs education about going on a low-sodium diet. He also needs instructions on taking his blood pressure at home and recording the results. ■

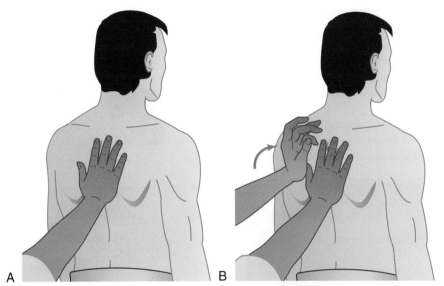

Figure 5-13. Percussion involves tapping the patient with the fingers. **A,** The nondominant hand is placed directly on the area to be assessed, with the fingers slightly separated. **B,** The fingers of the dominant hand are used to strike the joint of the middle finger to produce a sound vibration.

different parts of the body, handing the physician instruments and supplies, and reassuring the patient to reduce apprehension. When the examination is completed, the medical assistant should assist the patient off the examining table and provide additional information if needed, such as scheduling a return visit or patient education to promote wellness. Procedure 5-11 describes the procedure for assisting with the physical examination.

PROCEDURE 5-11 Assisting With the Physical Examination

Outcome Prepare the patient and assist with a physical examination.

Equipment/Supplies

- Examining table
- Equipment for the type of examination to be performed

1. **Procedural Step.** Prepare the examining room. Ensure that the room is clean, free of clutter, and well lit, and that the room temperature is comfortable for the patient.
2. **Procedural Step.** Sanitize your hands.
3. **Procedural Step.** Assemble the equipment according to the type of examination to be performed and the physician's preference. Arrange the instruments and supplies in a neat and orderly manner on a table or tray. Do not allow one item to be placed on top of another.
4. **Procedural Step.** Obtain the patient's medical record. Go to the waiting room and ask the patient to come back to the examining room.
5. **Procedural Step.** Escort the patient to the examining room.

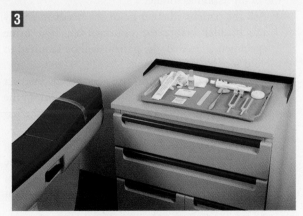

Assemble the equipment.

Continued

PROCEDURE 5-11   Assisting With the Physical Examination—cont'd

6. Procedural Step. Ask the patient to be seated. Greet the patient and introduce yourself using a calm and friendly manner. Identify the patient by his or her full name and date of birth.
Principle. Identifying the patient correctly avoids mistaking one patient for another. Using a calm and friendly manner helps to put the patient at ease.

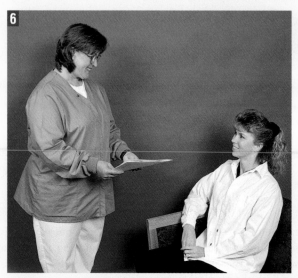

Greet and identify the patient by name and date of birth.

7. Procedural Step. Seat yourself so that you face the patient at a distance of 3 to 4 feet.

8. Procedural Step. Obtain and record the patient's symptoms while following the procedure outlined in Procedure 1-4 in Chapter 1.

9. Procedural Step. Measure the patient's vital signs, and chart the results.

10. Procedural Step. Measure the weight and height of the patient, and chart the results.

11. Procedural Step. Instruct and prepare the patient for the examination as follows:

a. Ask the patient whether he or she needs to empty the bladder before the examination. If a urine specimen is needed, the patient will be required to void into a urine container.

b. Provide the patient with a patient gown. Instruct the patient to remove all clothing and to put on the patient gown. Offer assistance if you sense the patient may have trouble undressing.

c. Tell the patient to have a seat on the examining table after putting on the patient gown. Inform the patient that the physician will be with him or her soon, and leave the room to provide the patient with privacy.
Principle. An empty bladder makes the examination easier and is more comfortable for the patient.

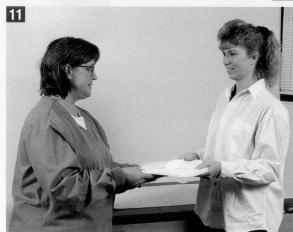

Instruct and prepare the patient for the examination.

12. Procedural Step. Make the medical record available to the physician. The medical office has a designated location where the record is placed, such as on a small shelf mounted on the wall next to the outside of the examining room door or in a chart holder on the outside of the examining room door. Position the medical record so that patient-identifiable information is not visible. Check to make sure that the patient is ready to be seen by the physician. Before entering a patient's room, knock lightly on the door to let the patient know that you are getting ready to enter the room. If a patient is ready to be seen, inform the physician. This may be done using a color-coded flagging system mounted on the wall next to the examining room.
Principle: HIPAA requires protection of a patient's health information.

13. Procedural Step. Assist the physician with examination of the body systems as follows:

a. Ensure that the patient is positioned correctly in a sitting position on the examining table. This allows the physician to examine the patient's head, eyes, ears, nose, mouth and pharynx, neck, chest, lungs, and heart.

b. Hand the physician the ophthalmoscope, otoscope, and tongue depressor.

c. Dim the light when the physician is ready to use the ophthalmoscope. The dim light helps dilate the patient's pupils, providing the physician better visualization of the interior of the eye.

d. After use, the tongue depressor should be transferred by holding it at the center to prevent contact with the patient's secretions, which may contain pathogens. Dispose of the tongue depressor in a regular waste container.

e. Offer reassurance to the patient to reduce apprehension.

PROCEDURE 5-11   Assisting With the Physical Examination—cont'd

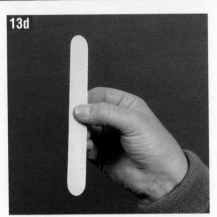

Transfer the tongue depressor by holding it at the center.

14. Procedural Step. Position the patient as required for examination of the remaining body systems. Place and drape the patient in the proper position for examination of a particular part of the body using proper body mechanics.

15. Procedural Step. Assist and instruct the patient as follows:

   a. Allow the patient to rest in a sitting position on the examining table before he or she gets off of it. Some patients become dizzy after being positioned on the examining table.

   b. Assist the patient off the examining table to prevent falls.

   c. Instruct the patient to get dressed. Provide assistance if needed.

   d. Provide the patient with any necessary instructions, such as patient education and scheduling a return visit. Give instructions involving medical care in terms the patient can understand; do not use medical terms.

   e. Sanitize the hands, and chart in his or her medical record any instructions given to the patient.

   f. Escort the patient to the reception area.

16. Procedural Step. Clean the examining room in preparation for the next patient as follows:

   a. Discard the paper on the examining table. If body secretions have gotten on the examining table, apply gloves, and clean and disinfect the table. Unroll a fresh length of paper on the table.

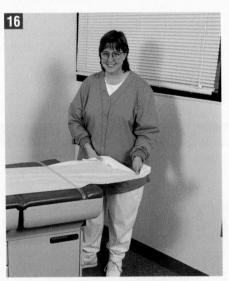

Unroll a fresh length of paper.

   b. Discard all disposable supplies into an appropriate waste container.

   c. Ensure that there are ample numbers of clean gowns and drapes and other supplies.

   d. Remove reusable equipment to a work area for sanitization, sterilization, or disinfection as required by the medical office policy.

CHARTING EXAMPLE	
Date	
11/20/12	11:30 a.m. CC. Shortness of breath x 2 days.
	T: 98.8° F AD, P: 78 reg and strong, R: 20
	even and reg, BP: 110/68, Wt: 126, Ht: 5' 6"
	———————— H. Fauber, CMA (AAMA)

evolve *Check out the Evolve site to access additional interactive activities.*

MEDICAL PRACTICE and the LAW

Activities involved in the physical examination can be sensitive for the patient. Information obtained while taking the patient history is confidential; revealing this information to anyone is unethical and illegal. A good rapport is essential for obtaining complete information, especially when asking sensitive questions. Complete information is necessary for accurate diagnosis and treatment.

Preparing the patient for a physical examination can be embarrassing for the patient. Keep in mind your duty to "do good" and "do no harm" to the patient. This involves proper knowledge and techniques and a professional, caring, and helpful attitude. Draping the patient correctly allows only minimal exposure. Incorrect draping or positioning that is unnecessarily uncomfortable could become a legal issue. Patients who are young, very old, or weak should never be left alone on an examining table. A fall from a table often results in harm and potential for a lawsuit.

Finally, while assisting the physician, be supportive of the patient as much as you are able. While the physician concentrates on the examination, you should continually assess the patient and provide for any needs, including assistance, encouragement, and physical comfort. Be patient, polite, and professional in all directions given to the patient. You may have done this many times, but this could be the first time for a frightened, ill patient. ∎

What Would You Do? What Would You *Not* Do? RESPONSES

Case Study 1
Page 178

What Did Hope Do?
- ❑ Empathized with Abbey and told her that a lot of patients feel just like she does about having their weight taken. Explained that the information in her medical record is strictly confidential.
- ❑ Told Abbey that weight is important so that the physician can properly diagnose and treat her condition, and that medication dosage is often based on a person's weight.
- ❑ Told Abbey that she could stand on the scale backward while her weight is being measured so that she would not see the reading on the scale.
- ❑ Returned the weights to zero before Abbey got off the scale.
- ❑ Recorded Abbey's weight in her chart without telling her the results.
- ❑ Encouraged Abbey to see the physician when she needs to so that she stays as healthy as possible.

What Did Hope Not Do?
- ❑ Did not make any comments about Abbey's body or weight after weighing her.
- ❑ Did not criticize Abbey for letting her weight stand in the way of coming in when she needed health care.

What Would You Do/What Would You *Not* Do? Review Hope's response and place a checkmark next to the information you included in your response. List the additional information you included in your response.

_____
_____
_____
_____

Case Study 2
Page 178

What Did Hope Do?
- ❑ Listened carefully to Mikayla and showed concern verbally and nonverbally.
- ❑ Carefully charted the information relayed by Mikayla so that the physician would be aware of all aspects of Mikayla's problem.
- ❑ Told Mikayla that she needs to talk to the physician about wanting some medicine for heartburn.
- ❑ Encouraged Mikayla to talk to her parents about what's been going on with her.

What Did Hope Not Do?
- ❑ Did not agree with Mikayla that she needs to lose more weight.
- ❑ Did not make comments about Mikayla being too thin.

What Would You Do/What Would You *Not* Do? Review Hope's response and place a checkmark next to the information you included in your response. List the additional information you included in your response.

_____
_____
_____
_____

Case Study 3
Page 206

What Did Hope Do?
- ❑ Greeted Chang-Yi first before greeting his son.
- ❑ Spoke clearly and slowly to Ben-Yi in a normal tone of voice.
- ❑ Gave them a brochure on low-sodium diets and went over the foods that are low in sodium.

❏ Asked Chang-Yi (via Ben-Yi's translating) to indicate the foods he likes that he thinks would be low in sodium. Determined whether these foods are low in sodium.

❏ Showed Ben-Yi how to take his father's blood pressure. Had Ben-Yi practice taking his father's blood pressure.

❏ Made sure that Chang-Yi and Ben-Yi understood all of the information before they left the office.

What Did Hope Not *Do?*

❏ Was careful not to ignore Chang-Yi.

What Would You Do/What Would You *Not* Do? Review Hope's response and place a checkmark next to the information you included in your response. List the additional information you included in your response.

_____

_____

_____

_____

CERTIFICATION REVIEW

❏ **A patient examination consists of three parts:** health history, physical examination, and laboratory and diagnostic tests. The physician uses the results to determine the patient's general state of health, to arrive at a diagnosis and prescribe treatment, and to observe any change in a patient's illness after treatment has been instituted.

❏ **Diagnosis** refers to the scientific method of determining and identifying a patient's condition through evaluation of the health history, physical examination, and results of laboratory tests and diagnostic procedures.

❏ **The clinical diagnosis** is obtained through evaluation of the health history and the physical examination without the benefit of laboratory or diagnostic tests. The prognosis is the probable course and outcome of a patient's condition.

❏ **The equipment and supplies** needed for the physical examination vary according to the type of examination and the physician's preference. The medical assistant should have the equipment and supplies ready for the examination. They should be arranged for easy access by the physician.

❏ **An adult patient's weight** is usually measured during every office visit, whereas an adult's height is typically measured only during the first visit or when a complete physical examination of the patient is requested. Children are weighed and measured during every office visit to observe their pattern of growth and to calculate medication dosage.

❏ **The scale** must be balanced before measuring a patient's weight to ensure an accurate weight measurement. The weight measurement should be recorded in pounds to the nearest quarter pound. The height measurement should be recorded in feet and inches to the nearest quarter inch.

❏ **Body mechanics** is the utilization of the correct muscles to maintain proper balance, posture, and body alignment to accomplish a task safely and efficiently without undue strain on any muscle or joint. Proper body mechanics should be used to prevent musculoskeletal injuries when the medical assistant performs tasks in the medical office.

❏ **Correct patient positioning** facilitates the examination by permitting better access to the part being examined or treated. Positions used in the medical office are sitting, supine, prone, dorsal recumbent, lithotomy, Sims, knee-chest, and Fowler's. The position used depends on the type of examination or procedure to be performed.

❏ **The patient is draped** during positioning to provide modesty, comfort, and warmth. The part to be examined is the only part that should be exposed.

❏ **Wheelchair transfer** may need to be performed by the medical assistant to transfer a patient safely and efficiently from a wheelchair to an examining table and back again. A transfer belt should be used to assist in the safe and comfortable transfer of the patient. Before transferring a patient, the medical assistant should carefully assess his or her ability to make the transfer. If factors exist that might cause strain to the medical assistant's musculoskeletal system, the medical assistant should ask for assistance or notify the physician that it is not possible to transfer the patient to the examining table.

❏ **A physical examination** is performed using an organized and systematic approach, starting with examination of the patient's head and proceeding toward the feet.

❏ **Assessment techniques** to obtain information during the physical examination include inspection, palpation, percussion, and auscultation. Inspection involves observation of the patient for signs of disease. Palpation is the examination of the body using the sense of touch. Percussion involves tapping the patient with the fingers and listening to the sounds produced to determine the size, density, and location of underlying organs. Auscultation involves listening with a stethoscope to the sounds produced within the body.

↻ TERMINOLOGY REVIEW

Medical Term	Word Parts	Definition
Audiometer	*audi/o:* hearing *-meter:* instrument used to measure	An instrument used to measure hearing.
Auscultation		The process of listening to the sounds produced within the body to detect signs of disease.
Bariatrics	*bar/o:* weight *-iatrics:* a branch of medicine	The branch of medicine that deals with the treatment and control of obesity and diseases associated with obesity.
Body mechanics		Utilization of the correct muscles to maintain proper balance, posture, and body alignment to accomplish a task safely and efficiently without undue strain on any muscle or joint.
Clinical diagnosis		A tentative diagnosis of a patient's condition obtained through evaluation of the health history and the physical examination, without the benefit of laboratory or diagnostic tests.
Diagnosis	*dia-:* through, complete *-gnosis:* knowledge	The scientific method of determining and identifying a patient's condition.
Differential diagnosis		A determination of which of two or more diseases with similar symptoms is producing a patient's symptoms.
Inspection		The process of observing a patient to detect signs of disease.
Mensuration		The process of measuring a patient.
Ophthalmoscope	*ophthalm/o:* eye *-scope:* to view, to examine	An instrument for examining the interior of the eye.
Otoscope	*ot/o:* ear *-scope:* to view, to examine	An instrument for examining the external ear canal and tympanic membrane.
Palpation		The process of feeling with the hands to detect signs of disease.
Percussion		The process of tapping the body to detect signs of disease.
Percussion hammer		An instrument with a rubber head, used for testing reflexes.
Prognosis	*pro-:* before *-gnosis:* knowledge	The probable course and outcome of a patient's condition and the patient's prospects for recovery.
Speculum		An instrument for opening a body orifice or cavity for viewing.
Symptom		Any change in the body or its functioning that indicates a disease might be present.

🖱 ON THE WEB

For information on nutrition:

American Dietetic Association: www.eatright.org

Ask the Dietitian: www.dietitian.com

For information on weight control and fitness:

American Obesity Association: www.obesity.org

Obesity Action Coalition: www.obesityaction.org

Weight Watchers: www.weightwatchers.com

E-Diets: www.ediets.com

Calorie Control Council: www.caloriecontrol.org

ON THE WEB—cont'd

For information on accessing health information:

InteliHealth: www.intelihealth.com

Mayo Clinic: www.mayoclinic.com

U.S. Department of Health and Human Services: www.os.dhhs.gov

American Academy of Family Physicians: Family Doctor: www.familydoctor.org

Healthfinder: www.health.gov

WebMD: www.webmd.com

Medline Plus: www.nlm.nih.gov/medlineplus

For information on cultural diversity:

National Geographic Society: www.nationalgeographic.com

U.S. Department of the Interior: Workforce Diversity: www.doi.gov/diversity/workforce

Generations United: www.gu.org

6

Eye and Ear Assessment and Procedures

astigmatism (uh-STIG-muh-tiz-em)
audiometer (aw-dee-OM-eh-ter)
canthus (KAN-thus)
cerumen
hyperopia (HYE-per-OP-ee-uh)
impacted
instillation (IN-still-AY-shun)

irrigation (EAR-ih-GAY-shun)
myopia (mye-OH-pee-uh)
otoscope (AH-toe-skope)
presbyopia (PRESS-bee-OH-pee-uh)
refraction (ree-FRAK-shun)
tympanic membrane (tim-PAN-ik MEM-brane)

Introduction to Eye and Ear Assessment

The medical assistant is responsible for performing a variety of assessments and procedures that involve the eye and the ear. An understanding of the structure and function of the eye and the ear is essential to mastering skills in these areas.

A visual acuity test is usually part of the routine physical examination. This test is a screening test to detect deficiencies in vision.

The medical assistant may be responsible for assessing color vision with the use of specially prepared colored plates. As a result of this testing, color blindness can be detected. Color blindness is an inability to distinguish certain colors; the most common problem is with the colors red and green. Color blindness is particularly significant if the patient is involved in an activity that relies on the ability to distinguish colors, such as electronics and interior decorating.

Hearing tests also may be part of the routine physical examination. During contact with the patient, the medical assistant should be alert to signs that indicate the patient might be having difficulty hearing what is being said. A whispered voice next to the patient's ear can be a screening test for hearing acuity. The use of tuning forks or an audiometer provides a more accurate determination of hearing acuity. An **audiometer** is an instrument that emits sound waves at various frequencies. The patient is instructed to indicate when a sound at a given frequency can be heard.

The medical assistant is responsible for performing or teaching the patient to perform eye and ear irrigations and instillations. **Irrigation** is washing a body canal with a flowing solution. **Instillation** is dropping a liquid into a body cavity. Eye and ear irrigations and instillations should be performed using the important principles of medical asepsis outlined in Chapter 2.

THE EYE

STRUCTURE OF THE EYE

The eye has three layers (Figure 6-1). The outer layer is the *sclera,* which is composed of tough, white fibrous connective tissue. The front part of the sclera is modified to form a transparent covering over the colored part of the eye; this covering is the *cornea.*

The middle layer of the eye is the *choroid,* which is composed of many blood vessels and is highly pigmented. The blood vessels nourish the other layers of the eye, and the pigment works to absorb stray light rays. The front part of the choroid is specialized into the ciliary body, the suspensory ligaments, and the iris. The *ciliary body* contains muscles that control the shape of the lens. The function of the *suspensory ligaments* is to suspend the lens in place. The *lens* is responsible for focusing the light rays on the retina. The colored part of the eye is the *iris,* which controls the size of the pupil. The *pupil* is the opening in the eye that permits the entrance of light rays.

The third and innermost layer of the eye is the *retina.* Light rays come to a focus on the retina and subsequently are transmitted to the brain, by way of the optic nerve, to be interpreted.

The *anterior chamber* is the area between the cornea and the iris, and the *posterior chamber* is the area between the iris and the lens. Both chambers are filled with a substance known as the *aqueous humor.* A transparent jelly-like material, known as *vitreous humor,* fills the eyeball between the lens and the retina. Its function is to help maintain the shape of the eyeball.

The *conjunctiva* is a membrane that lines the eyelids and covers the front of the eye except the cornea. The conjunctiva covering the sclera is transparent except for some capillaries, which allows the white sclera to show through.

VISUAL ACUITY

Visual acuity refers to acuteness or sharpness of vision. A person with normal visual acuity can see clearly and is able to distinguish fine details close up and at some distance.

Errors of refraction are the most common causes of defects in visual acuity (Figure 6-2). **Refraction** refers to the ability of the eye to bend the parallel light rays coming into it so that they can be focused on the retina. An *error of refraction* means that the light rays are not being refracted or bent properly and are not adequately focused on the retina. A defect in the shape of the eyeball can cause a refractive error. Errors of refraction can be improved with corrective lenses.

A person who is nearsighted has a condition termed **myopia.** The eyeball is too long from front to back, causing

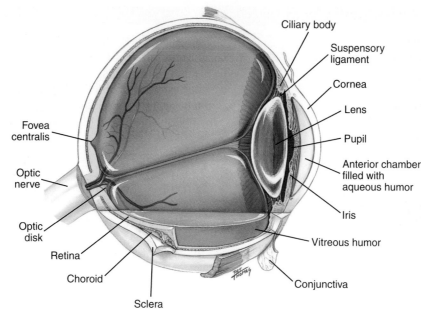

Figure 6-1. The internal structure of the eye. (From Applegate EJ: The anatomy and physiology learning system, ed 3, St Louis, 2006, Saunders.)

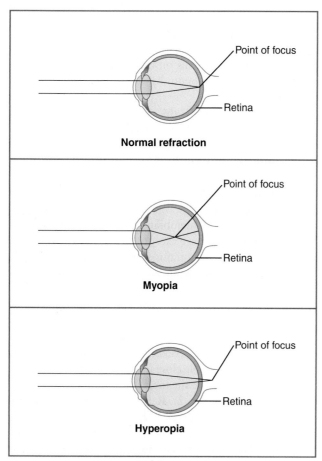

Errors of Refraction

Figure 6-2. Diagram of normal refraction compared with myopia (nearsightedness) and hyperopia (farsightedness), which are errors of refraction that cause visual defects.

the light rays to be brought to a focus in front of the retina. A myopic person has difficulty seeing objects at a distance and may squint and have headaches as a result of eyestrain. A corrective lens (e.g., eyeglasses, contact lenses) or laser eye surgery can correct this condition, which then allows the light rays to come to a focus on the retina.

A person who is farsighted has a condition known as **hyperopia.** The eyeball is too short from front to back, resulting in a different type of refractive error, in which the light rays are brought to a focus behind the retina. The individual has difficulty viewing objects at a reading or working distance. An individual with hyperopia may experience blurring, headaches, and eyestrain while performing up-close tasks. A corrective lens can correct this condition by causing the light rays to come to a focus on the retina.

Astigmatism is a refractive error that causes distorted and blurred vision for both near and far objects. A normal cornea has a round or spherical shape and is smooth. With astigmatism, the cornea is curved into an oval shape. This causes the light rays to focus on two different points on the retina, instead of just one, resulting in distorted and blurred vision. Astigmatism often occurs in combination with myopia or hyperopia and can be corrected with corrective lenses.

In most people, a decrease in the elasticity of the lens of the eye begins to occur after age 40 years. This condition, **presbyopia,** results in a decreased ability to focus clearly on close objects.

If a defect in visual acuity is detected, the patient is referred to an eye specialist for further evaluation. Several types of specialists are involved in the care of the eyes. An *ophthalmologist* is a physician who specializes in diagnosing and treating diseases and disorders of the eye. An ophthalmologist is qualified to prescribe ophthalmic and systemic medications and to perform eye surgery. An *optometrist* is a licensed primary health care provider who has expertise in measuring visual acuity and prescribing corrective lenses for the treatment of refractive errors. An optometrist also is qualified to diagnose and treat disorders and diseases of the eye and to prescribe ophthalmic medications. An optometrist is not a physician and is not permitted to prescribe systemic medications or to perform eye surgery. An *optician* is a professional who interprets and fills prescriptions for eyeglasses and contact lenses.

Assessment of Distance Visual Acuity (DVA)

Myopia can be diagnosed (in combination with other tests) by a distance visual acuity test. In the medical office, the Snellen eye chart is most often used. Two types of charts are commonly used. One type is used for school-age children and adults and consists of a chart of letters in decreasing sizes (Figure 6-3). The other type is used for preschool children, non–English-speaking people, and nonreaders; it is composed of the capital letter E in decreasing sizes and arranged in different directions (Figure 6-4). Visual acuity charts with pictures of familiar objects also are available for use with preschool children. Testing with these charts tends to be less accurate than with the Snellen charts. Some children are unable to identify the objects because of lack of recognition, not because of a defect in visual acuity. It is suggested that the Snellen Big E chart be used with preschool children.

Conducting a Snellen Test

The visual acuity test should be performed in a well-lit room that is free of distractions. The test is usually performed at a distance of 20 feet; this can be conveniently marked off in the medical office with paint or a piece of tape so that it does not have to be remeasured every time the test is performed.

Two numbers, separated by a line, appear at the side of each row of letters on the chart. The number above the line represents the distance (in feet) at which the test is conducted. It is usually 20 feet because most eye tests are conducted at this distance. The number below the line represents the distance from which a person with normal visual acuity can read the row of letters. The line marked 20/20 indicates normal distance visual acuity, or 20/20 vision. This means a person could read what he or she was supposed to read at a distance of 20 feet.

A visual acuity reading of 20/30 means this was the smallest line that the individual could read at a distance of 20 feet. People with normal acuity would be able to read this line at a distance of 30 feet.

A visual acuity reading of 20/15 means this was the smallest line that the individual could read at a distance of 20 feet. It indicates above-average acuity for distance vision. People with normal acuity would be able to read this line at 15 feet.

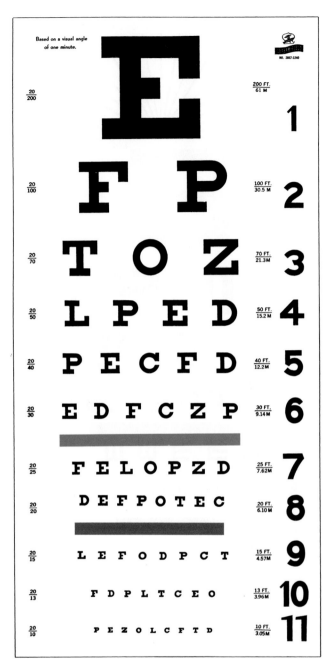

Figure 6-3. Snellen eye chart consisting of letters in decreasing sizes; this chart is used to measure distance visual acuity.

The acuity of each eye should be measured separately, traditionally beginning with the right eye. Most physicians prefer that the patient wear his or her contact lenses or glasses, except reading glasses, during the test; the medical assistant should record in the patient's chart that corrective lenses were worn by the patient during the test. An eye occluder should be held over the eye not being tested. The patient's hand should not be used to cover the eye because this may encourage peeking through the fingers, especially in the case of children. The patient should be instructed to leave open the eye not being tested because closing it causes squinting of the eye that is being tested. The proce-

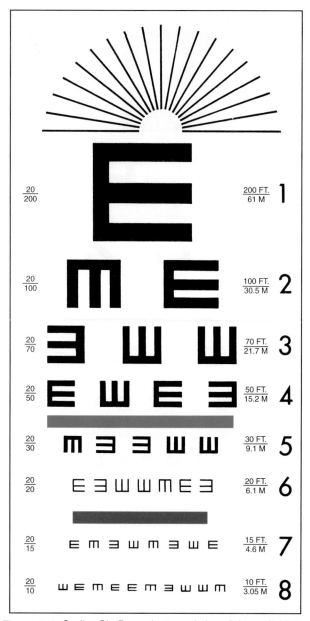

Figure 6-4. Snellen Big E eye chart consisting of the capital letter E in decreasing sizes and arranged in different directions; this chart is used to measure distance visual acuity.

dure for measuring distance visual acuity is outlined in Procedure 6-1.

Assessing Distance Visual Acuity in Preschool Children

With minor variations, Procedure 6-1 can be used to test distance visual acuity in preschool children. The Snellen Big E chart is used for this purpose.

A child needs a complete and thorough explanation of what is expected of him or her before beginning the test. Tell the child you will be playing a pointing game. Do not force the child to play the game because the results then tend to be inaccurate. Draw the capital letter E on an index card, and teach the child to point in the direction of the

open part of the E by turning the card in different directions (up, down, to the right, and to the left). Using such phrases as "fingers" or the "legs of the table" to describe the open part of the E helps the child understand what is expected (Figure 6-5). Allow the child to practice the pointing game with the index card until you are sure this level of skill has been mastered. Be sure to praise the child when the correct response is given.

The child might need help holding the eye occluder in place. The aid of another person such as the parent would then be required.

Assessment of Near Visual Acuity (NVA)

Near visual acuity testing assesses the patient's ability to read close objects (i.e., at a reading or working distance); the test results are used to detect hyperopia and presbyopia.

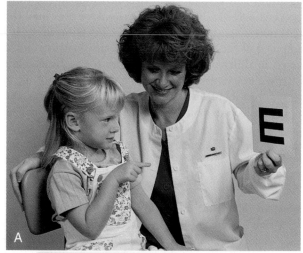

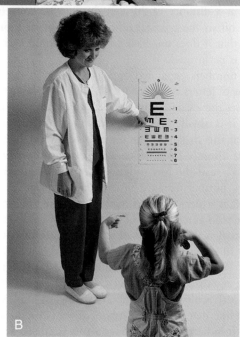

Figure 6-5. **A,** Cammie teaches a preschool child to point in the direction of the open part of the capital letter E. **B,** Cammie performs the Snellen Big E visual acuity test.

Highlight on Eye Assessment

Vision disorders are the fourth most common disability in the United States. Studies show that vision disorders are the most prevalent disabling condition in children. Because of this, both children and adults should have regular eye examinations.

For individuals at any age *with symptoms of, or at risk for, eye disease* (such as those with a family history of eye disease, diabetes, or high blood pressure), the American Academy of Ophthalmology (AAO) recommends that individuals see their ophthalmologist to determine how frequently their eyes should be examined. For individuals who *do not have eye conditions* requiring treatment, the AAO recommends eye examinations at the intervals listed below:

Age 3 and younger: Eye screening should be performed during regularly scheduled pediatric visits. At age 3, it is recommended that the child be checked for eye conditions including strabismus (crossed eyes), amblyopia (lazy eye), ptosis (drooping of the eye), and refractive errors.

Ages 3 to 19: Eye screening should be performed every 1 to 2 years during regularly scheduled health care visits.

Ages 20 to 39: A complete eye examination should be performed at least once between the ages of 20 and 29 and at least twice between the ages of 30 and 39. A complete eye examination consists of visual acuity testing and testing for errors of refraction and eye diseases. Most young adults have healthy eyes, but it is important for them to be aware that they need to protect their vision by wearing protective eyewear during sport activities, performing yard work, working with chemicals, or engaging in any activities that could cause injury to the eye. These individuals should also be instructed to contact their physician of any of the following symptoms that could indicate a problem:

- Visual changes or pain
- Flashes of light
- Seeing spots or ghostlike images
- Line edges that appear distorted or wavy
- Dry eyes with itching and burning

Ages 40 to 64: In July 2007, the AAO issued a new eye disease screening recommendation for this age group. The AAO recommends that adults with no signs or risk factors for eye disease obtain a baseline eye disease screening at age 40. This is the time when early signs of diseases and changes in vision may begin to occur. The examination allows for the opportunity for early treatment and preservation of vision. Based on the results of the baseline examination, the ophthalmologist will prescribe the necessary intervals for follow-up examinations (usually every 2 to 4 years for patients with no risk factors). This new recommendation does not replace regular visits to the ophthalmologist to treat ongoing diseases or injuries or for vision examinations for corrective lenses.

Age 65 and older: Individuals age 65 and older should have a complete eye examination every 1 to 2 years to check for cataracts, glaucoma, age-related macular degeneration, diabetic retinopathy, and other eye conditions.

Visual acuity is considered normal for the various age groups if it falls within the following values:

Newborn	20/500
Infant 1-6 mo	20/200 to 20/90
Infant 6-12 mo	20/60
Child 12-18 mo	20/40
Child 18 mo-3 yr	20/30
Child 3-18 yr	20/20
Adult 18 yr or older	20/20

Legal blindness is defined as a visual acuity measurement of 20/200 or less in both eyes with the use of corrective lenses.

The term *color blind* is not an accurate term to describe an individual with abnormal color vision because the inability to distinguish any colors at all is extremely rare. Most individuals with a color vision abnormality are unable to distinguish certain hues of color, such as red and green. A better term is *color vision defect.*

Defective color vision is usually congenital. It is found in 5% to 8% of men and in less than 1% of women.

Studies show that there is no significant correlation between defective color vision and increased automobile accidents. Most drivers who have a color vision defect are able to distinguish traffic lights by the different light intensities and by the positions of the lights on the traffic signal. ■

The test is conducted with a card similar to the Snellen eye chart; however, the size of the type ranges from the size of newspaper headlines down to considerably smaller print such as would be found in a telephone directory (Figure 6-6). The test card is available in a variety of forms, such as printed paragraphs, printed words, and pictures.

The test should be performed in a well-lit room free of distractions. It is conducted with the patient holding the test card at a distance between 14 and 16 inches. If the patient wears reading glasses, they should be worn during the test. The acuity should be measured in each eye separately, traditionally beginning with the right eye. An eye occluder should be held over the eye not being tested. The patient should be instructed to keep the covered eye open because closing it may cause squinting of the eye that is being tested.

The patient is asked to read or identify orally each line or paragraph of type. During the test, the patient should be observed for unusual symptoms, such as squinting, tilting the head, or watering of the eyes, which may indicate that the patient is having difficulty reading the card. The patient continues until reaching the smallest type that can be read.

The results are recorded as the smallest type that the patient could comfortably read with each eye at the distance at which the card is held (i.e., 14 to 16 inches). The recording is based on the type of test card used to conduct the test. One type of card uses a recording method similar to that used with the Snellen eye test. For this type of near visual acuity card, the results would be recorded as 14/14 for a patient with normal near visual acuity. This means the patient read what was supposed to be read at a distance of

No. 1.
.37M

In the second century of the Christian era, the empire of Rome comprehended the fairest part of the earth, and the most civilized portion of mankind. The frontiers of that extensive monarchy were guarded by ancient renown and disciplined valor. The gentle but powerful influence of laws and manners had gradually cemented the union of the provinces. Their peaceful inhabitants enjoyed and abused the advantages of wealth.

No. 2.
.50M

fourscore years, the public administration was conducted by the virtue and abilities of Nerva, Trajan, Hadrian, and the two Antonines. It is the design of this, and of the two succeeding chapters, to describe the prosperous condition of their empire; and afterwards, from the death of Marcus Antoninus, to deduce the most important circumstances of its decline and fall; a revolution which will ever be remembered, and is still felt by

No. 3.
.62M

the nations of the earth. The principal conquests of the Romans were achieved under the republic; and the emperors, for the most part, were satisfied with preserving those dominions which had been acquired by the policy of the senate, the active emulations of the consuls, and the martial enthusiasm of the people. The seven first centuries were filled with a rapid succession of triumphs; but it was

No. 4.
.75M

reserved for Augustus to relinquish the ambitious design of subduing the whole earth, and to introduce a spirit of moderation into the public councils. Inclined to peace by his temper and situation, it was very easy for him to discover that Rome, in her present exalted situation, had much less to hope than to fear from the chance of arms; and that, in the prosecution of

No. 5.
1.00M

the undertaking became every day more difficult, the event more doubtful, and the possession more precarious, and less beneficial. The experience of Augustus added weight to these salutary reflections, and effectually convinced him that, by the prudent vigor of

No. 6.
1.25M

his counsels, it would be easy to secure every concession which the safety or the dignity of Rome might require from the most formidable barbarians. Instead of exposing his person or his legions to the arrows of the Parthinians, he obtained, by an honor-

No. 7.
1.50M

able treaty, the restitution of the standards and prisoners which had been taken in the defeat of Crassus. His generals, in the early part of his reign, attempted the reduction of Ethiopia and Arabia Felix. They marched near a thou-

No. 8.
1.75M

sand miles to the south of the tropic; but the heat of the climate soon repelled the invaders, and protected the unwarlike natives of those sequestered regions

No. 9.
2.00M

The northern countries of Europe scarcely deserved the expense and labor of conquest. The forests and morasses of Germany were

No. 10.
2.25M

filled with a hardy race of barbarians who despised life when it was separated from freedom; and though, on the first

No. 11.
2.50M

attack, they seemed to yield to the weight of the Roman power, they soon, by a signal

Figure 6-6. Example of a near visual acuity card.

14 inches. Also included in the recording should be the date and time, corrective lenses worn, and any unusual symptoms exhibited by the patient.

ASSESSMENT OF COLOR VISION

Defects in color vision may be classified as congenital or acquired. *Congenital defects* are more common and refer to a color vision deficiency that is inherited and is present at birth. Congenital color vision deficiencies most often affect males. *Acquired defects* refer to a color vision deficiency that is acquired after birth, resulting from such factors as an eye or brain injury, disease, and certain drugs. Color vision tests, such as the Ishihara test (Figure 6-7), detect congenital color vision disturbances and are commonly performed in the medical office. A basic screening for color vision can be performed by asking the patient to identify the red and green lines on the Snellen eye chart.

Ishihara Test

The Ishihara test for color blindness is a convenient and accurate method to detect total congenital color blindness and red-green color blindness by assessing an individual's ability to perceive primary colors and shades of color. The Ishihara book contains a series of polychromatic plates of primary colored dots arranged to form a numeral against a background of similar dots of contrasting colors (see Figure 6-7). Patients with normal color vision are able to read the appropriate numeral; however, patients with color vision defects read the dots either as not forming a number at all or as forming a number different from the one identified by

---

What Would You Do? What Would You *Not* Do?

Case Study 1
Nicole Neason brings her daughter, Haley, to the office for a camp physical. Haley has just completed the fourth grade and is going to summer camp for 2 weeks with Tess, her best friend. Tess wears glasses and Haley thinks they are really cool. She often asks to try on Tess' glasses and wishes she could wear glasses just like her best friend. When Haley is measured for visual acuity, she misses a few letters on the 20/70 line, the 20/50 line, the 20/40 line, and the 20/20 line. She is unable to read any of the letters on the 20/15 line. After the examination, Haley wants to know if she's missed enough letters to be able to get glasses. ■

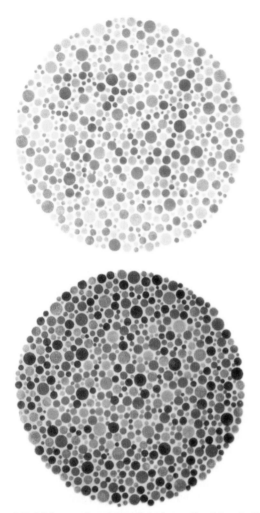

Figure 6-7. Ishihara color plates. Polychromatic plates. In the *upper figure,* a person with normal color vision reads 74, but a person with red-green color blindness reads 21. In the *lower figure,* a red-blind person (protanope) reads 2, but a green-blind person (deuteranope) reads 4. A normal-vision person reads 42. Reproduced plates are not good for testing for color deficiency. (From Ishihara J: Tests for color blindness, Tokyo, 1920, Kanehara.)

light as much as possible. Using light other than just described, such as bright sunlight, may change the appearance of shades of color on the plates, leading to inaccurate test results.

The medical assistant is responsible for performing the color vision test and for recording results in the patient's chart. The physician assesses the results to determine whether the patient has a deficiency in color vision.

The Ishihara test consists of 14 color plates. Plates 1 through 11 are used to conduct the basic test, and plates 12, 13, and 14 are used to further assess patients who exhibit a red-green color deficiency. It is unnecessary to include these plates (12, 13, and 14) in the test of patients who exhibit normal color vision. In interpreting the results, if 10 or more plates are read correctly, the patient's color vision is considered normal. If 7 or fewer of the 11 Ishihara plates are read correctly, the patient is identified as having a color vision deficiency. It would be unusual for the medical assistant to obtain results in which the patient has read eight or nine plates correctly. The test is structured so that a patient with a color vision defect generally does not read eight or nine plates correctly and the rest incorrectly.

If a defect in color vision is detected, the patient is referred for additional assessment of color vision to an ophthalmologist or optometrist, who would use more precise color vision tests. The procedure for assessing color vision using the Ishihara color plates is outlined in Procedure 6-2.

the individual with normal color vision. The first plate in the Ishihara book is designed to be read correctly by all individuals (with normal vision and exhibiting color vision deficiencies) and should be used to explain the procedure to the patient.

The book includes plates with winding colored lines for patients who are unable to identify the numbers by name, such as preschool children and non–English-speaking people. The patient should be asked to trace the line formed by the colored dots using a cotton swab or the eraser end of a pencil. The patient's finger should not be used to do the tracing because over time soiled fingers can degrade the polychromatic plates.

The Ishihara test should be conducted in a quiet room illuminated by natural daylight. If this is not feasible, a room lit with electric light may be used; however, the light should be adjusted to resemble the effect of natural day-

PROCEDURE 6-1   Assessing Distance Visual Acuity—Snellen Chart

Outcome Assess distance visual acuity.

Equipment/Supplies

- Snellen eye chart
- Eye occluder
- Antiseptic wipe

1. **Procedural Step.** Sanitize your hands.
2. **Procedural Step.** Assemble the equipment. Perform the test in a well-lit room that is free of distractions. Wipe the eye occluder with an antiseptic wipe, and allow it to dry completely.
   Principle. The eye occluder should be disinfected before use.
3. **Procedural Step.** Greet the patient and introduce yourself. Identify the patient and explain the procedure. Tell the patient that he or she will be asked to read several lines of letters. The patient should not have an opportunity to study or memorize the letters before beginning the test.
4. **Procedural Step.** Determine whether the patient wears contact lenses or glasses (other than reading glasses). If the patient wears such aids, he or she should be told to keep them on during the test.
5. **Procedural Step.** Ask the patient to stand on the marked line located 20 feet from the chart.
6. **Procedural Step.** Position the center of the Snellen chart at the patient's eye level. Stand next to the chart during the test to indicate to the patient the line to be identified.
   Principle. Ensure that the chart is at the patient's eye level rather than at your eye level, to provide the most accurate results.
7. **Procedural Step.** Test the acuity of each eye separately. Measure the visual acuity of the right eye first.
   Principle. The medical assistant should establish a pattern of beginning with the same eye (traditionally the right eye) every time the test is performed. This helps to reduce errors during the recording of results.
8. **Procedural Step.** Ask the patient to cover the left eye with the eye occluder. If the patient wears eyeglasses, tell him or her to place the occluder in front of the glasses gently to prevent the glasses from being moved out of their normal position. Instruct the patient to keep the left eye open. During the test, the medical assistant should check to make sure the patient is keeping the left eye open.
   Principle. Eyeglasses moved out of normal position may lead to inaccurate test results. Keeping the left eye open prevents squinting of the right eye, which temporarily improves vision, leading to inaccurate test results.

9. **Procedural Step.** Instruct the patient not to squint during the test because squinting temporarily improves vision. Ask the patient to identify orally one line at a time on the Snellen chart, starting with the 20/70 line (or a line that is several lines above the 20/20 line).
   Principle. It is best to start at a line above the 20/20 line to give the patient a chance to gain confidence and to become familiar with the test procedure.
10. **Procedural Step.** If the patient is able to read the 20/70 line, proceed down the chart until reaching the smallest line of letters the patient can read. If the patient is unable to read the 20/70 line, proceed up the chart until the smallest line of letters the patient can read is reached.
11. **Procedural Step.** While the patient is reading the letters, observe him or her for unusual symptoms, such as squinting, tilting of the head, or watering of the eyes.
    Principle. These symptoms may indicate that the patient is having difficulty identifying the letters.
12. **Procedural Step.** On a small piece of paper, jot down the numbers that are displayed next to the smallest line of letters that the patient is able to read. If one or two letters are missed, record the visual acuity with a minus sign next to the bottom number, along with the number of letters missed. If more than two letters are missed, the previous line is recorded.
13. **Procedural Step.** Ask the patient to cover the right eye with the eye occluder and to keep the right eye open. Measure the visual acuity in the left eye as de-

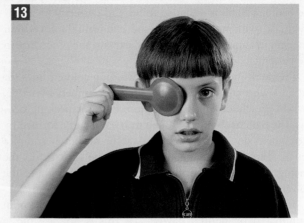

Ask the patient to cover the right eye and to keep the left eye open.

PROCEDURE 6-1   Assessing Distance Visual Acuity—Snellen Chart—cont'd

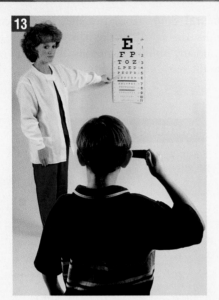

Ask the patient to identify one line at a time.

scribed in steps 9 through 12. During the test, check to make sure the patient is keeping the right eye open. *Principle.* Keeping the right eye open prevents squinting of the left eye.

14. Procedural Step. Chart the procedure. Include the date and time, the name of the test (Snellen test), the visual acuity results, and any unusual symptoms the patient exhibited during the test. Also chart whether the patient was wearing corrective lenses during the test. Use the following abbreviations: *s̄c* without correction or *c̄c* with correction. Latin abbreviations are used to record visual acuity. The abbreviation for the right eye is *OD (oculus dexter),* the abbreviation for the left eye is *OS (oculus sinister),* and the abbreviation for both eyes is *OU (oculus uterque).*

CHARTING EXAMPLE

Date	
11/5/12	3:30 p.m. Snellen test, s̄c: OD 20/20-1.
	OS 20/25. Exhibited squinting, OD. ————
	———————— C. Lindner, CMA (AAMA)

15. Procedural Step. Disinfect the eye occluder with an antiseptic wipe, and sanitize your hands.

PROCEDURE 6-2   Assessing Color Vision—Ishihara Test

Outcome Assess color vision.

Equipment/Supplies

• Ishihara book
• Cotton swab

1. Procedural Step. Sanitize your hands. Assemble the equipment.
2. Procedural Step. Conduct the test in a quiet room illuminated by natural daylight.
Principle. Using unnatural light may change the appearance of the shades of color on the plates, leading to inaccurate test results.
3. Procedural Step. Greet the patient and introduce yourself. Identify the patient and explain the procedure. Using the first (practice) plate as an example, instruct the patient to orally identify numbers formed by colored dots. Tell the patient that 3 seconds will be given to identify each plate.
Principle. The first plate is designed to be read correctly by all individuals and is used to explain the procedure to the patient.
4. Procedural Step. Hold the first color plate 30 inches (75 cm) from the patient, at a right angle to the pa-

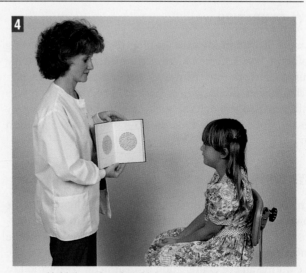

Hold the color plate 30 inches from the patient.

Continued

PROCEDURE 6-2 Assessing Color Vision—Ishihara Test—cont'd

tient's line of vision. The patient should keep both eyes open during the test.

5. **Procedural Step.** Ask the patient to identify the number on the plate. If the plate consists of a traceable winding colored line, ask the patient to trace the line using a cotton swab or the eraser end of a pencil. The patient's finger should not be used to make the tracing.
Principle. The patient's finger should not be used to trace the line because soiled fingers can degrade the plate over time.

6. **Procedural Step.** Record results after each plate. Continue until the patient has viewed all the plates. To record color vision results, use the plate identification number and the number given by the patient. If the patient is unable to identify a number, the mark "X" should be recorded to indicate that the patient could not read the plate. Examples:
Plate 5: 21. This means the patient read the number 21 on plate 5 (instead of 74).
Plate 6: X. This means the patient could not identify a number on plate 6.
Plate 11: Traceable. This means that the patient correctly traced a winding line on plate 11.
As you can see from the results of this patient's color vision test, the patient correctly identified all 11 plates, which indicates normal color vision. Because the patient has normal color vision, the medical assistant did not need to include plates 12, 13, and 14 in the color vision test.
Principle. Reading 10 or more plates correctly indicates normal color vision. If 7 or fewer of the plates are read correctly, the patient is identified as having a color vision deficiency.

7. **Procedural Step.** Complete the charting entry. Include the date and time, the name of the test (Ishihara test), and any unusual symptoms the patient exhibited during the test, such as squinting or rubbing the eyes.

7
CHARTING EXAMPLE

Plate No.	Normal Person	Results
1	12	12
2	8	8
3	5	5
4	29	29
5	74	74
6	7	7
7	45	45
8	2	2
9	X	X
10	16	16
11	Traceable	Traceable
11/6/12	10:00 a.m.	
	C. Lindner, CMA (AAMA)	

8. **Procedural Step.** Return the Ishihara book to its proper place. The book of color plates must be stored in a closed position to protect it from light.
Principle. Exposing the plates to excessive and unnecessary light results in fading of the color.

EYE IRRIGATION

An eye irrigation involves washing the eye with a flowing solution. Eye irrigations are performed for the following purposes: to cleanse the eye by washing away foreign particles, ocular discharges, or harmful chemicals; to relieve inflammation through the application of heat; and to apply an antiseptic solution. Procedure 6-3 shows how to perform an eye irrigation.

EYE INSTILLATION

An eye instillation involves the dropping of a liquid into the lower conjunctival sac of the eye. Eye instillations are performed to treat eye infections (with medication), to soothe an irritated eye, to dilate the pupil, and to anesthetize the eye during an eye examination or treatment. Medication to be instilled in the eye may come in the form of a liquid, as

What Would You Do? What Would You *Not* Do?

Case Study 2
Peter Mitchell comes in with his 5-year-old son, Clive. Clive is diagnosed with conjunctivitis ("pink eye"), and the physician prescribes Polytrim ophthalmic suspension. Mr. Mitchell says that Clive does not cooperate very well when having drops put in his eyes and asks for any ideas that might make it less of an ordeal. Mr. Mitchell has 7-year-old twin girls at home and wants to know what can be done so they don't get pink eye. He asks if it would be all right to instill the drops in the twins' eyes as a preventive measure. ■

ophthalmic drops, or as an ophthalmic ointment. Eye drops are usually dispensed in a flexible plastic container with an attached dropper. Eye ointment is dispensed in a small metal tube with a small tip for applying the medication. Procedure 6-4 shows how to perform an eye instillation.

PATIENT TEACHING Conjunctivitis

Answer questions that patients have about conjunctivitis.

What is conjunctivitis?

Conjunctivitis, often referred to as *pink eye,* is an inflammation of the conjunctiva (see illustration). The conjunctiva is a thin transparent membrane that covers the white of the eye. Conjunctivitis occurs when the conjunctiva becomes infected with a bacterium or virus. Other causes of conjunctivitis include allergies, prolonged wearing of contact lenses, and irritation from wind, dust, and smoke. Conjunctivitis is almost always harmless and clears up by itself within 2 weeks. If it is caused by a bacterium, the physician may prescribe antibiotic eye drops or ointment.

What are the symptoms of conjunctivitis?

Most types of conjunctivitis are relatively painless. The eye is red or pink because of irritation, and there is a feeling of sandiness or grittiness in the eye. A discharge is usually present, which dries at night when the eyes are closed. This may cause the eyelids to be stuck together in the morning. Other symptoms include tearing, itching, and sensitivity to light.

Is conjunctivitis contagious?

Conjunctivitis caused by a virus or bacterium is highly contagious. It can be spread easily from one eye to another and throughout a family or classroom in a matter of days.

How can we avoid spreading conjunctivitis?

The following measures help prevent the spread of conjunctivitis:
- Avoid touching or rubbing the infected eye, which can spread the infection to the other eye or to other people.

- Sanitize your hands frequently with soap, particularly after touching the eyes or face.
- Do not share washcloths, towels, or pillows with anyone.
- Do not wear contact lenses or eye makeup until the conjunctivitis is completely gone.
- Discard eye makeup that was used while you were infected to prevent reinfection.
- Encourage the patient to practice techniques that prevent the spread of conjunctivitis.
- If the physician has prescribed eye medication, teach the patient (or parent) the proper procedure for performing an eye instillation.
- Give the patient educational materials on conjunctivitis.

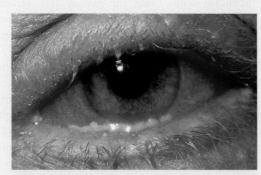

Bacterial conjunctivitis. (From Cuppett M, Walsh KM: General medical conditions in the athlete, St Louis, 2005, Mosby.)

 PROCEDURE 6-3 Performing an Eye Irrigation

Outcome Perform an eye irrigation.

Equipment/Supplies

- Disposable gloves (nonpowdered)
- Irrigating solution
- Solution basin
- Bath thermometer
- Disposable rubber bulb syringe
- Basin
- Moisture-resistant towel
- Gauze pads

1. **Procedural Step.** Sanitize your hands.
2. **Procedural Step.** Assemble the equipment. If both eyes are to be irrigated, two sets of equipment must be used to prevent cross-infection from one eye to the other. Normal saline is generally used to irrigate the eye. Perform the following:
   a. Carefully check the label of the irrigating solution three times to make sure you have the correct solution. The first time is after you remove the solution container from the shelf. Compare the label of the solution container with the physician's instructions.

   b. Check the expiration date of the solution.
   c. Warm the irrigating solution to body temperature (98.6° F [37° C]) by placing the solution container in a basin of warm water. Use a bath thermometer to make sure the temperature of the water used to warm the solution does not exceed body temperature.
   d. Check the solution label a second time before pouring the solution.
   e. Pour the solution as follows:
   Palm the label of the container and remove the cap. Place the cap on a flat surface with the open end

Continued

PROCEDURE 6-3   Performing an Eye Irrigation—cont'd

up. Pour the solution into the basin and replace the cap without contaminating it. Cover the basin to keep the solution warm.

f. Check the solution label a third time before returning the container to its storage area.

Principle. The solution label should be carefully checked three times to prevent an error. Outdated solutions may produce undesirable effects and should be discarded. If the solution is too cold or too warm, it will be uncomfortable for the patient. Palming the label prevents solution from dripping on the label and obscuring it or loosening the label. Placing the cap open end up prevents contamination.

3. **Procedural Step.** Greet the patient and introduce yourself. Identify the patient and explain the procedure and the irrigation. If the patient wears glasses or contact lenses, ask him or her to remove them.

4. **Procedural Step.** Position the patient. The patient may be placed in a sitting or lying position. Place a moisture-resistant towel on the patient's shoulder to protect the patient's clothing. Position a basin tightly against the patient's cheek under the affected eye to catch the irrigating solution, and ask the patient to hold it in place. Ask the patient to tilt the head in the direction of the affected eye.

Principle. The patient is positioned so that the solution flows away from the unaffected eye to prevent cross-infection.

5. Procedural Step. Apply nonpowdered gloves. Cleanse the eyelids from inner to outer canthus with a moistened gauze pad to remove any discharge or debris on the lids. The inner canthus is the inner junction of the eyelids next to the nose. The outer canthus is the junction of the eyelids farthest from the nose. Normal saline or the solution ordered for the irrigation may be used. Discard the gauze pad after each wipe.

Principle. Nonpowdered gloves avoid irritation of the patient's eye with powder that may have gotten on the outside of the glove. The eyelids should be clean to prevent foreign particles from entering the eye dur-

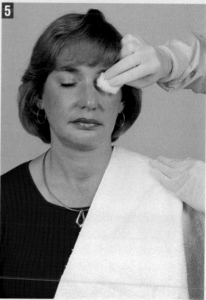

Cleanse the eyelids from inner to outer canthus.

ing the irrigation. Cleansing from inner to outer canthus prevents cross-infection.

6. **Procedural Step.** Fill the irrigating syringe with the solution by squeezing the bulb and slowly releasing it until the desired amount of solution enters the bulb. Instruct the patient to keep both eyes open and to find a focal point in the room and focus on it.

Principle. Looking at a focal point helps the patient keep the irrigated eye open during the procedure.

7. Procedural Step. Separate the eyelids with the index finger and thumb to expose the lower conjunctiva and to hold the upper eyelid open.

Principle. The medical assistant must hold the eye open during the procedure because the patient has a tendency to close it.

8. **Procedural Step.** Hold the tip of the syringe approximately 1 inch above the eye. Gently release the solution onto the eye at the inner canthus. This allows the solution to flow over the eye at a moderate rate from the inner to the outer canthus. Direct the solution to the lower conjunctiva. To prevent injury, do not allow the tip of the syringe to touch the eye.

Principle. The solution flows away from the unaffected eye to prevent cross-infection. The cornea is sensitive and can be harmed easily. The irrigating solution must be directed to the lower conjunctiva to prevent injury to the cornea.

9. **Procedural Step.** Refill the syringe, and continue irrigating until the desired results have been obtained or all the solution is used, depending on the purpose of the irrigation.

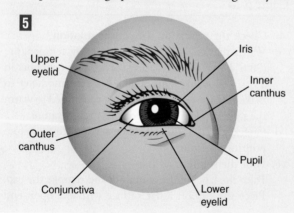

5

Upper eyelid

Outer canthus

Conjunctiva

Iris

Inner canthus

Pupil

Lower eyelid

PROCEDURE 6-3 Performing an Eye Irrigation—cont'd

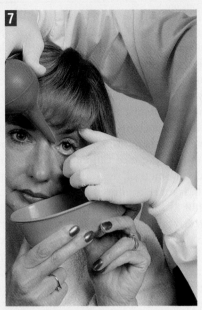

Separate the eyelids, and hold the tip of the syringe 1 inch above the eye.

10. Procedural Step. Dry the eyelids from inner to outer canthus with a gauze pad.

11. Procedural Step. Remove the gloves, and sanitize your hands.

12. Procedural Step. Chart the procedure. Include the following: the date and time; which eye was irrigated; the type, strength, and amount of solution used; and any significant observations and patient reactions. Use one of these abbreviations to indicate which eye was irrigated:

OU—Both eyes
OD—Right eye
OS—Left eye

CHARTING EXAMPLE	
Date	
11/5/12	10:30 a.m. Irrigated OS c̄ sterile saline at
	98.6° F. No complaints of discomfort.
	——————— C. Lindner, CMA (AAMA)

13. Procedural Step. Remove reusable equipment to a work area for sanitization, sterilization, or disinfection as required by the medical office policy.

PROCEDURE 6-4

PROCEDURE 6-4 Performing an Eye Instillation

Outcome Perform an eye instillation.

Equipment/Supplies

- Disposable gloves (nonpowdered)
- Ophthalmic drops or ophthalmic ointment as ordered by the physician
- Tissues
- Gauze pads

1. Procedural Step. Sanitize your hands.

2. Procedural Step. Assemble the equipment, and perform the following:

  a. Check the drug label three times to make sure you have the correct medication. The first time should be when you remove the medication from the shelf. The medication label must bear the word *ophthalmic.*

  b. Check the medication label a second time against the physician's instructions. Also check the dosage ordered by the physician.

  c. Check the expiration date.

  d. Check the medication label a third time before the cap is removed to instill the medication.

Principle. The drug label should be carefully checked three times to prevent a medication error. Medication

not bearing the word *ophthalmic* must never be placed in the eye because it could injure the eye. An outdated medication may produce undesirable effects and should be discarded.

3. Procedural Step. Greet the patient and introduce yourself. Identify the patient and explain the procedure and the purpose of the instillation. If the patient wears glasses or contact lenses, ask him or her to remove them.

4. Procedural Step. Help the patient into a sitting or supine position.

5. Procedural Step. Apply nonpowdered gloves. Prepare the medication. **Eye drops:** If the medication requires mixing, shake the container well. Check the medication label for the third time, and remove the cap from the container. **Eye ointment:** Check the medication

Continued

PROCEDURE 6-4   *Performing an Eye Instillation—cont'd*

label for the third time, and remove the cap from the tip of the tube.

Principle. Nonpowdered gloves avoid irritation of the patient's eyes with powder that may have gotten on the outside of the gloves.

6. **Procedural Step.** Ask the patient to look up at the ceiling, and expose the lower conjunctival sac by using the fingers of the nondominant hand placed over a tissue. The fingers should be placed on the patient's cheekbone just below the eye, and the skin of the cheek should be drawn gently downward.

Principle. Looking up helps keep the patient from blinking when the drops are instilled.

7. **Procedural Step.** Insert the medication. **Eye drops:** Invert the container and hold the tip of the dropper approximately ½ inch above the eye sac. Do not allow the dropper to touch the eye or any other surface. Gently squeeze the container and place the correct number of eye drops in the center of the lower conjunctival sac. Never place the drops directly on the

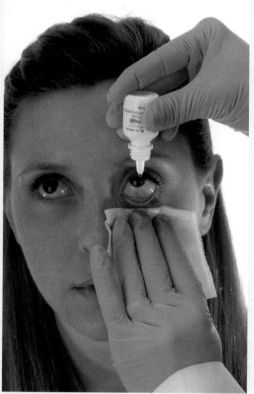

7

Ask the patient to look up, and insert the medication.

eyeball. Replace the cap on the container. **Eye ointment:** Gently squeeze the tube and place a thin ribbon of ointment along the length of the lower conjunctival sac from inner to outer canthus. Be careful not to touch the tip of the ointment tube to the eye or any other surface. Discontinue the ribbon by twisting the tube. Replace the cap on the tube.

Principle. Touching the dropper or tip of the tube to the eye (or other surfaces) could injure the eye and contaminate the medication. Placing the medication in the conjunctival sac, rather than directly on the eyeball, is more comfortable for the patient.

8. **Procedural Step.** Ask the patient to close his or her eyes gently and move the eyeballs. Instruct the patient not to shut the eyes tight or to blink and to keep the eyes closed for 1 to 2 minutes. Tell the patient that the instillation may blur the vision temporarily.

Principle. Moving the eyeballs helps distribute the medication over the entire eye. Keeping the eyes closed allows the medication to be absorbed. If the eyes are shut tightly or if the patient blinks, the drops or ointment may be pushed out of the eye.

9. **Procedural Step.** Dry the eyelid from inner to outer canthus with a gauze pad to remove excess medication.

10. **Procedural Step.** Remove the gloves, and sanitize your hands.

11. **Procedural Step.** Chart the procedure. The medication dosage for eye drops is recorded in the number of drops instilled. The abbreviation for drop is *gtt;* for drops, *gtts.* The number of drops must be recorded in Roman numerals (e.g., i, ii) following the *gtt* abbreviation. The recording should include the date and time, the name and strength of the medication, the number of drops or amount of ointment, which eye received the instillation, your observations, and the patient's reaction.

CHARTING EXAMPLE

Date	
11/5/12	2:30 p.m. Atropine sulfate 1%, gttsii OU.
	Pt states a temporary blurring of vision. ——
	——————————— C. Lindner, CMA (AAMA)

12. **Procedural Step.** Return the medication to its proper storage area.

THE EAR

STRUCTURE OF THE EAR

The ear functions in hearing and in maintaining equilibrium. It consists of three divisions: the *external ear,* the *middle ear,* and the *inner ear.* The structures in the ear are illustrated in Figure 6-8 and are described next.

The external ear is composed of the auricle (or pinna) and the external auditory canal, also known as the *external ear canal.* The opening into this canal is the *external auditory meatus.*

The *auricle* is a flap of cartilage covered with skin that projects from the side of the head. Its function is to receive and collect sound waves and to direct them toward the external auditory canal.

The *external auditory canal* is approximately 1 inch long in an adult and extends from the auricle to the tympanic membrane. It is lined with skin that contains fine hairs, nerve endings, and glands. The glands secrete earwax, or **cerumen,** which lubricates and protects the ear canal. The canal has an S-shaped curve as it leads inward. The canal must be straightened during examination with an otoscope, ear instillation or irrigation, or aural temperature measurement.

The **tympanic membrane** is at the end of the external auditory canal. It is a pearly gray, semitransparent membrane that receives sound waves.

The middle ear is an air-filled cavity that contains three small bones, or *ossicles:* the malleus, the incus, and the stapes. The *eustachian tube* connects the middle ear to the nasophar-

ynx. Air pressure between the external atmosphere and the middle ear is stabilized through the eustachian tube.

The inner ear contains the *cochlea,* which is the essential organ of hearing. The *semicircular canals* also are located in the inner ear and help to maintain equilibrium.

ASSESSMENT OF HEARING ACUITY

The assessment of hearing acuity is an integral part of a complete physical examination. It is possible for an individual to have hearing loss and not be aware of it. Early detection and treatment of hearing problems help prevent permanent hearing loss.

What Would You Do? *What Would You Not Do?*

Case Study 3

Willow Basil brings in her 6-year-old daughter, Jade. For the past 3 days, Jade has been running a fever and has had persistent pain and hearing loss in her left ear. Mrs. Basil practices alternative medicine and uses prescription medications as little as possible. She says that she has been trying herbal therapy and aromatherapy to make Jade better, but it does not seem to be helping. Jade is diagnosed with acute otitis media, and the physician prescribes amoxicillin for 10 days. Mrs. Basil wants to know if she has to give Jade the amoxicillin for the entire 10 days. She asks if she can stop using it when Jade starts feeling better. Mrs. Basil also wants to know if the ear infection will cause a permanent problem with Jade's hearing. ■

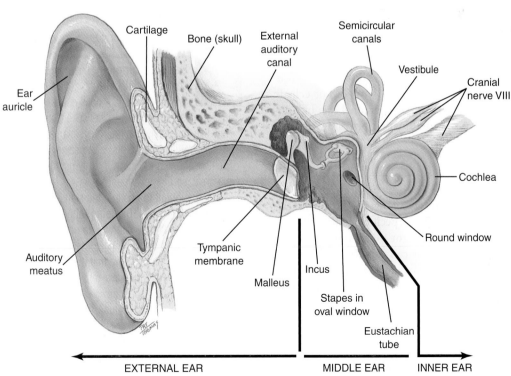

Figure 6-8. Structure of the ear. (From Applegate EJ: The anatomy and physiology learning system, ed 3, St Louis, 2006, Saunders.)

An individual with normal hearing should be able to hear the frequencies of normal speech, which range from 300 to 4000 Hz (hertz, or cycles per second) at a normal sound intensity. Patients who exhibit hearing loss are referred to an otolaryngologist or an audiologist for further evaluation.

Types of Hearing Loss

There are three types of hearing loss: conductive, sensorineural, and mixed. *Conductive hearing loss* results when there is a physical interference with the normal conduction of sound waves through the external and middle ear. Because of the interference, the amount of sound reaching the inner ear is less than normal, resulting in hearing impairment. Conductive loss in the external ear may be caused by an obstruction in the external ear canal, such as impacted cerumen, swelling from external otitis (swimmer's ear), foreign bodies, and benign growths such as polyps. Conductive loss in the middle ear may be caused by serous otitis media (fluid in the middle ear) or acute otitis media (infection in the middle ear), a perforated tympanic membrane, or otosclerosis. The cause of conductive hearing loss often can be detected by examining the external ear canal with an otoscope. Hearing is frequently restored by removing the obstruction (e.g., impacted cerumen) or treating the disorder (e.g., serous otitis media).

Sensorineural hearing loss results from damage to the inner ear or auditory nerve. With this type of hearing loss, sound is conducted normally through the outer and middle ear structures, but because of a problem with the perception of sound waves, a hearing deficit occurs. Specific causes of sensorineural loss include hereditary factors, degenerative changes from the normal aging process known as *presbycusis*, intense noise exposure over time, tumors, ototoxicity caused by certain medications, and infectious diseases, such as measles, mumps, and meningitis. The most common cause of sensorineural hearing loss in an adult is presbycusis. As an individual ages, nerves and sensory receptor cells in the inner ear deteriorate, leading to a gradual loss of hearing. *Mixed hearing loss* is a combination of conductive and sensorineural loss.

Hearing Acuity Tests

Numerous tests can be used to assess hearing acuity. Tests range from the simple gross screening test to qualitative tests using a tuning fork to highly specific quantitative tests using an audiometer. It is important to test only one ear at a time because a hearing deficit can exist in one ear only. The ear not being tested should be blocked by an earplug or masked. *Masking* involves the presentation of sound (usually noise) to the ear not being tested so that the patient's response is based only on hearing in the ear being tested.

Gross Screening Test

The gross hearing test is a simple and quick screening test used to identify a large hearing impairment. The physician performs the screening test during the physical examination. Hearing is assessed by asking the patient to repeat a simple word or series of numbers whispered from a distance of 1 to 2 feet from the ear. When a hearing loss is discovered, a tuning fork or audiometer is used for a more precise assessment of hearing.

Tuning Fork Tests

Tuning fork tests provide a general assessment of hearing acuity and may be part of the physical examination. A tuning fork with a frequency of 512 Hz or 1024 Hz is generally used because these frequencies fall within the range of normal speech. The Weber and Rinne tests are the tuning fork tests most commonly performed by the physician; they are used to identify conductive and sensorineural hearing loss.

The *Weber test* is a useful assessment of hearing loss when one ear hears better than the other. The tuning fork is set in vibration, and the base of the fork is placed on the center of the patient's head. The patient is asked to indicate where the sound is heard best. A patient with normal hearing would hear the sound equally in both ears or in the center of the head. Figure 6-9 illustrates the Weber test and describes the interpretation of results.

The *Rinne test* compares the duration of sound perception by air conduction with that of bone conduction. The tuning fork is set in vibration, and the base of the fork is placed against the bone of the mastoid process. The patient is instructed to indicate when the sound is no longer heard. The prongs of the fork (still vibrating) are placed in the air about 1 inch from the opening of the patient's ear canal, and the patient indicates when the sound is no longer heard. An individual with normal hearing is able to hear the sound at least twice as long through air conduction as

Memories *from* **Externship**

Cammie Lindner: There is one characteristic that is shared by all patients. I first noticed this during my externships, and it does not seem to matter what type of practice it is. Patients like to feel special and to be treated that way. They like consistency in their physician and in the office staff, and seeing familiar faces. This is especially hard during externship. The time spent is too short to truly get to know the patients, but it is a great learning experience.

It is important to observe the staff and patient communication and interaction skills. By doing this, you can decide which ones you admire and those that you do not wish to copy. The following are just a few of the guidelines that have helped me: (1) Call patients by name, and be sure that they know your name. (2) Follow through with what you have told patients you will do, and keep them updated if circumstances change. (3) Smile, and do not let one patient's negative attitude interfere with your care of others. (4) Take time to listen.

When you do begin your career, it does not take long to get into a routine and to start knowing your patients. When patients see a familiar face, they are more willing to share information that can contribute to improved communication and good health care. ∎

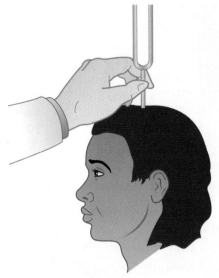

Normal Hearing
The patient hears the sound equally
in both ears or in the center of the head.

Conductive Hearing Loss
The patient hears the sound better in
the problem ear.

Sensorineural Hearing Loss
The patient does not hear the sound as
well in the problem ear.

Figure 6-9. Weber test.

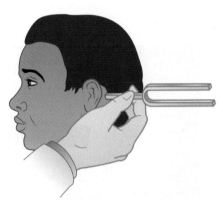

Bone conduction

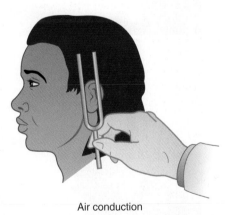

Normal Hearing
The patient hears the sound at least
twice as long through air conduction as
through bone conduction.

Conductive Hearing Loss
The patient hears the sound longer by
bone conduction than by air conduction.

Sensorineural Hearing Loss
The sound is reduced. The patient will
also hear the sound longer through air
conduction than through bone
conduction but not twice as long.

Air conduction

Figure 6-10. Rinne test.

through bone conduction. Figure 6-10 illustrates the Rinne test and describes the interpretation of results.

Audiometry

Audiometry is the measurement of hearing acuity using a special instrument called an **audiometer.** An audiometer quantitatively measures hearing for the various frequencies of sound waves. Audiometry is a more specific hearing acuity test because it provides information on how extensive a hearing loss is and which frequencies are involved. It is important that the test be conducted in a quiet room because outside noise may affect the results, especially in the lower frequencies. The patient wears headphones placed snugly over the ears (Figure 6-11). The audiometer delivers

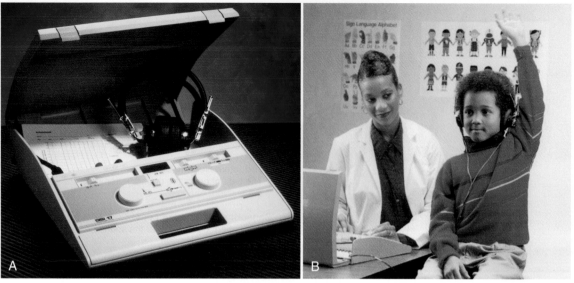

Figure 6-11. **A,** Audiometer. **B,** The patient signals when he hears a sound. (Courtesy GSI [Grayson-Stadler], Milford, NH.)

a single frequency at a time at specific intensities, starting with low-frequency tones of 250 to 500 Hz and going to very high frequencies of 6000 to 8000 Hz. The patient is asked to signal when he or she hears a sound so that the patient's hearing threshold for each frequency can be determined. The hearing acuity in each ear is assessed separately, and the results are plotted on a graph known as an *audiogram*. The medical assistant may be responsible for performing audiometry in the medical office. Before operating an audiometer, however, the medical assistant must receive extensive on-site training by an audiologist to ensure that proper technique is used to conduct the test.

Tympanometry

Tympanometry is not a hearing test, but it does help determine the cause of hearing loss, so it is presented in this section. The tympanometer consists of an earpiece attached to an electronic device (Figure 6-12). The earpiece is placed snugly in the patient's ear, and low-frequency sound waves are directed against the eardrum while pressure is applied in the ear canal. With a normal ear, the eardrum exhibits mobility in response to the pressure, as indicated on a graphic readout known as a *tympanogram*. If there is fluid in the middle ear, the eardrum does not move but remains stiff, as indicated on the tympanogram. Tympanometry is useful in diagnosing serous otitis media (fluid in the middle ear), which is a common cause of temporary hearing loss in children.

EAR IRRIGATION

Ear irrigation is the washing of the external auditory canal with a flowing solution. Ear irrigations are performed for the following purposes: to cleanse the external auditory ca-

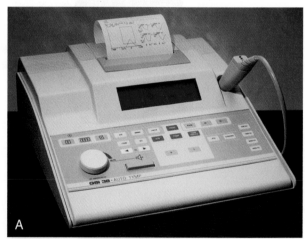

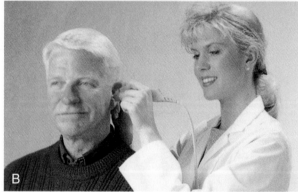

Figure 6-12. **A,** Tympanometer. **B,** The earpiece is placed snugly in the patient's ear. (Courtesy GSI [Grayson-Stadler], Milford, NH.)

PATIENT TEACHING Acute Otitis Media

Answer questions patients have about otitis media.

What is a middle ear infection?
An infection of the middle ear is medically referred to as *acute otitis media*. It is an inflammation of the middle ear caused by an infection and can occur in one or both ears. It is common in young children 3 months to 3 years old, but is unusual in adults. A middle ear infection is not serious if treated promptly and effectively. If not treated, however, middle ear infections can lead to serious complications, such as acute mastoiditis, meningitis, and permanent hearing loss.

What causes a middle ear infection?
A middle ear infection is often due to an upper respiratory infection or allergy that causes the eustachian tube to swell and become blocked. The blockage causes fluid to build up in the middle ear. This fluid is an ideal place for bacteria to grow. If this occurs, the result is acute otitis media.

What are the symptoms of a middle ear infection?
The most common symptoms are intense pain, fever, and temporary hearing loss. Other symptoms may include dizziness, nausea and vomiting, and (if the eardrum ruptures) drainage from the ear.

How does the physician know whether a middle ear infection is present?
The physician examines the ears with an otoscope. If a middle ear infection is present, the eardrum is red and swollen (see illustration) as a result of irritation from the infection, and pus and mucus can be seen behind the eardrum.

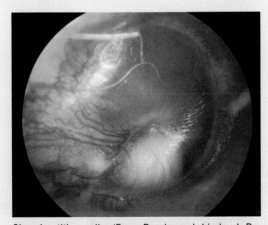

Chronic otitis media. (From Damjanov I, Linder J: Pathology: a color atlas, St Louis, 1999, Mosby.)

How is the infection treated?
A middle ear infection is usually treated with an oral antibiotic for 10 to 14 days. It is important to take all of the antibiotic prescribed; otherwise, the ear infection may recur. The physician also may recommend a decongestant to help open the blocked eustachian tube. After the acute infection is over, fluid may remain trapped in the middle ear. This condition is known as *serous otitis media* (see illustration) and, if not treated, may last for days, weeks, months, or even a year. Although fluid in the middle ear is painless, it may result in a feeling of fullness or pressure in the ears and temporary hearing loss.

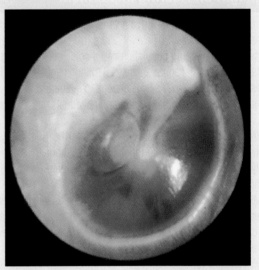

Serous otitis media. (From Swartz MH: Textbook of physical diagnosis, ed 5, Philadelphia, 2006, Saunders.)

Why are middle ear infections so common in children?
In children, the eustachian tube is positioned horizontally and is shorter and narrower than in adults. When a child has an upper respiratory infection, bacteria can travel easily to the middle ear. In addition, swelling from the respiratory infection can block this narrow tube, which causes fluid to build up in the middle ear.
- Encourage the patient to complete the entire prescribed course of antibiotics.
- If the physician has prescribed ear drops, teach the patient (or parent) the proper procedure for performing an ear instillation.
- Encourage early treatment of upper respiratory infections.
- Give the patient educational materials on otitis media.

nal to remove cerumen, discharge, or a foreign body; to relieve inflammation by applying an antiseptic solution; and to apply heat to the ear. Before irrigating, impacted cerumen must be softened by instilling warm mineral oil or hydrogen peroxide for 10 to 15 minutes. Procedure 6-5 shows how to perform an ear irrigation. An ear irrigation should not be performed if the tympanic membrane is perforated because this could result in severe irritation or infection of the middle ear.

EAR INSTILLATION

An ear instillation involves dropping a liquid into the external auditory canal. Ear instillations are performed to soften impacted cerumen, to combat infection with the use of antibiotic ear drops, and to relieve pain. The ear drops are usually dispensed in a flexible plastic container with an attached dropper. Procedure 6-6 shows how to perform an ear instillation.

Highlight on Hearing Impairment

The number of individuals with a hearing impairment has gradually increased over the past 20 years. Factors that contribute to this increase include an aging population and a noisier environment.

It is estimated that approximately 28 million people in the United States have a hearing loss severe enough to interfere with their daily activities, whereas another 2 million individuals are profoundly deaf.

Precise screening of preschool children for hearing loss is difficult. This is because tuning fork tests and audiometry require the ability to signal in response to sound, and children up to age 4 or 5 years have trouble mastering this skill.

Most state, county, and local school systems require hearing screening as a prerequisite for entrance to school and again at periodic intervals, usually during the first, third, fifth, and seventh grades.

Risk factors for hearing impairment in children include family history of deafness, premature birth, low birth weight, measles, mumps, high fevers, meningitis, recurrent or chronic ear infections, and the maternal rubella infection during pregnancy.

Signs of hearing impairment in children are poor attentiveness, delayed speech development, and persistent problems with articulation. Signs of hearing impairment in adults include frequent requests for words or statements to be repeated, leaning toward the speaker, turning the head, cupping the ears, and speaking in a loud or unvaried tone of voice.

The most common cause of conductive hearing loss in children is fluid in the middle ear, which prevents the tympanic membrane from vibrating freely. In adults, the most common cause of conductive loss is otosclerosis, a condition in which the stapes becomes fixed because of calcium deposits and less able to pass on vibrations when sound enters the ear.

The loudness of sound is measured in units called *decibels* (dB). Sounds of less than 75 dB, even after long exposure, are unlikely to cause hearing loss. Normal conversation is approximately 60 dB, and a whisper in a quiet library is 30 to 40 dB.

Permanent sensorineural hearing loss can result when the ear is repeatedly bombarded with loud sounds over time. Standards set by the Occupational Safety and Health Administration (OSHA) indicate that continued exposure to noise louder than 85 dB eventually harms an individual's hearing by damaging the tiny hair cells in the organ of Corti. The organ of Corti is a structure in the cochlea (inner ear) that converts sound waves into nerve impulses for transmission to the brain. This type of sensorineural hearing loss is known as *noise-induced hearing loss*. It is most often seen in individuals who frequently listen to loud music, fire guns without wearing ear protection, or are exposed to loud noise as part of their jobs. The following are examples of common noises and the decibel level of each:

Noise	Decibels
Normal breathing	10
Humming of a refrigerator	40
Television	70
Vacuum cleaner	60-85
Motorcycle	95-100
Personal stereo system with earphones (on high)	115
Rock concert	120
Chain saw	120
Auto stereo on high	125
Jet taking off	140
Firecracker	150
Firearms	140-170

Many hearing impairments can be helped with the use of a hearing aid. Individuals who benefit most from a hearing aid have mild to moderate conductive hearing loss. Individuals with sensorineural or mixed hearing loss have more trouble finding a suitable hearing aid and often get less satisfactory results. ∎

PROCEDURE 6-5   Performing an Ear Irrigation

Outcome Perform an ear irrigation.

Equipment/Supplies

- Disposable gloves
- Irrigating solution
- Solution basin
- Bath thermometer
- Irrigating syringe

- Ear basin
- Moisture-resistant towel
- Gauze pads
- Ear wick

1. Procedural Step. Sanitize your hands.

2. Procedural Step. Assemble the equipment. If both ears are to be irrigated, two sets of equipment must be used to prevent cross-infection from one ear to the other. Perform the following:

a. Carefully check the label of the irrigating solution three times to make sure you have the correct solution. The first time is after you remove the solution container from the shelf. Compare the label of the solution container with the physician's instructions.

b. Check the expiration date of the solution.

c. Warm the irrigating solution to body temperature (98.6° F [37° C]) by placing the solution container in a basin of warm water. Use a bath thermometer to make sure the temperature of the water used to warm the solution does not exceed body temperature.

d. Check the solution label a second time before pouring the solution.

e. Pour the solution as follows:
Palm the label of the container and remove the cap. Place the cap on a flat surface with the open end up. Pour the solution into the basin and replace the cap without contaminating it. Cover the basin to keep the solution warm.

f. Check the solution label a third time before returning the container to its storage area.

Principle. The solution label should be carefully checked three times to prevent an error. An outdated

solution may produce undesirable effects. If the solution is too cold or too warm, it might stimulate the inner ear and the patient may become dizzy. Palming the label prevents the solution from dripping on the label and obscuring it or loosening the label. Placing the cap open end up prevents contamination.

3. Procedural Step. Greet the patient and introduce yourself. Identify the patient and explain the procedure. Explain the purpose of performing the irrigation—for example, to remove cerumen. Tell the patient the procedure is not painful; however, he or she may feel a minimal amount of discomfort and occasional dizziness, fullness, and warmth as the ear solution comes in contact with the tympanic membrane.

4. Procedural Step. Position the patient in a sitting position. Place a moisture-resistant towel on the patient's shoulder under the ear to be irrigated to protect clothing and to prevent water from running down the neck. Position a basin tightly against the patient's neck under the affected ear to catch the irrigating solution, and ask the patient to hold it in place. Ask the patient to tilt the head in the direction of the affected ear.
Principle. The patient is positioned so that gravity aids the flow of the solution out of the ear and into the basin.

5. Procedural Step. Apply gloves. Cleanse the outer ear with a moistened gauze pad to remove any discharge or debris present. Normal saline or the solution ordered for the irrigation may be used.
Principle. The outer ear should be clean to prevent foreign particles from entering the ear canal during the irrigation.

6. Procedural Step. Fill the syringe with the irrigating solution (approximately 50 ml). Expel air from the syringe.
Principle. Air forced into the ear is uncomfortable for the patient.

7. Procedural Step. Straighten the external ear canal. The canal is straightened by gently pulling the ear upward and backward for adults and children older than 3 years old and downward and backward for children 3 years old and younger.
Principle. Straightening the canal permits the irrigating solution to reach all areas of the canal.

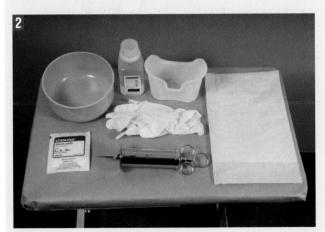

Assemble the equipment.

Continued

PROCEDURE 6-5   Performing an Ear Irrigation—cont'd

8. Procedural Step. Insert the syringe tip into the ear, but not too deeply. Make sure that the tip of the syringe does not obstruct the canal opening so that the solution can flow freely out of the canal.

Principle. Inserting the tip of the syringe too deeply causes discomfort for the patient.

Obstruction of the canal causes pressure to build up in the canal, resulting in patient discomfort and possible injury to the tympanic membrane.

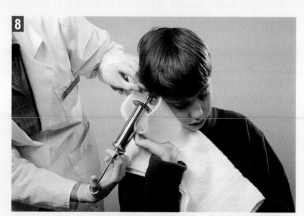

Inject the irrigating solution toward the roof of the ear canal.

9. Procedural Step. Inject the irrigating solution toward the roof of the ear canal. It is important that the solution be injected toward the roof of the canal to prevent it from being injected directly onto the tympanic membrane.

Principle. The tip of the syringe should be directed at the roof of the canal to prevent injury to the tympanic membrane and to aid in the removal of foreign particles by allowing the solution to flow down the length of the canal and out the bottom. In addition, severe patient discomfort and dizziness may occur if the solution is injected directly onto the tympanic membrane.

10. Procedural Step. Refill the syringe, and continue irrigating until the desired results have been obtained or all the solution is used, depending on the purpose of

the irrigation. Observe the returning solution to note the material present (e.g., cerumen, discharge, a foreign object) and the amount (small, moderate, or large).

11. Procedural Step. Dry the outside of the ear with a gauze pad. Have the patient lie on the affected side on the treatment table. Tell the patient that the ear will feel sensitive for a short time. Place a cotton wick loosely in the ear canal for 15 minutes if instructed to do so by the physician.

Principle. Any solution remaining in the ear canal should be allowed to drain out. A cotton wick makes the patient's ear feel less sensitive after the irrigation.

12. Procedural Step. Remove the gloves, and sanitize your hands.

13. Procedural Step. Chart the procedure. Include the following: the date and time; which ear was irrigated; the type, strength, and amount of solution used; the amount and type of material returned in the irrigating solution; any significant observations; and patient reactions. Use one of these abbreviations to indicate which ear was irrigated:

AU—Both ears
AD—Right ear
AS—Left ear

CHARTING EXAMPLE

Date	
11/15/12	2:15 p.m. Irrigated AD c̄ saline, 200 ml at 98.6° F. Mod amt of cerumen present in returned solution. Cotton wick placed in ear canal × 15 min. No complaints of discomfort.
	———————— C. Lindner, CMA (AAMA)

14. Procedural Step. Remove reusable equipment to a work area for sanitization, sterilization, or disinfection as required by the medical office policy.

PROCEDURE 6-6 **Performing an Ear Instillation**

Outcome Perform an ear instillation.

Equipment/Supplies

- Disposable gloves
- Otic drops
- Gauze pad

1. **Procedural Step.** Sanitize your hands.
2. **Procedural Step.** Assemble the equipment, and perform the following:
   a. Check the drug label three times to make sure you have the correct medication. The first time should be when you remove the medication from the shelf. The medication label must bear the word *otic*.
   b. Check the medication label a second time against the physician's instructions. Also check the dosage ordered by the physician.
   c. Check the expiration date.
   d. Check the medication label a third time before the cap is removed to instill the medication.
   Principle. The drug label should be carefully checked three times to prevent a medication error. Medication not bearing the word *otic* must never be placed in the ear because it could injure the ear. An outdated medication may produce undesirable effects and should be discarded.
3. **Procedural Step.** Greet the patient and introduce yourself. Identify the patient and explain the procedure and the purpose of the instillation.
4. **Procedural Step.** Position the patient in a sitting position.
5. **Procedural Step.** Warm the drops to body temperature by holding the medication container in the palms of your hands for a few minutes. Do not warm the drops by placing them in hot water.
   Principle. If the drops are too cold or too warm, they might stimulate the inner ear, causing the patient to become dizzy.
6. **Procedural Step.** Apply gloves. If the medication requires mixing, shake the container well. Check the medication label for the third time, and remove the cap from the container.
   Principle. Gravity aids in the flow of medication into the ear canal.
7. **Procedural Step.** Ask the patient to tilt his or her head in the direction of the unaffected ear. Straighten the external auditory canal. The canal is straightened by pulling the ear upward and backward for adults and children older than 3 years old and downward and backward for children 3 years old and younger.
   Principle. Straightening the canal permits the medication to reach all areas of the canal.

8. **Procedural Step.** Invert the container and place the tip of the dropper at the opening of the ear canal. Gently squeeze the container and instill the correct number of drops along the side of the canal. Replace the cap on the container.

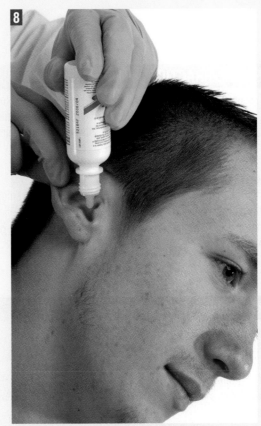

Instill the medication along the side of the ear canal.

9. **Procedural Step.** Instruct the patient to lie on the unaffected side for 2 to 3 minutes.
   Principle. Lying on the unaffected side prevents the medication from running out and allows complete distribution of the medication.
10. **Procedural Step.** Place a moistened cotton wick loosely in the ear canal for 15 minutes if instructed to do so by the physician.
    Principle. The cotton wick prevents the medication from running out when the patient is upright. Moist-

Continued

PROCEDURE 6-6

PROCEDURE 6-6   Performing an Ear Instillation—cont'd

ening the wick prevents the medication from being absorbed by the cotton.

11. Procedural Step. Remove the gloves, and sanitize your hands.

12. Procedural Step. Chart the procedure. Include the date and time, the name and strength of the medication, the number of drops, which ear received the instillation, any significant observations, and the patient's reaction.

13. Procedural Step. Return the medication to its storage area.

CHARTING EXAMPLE

Date	
11/20/12	9:30 a.m. Auralgan, gttsïï, AD. No discharge
	present. Pt states a relief of pain. ———
	————— C. Lindner, CMA (AAMA)

⊝volve *Check out the Evolve site to access additional interactive activities.*

MEDICAL PRACTICE *and the* LAW

Legal issues concerning eye and ear assessment are similar to the legal issues that concern any assessment. Accurate assessments done properly are necessary for accurate diagnoses and treatment and to prevent injuries to these structures.

Patient Rights

Patients entering the office have six major rights, which are enforceable by law, as follows:

1. The right to have the physician and medical assistant *do good for them.*

2. The right to *be treated fairly.*
3. The right to *be free.*
4. The right *not to be harmed.*
5. The right of fidelity, or *being true.*
6. The right to *life.*

If any of these rights is violated, the patient has the right to sue. ■

What Would You Do? What Would You *Not* Do? RESPONSES

Case Study 1
Page 220

What Did Cammie Do?

❑ Talked with Haley (on her level) about why someone needs to wear glasses.

❑ Retested Haley with the Snellen chart to see if she missed the same letters.

❑ Tested Haley with the Big E chart to give the physician an additional measurement to make an interpretation of Haley's visual acuity.

What Did Cammie Not *Do?*

❑ Did not tell Haley that she needs glasses.

❑ Did not scold Haley for trying to miss letters on the test.

What Would You Do/What Would You *Not* Do? Review Cammie's response and place a checkmark next to the information you included in your response. List the additional information you included in your response.

Case Study 2
Page 224

What Did Cammie Do?

❑ Gave Mr. Mitchell some suggestions on how to put drops in Clive's eyes so it is less scary. One idea is to have Clive lie down flat and close his eyes. Place the drops in the inner corner of his eye next to the bridge of his nose, letting them make a little lake there. When Clive relaxes and opens his eye, the drops will gently flow into his eye.

❑ Talked with Clive (on his level) about why he needs eye drops.

❑ Told Mr. Mitchell that the eye drops were prescribed for Clive, and they should be used only for Clive. Told him that if the twins developed conjunctivitis, he should call the office.

What Would You Do? What Would You *Not* Do? RESPONSES—cont'd

❑ Gave Mr. Mitchell suggestions for preventing the twins from getting conjunctivitis (not touching the infected eye, frequent handwashing, not sharing toys or towels).

What Did Cammie Not Do?

❑ Did not tell Mr. Mitchell to hold Clive down or force drops in his eyes.

❑ Did not tell Mr. Mitchell that he should know better than to think about giving the twins a medication not prescribed for them

What Would You Do/What Would You *Not* Do? Review Cammie's response and place a checkmark next to the information you included in your response. List the additional information you included in your response.

_____

_____

_____

_____

Case Study 3
Page 229

What Did Cammie Do?

❑ Explained to Mrs. Basil that Jade may begin to feel better after several days of antibiotics, but not all of the germs causing her

ear infection will have been killed by then. If she does not give Jade the full course of antibiotics, the infection could come back.

❑ Documented all the medications that Mrs. Basil has administered to Jade.

❑ Gave Mrs. Basil a patient information brochure on acute otitis media.

❑ Told Mrs. Basil that she needs to talk to the physician about her concern regarding hearing loss because he is most qualified to answer that question.

❑ Encouraged Mrs. Basil to bring Jade in sooner when she develops fever and ear pain.

What Did Cammie Not Do?

❑ Did not criticize Mrs. Basil for waiting so long to bring Jade in.

❑ Did not offer a personal opinion about alternative medicine.

What Would You Do/What Would You *Not* Do? Review Cammie's response and place a checkmark next to the information you included in your response. List the additional information you included in your response.

_____

_____

_____

_____

CERTIFICATION REVIEW

❑ **Visual acuity** refers to acuteness or sharpness of vision. A person with normal visual acuity can see clearly and is able to distinguish fine details close up and at some distance.

❑ **Errors of refraction** are the most common cause of defects in visual acuity. A nearsighted person has a condition termed *myopia* and has difficulty seeing objects at a distance. A farsighted person has a condition known as *hyperopia* and has difficulty viewing objects at a reading or working distance. *Astigmatism* causes distorted and blurred vision for both near and far objects due to a cornea that has an oval shape. *Presbyopia* is a decrease in the elasticity of the lens that occurs with aging; it results in a decreased ability to focus clearly on close objects.

❑ **A distance visual acuity test** assesses an individual's ability to see objects at a distance. The Snellen test is generally used in the medical office to screen for distance visual acuity. A reading of 20/20 indicates normal distance visual acuity.

❑ **Near visual acuity testing** assesses an individual's ability to read close objects. The test results are used to detect hyperopia and presbyopia. The results are recorded as the smallest type the patient can comfortably read.

❑ **Congenital color defects** are color vision deficiencies that are inherited and present at birth. Acquired defects are color vision deficiencies that are acquired after birth. Color vision tests, such as the Ishihara test, detect congenital color vision disturbances.

❑ **An eye irrigation** involves washing the eye with a flowing solution. Eye irrigations are performed to cleanse the eye of ocular discharges or harmful chemicals, to relieve inflammation through the application of heat, and to apply an antiseptic solution.

❑ **An eye instillation** involves the dropping of a liquid into the lower conjunctival sac of the eye. Eye instillations are performed to treat eye infections, to soothe an irritated eye, and to dilate the pupil or anesthetize the eye during an eye examination or treatment. Eye medications come in the form of ophthalmic drops and an ophthalmic ointment.

❑ **There are three types of hearing loss: conductive, sensorineural, and mixed.** A conductive loss results from interference with the conduction of sound waves through the external and middle ear. Sensorineural loss results from damage to the inner ear or auditory nerve. Mixed loss is a combination of conductive and sensorineural loss.

Continued

CERTIFICATION REVIEW—cont'd

❑ **Tests to assess** hearing acuity include gross screening, tuning fork, audiometric, and tympanometric tests. Of these, audiometry is the most specific hearing acuity test because it provides information on how extensive a patient's hearing loss is and which frequencies are involved.

❑ **An ear irrigation** is the washing of the external auditory canal with a flowing solution. Ear irrigations are performed to remove cerumen, discharge, or a foreign body; to relieve inflammation by applying an antiseptic solution; and to apply heat to the ear.

❑ **An ear instillation** involves the dropping of a liquid into the external auditory canal. Ear instillations are performed to soften impacted cerumen, to combat infection with the use of antibiotic drops, and to relieve pain.

TERMINOLOGY REVIEW

Medical Term	Word Parts	Definition
Astigmatism	*a-*: without *stigma/a*: point *-ism*: state of	A refractive error that causes distorted and blurred vision for both near and far objects due to a cornea that is oval shaped.
Audiometer	*audi/o*: hearing *-meter*: instrument used to measure	An instrument used to measure hearing acuity quantitatively for the various frequencies of sound waves.
Canthus		The junction of the eyelids at either corner of the eye.
Cerumen		Earwax.
Hyperopia	*hyper-*: above, excessive *-opia*: vision	Farsightedness.
Impacted		Wedged firmly together so as to be immovable.
Instillation		The dropping of a liquid into a body cavity.
Irrigation		The washing of a body canal with a flowing solution.
Myopia	*-opia*: vision	Nearsightedness.
Otoscope	*ot/o*: vision *-scope*: to view	An instrument used to examine the external ear canal and tympanic membrane.
Presbyopia	*-opia*: vision	A decrease in the elasticity of the lens that occurs with aging, resulting in a decreased ability to focus on close objects.
Refraction		The deflection or bending of light rays by a lens.
Tympanic membrane	*tympan/o*: eardrum *-ic*: pertaining to	A thin, semitransparent membrane between the external ear canal and the middle ear that receives and transmits sound waves. Also known as the *eardrum*.

ON THE WEB

For information on the eye:

American Optometric Association: www.aoa.org

American Academy of Ophthalmology: www.aao.org

National Eye Institute: www.nei.nih.gov

All About Vision: www.allaboutvision.com

Sight and Hearing Association: www.sightandhearing.org

American Academy of Optometry: www.aaopt.org

American Association for Pediatric Ophthalmology and Strabismus: www.aapos.org

The Eyes Have It: http://www.aboutcataractsurgery.com/

About Cataract Surgery: http://www.kellogg.umich.edu/theeyeshaveit/index.html

ON THE WEB—cont'd

For information on the ear:

American Academy of Audiology: www.audiology.org

National Institute on Deafness and Other Communication Disorders: www.nidcd.nih.gov

Healthy Hearing: www.healthyhearing.com

Hear It: www.hear-it.org

League for the Hard of Hearing: www.lhh.org

7

Physical Agents to Promote Tissue Healing

LEARNING OBJECTIVES	PROCEDURES

Local Application of Heat and Cold

1. State examples of moist and dry applications of heat and cold.
2. State the factors to consider when applying heat and cold.
3. List the effects of local application of heat, and state reasons for applying heat.
4. List the effects of local application of cold, and state reasons for applying cold.

Apply each of the following heat treatments:
- Heating pad
- Hot soak
- Hot compress
- Chemical hot pack

Apply each of the following cold treatments:
- Ice bag
- Cold compress
- Chemical cold pack

Casts

1. List reasons for applying a cast.
2. Identify the advantages and disadvantages of synthetic casts.
3. Explain the purpose of each step in the cast application procedure.

Assist with the application of a cast.
Assist with the removal of a cast.
Instruct a patient in proper cast care.

Splints and Braces

1. Describe a splint and explain its use.
2. Explain the purpose of a brace.

Apply a splint following the manufacturer's instructions.
Apply a brace following the manufacturer's instructions.

Ambulatory Aids

1. List factors that are taken into consideration when ambulatory aids are prescribed.
2. Explain the difference between an axillary crutch and a forearm crutch.
3. State conditions that may result when axillary crutches are not fitted properly.
4. List the guidelines that should be followed by the patient to ensure safe use of crutches.
5. State the use of each of the following crutch gaits: four-point gait, two-point gait, three-point gait, swing-to gait, and swing-through gait.
6. List and describe the three types of canes.
7. Identify the patient conditions that warrant the use of a cane or walker.

Measure a patient for axillary crutches.
Instruct a patient in the proper use of crutches.
Instruct a patient in the proper procedure for each of the following crutch gaits:
- Four-point
- Two-point
- Three-point
- Swing-to
- Swing-through

Instruct a patient in the use of a cane.
Instruct a patient in the proper use of a walker.

KEY TERMS

ambulation (AM-byoo-LAY-shun)
ambulatory
brace
compress (KOM-press)
edema (uh-DEE-muh)
erythema (err-uh-THEE-muh)
exudate (EKS-oo-date)
long arm cast
long leg cast

maceration (mass-er-AY-shun)
orthopedist (OR-thoe-PEE-dist)
short arm cast
short leg cast
soak
splint
sprain
strain
suppuration (SUP-er-AY-shun)

Introduction to Tissue Healing

Physical agents are often employed in the medical office to promote tissue healing for individuals who experience a disability as a result of injury, disease, or loss of a body part. Physical agents are used therapeutically to improve circulation, provide support, and promote the return of motion so that the individual can perform the activities of daily living. Physical agents frequently used in the medical office include heat and cold applied locally; casts; and ambulatory aids, such as crutches, canes, and walkers.

LOCAL APPLICATION OF HEAT AND COLD

The application of heat and cold is used therapeutically to treat conditions such as infection and trauma. The medical assistant may be responsible for applying various forms of heat and cold at the medical office or for instructing patients in the proper procedure for applying heat or cold at home. The medical assistant should have a basic understanding of the physiologic effects of heat and cold on the body and of possible adverse reactions if they are not administered correctly.

Heat and cold can be applied in moist or dry forms. Common applications of dry and moist heat and cold are as follows:

1. *Dry heat:* heating pad, chemical hot pack
2. *Moist heat:* hot soak, hot compress
3. *Dry cold:* ice bag, chemical cold pack
4. *Moist cold:* cold compress

Heat and cold are applied for short periods (generally 15 to 30 minutes) to produce the desired therapeutic results. The application may be repeated at time intervals specified by the physician. Prolonged application of heat or cold is not recommended because it can result in adverse secondary effects. The type of heat or cold application used for a particular condition depends on the purpose of the application, the location and condition of the affected area, and the age and general health of the patient. The physician instructs the medical assistant to apply a heat or cold treatment based on these factors.

Heat and cold receptors in the skin readily adapt to changes in temperature, eventually resulting in diminished heat or cold sensations. The temperature actually remains the same and is providing the intended therapeutic effects. The patient, not perceiving the same degree of temperature, may want to increase the intensity of the application, however, without realizing the inherent dangers. Excessive heat or cold could result in tissue damage. A common example of this situation is a patient who turns up the setting of a heating pad from medium to high when the heating pad no longer feels warm. The medical assistant should fully explain to the patient the necessity of maintaining a safe temperature range during the application.

Factors Affecting the Application of Heat and Cold

Before applying heat or cold, certain factors must be taken into consideration to prevent unfavorable reactions, such as tissue necrosis. The temperature may need to be adjusted based on the following conditions:

1. **The age of the patient.** Young children and elderly patients tend to be more sensitive to the application of heat or cold.

2. **Location of the application.** Certain areas of the body are more sensitive to the application of heat or cold, especially thin areas of the skin and areas that are usually covered by clothing, such as the chest, back, and abdomen. The skin on the hands and face is not as sensitive and is better able to tolerate temperature change. Broken skin, such as is found with an open wound, is more sensitive to heat and cold and is more prone to tissue damage.

3. **Impaired circulation.** Patients with impaired circulation tend to be more sensitive to heat and cold. This impairment may be at the site of the application or may be a systemic problem involving the entire body that is a result of certain conditions, such as peripheral vascular disease, diabetes mellitus, or congestive heart failure.

4. **Impaired sensation.** Patients with impaired sensation, such as diabetic patients, must be watched carefully because tissue damage may occur from the application of heat or cold without the patient's awareness.

5. **Individual tolerance to change in temperature.** Some individuals cannot tolerate temperature change as easily as others.

The medical assistant should observe the area to which the heat or cold has been applied before, during, and after treatment for signs indicating that a modification of temperature is needed. Prolonged erythema or paleness, pain, swelling, and blisters should be reported to the physician. The medical assistant also should ask the patient whether the application feels comfortable or is too hot or too cold.

Heat

Local Effects of Heat

The application of moderate heat to a localized area of the body for a short time (approximately 15 to 30 minutes) produces *dilation,* or an increase in diameter, of the blood vessels in the area as the body tries to rid itself of excess heat (Figure 7-1). This results in an increased blood supply to the area, and tissue metabolism increases. Nutrients and oxygen are provided to the cells at a faster rate, and wastes and toxins are carried away faster. The skin in the area becomes warm and exhibits erythema. **Erythema** is reddening of the skin caused by dilation of superficial blood vessels in the skin.

These physiologic effects of moderate heat applied to a localized area promote healing. Prolonged application of heat (longer than 1 hour) produces secondary effects, however, that reverse this healing process. Blood vessels constrict, and blood supply to the area decreases. The medical assistant must be careful to apply heat for the length of time specified by the physician.

Purpose of Applying Heat

Heat functions in relieving pain, congestion, muscle spasms, and inflammation. Conditions for which the local application of heat is often prescribed are low back pain, arthritis, menstrual cramping, and localized abscesses.

Heat promotes muscle relaxation and is often used for the relief of pain caused by excessive contraction of muscle fibers. **Edema,** or swelling, in the tissues can be reduced through the application of heat because the increased blood supply functions to increase the absorption of fluid from the tissues through the lymphatic system.

Heat, usually in the form of a hot **compress,** can be used to soften exudates. An **exudate** is a discharge produced by the body's tissues. Exudates may sometimes form a hard crust over an area and require removal. Heat also increases **suppuration,** or the process of pus formation, to help in the relief of inflammation by breaking down infected tissues. Heat is not recommended, however, for the initial treatment of acute inflammation or trauma.

Types of Heat Applications

The most common types of heat applications are described next, along with the conditions they are often used to treat.

Heating Pad

The electric heating pad consists of a network of wires that function to convert electric energy into heat to provide a constant and even heat application. The wires must not be bent or crushed. This could damage the pad, resulting in

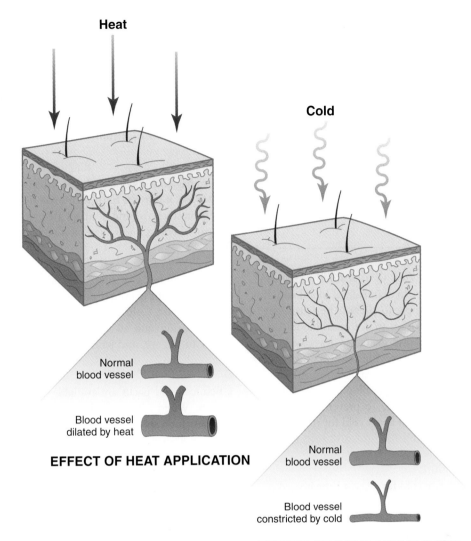

Figure 7-1. Effects of the local application of heat and cold. (From Wood LA, Rambo BJ: Nursing skills for allied health services, vol 2, Philadelphia, 1980, Saunders.)

overheating of parts of the pad and leading to burns or fire. Pins must not be inserted into the pad as a means of securing it; if a pin comes in contact with a wire, an electric shock could result. To prevent electric hazards, heating pads should not be used over areas that contain moisture, such as wet dressings. Heating pads are often used to relieve pain and muscle spasms.

Hot Soak

A **soak** is the direct immersion of a body part in water or a medicated solution. A soak can be applied to an extremity or a part of the torso. Hot soaks are used to cleanse open wounds, increase suppuration, increase the blood supply to an area to hasten the healing process, and apply a medicated solution to an area.

Hot Compress

A hot compress is a soft, moist, absorbent cloth, such as a washcloth, that is immersed in a warm solution and applied to a body part. Hot compresses are used to increase suppuration, to improve circulation to a body part to aid in healing, to promote drainage from infection, and to soften exudates. Applying a hot compress to an open wound requires the use of sterile technique.

Chemical Hot Pack

Chemical hot packs are available in a variety of sizes and shapes. When activated, they provide a specific degree of heat for a specific period of time (usually 30 to 60 minutes), as indicated on the package label. A chemical hot pack consists of a vinyl bag containing calcium chloride crystals and a smaller bag (encased in the vinyl bag) containing water. Pressure is applied with the hands to break the inner bag. The water in the inner bag combines with the calcium chloride crystals to produce heat. After using the pack, it should be discarded in an appropriate receptacle. Chemical hot packs should be stored at room temperature and are used as an alternative to a heating pad to relieve pain and muscle spasms.

Procedures 7-1, 7-2, 7-3, and 7-6 (see later) present the proper application of heat with a heating pad, a hot soak, a hot compress, and a chemical hot pack.

What Would You Do? What Would You *Not* Do?

Case Study 1

Aaron Collins is at the office. Aaron recently helped a friend move, and the next day he developed intense pain in his lower back. To alleviate the pain, he slept on a heating pad, but when he woke up, his back was red and blistered. Aaron says he turned the setting on the heating pad to high because his back was hurting so much and he thought that it would help his back feel better sooner. Aaron wants to know the best way to apply heat using a heating pad. He also wants to know what he can do to prevent low back pain in the future. ■

Cold

Local Effects of Cold

The application of moderate cold to a localized area produces *constriction,* or a decrease in diameter, of blood vessels in the area as the body attempts to prevent heat loss (see Figure 7-1). This constriction leads to decreased blood supply to the area. Tissue metabolism decreases, less oxygen is used, and fewer wastes accumulate. The skin becomes cool and pale. Prolonged application of cold (longer than 1 hour) has a reverse secondary effect. Blood vessels dilate, and tissue metabolism is increased. To prevent secondary effects, the medical assistant must apply cold for the recommended length of time only.

Purpose of Applying Cold

The application of moderate cold for a short time is used to prevent edema. Cold may be applied immediately after an individual has suffered direct trauma, such as a bruise, minor burn, **sprain, strain,** joint injury, or fracture. The cold limits the accumulation of fluid in the body tissues by constricting blood vessels and reducing the leakage of fluid into the tissues. Through constriction of peripheral blood vessels, cold can be used to control bleeding. Cold temporarily relieves pain through its anesthetic, or numbing, effect, which reduces stimulation of the pain receptors. Cold also slows the movement of blood and tissue fluids in the affected area, resulting in less pressure against pain receptors

and therefore less pain. In the early stages of an infection, the local application of cold inhibits the activity of microorganisms. In this way, suppuration is decreased and inflammation is reduced. Cold applications should always be placed in a protective covering because applying cold directly to the skin could result in a skin burn.

Types of Cold Applications

Ice Bag

An ice bag consists of a waterproof bag with a screw-on cap. Before use, it must be filled with small pieces of ice and placed in a protective covering. Ice bags are used to prevent swelling, control bleeding, and relieve pain and inflammation.

Cold Compress

A cold compress is a soft, moist, absorbent cloth, such as a washcloth, that is immersed in a cold solution and applied to a body part. Cold compresses are used to relieve pain and inflammation and to treat conditions such as headache, injury to the eye, and pain after tooth extraction.

Chemical Cold Pack

Chemical cold packs are available in a variety of sizes and shapes. When activated, they provide a specific degree of coldness for a specific period of time (usually 30 to 60 minutes), as indicated on the package label. Most cold packs consist of a vinyl bag of ammonium nitrate crystals. Enclosed in this bag is a smaller vinyl bag of water. The cold pack is activated by applying pressure until the inner bag ruptures. This releases the water into the larger bag, and a chemical reaction occurs between the crystals and the water, producing coldness. These packs are disposable, and when the coldness diminishes, they should be discarded in an appropriate receptacle. Chemical cold packs should be stored at room temperature. They are used as an alternative to ice bags for the local application of cold to prevent swelling, control bleeding, and relieve pain and inflammation.

Procedures 7-4, 7-5, and 7-6 present proper application of cold with an ice bag, a cold compress, and a chemical cold pack.

PROCEDURE 7-1   Applying a Heating Pad

Outcome Apply a heating pad.

Equipment/Supplies

- Heating pad with a protective covering

1. **Procedural Step.** Sanitize your hands.
2. **Procedural Step.** Assemble the equipment.
3. **Procedural Step.** Greet the patient and introduce yourself. Identify the patient and explain the procedure. Explain the purpose of the application (e.g., to relieve pain).

4. **Procedural Step.** Place the heating pad in the protective covering.
   Principle. The protective covering provides more comfort for the patient and absorbs perspiration.

PROCEDURE 7-1   Applying a Heating Pad—cont'd

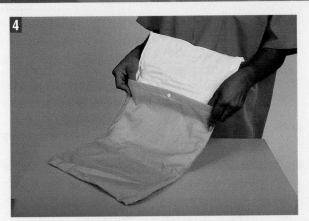

Place the heating pad in a protective covering.

5. **Procedural Step.** Connect the plug to an electric outlet. Set the selector switch at the proper setting, as designated by the physician (usually low or medium).

6. **Procedural Step.** Place the heating pad on the patient's affected body area. Ask the patient how the temperature feels. The heating pad should feel warm but not uncomfortable.

7. **Procedural Step.** Instruct the patient not to lie on the pad or turn the control higher to prevent burns. *Principle.* Lying on the pad causes heat to accumulate and burn the patient. The patient's heat receptors eventually become adjusted to the temperature change, resulting in a decreased heat sensation, and the patient may be tempted to increase the temperature. Turning

the control higher results in excessive heat on the patient's skin, which could burn the patient.

8. **Procedural Step.** Check the patient periodically for signs of an increase or decrease in redness or swelling, and ask the patient whether the site is painful. Administer the treatment for the proper length of time as designated by the physician.

9. **Procedural Step.** Sanitize your hands, and chart the procedure. Include the date and time, method of heat application (heating pad), temperature setting of the pad, location and duration of the application, appearance of the application site, and the patient's reaction. Also, chart any instructions provided to the patient on applying a heating pad at home.

10. **Procedural Step.** Properly care for equipment, and return it to its storage location.

CHARTING EXAMPLE

Date	
12/10/12	10:15 a.m. Heating pad on medium setting applied to lower back x 20 min. Area appears pink following application. Pt states a relief of pain and better mobility. Provided instructions on the application of a heating pad at home. ———— M. Cooper, CMA (AAMA)

PROCEDURE 7-2   Applying a Hot Soak

Outcome Apply a hot soak.

Equipment/Supplies

- Soaking solution ordered by the physician
- Bath thermometer
- Basin
- Bath towels

1. **Procedural Step.** Sanitize your hands.

2. **Procedural Step.** Assemble the equipment. Check the label on the solution container to make sure you have the correct solution as ordered by the physician. Place the solution containers in a basin of warm water. Warm the soaking solution to a temperature between 105° F and 110° F (41° C and 44° C).

3. **Procedural Step.** Greet the patient and introduce yourself. Identify the patient and explain the procedure. Explain the purpose of the application (e.g., to apply a medicated solution).

4. **Procedural Step.** Fill the basin one-third to two-thirds full with the warmed soaking solution.

5. **Procedural Step.** Check the temperature of the solution with a bath thermometer. The temperature for an adult should be 105° F to 110° F (41° C to 44° C).

6. **Procedural Step.** Assist the patient into a comfortable position to avoid fatigue and muscle strain. Pad the side of the basin with a towel for the patient's comfort.

Continued

PROCEDURE 7-2

PROCEDURE 7-2   Applying a Hot Soak—cont'd

7. Procedural Step. Slowly and gradually immerse the patient's affected body part in the solution. Ask the patient how the temperature feels.

Principle. The affected body part should gradually become accustomed to the change in temperature.

8. Procedural Step. Test the temperature of the solution frequently. To keep the solution at a constant temperature, remove cooler fluid every 5 minutes, and replace it with hot solution. Pour the hot solution in near the edge of the basin by placing your hand between the patient and the solution. Stir the solution as you pour.

Principle. The solution should be added away from the patient's body part to prevent splashing hot fluid

on the patient. Stirring in the solution helps distribute the heat and keep the temperature constant.

9. Procedural Step. Check the patient's skin periodically for signs of an increase or decrease in redness or swelling, and ask the patient whether the site is painful. Apply the hot soak for the proper length of time as designated by the physician (usually 15 to 20 minutes).

10. Procedural Step. Dry the affected part completely and gently.

11. Procedural Step. Sanitize your hands, and chart the procedure. Include the date and time, method of heat application (hot soak), name and strength of the solution, temperature of the soak, location and duration of the application, appearance of the application site, and the patient's reaction.

12. Procedural Step. Properly care for equipment, and return it to its storage location.

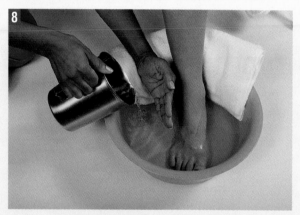

Replace cooler solution with hot solution.

CHARTING EXAMPLE

Date	
12/12/12	1:15 p.m. Normal saline hot soak at 105° F applied to Ⓡ ankle x 20 min. Area appears pink following application. Pt states less stiffness in ankle. ——————————
	———————— M. Cooper, CMA (AAMA)

PROCEDURE 7-3   Applying a Hot Compress

Outcome Apply a hot compress.

Equipment/Supplies

- Solution ordered by the physician
- Bath thermometer
- Basin

- Washcloths
- Waterproof covering
- Towel

1. Procedural Step. Sanitize your hands.

2. Procedural Step. Assemble the equipment. Check the label on the solution container to make sure you have the correct solution as ordered by the physician. Place the solution containers in a basin of warm water. Warm the soaking solution to a temperature between 105° F and 110° F (41° C and 44° C).

3. Procedural Step. Greet the patient and introduce yourself. Identify the patient and explain the procedure. Explain the purpose of the application (e.g., to soften an exudate).

4. Procedural Step. Fill the basin half full with warmed solution. Check the temperature of the solution with the bath thermometer. The temperature for an adult should be 105° F to 110° F (41° C to 44° C).

5. Procedural Step. Completely immerse the compress in the solution. Wring the compress to remove excess moisture. The compress should be wet but not dripping. Apply it lightly at first to the affected site to allow the patient to become used to the heat gradually. You may want to cover the compress with a waterproof cover to help hold in the heat. Ask the patient

PROCEDURE 7-3   Applying a Hot Compress—cont'd

how the temperature feels. The compress should be as hot as the patient can comfortably tolerate.

Principle. The waterproof cover prevents cool air currents from coming into contact with the compress and reduces the number of times the compress needs to be changed.

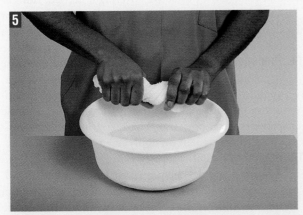

Wring out the compress.

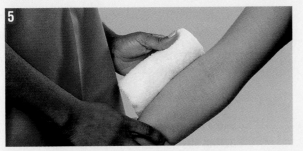

Apply the compress to the affected site.

6. Procedural Step. Place additional compresses in the solution so that they are ready for use.

7. Procedural Step. Repeat the application of the compress every 2 to 3 minutes for the duration of time specified by the physician (usually 15 to 20 minutes). Check the patient's skin periodically for signs of an increase or decrease in redness or swelling, and ask the patient whether the site is painful.

8. Procedural Step. Check the temperature of the solution periodically. Remove cooler fluid and replace it with hot solution if needed. Administer the treatment for the proper length of time as designated by the physician.

9. Procedural Step. Dry the affected part thoroughly and gently.

10. Procedural Step. Sanitize your hands, and chart the procedure. Include the date and time, method of heat application (hot compress), name and strength of the solution, temperature of the solution, location and duration of the application, appearance of the application site, and the patient's reaction.

11. Procedural Step. Properly care for equipment, and return it to its storage location.

CHARTING EXAMPLE

Date	
12/20/12	10:30 a.m. Normal saline hot compress at 110° F applied to ℝ forearm x 20 min.
	No complaints of discomfort. ————
	———————— M. Cooper, CMA (AAMA)

PROCEDURE 7-4   Applying an Ice Bag

Outcome Apply an ice bag.

Equipment/Supplies

- Ice bag with a protective covering
- Small pieces of ice (ice chips or crushed ice)

1. Procedural Step. Sanitize your hands.

2. Procedural Step. Assemble the equipment.

3. Procedural Step. Greet the patient and introduce yourself. Identify the patient and explain the procedure. Explain the purpose of applying the ice bag (e.g., to prevent swelling).

4. Procedural Step. Check the ice bag for leakage.

Principle. A leaking bag would get the patient wet and cause chilling.

5. Procedural Step. Fill the bag one-half to two-thirds full with small pieces of ice.

Continued

PROCEDURE 7-4   Applying an Ice Bag—cont'd

Principle. Small pieces of ice work better than large pieces because they reduce the air spaces in the bag, resulting in better conduction of cold. In addition, small pieces of ice allow the bag to mold better to the body area.

6. Procedural Step. Expel air from the bag by squeezing the empty top half of the bag together and screwing on the stopper.

Principle. Air is a poor conductor of cold and makes it difficult to mold the ice bag to the body area.

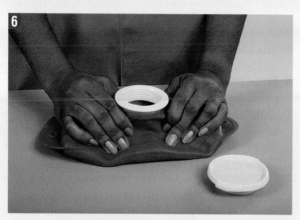

Expel air from the bag.

7. Procedural Step. Place the bag in the protective covering.

Principle. The protective covering provides for patient comfort and absorbs the moisture that condenses on the outside of the bag.

8. Procedural Step. Place the bag on the patient's affected body area. Ask the patient how the temperature feels. The application of ice is usually uncomfortable, but most patients tolerate it when they know how much benefit may be derived from it.

Principle. Individuals vary in their ability to tolerate cold.

9. Procedural Step. Check the patient's skin periodically for signs of an increase or decrease in redness or swelling, and ask the patient whether the site is painful. If extreme paleness and numbness or a mottled blue appearance occur at the application site, remove the bag, and notify the physician.

10. Procedural Step. Refill the bag with ice as necessary, and change the protective covering if needed. Administer the treatment for the proper length of time, as designated by the physician (usually until the area feels numb, approximately 15 to 30 minutes).

11. Procedural Step. Sanitize your hands, and chart the procedure. Include the date and time, method of cold application (ice bag), location and duration of the application, appearance of the application site, and the patient's reaction. Also, chart any instructions provided to the patient on applying an ice bag at home.

12. Procedural Step. Properly care for the ice bag. Dispose of or launder the protective covering as required. Cleanse the ice bag with a warm detergent solution, rinse thoroughly, and dry by hanging the bag upside down with the top removed. Store the bag by screwing on the stopper, leaving air inside to prevent the sides from sticking together.

CHARTING EXAMPLE

Date	
12/22/12	11:30 a.m. Ice bag applied to Ⓡ knee x 20 min. Pt complained of slight discomfort during the application. Area appears less swollen following application. Provided instructions on the application of an ice bag at home.———M. Cooper, CMA (AAMA)

PROCEDURE 7-5   Applying a Cold Compress

Outcome Apply a cold compress.

Equipment/Supplies

- Ice cubes
- Basin
- Washcloths

- Towel
- Ice bag

1. Procedural Step. Sanitize your hands.

2. Procedural Step. Assemble the equipment. Check the label on the solution container to make sure you have the correct solution as ordered by the physician.

3. Procedural Step. Greet the patient and introduce yourself. Identify the patient and explain the procedure. Explain the purpose of the application (e.g., to treat an eye injury).

PROCEDURE 7-5   Applying a Cold Compress—cont'd

4. Procedural Step. Place large ice cubes in the basin. Add the solution until the basin is half full.
Principle. Using larger pieces of ice prevents them from sticking to the compress and slows the rate at which they melt in the solution.

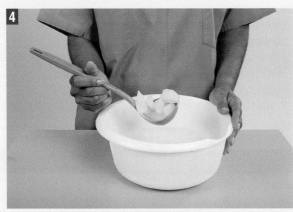

Place large ice cubes in the basin.

5. Procedural Step. Completely immerse the compress in the solution. Wring the compress to rid it of excess moisture. The compress should be wet but not dripping. Apply it lightly at first to the affected site to allow the patient to become used to the cold gradually. The compress can be covered with an ice bag to help keep it cold and to reduce the number of times it needs to be changed. Ask the patient how the temperature feels.

6. Procedural Step. Place additional compresses in the solution to be ready for use.

7. Procedural Step. Repeat the application of the compress every 2 to 3 minutes for the duration of time specified by the physician (usually 15 to 20 minutes). Check the patient's skin periodically for signs of an increase or decrease in redness or swelling, and ask the patient whether the site is painful.

8. Procedural Step. Add ice if needed to keep the solution cold. Administer the treatment for the proper length of time designated by the physician.

9. Procedural Step. Thoroughly dry the affected part.

10. Procedural Step. Sanitize your hands, and chart the procedure. Include the date and time, method of cold application (cold compress), location and duration of the application, appearance of the application site, and the patient's reaction.

11. Procedural Step. Properly care for equipment, and return it to its storage location.

CHARTING EXAMPLE

Date	
12/27/12	9:15 a.m. Normal saline cold compress applied to bridge of nose x 15 min. Nose appears less swollen following application. Tolerated application well ———— M. Cooper, CMA (AAMA)

PROCEDURE 7-6   Applying a Chemical Pack

Outcome Apply a chemical cold pack and a chemical hot pack.
The procedure for applying a chemical cold or hot pack is as follows:

1. Procedural Step. Shake the crystals to the bottom of the bag.

2. Procedural Step. Squeeze the bag firmly with your hands to break the inner water bag.

3. Procedural Step. Shake the bag vigorously to mix the contents.

4. Procedural Step. Cover the bag with a protective covering.

5. Procedural Step. Apply the bag to the affected area. Check the patient's skin periodically.

6. Procedural Step. Administer the treatment for the proper length of time.

7. Procedural Step. Discard the bag in an appropriate receptacle.

8. Procedural Step. Sanitize your hands, and chart the procedure. Include the date and time, method of application (chemical cold or hot pack), location and

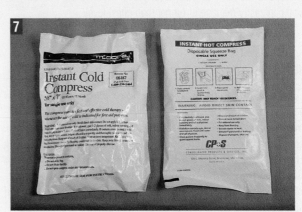

Chemical packs.

duration of the application, appearance of the application site, and the patient's reaction.

PATIENT TEACHING   Low Back Pain

Answer questions patients have about low back pain.

What causes low back pain?
Low back pain is one of the most common health problems in the United States. Approximately 80% of Americans are affected by low back pain at some time during their life. The most frequent cause of low back pain is poor posture and poor body mechanics, which strain the muscles and ligaments that support the back. Other causes include physical inactivity, excessive body weight, disc damage, osteoarthritis, spondylitis, and congenital deformities.

How might the physician treat low back pain?
To treat low back pain caused by strain, the physician might prescribe bed rest, local application of heat or cold, massage, medica-tions, back manipulation, use of back-supporting devices, deep-heating treatments such as ultrasound, and exercises to strengthen the supporting structures of the back and prevent the back pain from recurring or becoming chronic.

What can be done to prevent low back pain?
Most cases of low back pain can be prevented by practicing good body mechanics.
- Encourage patients to maintain correct posture while sitting, standing, and sleeping.
- Encourage patients to follow practices that prevent strain to the lower back, such as using correct lifting techniques.
- Encourage patients to maintain a healthy body weight.
- Provide the patient with educational materials on low back pain.

PATIENT TEACHING   Body Mechanics

Teach patients the essentials of good body mechanics as follows.

Standing and Walking
Wear comfortable low-heeled shoes that offer good support. Hold the head erect at the midline of the body, with the back as straight as possible and the pelvis tucked inward, the chest forward with the shoulders back, and the abdomen drawn in and kept flat. This helps to maintain appropriate alignment of the vertebral column.

Lifting
Determine the weight of the object first to determine if you can safely lift it. Pushing the object with one foot can help you determine if you can lift it without assistance. Never lift anything heavier than you can easily manage. Stand in front of the object and balance yourself with the feet about 6 to 8 inches apart, toes pointed outward, and one foot slightly forward to provide a wide base of support. Tighten the stomach and gluteal muscles in preparation for lifting the object. To lift an object, always bend the body at the knees and hips. Never bend from the waist. Lift the object with the leg muscles, and hold it close to the body at waist level. Never lift anything heavier than you can easily manage or higher than chest level.

Sitting
Sit in a chair with a firm back. Sit firmly with the back and buttocks supported against the back of the chair; avoid slumping. The body weight should be evenly distributed over the buttocks and thighs. Use a small pillow or a rolled towel to support the lower back. The feet should be flat on the floor, and the knees should be level with the hips. If you need to sit for a prolonged period of time, use a footstool to raise one knee to reduce strain on the back. Take frequent stretch breaks.

Driving
Ensure that the car seat is not too far back. Stretching for the pedals strains the back. The car seat should be positioned so that the driver's back is straight and the knees are raised.

Sleeping
Sleep on a firm, comfortable mattress that supports the back and does not allow it to sag. Sleep on your side with knees bent or on your back with a pillow under the knees. Do not sleep on your stomach because this causes the body to sag into the mattress, which results in strain to the back, neck, and shoulders. ■

CASTS

A cast is a stiff cylindrical synthetic or plaster casing that is used to immobilize a body part. Casts are applied most often when an individual sustains a fracture (Figure 7-2). The cast keeps the fractured bones aligned until proper healing occurs. Casts also are used to support and stabilize weak or dislocated joints; to promote healing after a surgical correction, such as knee surgery; and to aid in the nonsurgical correction of deformities, such as congenital dislocation of the hip.

Casts are applied by an orthopedist, also known as an *orthopedic surgeon*. An **orthopedist** is a physician who specializes in the diagnosis and treatment of disorders of the musculoskeletal system. An orthopedist treats patients with deformities, injuries, and diseases of the bones, joints, ligaments, tendons, muscles, nerves, and skin. The role of the medical assistant in cast application is to assemble the equipment and supplies, prepare the patient for the procedure, assist the physician during the application, provide or reinforce cast care instructions, and clean the examining room after the application.

An important goal of cast management is the prevention of pressure areas, which are most apt to occur over bony prominences. A *pressure area* occurs when the cast presses or rubs against the patient's skin and prevents adequate circulation to the area. When this occurs, the patient usually feels a painful rubbing, burning, or stinging sensation un-

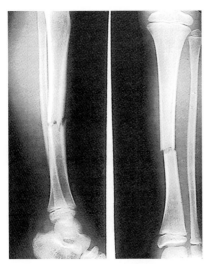

Figure 7-2. A fracture of the tibia in the left lower leg. (From McRae R, Esser M: Practical fracture treatment, ed 4, Philadelphia, 2002, Churchill Livingstone.)

Memories *from* **Externship**

Marlyne Cooper: At my first externship site, I was scared to death about having to give injections to small children. I didn't want to hurt them. A 6-month-old infant was brought to the office for her immunizations. My externship supervisor wanted me to give the injections. The infant was so small, and she was crying before I even gave her the first injection. I knew that when I gave the injection, she was going to cry even more, and that made me feel bad. My supervisor was there with me, and she talked me through it. It turned out that it wasn't as bad as I had thought it would be. My supervisor was very helpful in keeping me calm. After that first experience, I felt much more comfortable when I had to give an injection to a small child. ■

der the cast. If permitted to continue, the pressure can cause the skin to break down, leading to the development of a *pressure ulcer* (Figure 7-3). If not treated, a pressure ulcer progresses from a simple red patch of skin to erosion into the subcutaneous tissue and eventually erosion into the muscle and bone. Deep pressure ulcers often become infected by invading organisms and develop gangrene. It is important to detect the occurrence of a pressure area early so that prompt treatment can be instituted to prevent serious complications.

Plaster Casts

Since the development of synthetic casts, plaster casts are not used as much as they once were. A plaster cast consists of powdered calcium sulfate crystals formed into a bandage. The bandage roll must be soaked in tepid water to activate the crystals. When wet, the plaster bandage becomes pliable and self adhering, allowing it to be molded to the body part. Plaster bandages are available in individual rolls of widths ranging from 2 to 6 inches. The width used depends on the body part to be casted. Bandages with a smaller

width are used for the arms, and bandages with a larger width are used for the legs and trunk.

Some orthopedists initially apply a plaster cast after a patient sustains a fracture. This is because a plaster cast can be molded easily to allow for swelling of the extremity beneath the cast. After the swelling has gone down (several days to 1 week), the orthopedist removes the plaster cast and applies a synthetic cast, which weighs less and is more durable than a plaster cast.

Synthetic Casts

Synthetic casts consist of a knitted fabric tape made of fiberglass, polyester and cotton, or plastic. The tape is impregnated with polyurethane resin that is activated when soaked in water. Of the three kinds of synthetic material, fiberglass is used most. Synthetic tape comes in different colors and is packaged as an individual roll in an airtight pouch (Figure 7-4). Synthetic tape is available in widths ranging from 2 to 8 inches.

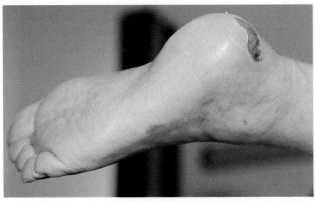

Figure 7-3. Pressure ulcer. (From Patton KT: Anatomy and physiology, ed 7, St Louis, 2010, Mosby.)

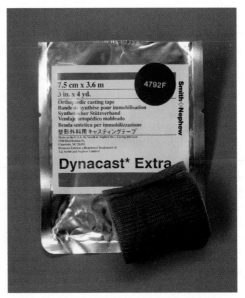

Figure 7-4. A roll of synthetic tape comes packaged in an airtight pouch.

Advantages of Synthetic Casts

The advantages of synthetic casts compared with plaster casts are as follows:

- Synthetic casts dry and set much more quickly than plaster casts. Because of this, they are able to bear weight soon after application.
- Synthetic casts are less likely to become indented because of their fast drying time. Indentations can result in pressure areas.
- Synthetic casts weigh less than plaster casts and are less restrictive, which allows the patient greater mobility.
- Synthetic casts are less bulky than plaster casts; patients usually can wear regular clothing over them.
- Synthetic casts are moisture resistant and do not break down when they get wet; plaster casts may break down when wet.

Disadvantages of Synthetic Casts

Disadvantages of synthetic casts compared with plaster casts are as follows:

- Synthetic casts cannot be molded to the body part as easily as plaster casts, so they are less effective for immobilizing severely displaced bones or unstable fractures.
- Because of the cost of synthetic casting materials, synthetic casts are more expensive than plaster casts.
- The surface of a synthetic cast is rougher than that of a plaster cast; there are increased chances of snagging clothes, scratching furniture, and causing abrasions on other parts of the body with the cast. A newer type of synthetic casting material is available that is tightly woven, which provides a smoother cast surface to help alleviate this problem.

Cast Application

The physician applies the cast so that it fits snugly but still allows adequate circulation necessary for proper healing. Four to 6 weeks are usually required for the complete healing of a fracture.

Casts are classified according to the body part they cover. The types of casts most frequently applied in the medical office and common uses of each are illustrated and described in Figure 7-5. The type of cast applied depends on the nature of the patient's injury or condition. A **short arm cast** is used for a dislocated wrist, and a **long arm cast** is used for a fracture of the humerus.

Regardless of the casting material used (plaster or synthetic), the following steps are performed in applying a cast:

1. **Inspect the skin.** The area to which the cast is to be applied must be clean and dry. The patient's skin should be inspected for redness, bruises, and open areas. This information should be recorded in the patient's chart, which may assist in evaluating patient complaints after the cast has been applied.
2. **Apply the stockinette.** Before applying the cast, the physician covers the body part with a stockinette (Figure 7-6). A stockinette consists of a soft, tubular, knitted cotton material that stretches up to three times its original

Short arm cast

Extends from below the elbow to the fingers.

Use:
- Fracture of the hand or wrist
- Postoperative immobilization

Long arm cast

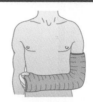

Extends from the upper arm to the fingers, usually with a bend in the elbow.

Use:
- Fracture of the humerus, forearm, or elbow
- Postoperative immobilization

Short leg cast

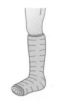

Begins just below the knee and extends to the toes.

Use:
- Fracture of the foot, ankle, or distal tibia or fibula
- Severe sprain or strain
- Postoperative immobilization
- Correction of a deformity

Long leg cast

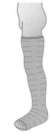

Extends from the midthigh to the toes.

Use:
- Fracture of the distal femur, knee, or lower leg
- Soft tissue injury to the knee or knee dislocation
- Postoperative immobilization

Figure 7-5. Types of casts.

width to accommodate the diameter of the body part. It is put on like a stocking. The purpose of the stockinette is to provide patient comfort and to cover the rough edges at the ends of the cast. Stockinettes come in widths ranging from 2 to 12 inches; the width used depends on the diameter of the part to be covered. Typically, a 3-inch width is used for arm casts, a 4-inch width is used for leg casts, and a 10- to 12-inch width is used for body casts.

3. **Apply the cast padding.** Cast padding consists of a soft cotton material that comes in a roll in widths ranging from 2 to 4 inches. The purpose of cast padding is to prevent pressure areas and to shield the patient's skin when the cast is removed. Two or three layers are applied directly over the stockinette, using a spiral turn. Each turn overlaps the preceding one by one-half the width of the roll. Extra layers of padding are applied over bony prominences to prevent pressure areas (Figure 7-7).
4. **Apply the cast bandage or tape.** The plaster cast bandage or synthetic tape is applied over the cast padding. The number of rolls used depends on the desired

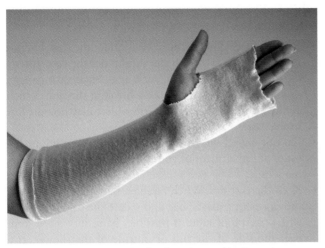

Figure 7-6. Application of a stockinette.

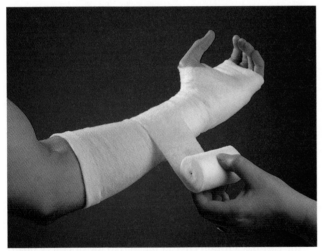

Figure 7-7. Application of cast padding. (Courtesy 3M Health Care, St Paul, Minn.)

strength of the finished cast. A nonweight-bearing cast requires fewer rolls than a weight-bearing cast.

The physician wears rubber gloves during the procedure to protect the hands from the casting material. After application, the cast must be allowed to dry. The drying time varies based on the type of casting material. Because of their porous nature, plaster casts require a longer drying period than synthetic casts. Only when a cast is completely dry does it become hard and inflexible and able to bear weight. The physician usually prescribes a supportive device, such as a sling or crutches, to prevent unnecessary strain and to minimize swelling during the healing process. Specific information on applying plaster casts and synthetic casts is presented next.

Plaster Cast

To activate the plaster, the bandage roll must be completely immersed in tepid water (70° F to 95° F [21° C to 35° C]) until bubbles no longer rise from the roll. The edges of the

roll are gently squeezed (but not wrung) toward the center to remove excess water. A properly squeezed roll should be saturated with water but not dripping.

The physician wraps the body part with the plaster bandage, using a spiral turn, until the desired number of layers has been applied (usually four to six). The stockinette is folded over the edges of the cast and anchored with the cast bandage to produce a smooth, comfortable edge on the cast. The physician molds and smoothes the plaster to conform to the contours of the body part until the cast is firmly set. Finally, the physician trims the ends of the cast with a cast knife to remove rough edges and to provide freedom of movement for the uninvolved part of the extremity, such as the thumb, fingers, or toes.

As the plaster begins to harden, a chemical reaction occurs that releases heat. Because of this reaction, the patient may feel warmth during and after the application. The patient should be told that this is normal; most patients find that the warmth has a soothing effect. The patient should not put weight on the cast until it is completely dry; otherwise the cast may break down. It takes approximately 24 hours for the standard plaster cast to dry completely.

Synthetic Cast

A synthetic cast is applied in a similar manner to that used for a plaster cast. The airtight pouch containing a roll of synthetic tape should remain sealed until just before it is time to immerse the roll in water. This is because air causes the resin in the tape to begin to harden and become rigid, making it unacceptable for use.

The roll of synthetic tape is fully immersed in cool, room-temperature water (68° F to 75° F [20° C to 24° C]) for a period of time recommended by the manufacturer. Fiberglass tape is immersed for 5 to 15 seconds. The tape is wrapped over the body part, using a spiral turn, until the desired number of layers has been applied (Figure 7-8). Generally three or four layers are applied for a nonweight-bearing cast (e.g., short or long arm cast), and five to eight layers are applied for a weight-bearing cast (e.g., short or long leg cast). The cast is allowed to dry for a period of

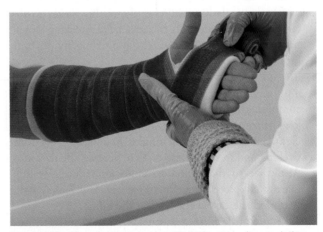

Figure 7-8. Wrapping the tape over the body part, using a spiral turn.

time specified by the manufacturer. A fiberglass cast usually dries within 30 minutes.

Precautions

The following precautions should be observed during and after cast application.

Plaster Casts

- Ensure that the temperature of the water used to activate a plaster bandage roll does not exceed 95° F (35° C). If a thick cast is being applied, water that is too warm can result in a serious burn to the patient's skin.
- Do not cover a wet cast with a towel, plastic, or other material. Covers prevent heat from escaping, which could burn the patient's skin.
- Take precautions to prevent indentations, which could lead to pressure areas. This is accomplished by not allowing the cast to come in contact with a hard surface while it is drying and by handling a wet cast with the palms of the hands rather than the fingertips.

Plaster Casts and Synthetic Casts

- Remove excess casting particles. Remove any crumbs of plaster from the patient's skin, using a cloth dampened with warm water. Remove synthetic casting material with a swab moistened with alcohol or acetone. If cast particles are not removed, they may work their way under the cast, resulting in irritation and infection.
- Before the patient leaves the medical office, the physician checks the circulation, sensation, and movement of the exposed extremity to ensure that the cast is not too tight. The physician also ensures that all joints excluded from the cast are free to move.

Guidelines for Cast Care

The medical assistant is often responsible for explaining or reinforcing the guidelines that should be followed by a patient with a cast to promote the healing process. These guidelines are often presented on an instruction sheet that is signed by the patient, with a copy filed in the patient's chart. Guidelines for cast care include the following:

- Wait at least 24 hours before putting any pressure or weight on a plaster cast. This allows the plaster to dry completely and prevents the cast from breaking down. Synthetic casts can bear weight approximately 30 minutes to 1 hour after application.
- Elevate the cast above heart level for the first 24 to 48 hours to decrease swelling and pain. This can be accomplished by propping the casted extremity up on pillows or some other type of support.
- Gently move the toes or fingers frequently to prevent swelling and joint stiffness and to increase circulation.
- Apply ice to the casted extremity to reduce swelling. Place small pieces of ice in an ice bag, and loosely wrap it around the cast at the level of the injury.
- Take precautions to prevent dirt, sand, powder, and other foreign particles from becoming trapped under the cast. They can cause irritation to the skin, leading to infection.
- Do not apply powder for itching under the cast. Do not use any object to scratch the skin under the cast. Inserting anything into the cast, such as a pencil, coat hanger, or knitting needle, may cause a break in the skin, which could become infected. Also, the object may become lost in the cast.
- Do not engage in activities that could cause injury because of impairment of your physical abilities (e.g., driving a car).
- Keep the cast dry. When taking a bath or shower, cover the cast with a plastic bag and secure the bag to the skin with waterproof tape. If possible, hang the casted limb over the side of the tub or outside of the shower. If a plaster cast becomes wet, it loses its shape and may break down. Although the material making up a synthetic cast is moisture resistant, the cast padding is not. If a synthetic cast becomes wet, it must be dried as soon as possible to prevent maceration. **Maceration** is the softening and breaking down of the skin, which can lead to infection.
- To dry a wet cast, first blot the outside of the cast with an absorbent towel. This should be followed by the application of a blow dryer on a low setting using a sweeping motion over the entire cast until it is completely dry. The patient should be instructed not to use the high setting on the blow dryer because this amount of heat could burn the skin.
- Inspect the skin around the cast at regular intervals to check for redness, sores, or swelling.
- Do not trim the cast or break off any rough edges because this may weaken or break the cast. If the surface of the cast has a rough edge, a metal nail file or emery board can be used to smooth it. Notify the physician if the cast becomes loose, broken, or cracked, because the cast may need to be replaced.
- Synthetic casts cannot be signed with a ballpoint pen; only permanent markers can be used to write on them.

Symptoms to Report

The patient should report the following symptoms *immediately* to the physician; they may indicate that the cast is too tight or an infection is developing:

- Increased pain or swelling that does not go away with application of an ice bag medication, elevation, or rest
- A feeling that the cast is too tight. Slight pressure applied with the thumbnail to the fingernail or toenail should cause it to blanch white, and then when the pressure is released, the nail should immediately return to its normal color. If this does not occur, it could indicate insufficient blood flow to the extremity from a cast that is too tight.
- Tingling, numbness, or loss of movement of the fingers or toes
- Coldness, paleness, or blueness of the fingers or toes
- Painful rubbing, burning, or stinging under the cast

- Foul odor or drainage coming from the cast
- Sore areas around the edge of the cast
- Chills, fever, nausea, or vomiting

Cast Removal

The easiest and safest way to remove a cast is to bivalve it—this means cutting the cast into two halves, resulting in an anterior shell and a posterior shell. To bivalve a cast, the physician cuts the entire length of the cast on two opposite sides down to the level of the cast padding. The cuts are made with a cast cutter. A cast cutter is a handheld electric saw with a circular blade that oscillates, which means that the saw vibrates but does not rotate (Figure 7-9, *A*). The medical assistant should reassure the patient that, although the saw is noisy, only a tickling sensation and some heat are felt from the saw's vibration. After cutting the cast, the physician pries it apart with a cast spreader (Figure 7-9, *B*). Next, the physician uses bandage scissors to cut through the cast padding and stockinette (Figure 7-9, *C*). The cast is carefully removed from the patient's extremity.

The skin of the affected extremity typically appears yellow and scaly. The extremity also appears thinner, and the muscles are flabby. The medical assistant should explain to the patient that this is normal and results from lack of use of the extremity. The physician may recommend exercises

or physical therapy or both to help the patient regain strength and function of the body part.

SPLINTS AND BRACES

Along with casts, splints and braces are used to assist in the treatment of fractures. A **splint** is a rigid removable device used to support and immobilize a displaced or fractured

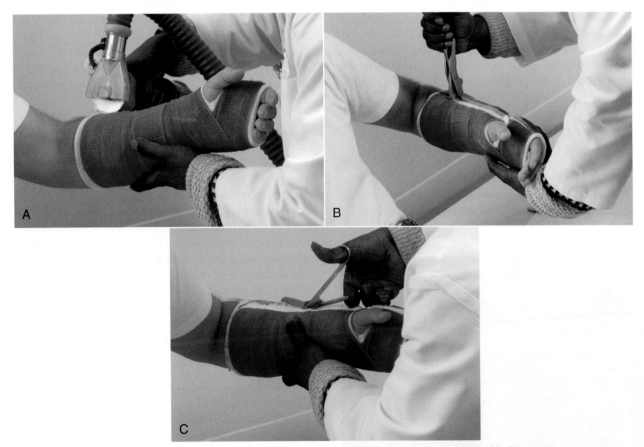

Figure 7-9. Cast removal. **A,** A cast cutter is used to cut the entire length of the cast. **B,** The cast is pried open with a cast spreader. **C,** Bandage scissors are used to cut through the cast padding and stockinette.

PATIENT TEACHING Cast Care

- Teach the patient the important guidelines of cast care.
- Emphasize the importance of contacting the physician immediately if any signs of circulatory impairment or infection occur.
- If the physician has prescribed cold to reduce swelling, teach the patient the procedure for applying an ice bag to the casted extremity.
- Emphasize the importance of returning to have the cast checked by the physician.
- If the physician prescribes isometric exercises to maintain the muscle tone of the affected extremity, provide the patient with a sheet that illustrates the exercises.
- Provide the patient with printed materials on cast care.

part of the body. Splints also are commonly used to protect areas that are sprained or strained. Splints are molded to fit specific parts of the body and are well padded to provide patient comfort and to prevent pressure areas. A splint can be custom made by an orthopedist using plaster or fiberglass casting materials. Splints also are commercially available and consist of two parts: a rigid material such as plastic or fiberglass and straps with Velcro that hold the splint in place (Figure 7-10).

A splint may be applied initially to a fractured limb because it can be adjusted to accommodate swelling from injuries more easily than a cast. After the swelling subsides, a cast is usually applied. When the fracture is almost healed, the cast may be removed and another splint applied. This allows for bathing of the extremity and easy removal for therapy until the fracture heals completely and the splint is no longer needed.

A **brace** is designed to support a part of the body and hold it in its correct position to allow for functioning of the body part while healing takes place. An example of a brace is a *short leg walker*, which consists of a rigid lightweight frame with a removable padded liner (Figure 7-11). A short leg walker is often used, instead of a cast, to heal a stable fracture (e.g., stress fracture) of the lower leg. A short leg

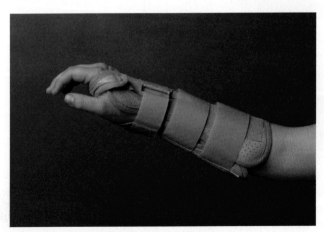

Figure 7-10. Arm splint.

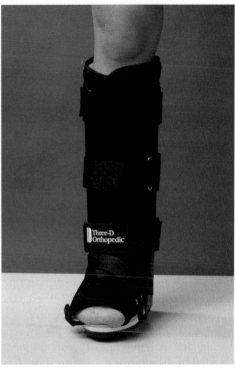

Figure 7-11. Short leg walker, which is an example of a leg brace.

walker is available in different sizes so it can be properly fitted to extend from just below the patient's knee to the toes. Special fasteners or straps with Velcro are used to hold the walker in place and allow for adjustment of it (see Figure 7-11). A short leg walker permits walking and standing, which encourage healing. It also can be removed to permit bathing of the leg.

AMBULATORY AIDS

Mechanical assistive devices are used by individuals who require aid in ambulation. The word **ambulation** means walking; patients who are **ambulatory** are able to walk as opposed to being confined to a wheelchair or a bed. Ambulatory aids include crutches, canes, and walkers. The device used depends on factors such as the type and severity of the disability, the amount of support required, and the patient's age and degree of muscular coordination. The ambulatory aid may be prescribed for a temporary condition, such as a fracture, a sprain to a lower extremity, and disability after orthopedic surgery. It also may be prescribed for a long-term condition, such as paralysis, deformity, and permanent weakness of the lower extremities.

Crutches

Crutches are artificial supports that consist of wood or tubular aluminum. They are used for patients who require assistance in walking as a result of disease, injury, or birth defects of the lower extremities. Crutches function by removing weight from the legs and transferring it to the arms. The two main crutch types are the axillary crutch and the

Highlight on Ambulatory Aids

Many people who could benefit from ambulatory aids are not using them. The primary reason is that they do not know how to use them correctly, become discouraged, and quit using them.

Other types of aids available to assist individuals with physical disabilities include raised toilet seats, handle bars, carrying devices, tub seats, over-bed tables, and swivel cushions for assistance in getting into and out of cars.

If an individual needs help in learning to drive with a physical disability, the local bureau of vocational rehabilitation or the state motor vehicle department can provide information on qualified instruction available in the community.

Walking with an ambulatory aid is a physiologic stressor to the body because it requires more energy than normal walking. Because of this, individuals need to rest frequently when using an ambulatory aid.

Many people need to have their crutches lengthened after they have had them for a while. This is because their posture improves as they gain confidence in walking with them. Children and teenagers who use crutches for a long time also need frequent adjustments as they grow.

A cane can provide security to the individual using it; however, it can be more trouble than it is worth if it is the incorrect size. It is estimated that two thirds of people who buy canes select one that is too long.

Some walkers are designed to fit over chairs and toilets, allowing the user additional support when rising or sitting. Folding walkers are available, and they are easy to store and transport. ■

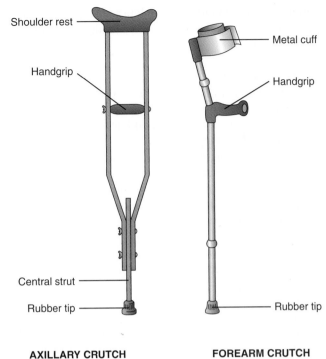

Figure 7-12. Types of crutches.

the axillae and palms of the hands. Procedure 7-7 presents the correct way to measure a patient for axillary crutches.

If the crutches are too long, the shoulder rests exert pressure on the patient's axillae. This can injure the radial nerve in the brachial plexus, which eventually may lead to *crutch palsy,* a condition of muscular weakness in the forearm, wrist, and hand. In addition, crutches that are too long force the patient's shoulders forward, preventing the patient from pushing his or her body off the ground. Crutches that are too short force the patient to be bent over and uncomfortable, also making them awkward to use. If the handgrips are too low, pressure is put on the patient's axillae, whereas handgrips that are too high are awkward.

Wooden crutches are made with bolts and wing nuts, which allow proper adjustment of the length and handgrip level. Aluminum crutches consist of aluminum tubes.

forearm crutch (Figure 7-12). The axillary crutch and the forearm crutch require rubber tips, which increase surface tension to prevent the crutches from slipping on the floor.

The *axillary crutch* is used most frequently and is made of wood or tubular aluminum. This type of crutch has a shoulder rest and handgrips and extends from the ground almost to the patient's axilla.

The *forearm crutch,* also known as a *Lofstrand crutch,* consists of a single adjustable tube of aluminum that extends to the forearm. A metal cuff attached to the crutch fits securely around the patient's forearm, and a handgrip covered with rubber extends from the crutch for weight bearing. The metal cuff and the handgrip stabilize the patient's wrists to make walking safer and easier. One advantage of the forearm crutch is that the individual can release the handgrip, enabling use of the hand, while the metal cuff holds the crutch in place. Individuals who are paraplegic or have cerebral palsy use the forearm crutch most often.

Axillary Crutch Measurement

The patient must be measured for axillary crutches to ensure the correct crutch length and proper placement of the handgrip. Incorrectly fitted crutches increase the patient's risk of developing back pain, nerve damage, and injuries to

PATIENT TEACHING Crutches

- Teach patients the guidelines for the proper use of crutches.
- Provide the patient with an exercise sheet that illustrates exercises to strengthen arm muscles before beginning crutch walking.
- Teach the patient the crutch gaits prescribed by the physician, and have the patient demonstrate the gaits before leaving the office.
- Provide the patient with a list of local vendors who provide crutch services, such as repairs and supplies (e.g., rubber tips, crutch pads).
- Provide the patient with printed educational materials on the use of crutches and crutch gaits.

Spring-loaded pushbuttons on an inner tube "pop out" into holes on an outer tube to allow proper adjustment of the crutch length.

Crutch Guidelines

It is important that the patient receive specific guidelines to ensure safety while using crutches, to prevent injuries and falls. The medical assistant is responsible for instructing the patient in the following guidelines:

1. Wear well-fitting flat shoes with firm, nonskid soles to provide good traction and stability.
2. Use correct posture to prevent strain on muscles and joints and to maintain proper body balance.
3. Support your weight with your hands on the handgrips and the axillary pads pressing against the sides of the rib cage. The body weight should not be supported by the axillae because pressure on the axillae may cause crutch palsy.
4. Look ahead when walking, rather than down at your feet.
5. Be aware of the surface on which you are walking. It should be clean, flat, dry, and well lighted. Throw rugs and objects serving as obstacles should temporarily be removed from your environment to prevent falls.
6. Keep the crutches about 4 to 6 inches out from the sides of your feet when walking to prevent obstruction of the pathway for the feet.
7. Take steps by moving the crutches forward a safe and comfortable distance, preferably 6 inches. When first learning to use the crutches, take small steps rather than large ones. Do not move forward more than 12 to 15 inches with each step. A greater distance might cause the crutches to slide forward and you to lose your balance.
8. Report tingling or numbness in the upper body to the physician. You might be using the crutches incorrectly, or they might be the wrong size for you.
9. Extra padding can be added to the shoulder rests of your crutches to make them more comfortable. If you do this, ensure that the extra padding does not press against your axillae, but rather against your lateral rib cage. The handgrips also can be padded for increased comfort.
10. To prevent slipping, keep the crutch tips dry to maintain their surface friction. If they become wet, dry them completely before use.
11. Inspect the crutch tips regularly. They should be securely attached. If the crutch tips are worn down, they should be replaced with tips of the proper size.
12. For wooden crutches, periodically check the wing nuts holding the central strut and handgrips in place to ensure that they are tight.

Crutch Gaits

The type of crutch gait used depends on the amount of weight the patient is able to support with one or both legs and the patient's physical condition and muscular coordina-

tion. The patient should learn a fast and a slow gait. The faster gait is used for making speed in open areas, and the slower one is used in crowded places. In addition, learning more than one gait reduces patient fatigue because a different combination of muscles is used for each gait. Procedure 7-8 provides guidelines and charts for use in instructing the patient on how to walk with crutches.

Canes

A cane is a lightweight, easily movable device made of wood or aluminum with a rubber tip and is used to help provide balance and support. Canes are generally used by patients who have weakness on one side of the body, such as patients with hemiparesis, joint disabilities, or defects of the neuromuscular system. The three main types of canes are the *standard cane,* the *tripod cane,* and the *quad cane* (Figure 7-13). The standard cane provides the least amount of support and is used by patients who require only slight assistance in walking. The tripod and quad canes have three and four legs, respectively, a bent shaft, and a T-shaped handle with grips. They are easier to hold and provide greater stability than a standard cane because of the wider base of support. In addition, multilegged canes are able to stand alone, which frees the arms when the patient is getting up from a chair. The disadvantage of a multilegged cane is that it is bulkier and more difficult to move.

A cane is held on the side of the body that is opposite to the side that needs support. The cane length must be properly adjusted to ensure optimal stability. The cane handle should be approximately level with the greater trochanter, and the elbow should be flexed at a 25- to 30-degree angle. The patient should be instructed to stand erect and not lean on the cane to ensure good balance. Procedure 7-9 presents guidelines on instructing the patient on how to walk with a cane.

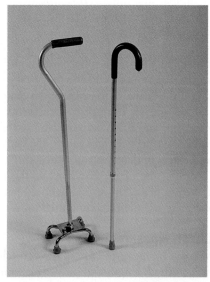

Figure 7-13. Examples of a quad cane *(left)* and a standard cane *(right)*. (Courtesy 3M Health Care, St Paul, MN.)

Walkers

A walker is an ambulatory aid consisting of an aluminum frame with handgrips and four widely placed legs with rubber suction tips and one open side (Figure 7-14). A walker is light and easily movable. Walkers are available with wheels that facilitate movement of the walker. They are also available with a fold-up feature that allows them to be easily transported in a vehicle. For proper ambulation, the walker should extend from the ground to approximately the level of the patient's hip joint. Procedure 7-10 presents guide-lines on instructing the patient on how to walk with a walker.

Walkers are used most often by geriatric patients with weakness or balance problems. Walkers also are used during the healing process for patients who have had knee or hip joint replacement surgery. These patients need more help with balance and walking than can be provided by crutches or a cane. Because of its wide base, a walker provides the patient with a great amount of stability and security. Disadvantages of a walker include a slow pace and difficulty in maneuvering the walker in a small room.

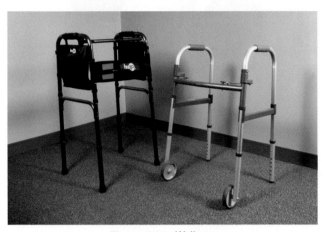

Figure 7-14. Walkers.

What Would You Do? What Would You *Not* Do?

Case Study 3

Thaddeus Bernard calls the office. Thaddeus fractured the femur of his left leg 2 weeks ago in a skiing accident. The physician applied a long leg fiberglass cast, and Thaddeus was properly fitted with aluminum crutches. Thaddeus says that he is having some problems with his crutches. He is complaining of weakness in his forearms and hands and some tingling and numbness in his fingers. He also says that he has bruises under his arms. Thaddeus says that after he got home, his crutches didn't seem to fit right, so he readjusted them. Thaddeus is getting ready to return to college and wants to know the best way to carry his books while using crutches. ∎

PROCEDURE 7-7   Measuring for Axillary Crutches

Outcome Measure an individual for axillary crutches.

Determining Crutch Length

For you to determine crutch length correctly, the patient must wear shoes while being measured. The measurement can be taken while the patient is standing.

1. **Procedural Step.** Ask the patient to stand erect.
2. **Procedural Step.** Position the crutches with the crutch tips at a distance of 2 inches (5 cm) in front of and 4 to 6 inches (15 cm) to the side of each foot. (The large dots in the figure represent crutch tips.)
3. **Procedural Step.** Adjust the crutch length so that the shoulder rests are approximately 1½ to 2 inches (about 2 finger widths) below the axillae.
   Wooden Crutches. The length of the crutch is adjusted by removing the bolt and wing nut and sliding the central strut (support piece) at the bottom upward or downward as necessary to attain the proper length. The strut is secured by replacing the bolt and securely fastening the wing nut.
   Tubular Aluminum Crutches. The length of the crutch is adjusted by pressing the spring-loaded push button with your thumb and sliding the outer tube upward or downward as necessary to attain the proper length. The spring-loaded button on the inner tube should be allowed to "pop out" into the appropriate hole on the outer tube.

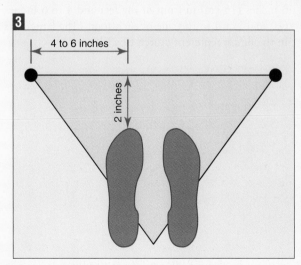

Position for measuring for crutches.

Continued

PROCEDURE 7-7   Measuring for Axillary Crutches—cont'd

Handgrip Positioning

When the crutch length has been adjusted, correct placement of the handgrips must be determined.

1. **Procedural Step.** Ask the patient to stand erect with a crutch under each arm and to support his or her weight by the handgrips.

2. **Procedural Step.** Adjust the handgrips on the crutches so that the patient's elbow is flexed to an angle of approximately 30 degrees. The handgrip level is adjusted by removing the bolt and wing nut and sliding the handgrip upward or downward, as required. The handgrip is secured by replacing the bolt and tightly fastening the wing nut. The angle of elbow flexion can be verified by using a measuring device known as a *goniometer*. A *goniometer* is an instrument that measures the angle of a joint.

3. **Procedural Step.** Check the fit of the crutches. If the crutches are measured correctly, the medical assistant should be able to insert two fingers between the top of

the crutches and the axillae when the patient is standing erect with the crutches under the arms.

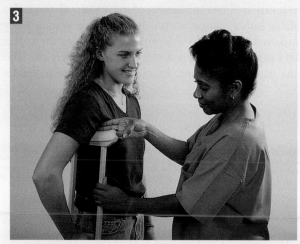

Insert two fingers between the top of the crutch and the axilla.

PROCEDURE 7-8   Instructing a Patient in Crutch Gaits

Outcome Instruct a patient in the following crutch gaits: four-point, two-point, three-point, swing-to, and swing-through.

Tripod Position

The tripod position is the basic crutch stance used before crutch walking. It provides a wide base of support and enhances stability and balance.

Instruct the patient in the tripod position as follows:

1. **Procedural Step.** Stand erect, and face straight ahead.

2. **Procedural Step.** Place the tips of the crutches 4 to 6 inches (15 cm) in front of the feet and 4 to 6 inches (10 to 15 cm) to the side of each foot. (The large dots in the figure represent crutch tips.)

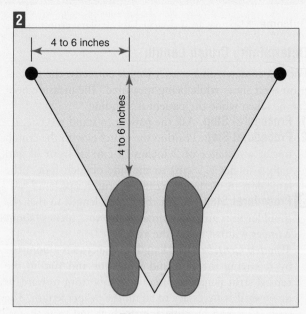

Tripod position.

PROCEDURE 7-8   Instructing a Patient in Crutch Gaits—cont'd

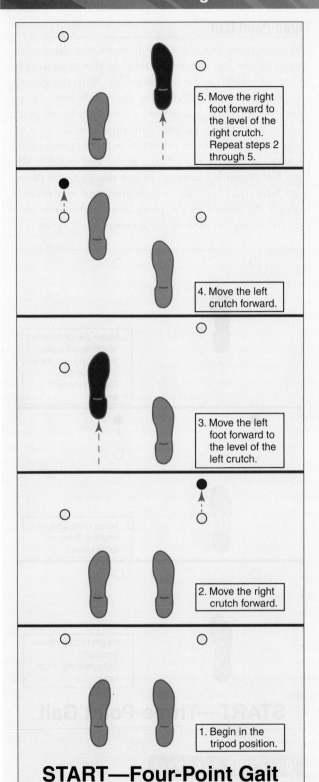

5. Move the right foot forward to the level of the right crutch. Repeat steps 2 through 5.

4. Move the left crutch forward.

3. Move the left foot forward to the level of the left crutch.

2. Move the right crutch forward.

1. Begin in the tripod position.

START—Four-Point Gait

Four-Point Gait

The four-point gait is a basic and slow gait. To use this gait, the patient must be able to bear considerable weight on both legs. The four-point gait is the most stable and the safest of the crutch gaits because it provides at least three points of support at all times. It is used most often by patients who have leg muscle weakness or spasticity, poor muscular coordination or balance, or degenerative leg joint disease. Instruct the patient in the procedure for the four-point gait, following the steps in the accompanying figure.

CHARTING EXAMPLE	
Date	
12/15/12	1:30 p.m. Instructed pt in four-point gait. Pt was able to demonstrate four-point gait. ——— ————————— M. Cooper, CMA (AAMA)

PROCEDURE 7-8

Continued

PROCEDURE 7-8   Instructing a Patient in Crutch Gaits—cont'd

Two-Point Gait

The two-point gait is similar to, but faster than, the four-point gait. This gait requires better balance because only two points support the body at one time. The two-point gait is used when the patient is capable of partial weight bearing on each foot and has good muscular coordination. Instruct the patient in the procedure for the two-point gait, following the steps in the accompanying figure.

Three-Point Gait

The three-point gait is used by patients who cannot bear weight on one leg. The patient must be able to support his or her full weight on the unaffected leg. With this gait, the crutches and the unaffected leg alternately bear the patient's weight. This gait is used most often by amputees without a prosthesis, patients with musculoskeletal or soft tissue trauma to a lower extremity (e.g., fracture, sprain), patients with acute leg inflammation, and patients who have had recent leg surgery. To use this gait, the patient must have good muscular coordination and arm strength. Instruct the patient in the procedure for the three-point gait, following the steps in the accompanying figure.

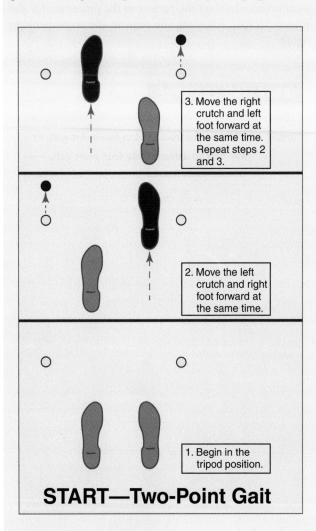

3. Move the right crutch and left foot forward at the same time. Repeat steps 2 and 3.

2. Move the left crutch and right foot forward at the same time.

1. Begin in the tripod position.

START—Two-Point Gait

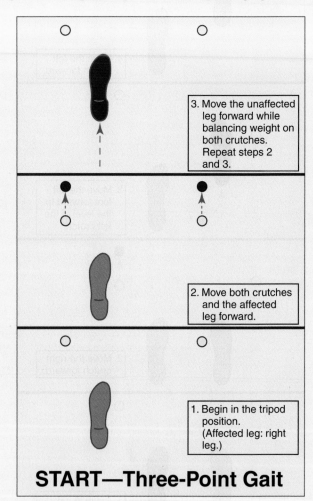

3. Move the unaffected leg forward while balancing weight on both crutches. Repeat steps 2 and 3.

2. Move both crutches and the affected leg forward.

1. Begin in the tripod position. (Affected leg: right leg.)

START—Three-Point Gait

CHARTING EXAMPLE

Date	
12/16/12	2:30 p.m. Instructed pt in two-point gait. Pt was able to demonstrate two-point gait. ——— ——— M. Cooper, CMA (AAMA)

CHARTING EXAMPLE

Date	
12/17/12	2:30 p.m. Instructed pt in three-point gait. Pt was able to demonstrate three-point gait. ——— ——— M. Cooper, CMA (AAMA)

PROCEDURE 7-8   Instructing a Patient in Crutch Gaits—cont'd

Swing Gaits

The swing gaits include the swing-to gait and the swing-through gait and are used by patients with severe lower extremity disabilities, such as paralysis, and by patients who wear supporting braces on their legs.

Instruct the patient in the procedures for the swing-to and the swing-through crutch gaits, following the steps in the accompanying figures.

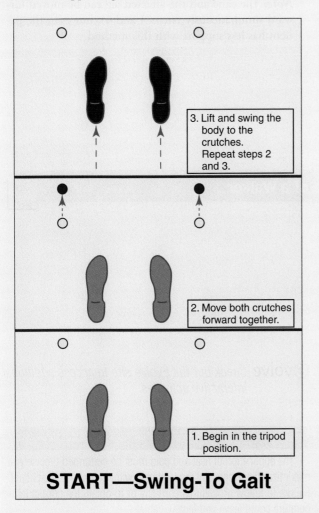

3. Lift and swing the body to the crutches. Repeat steps 2 and 3.

2. Move both crutches forward together.

1. Begin in the tripod position.

START—Swing-To Gait

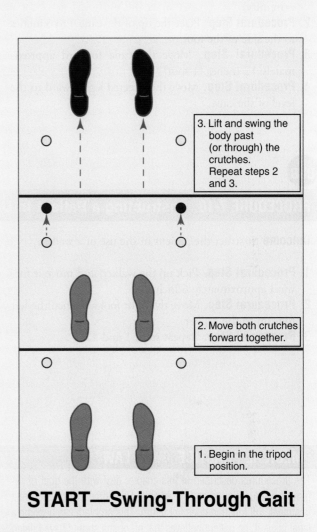

3. Lift and swing the body past (or through) the crutches. Repeat steps 2 and 3.

2. Move both crutches forward together.

1. Begin in the tripod position.

START—Swing-Through Gait

PROCEDURE 7-9

CHARTING EXAMPLE	
Date	
12/18/12	3:30 p.m. Instructed pt in swing-to and swing-through gaits. Pt was able to demonstrate swing gaits.— M. Cooper, CMA (AAMA)

PROCEDURE 7-9   Instructing a Patient in Use of a Cane

Outcome Instruct the patient in the use of a cane.

1. **Procedural Step.** Hold the cane on the strong side of the body (i.e., in the hand opposite the affected extremity).
2. **Procedural Step.** Place the tip of the cane 4 to 6 inches to the side of the foot.
3. **Procedural Step.** Move the cane forward approximately 12 inches (1 foot).
4. **Procedural Step.** Move the affected leg forward to the level of the cane.

5. **Procedural Step.** Move the strong leg forward and ahead of the cane and weak leg.
6. **Procedural Step.** Repeat steps 3 through 5.
   Note: The cane and the affected leg can be moved forward simultaneously (steps 3 and 4); however, the patient has less support with this method.

PROCEDURE 7-10   Instructing a Patient in Use of a Walker

Outcome Instruct the patient in the use of a walker.

1. **Procedural Step.** Pick up the walker, and move it forward approximately 6 inches.
2. **Procedural Step.** Move the right foot and then the left foot up to the walker.
3. **Procedural Step.** Repeat steps 1 and 2.

evolve *Check out the Evolve site to access additional interactive activities.*

MEDICAL PRACTICE and the LAW

The procedures described in this chapter deal with the goal of returning full function to an injured area. Sometimes, despite correct treatment, full function does not return. This problem can become a legal issue if the patient believes that he or she should have healed fully or cannot return to work. To protect yourself, follow each procedure to the letter, and record the patient's progress (or lack of progress) carefully in the medical record. Sometimes the patient is involved in insurance fraud and falsely complains of pain or impaired function to continue receiving disability benefits. If you suspect this is the case, objectively document the functions you have seen the patient perform.

The application of heat and cold must be performed precisely to maximize effectiveness of the treatment without injury to the patient. Failure to follow procedures correctly or to obtain the correct temperature could leave you legally liable.

Ambulatory aids used correctly can help the patient regain mobility. If crutches are used improperly, the patient could fall or develop nerve or other injuries. When instructing about ambulation aid use, allow enough time for the patient to give a return demonstration, and send home written instructions in case the patient forgets what was taught. ■

What Would You Do? What Would You *Not* Do? RESPONSES

Case Study 1
Page 246

What Did Marlyne Do?
- ❏ Empathized with Aaron for being in so much pain.
- ❏ Explained to Aaron that he should never sleep on a heating pad because the heat builds up and causes the type of burn he experienced.
- ❏ Explained to Aaron that it is best to apply heat for 15 to 30 minutes at a time with the pad set no higher than the medium setting. Told him the pad may not feel warm after his body gets used to it, but that it is still helping him. Told Aaron that the high setting could burn his skin.
- ❏ Told Aaron how to prevent low back pain by using good body mechanics, especially during lifting.

What Did Marlyne Not *Do?*
- ❏ Did not criticize Aaron for sleeping on the heating pad or turning the pad to the high setting.

What Would You Do?/What Would You *Not* Do? Review Marlyne's response and place a checkmark next to the information you included in your response. List the additional information you included in your response.

_____

_____

_____

_____

Case Study 2
Page 257

What Did Marlyne Do?
- ❏ Reassured Christina that the medical staff is there to help her, and she should never hesitate to call when she needs information or is having a problem.
- ❏ Asked Christina what she did to try to make her arm feel better and recorded this information in her chart. Checked with the physician to determine whether he wanted to see Christina.
- ❏ Reeducated Christina in proper cast care instructions over the phone and mailed her another cast care instruction sheet.
- ❏ Explained to Christina how to dry her cast properly by first blotting it and then using a hair dryer. Told her that if she is unable to dry her cast completely, she will need to come in to have it replaced.
- ❏ Explained to Christina that the physician applied the type of cast that would best treat her injury and help her to heal.

What Did Marlyne Not *Do?*
- ❏ Did not criticize Christina for waiting so long to call the office.
- ❏ Did not tell Christina it would be a good idea for her to have a "removable cast."

What Would You Do?/What Would You *Not* Do? Review Marlyne's response and place a checkmark next to the information you included in your response. List the additional information you included in your response.

_____

_____

_____

_____

Case Study 3
Page 261

What Did Marlyne Do?
- ❏ Listened carefully and empathetically to Thaddeus' problems with and concerns about his crutches.
- ❏ Explained to Thaddeus that the crutches were adjusted to fit him properly at the office and that he may have caused some problems by readjusting them.
- ❏ Scheduled an appointment for Thaddeus to come in that day so the physician could examine him and his crutches could be checked for proper length.
- ❏ Went over crutch guidelines and crutch gaits with Thaddeus again when he came to the office for his appointment.
- ❏ Told Thaddeus that he should use a backpack to carry his books to keep his hands free to move on his crutches. Stressed that he should keep his backpack as light as possible and keep the weight evenly distributed on his back (i.e., use both straps).

What Did Marlyne Not *Do?*
- ❏ Did not tell Thaddeus to readjust the crutches himself.
- ❏ Did not tell Thaddeus that he should have paid more attention when he was being instructed in crutch guidelines.

What Would You Do?/What Would You *Not* Do? Review Marlyne's response and place a checkmark next to the information you included in your response. List the additional information you included in your response.

_____

_____

_____

CERTIFICATION REVIEW

❑ **The application of heat or cold** is used to treat pathologic conditions such as infection and trauma. Heat and cold are applied for short periods, usually ranging from 15 to 30 minutes. The type of heat or cold application depends on the purpose of the application, the location and condition of the affected area, and the age and general health of the patient.

❑ **The local effects of applying heat** to the body include the dilation of blood vessels in the area. Nutrients and oxygen are provided to the cells at a faster rate, and wastes are carried away faster. Erythema is redness of the skin caused by congestion of capillaries in the lower layers of the skin. Heat functions in relieving pain, congestion, muscle spasms, and inflammation.

❑ **The local application of cold** constricts the blood vessels. As a result, tissue metabolism decreases, less oxygen is used, and fewer wastes accumulate. Local application of cold is used to prevent edema and may be done immediately after an individual has experienced direct trauma, such as a bruise, sprain, muscle strain, joint injury, or fracture.

❑ **Factors that affect the local application of heat and cold** include the age of the patient, the location of the application, impaired circulation and sensation, and individual tolerance to change in temperature.

❑ **A cast is a stiff cylindrical casing** that is used to immobilize a body part. Casts are applied most often when an individual sustains a fracture. Other uses of a cast are to support and stabilize weak or dislocated joints, to promote healing after a surgical correction, and to aid in the nonsurgical correction of deformities.

❑ **Casts are classified** according to the body part they cover. The types of casts most frequently applied are short arm cast, long arm cast, short leg cast, and long leg cast. The type of cast applied depends on the nature of the patient's injury or condition.

❑ **Splints and braces** are used to assist in the treatment of musculoskeletal injuries. A splint is a rigid removable device used to support and immobilize a displaced or fractured part of the body and to protect areas that are sprained or strained. A brace is designed to support a part of the body and hold it in its correct position to allow functioning of the body part while healing takes place.

❑ **Mechanical assistive devices** are used by individuals who require help to walk. Ambulatory aids include crutches, canes, and walkers. The device used depends on factors such as the type and severity of the disability, the amount of support required, and the patient's age and degree of muscular coordination.

❑ **Crutches are artificial supports** consisting of wood or tubular aluminum. They are used for patients who require assistance in walking as a result of disease, injury, or birth defects of the lower extremities. Crutches function by removing weight from the legs and transferring it to the arms.

❑ **The type of crutch gait** used depends on the amount of weight the patient is able to support with one or both legs, the patient's physical condition, and the patient's muscular coordination. Crutch gaits include the four-point gait, the two-point gait, the three-point gait, and the swing-through gait.

❑ **A cane** is a lightweight, easily movable device used to provide balance and support. Canes are generally used by patients who have weakness on one side of the body.

❑ **A walker** is an ambulatory aid that is most often used by geriatric patients with weakness or balance problems.

TERMINOLOGY REVIEW

Medical Term	Word Parts	Definition
Ambulation		Walking or moving from one place to another.
Ambulatory		Able to walk as opposed to being confined to bed or a wheelchair.
Brace		An orthopedic device used to support and hold a part of the body in the correct position to allow functioning and healing.
Compress		A soft, moist, absorbent cloth that is folded in several layers and applied to a part of the body in the local application of heat or cold.
Edema		The retention of fluid in the tissues, resulting in swelling.
Erythema	*hem/o:* blood	Reddening of the skin caused by dilation of superficial blood vessels in the skin.
Exudate		A discharge produced by the body's tissues.
Long arm cast		A cast that extends from the axilla to the fingers of the hand, usually with a bend in the elbow.
Long leg cast		A cast that extends from the midthigh to the toes.
Maceration		The softening and breaking down of the skin as a result of prolonged exposure to moisture.
Orthopedist	*orth/o:* straight *-ist:* specialist	A physician who specializes in the diagnosis and treatment of disorders of the musculoskeletal system, which includes the bones, joints, ligaments, tendons, muscles, and nerves.
Short arm cast		A cast that extends from below the elbow to the fingers.
Short leg cast		A cast that begins just below the knee and extends to the toes.
Soak		The direct immersion of a body part in water or a medicated solution.
Splint		An orthopedic device used to support and immobilize a part of the body.
Sprain		Trauma to a joint that causes injury to the ligaments.
Strain		An overstretching of a muscle caused by trauma.
Suppuration		The process of pus formation.

ON THE WEB

For Information on Rehabilitation and Disability:

National Rehabilitation Information Center (NARIC): www.naric.com

American Academy of Orthopaedic Surgeons: www.aaos.org

About.Com: Orthopedics: orthopedics.about.com

American Physical Therapy Association: www.apta.org

American Chiropractic Association: www.amerchiro.org

American Occupational Therapy Association: www.aota.org

National Stroke Association (NSA): www.stroke.org

Arthritis Foundation: www.arthritis.org

National Institute of Arthritis and Musculoskeletal and Skin Diseases: www.niams.nih.gov

American Academy of Physical Medicine and Rehabilitation: www.aapmr.org

8

The Gynecologic Examination and Prenatal Care

LEARNING OBJECTIVES	PROCEDURES
Gynecologic Examination	
1. State the purpose of the gynecologic examination.	
2. Identify the components of the gynecologic examination.	
Breast Examination	
1. Explain the purpose of a breast examination.	Instruct patient in the procedure for a breast self examination.
Pelvic Examination	
1. Explain the purpose of a pelvic examination.	Prepare patient for a gynecologic examination.
2. List and describe the four parts of the pelvic examination.	Assist the physician with a gynecologic examination.
3. State the purpose of a Pap test.	Complete a cytology requisition form.
4. List the advantages and disadvantages of the liquid-based Pap test.	
5. List and describe each category on a cytology request for a Pap test.	
Vaginal Infections	
1. Identify the symptoms of each of the following:	Assist in the collection of a vaginal microbiologic specimen.
• Trichomoniasis	
• Candidiasis	
• Chlamydia	
• Gonorrhea	
2. Explain how each of the above-listed infections is diagnosed and treated.	
Prenatal Visits	
1. Explain the purpose of each part of the prenatal record.	Record the patient's pregnancy in terms of gravidity and parity.
2. List and explain the purpose of each procedure included in the initial prenatal examination.	Calculate the expected date of delivery (EDD).
3. List and explain the purpose of each prenatal laboratory test.	Complete a prenatal health history.
4. Explain the purpose of return prenatal visits.	Assist with an initial prenatal examination.
5. Explain the purpose of each of the following:	Assist with a return prenatal examination.
• Triple screen test	
• Ultrasound scan	
• Amniocentesis	
• Fetal heart rate monitoring	
6 Weeks Postpartum Visit	
1. Explain the purpose of the 6 weeks postpartum visit.	Assist with a 6 weeks postpartum examination.
2. List and explain the purpose of each of the procedures included in the postpartum examination.	

KEY TERMS

Gynecology

adnexal (ad-NEKS-al)
amenorrhea (AY-men-ah-REE-ah)
atypical (ay-TIP-ih-kul)
cervix (SER-viks)
colposcopy (kol-POS-koe-pee)
cytology (sy-TOL-oh-jee)
dysmenorrhea (DIS-men-ah-REE-ah)
dyspareunia (DIS-pah-ROO-nee-ah)
dysplasia (dis-PLAY-shah)
ectocervix (EK-toe-SER-viks)
endocervix (EN-doe-SER-viks)
external os (eks-TER-nal AHS)
gynecology (gie-nuh-KOL-oh-jee)
internal os (in-TER-nal AHS)
menopause (MEN-oh-paws)
menorrhagia (men-uh-RAY-jee-ah)
metrorrhagia (met-ro-RAY-jee-ah)
perimenopause (PEAR-ee-MEN-oh-paws)
perineum (pear-ih-NEE-um)
risk factor
vulva (VUL-va)

Obstetrics

abortion (ah-BOR-shun)
Braxton Hicks contractions (BRAK-stun HIKS con-TRAK-shuns)
dilation (of the cervix) (die-LAY-shun)
effacement (eh-FAYS-ment)
embryo (EM-bree-oh)

engagement
expected date of delivery (EDD)
fetal heart rate
fetal heart tones
fetus (FEE-tus)
fundus (FUN-dus)
gestation (jess-TAY-shun)
gestational age (jess-TAY-shun-al)
gravidity (gra-VID-ih-tee)
infant
lochia (LOE-kee-uh)
multigravida (MUL-tee-GRAV-ih-duh)
multipara (mul-TIH-pear-uh)
nullipara (nul-IH-pear-uh)
obstetrics (ob-STEH-triks)
parity (PEAR-ih-tee)
position
postpartum (poest-PAR-tum)
preeclampsia (PREE-ih-KLAMP-see-ah)
prenatal (pree-NAY-tul)
presentation
preterm birth
primigravida (PRIH-mih-GRAV-ih-duh)
primipara (prih-MIH-pear-uh)
puerperium (PYOO-ur-PEER-ee-um)
quickening
term birth
toxemia (tok-SEE-mee-uh)
trimester (try-MES-ter)

Introduction to the Gynecologic Examination and Prenatal Care

The medical assistant should have knowledge of gynecology and obstetrics to assist in examinations and treatments in these specialties. Gynecologic examinations are frequently and routinely performed in the medical office. Prenatal care consists of a series of scheduled medical office visits for the promotion of the health of the mother and fetus during the pregnancy. Obtaining the patient's cooperation makes the gynecologic or prenatal examination proceed more smoothly and, as a result, makes the patient feel more comfortable. The medical assistant can help by explaining the purpose of the procedure to the patient. If the patient understands the beneficial results to be derived from the examination, she is more likely to participate as required. This chapter discusses the gynecologic examination and prenatal care and the procedures involved in both.

GYNECOLOGIC EXAMINATION
GYNECOLOGY

Gynecology is the branch of medicine that deals with diseases of the reproductive organs of women. The gynecologic examination is frequently and routinely performed in the medical office and generally includes a *breast examination* and a *pelvic examination.*

The purpose of the gynecologic examination is to assess the health of the female reproductive organs to detect early signs of disease, leading to early diagnosis and treatment.

This examination may be part of a general physical examination, or it may be performed by itself. Although assisting with the gynecologic examination is a routine procedure for the medical assistant, the patient may not consider it a routine examination. To reduce apprehension or embarrassment, the medical assistant should fully explain the procedure to the patient and offer to answer any questions.

Terms Related to Gynecology

The medical assistant should have a thorough knowledge of the female reproductive system (Figure 8-1) and the following terms associated with the female reproductive system:

Amenorrhea   Absence or cessation of the menstrual period. Amenorrhea occurs normally before puberty, during pregnancy, and after menopause.

Cervix   The lower narrow end of the uterus that opens into the vagina.

Colposcopy   Examination of the cervix using a colposcope (a lighted instrument with a magnifying lens).

Dysmenorrhea   Pain associated with the menstrual period.

Dyspareunia   Pain in the vagina or pelvis experienced by a woman during sexual intercourse.

Dysplasia   The growth of abnormal cells. Dysplasia is a precancerous condition that may or may not develop into cancer.

Menopause   The permanent cessation of menstruation, which usually occurs between the ages of 45 and 55 with an average age of 51.

Menorrhagia   Excessive bleeding during a menstrual period, in the number of days, the amount of blood, or both. Also called *dysfunctional uterine bleeding* (DUB).

Metrorrhagia   Bleeding between menstrual periods.

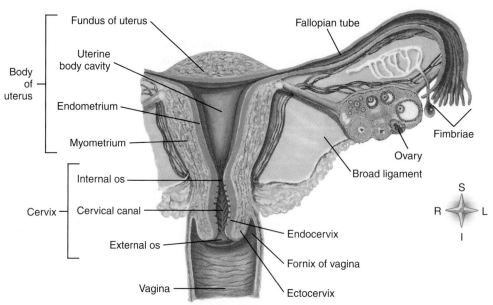

Figure 8-1. The female reproductive system. (Modified from Thibodeau GA, Patton KT: Anatomy and physiology, ed 5, St Louis, 2003, Mosby.)

Perimenopause   Before the onset of menopause, the phase during which a woman with regular periods changes to irregular cycles and increased periods of amenorrhea.

Perineum   The external region between the vaginal orifice and the anus in a female and between the scrotum and the anus in a male.

Risk factor   Anything that increases an individual's chance of developing a disease. Some risk factors (e.g., smoking) can be avoided, but others cannot (e.g., age and family history).

BREAST EXAMINATION

The physician usually begins the gynecologic examination with the breast examination. The medical assistant is responsible for assisting the patient into the supine position. The physician inspects the breasts and nipples for swelling, dimpling, puckering, and change in skin texture. The nipples are checked for abnormalities such as bleeding and discharge. The breasts and axillary lymph nodes are palpated for lumps, hard knots, and thickening.

The patient should know how to examine her breasts at home for the presence of lumps and other changes with a breast self-examination (BSE). Most breast cancers are first discovered by women themselves. The American College of Obstetricians and Gynecologists recommends that women 20 years of age and older examine their breasts once every month. The medical assistant may be responsible for instructing the patient in this procedure at the medical office (Procedure 8-1). If a lump or other change is discovered,

Putting It All into Practice

My Name is Yin-Ling Wu, and I am a Registered Medical Assistant. I work with 10 physicians in a large clinic. My primary job responsibilities include documenting patient histories and complaints, taking vital signs, and assisting physicians with patient examinations and procedures.

One experience that has probably affected me more than any other occurred while I was working in obstetrics and gynecology. A full-term prenatal patient came in for a routine weekly appointment late one afternoon. By this stage of the pregnancy, you have seen the patients often enough to develop a more personal relationship. I was obtaining her vital signs and asking the routine questions when she said, "I haven't felt the baby move for 2 days." This immediately sent up a red flag, but I was careful to hide my concern until I was out of her room. The physician was unable to pick up any fetal heart tones, so she immediately did an ultrasound. It showed that the fetus had died. The patient was alone and extremely upset. I stayed with her until her family came.

Although little medical treatment was given during this time, I do believe that my medical assisting training and experience made a difference in my knowing what to do and say to help comfort the patient through this crisis. ■

Answer questions patients have about breast self-examination.

When should I examine my breasts?
Beginning at age 20, the American College of Obstetricians and Gynecologists recommends that you examine your breasts once a month according to your reproductive status as follows:

- **Regular periods:** Approximately 2 to 3 days after your menstrual period has ended. At this time, your breasts are least likely to be tender or swollen, and it will be easier to perform the examination.
- **No periods (because of menopause or hysterectomy):** Any day of the month is fine; however, it helps to choose a particular day, such as the first day of the month or an easy-to-remember date such as your birthday.
- **Hormone therapy:** If you are taking hormones, talk to your physician about when to examine your breasts.

Why is it important to examine my breasts every month?
The purpose of a breast self-examination is not just to find lumps, but also to notice when there are changes in your breasts. The best way to do this is to become as familiar as possible with your breasts. By examining your breasts once every month, you will learn what is normal for you, and it will be easier to notice changes.

What is considered normal?
Breast tissue normally feels a little lumpy and uneven. The left and right breasts may not be the same size; most women's breasts are slightly different in size. Many women have a normal thickening or ridge of firm tissue under the lower curve of the breast where it attaches to the chest wall. Throughout your life, changes also can occur in the size, shape, and feel of your breasts because of aging, weight changes, the menstrual cycle, pregnancy, breastfeeding, and use of birth control pills or other hormones.

What should be reported to the physician?
Early breast cancer does not usually cause pain. When breast cancer first develops, there may be no symptoms at all. As the cancer grows, it can cause changes that should be reported to the physician. Contact your physician immediately if any of the following changes occurs:

- Any new lump, hard knot, or thickening in the breast or underarm area
- A change in the size or shape of the breast
- A puckering or dimpling of the skin of the breast or nipple
- A change in skin texture of the breast or nipple
- A nipple that becomes retracted (pulled in)
- A discharge or bleeding from the nipple

the woman should schedule an appointment with her physician as soon as possible. Most breast lumps are not cancerous, but the physician must make that diagnosis.

PELVIC EXAMINATION

The purpose of the pelvic examination is to assess the size, shape, and location of the reproductive organs and to detect the presence of disease. The pelvic examination consists of the following components:

- Inspection of the external genitalia, vagina, and cervix
- Collection of a specimen for a Pap test
- Bimanual pelvic examination
- Rectal-vaginal examination

For the pelvic examination, the patient is positioned in the lithotomy position. The patient lies on the table on her back, with her feet in the stirrups and her buttocks at the bottom edge of the table. The stirrups should be level with the examining table and pulled out approximately 1 foot from the edge of the table. The patient's knees should be bent and relaxed, and her thighs should be rotated outward as far as is comfortable. This position helps relax the vulva and perineum and facilitates insertion of the vaginal speculum. The patient should be properly draped to reduce exposure and to provide warmth. The lithotomy position is difficult to maintain, and the patient should not be placed in this position until the physician is ready to begin the examination.

The medical assistant can help the patient relax during the examination by telling her to breathe deeply, slowly, and evenly through the mouth. If the patient is relaxed, it is easier for the physician to insert the vaginal speculum and to perform the bimanual pelvic examination; it also is more comfortable for the patient. It is recommended that the medical assistant remain in the room during the pelvic examination to provide legal protection for the physician, to reassure the patient, and to assist the physician. Procedure

8-2 outlines the medical assistant's role in assisting the physician with a gynecologic examination.

Inspection of External Genitalia, Vagina, and Cervix

The physician begins the pelvic examination with inspection of the external genitalia. The **vulva** is inspected for swelling, ulceration, and redness.

Next, the physician inserts a vaginal speculum into the vagina. Specula are available in two forms—metal and plastic. Metal specula are reusable and must be sanitized and sterilized after each use. Plastic specula are disposable and are designed to be used only once. Vaginal specula come in three sizes—small, medium, and large. The physician determines the size required based on the physical and sexual maturity of the patient. The function of the speculum is to hold the walls of the vagina apart to allow visual inspection of the vagina and cervix (Figure 8-2).

A metal vaginal speculum is cold and should be warmed before use by placing it on a heating pad or by storing it in a warming drawer. A warmed speculum is more comfortable for the patient. It is important not to overheat the speculum, however; one that is too hot is just as uncomfortable as one that is too cold. A disposable plastic speculum does not hold the cold and does not need to be warmed.

The physician inspects the vagina and cervix for color, lacerations, ulcerations, redness, nodules, and discharge. If an abnormal discharge is present, the physician obtains a specimen for microbiologic examination. Examples of pathologic conditions that produce a discharge include vaginal infections such as *trichomoniasis, candidiasis, chlamydia,* and *gonorrhea,* which are discussed in detail later.

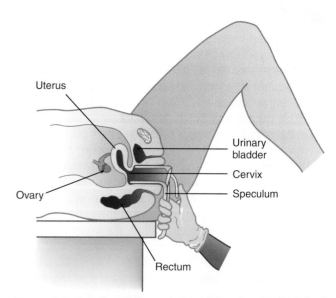

Figure 8-2. Insertion of the vaginal speculum for visualization of the vagina and cervix.

Highlight on Breast Cancer

Breast cancer is one of the most common types of cancer among American women. The American Cancer Society estimates that one of every nine women in the United States develops breast cancer at some point in her lifetime. Every year, more than 200,000 women learn they have breast cancer, and about 40,000 of them die from the disease. Most women (82%) diagnosed with breast cancer are older than 50 years old, but breast cancer does occur in younger women.

Survival Rate

The 5-year survival rate for breast cancer that has spread to a distant site in the body (metastasized) is only 21%. The 5-year survival rate for small, localized tumors is 94%. If the cancer has spread to lymph nodes in the region of the breast, the 5-year survival rate is 73%. These encouraging statistics are the result of advances in the early detection of breast cancer and better treatment, including improved surgical procedures, radiation therapy, chemotherapy, hormonal therapy, and biologic therapy.

Recommendations for Early Detection

A three-point program is recommended for the early detection of breast cancer: (1) monthly breast self-examination, (2) periodic clinical breast examination by a physician, and (3) screening mammography.

Risk Factors

Breast cancer results from the abnormal growth of cells in breast tissue. It occurs more often in the left breast than in the right, and more often in the upper outer quadrant of the breast. The cause of abnormal growths in the breasts is unknown; therefore, every woman should consider herself at risk for breast cancer. Certain factors seem to place a woman at higher than normal risk for breast cancer, however, including the following:

- **Gender.** Women are much more likely than men to develop breast cancer.
- **Age.** The risk of breast cancer increases as women get older. Most women diagnosed with breast cancer are older than age 50.
- **Personal history.** Women with cancer in one breast have a greater chance of developing a new cancer in the other breast or in another part of the same breast.
- **Family history.** A woman's risk of developing breast cancer increases if her mother, sister, or daughter had breast cancer, especially at a young age.
- **Dense breast tissue.** Women with dense breast tissue (meaning they have more glandular tissue than fat tissue as seen on a mammogram) have a higher risk of developing breast cancer.
- **Breast biopsy.** Women who have had a breast biopsy that indicated certain types of benign breast disease (characterized by atypical hyperplasia) have an increased risk of developing breast cancer.
- **Breast cancer genes.** A woman who has inherited mutations in breast cancer genes (mutations of the *BRCA1* and *BRCA2* genes) from either parent is more likely to develop breast cancer.
- **Reproductive history.** Women who began menstruating at an early age (before age 12) or who went through menopause at a late age (after age 55) have a slightly increased risk of breast cancer.
- **Childbearing.** Women who have never had a child or women who had their first child late (after age 30) have a slightly increased risk of developing breast cancer.
- **Hormone replacement therapy (HRT).** Studies indicate that the long-term use of estrogen and progesterone combination hormone replacement therapy for relief of menopausal symptoms increases the risk of breast cancer.
- **Radiation treatment.** Women who have had radiation of the chest before age 30 as treatment for another type of cancer (e.g., Hodgkin's disease) have a significantly increased risk of developing breast cancer.
- **Race.** Caucasian women are diagnosed more frequently than Hispanic, Asian, or African American women.
- **Lifestyle factors.** Studies suggest that the use of alcohol (more than two drinks per day) increases the risk of breast cancer. Obesity, especially for women after menopause, also may increase the risk of breast cancer.

Warning Signs

The warning signs of possible breast cancer include a lump, hard knot, or thickening in the breast or armpit; a change in breast color or texture; dimpling or puckering; nipple discharge; changes in the size or shape of the breast; and an enlargement of the lymph nodes.

Diagnosis

A biopsy is the only conclusive method of determining whether a breast lump or suspicious area seen on a mammogram is benign or malignant. A biopsy involves the surgical removal and analysis of all or part of the lump. Biopsy methods include fine needle aspiration biopsy, core needle biopsy (removal of a core of tissue from the lump), vacuum-assisted biopsy (Mammotome), large core biopsy, and open surgical excisional biopsy (removal of all or part of the entire lump). The physician may recommend one or more of these procedures to evaluate a lump or other change in the breast.

Eighty percent of breast lumps are benign. A lump or suspicious area is often the result of a benign breast condition, such as normal hormonal changes, fibrocystic breast disease, or a fibroadenoma. ∎

Pap Test

A Pap test is usually part of the pelvic examination. It is a simple and painless **cytology** evaluation named after its developer, Dr. George Papanicolaou (1883–1962). It is used for the early detection of cervical cancer. Almost all cancers of the cervix can be cured if detected early enough. The Pap test also is used to detect abnormal (**atypical**) cells of the cervix that might develop into cancer if not treated. In some cases, the Pap test can detect cancer of the endometrium; however, it is less reliable in doing so.

The American Cancer Society (ACS) recommends a woman have her first Pap test beginning within 3 years of having vaginal intercourse or at 21 years of age, whichever is earlier. Screening should be performed every year with the direct smear Pap test or every 2 years with the liquid-based Pap test. The ACS guidelines further state that beginning at age 30, women who have tested negative for three or more consecutive Pap tests may be screened every 2 to 3 years. Women who are at high risk for cervical cancer or who have had abnormal Pap test results should continue to be screened annually. Factors that place a woman at a higher risk for cervical cancer include diethylstilbestrol (DES) exposure before birth, human immunodeficiency virus (HIV) infection, and a weakened immune system due to organ transplantation, chemotherapy, or long-term steroid use.

Patient Instructions

A Pap specimen must not be collected from a woman during her menstrual period because the red blood cells obscure the specimen and interfere with an accurate evaluation. The patient should be instructed to schedule her Pap test 10 to 20 days after the first day of her last menstrual period. The patient should be told not to douche or insert tampons, medications, or contraceptive spermicides into the vagina for 2 days before having a Pap test. Douching and tampon insertion reduce the number of cells available for analysis, and vaginal medications and spermicides change the pH of the vagina, making the specimen nonrepresentative or invalid. The patient also should be told to abstain from sexual intercourse for 2 days before the Pap test. Recent sexual intercourse can produce inflammatory changes that can interfere with visualization of abnormal cells that may be present.

Specimen Collection

The outermost layer of the cervix consists of a thin, flat layer of cells, approximately 10 layers thick, known as *squamous epithelial cells*. With the speculum in place, the physician collects a sampling of these cells for evaluation by the laboratory. A scraping of epithelial cells is taken from the ectocervix and the endocervix (see Figure 8-1). A scraping of cells also can be collected from the vagina; however, this is not usually done unless the physician has observed a lesion on the vaginal wall, or the maturation index is to be determined. The technique used by the physician to collect the epithelial cells is described next.

Vaginal Specimen

If a vaginal specimen is needed, it is collected first, before the cervical and endocervical specimens are obtained. The rounded end of the plastic spatula is used to collect the specimen. If a routine vaginal specimen is being obtained, it is collected from the vaginal pool in the posterior fornix of the vagina, which is located just below the cervix (Figure 8-3, *A*). If the physician is collecting a specimen from a lesion on the vaginal wall, a scraping of cells is taken from the area of the lesion. To obtain a specimen for determination of the maturation index (discussed later), the physician obtains the vaginal specimen from the upper one third of the lateral vaginal wall.

Cervical Specimen

The physician obtains the cervical specimen by placing the S-shaped end of the plastic spatula just inside the cervical canal at the **external os** and rotating the blade 360 degrees over the surface of the ectocervix at the squamocolumnar junction, where cervical cancer is most often found (Figure 8-3, *B*). The ectocervix is the part of the cervix that projects into the vagina and is lined with stratified squamous epithelium.

Endocervical Specimen

The physician collects this specimen from the endocervix. The endocervix consists of the mucous membrane lining the endocervical canal. This is accomplished by inserting an endocervical brush into the endocervical canal and rotating the brush (Figure 8-3, *C*). The endocervical brush is made up of soft bristles designed to be inserted into the canal without causing damage to it.

Preparation Methods

Two methods are used to prepare a specimen for a Pap test. The traditional method is the *direct smear* (Pap smear), and the newer method is the *liquid-based preparation*.

Direct Smear

With the direct smear method, a thin smear of each specimen is spread on a glass slide that has a frosted edge. The medical assistant must label each slide on its frosted edge with a lead pencil according to the source of the specimen as follows: *V (vaginal)*, *C (cervical)*, or *E (endocervical)*. Slides on which all three specimens can be placed also are available. These slides are divided into thirds and are prelabeled with *V*, *C*, and *E*.

The smears must be fixed immediately by flooding the slides with 95% ethyl alcohol or by lightly spraying the slides with a commercial cytology spray fixative. The slides must be fixed before they dry to avoid inaccurate results. The purposes of the fixative are to maintain the normal appearance of the cells; to protect the slides from contaminants in the air, such as dust and bacteria; and to attach the smear firmly to the slide. The cytology fixative must be allowed to dry thoroughly; the slides are then ready for transport to a laboratory for evaluation. To protect the slides

Vaginal Specimen

Vaginal speculum

Posterior fornix

The rounded end of the spatula is used to obtain the vaginal specimen from the posterior fornix of the vagina.

A

Cervical Specimen

External os

Ectocervix

The S-shaped end of the spatula is placed inside the cervical canal and rotated 360 degrees over the surface of the cervix.

B

Endocervical Specimen

Endocervical canal

An endocervical brush is inserted into the endocervical canal and rotated to obtain a specimen.

C

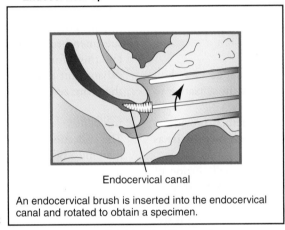

Figure 8-3. Obtaining the Pap specimen.

during transport, they must be placed in a slide container designed especially for this purpose.

Liquid-Based Preparation

A newer method to prepare the specimen for evaluation is the liquid-based preparation. Brand names include Thin-Prep, AutoCyte, and SurePath. Using the liquid-based method improves the quality of the specimen, resulting in fewer slides that are unsatisfactory for evaluation. A better quality specimen also reduces the occurrence of false-negative test results.

The specimen for a liquid-based preparation can be obtained by using the specimen collection technique described earlier. A plastic spatula (S-shaped end) is used to collect the ectocervical specimen, and an endocervical brush is used to collect the endocervical specimen. If a vaginal specimen is needed, it is collected first using the rounded end of the spatula as previously described.

The Pap specimen also can be collected using a broom, a collection device made of flexible plastic. The physician inserts the central bristles of the broom into the endocervical canal deep enough to allow the shorter bristles to contact the outside of the cervix fully. The broom is gently pushed and rotated in a clockwise direction (Figure 8-4). In this way, specimens from the ectocervix and the endocervix can be collected at the same time.

When the Pap specimen has been collected, the medical assistant is responsible for performing one of the following steps depending on the brand of liquid-based preparation being used:

1. Rinse the collection device in the vial of liquid preservative, and discard the collection device (performed with ThinPrep).

2. Remove the tip of the collection device, and deposit it in the vial of preservative. Discard the handle (performed with SurePath).

The preservative maintains the specimen and prevents it from drying out during transport to the laboratory. After it is received by the laboratory, the vial is placed in an automated slide preparation processor. The automated processor performs several important functions. First, it separates the cells from debris present in the specimen, and then it dis-

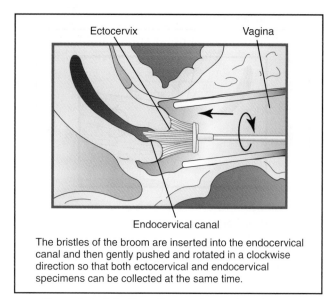

Ectocervix   Vagina

Endocervical canal

The bristles of the broom are inserted into the endocervical canal and then gently pushed and rotated in a clockwise direction so that both ectocervical and endocervical specimens can be collected at the same time.

Figure 8-4. Collecting a Pap specimen using a broom.

perses a representative cell sample onto a slide in a thin, uniform layer. The slide is next immersed in a fixative to maintain the normal appearance of the cells.

The ways in which the liquid-based method provides a better quality specimen than the direct smear method are as follows:

- With the direct smear method, only a small portion of the specimen is smeared on the slide; most of it is thrown away with the collection device. With the liquid-based method, the collection device is rinsed or the tip is deposited in a vial of liquid that preserves all or most of the specimen. Having more of the specimen available allows the laboratory to evaluate it better.
- When a Pap specimen is collected, it includes unnecessary debris, such as blood, mucus, and inflammatory cells. With the direct smear method, the debris is smeared on the slide along with the cells. This debris may obscure the cells in the specimen, making it difficult to evaluate them. With the liquid-based method, the automated processor removes a large portion of the debris from the specimen and transfers the cells to a glass slide. This provides the cytotechnologist with a clear, unobstructed view of the epithelial cells.
- With the direct smear method, the cells have a tendency to clump together when they are smeared on the slide, making them more difficult to evaluate. With the liquid-based method, the automated processor disperses the cells onto the slide in a thin, even layer. In this way, the cells are spread out, making it easier for the cytotechnologist to evaluate them.

Cytology Request

A cytology request must accompany all Pap specimens. Figure 8-5 is an example of a cytology request form. The medical assistant is responsible for completing the request, which includes the following categories.

General Information

General information includes the physician's name, address, and phone number and the patient's name, address, identification number, date of birth, and date of last menstrual period (LMP). Insurance information also is required in this section for third-party billing.

Date and Time of Collection

The date and time of collection indicate to the laboratory the number of days that have passed since the collection, providing the laboratory with information regarding the freshness of the specimen.

Collection Method

Under the collection method category, the medical assistant must indicate whether the specimen is a direct smear (Pap smear) or a liquid-based preparation.

Source of the Specimen

The purpose of this category is to identify the origin of the specimen because it is impossible for the laboratory to obtain this information by looking at the specimen. The medical assistant checks one or more of the following boxes on the form: cervical, endocervical, or vaginal.

Collection Technique

The collection device or devices used to obtain the specimen must be indicated. The medical assistant checks one or more of the following boxes on the form: spatula, brush, or broom.

Patient History

Information on the present and past health status of the patient is specified under the patient history category. The medical assistant must check the following boxes that apply to the patient: pregnant, lactating, oral contraceptives, postmenopausal, hormone replacement therapy, postmenopausal bleeding, postpartum, intrauterine device (IUD), postcoital bleeding, DES (diethylstilbestrol) exposure, and previous abnormal smear. This information assists the laboratory in evaluating the specimen.

Previous Treatment

Any previous treatment for a precancerous or cancerous condition of the cervix is indicated under this category. The medical assistant checks the appropriate box on the form if any of the following procedures have been performed on the patient: colposcopy and biopsy, cryosurgery, loop electrocautery excision procedure (LEEP), laser vaporization, conization, hysterectomy, radiation, and chemotherapy.

Evaluation of the Pap Specimen

Before a Pap slide can be evaluated, it must be stained by a laboratory technician. Staining is performed on slides prepared by the direct smear method and the liquid-based method. The purpose of staining is to allow better viewing of the morphology of the epithelial cells. The slide is studied under a microscope for evidence of abnormalities by a spe-

GYN CYTOLOGY REQUISITION

THOMAS WOODSIDE, MD
501 MAIN ST
ST. LOUIS, MO 63146
(314) 555-0093

PATIENT INFO

| Patient's Name (Last) | (First) | (MI) | Date of Birth MO | DAY | YR | Collection Time : AM PM | Collection Date MO | DAY | YR | Patient's ID # |

Patient's Address   Phone

City   State   ZIP

RESP. PARTY

Name of Responsible Party (if different from patient)

Address of Responsible Party   APT #

City   State   ZIP

INSURANCE

Patient's Relationship to Responsible Party   ☐ 1. Self   ☐ 2. Spouse   ☐ 3. Child   ☐ 4. Other

Insurance Comany Name	Plan	Carrier Code
Subscriber/Member #	Location	Group #
Insurance Address		Physician's Provider #
City	State	ZIP
Employer's Name or Number	Insured SSN	

Diagnosis/Signs/Symptoms in ICD-9 Format (Highest Specificity)

REQUIRED

ICD-9 codes are the internationally accepted method of describing the clinical picture of the patient. All diagnoses should be provided by the ordering physician or his or her authorized designee. The following is a partial list of of common diagnoses in ICD-9 format. Most third party payers require an ICD-9 code to indicate the medical necessity of the test(s) and or profile(s) ordered. For a complete list of all ICD-9 codes, please refer to a current ICD-9 manual.

V76.2	Routine Cervical Pap Smear	616.0	Cervicitis	626.8	Abnormal Bleeding
V15.89	High Risk Cervical Screening	616.10	Vaginitis	627.1	Postmenopausal Bleeding
V22.2	Pregnancy	617.0	Endometriosis, Uterus	627.3	Atrophic Vaginitis
079.4	Human Papillomavirus	622.1	Dysplasia, Cervix	795.0	Abnormal Cervical Pap Smear
180.0	Malignant Neoplasm, Cervix	623.0	Dysplasia, Vagina		

COLLECTION METHOD

Liquid-Based Prep

192055 ☐ ThinPrep Pap Test

192039 ☐ ThinPrep Pap Test w/reflex to HPV Hybrid Capture when ASC-US or SIL

192047 ☐ ThinPrep Pap Test w/reflex to high-risk only HPV Hybrid Capture when ASC-US

Pap Smear
009100 ☐ 1 Slide   009191 ☐ 2 Slides

Pap Smear and Maturation Index
009209 ☐ 1 Slide   190074 ☐ 2 Slides

SOURCE OF SPECIMEN

☐ Cervical
☐ Endocervical
☐ Vaginal

Date LMP

___/___/___
Mo   Day   Year

COLLECTION TECHNIQUE

☐ Spatula
☐ Brush
☐ Broom
☐ Other _____

PATIENT HISTORY

☐ Pregnant
☐ Lactating
☐ Oral Contraceptives
☐ Postmenopausal
☐ Hormone Replacement Therapy

☐ PMP Bleeding
☐ Postpartum
☐ IUD
☐ Postcoital Bleeding
☐ DES Exposure
☐ Previous Abnormal Pap Test

☐ Other _____

PREVIOUS TREATMENT   Date/Results

☐ None
☐ Colposcopy and Bx   _____
☐ Cryosurgery   _____
☐ LEEP   _____
☐ Laser Vaporization   _____
☐ Conization   _____
☐ Hysterectomy   _____
☐ Radiation   _____
☐ Chemotherapy   _____

Figure 8-5. Cytology request form.

cially trained technician, known as a *cytotechnologist.* When an abnormality is detected, it is reviewed by a *cytopathologist* (a physician specializing in pathology), who makes a final evaluation. The findings are recorded on a cytology report and returned to the medical office.

A more recent development in the evaluation of Pap slides is the use of automated cytology computer-imaging devices. An abnormal slide may contain only a few abnormal cells among thousands of normal cells. Because of this, these abnormal cells may be missed during the evaluation by the cytotechnologist. A cytology computer-imaging device is able to examine every cell on the slide and select and display cells that appear "most abnormal." The cytotechnologist can evaluate these cells further under a microscope. In this way, the cytotechnologist is able to focus his or her expertise and decision making on preselected areas of the slide.

Maturation Index

The maturation index must be performed on a sampling of cells taken from the upper third of the lateral vaginal wall. The *maturation index* refers to the percentage of parabasal, intermediate, and superficial cells present in the specimen. The maturation index provides the physician with an endocrine evaluation of the patient, which can assist in evaluating the cause of infertility, menopausal or postmenopausal bleeding, or amenorrhea and can help assess the results of treatment with hormones. If the physician orders a maturation index along with the Pap test, the medical assistant must indicate this on the cytology request by checking the box labeled *Maturation Index* (see Figure 8-5). Numerous factors affect the results of the maturation index; it is important to indicate on the cytology request the presence of abnormal bleeding; hormone treatment; or treatment with digitalis, corticosteroids, or thyroid medication.

Cytology Report

The Bethesda System (TBS) is the standard for reporting the results of a Pap test on the cytology report (Figure 8-6). The National Cancer Institute in Bethesda, Maryland, developed this system. It provides a detailed cytologic description, rather than a numerical result (as with the previous

---

GYN CYTOLOGY REPORT

RIVERVIEW MEDICAL LABORATORY
DEPARTMENT OF PATHOLOGY
2501 GRANT AVENUE
ST. LOUIS, MO 63146
(314) 555–3443

PATIENT:	Heather Jones
PATIENT NO:	45876
DOB:	10/20/65
SUBMITTING:	T. Woodside, MD

Date of Specimen: 7/01/12

Date Received: 7/02/12

Date Reported: 7/06/12

SPECIMEN TYPE

[X] ThinPrep   [ ] Conventional Pap Smear

Performed By: Richard McVay, Cytotechnologist   **Checked By:** Melissa Wagner, Pathologist

SPECIMEN ADEQUACY

[X] Satisfactory for Evaluation
[ ] Unsatisfactory for Evaluation

GENERAL CATEGORIZATION

[ ] Negative for Intraepithelial Lesion or Malignancy (*see Interpretation/Result*)
[X] Epithelial Cell Abnormality (*see Interpretation/Result*)
[ ] Other (*see Interpretation/Result*)

INTERPRETATION/RESULT

A. BENIGN CELLULAR CHANGES

[ ] Infection:
    [ ] Trichomonas vaginalis
    [ ] Fungal organisms morphologically compatible w/ Candida species
    [ ] Cellular changes associated with herpes simplex virus
    [ ] Bacterial infection morphologically compatible with gardnerella
    [ ] Cytoplasmic inclusions suggestive of chlamydia

[ ] Reactive changes
    [ ] Without inflammation
    [ ] With inflammation
    [ ] Atrophy with inflammation (atrophic vaginitis)
    [ ] Radiation effect
    [ ] Repair
    [ ] Hyperkeratosis
    [ ] Parakeratosis

B. EPITHELIAL CELL ABNORMALITIES

[X] Squamous Cell
    [X] Atypical Squamous Cells of Undetermined Significance (ASC-US)
    [ ] Atypical Squamous Cells of Higher Risk (ASC-H)
    [ ] Low-Grade Squamous Intraepithelial Lesion (LSIL)
    [ ] High-Grade Squamous Intraepithelial Lesion (HSIL)
    [ ] Squamous Cell Carcinoma
[ ] Glandular Cell
    [ ] Atypical Glandular Cells of Undetermined Significance (AGUS)
    [ ] Adenocarcinoma

Figure 8-6. Cytology report form (The Bethesda System).

class I through V system). For this reason, TBS is a more effective means of communicating the results of the Pap test to the physician. TBS separates the cytology report into the following categories:

1. **Specimen Type.** This category identifies whether the specimen is a conventional cell sample (Pap smear) or a liquid-based cell sample (ThinPrep).

2. **Specimen Adequacy.** This category refers to the quality of the specimen collected by the physician. The specimen is described using one of the following classifications:
   - **Satisfactory for Evaluation.** This indicates that the specimen was of sufficient sampling and quality for a comprehensive assessment of the cells.
   - **Unsatisfactory for Evaluation.** This indicates that the overall sampling or quality of the specimen was inadequate. A reason is given for the inability to evaluate the Pap slide, such as too few cells were collected or the presence of blood or inflammation is obscuring the cells.

3. **General Categorization.** This category provides the medical office with a quick review of the report. The following classifications are used to categorize the specimen:
   - **Negative for Intraepithelial Lesion or Malignancy.** This indicates that the epithelial cells were normal and that there were no precancerous or cancerous findings. This classification also is assigned to a specimen that exhibits certain benign (noncancerous) changes. Benign changes can be caused by vaginal infections, such as bacterial vaginosis, chlamydia, trichomoniasis, candidiasis, and herpes. Benign changes also can be caused by inflammation resulting from the normal cell repair process, radiation, and chemotherapy. Any benign findings of importance (e.g., vaginal infections) are described in detail

in the Interpretation/Result section of the cytology report.
   - **Epithelial Cell Abnormality.** This classification indicates abnormal cell changes. The abnormality is described in detail in the Interpretation/Result section of the report.
   - **Other.** This classification is used to indicate that no abnormality was found in the cells, but the findings indicate some increased risk. The presence of normal-appearing endometrial cells in a postmenopausal woman may indicate an abnormality of the endometrium. These findings are described in detail in the Interpretation/Result section of the report.

4. **Interpretation/Result.** This part of the report provides the physician with a detailed description of findings. This includes any significant benign changes (e.g., vaginal infections) and any abnormal changes in the epithelial cells. Table 8-1 lists and describes the findings most frequently reported.

5. **Automated Review.** This category indicates whether the specimen was evaluated using an automated computer-imaging device. The name of the device and the results are specified in this section.

6. **Ancillary Testing.** This category is used if an additional test method is used to evaluate the specimen. If abnormal cells are detected on the Pap slide, a human papillomavirus (HPV) test may be performed. The name of the test method and the results would be reported under this category.

Bimanual Pelvic Examination

After obtaining the smear for the Pap test, the physician withdraws the speculum and performs a bimanual pelvic examination. The physician inserts the index and middle

Table 8-1 Pap Test Results

Test Result	Interpretation
Negative for intraepithelial lesion or malignancy	Epithelial cells were normal, and there were no precancerous or cancerous findings.
Atypical squamous cells of undetermined significance (ASC-US)	Cells are only slightly abnormal. Nature and cause of abnormality cannot be determined. These slightly altered cells usually return to normal on their own, resulting in negative results on subsequent Pap tests.
Atypical squamous cells of higher risk (ASC-H)	Minor abnormal changes in cells with unknown causes, but at risk of progressing to high-grade lesion (HSIL). Further testing is required to determine whether this is a minor condition or one that may progress to HSIL.
Low-grade squamous intraepithelial lesion (LSIL)	Abnormal cells that show definite minor changes but are unlikely to progress to cancer (general term for this is *mild dysplasia*). LSIL may be caused by HPV infection, but of a type that is not likely to lead to cervical cancer.
High-grade squamous intraepithelial lesion (HSIL)	Abnormal cell changes that have a higher likelihood of progressing to cancer. Although not cancerous yet, abnormal cells may become cancerous if treatment is not obtained (general term for this is *moderate-to-severe dysplasia*). HSIL is often caused by HPV infection of a type associated with cervical cancer.
Carcinoma	Usually means patient has cervical cancer. Most women with cervical cancer also test positive for HPV infection.

HPV, Human papillomavirus.

fingers of a lubricated gloved hand into the vagina. The fingers of the other hand are placed on the woman's lower abdomen. Between the two hands, the physician can palpate the size, shape, and position of the uterus and ovaries and can detect tenderness or lumps (Figure 8-7).

Rectal-Vaginal Examination

The last part of the pelvic examination is a rectal-vaginal examination. The physician inserts one gloved finger into the vagina and another gloved finger into the rectum to obtain information about the tone and alignment of the pelvic organs and the **adnexal** region (ovaries, fallopian tubes, and ligaments of the uterus). The presence of hemorrhoids, fistulas, and fissures also can be noted. During this examination, the physician may want to obtain some fecal material from the rectum to test for occult blood in the stool, which requires a guaiac slide test (e.g., Hemoccult). This is typically performed on women beginning at 40 years of age. The medical assistant is responsible for assisting with the collection and testing the specimen for occult blood. This procedure (fecal occult blood testing) is presented in detail in Chapter 13.

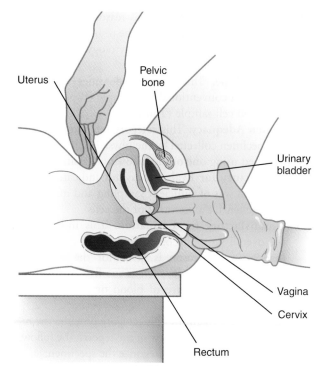

Figure 8-7. The bimanual pelvic examination.

 PROCEDURE 8-1   Breast Self-Examination Instructions

Outcome Instruct a patient in the procedure for performing a breast self-examination.

Equipment/Supplies

- Small pillow

1. **Procedural Step.** Greet the patient and introduce yourself. Identify the patient and inform the patient that you will be showing her how to perform a breast self-examination. Discuss with her the purpose of a breast self-examination and when to examine the breasts (see the box *Patient Teaching: Breast Self-Examination*).

2. **Procedural Step.** Explain to the patient that a complete breast self-examination should be performed in three ways—before a mirror, lying down, and in the shower.
   Principle. Using three methods results in a thorough examination, making it more likely that breast changes will be detected.

   Instruct the patient in the procedure for performing a breast self-examination as follows:

Before a Mirror

3. **Procedural Step.** Remove clothing from the waist up. Stand in front of a large mirror with your arms relaxed at your sides. Observe each breast for the following:
   a. Change in size or shape
   b. Swelling, puckering, or dimpling of the skin

   c. Change in skin texture
   d. Retraction of the nipple
   e. Changes in size or position of one nipple compared with the other
   Principle. Puckering and dimpling of the skin or retraction of the nipple may mean that a tumor is pulling the skin inward.

4. **Procedural Step.** Slowly raise your arms over your head, and repeat the same inspection listed in Procedural Step 3.

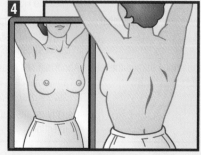

Raise your arms over your head.

PROCEDURE 8-1   Breast Self-Examination Instructions—cont'd

Principle. When the arms are moved at the same time into the same positions, both breasts and nipples should react to the movement in the same way. A change in one breast (e.g., dimpling or puckering of the skin) and not the other should be reported to your physician.

5. Procedural Step. Rest your palms on your hips and press down firmly to flex your chest muscles. Repeat the inspection in Procedural Step 3.

Principle. Flexing the chest muscles allows abnormalities to become more apparent.

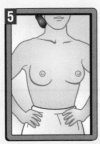

Press down firmly to flex the chest muscles.

6. Procedural Step. Gently squeeze the nipple of each breast with your fingertips and look for a discharge.

Lying Down

7. Procedural Step. To examine the right breast, lie on your back and place a small pillow (or folded towel) under your right shoulder. Place your right hand behind your head.

Principle. The purpose of this step is to flatten the breast and distribute the breast tissue more evenly on the chest, making it easier to palpate the breast tissue.

8. Procedural Step. Extend your left hand with the fingers held flat. The pads of the middle three fingers of the left hand are used to perform the examination. The finger pads include the top third of each finger. Do not use the tips of the fingers. Use small rotating motions (about the size of a dime) and continuous firm pressure with the finger pads.

Principle. The finger pads are more sensitive than the fingertips, making it easier to detect an abnormality.

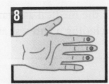

Use the pads of the middle three fingers.

9. Procedural Step. Use one of the following patterns to move around the breast: circular, vertical strip, or wedge. Choose the pattern that is easiest for you. When you have chosen a pattern, use the same pattern each time you examine your breasts.

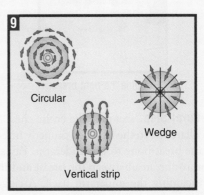

Use one of three patterns to examine the breasts.

Circular
a. Visualize the breast as a clock face.
b. Start at the outside top edge of the breast.
c. Proceed clockwise around the entire outer rim of the breast until your fingers return to the starting point.
d. Move in about 1 inch toward the nipple, and make the same circling motion again.
e. Move around the breast in smaller and smaller circles until you reach the nipple.

Vertical Strip
a. Mentally divide the breast into strips.
b. Start in the underarm area and slowly move your fingers downward until they are below the breast.
c. Move your fingers about 1 inch toward the middle, and slowly move back up.
d. Repeat until the entire breast has been examined.

Wedge
a. Mentally divide your breast into wedges, similar to the pieces of a pie.
b. Starting at the outer edge of the breast, move your fingers toward the nipple and back to the edge of the breast.
c. Check your entire breast, covering one small wedge-shaped section at a time.

Principle. Using a specific pattern ensures that the entire breast is examined.

10. Procedural Step. Holding the middle three fingers of your hand together with the thumb extended, use your finger pads and the pattern you selected to examine the right breast thoroughly. Press firmly enough to feel the different breast tissues. The breast should be palpated for lumps, hard knots, and thickening. Breast tissue normally feels a little lumpy and uneven.

Continued

PROCEDURE 8-1   Breast Self-Examination Instructions—cont'd

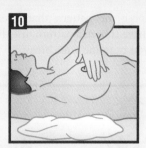

Examine the right breast.

11. Procedural Step. Examine the entire chest area from your collarbone to the base of a properly fitted bra and from the breastbone to the underarm. Pay special attention to the area between the breast and the underarm, including the underarm itself. A ridge of firm tissue in the lower curve of the breast is normal. Continue the examination until every part of the breast has been examined, including the nipple.
Principle. An enlarged node in the armpit also can be a sign of breast cancer even if nothing can be felt in the breast.

12. Procedural Step. Repeat this procedure on the left breast. Place a small pillow (or folded towel) under the left shoulder, and place your left hand behind your head. Use the finger pads of the right hand to examine the left breast.

In the Shower

13. Procedural Step. Gently lather each breast.
Principle. Fingers glide easily over wet, soapy skin, making it easier to detect changes in the breast.

14. Procedural Step. Place your right hand behind your head. Extend your left hand with the fingers held flat. With the finger pads of the middle three fingers, use small rotating motions (about the size of a dime) and continuous firm pressure with the finger pads to examine the right breast. Use your preferred pattern (circular, vertical strip, or wedge) to palpate for lumps, hard knots, and thickening. Examine the area between

the breast and the underarm, including the underarm itself.
Principle. The upright position makes it easier to examine the upper and outer portions of the breast.

15. Procedural Step. Repeat the procedure on the left breast. Place the left arm behind the head, and use the right fingers to examine the left breast.

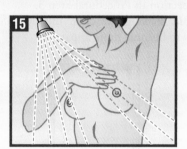

Examine the breasts in the shower.

16. Procedural Step. Instruct the patient to report lumps and other changes to the physician immediately. Reassure the patient that most breast lumps are not cancerous, but the only way to know for sure is to see the physician as soon as possible.

17. Procedural Step. Chart the procedure. Include the date and time and the type of instructions given to the patient. If you gave a printed instruction sheet or educational brochure to the patient, document this as well.

CHARTING EXAMPLE

Date	
9/7/12	11:00 a.m. Instructions provided for a
	BSE. Pt given a BSE educational brochure.
	———————————— Y. Wu, RMA

PROCEDURE 8-2   Assisting with a Gynecologic Examination

Outcome Assist with a gynecologic examination. The following procedure describes the medical assistant's role in assisting with a gynecologic examination consisting of breast and pelvic examinations, including a Pap test and a fecal occult blood test.

Equipment/Supplies

- Disposable gloves
- Examining gown and drape
- Disposable vaginal speculum
- Water-based lubricant
- Gauze pads

- Hemoccult slide and developing solution
- Tissues
- Cytology request form
- Biohazard specimen transport bag

PROCEDURE 8-2 Assisting with a Gynecologic Examination—cont'd

Direct Smear Method

- Glass slides with frosted edge
- Cytology fixative
- Plastic spatula
- Endocervical brush
- Slide container

Liquid-Prep Method

- Vial with preservative (ThinPrep, SurePath)
- Plastic spatula and endocervical brush or cytology broom

1. **Procedural Step.** Sanitize your hands.
2. **Procedural Step.** Assemble the equipment. Complete as much of the cytology request form as possible. Some information on the form, such as the last menstrual period (LMP), requires input from the patient and must be completed later. Prepare the collection materials as follows:

   Pap Smear Method. Using a lead pencil, identify the slides on the frosted edge with the patient's name and date of birth, the date, and the source of the specimen using the following abbreviations: *V (vaginal)*, *C (cervical)*, and *E (endocervical)*.

   Liquid-Prep Method. Check the expiration date on the vial. Label the vial with the date and the patient's name, date of birth, and identification number. The identification number is located on the cytology request form.

   Principle. If the vial is outdated, it should be discarded because it may lead to inaccurate test results.

3. **Procedural Step.** Greet the patient and introduce yourself.

4. **Procedural Step.** Escort the patient to the examining room and ask her to be seated. Identify the patient. Seat yourself so that you are facing the patient. Ask the patient whether she has any problems or concerns, and record the information in the patient's chart. Ask the patient the necessary questions to complete the rest of the cytology request form.

5. **Procedural Step.** Measure the patient's vital signs, height, and weight, and chart the results.

6. **Procedural Step.** Instruct and prepare the patient for the examination as follows:

   a. Ask the patient whether she needs to empty the bladder before the examination. If a urine specimen is needed, instruct the patient in the proper collection of the specimen.

   b. Provide the patient with a patient gown. Instruct the patient to remove all clothing and to put on the patient gown with the opening in front. If the patient is wearing socks, tell her she can keep them on. Offer assistance if you sense the patient may have trouble undressing.

   c. Tell the patient to have a seat on the examining table after she has put on the examining gown.

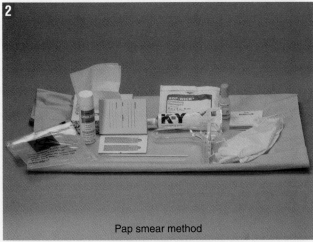

Pap smear method

Assemble equipment.

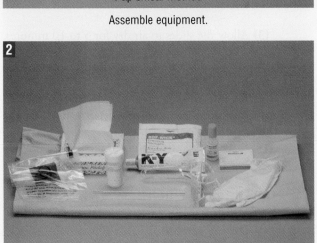

Liquid-prep tray set-up

Assemble equipment.

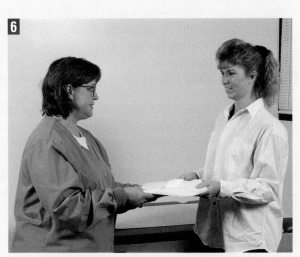

Instruct and prepare the patient for the examination.

Continued

PROCEDURE 8-2   Assisting with a Gynecologic Examination—cont'd

d. Inform the patient that the physician will be with her soon, and leave the room to give her privacy.

Principle. An empty bladder makes the examination easier and is more comfortable for the patient. Wearing socks helps keep the patient's feet warm during the examination.

7. Procedural Step. Make the medical record available for review by the physician. The medical office has a designated location where the record is placed, such as a small shelf mounted on the wall next to the outside of the examining room door or a chart holder on the outside of the examining room door. Position the medical record so that patient-identifiable information is not visible.

Principle: Before going into the room, the physician will want to review the patient's measurements and urine test results documented by the medical assistant. The Health Insurance Portability and Accountability Act (HIPAA) requires protection of a patient's health information.

8. Procedural Step. Check to make sure the patient is ready to be seen by the physician. Before entering a patient's room, always knock lightly on the door to let the patient know you are getting ready to enter the room. Inform the physician that the patient is ready. This may be done using a color-coded flagging system mounted on the wall next to the examining room.

9. Procedural Step. Assist the patient into a supine position, and properly drape her for the breast examination.

10. Procedural Step. Assist the patient into the lithotomy position for the pelvic examination.

11. Procedural Step. Prepare the vaginal speculum by removing it from the warming drawer and performing one of the following:

Pap Smear Method: Moisten the blades of the speculum with warm water.

Liquid Prep Method: Thinly lubricate the blades of the speculum with a water-based lubricant. Never apply lubricant to the tip of the speculum.

Principle. Preparing the vaginal speculum facilitates its insertion into the vagina.

12. Procedural Step. Prepare the light for the physician as follows:

a. *Overhead examination lamp:* Adjust and focus the light for the physician.

b. *Speculum-illumination system:* Snap the light source device into the light holder on the vaginal speculum and turn it on. The lighting system produces a beam of light that shines through the blades of the speculum for visualization of the vagina and cervix.

Principle. Visualization of the vagina and cervix requires direct light.

13. Procedural Step. Hand the vaginal speculum to the physician. Reassure the patient, and help her relax the abdominal muscles during the examination by telling her to breathe deeply, slowly, and evenly through the mouth.

Principle. If the patient is relaxed, the examination proceeds more smoothly and is more comfortable for her.

14. Procedural Step. Apply gloves, and assist with the collection of the Pap specimen as follows:

a. **Direct Smear Method**

  (1) Hold each slide so that the physician can smear the specimen on it.

  [2] Fix each slide immediately after collection by flooding it with 95% ethyl alcohol or by spraying it with a cytology fixative. The slide should be sprayed lightly with a continuous motion from a distance of 5 to 6 inches.

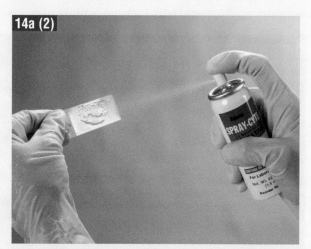

14a (2)

Spray lightly from a distance of 5 to 6 inches.

  (3) Allow the slides to air dry for 5 to 10 minutes, and place them in a protective slide container.

b. **Liquid-Prep Method (ThinPrep) Spatula and Brush Method**

  (1) Remove the cap from the ThinPrep vial, and hold it so that the physician can insert the spatula into the vial.

  [2] Rinse the plastic spatula in the liquid preservative by vigorously swirling it around in the solution 10 times.

  (3) Discard the spatula in a biohazard waste container.

  (4) Hold the vial so that the physician can insert the endocervical brush into the vial.

  [5] Rinse the brush in the liquid preservative by vigorously rotating it in the solution 10 times while pushing the brush against the vial wall.

PROCEDURE 8-2   Assisting with a Gynecologic Examination—cont'd

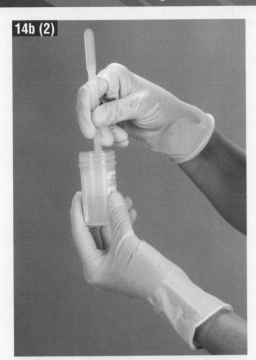

Vigorously swirl the spatula in the preservative.

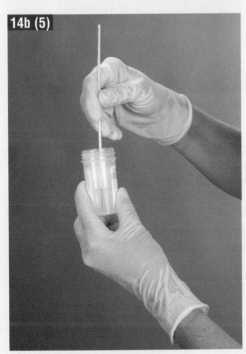

Rotate the brush in the preservative.

Swirl the brush in the solution to further release cellular material.

(6) Discard the brush in a biohazard waste container. Securely tighten the cap so that the torque line on the cap passes the torque line on the vial.

c. **Broom Method**

(1) Remove the cap from the ThinPrep vial, and hold it so that the physician can insert the broom into the vial.

[2] Rinse the broom in the liquid preservative by pushing the broom vigorously into the bottom of the vial 10 times. This motion forces the broom bristles apart, releasing cervical cells into the solution. Swirl the broom vigorously in the liquid preservative to further release cellular material.

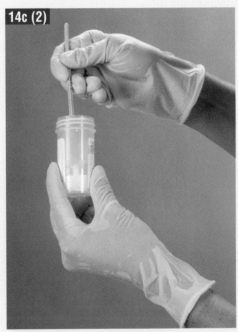

Push the broom vigorously into the bottom of the vial.

(3) Discard the broom in a biohazard waste container. Tighten the cap so that the torque line on the cap passes the torque line on the vial.

d. **Liquid-Prep Method (SurePath)**

(1) Remove the cap from the SurePath vial, and hold it so that the physician can insert the collection device into the vial.

(2) Break off or disconnect the tip of the collection device from the handle.

(3) Discard the handle of the collection device in a waste container.

(4) Repeat the above steps until the physician has collected all of the specimens needed for the Pap test.

(5) Securely tighten the cap on the vial.

Continued

PROCEDURE 8-2

PROCEDURE 8-2   Assisting with a Gynecologic Examination—cont'd

15. Procedural Step. Turn off the examining lamp or disconnect the light source from the vaginal speculum. Discard the disposable vaginal speculum in a biohazard waste container. Apply lubricant to a gauze square. Hold it out so that the physician can apply lubricant to his or her gloves to perform the bimanual and rectal-vaginal examinations. Assist with the collection of the fecal specimen for the fecal occult blood test.
Principle. Applying lubricant to a gauze square (rather than directly to the physician's gloved fingers) prevents the opening of the tube of lubricant from touching the physician's gloves and contaminating the contents of the tube.

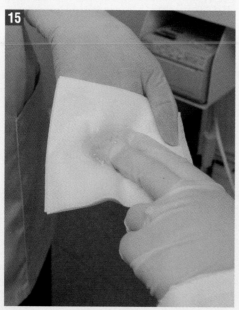

Hold the gauze with the lubricant for the physician.

16. Procedural Step. After the examination, assist the patient into a sitting position, and allow her the opportunity to rest for a moment. Offer the patient tissues to remove excess lubricant from the perineum. Assist the patient off the examining table.
Principle. Some patients (especially geriatric) become dizzy after lying on the examining table and should be allowed to rest after sitting up.

17. Procedural Step. Instruct the patient to get dressed. Tell the patient how and when she will be notified of Pap test results.

18. Procedural Step. Test the fecal occult blood specimen, and chart the results.

19. Procedural Step. Prepare the Pap specimen for transport to the laboratory. Place the specimen (slide container or vial) in a biohazard specimen transport bag, and seal the bag. Insert the cytology requisition into the outside pocket of the bag, and tuck the top of the requisition under the flap. Place the bag in the appropriate location for pickup by the laboratory.

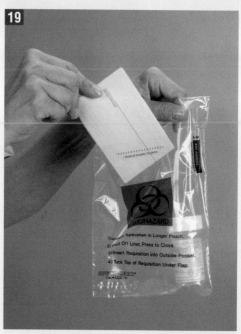

Insert the laboratory request into the outside pocket.

20. Procedural Step. Chart the transport of the Pap specimen to an outside laboratory.

21. Procedural Step. Clean the examining room.

CHARTING EXAMPLE	
Date	
9/7/12	10:00 a.m. Hemoccult: negative.
	Instructions provided for BSE. ThinPrep
	Pap specimen to Medical Center Laboratory
	for cytology. —————————— Y. Wu, RMA

VAGINAL INFECTIONS

The vagina provides a warm, moist environment, which tends to encourage the growth of various organisms that can result in a vaginal infection, or *vaginitis*. If an unusual vaginal discharge is present, suggesting a vaginal infection, a specimen is obtained to identify the invading organism. A specimen of the discharge is collected at the medical office and is evaluated there or placed in a transport medium that is picked up by a laboratory courier and transported to an outside medical laboratory for evaluation. The patient should be instructed not to douche before coming to the medical office because the physician won't be able to observe the discharge or to obtain a specimen for microbiologic analysis.

The medical assistant is responsible for assembling the appropriate supplies for the collection and evaluation of the suspected invading organism. The medical assistant must label all specimens with the patient's name and date of birth, the date, and the source of the specimen. If the specimen is to be transported to an outside medical laboratory for evaluation, a laboratory request form must be completed. The request form indicates the source of the specimen, the physician's clinical diagnosis, the microbiologic examination requested, and other pertinent information, such as medications the patient is taking. The physician's clinical assessment of the patient's signs and symptoms, along with the results of the laboratory evaluation of the specimen, are used to diagnose the presence of a vaginal infection.

Medical assistants should protect themselves from infection with a pathogen while assisting with the collection and evaluation of the specimen by practicing good techniques of medical asepsis. Methods used to identify the invading organism and supplies required for the collection and evaluation of organisms that cause common vaginal infections are presented next.

Trichomoniasis

Trichomonas vaginalis, the causative agent of trichomoniasis (trich), is a pear-shaped protozoan with four flagella, which allow for the motility of the organism (Figure 8-8). Trichomoniasis is usually, but not always, spread through sexual intercourse. Symptoms of this infection include a profuse, frothy vaginal discharge that is usually yellowish green and has an unpleasant odor; itching and irritation of the vulva and vagina; dyspareunia; and dysuria. The cervix may exhibit small red spots, a condition known as "strawberry cervix."

Trichomonas may be identified at the medical office by a wet preparation, which involves placing a small amount of the discharge on a microscope slide using a sterile swab, adding a drop of isotonic saline to it, and placing a coverslip over the mixture to protect it (Figure 8-9). The slide is examined under the microscope and observed for the presence of the lashing movements of the flagella and the motility of the organism.

If the physician prefers to have an outside laboratory evaluate the specimen, it must be placed in a tube containing a transport medium. The specimen must be transported

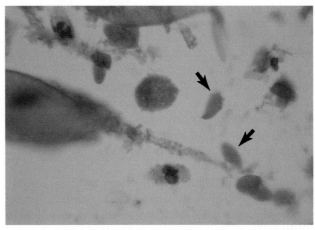

Figure 8-8. *Trichomonas vaginalis* under a microscope. (Modified from Mahon C, Manuselis G: Textbook of diagnostic microbiology, ed 3, St Louis, 2007, Saunders.)

Wet Preparation

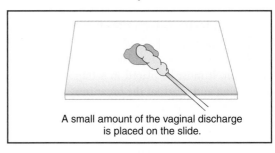

A small amount of the vaginal discharge is placed on the slide.

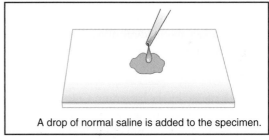

A drop of normal saline is added to the specimen.

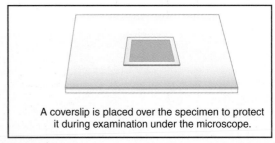

A coverslip is placed over the specimen to protect it during examination under the microscope.

Figure 8-9. Preparing a wet preparation for the identification of *Trichomonas vaginalis.*

as soon as possible (within 24 hours) to prevent it from dying, which would impede visualization of the motility of the organism.

Trichomoniasis is treated with the oral administration of metronidazole (Flagyl). The woman and her sexual partner must be treated at the same time to prevent reinfection because her partner may harbor the organism without displaying noticeable symptoms.

Candidiasis

Candida albicans is a yeastlike fungus normally found in the intestinal tract and is a frequent contaminant of the vagina; however, it usually does not produce symptoms indicating a vaginal infection. Conditions such as pregnancy, diabetes mellitus, and prolonged antibiotic therapy produce changes in the vagina that may precipitate a candidal infection of the vagina, commonly referred to as a "yeast infection." Symptoms of candidiasis include white patches on the mucous membrane of the vagina; a thick, odorless, cottage cheese–like discharge; vulval irritation; and dysuria. The discharge is extremely irritating and usually results in burning and intense itching.

Candida may be identified microscopically in the medical office by placing a specimen of the vaginal discharge on a slide using a sterile swab and adding a drop of a 10% solution of potassium hydroxide (KOH). The KOH dissolves cellular debris present in the smear and allows better visualization of yeast buds, spores, or hyphae (fungus filaments) indicating the presence of *C. albicans* (Figure 8-10). If the specimen is to be transported to a medical laboratory for identification, it must be placed in a transport medium to prevent drying and death of the organism.

Candidiasis is treated with the application of vaginal ointments or suppositories, such as miconazole (Monistat), clotrimazole (Gyne-Lotrimin), and nystatin (Mycostatin), or the oral administration of fluconazole (Diflucan). Candidiasis has a tendency to recur; the patient should be instructed to contact the medical office if symptoms of the yeast infection reappear.

Chlamydia

Chlamydia is caused by the bacterium *Chlamydia trachomatis.* It is a gram-negative intracellular bacterium that grows and multiplies in the cytoplasm of the host cell. Chlamydia

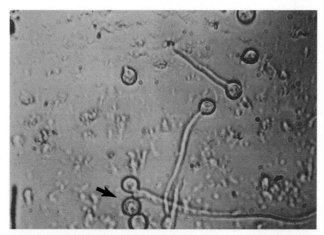

Figure 8-10. *Candida albicans* under a microscope. (Modified from Mahon C, Manuselis G: Textbook of diagnostic microbiology, ed 3, St Louis, 2007, Saunders.)

is the most frequently reported and fastest spreading sexually transmitted disease in the United States, particularly among adolescent girls and young women.

Most women with chlamydia have no symptoms and are not aware of having the condition. Because of this, many women do not seek medical care until serious complications have occurred. After infection, chlamydia first attacks the cervix, resulting in cervicitis. If symptoms do occur, they may include one or more of the following: dysuria, itching and irritation of the genital area, and a yellowish, odorless vaginal discharge. These symptoms usually appear 1 to 3 weeks after the patient has been infected.

If not treated, chlamydia can spread further into the female reproductive tract and cause *pelvic inflammatory disease* (PID). The symptoms of PID include lower abdominal pain, fever, nausea and vomiting, dyspareunia, vaginal discharge, and bleeding between periods. Complications of PID are serious and include chronic pelvic pain, scarring of the fallopian tubes, ectopic pregnancy, and infertility.

Symptoms of a chlamydial infection in men include mild dysuria and a thin, watery discharge from the penis. Men are more likely to have symptoms than women; however, the symptoms may appear only early in the day and be so mild that they are ignored. If the infection is not treated, it can cause *epididymitis,* a painful condition of the testicles that could result in infertility.

When diagnosed early, chlamydia can be treated successfully with antibiotics. The antibiotics most often used are azithromycin (Zithromax) and doxycycline. The patient's partner also should be tested for chlamydia so that if treatment is needed, it can be administered as soon as possible.

Chlamydia is most frequently diagnosed using a nuclei acid amplification test (NAAT) or a nuclei acid hybridization test known as the *DNA-probe test.* These tests are able to detect the presence of the genes (DNA) of chlamydia bacteria. The physician collects a specimen using a sterile swab. The specimen is collected from the endocervical canal of a female patient and from the urethra of a male patient. Male patients should be instructed not to void for 1 hour before the collection of the specimen to prevent chlamydia organisms from being washed out of the urethra. After collection, the specimen is placed in a tube containing a transport medium to preserve the specimen until it reaches the laboratory. See the box *Chlamydia and Gonorrhea Specimen Collection* for detailed instructions on how to assist with the collection of a chlamydia specimen.

Gonorrhea

Gonorrhea is caused by the bacterium *Neisseria gonorrhoeae,* which is a gram-negative diplococcus. Gonorrhea is an infection of the genitourinary tract that is transmitted through sexual intercourse. Chlamydia often occurs in association with gonorrhea; approximately 25% to 40% of patients infected with gonorrhea also have chlamydia.

Women who have contracted gonorrhea may have no symptoms or may exhibit dysuria and a yellow vaginal discharge. The symptoms of gonorrhea (if they occur) appear

2 to 10 days after infection and may be so mild that they are ignored. As the disease progresses, it can spread farther into the reproductive tract, resulting in PID. As mentioned previously, PID can lead to serious complications such as infertility.

Men who have contracted gonorrhea exhibit more symptoms than women, including dysuria and a whitish discharge from the penis, which may progress to a thick and creamy discharge. The burning and pain experienced during urination are often severe, which usually prompts an infected man to seek early treatment. If not treated, gonorrhea may cause epididymitis, which could lead to infertility.

Gonorrhea can be treated effectively with antibiotics. In recent years, gonorrhea bacteria have become resistant to the antibiotics typically used to treat the disease. Because of this, newer types of antibiotics have been developed. One of the most effective antibiotics used to treat gonorrhea is ceftriaxone, which is administered in one dose by injection.

The medical office most frequently uses a DNA-probe test or a nucleic acid amplification test (NAAT) to diagnose gonorrhea. These tests detect the presence of the genes of the gonorrhea bacterium. Before the development of the DNA-probe test and the NAAT test, a culture test was most often used to diagnose gonorrhea. Although occasionally still used, the disadvantage of this method is that gonorrhea is difficult to culture. Special procedures must be performed after collection of the specimen to ensure that the organism remains alive during transport to the laboratory. This includes an atmosphere of carbon dioxide and a specially enriched Thayer-Martin culture medium. Most offices now prefer the DNA-probe or NAAT test, both of which are just as accurate as the culture test but are much easier in terms of specimen preparation for transport to the laboratory. The

Highlight on Sexually Transmitted Diseases

Sexually transmitted diseases (STDs) are among the most common infectious diseases in the United States today. Each year, more than 19 million new cases of STDs are reported in the United States. If this trend continues, at least one in four Americans will contract an STD at some time in his or her life. STDs are most prevalent among teenagers and young adults; more than half of STDs are contracted by individuals 15 to 25 years old.

Transmission

STDs are spread most often by sexual contact (vaginal, anal, or oral) with an infected person. They are less commonly spread by skin-to-skin contact and by the use of contaminated needles among drug users. More than 20 STDs have been identified. The most common STDs are chlamydia, gonorrhea, herpes, human papillomavirus (HPV), hepatitis B, human immunodeficiency virus (HIV), and syphilis. Currently, a preventive vaccine is available for HPV and hepatitis B.

Symptoms

An STD sometimes causes no symptoms at all, particularly in women. If symptoms do occur, they include one or more of the following: an unusual discharge from the penis or vagina; itching, redness, or soreness of the genitals; sores or blisters on or around the genitals, anus, or both; and pain or burning during urination.

With or without symptoms, an STD can be spread to someone else. If symptoms develop, they may be so mild that they go unnoticed, or they may be confused with symptoms of other diseases. Because of this, STDs may go undetected and untreated. If not treated, many STDs result in serious complications, such as infertility. In addition, some STDs can be passed from an infected mother to her infant before or during birth.

Treatment

When diagnosed early, most STDs can be treated effectively, and many can be cured. Antibiotics can cure STDs caused by bacteria, such as chlamydia, gonorrhea, and syphilis. Medications have been developed to control the symptoms of STDs caused by viruses, such as herpes and HPV; however, they cannot eliminate the virus from the body.

Prevention and Control

All STDs can be prevented. The best way to prevent STDs is to practice abstinence or to have a mutually monogamous sexual relationship with an uninfected partner. If an individual's lifestyle does not follow one of these patterns, the following can be done to reduce the risk of contracting an STD:

- Before having a sexual relationship, partners should discuss their sexual histories with each other and get tested for STDs.
- Use a condom during sexual intercourse. If the condom is not used correctly, however, an individual still could contract an STD.
- Limit the number of sexual partners. The risk of an STD increases with each new partner, particularly if it is unknown how many previous partners that person has had.

Plan of Action

Sexually active individuals who are not in a monogamous relationship should have regular health checkups and ask to be tested for STDs. These individuals also should learn to recognize the symptoms of STDs and check themselves for signs of STD infection once a month.

If an individual thinks he or she has an STD, a physician should be consulted as soon as possible. If an individual has been treated for an STD and still has symptoms, he or she should return to the physician for further evaluation. It is possible to have more than one STD at a time and to become reinfected with the same STD.

An individual diagnosed with an STD should inform his or her partner immediately so that the partner can be tested. It also is important for an infected person to take all prescribed medication and to abstain from intercourse until a physician has determined that he or she is no longer contagious. ∎

Chlamydia and Gonorrhea Specimen Collection

DNA-Based Detection Test

The procedure for collecting a specimen for the DNA test is outlined below. Chlamydia and gonorrhea tests can be performed on the same specimen.

1. The medical assistant assembles supplies needed to collect the specimen, including a vaginal speculum, clean disposable gloves, and the DNA-probe collection kit. The collection kit includes cotton-tipped swabs and a tube of transport medium.
2. The transport tube must be labeled with the following information: patient's name, date of birth, and identification number, date and time of collection, and physician's name and telephone number.

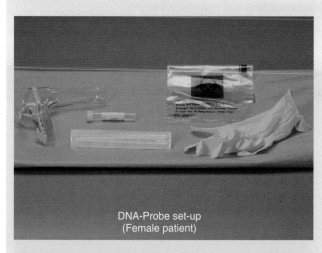

DNA-Probe set-up
(Female patient)

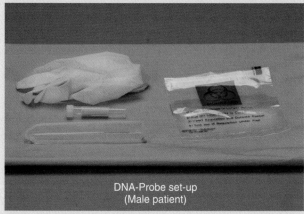

DNA-Probe set-up
(Male patient)

3. The physician collects the specimen as follows:
   - **Female Patient:** The physician inserts a vaginal speculum into the vagina. Using a cotton-tipped swab, the physician first removes excess mucus or discharge from the cervix. Next, the physician collects the specimen by inserting another cotton-tipped swab into the endocervical canal and rotating it for 5 to 10 seconds. This ensures a good sampling of the specimen.
   - **Male Patient:** The patient must not urinate for 1 hour before the collection to prevent any urethral discharge from being washed away. The physician inserts a small-tipped cotton swab 2 to 4 cm into the penis. The swab is gently rotated for 3 to 5 seconds to dislodge cells and to ensure contact with all urethral surfaces.
4. The physician withdraws the swab.
5. The medical assistant should ensure that the transport medium is at the bottom of the tube. The medical assistant unscrews the cap and holds the tube for the physician.
6. The physician inserts the swab into the transport tube and breaks off the shaft of the swab at the score line.

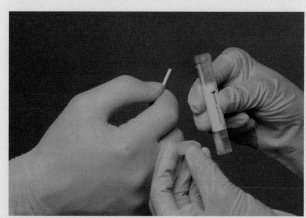

The physician inserts the swab into the tube and breaks off the shaft.

7. The medical assistant places the cap on the tube and twists it until it clicks into place. The tube is placed in a biohazard specimen transport bag along with the laboratory requisition for pickup by the laboratory.

What Would You Do? What Would You *Not* Do?

Case Study 2

Dagny Fairchild comes to the office. She is 16 years old, and her father is a lawyer and her mother is a chemical engineer. Her boyfriend was diagnosed 2 weeks ago with chlamydia. Dagny was hesitant to come in because she does not have any symptoms and her boyfriend always uses a condom. She is worried about her parents finding out that she is sexually active and what they will think if she has one of "those diseases." Dagny also is afraid and extremely embarrassed about what will be "done to her" to determine whether she has chlamydia. She tells Yin-Ling that she is thinking of leaving the office and not seeing the physician at all. (*Note:* Dagny lives in a state that allows minors to receive health care services without parental consent.) ■

Memories *from* Externship

Yin-Ling Wu: During my externship, I was assigned to an OB/GYN clinic. They had an ultrasound technician working there who ran all the scans on prenatal patients. She would always bring the pictures out so we could all look at them. They always looked like a big blob to me—I could never see anything.

One day, a patient that one of the medical assistants knew really well came into the office. The patient agreed to let us all come in for her ultrasound. It was her first time getting an ultrasound. When the technician put the ultrasound probe on her abdomen, we could see the outline of the whole baby. You could even see a tiny arm and fingers, and it looked like the baby was waving. The look of joy and amazement on the mom's face was unforgettable. After that, I knew I was in the right profession. ∎

procedure for obtaining a specimen for the DNA-probe test is outlined in the box *Chlamydia and Gonorrhea Specimen Collection.*

PRENATAL CARE

OBSTETRICS

Obstetrics is the Labranch of medicine that deals with the supervision of women's health during pregnancy, childbirth, and the puerperium. **Prenatal** refers to the care of a pregnant woman before delivery of the infant. Prenatal care consists of a series of scheduled medical office visits for promotion of the health of the mother and fetus through prevention of disease and early detection, diagnosis, and treatment of problems common to pregnancy (e.g., anemia, urinary tract infection, and preeclampsia). Early detection of medical problems helps prevent serious complications in the mother and the fetus.

Obstetric Terminology

The medical assistant should know the common terms related to obstetrics, as follows:

Braxton Hicks contractions   Intermittent and irregular painless uterine contractions that occur throughout pregnancy. They occur more frequently toward the end of pregnancy and are sometimes mistaken for true labor pains.

Dilation   Stretching of the external os (of the cervix) from an opening of a few millimeters to an opening large enough to allow the passage of an infant (approximately 10 cm).

Effacement   Thinning and shortening of the cervical canal from its normal length of 1 to 2 cm to a structure with paper-thin edges in which there is no canal at all. Effacement occurs late in pregnancy, during labor, or both. The purpose of effacement, along with dilation, is to permit the passage of the infant into the birth canal.

Embryo   The child in utero from the time of conception to the beginning of the first trimester (i.e., the first 2 months of development).

Engagement   The entrance of the fetal head or the presenting part into the pelvic inlet.

Fetus   The child in utero, from the third month after conception to birth; during the first 2 months of development, it is called an *embryo.*

Fundus   The dome-shaped upper portion of the uterus between the fallopian tubes.

Gestation   The period of intrauterine development from conception to birth; the period of pregnancy. The average pregnancy lasts about 280 days, or 40 weeks, from the date of conception to childbirth.

Gestational age   The age of the fetus between conception and birth.

Infant   A child from birth to 12 months old.

Multigravida   A woman who has been pregnant more than once.

Multipara   A woman who has completed two or more pregnancies to the age of viability regardless of whether they ended in live infants or stillbirths.

Nullipara   A woman who has not carried a pregnancy to the point of fetal viability (20 weeks of gestation).

Position   The relation of the presenting part of the fetus to the maternal pelvis.

Postpartum   Occurring after childbirth.

Preeclampsia   A major complication of pregnancy, the cause of which is unknown, characterized by increasing hypertension, albuminuria, and edema. If the condition is neglected or is not treated properly, preeclampsia may develop into eclampsia, which could cause maternal convulsions and coma. Preeclampsia generally occurs between the 20th week of pregnancy and the end of the first week postpartum.

Presentation   Indication of the part of the fetus that is closest to the cervix and is delivered first. A cephalic presentation is a delivery in which the fetal head is presenting against the cervix. A breech presentation is a delivery in which the buttocks or feet are presented instead of the head.

Primigravida   A woman who is pregnant for the first time.

Primipara   A woman who has carried a pregnancy to fetal viability (20 weeks of gestation) for the first time regardless of whether the infant was stillborn or alive at birth.

Puerperium   The period of time (usually 4 to 6 weeks) after delivery in which the uterus and the body systems are returning to normal.

Quickening   The first movements of the fetus in utero as felt by the mother, which usually occurs between 16 and 20 weeks of gestation and is felt consistently thereafter.

Toxemia   A condition that can occur in pregnant women that includes preeclampsia and eclampsia. If preeclampsia goes undiagnosed or is not satisfactorily controlled, it could develop into eclampsia, which is characterized by convulsions and coma.

Trimester   Three months, or one third, of the gestational period. The 9 months of pregnancy are divided into three trimesters, each consisting of 3 months. From conception to 3 months is the first trimester, from 4 to 6 months is the second trimester, and from 7 to 9 months is the third trimester.

PRENATAL VISITS

Medical office visits for prenatal and postpartum care of the pregnant woman can be grouped into three major categories as follows:
1. First prenatal visit
2. Return prenatal visits
3. 6 weeks postpartum visit

First Prenatal Visit

The first prenatal visit generally occurs after the woman has missed her second menstrual period; if problems exist, the woman is seen after missing her first menstrual period. Regardless of whether or not the patient is happy and excited about the pregnancy, the first visit is often a stressful experience for the patient. The medical assistant plays an important role in relaxing the patient and relieving her anxiety.

The first prenatal visit requires more time than subsequent prenatal visits; sufficient time should be scheduled to allow a complete and accurate initial assessment of the pregnant woman. The components of the first prenatal visit vary depending on the medical office, but they generally include the following:
- Completion of a prenatal record form.
- Initial prenatal examination, consisting of a complete physical examination. Of particular importance are the breast, abdominal, and pelvic examinations. Pelvic measurements may be taken at this time or during a return prenatal visit.
- Prenatal patient education.
- Laboratory tests.

Prenatal Record

The prenatal record provides information regarding the past and present health of the patient and serves as a database and flow sheet for subsequent prenatal visits. The prenatal record is essential in helping identify high-risk patients. The medical assistant is usually responsible for collecting a portion of the information required for the prenatal record. Many types of printed prenatal record forms are available (Figure 8-11). The specific form used in the medical office is based on the physician's preference and the method used for conducting the prenatal examination.

Obtaining and recording information in the prenatal record from one visit to the next provides an opportunity for the medical assistant to develop a rapport with the patient. It is also an excellent time to relay information to her regarding various aspects of the prenatal and postnatal periods, such as an explanation of the changes occurring in her body, the signs and symptoms of labor, nutrition of the infant (breastfeeding and bottle feeding), and care of the newborn infant. The prenatal record form should be completed in a quiet setting that is free from distractions. This gives the patient the confidence to discuss areas of concern openly, which helps ensure a complete and accurate prenatal history.

During the first prenatal visit, the medical assistant should relay his or her name and position to the patient to help build a supportive relationship with her and to allow her to ask for the medical assistant by name when contacting the medical office. The prenatal record is similar to and contains much of the same information as the health history described in Chapter 1. Particular attention is given to factors that may influence the course of pregnancy, as described in the following paragraphs.

Past Medical History

The past medical history focuses on conditions that could affect the health of the mother and fetus, such as diabetes, hypertension, heart disease, autoimmune disorders, kidney disease, liver disease, varicosities or phlebitis, alcohol and tobacco intake, drug addiction, Rh sensitization, pulmonary disease (e.g., tuberculosis, asthma), bleeding tendencies, surgeries, anesthetic complications, previous abnormal Pap tests, infertility problems, sexually transmitted diseases, and drug allergies. In addition, the medical assistant solicits information from the patient regarding immunizations and childhood diseases to provide the physician with the information needed to assess her antibody protection against such diseases.

Rubella, if contracted during pregnancy, can be dangerous to the developing fetus; the earlier in pregnancy the infection occurs, the greater is the chance of birth defects. The infant may be born with heart defects, cataracts, mental retardation, and deafness. Patients who do not have antibody protection against rubella are given a rubella immunization within 6 weeks of delivery. The rubella vaccination cannot be given to a pregnant woman because it may be harmful to the fetus. These patients should be told to avoid exposure to children with rubella during their pregnancy.

Menstrual History

A menstrual history is obtained from the patient. It includes the date of onset of menstruation, the menstrual interval cycle, the duration, the amount of flow (recorded as small, moderate, or large), and any gynecologic disorders. The form also includes a space for the patient to indicate whether or not she was using a method of contraception when she became pregnant.

Obstetric History

A thorough obstetric history is a component of the prenatal record and provides the opportunity to obtain information from the patient related to previous pregnancies. Information that is obtained and explored includes gravidity, parity, and other information related to previous pregnancies.

PRENATAL HEALTH HISTORY

PATIENT INFORMATION

Date: _____   EDD: _____   Referred By: _____

Name: _____   Phone (home): _____

      LAST   FIRST   MIDDLE   Phone (work): _____

Address: _____   Emergency Contact: _____

      CITY   STATE   ZIP   Phone: _____

Date of Birth: ____/____/____ Age: ____ Marital Status: _____

Occupation: _____

Education: ☐ High School   ☐ College   ☐ Post-graduate

PAST MEDICAL HISTORY

	○ Neg + Pos	DETAIL POSITIVE REMARKS INCLUDE DATE AND TREATMENT		○ Neg + Pos	DETAIL POSITIVE REMARKS INCLUDE DATE AND TREATMENT
1. DIABETES			16. D (Rh) SENSITIZED		
2. HYPERTENSION			17. PULMONARY (TB, ASTHMA)		
3. HEART DISEASE			18. RHEUMATIC FEVER		
4. AUTOIMMUNE DISORDER			19. BLEEDING TENDENCY		
5. KIDNEY DISEASE/UTI			20. GYN SURGERY		
6. NEUROLOGIC/EPILEPSY					
7. PSYCHIATRIC			21. OPERATIONS/HOSPITALIZATIONS (YEAR AND REASON)		
8. HEPATITIS/LIVER DISEASE					
9. VARICOSITIES/PHLEBITIS					
10. THYROID DYSFUNCTION			22. ANESTHETIC COMPLICATIONS		
11. TRAUMA/DOMESTIC VIOLENCE			23. HISTORY OF ABNORMAL PAP		
12. BLOOD TRANSFUSION			24. UTERINE ANOMALY/DES		

	AMT/DAY PREPREG.	AMT/DAY PREG.	# YEARS USE			
				25. INFERTILITY		
				26. SEXUALLY TRANSMITTED DISEASE		
13. TOBACCO						
14. ALCOHOL						
15. STREET DRUGS				27. OTHER		

IMMUNIZATIONS:

Mark an X next to those you have had.

☐ Influenza   ☐ Chickenpox

☐ Hepatitis B   ☐ Pneumococcal

☐ Hib   ☐ Tuberculin Test

☐ Polio   ☐ Tetanus Booster

☐ MMR

ALLERGIES:

List all allergies (foods, drugs, environment).   ☐ None

_____

_____

_____

_____

MENSTRUAL HISTORY

Menarche: Age at Onset _____

Frequency: Q _____ Days

Duration: _____ Days

Amount of Flow: ☐ Small   ☐ Moderate   ☐ Large

GYN Disorders (List): _____

_____

On contraceptive at conception? ☐ Yes ☐ No

Figure 8-11. Example of a prenatal record form.   *Continued*

Gravidity and parity provide data with respect to the pregnancy, and the medical assistant should develop skill in recording this information. **Gravidity (G)** is recorded using one digit, which indicates the number of times a woman has been pregnant regardless of the duration of the pregnancy and including the current pregnancy. A woman who is pregnant for the second time but had a spontaneous abortion during the first pregnancy would be recorded as *G: 2.* A woman who is pregnant for the second time (and did not have a spontaneous abortion) also would be recorded as *G: 2.*

Parity refers to the condition of having borne offspring regardless of the outcome. It is recorded using four abbreviations and digits, which represent the following pregnancy outcomes:

1. **Term birth (T).** Delivery after 37 weeks regardless of whether the child was born alive or stillborn.
2. **Preterm birth (P).** Delivery between 20 and 37 weeks regardless of whether the child was born alive or stillborn.
3. **Abortion (A).** Termination of the pregnancy before the fetus reaches the age of viability (20 weeks). An abortion can be spontaneous or elective.

OBSTETRIC HISTORY

G _____ T _____ P _____ A _____ L _____
(Total Pregnancies) (Term) (Preterm) (Abortions) (Living Children)

PREVIOUS PREGNANCIES:

DATE MONTH/ YEAR	WEEKS GEST.	LENGTH OF LABOR	BIRTH WEIGHT	SEX M/F	TYPE DELIVERY	ANES.	MATERNAL COMPLICATIONS	INFANT COMPLICATIONS

PRESENT PREGNANCY HISTORY

NAUSEA			ABDOMINAL PAIN		
VOMITING			URINARY COMPLAINTS		
FATIGUE			VAGINAL BLEEDING		
BREAST CHANGES			VAGINAL DISCHARGE		
INDIGESTION			PRURITIS		
CONSTIPATION			ACCIDENTS		
PERSISTENT HEADACHES			SURGERY		
DIZZINESS			X-RAYS		
VISUAL DISTURBANCE			RUBELLA EXPOSURE		
EDEMA (SPECIFY AREA)			OTHER VIRAL INFECTIONS		

LMP _____ / _____ / _____   Amount of Flow: ☐ Small ☐ Moderate ☐ Large
Mo   Day   Year

CURRENT MEDICATIONS: (Include prescription, OTC, herbal, and vitamins). ☐ None

Medication   **Frequency**

_____

_____

INITIAL PHYSICAL EXAMINATION

DATE ____ / ____ / ____

1. HEENT	☐ NORMAL	☐ ABNORMAL	12. VULVA	☐ NORMAL	☐ CONDYLOMA	☐ LESIONS
2. FUNDI	☐ NORMAL	☐ ABNORMAL	13. VAGINA	☐ NORMAL	☐ INFLAMMATION	☐ DISCHARGE
3. TEETH	☐ NORMAL	☐ ABNORMAL	14. CERVIX	☐ NORMAL	☐ INFLAMMATION	☐ LESIONS
4. THYROID	☐ NORMAL	☐ ABNORMAL	15. UTERUS SIZE	_____ WEEKS		☐ FIBROIDS
5. BREASTS	☐ NORMAL	☐ ABNORMAL	16. ADNEXA	☐ NORMAL	☐ MASS	
6. LUNGS	☐ NORMAL	☐ ABNORMAL	17. RECTUM	☐ NORMAL	☐ ABNORMAL	
7. HEART	☐ NORMAL	☐ ABNORMAL	18. DIAGONAL CONJUGATE	☐ REACHED	☐ NO	_____ CM
8. ABDOMEN	☐ NORMAL	☐ ABNORMAL	19. SPINES	☐ AVERAGE	☐ PROMINENT	☐ BLUNT
9. EXTREMITIES	☐ NORMAL	☐ ABNORMAL	20. SACRUM	☐ CONCAVE	☐ STRAIGHT	☐ ANTERIOR
10. SKIN	☐ NORMAL	☐ ABNORMAL	21. SUBPUBIC ARCH	☐ NORMAL	☐ WIDE	☐ NARROW
11. LYMPH NODES	☐ NORMAL	☐ ABNORMAL	22. GYNECOID PELVIC TYPE	☐ YES	☐ NO	

COMMENTS (Number and explain abnormals): _____

_____

_____

EXAM BY _____

Figure 8-11, cont'd. Example of a prenatal record form.

4. **Living children (L).** Number of living children.
   Example: A woman has been pregnant four times with the following outcomes: a spontaneous abortion, a full-term stillbirth, a preterm birth of a healthy child, and a full-term birth of a healthy child. The recording would be as follows:
   G: 4 *(pregnancies);* **T: 2** *(term);* **P: 1** *(preterm);* **A: 1** *(abortion);* **L: 2** *(living children)*

Multiple births (twins, triplets) count as one pregnancy and one delivery. If a woman had been pregnant two times and had a set of full-term healthy twins and a set of preterm healthy triplets, the recording would be **G: 2 T: 1 P: 1 A: 0 L: 5.**

If a woman is a multigravida, information about each pregnancy is obtained, including the date of delivery, gestation in weeks, length of labor in hours, birth weight and sex of the newborn, type of delivery (vaginal or cesarean section), type of anesthesia, and any maternal or infant complications. The obstetric history assists in identifying areas that may need to be investigated further or monitored during the prenatal period. Women with previous complications, such as premature labor, gestational diabetes, or

PATIENT'S NAME _____

INTERVAL PRENATAL HISTORY

Date 20__	Weeks Gestation	Height of Fundus (cm)	Weight	B/P	Urine Glucose	Urine Protein	FHT	Vaginal Examination	Presentation	Edema	Discharge	Bleeding	Contractions	Fetal Activity	NST	Next Appt.	Initials

PLANS/EDUCATION   (COUNSELED ☑)

☐ ANESTHESIA PLANS _____

☐ TOXOPLASMOSIS PRECAUTIONS (CATS/RAW MEAT) _____

☐ CHILDBIRTH CLASSES _____

☐ PHYSICAL/SEXUAL ACTIVITY _____

☐ LABOR SIGNS _____

☐ NUTRITION COUNSELING _____

☐ BREAST OR BOTTLE FEEDING _____

☐ NEWBORN CAR SEAT _____

☐ POSTPARTUM BIRTH CONTROL _____

☐ ENVIRONMENTAL/WORK HAZARDS _____

☐ TUBAL STERILIZATION _____

☐ VBAC COUNSELING _____

☐ CIRCUMCISION _____

☐ TRAVEL _____

☐ LIFESTYLE, TOBACCO, ALCOHOL _____

REQUESTS _____

_____

_____

TUBAL STERILIZATION   DATE   INITIALS
CONSENT SIGNED   ___/___/___   _____

Figure 8-11, cont'd. Example of a prenatal record form.   *Continued*

postpartum hemorrhaging, are at risk for having these problems again.

Present Pregnancy History

The present pregnancy history establishes a baseline for the present health status of the prenatal patient. In addition, the patient is queried regarding any warning signs that may be present and that may place the mother or fetus in jeopardy, such as persistent headaches, visual disturbances, abdominal pain, vaginal bleeding, or discharge. The patient also is asked whether she has experienced any of the early signs of pregnancy, such as nausea, vomiting, fatigue, and breast changes.

All prescribed or over-the-counter medications (including vitamin supplements and herbal products) the patient is taking must be recorded. Certain medications cross the placental barrier and could be harmful to the developing fetus. The patient should be instructed not to take any medications without first checking with the physician.

In the space provided under the present pregnancy history, the medical assistant needs to record the date of the first day of the patient's last menstrual period (LMP). The LMP is used to calculate due date, or **expected date of delivery (EDD),** by using Nägele's rule: Add 7 days to the date of the LMP, subtract 3 months, and add 1 year (EDD = LMP + 7 days − 3 months + 1 year). For example, if the date of the patient's LMP was June 10, 2011, the EDD is March 17, 2012. The problem is set up as follows:

$$
\begin{array}{rrl}
6 & 10 & 2011 \text{ (LMP)} \\
-3 & +7\;+ & 1 \text{ (Applying Nägele's rule)} \\
\hline
3 & 17 & 2012 \text{ (Delivery Date)}
\end{array}
$$

LABORATORY		PATIENT'S NAME _____			
INITIAL LABS	**DATE**	**RESULTS**		**REVIEWED**	**COMMENTS**
BLOOD TYPE	/ /	A B AB O			
Rh FACTOR	/ /	☐ Pos ☐ Neg			
Rh ANTIBODY SCREEN	/ /	☐ Pos ☐ Neg			
HCT/HGB	/ /	_____% _____ g/dL			
RUBELLA ANTIBODY TITER	/ /	Immune Nonimmune			
VDRL	/ /	☐ NR ☐ R			
HBsAg (HEPATITIS B)	/ /	☐ Pos ☐ Neg			
HIV	/ /	☐ Pos ☐ Neg ☐ Declined			
URINE CULTURE/SCREEN	/ /				
PAP TEST	/ /	☐ Normal ☐ Abnormal			
CHLAMYDIA	/ /	☐ Pos ☐ Neg			
GONORRHEA	/ /	☐ Pos ☐ Neg			
7–20 WEEK LABS (WHEN INDICATED/ELECTED)	**DATE**	**RESULTS**		**REVIEWED**	**COMMENTS**
ULTRASOUND #1 (7–12 WEEKS)	/ /	EDD:			
ULTRASOUND #2 (18–20 WEEKS)	/ /	EFW:			
TRIPLE SCREEN (15–20 WEEKS)	/ /				
CVS	/ /				
AMNIOCENTESIS	/ /				
24–28 WEEK LABS (WHEN INDICATED)	**DATE**	**RESULTS**		**REVIEWED**	**COMMENTS**
HCT/HGB	/ /	_____ % _____ g/dL			
GCT (24–28 WKS)	/ /	1 Hour _____			
GTT (IF SCREEN ABNORMAL)	/ /	_____ FBS _____ 1 Hour _____ 2 Hour _____ 3 Hour			
D (Rh) ANTIBODY SCREEN	/ /				
D IMMUNE GLOBULIN (RhIG) GIVEN (28 WKS)	/ /	SIGNATURE			
32–36 WEEK LABS	**DATE**	**RESULTS**		**REVIEWED**	**COMMENTS**
HCT/HGB (32 WKS)	/ /	_____ % _____ g/dL			
ULTRASOUND #3 (34 WKS)	/ /	EFW:			
GROUP B STREP (35–37 WKS)	/ /	☐ Pos ☐ Neg			
ADDITIONAL LAB TESTS	**DATE**	**RESULTS**		**REVIEWED**	**COMMENTS**
	/ /				
	/ /				
	/ /				
	/ /				
	/ /				

Figure 8-11, cont'd. Example of a prenatal record form.

Using Nägele's rule, approximately 4% of patients deliver spontaneously on the EDD; most patients deliver during the period extending from 7 days before to 7 days after the EDD.

Gestation calculators are commercially available that can be used to determine the delivery date by lining up an arrow and the date of the LMP, using a movable inner cardboard wheel (Figure 8-12). These calculators require less time to determine the EDD than using Nägele's rule, and they provide information on the probable size (length and weight) of the fetus on any given date. The accuracy of gestation calculators is comparable with that of Nägele's rule. If the patient is unsure of the date of her LMP, the physician estimates the length of gestation by other methods, such as fundal height measurement and sonography.

Interval Prenatal History

The interval prenatal history also is included in the prenatal record form; its purpose is to update the record. During every return visit, essential data, including weight, blood pressure, urine testing results, fundal height measurement, and fetal heart rate, are collected and recorded in this section. A general inquiry is made regarding the occurrence of additional signs of pregnancy, such as fetal movement or Braxton Hicks contractions, and how the patient is feeling and any concerns or symptoms since the last prenatal visit.

This information is recorded and assists the medical staff in planning, implementing, and evaluating individual needs. Particular attention is focused on risk factors, such as hypertension, thrombophlebitis, and uterine bleeding, which could influence the course of the pregnancy.

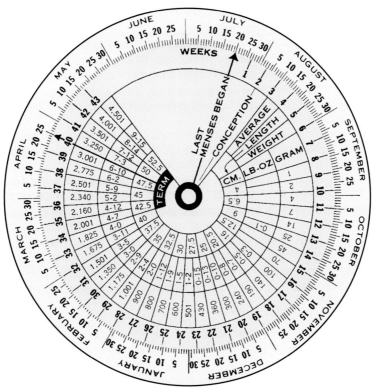

Figure 8-12. Gestation calculator. The last menstrual period is July 20, and the expected date of delivery is April 25.

Initial Prenatal Examination

Purpose

The initial prenatal examination is of particular importance because it results in confirmation of the pregnancy and establishes a baseline for the woman's state of health. It includes a thorough gynecologic examination (breast and pelvic examinations) and a general physical examination of the other body systems, although the latter may be performed during a subsequent prenatal visit, depending on the medical office routine.

Women often have little or no medical supervision during their childbearing years; the physical examination is of particular importance in establishing a baseline for the woman's general state of health and in identifying high-risk prenatal patients. Conditions such as obesity, hypertension, severe varicosities, and uterine size inappropriate for the due date can be diagnosed by the physician, and necessary treatment or monitoring can be instituted to help prevent complications.

Preparation of the Patient

When the patient arrives at the medical office and the prenatal record form has been completed, the medical assistant is responsible for taking and recording the patient's vital signs, height, and weight to provide a database for subsequent prenatal visits. The patient is asked to disrobe com-

pletely and put on an examining gown with the opening in front. The medical assistant must give complete and thorough instructions so the patient knows exactly what is expected. The patient should be asked whether she needs to empty her bladder because an empty bladder facilitates the examination and is more comfortable for her. If the office policy is such that a specimen is needed for urine testing at the initial prenatal visit, the patient will be required to void.

Special precautions should be taken in assisting the prenatal patient. The medical assistant should support the patient as she gets onto and off the scale and examining table to ensure her safety and comfort. This is especially important as the pregnancy progresses and the patient becomes more awkward and off balance.

The medical assistant is responsible for setting up the tray required for the examination. The setup includes the equipment and supplies required for the procedures to be performed. During the prenatal examination, the medical assistant is responsible for positioning the patient as required for each aspect of the examination and assisting the physician as necessary. Table 8-2 lists the procedures commonly included in the prenatal examination and the purpose, the implications, and (when applicable) the patient's position. Most of the procedures included in the initial prenatal examination are presented elsewhere in this book; the number of the chapter that contains the step-by-step procedure is included in Table 8-2.

Table 8-2 Components of the Initial Prenatal Examination

Procedure	Purpose and Implications
Vital signs (see Chapter 4)	To provide a baseline for subsequent prenatal visits. Blood pressure decreases slightly during the first and second trimesters and returns to normal or slightly above normal during the last trimester.
Temperature Pulse Respiration Blood pressure Weight (see Chapter 5)	Elevation in blood pressure during pregnancy in conjunction with other signs and symptoms indicates possible problems, such as pregnancy-induced hypertension or preeclampsia. Patient position: sitting. To provide baseline weight measurement for comparison with all future weight measurements at subsequent prenatal visits. Medical assistant charts patient's weight on flow sheet at each prenatal visit, and any deviations from expected progressions are evaluated by the physician. Measuring and recording maternal weight gain or loss is helpful in assessing fetal development and, to some extent, mother's nutrition and state of health. Sudden unexplained weight gain may indicate preeclampsia of pregnancy.
Physical examination (see Chapter 5)	To establish a baseline for woman's general state of health to ensure patient is entering pregnancy in best possible physical condition. Physical examination includes examination of patient's eyes, ears, nose, and throat; chest, lungs, and heart; breasts; abdomen; reproductive organs; rectum; and extremities. Of particular importance are the breast, abdominal, and pelvic examinations.
Breast examination (see Chapter 8)	To check for lumps, swelling, dimpling, puckering, and changes in skin texture. To check for breast changes that occur during pregnancy, such as tenderness and fullness and darkening of nipples and areolae. Patient position: supine.
Abdominal examination (see Chapter 8)	To detect masses or lumps other than the developing fetus. Abdomen is inspected for scars and striations, and initial measurement of fundal height is made to provide a baseline for future fundal height measurements. Patient position: supine.
Pelvic examination (see Chapter 8)	To provide data to confirm pregnancy and to determine length of gestation. To estimate gestational age of developing embryo (at 7 weeks, the uterus is the size of an egg; at 10 weeks, it is the size of an orange; and at 12 weeks, it is the size of a grapefruit). To identify pelvic characteristics and any abnormalities that may result in complications during pregnancy or delivery. Pelvic examination generally includes the following: • Inspection of external genitalia • Speculum examination of vagina and cervix • Pap test • Specimen for chlamydia and gonorrhea tests • Vaginal specimen if infection is suspected • Bimanual examination Patient position: lithotomy.
Rectal-vaginal examination (see Chapter 8)	To assess strength and irregularity of posterior vaginal wall and posterior cervix. Anus is inspected for hemorrhoids and fissures, and rectum is inspected for herniation and masses. Patient position: lithotomy.
Pelvic measurements (see Chapter 8)	To verify that size and shape of the pelvis are within normal limits to allow full-term fetus to pass safely through pelvic inlet in normal vaginal route of delivery; if not, cesarean section will be required. Some physicians delay taking pelvic measurements until later in pregnancy. At that time, the prenatal patient's perineal muscles are more relaxed, allowing pelvic measurements to be taken with less patient discomfort and greater accuracy.

Patient Education

At the conclusion of the initial prenatal examination and after the patient is dressed, the physician talks with her regarding instructions on diet, weight gain, rest, sleep, employment, exercise, travel, sexual intercourse, dental care, smoking, alcohol, and drugs. Many offices have a prenatal guidebook designed especially for this purpose that is given to each patient to use as a reference. Some offices also use a series of teaching films that the patient views during the return prenatal visit while waiting to see the physician. The physician also prescribes a daily vitamin supplement to be

taken during the prenatal period to ensure that the mother and fetus obtain an adequate supply of vitamins and minerals.

When the physician is finished talking with the patient, the medical assistant is responsible for scheduling the next prenatal visit and for ensuring that the patient understands the instructions for maintaining health and preventing disease during the pregnancy. The medical assistant should tell the patient to report the occurrence of any warning signs during the pregnancy (see the *Warning Signs During Pregnancy* box) and not to take any medications without first

Warning Signs During Pregnancy

Signs of Infection
- Fever
- Vaginal discharge
- Dysuria
- Increased frequency of urination
- Marked decrease in urinary output

Signs of Spontaneous Abortion
- Vaginal bleeding
- Persistent low back pain
- Abdominal pain and cramping

Signs of Preeclampsia
- Severe, persistent headache
- Dizziness
- Blurred vision
- Sudden swelling of hands, feet, or face
- Sudden rapid weight gain
- Abdominal pain

Signs of Placental or Fetal Problems
- Vaginal spotting or bleeding
- Abdominal pain and cramping
- Back pain
- Noticeable decrease in fetal activity
- No fetal movement

Signs of Preterm Labor
- Regular or frequent contractions (more than four to six per hour)
- Recurring low, dull backache
- Menstrual-like cramping
- Unusual pressure in the pelvis, low back, abdomen, or thighs

checking with the physician. The patient also should be encouraged to contact the medical office should any questions or problems arise.

Laboratory Tests

The physician orders many laboratory tests to assist in the assessment of the patient's state of health and to detect problems that may put the pregnancy at risk. Several tests, such as the Pap test and the chlamydia and gonorrhea tests, require the physician to collect the specimens at the medical office and have them transported by laboratory courier to an outside laboratory for evaluation. The specimen required for the prenatal blood tests (known as a *prenatal profile*) must be obtained through a venipuncture to provide a sufficient quantity of blood for the number of tests ordered. The blood specimen is collected at the medical office or at an outside laboratory.

It is important to have these initial tests completed as soon as possible to provide the physician with the test re-

sults by the time of the next scheduled prenatal visit. Based on the results of the prenatal examination and the laboratory tests, the physician may order additional tests to assess the patient's condition. Certain tests and procedures, such as the glucose challenge test (GCT) and the group B streptococcus (GBS) test, are scheduled later in the pregnancy. The prenatal laboratory tests that are usually performed on a pregnant woman are described next.

Urine Tests

Urinalysis

A complete urinalysis, including physical, chemical, and microscopic analyses of the urine, is performed; a clean-catch midstream urine specimen is generally required for the test. If bacteria are found in the urine specimen, the physician usually requests a urine culture and sensitivity test to determine the possible presence of a urinary tract infection. A pregnancy test also may be performed on the urine specimen, if ordered by the physician.

Swab Tests

Pap Test

A Pap test is done for the detection of abnormalities of cell growth to diagnose precancerous or cancerous conditions of the cervix. This test also can be used for hormonal assessment (maturation index) and to assist in the detection of vaginal infections.

Chlamydia and Gonorrhea

Specimens are taken from the endocervical canal and sent to the laboratory to rule out chlamydia and gonorrhea. Chlamydia can be passed from an infected woman to her infant during childbirth, resulting in conjunctivitis and pneumonia in the newborn. If a gonorrheal infection is present at the time of delivery, the *N. gonorrhoeae* organism could infect the infant's eyes during passage through the birth canal. This may result in *ophthalmia neonatorum*, which, if not treated, could lead to blindness. For this reason, most states require that pregnant women be tested for gonorrhea, and that the eyes of newborns be treated with antibiotic drops immediately after birth to kill any gonococcal bacteria that may be present. A patient who is diagnosed with chlamydia or gonorrhea requires immediate treatment with an appropriate antibiotic to prevent problems for herself and her child.

Trichomoniasis and Candidiasis

If an excessive irritating vaginal discharge is present, the physician obtains a specimen to rule out trichomoniasis and candidiasis. It is important to control candidiasis before delivery to prevent the development of thrush, a yeastlike infection of the infant's mucous membranes of the mouth or throat.

Group B Streptococcus

Group B streptococcus (GBS) is a common bacterium often found in the vagina and rectum of healthy women. Normally, one in four pregnant women carries GBS. GBS is not harmful to a pregnant woman, but it can cause life-threatening infections in the newborn. While passing through the birth canal, a newborn can become infected with the bacteria carried by the mother. When infected, the infant may develop an infection of the blood (septicemia), pneumonia, or meningitis.

To prevent GBS infection of the newborn, a pregnant woman is tested for the bacteria between 35 and 37 weeks of gestation. Using two swabs, the physician collects specimens from the vagina and the rectum. The specimen swabs are placed in a transport tube and sent to the laboratory to be cultured for GBS. If GBS is found, intravenous antibiotics are administered to the woman every 4 hours during labor until delivery. In most cases, this antibiotic administration prevents the newborn from becoming infected with GBS. In situations in which the newborn does become infected with GBS, antibiotics are administered immediately, and the infant is closely monitored.

Blood Tests

Complete Blood Count

The complete blood count (CBC) is a basic screening test used to assist in assessing the patient's state of health. It includes a hemoglobin, hematocrit, white blood cell count, red blood cell count, differential white blood cell count, platelet count, and red blood cell indices. Of particular importance with respect to the prenatal patient are the hemoglobin and hematocrit evaluations, which are described here.

Hemoglobin and Hematocrit

Low hemoglobin or hematocrit values are seen in cases of anemia. Prenatal patients have a tendency to develop anemia because there is an increased demand for and correlating increased production of red blood cells during pregnancy; the physician carefully reviews the results of these tests. If the hemoglobin or hematocrit value is low, further hematologic evaluation is usually required. If necessary, therapy is instituted, which usually consists of an iron supplement and nutritional counseling. The hemoglobin and hematocrit values are checked again at approximately 32 weeks of gestation as a precaution against anemia before delivery.

What Would You Do? What Would You *Not* Do?

Case Study 3

Johanna Kruger is 24 years old and pregnant with her first child. She is at the office for her first prenatal visit. She is quite upset. Her best friend just had her first baby, and the baby died 24 hours later from a group B strep infection. Johanna is afraid that the same thing will happen to her baby. She wants to be tested for GBS as soon as possible. She has some antibiotics at home and is thinking of taking them. Johanna is worried because she has been experiencing some problems with her pregnancy. She is sick all day, her breasts hurt, and yesterday she had some spotting. Johanna is hesitant to tell all of this to the physician because he might think she worries too much. ■

Rh Factor and ABO Blood Type

Tests are performed to anticipate ABO blood type and Rh factor incompatibilities. If the patient is Rh-negative, the father's blood type also must be evaluated. If the father's blood type is Rh-positive, the possibility of an Rh incompatibility exists. This situation warrants the performance of an Rh antibody titer test and repeat antibody titers throughout the pregnancy to determine whether the mother's antibody level is increasing. An increased Rh antibody level could be dangerous to the developing fetus. It can result in severe anemia, jaundice, brain damage, heart failure, and sometimes death of the fetus.

Glucose Challenge Test

A glucose challenge test is performed between 24 and 28 weeks of gestation to screen for gestational diabetes mellitus (GDM). This test works by assessing the body's response to a measured glucose solution. The patient does not need to fast for this test, and no preparation is required other than arriving at the laboratory at the scheduled time. To perform the glucose challenge test, the patient is asked to drink 50 g of a glucose solution, and her glucose level is measured 1 hour later. A woman with a glucose level of less than 140 mg/dL does not have GDM and requires no further testing. If the glucose level is greater than 140 mg/dL, the test is abnormal. Not all women with elevated results have diabetes, however, and further testing using the 3-hour oral glucose tolerance test (OGTT) must be performed before a final diagnosis can be made. (NOTE: Refer to Chapter 19 for information on the OGTT.)

Syphilis Test

The microorganism that causes syphilis, *Treponema pallidum,* is able to cross the placental barrier and infect the fetus; this could result in intrauterine death or could cause the fetus to be born with congenital syphilis. Infants with congenital syphilis are often born with deformities and may become blind, deaf, paralyzed, or insane. The tests most commonly employed to screen for the presence of syphilis are the Venereal Disease Research Laboratory (VDRL) test and the rapid plasma reagin (RPR) test. The test results are reported as nonreactive, weakly reactive, or reactive. Because these tests are screening tests, a weakly reactive or reactive test result warrants more specific testing to arrive at a diagnosis for syphilis. Examples of these tests are the fluorescent treponemal antibody absorption (FTA-ABS) test and the *Treponema pallidum* particle agglutination assay (TPPA) test.

A prenatal test for syphilis is mandated by most states and should be performed early in the pregnancy, before fetal damage occurs. A patient who has contracted syphilis requires treatment with an appropriate antibiotic.

Rubella Antibody Titer

The rubella antibody titer assesses the level of antibody against rubella (German measles) in the patient's blood and is used to determine whether the woman is immune to rubella. If the mother contracts rubella during pregnancy, serious congenital abnormalities can occur in the fetus. Patients who lack immunity should be immunized against rubella within 6 weeks of delivery.

Highlight on Gestational Diabetes Mellitus

Definition of Gestational Diabetes Mellitus

Gestational diabetes mellitus (GDM) is a condition in which a pregnant woman who has never had diabetes mellitus develops an elevated glucose level (hyperglycemia). Every year, approximately 3% to 5% of pregnant women in the United States are diagnosed with GDM. Because most women with GDM have no symptoms, the American Diabetes Association recommends that all pregnant women be screened for GDM during the second trimester of the pregnancy. The screening test used is the glucose challenge test, which is performed at between 24 and 28 weeks of gestation.

Cause of Gestational Diabetes Mellitus

GDM develops from a physical interaction between the mother and the fetus. The placenta of the fetus produces hormones to preserve the pregnancy. These hormones are excreted into the mother's circulatory system in increasing amounts during the second trimester of pregnancy. These hormones counteract the effect of the mother's insulin, which results in a condition known as *insulin resistance*. In most cases, the mother's pancreas responds to insulin resistance by producing additional insulin to keep the blood glucose at a normal level. Some women are unable to produce enough extra insulin, however, which causes an elevation of their blood glucose level and results in GDM.

Problems for the Child

If GDM is not treated or if it is poorly controlled, problems can occur in the unborn child. The extra glucose crosses the placenta and enters the fetus' circulatory system. To decrease the elevated glucose level, the fetus' pancreas produces large amounts of insulin. The increased insulin converts the extra glucose into fat, resulting in the development of a large infant with a condition known as *macrosomia*. Infants with macrosomia may be too large to be born vaginally and may require a cesarean birth. Although the infant does not have diabetes, he or she is at risk for developing type 2 diabetes later in life. Other problems that can occur at birth include hypoglycemia, breathing difficulties, and jaundice.

Problems for the Mother

Problems that a mother with GDM can develop include an increased incidence of preeclampsia, infection, postpartum bleeding, and injury to the birth canal if the infant is delivered vaginally. Another problem is the development of polyhydramnios (excess amount of amniotic fluid), which causes the uterus to stretch and take up more space in the abdominal cavity. This can result in breathing difficulties for the mother during the pregnancy. GDM almost always resolves after delivery. This is because when the placenta is removed, the hormones causing the problem also are removed. The mother's insulin can work normally without resistance. Some women go on to develop type 2 diabetes later in life, however.

Risk Factors for Gestational Diabetes Mellitus

Certain factors put some women at greater risk for developing GDM. These women are usually screened earlier and more often for GDM during the pregnancy. Risk factors for GDM include the following:

- Obesity
- Family history of diabetes mellitus
- Previous birth of an infant weighing more than 9 lb
- Previous birth of an infant who was stillborn or had a birth defect
- Previous GDM diagnosis
- Age older than 25 years
- Polyhydramnios
- Belonging to an ethnic group known to have higher rates of GDM (Hispanic, African American, Native American, Asian, Pacific Islander)

Treatment

If a woman is diagnosed with GDM, the treatment is focused on keeping her glucose at a safe level. This includes special meal plans, exercise, daily blood glucose testing, and insulin injections, if needed. If the blood glucose is controlled during pregnancy, most women with GDM are able to prevent maternal or fetal complications. ∎

Rh Antibody Titer (on Rh-Negative Blood Specimens)

An Rh antibody titer detects the quantity of circulating Rh antibodies against red blood cells. These antibodies can occur in a pregnant woman who is Rh-negative and is carrying an Rh-positive fetus; an Rh antibody titer is performed on all Rh-negative blood specimens. Repeat antibody titer levels also are performed during the pregnancy to determine whether the woman's antibody level is increasing. As was previously indicated, an increased Rh antibody level could be dangerous to the developing fetus. As a preventive measure, Rh-negative women with the potential of having an Rh-positive infant and who test negative for Rh antibodies are given two injections of Rh immune globulin (Rho-GAM). The Rh immune globulin prevents the formation of Rh antibodies in the mother, which avoids Rh incompatibility complications during the next pregnancy. The first injection is given at 28 weeks of gestation, and the second injection is administered within 72 hours of delivery.

Hepatitis B and Human Immunodeficiency Virus

The Centers for Disease Control and Prevention (CDC) recommends that pregnant women have the hepatitis B surface antigen (HBsAg) test to screen for hepatitis B virus. Women who have positive HBsAg test results have an increased risk of spontaneous abortion or preterm labor. In addition, the mother may transmit hepatitis B to the infant, particularly during delivery or in the first few days of life. This risk can be greatly reduced by administering hepatitis B immune globulin (HBIG) and the hepatitis B vaccine within 12 hours of birth to the newborns of women who have tested positive for hepatitis B.

Infants born to women who are human immunodeficiency virus (HIV) positive are at risk of developing the disease. If antiretroviral drugs are taken during pregnancy and the infant is delivered by cesarean section, the chance of transmitting HIV to the infant is reduced significantly. Because of this, the CDC recommends that testing for HIV be included in the routine panel of prenatal screening tests for all pregnant women, and that separate written consent is not required. The CDC further recommends that the patient should be notified that HIV testing will be performed unless the patient declines the test. The CDC recommends that repeat HIV screening be performed in the third trimester in geographic areas that have elevated rates of HIV infection among pregnant women.

Return Prenatal Visits

Return prenatal visits provide the opportunity for a continuous assessment of the health of the mother and the fetus. During each visit, essential data are collected and recorded in the prenatal record, resulting in an updated record at each visit, as is discussed in this section. If signs or symptoms of a pathologic condition are present, the physician performs select aspects of the physical examination as necessary to diagnose and treat the condition. In addition, diagnostic and laboratory tests may be ordered to assist in diagnosis and treatment. The usual schedule of visits for prenatal care is listed below. A patient who exhibits complications is seen more frequently for closer monitoring.

- 0 to 28 weeks of gestation: Every 4 weeks
- 29 to 35 weeks: Every 2 weeks
- 36 weeks until delivery: Every week

The return prenatal visit also provides the opportunity for the physician and the medical assistant to lend support to the mother, to provide her with ongoing prenatal education to reduce apprehension and anxiety, and to ensure that the mother is well informed and prepared during her pregnancy, childbirth, and the postpartum period. The medical assistant plays an important role in prenatal education and should take the necessary time with each patient to provide appropriate information and to allow the patient to ask questions. Procedure 8-3 outlines the medical assistant's role in the return prenatal visit.

The patient is asked to provide a urine specimen during each return prenatal visit. The medical assistant is responsible for testing the specimen for glucose and protein using a reagent strip and for recording results in the prenatal record. A positive reaction to glucose may indicate the development of gestational diabetes mellitus or a prediabetic condition, and a positive reaction to protein may indicate a urinary tract infection or preeclampsia. Further testing usually is needed to arrive at a final diagnosis and to institute treatment. Hypertension is the most common medical disorder of pregnancy and occurs in 10% to 12% of all pregnancies. Because of this, the medical assistant must make sure to obtain an accurate blood pressure measurement.

During the return visit, the physician performs one or more of the following procedures, depending on the stage of the pregnancy: (1) palpation of the woman's abdomen to measure fundal height, (2) measurement of the fetal heart rate, and (3) a vaginal examination. These procedures are discussed in detail next.

Fundal Height Measurement

The pregnant uterus rises gradually into the abdominal cavity, and the fundus is palpable between 8 and 13 weeks of gestation. The first fundal height measurement, which is usually performed during the first prenatal visit, is used as a guideline for all subsequent measurements. The physician measures the fundal height by placing one end of a flexible, nonstretchable centimeter tape measure on the superior aspect of the symphysis pubis and measuring to the crest or top of the uterine fundus (Figure 8-13). The measurement is recorded on a flow chart in the patient's prenatal record. By 20 weeks, the fundus reaches the lower border of the umbilicus, and between 36 and 37 weeks, it reaches the tip of the sternum. During the first and second trimesters, measuring the fundal height provides a rough estimate of the duration of the pregnancy (Figure 8-14). The fundal height measurement is considered accurate to within 4 weeks using McDonald's rule.

Calculation of the duration of the pregnancy using McDonald's rule is as follows:

Height of fundus (in centimeters) $\times$ 8/7 = Duration of the pregnancy in weeks

Example: 21 cm $\times$ 8/7 = 24 weeks

Height of fundus (in centimeters) $\times$ 2/7 = Duration of the pregnancy in lunar months

Example: 21 cm $\times$ 2/7 = 6 months

Because fetal weights vary considerably during the third trimester, it is difficult to use fundal height measurements as an estimate of the duration of the pregnancy in the last trimester.

In addition to assessing the duration of the pregnancy, the fundal height measurements permit variations from normal to become apparent and are used to assess whether fetal growth is progressing normally. Growth that is too rapid or too slow must be evaluated further by the physician as a possible indication of high-risk conditions, such as multiple pregnancies, polyhydramnios, ovarian tumor, and intrauterine growth retardation, intrauterine death, or an error in estimating the fetal progress.

Fetal Heart Tones

The normal **fetal heart rate** is between 120 and 160 beats per minute with a regular rhythm. A very slow or rapid fetal heart rate usually indicates fetal distress. The term **fetal heart tones** refers to the heartbeat of the fetus as heard through the mother's abdominal wall. The fetal heart tones can be heard with a Doppler fetal pulse detector between 10 and 12 weeks of gestation. The Doppler fetal pulse detector converts ultrasonic waves into audible sounds of the fetal pulse.

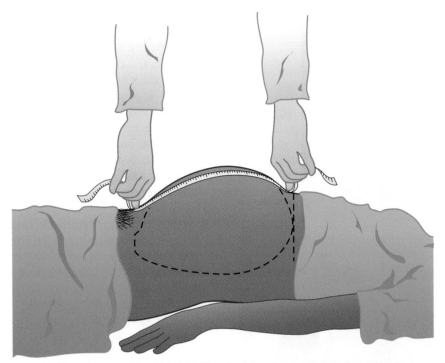

Figure 8-13. Measurement of fundal height. The physician places one end of a centimeter tape measure on the superior aspect of the symphysis pubis and measures to the top of the uterine fundus.

The Doppler device consists of a main control unit and a probe (Figure 8-15, *A*). The probe head contains a transducer and electronic components, which generate the sound waves. The probe head is delicate and must be handled carefully, making sure not to drop or knock the head to prevent damaging it.

Because air is a poor conductor of sound, an ultrasound coupling gel must first be spread on the mother's abdomen in the area to be examined. The gel is usually applied by the medical assistant, and its purpose is to increase conductivity of the sound waves between the abdomen and the transducer.

The physician places the head of the probe into the gel on the mother's abdomen and slowly moves it until the fetal heart tones are located. The Doppler device amplifies the fetal heart tones, and they are broadcast through a built-in loudspeaker in the main unit. A volume control provides adjustment of the sound level as required. (Fetal heart tones sound like the hoofbeats of a galloping horse, and when the probe is over the placenta, a windlike sound is heard.) The Doppler device also may have an LCD screen, which provides a digital display of the fetal pulse rate. Stereo headphones come with the Doppler device to allow private listening. The loudspeaker is muted when the headphones are connected (Figure 8-15, *B*).

After the procedure, the medical assistant should remove excess gel from the mother's abdomen with a paper towel. The probe head is cleaned using a damp cloth or a paper towel. The Doppler device should be properly stored in its carrying case to prevent it from becoming damaged.

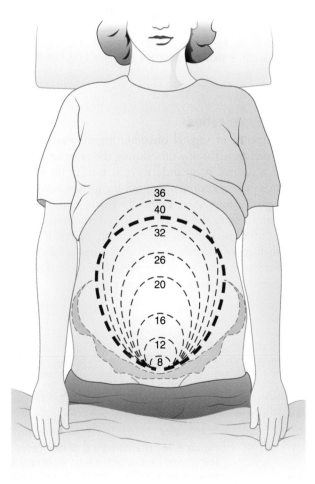

Figure 8-14. Fundal height showing gestational age in weeks.

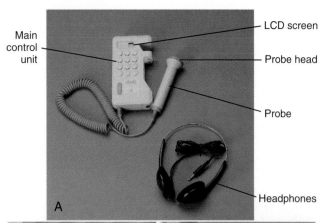

Main control unit

LCD screen

Probe head

Probe

Headphones

A

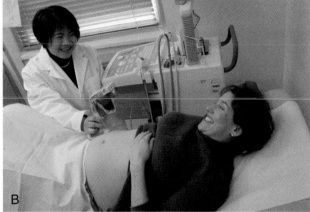

B

Figure 8-15. **A,** Parts of a Doppler device. **B,** The probe of the Doppler device is moved across the abdomen to detect the fetal pulse.

Vaginal Examination

In the absence of vaginal bleeding, vaginal examinations may be performed at any time during the pregnancy; however, in a normal pregnancy, there is usually no need to perform a vaginal examination until the patient nears term. The vaginal examination is usually begun approximately 2 to 3 weeks from the EDD and is performed to confirm the presenting part and to determine the degree, if any, of cervical dilation and effacement. The purpose of dilation and effacement is to permit the passage of the infant from the uterus into the birth canal (Figure 8-16).

Case Study 4

Wynita Lopez is at the office with her husband. She is 32 years old and 18 weeks pregnant. It took Wynita a long time—almost 6 years—to get pregnant. She is excited and happy about being pregnant but, at the same time, sad and confused. Her test results on her triple screen test came back indicating the possibility that her baby has Down syndrome. A repeat test was done with the same results. Wynita just got finished having an ultrasound that showed a normal baby, but Wynita and her husband understand that the only way to know for sure is to have an amniocentesis. Wynita does not know what to do. She is afraid of having an amniocentesis because of the chance of miscarriage. She also knows her triple screen test could be a false-positive. Wynita is unsure what her decision would be if the baby did have Down syndrome. Her husband is visibly distressed and wants Wynita to make all the decisions, saying he will be supportive of whatever she decides. Right now she wants as much information as she can get about all of this before she makes a decision. She feels "safer" being at the medical office and does not want to go home just yet. ■

Special Tests and Procedures

The pregnancy can be evaluated with one or more of the following special tests and procedures: triple screen test, obstetric ultrasound scan, amniocentesis, and fetal heart rate monitoring. These are not considered routine procedures; however, they involve little or no risk to the mother or the fetus. Because some of these tests may be performed in the obstetric medical office, the medical assistant should have a general knowledge of these procedures.

Triple Screen Test

The triple screen test (also known as the multiple marker test) is a laboratory test available to pregnant women between 15 and 20 weeks of gestation. Its purpose is to screen for the presence of certain fetal abnormalities, which include neural tube defects, Down syndrome, trisomy 18, and ventral wall defect. Because the triple screen test has a high incidence of false-positive test results, it is not a mandatory prenatal test; however, the American College of

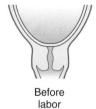
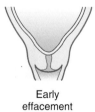
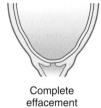
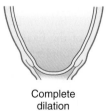

Before labor

Early effacement

Complete effacement

Complete dilation

Figure 8-16. Effacement and dilation occur to permit the passage of the infant into the birth canal. The cervical canal shortens from its normal length of 1 to 2 cm to a structure with paper-thin edges in which there is no canal at all. The cervix dilates from an opening a few millimeters wide to an opening large enough to allow the passage of the infant (approximately 10 cm).

Obstetricians and Gynecologists believes that this test should be offered to all pregnant women regardless of maternal age.

The triple screen test measures the level of the following three substances normally produced by the fetus and placenta and excreted into the mother's blood in the second trimester of pregnancy: alpha-fetoprotein (AFP), unconjugated estriol (uEST), and human chorionic gonadotropin (hCG).

AFP is a glycoprotein produced by the fetus. During pregnancy, some AFP crosses from the amniotic fluid into the mother's bloodstream. When the neural tube of the fetus is not properly formed, increased amounts of AFP appear in the maternal blood. Elevated AFP levels indicate the possibility of a neural tube defect in the fetus, such as spina bifida (incomplete closure of the spinal column) and anencephaly (incomplete closure of the brain).

A lower serum level of AFP and estriol, along with a higher level of hCG, is associated with an increased risk of having an infant with Down syndrome. A woman who is carrying a fetus with trisomy 18 may have lower blood levels of AFP, estriol, and hCG than women with unaffected fetuses.

The triple screen test is a screening test. Abnormal test results always require further testing, such as an ultrasound or amniocentesis, to determine whether a fetal abnormality actually exists.

Obstetric Ultrasound Scan

An obstetric ultrasound scan is a diagnostic imaging technique, similar to sonar, used to view the fetus in utero. It allows continuous viewing of the fetus and shows fetal movement. The physician or an ultrasound technologist performs the procedure. The primary purpose of an ultrasound scan is to evaluate the health of the fetus and to determine gestational age. This is accomplished by viewing the image of the fetus and by taking various measurements of the image, such as crown-rump length; biparietal diameter, which is a side-to-side measurement of the fetal head; femur length; and abdominal circumference.

Obstetric ultrasound scanning uses high-frequency sound waves that are directed into the uterus through a transducer. When the sound waves reach the uterus, they "bounce" back to the transducer, similar to an echo. These reflected sound waves are converted into an image, or *sonogram* (Figure 8-17), which is displayed on a monitor screen. The monitor is usually positioned so the mother can observe the image on the screen if she wishes. There are two methods for performing an ultrasound scan—the transabdominal method and the endovaginal method.

Although an obstetric ultrasound scan can be performed at any time during the pregnancy, it is often performed at between 7 and 12 weeks of gestation and again at between 18 and 20 weeks. A third scan is sometimes done around 34 weeks of gestation. Box 8-1 outlines this schedule and what can be assessed at these times.

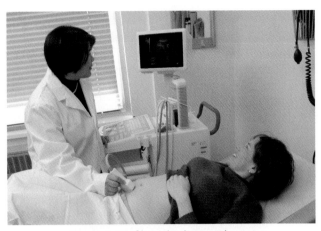

Figure 8-17. Obstetric ultrasound scan.

Transabdominal Ultrasound Scan

Transabdominal ultrasound is the scanning method performed most often. The patient must have a full bladder for this examination. This is accomplished by instructing the patient to consume 32 oz of fluid approximately 1 hour before the procedure. A full bladder acts as an "acoustic window" through which the sound waves can travel to provide a clear visualization of the uterus. In addition, a full bladder holds the uterus stable and pushes away any bowel that might interfere with the image. The patient lies on an examining table in a supine position and is draped with the abdomen exposed. A coupling agent, in the form of a liquid gel, is applied to the patient's abdomen to increase the transmission of the sound waves. An abdominal probe (containing a transducer) is placed into the gel, and the probe is moved slowly over the patient's abdomen; the image of the fetus is displayed on the screen of the monitor (see Figure 8-17).

Endovaginal Ultrasound Scan

In the early stages of the pregnancy (up to 12 weeks), endovaginal scanning is preferred over transabdominal scanning. The patient must have an empty bladder for this scan, which makes the examination more comfortable. The patient is placed in the lithotomy position, and a vaginal probe is placed in the patient's vagina. The image of the embryo is displayed on the screen of the monitor. An endovaginal ultrasound scan provides clearer visualization of the uterus at the beginning of the pregnancy because the probe is situated in the vagina, which places it closer to the uterus.

Amniocentesis

Amniocentesis is a diagnostic procedure that can be performed between 15 and 18 weeks of gestation. Amniocentesis aids in prenatal diagnosis of certain genetically transmitted errors of metabolism, congenital abnormalities, and chromosomal disorders such as Down syndrome. It also is used to detect fetal jeopardy or distress and, later in the pregnancy, to assess fetal lung maturity. Amniocentesis also can determine whether the fetus is a boy or a girl.

BOX 8-1 Purpose of Obstetric Ultrasound Scanning

Between 7 and 12 Weeks
- To confirm pregnancy by detecting fetal heart motion
- To determine gestational age by taking measurements of the embryo and embryonic sac
- To detect an ectopic pregnancy

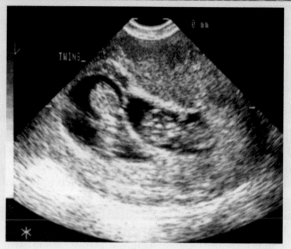

Twins.

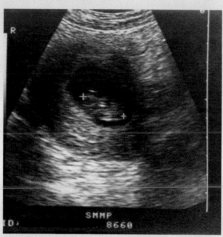

Embryo at approximately 9 weeks of gestation. (From Greer I, et al: Mosby's color atlas and text of obstetrics and gynecology, St Louis, 2001, Mosby.)

Between 18 and 20 Weeks
- To determine fetal growth, size, and weight by taking measurements of the fetus
- To detect the presence of multiple fetuses
- To examine the brain, spinal cord, heart, lungs, gastrointestinal tract, reproductive organs, kidneys, bladder, bowel, and extremities of the fetus
- To detect congenital abnormalities
- To determine the location of the placenta
- To determine the cause of bleeding or spotting

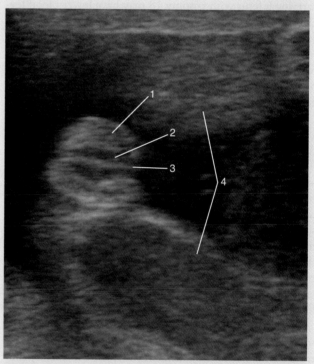

External female genitalia. *1*, major labium; *2*, minor labium; *3*, vaginal cleft; *4*, thighs. (From Callen P: Ultrasonography in obstetrics and gynecology, ed 4, Philadelphia, 2000, Saunders.)

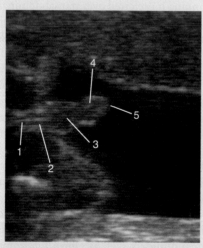

Erect fetal penis. *1*, urethra; *2*, corpus cavernosum; *3*, shaft; *4*, glans; *5*, foreskin. (From Callen P: Ultrasonography in obstetrics and gynecology, ed 4, Philadelphia, 2000, Saunders.)

BOX 8-1 Purpose of Obstetric Ultrasound Scanning—cont'd

At 34 Weeks
- To evaluate fetal growth, size, and weight by taking measurements of the fetus
- To verify the location of the placenta
- To confirm fetal presentation in uncertain cases

Other Purposes
- To diagnose uterine and pelvic abnormalities during pregnancy
- To view the fetus, placenta, and amniotic fluid during tests such as amniocentesis and chorionic villus sampling
- To confirm intrauterine death

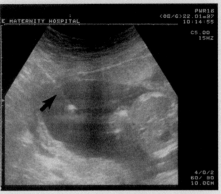

Amniocentesis being performed under ultrasound guidance. (From Greer I, et al: Mosby's color atlas and text of obstetrics and gynecology, St Louis, 2001, Mosby.)

To perform the procedure, the physician inserts a long, thin needle through the mother's abdomen and into the amniotic sac surrounding the fetus (Figure 8-18). An obstetric ultrasound scan is always performed in conjunction with amniocentesis so that the physician can view the position of the fetus, placenta, and amniotic fluid. This allows the physician to know the exact place to insert the needle. The physician withdraws a sample (about 1 tablespoon) of fluid, which contains fetal cells. The fluid is sent to a laboratory for study. It usually takes 1 to 3 weeks to evaluate the amniotic fluid and report the results.

Although the complication rate for an amniocentesis is extremely low, the procedure is not risk free. There is a slight risk of bleeding, leakage of fluid, and infection of the amniotic fluid. There also is a slight possibility of miscarriage. Because of these risks, amniocentesis is offered only to women whose pregnancies are at risk for fetal abnormalities. This includes women who are 35 years old or older, women who have a child with a genetic or neural tube defect, women who have abnormal triple screen test results, women who have or whose partner has a chromosomal abnormality, and women who are or whose partner is a carrier for a metabolic disease.

Fetal Heart Rate Monitoring

Fetal heart rate (FHR) monitoring is performed later in the pregnancy to obtain information on the physical condition of the fetus. Specific conditions that may warrant this procedure are fetal growth that is not progressing well, decreased amniotic fluid, decreased fetal activity, elevation of the mother's blood pressure, gestational diabetes, and an overdue infant.

To perform the procedure, an electronic microphone is strapped to the mother's abdomen to amplify the fetal heartbeat. A gel is usually applied under the microphone to make the sounds clearer. The fetal heartbeat is heard and displayed on a screen and printed on special paper.

There are two kinds of fetal heart rate monitoring procedures—the nonstress test and the contraction stress test. The *nonstress test* (NST) monitors changes in the fetal heart rate in response to the fetus' spontaneous movements. The mother is instructed to press a button when she feels the fetus move. In a normal test, the fetus' heart rate increases when the fetus moves. To prepare for the nonstress test, the mother must be instructed to eat a light meal within 2 hours of the procedure to stimulate fetal movement.

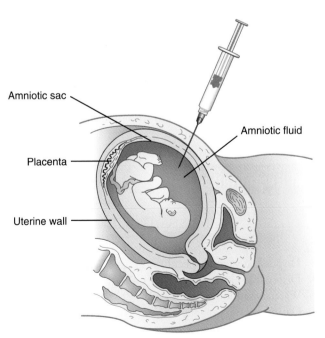

Amniotic sac

Amniotic fluid

Placenta

Uterine wall

Figure 8-18. Amniocentesis.

If the results of the nonstress test are abnormal, a *contraction stress test* (CST) may be performed. This test is similar to the nonstress test except that mild contractions of the uterus are stimulated for a short period of time. The contraction stress test is used to evaluate the response of the fetus' heart rate to the contractions to determine whether the fetus would be able to withstand the stress of repeated contractions during labor. If the results of the test are abnormal, further evaluation is required to evaluate the well-being of the fetus and to determine how and when delivery of the fetus should be carried out.

PATIENT TEACHING   Obstetric Ultrasound Scan

1. Emphasize the importance of preparing properly for the examination.
2. Provide the patient with educational materials on the obstetric ultrasound.
3. Answer questions patients have about an obstetric ultrasound scan.

What is an ultrasound scan?
An ultrasound scan is performed to look at the fetus in the uterus with the use of sound waves. During the examination, a gel is spread over your abdomen, and a scanning device is moved lightly over the area. The baby's image is displayed on a monitor similar to a television screen. During the examination, pictures of your baby will be taken, and you will be given a copy for your baby album. The ultrasonographer may also provide you with a video recording of the scan on a DVD. The ultrasound examination usually takes about 30 minutes.

Why is an ultrasound scan performed?
Ultrasound scanning is used to determine the age and position of the fetus, the location of the placenta, and the number of babies present, and overall to help the physician monitor and manage the pregnancy.

What preparation is needed?
To prepare for an obstetric (transabdominal) ultrasound scan, you will need to drink 32 oz of fluid 1 hour before the examination. Drink all the water within 15 to 20 minutes, and do not void until the examination has been completed. You should wear comfortable clothing. A two-piece outfit is recommended so that you do not have to undress completely.

Is an ultrasound scan safe?
There are no known side effects or risks to either mother or fetus during an ultrasound examination. Ultrasound does not use x-rays. No long-term risks have been detected. The procedure is painless, and the only discomfort is from a full bladder, which will make you want to go to the bathroom. When the examination is completed, you will have the opportunity to do so.

Can I learn the sex of my baby through an ultrasound scan?
Although an ultrasound scan is not performed only to determine the sex of the baby, it is sometimes possible (usually by 20 weeks) to tell whether the baby is a boy or girl, depending on the position of the baby in the uterus. Because not all parents want to know their baby's sex in advance, you will not automatically be told the baby's sex if it is determined, but you will be given the opportunity to make the choice of knowing or not knowing.

Medical Assisting Responsibilities
The medical assistant has many important responsibilities in the return prenatal examination, which are outlined in Procedure 8-3. The medical assistant is responsible for assembling the equipment and supplies required for the examination, for obtaining information to update the prenatal record, for preparing the patient for the examination, and for assisting the physician during the examination. The physician depends on the medical assistant to have the urine test results and certain measurements, such as blood pressure and weight, completed and recorded in advance to allow him or her the opportunity to review these measurements before examining the patient. ■

 PROCEDURE 8-3   Assisting With a Return Prenatal Examination

Outcome   Assist with a return prenatal examination.

Equipment/Supplies

- Urine specimen container
- Centimeter tape measure
- Doppler fetal pulse detector
- Ultrasound coupling gel
- Paper towel

- Disposable vaginal speculum
- Disposable gloves
- Water-based lubricant
- Gauze pads
- Examining gown and drape

PROCEDURE 8-3   Assisting With a Return Prenatal Examination—cont'd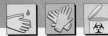

1. **Procedural Step.** Sanitize your hands.
2. **Procedural Step.** Set up the tray for the prenatal examination. The equipment and supplies depend on the procedures to be included in the examination, which may include one or more of the following:
   a. Fundal height measurement
   b. Measurement of fetal heart tones
   c. Examination of the legs, feet, and face for edema and development of varicosities
   d. Taking a specimen for the diagnosis of a vaginal infection
   e. Vaginal examination

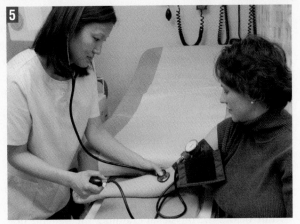

Measure the patient's blood pressure.

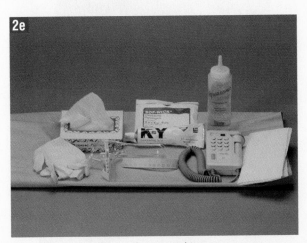

Set up the prenatal tray.

3. **Procedural Step.** Greet the patient and introduce yourself. Identify the patient and explain the procedure. Provide the patient with a urine specimen container, and ask her to obtain a urine specimen.
   Principle. A urine specimen is needed to test for glucose and protein at each prenatal visit. In addition, an empty bladder makes the examination easier and is more comfortable for the patient.
4. **Procedural Step.** Escort the patient to the examining room, and ask her to be seated. Seat yourself so that you are facing the patient. Ask the patient whether she has experienced any problems since the last prenatal visit, and record information in the appropriate section in her prenatal record.
   Principle. The physician investigates any unusual or abnormal signs or symptoms relayed by the patient.
5. **Procedural Step.** Measure the patient's blood pressure, and chart the results in the prenatal record. If the blood pressure is elevated, allow the patient to relax, and then measure the blood pressure again.
   Principle. Taking the blood pressure again gives the opportunity to determine whether the elevation was due to emotional excitement.

6. **Procedural Step.** Weigh the patient, and chart the results in the prenatal record.
   Principle. Maternal weight gain or loss assists in assessing fetal development, as well as the mother's nutrition and state of health.

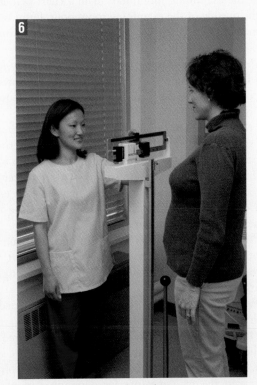

Weigh the patient.

Continued

PROCEDURE 8-3

PROCEDURE 8-3   Assisting With a Return Prenatal Examination—cont'd

7. Procedural Step. Instruct and prepare the patient for the examination. Have her remove or pull up her outer clothing to expose the abdominal area. If the physician will be performing a vaginal examination, the patient also must remove her panties; otherwise, she may leave them on. Tell the patient to have a seat on the examining table when she is finished getting ready for the examination. Inform the patient that the physician will be with her soon, and leave the room to give her privacy.

8. Procedural Step. Using a reagent strip, test the urine specimen for glucose and protein, and chart the results. *Note:* The urine specimen may be tested at any time before the physician examines the patient; however, a convenient time to test the specimen is while the patient is disrobing.
Principle. The prenatal patient's urine must be tested at every visit to assist in early detection and prevention of disease.

9. Procedural Step. Make the medical record available for review by the physician. The medical office has a designated location where the record is placed, such as a small shelf mounted on the wall next to the outside of the examining room door or in a chart holder on the outside of the examining room door. Position the medical record so that patient-identifiable information is not visible.
Principle. Before going into the room, the physician will want to review the patient's chart and information documented by the medical assistant. HIPAA requires protection of a patient's health information.

10. Procedural Step. Check to make sure the patient is ready to be seen by the physician. Before entering a patient's room, always knock lightly on the door to let the patient know you are getting ready to enter the room. Inform the physician. This may be done using a color-coded flagging system mounted on the wall next to the examining room.

11. Procedural Step. Assist the patient into a supine position, and properly drape her. Provide support and reassurance to the patient to help her relax during the examination.
Principle. The patient should be properly draped so that she is warm and comfortable.

12. Procedural Step. Assist the physician as required for the prenatal examination, as follows:
a. **Fundal Height Measurement:** Hand the physician the tape measure for determination of the fundal measurement.

b. **Fetal Heart Tones:** Apply a liberal amount of coupling gel to the patient's abdomen. Turn on the Doppler fetal pulse detector and hand it to the physician. When the physician is finished, remove excess gel from the patient with a paper towel. Clean the probe head of the Doppler device with a damp cloth or a paper towel. Place the probe head back in its holder.

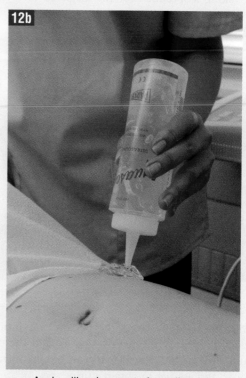

Apply a liberal amount of coupling gel.

c. **Vaginal Specimen:** Assist the patient into the lithotomy position if a specimen is to be taken for the detection of a vaginal infection. Assist with collection of the specimen as required.

d. **Vaginal Examination:** Assist the patient into the lithotomy position if a vaginal examination is to be performed.

PROCEDURE 8-3   Assisting With a Return Prenatal Examination—cont'd

13. Procedural Step. After the examination, assist the patient into a sitting position, and allow her the opportunity to rest for a moment. If a vaginal examination was performed, offer the patient tissues to remove excess lubricating jelly from the perineum. Assist her off the examining table to prevent falls. Instruct the patient to get dressed. Leave the room to provide the patient with privacy.

Principle. The patient may become dizzy after being on the examining table and should be allowed to rest before getting off the table. The medical assistant must provide for the safety of the prenatal patient while she is getting off the examining table.

14. Procedural Step. Provide the prenatal patient teaching and further explanation of the physician's instructions as required to meet individual patient needs. Escort the patient to the reception area.

15. Procedural Step. Clean the examining room in preparation for the next patient, and, if necessary, prepare specimens for transport to an outside medical laboratory.

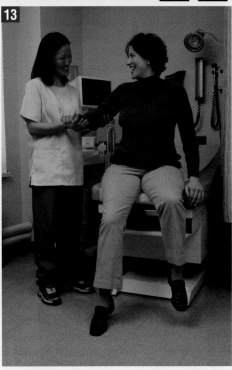

Assist the patient off the examining table.

SIX WEEKS POSTPARTUM VISIT

The **puerperium** includes the period of time in which the body systems are returning to their prepregnant or nearly prepregnant state, which usually is 4 to 6 weeks after delivery. During this time, numerous changes occur in the woman's body. The *involution of the uterus* (i.e., the process by which it returns to its normal size and state) occurs; this includes healing of any injuries sustained to the birth canal during delivery.

During the puerperium, the patient experiences a vaginal discharge shed from the lining of the uterus, known as **lochia.** Lochia consists of blood, tissue, white blood cells, mucus, and some bacteria. The color of the lochia is an indication of the progress of the healing of the uterus. For the first 3 days after delivery, the lochia consists almost entirely of blood and, because of its red color, is termed *lochia rubra.* By approximately 4 days postpartum, the amount of blood decreases, and the discharge becomes pink or brownish and is known as *lochia serosa.* By 10 days postpartum, the flow should decrease, and the lochia should become yellowish white; this is known as *lochia alba.* Lochia usually continues in consistently decreasing amounts (from moderate to scant to occasional spotting) and becomes paler in color until the third week after delivery, when it usually disappears altogether. It would not be considered unusual for the discharge to last the entire 6 weeks, however.

The patient should be instructed to contact the medical office under the following circumstances: if the amount of discharge increases rather than decreases; if the discharge is absent within the first 2 weeks after delivery; if it changes to red after having been yellowish white, which indicates bleeding; or if it takes on a foul odor, which indicates infection. Menstruation usually begins approximately 2 months after delivery in a nonnursing mother and 3 to 6 months after delivery in a nursing mother.

During the puerperium, the patient should be encouraged to avoid fatigue, to avoid lifting heavy objects, and to consume a nutritious, well-balanced diet that helps maintain health and promote healing. The physician will want to see the patient at the medical office at the end of the 6-week period. The purpose of the 6 weeks postpartum visit is to evaluate the general mental and physical condition of the patient, to ensure there are no residual problems from childbearing, and to provide the patient with education regarding postpartum depression and methods of contraception and infant care. During this visit, the patient is queried about problems or abnormalities related to postpartum depression, vaginal discharge, urinary or bowel function, and breastfeeding if she is nursing. This information is recorded in the patient's chart. The postpartum visit provides an excellent opportunity for the medical assistant to instruct the patient in the technique for performing a breast self-examination and to educate

Table 8-3 Six Weeks Postpartum Examination

Procedure	Purpose

Vital signs (see Chapter 4)
    Temperature
    Pulse
    Respiration
    Blood pressure
	To ensure vital signs fall within normal limits and that blood pressure has returned to normal prepregnant level.

Weight (see Chapter 5)	To determine whether patient's weight has returned to prepregnant measurement. If not, nutritional counseling may be indicated.
Breast examination (see Chapter 8)	To ensure breasts are not sore or tender and no cysts or lumps are present. In nonnursing mother, breasts are examined to determine whether they have returned to their prepregnant size. In nursing mother, nipples are examined for cracks, redness, soreness, and fissures.
Pelvic examination (see Chapter 8)	To ensure that involution of uterus is complete and to determine whether the cervix has healed. To ensure that episiotomy (if performed) and any injuries sustained by the birth canal have healed. To ensure that no abnormal vaginal discharge is present.
Rectal-vaginal examination (see Chapter 8)	To ensure pelvic floor has regained its muscle tone. To determine whether hemorrhoids are present.
Evaluation of patient's general mental and physical condition (see Chapter 5)	To ensure body systems have returned to their prepregnant state. To discuss and evaluate signs and symptoms of postpartum depression.

her on the importance of returning to the medical office annually for a Pap test.

During the postpartum examination, the physician evaluates the patient's general mental status and physical appearance, performs breast and pelvic examinations, and checks to determine whether the muscle tone has returned to the muscles of the abdominal wall. During the puerperium, atypical cells may be sloughed off into the cervical and vaginal mucus as part of the normal healing process. Because of this, the Pap test is not included in the postpartum visit. If the patient has problems with hemorrhoids or varicosities, the physician discusses any further treatment required. If the patient does not have antibody protection to rubella, as has been evidenced through the prenatal laboratory tests, she receives rubella immunization at this time (if it was not administered in the hospital). In addition,

hemoglobin and hematocrit determinations usually are performed on the postpartum patient to screen for anemia caused by blood loss during delivery and the puerperium.

Responsibilities of the medical assistant during the postpartum visit include measuring and recording the patient's vital signs and weight and preparing the patient for the examination. The patient is required to disrobe completely for this examination and to put on an examining gown with the opening in front. Table 8-3 lists the procedures commonly included in the 6 weeks postpartum visit and the purpose of each.

evolve *Check out the Evolve site to access additional interactive activities.*

MEDICAL PRACTICE and the LAW

Mature Minor

A difficult and complex issue facing policymakers today involves whether a minor should be able to obtain health care services without a parent's consent. A minor is an individual who has not reached the age of majority; in most states, minors reach majority at 18 years old (at that time, individuals are legally able to make their own decisions regarding health care).

Over the past 3 decades, many states have passed legislation permitting minors to receive some health care services without parental consent. These include contraceptive services, testing and treatment for sexually transmitted diseases, prenatal care and delivery services, treatment for alcohol and drug abuse, and outpatient

mental health care. States that have passed such legislation reason that some minors might avoid seeking the care that they need for certain conditions if they have to have parental consent. The one major exception to this is abortion. Most states have laws that require the involvement of at least one parent in a minor's decision to have an abortion.

In recent years, some states have given minors even greater authority to make health care decisions for themselves by adopting what is known as the *mature minor rule.* This allows an individual in the middle to late teens who exhibits the intelligence and maturity to understand the nature and consequences of a medical treatment to consent to such treatment without parental consent.

MEDICAL PRACTICE and the LAW—cont'd

It is important for the medical assistant to become familiar with the laws in his or her state regarding a minor's right to consent to health care to help the medical assistant in making appropriate decisions with respect to minors. For example, if a state does not allow a minor to obtain prenatal care without parental consent, the medical assistant would not be permitted to make an appointment for a minor who is pregnant; rather, the appointment would have to be scheduled by the minor's parent. Consent by minors to health care services will continue to be a complex issue; the medical assistant must keep up-to-date with changes in his or her state. ■

What Would You Do? What Would You *Not* Do? RESPONSES

Case Study 1
Page 274

What Did Yin-Ling Do?
❑ Reassured Mrs. Wooster that the physician is there to help her and stressed that he will be pleased that she has come to the office for an examination.
❑ Commended Mrs. Wooster on performing a breast self-examination at home and encouraged her to continue performing a BSE each month. Asked her whether she had any questions on how to perform a BSE.
❑ Told Mrs. Wooster that some breast changes are normal and others are not normal, and the only way to know for sure is to be examined by the physician.
❑ Told Mrs. Wooster that it is important to have a periodic gynecologic examination even if her periods are normal. Explained to her that some conditions can be present without symptoms. Took plenty of time with her so that she would feel comfortable coming back again in the future for a gynecologic examination. Gave Mrs. Wooster a patient information brochure on gynecologic examinations.
❑ Gave Mrs. Wooster a patient information brochure on mammograms, and explained the mammogram procedure to reduce her apprehension. Explained that the procedure is not painful, but there may be some minor discomfort. Provided her with some tips on reducing discomfort that may occur, such as avoiding caffeine several days before the procedure and having the office schedule the mammogram a week after her menstrual period.

What Did Yin-Ling Not Do?
❑ Did not criticize Mrs. Wooster for waiting so long to schedule a gynecologic examination.
❑ Did not tell Mrs. Wooster that there is no discomfort involved with a mammogram.

What Would You Do?/What Would You *Not* Do? Review Yin-Ling's response and place a checkmark next to the information you included in your response. List additional information you included in your response.

_____
_____
_____
_____

Case Study 2
Page 292

What Did Yin-Ling Do?
❑ Stressed to Dagny how important it is that she be seen by the physician. Explained that she could be infected with chlamydia and not know it because chlamydia often has no symptoms, especially in women.
❑ Explained to Dagny that state law allows her to be treated for a sexually transmitted disease without permission from her parents. Told her the law was created to encourage minors to seek treatment for sexually transmitted diseases.
❑ Commended Dagny on practicing safe sex. Relayed to her that if a condom is not used correctly, or if it tears, she might not be protected from getting a sexually transmitted disease. That is another reason she should be tested.
❑ Explained to Dagny what will occur during the examination and what the physician will be doing. Relayed techniques that Dagny could use to relax during the procedure.

What Did Yin-Ling Not Do?
❑ Did not tell Dagny everything would be all right and that she probably does not have chlamydia.
❑ Did not ask Dagny whether she knew how her boyfriend got chlamydia.
❑ If Dagny still insisted on leaving, did not try to prevent her from doing so.

What Would You Do?/What Would You *Not* Do? Review Yin-Ling's response and place a checkmark next to the information you included in your response. List additional information you included in your response.

_____
_____
_____
_____

Case Study 3
Page 302

What Did Yin-Ling Do?
❑ Tried to calm Johanna by telling her that it is normal for her to be worried and concerned. Explained that the purpose of her

Continued

What Would You Do? What Would You *Not* Do? RESPONSES—cont'd

prenatal visits is so that the physician can keep a close watch on her and detect any problems that might occur.

❑ Reassured Johanna that she does not need to be afraid to tell the physician any of her concerns because he is there to help her and her baby.

❑ Told Johanna that it is important not to take any medications during her pregnancy without first checking with the physician because some medications could be harmful to her baby.

❑ Told Johanna that her problems and concerns would be relayed to the physician and that he would want to talk to her about them. Explained that the physician also would talk with her about being tested for group B streptococcus.

What Did Yin-Ling Not Do?

❑ Did not tell Johanna that it was all right to take the antibiotics.

What Would You Do?/What Would You *Not* Do? Review Yin-Ling's response and place a checkmark next to the information you included in your response. List additional information you included in your response.

_____

_____

_____

_____

Case Study 4
Page 306

What Did Yin-Ling Do?

❑ Escorted Mr. and Mrs. Lopez to a private room in the office. Tried to relax them and told them that whatever they choose to do will be the right decision for them. Reassured them that they could stay at the office for as long as they wanted.

❑ Gave Mrs. Lopez the information she requested that was available at the office and provided her with a list of resources approved by the physician that she could contact for further information.

❑ Asked Mr. and Mrs. Lopez whether they had any more questions they wanted to ask the physician.

What Did Yin-Ling Not Do?

❑ Did not give Mr. and Mrs. Lopez advice on what they should do.

What Would You Do?/What Would You *Not* Do? Review Yin-Ling's response and place a checkmark next to the information you included in your response. List additional information you included in your response.

_____

_____

_____

_____

CERTIFICATION REVIEW

❑ **Gynecology** is the branch of medicine that deals with diseases of female reproductive organs. A gynecologic examination includes breast and pelvic examinations. The purpose of the examination is to assess the health status of the female reproductive organs and to detect early signs of disease, leading to early diagnosis and treatment.

❑ **During the breast examination,** the physician inspects the breasts and nipples for swelling, dimpling, puckering, and change in skin texture. The nipples are checked for abnormalities, and the breasts and axial lymph nodes are palpated for lumps. Women should perform a breast self-examination at home each month starting at age 20, approximately 2 to 3 days after the menstrual period ends.

❑ **The purpose of the pelvic examination** is to assess the size, shape, and location of the reproductive organs and to detect the presence of disease. The pelvic examination consists of an inspection of the external genitalia, vagina, and cervix; collection of a specimen for a Pap test; bimanual pelvic examination; and rectal-vaginal examination.

❑ **The purpose of the Pap test** is early detection and treatment of cervical cancer. It also is used to detect abnormal cells that might develop into cancer if not treated. Abnormal cytologic findings on the Pap test indicate the need for additional tests, such as colposcopy, cervical biopsy, and endocervical curettage.

❑ **The purpose of the bimanual pelvic examination** is to determine the size, shape, and position of the uterus and ovaries and detect tenderness or lumps. The purpose of the rectal-vaginal examination is to obtain information about the tone and alignment of the pelvic organs and the adnexal region and to collect a fecal specimen for occult blood testing. The presence of hemorrhoids, fistulas, and fissures also can be noted during this examination.

❑ **Trichomoniasis** is a vaginal infection caused by a protozoan and is most commonly spread through sexual intercourse. Symptoms include a profuse, frothy, yellowish-green vaginal discharge with an unpleasant odor; itching and irritation of the vulva and vagina; and dysuria. The cervix may exhibit small red spots; this is known as "strawberry cervix."

❑ **Candidiasis** is a vaginal infection caused by a yeastlike fungus. Conditions such as pregnancy, diabetes mellitus, and prolonged antibiotic therapy may precipitate a candidal infection, commonly referred to as a "yeast infection." Symptoms of candidiasis include white patches on the mucous membrane of the vagina, along with a thick, odorless, cottage cheese–like discharge that results in burning and intense itching.

❏ **Chlamydia** is caused by a bacterium and is the most frequently reported and fastest spreading sexually transmitted disease in the United States. Most women with chlamydia have no symptoms. Women with symptoms have dysuria; itching and irritation of the genital area; an odorless, thick, yellowish-white vaginal discharge; dull abdominal pain; and bleeding between menstrual periods. If not treated, chlamydia can lead to pelvic inflammatory disease (PID), which can result in infertility.

❏ **Gonorrhea** is an infection of the genitourinary tract and is caused by a bacterium that is transmitted through sexual intercourse. Women who have contracted gonorrhea may be asymptomatic or may exhibit dysuria and a yellow vaginal discharge. As the disease progresses, it may spread to the lining of the uterus, resulting in PID.

❏ **Obstetrics** is the branch of medicine that deals with the supervision of women during pregnancy, childbirth, and the puerperium. *Prenatal* refers to the care of the pregnant woman before delivery of the infant to promote the health of the mother and fetus through the prevention of disease and early detection, diagnosis, and treatment of problems common to pregnancy.

❏ **The first prenatal examination** consists of the completion of a prenatal record form, an initial prenatal examination, prenatal patient education, and laboratory tests.

❏ **The prenatal record** provides information regarding the past and present health of the patient and serves as a database and flow sheet for subsequent prenatal visits. The past medical history focuses on conditions that could affect the health of the mother and fetus. The menstrual history provides information on the patient's menstrual cycle. The obstetric history provides information from the patient related to previous pregnancies. The present pregnancy history establishes a baseline for the present health status of the patient. The purpose of the interval prenatal history is to update the prenatal record at each return visit.

❏ **The expected date of delivery (EDD)** can be determined using Nägele's rule and a gestation calculator. Approximately 4% of patients deliver spontaneously on the EDD, and most patients deliver during the period from 7 days before to 7 days after the EDD.

❏ **The purpose of the initial prenatal examination** is to confirm the pregnancy and to establish a baseline for the woman's state of health. It includes a thorough gy-

necologic examination (breast and pelvic) and a general physical examination of the other body systems.

❏ **Numerous laboratory tests** are ordered to assist in the overall initial assessment of the patient's health and to detect problems that might put the pregnancy at risk. Prenatal laboratory tests that are performed include a complete urinalysis, Pap test, chlamydia and gonorrhea tests, tests for trichomoniasis and candidiasis (if warranted), group B streptococcus (GBS) test, complete blood count (CBC), Rh factor and ABO blood type, glucose challenge test (GCT), syphilis test, rubella antibody titer, Rh antibody titer, hepatitis B test, and HIV test.

❏ **Return prenatal visits** provide the opportunity for continuous assessment of the health of the mother and fetus. During each return prenatal visit, the medical assistant is responsible for measuring the patient's blood pressure and weight and testing the patient's urine for glucose and protein. During the return visit, the physician performs one or more of the following procedures: palpation of the woman's abdomen to measure fundal height, measurement of the fetal heart rate, and a vaginal examination.

❏ **The triple screen test** is performed between 15 and 20 weeks of gestation to screen for certain fetal abnormalities. Abnormal test results may indicate the possibility of a neural tube defect, Down syndrome, trisomy 18, and ventral wall defect.

❏ **Obstetric ultrasound scanning** is used to view the fetus in utero. It is used most frequently to evaluate the health of the fetus and to determine gestational age. There are two methods for performing an ultrasound scan based on gestational age—endovaginal scan (up to 12 weeks of gestation) and transabdominal scan (after 12 weeks of gestation).

❏ **Amniocentesis** is performed to diagnose certain genetically transmitted errors of metabolism, congenital abnormalities, and chromosomal disorders such as Down syndrome. Fetal heart rate monitoring is performed to obtain information on the physical condition of the fetus.

❏ **The puerperium** includes the period of time in which the body systems are returning to the prepregnant or nearly prepregnant state, which usually is 4 to 6 weeks after delivery. The physician will want to see the patient at the medical office at the end of the 6-week period. The purpose of this postpartum visit is to evaluate the general physical condition of the patient, to ensure that there are no residual problems from childbearing, and to provide the patient with education regarding methods of birth control and infant care.

⟲ TERMINOLOGY REVIEW

Medical Term	Word Parts	Definition
Abortion		The termination of the pregnancy before the fetus reaches the age of viability (20 weeks).
Adnexal		Adjacent.
Amenorrhea	*a-:* without *men/o:* menstruation *-orrhea:* flow, excessive discharge	The absence or cessation of the menstrual period. Amenorrhea occurs normally before puberty, during pregnancy, and after menopause.
Atypical	*a-:* without	Deviation from the normal.
Braxton Hicks contractions		Intermittent and irregular painless uterine contractions that occur throughout pregnancy. They occur more frequently toward the end of pregnancy and are sometimes mistaken for true labor pains.
Cervix		The lower narrow end of the uterus that opens into the vagina.
Colposcopy	*colp/o:* vagina *-scopy:* visual examination	Examination of the cervix using a colposcope (a lighted instrument with a magnifying lens).
Cytology	*cyt/o:* cell *-ology:* study of	The science that deals with the study of cells, including their origin, structure, function, and pathology.
Dilation (of the cervix)		The stretching of the external os from an opening a few millimeters wide to an opening large enough to allow the passage of an infant (approximately 10 cm).
Dysmenorrhea	*dys-:* difficult, painful, abnormal *men/o:* menstruation *-orrhea:* flow, excessive discharge	Pain associated with the menstrual period.
Dyspareunia	*dys-:* difficult, painful, abnormal	Pain in the vagina or pelvis experienced by a woman during sexual intercourse.
Dysplasia	*dys-:* difficult, painful, abnormal *plasia:* a growth	The growth of abnormal cells. Dysplasia is a precancerous condition that may or may not develop into cancer.
Ectocervix	*ecto-:* outside, outer	The part of the cervix that projects into the vagina and is lined with stratified squamous epithelium.
Effacement		The thinning and shortening of the cervical canal from its normal length of 1 to 2 cm to a structure with paper-thin edges in which there is no canal at all. Effacement occurs late in pregnancy, during labor, or both. The purpose of effacement along with dilation is to permit the passage of the infant into the birth canal.
Embryo		The child in utero from the time of conception to the beginning of the first trimester.
Endocervix	*endo-:* within	The mucous membrane lining the cervical canal.
Engagement		The entrance of the fetal head or the presenting part into the pelvic inlet.
Expected date of delivery (EDD)		Projected birth date of the infant.
External os		The opening of the cervical canal of the uterus into the vagina.
Fetal heart rate		The number of times per minute the fetal heart beats.
Fetal heart tones		The sounds of the heartbeat of the fetus heard through the mother's abdominal wall.
Fetus		The child in utero from the third month after conception to birth; during the first 2 months of development, it is called an *embryo*.

↻ TERMINOLOGY REVIEW—cont'd

Medical Term	Word Parts	Definition
Fundus		The dome-shaped upper portion of the uterus between the fallopian tubes.
Gestation		The period of intrauterine development from conception to birth; the period of pregnancy. The average pregnancy lasts about 280 days, or 40 weeks, from the date of conception to childbirth.
Gestational age		The age of the fetus between conception and birth.
Gravidity	*gravid/o:* pregnancy	The total number of pregnancies a woman has had regardless of duration, including a current pregnancy.
Gynecology	*gynec/o:* woman *-ology:* study of	The branch of medicine that deals with the diseases of reproductive organs of women.
Infant		A child from birth to 12 months of age.
Internal os		The internal opening of the cervical canal into the uterus.
Lochia		A discharge from the uterus after delivery that consists of blood, tissue, white blood cells, and some bacteria.
Menopause	*men/o:* menstruation	The permanent cessation of menstruation, which usually occurs between the ages of 45 and 55.
Menorrhagia	*men/o:* menstruation *-orrhagia:* rapid flow of blood	Excessive bleeding during a menstrual period, in the number of days or the amount of blood or both. Also called *dysfunctional uterine bleeding (DUB).*
Metrorrhagia	*metr/o:* uterus *-orrhagia:* rapid flow of blood	Bleeding between menstrual periods.
Multigravida	*multi-:* many *gravid/o:* pregnancy	A woman who has been pregnant more than once.
Multipara	*multi-:* many *par/o:* bear, give birth to	A woman who has completed two or more pregnancies to the age of fetal viability regardless of whether they ended in live infants or stillbirths.
Nullipara	*nulli-:* none *par/o:* bear, give birth to	A woman who has not carried a pregnancy to the point of fetal viability (20 weeks of gestation).
Obstetrics		The branch of medicine concerned with the care of the woman during pregnancy, childbirth, and the postpartal period.
Parity	*par/o:* bear, give birth to	The condition of having borne offspring regardless of the outcome.
Perimenopause	*peri-:* surrounding *men/o:* menstruation	Before the onset of menopause, the phase during which the woman with regular periods changes to irregular cycles and increased periods of amenorrhea.
Perineum		The external region between the vaginal orifice and the anus in a female and between the scrotum and the anus in a male.
Position		The relation of the presenting part of the fetus to the maternal pelvis.
Postpartum	*post-:* after *par/o:* bear, give birth to	Occurring after childbirth.
Preeclampsia		A major complication of pregnancy, the cause of which is unknown, characterized by increasing hypertension, albuminuria, and edema. If this condition is neglected or is not treated properly, it may develop into eclampsia, which could cause maternal convulsions and coma. Preeclampsia generally occurs between the 20th week of pregnancy and the end of the first week postpartum.

Continued

↻ TERMINOLOGY REVIEW—cont'd

Medical Term	Word Parts	Definition
Prenatal	*pre-:* in front of, before *nat/o:* birth *-al:* pertaining to	Before birth.
Presentation		Indication of the part of the fetus that is closest to the cervix and is delivered first. A cephalic presentation is a delivery in which the fetal head is presenting against the cervix. A breech presentation is a delivery in which the buttocks or feet are presented instead of the head.
Preterm birth	*pre-:* in front of, before	Delivery occurring between 20 and 37 weeks of gestation regardless of whether the child was born alive or stillborn.
Primigravida	*prim/i:* first *gravid/o:* pregnancy	A woman who is pregnant for the first time.
Primipara	*prim/i:* first *par/o:* bear, give birth to	A woman who has carried a pregnancy to fetal viability (20 weeks of gestation) for the first time regardless of whether the infant was stillborn or alive at birth.
Puerperium		The period of time, usually 4 to 6 weeks after delivery, in which the uterus and the body systems are returning to normal.
Quickening		The first movements of the fetus in utero as felt by the mother, which usually occur between 16 and 20 weeks of gestation and are felt consistently thereafter.
Risk factor		Anything that increases an individual's chance of developing a disease. Some risk factors (e.g., smoking) can be avoided, but others cannot (e.g., age and family history).
Term birth		Delivery occurring after 37 weeks of gestation regardless of whether the infant was born alive or stillborn.
Toxemia		A condition that can occur in pregnant women that includes preeclampsia and eclampsia. If preeclampsia goes undiagnosed or is not satisfactorily controlled, it could develop into eclampsia, characterized by convulsions and coma.
Trimester	*tri-:* three	Three months, or one third, of the gestational period of pregnancy.
Vulva		The region of the external female genital organs.

🖐 ON THE WEB

For Information on Sexually Transmitted Diseases:

National Institute of Allergy and Infectious Diseases: Sexually Transmitted Infections: www3.niaid.nih.gov/topics/sti

Centers for Disease Control and Prevention: Sexually Transmitted Diseases: www.cdc.gov/std

Planned Parenthood: www.plannedparenthood.org

Medline Plus Sexually Transmitted Diseases: www.nlm.nih.gov/medlineplus/sexuallytransmitteddiseases.html

WebMD Sexual Conditions: www.webmd.com/sexual-conditions

Your STD Help: yourstdhelp.com

STD Support Website: herpes-coldsores.com/support/std.htm

American Social Health Association: www.ashastd.org

ON THE WEB—cont'd

Herpes Information: www.gotherpes.com

HPV Information: www.gothpv.com

For Information on Women's Health:

The National Women's Health Information Center: www.4women.gov

The Universe of Women's Health: www.obgyn.net

Women's Health: www.womenshealth.gov

For Information on Contraceptives:

Planned Parenthood: www.plannedparenthood.org

Mayo Clinic Birth Control Options: www.mayoclinic.com/health/birth-control/BI99999

Ultimate Birth Control Links: www.ultimatebirthcontrol.com

Reproductive Health Online: www.reproline.jhu.edu/index.htm

For Information on Menopause:

North American Menopause Society: www.menopause.org

Everything Menopause: www.menopauseinfo.org

Power Surge: www.power-surge.com

Project Aware: www.project-aware.org

Mayo Clinic Menopause Information: www.mayoclinic.com/health/menopause/DS00119

WebMD Menopause Health Center: www.webmd.com/menopause

Medline Plus Menopause: www.nlm.nih.gov/medlineplus/menopause.html

For Information on Pregnancy and Childbirth:

Pregnancy and Childbirth: www.childbirth.org

Pregnancy and Childbirth: pregnancy.about.com

Childbirth Connection: www.childbirthconnection.org

Pregnancy: www.pregnancy.org

My Pregnancy Guide: www.mypregnancyguide.com/

WebMD Health and Pregnancy: www.webmd.com/baby

StorkNet's Pregnancy Guide: www.pregnancyguideonline.com

What to Expect: www.whattoexpect.com

The American College of Obstetricians and Gynecologists: www.acog.com

American Baby: www.americanbaby.com

Baby Zone: www.babyzone.com

Baby Center: www.babycenter.com

Lamaze International: www.lamaze.org

LaLeche League International: http://www.llli.org

9

The Pediatric Examination

Pediatric Office Visits

1. List the components of the well-child visit.
2. State the usual schedule for well-child visits.
3. Explain the purpose of the sick-child visit.
4. List the procedures performed by the medical assistant during pediatric office visits.
5. Explain why it is important to develop a rapport with the pediatric patient.

Carry an infant using the following positions:
- Cradle
- Upright

Growth Measurements

1. State the importance of measuring the child's weight, height (or length), and head circumference during each office visit.
2. State the functions served by a growth chart.

Plot pediatric growth values on a growth chart.
Measure the weight and length of an infant.
Measure the head and chest circumference of an infant.

Pediatric Blood Pressure Measurement

1. State the importance of measuring a child's blood pressure.
2. List the three factors that determine whether a child has hypertension.

Measure the blood pressure of a child.

Collection of a Urine Specimen

1. List the reasons for collecting a urine specimen from a child.

Collect a urine specimen using a pediatric urine collector.

Pediatric Injections

1. State the range for the gauge and length of needles used for intramuscular and subcutaneous pediatric injections.
2. Explain the use of each of the following pediatric injection sites: vastus lateralis and deltoid.

Locate the following pediatric intramuscular injection sites:
- Vastus lateralis
- Deltoid

Administer an intramuscular injection to an infant.
Administer a subcutaneous injection to an infant.

Immunizations

1. Describe the schedule for immunization of infants and children recommended by the American Academy of Pediatrics.
2. State the information that must be provided to parents as required by the National Childhood Vaccine Injury Act.
3. List the information that must be recorded in the medical record after administering an immunization.

Read and interpret a vaccine information statement.
Record information on an immunization administration record.

Newborn Screening Test

1. Explain the purpose of a newborn screening test.
2. List the symptoms of phenylketonuria.
3. State what occurs if phenylketonuria is left untreated.

Collect a specimen for a newborn screening test.

KEY TERMS

adolescent
immunity (ih-MYOO-nih-tee)
immunization (IM-yoo-nih-ZAY-shun)
infant
length
pediatrician (PEE-dee-uh-TRIH-shun)
pediatrics (pee-dee-AT-riks)

preschool (PREE-skool) child
school-age child
toddler (TOD-ler)
toxoid (TOKS-oid)
vaccine (vak-SEEN)
vertex (VER-teks)

Introduction to the Pediatric Examination

Pediatrics is the branch of medicine that deals with the care and development of children and the diagnosis and treatment of diseases in children. A **pediatrician** is a physician who specializes in pediatrics. Many physicians in general practice accept pediatric patients. It is essential that the medical assistant develop the skills needed to assist the physician in the care and treatment of children.

PEDIATRIC OFFICE VISITS

There are two broad categories of pediatric patient office visits. The first is the *well-child visit* (also termed *health maintenance visit*), in which the physician progressively evaluates the growth and development of the child. A physical examination is performed during each well-child visit and is directed toward discovering any abnormal conditions commonly associated with the stage of development reached by the child. Table 9-1 provides an outline of normal development during infancy. The child also receives necessary immunizations during these visits.

Another important component of the well-child visit is *anticipatory guidance.* Anticipatory guidance is the process of providing parents with information to prepare them for anticipated developmental events and to assist them in promoting their children's well-being. Topics that are commonly included are safety, nutrition, sleep, play, exercise, development, and discipline.

What Would You Do? What Would You *Not* Do?

Case Study 1
My-Lai Chang comes into the office with Christopher Chang, her 2-month-old son. Christopher is here for his 2-month well-child visit. Mrs. Chang is very distraught. She says that Christopher has episodes of nonstop crying every day that last 2 to 3 hours at a time. She is breastfeeding Christopher and says that the crying is worse after he nurses. Although Mrs. Chang realizes that Christopher has colic, she feels guilty because it seems "her milk" is making it worse. She also is having problems with sore nipples and engorgement. She really wanted to breastfeed Christopher, but she is thinking of stopping because it just seems too hard to do. Christopher measures in the 50th percentile for weight and length. Mrs. Chang is worried that he is not growing enough and thinks it is because she is not producing enough milk. ∎

Table 9-1 Milestones of Gross and Fine Motor Development in Infancy

Average Age (mo)	Gross Motor	Fine Motor
1	Turns head from side to side	Grasping reflex present
2	Holds head at 45-degree angle when prone	Holds rattle briefly
3	Begins rolling over	Grasps rattle or dangling objects
4	Slight head lag when pulled to sitting position	Brings objects to mouth
5	No head wobble when held in sitting position	Transfers objects from hand to hand
6	Sits without support	Manipulates and examines large objects with hands
7	Stands while holding on	Reaches for, grabs, and retains object
8	Pulls self to stand	Grasps objects with thumb and finger
9	Crawls backward	Begins to show hand preference
10	Creeps on hands and knees	Hits cup with spoon
11	Walks using furniture for support	Picks up small objects with thumb and forefinger (pincer grasp)
12	Stands alone easily	Puts three or more objects into container
12-16	Walks alone easily	Turns two or three pages in large cardboard book

From Leahy JM, Kizilay PE: Foundations of nursing practice, Philadelphia, 1998, Saunders.

The interval between well-child visits depends on the medical office, but it frequently follows this schedule after birth: 1 month, 2 months, 4 months, 6 months, 9 months, 12 months, 15 months, 18 months, 24 months, and yearly thereafter.

The second category of pediatric patient office visits is the *sick-child visit*. The child is exhibiting the signs and symptoms of disease, and the physician evaluates the patient's condition to arrive at a diagnosis and to prescribe treatment.

During well-child and sick-child visits, the medical assistant performs many of the same procedures that have been presented in previous chapters (e.g., measurement of temperature, pulse, respiration, and blood pressure; measurement of weight and height; measurement of visual acuity; assisting with the physical examination). This chapter discusses procedures specifically related to the pediatric patient and variations in procedures previously presented.

DEVELOPING A RAPPORT

The medical assistant must establish a rapport with the pediatric patient. If the medical assistant gains the child's trust and confidence, the child is likely to cooperate during an

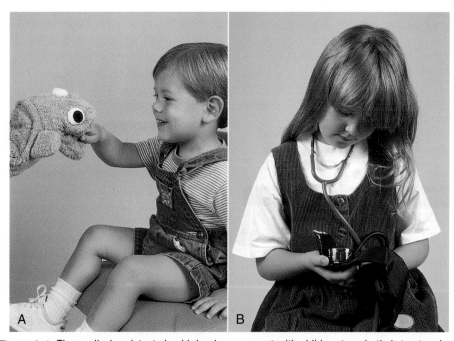

Figure 9-1. The medical assistant should develop a rapport with children to gain their trust and cooperation. Making a game of the procedure **(A)** and explaining the purpose of the stethoscope and allowing the child to hold it **(B)** help the child overcome fears.

examination or procedure. Interacting with children requires special techniques. The techniques employed depend on the age of the child. Toddlers and preschool children often respond well to making a game of the procedure. Explaining the purpose of an instrument (e.g., the stethoscope) to a school-age child and allowing him or her to hold the instrument or even to help during the procedure may overcome fears in that age group (Figure 9-1).

The medical assistant should always explain the procedure to children who are able to understand. Each child must be approached at his or her level of understanding. To do this, the medical assistant should know what to expect from a child at a particular age, in terms of motor and social development. Each child has his or her own individual rate of development; the descriptions of normal development based on age are meant to serve as a guide only and may have to be modified to meet individual needs. In addition,

it is normal for an ill child to regress to an earlier level of behavior. Table 9-2 outlines techniques that can be used with various age groups to gain their cooperation during an examination or procedure.

CARRYING THE INFANT

The medical assistant needs to lift and carry the infant to perform various procedures, such as measurement of length and weight. The infant should be lifted and carried in a manner that is safe and comfortable. Proper positions include the cradle and upright positions.

Cradle Position

The medical assistant slides the left hand and arm under the infant's back and grasps the infant's arm from behind. The thumb and fingers should encircle the infant's forearm.

Table 9-2 Techniques for Interaction With Children

Technique	Infant (Birth-1 yr)	Toddler (1-3 yr)	Preschool (3-6 yr)	School Age (6-12 yr)	Adolescent (12-18 yr)
Avoid sudden motion and loud or abrupt noises.	♥		♥		
Limit number of strangers in room.	♥				
Use distractions, bright objects, rattles, and talking to gain cooperation.	♥				
Physically restrain child if necessary to ensure safety.	♥	♥	♥		
Allow physical contact with parent during procedure.	♥	♥	♥		
Encourage parent to comfort child after procedure.	♥	♥	♥		
Use play to explain procedure (e.g., dolls, puppets).		♥	♥		
Perform procedures quickly, if possible.		♥	♥		
Use concrete terms, rather than abstract terms.		♥	♥		
Avoid words that have more than one meaning (e.g., shot).		♥	♥		
Give child permission to cry, yell, or otherwise express pain verbally.		♥	♥		
Praise child for cooperative behavior.		♥	♥	♥	
Allow child to handle equipment, if possible.			♥	♥	
Make sure child understands body part to be involved.			♥	♥	
Try to describe how procedure will feel.			♥	♥	
Tell child about any discomfort that may be felt, but don't dwell on it.			♥	♥	
Stress benefits of anything child may find pleasurable afterward (e.g., stickers, feeling better).			♥	♥	
Give child choices when possible (e.g., arm to use).			♥	♥	
Suggest ways to maintain control (e.g., counting, deep breathing, relaxation).			♥	♥	
Use drawing and diagrams to illustrate parts of body that will be involved.			♥	♥	
Encourage participation such as holding instrument during procedure.			♥	♥	
Include child in decision-making process.				♥	♥
Discuss risks of procedure.					♥
Provide information about appearance changes that might result.					♥
Give child educational brochures or have him or her view videos about procedure.					♥
Ask parent to step out if child does not want parent in examining room.					♥

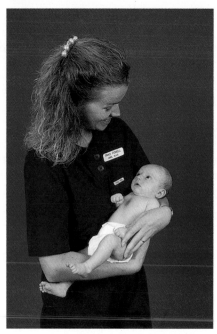

Figure 9-2. Traci holds the infant in the cradle position.

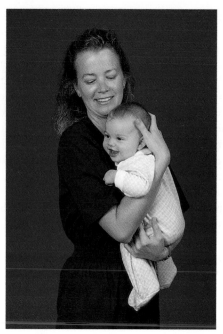

Figure 9-3. Traci holds the infant in the upright position.

The infant's head, shoulders, and back are supported by the medical assistant's arm. Next, the medical assistant slips the right arm up and under the infant's buttocks. The infant is cradled in the arm with his or her body resting against the medical assistant's chest (Figure 9-2).

Upright Position

The medical assistant slips the right hand under the infant's head and shoulders. The fingers should be spread apart to support the infant's head and neck. The left forearm is slipped under the infant's buttocks to help support the infant's weight. The infant should be allowed to rest against the medical assistant's chest with the cheek resting on the medical assistant's shoulder (Figure 9-3).

GROWTH MEASUREMENTS

One of the best methods to evaluate the progress of a child is to measure his or her growth. The weight, height (or length), and head circumference (up to age 3 years) of a child should be measured during each office visit and plotted on a growth chart.

Weight

A child's weight is often used to determine nutritional needs and the proper dosage of a medication to administer to the child. The medical assistant should exercise care in measuring weight. Infants are weighed in a recumbent position, as outlined in Procedure 9-1. Older children are weighed in a standing position, as presented in Chapter 5.

Length and Height

Another measure of a child's growth is **length,** or height (stature). Length is measured in children younger than 24 months. The recumbent length is a measurement from the **vertex** of the head to the heel of the infant in a supine position, as outlined in Procedure 9-1. Two people are often needed to determine the length of an infant accurately. The parent's help can be requested; the medical assistant must provide the parent with thorough instructions on what is to be done. Older children have their height measured in a standing position (Figure 9-4), as presented in Chapter 5.

Head and Chest Circumference

Infancy is a period of rapid brain growth. Because of this, the head circumference is an important measurement. The head circumference for a newborn ranges from 32 to 38 cm,

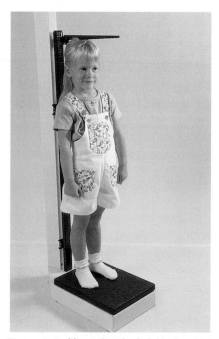

Figure 9-4. Measuring the height of a child.

Putting It All into Practice

My Name is Traci Powell, and I am a Certified Medical Assistant. I work in the pediatrics department of a large multispecialty clinic. My job responsibilities are mostly clinical; however, I do assist in the front office when needed. I love working with the children and have enjoyed watching them grow over the years.

A coworker and I recently organized a local AAMA (American Association of Medical Assistants) chapter. Our chapter provides AAMA continuing education units (CEUs). Our members attend state and national conventions every year, and they hold state and national leadership positions. It is my goal to see the medical assisting profession continue to grow and advance in the health care field.

It is interesting how your education, training, and experience all come together, especially in a crisis. Early one morning when I arrived at work, a mother was waiting with a small child who was approximately 2 years old. The child was dusky in color, panicky, and having trouble breathing. Apparently the child had gotten into some dry beans the previous night and had inhaled one into her lung. None of the physicians was in the building yet, and this child was in respiratory distress. We immediately called a Code Blue, put her on oxygen, and made arrangements for a squad car to take her to Children's Hospital, where a surgeon was waiting. All went well, and she is a healthy little girl today.

Looking back, I am grateful for a good, solid medical assisting education; a PALS (Pediatric Advance Life Support) certification; and experience in working with children so that I was able to help that child through a life-threatening experience. I firmly believe that no matter how long a person has been in the medical field or what his or her profession is, continuing education is essential to stay current in the ever-changing health care field. ■

---

or 12½ to 15 inches. A 10-cm (4-inch) increase in head circumference occurs within the first year of life.

The head circumference of children younger than 3 years old should be routinely measured and plotted on a head circumference growth chart. Measurement of head circumference is an important screening measure for microencephaly and macroencephaly.

At birth, a newborn's head circumference is about 2 cm larger than his or her chest circumference. The chest grows at a faster rate than the cranium, and between 6 months

---

Highlight on Childhood Obesity

Statistics

An epidemic of childhood obesity is occurring in the United States; the incidence of obesity in children has doubled over the past 20 years. Approximately 25% of Americans younger than age 19 are overweight or obese, which equates to one of every four children. A child is considered overweight if his or her weight falls in the 85th to 95th percentile for age, gender, and height on the National Center for Health Statistics growth charts. When a child's weight exceeds the 95th percentile for age, gender, and height, he or she is considered obese.

Causes

The primary causes of childhood obesity are overeating and inadequate exercise. Other causes include hormonal and genetic problems, but these are much less likely, occurring in only 5% of obese children. The risk of obesity tends to be greater among children who have obese parents. After age 3, the likelihood that obesity will persist into adulthood increases as an obese child gets older. When an obese child reaches age 6, the probability is more than 50% that obesity will persist into adulthood. Of obese adolescents, 70% to 80% remain obese as adults.

Related Problems

Problems associated with childhood obesity include high blood pressure, type 2 diabetes, orthopedic problems caused by increased stress on weight-bearing joints, skin disorders such as dermatitis, sleep apnea, low self-esteem, social isolation, and feelings of rejection and depression. Some authorities believe that the social and psychological problems are the most significant consequences of childhood obesity.

Prevention

It is much easier to prevent childhood obesity than to treat it after it has occurred. Authorities believe that the primary focus should be on educating parents about the problems associated with childhood obesity and helping them employ preventive measures. Guidelines for preventing childhood obesity include the following:

- Provide a healthy diet, with 30% or fewer calories coming from fat.
- Encourage active play.
- Do not use food for reward, comfort, or bribes.
- Limit television, video, and computer time.
- Limit the amount of "junk" food kept in the home.
- Do not make the child eat when he or she is not hungry.
- Do not offer dessert as a reward for finishing a meal.
- Encourage the child to drink water instead of sweet beverages.
- Do not frequently eat at fast-food restaurants.

Treatment

The treatment of childhood obesity is difficult, and the success rate is not particularly high. Children seem to be most successful at losing weight and keeping it off when the entire family is involved. Parents should eat healthy meals and snacks with their children. The most successful diets are those that use ordinary foods in controlled portions, rather than diets that require the avoidance of specific foods. Parents also should spend time being active with their children. Activities should stress self-improvement rather than competition. ■

and 2 years of age, the measurements are about the same. After age 2 years, the chest circumference is greater than the head circumference. The measurement of the chest circumference is valuable in a comparison with the head circumference, but not by itself. The chest circumference is not typically measured on a routine basis; this measurement is done only when a heart or lung abnormality is suspected. Procedure 9-2 outlines the procedure for measuring the head and chest circumference of an infant.

Growth Charts

Growth charts should be part of every child's permanent record. The National Center for Health Statistics developed growth charts to assist physicians in determining whether the growth of a child is normal. The charts can be used to identify children with growth or nutritional abnormalities. The medical assistant is usually responsible for plotting the child's measurements on the growth chart (Procedure 9-3).

Growth charts provide a means of comparing a child's weight and length (or height) with those of other children of the same age. For example, the medical assistant calculates the growth percentile of an 18-month-old boy and finds that he is in the 25th percentile for weight and the 80th percentile for length. This means that 75% of 18-month-old boys weigh more than he does, and 25% weigh less than he does. It also means that 20% of 18-month-old boys are taller, and 80% are shorter. Although comparing a child with other children of the same age is one use of growth charts (particularly by parents), it is not the most important use.

The primary use of growth charts is to look at the child's growth pattern. If a child has always hovered around a certain percentile in height and weight, there is no need for concern. If a child is in the 20th percentile for weight but has always been in this percentile, he is likely growing normally. It would be more of a concern if the child had been in the 75th percentile and dropped to the 20th percentile. The physician investigates any significant change or rapid increase or decrease in a child's growth pattern.

PROCEDURE 9-1   Measuring the Weight and Length of an Infant

Outcome Measure the weight and length of an infant.

Equipment/Supplies

- Pediatric balance scale (table model)

1. Procedural Step. Sanitize your hands.

2. Procedural Step. Greet the infant's parent and introduce yourself. Identify the infant and explain the procedure to the parent. The weight of the infant is usually measured first. Depending on the medical office policy, ask the parent to perform one of the following:

  a. Remove the infant's clothing and put a dry diaper on the infant.

  b. Remove the infant's clothing, including the diaper.

  Principle. The infant should not be weighed with a wet diaper because it could increase the infant's weight considerably. Also, growth charts for infants and young children base their percentiles on the weight of the child without clothing.

3. Procedural Step. Unlock the pediatric scale, and place a clean paper protector on it. Check the balance scale for accuracy, making sure to compensate for the weight of the paper.

  Principle. The paper protector prevents cross-contamination and reduces the spread of disease from one patient to another.

4. Procedural Step. Gently place the infant on his or her back on the table of the scale. Place one hand slightly above the infant as a safety precaution.

5. Procedural Step. Balance the scale as follows:

  a. Move the lower weight to the notched groove that does not cause the indicator point to drop to the bottom of the calibration area. Ensure that the lower weight is seated firmly in its groove.

  b. Slowly slide the upper weight along its calibration bar by tapping it gently until the indicator point comes to rest at the center of the balance area.

  Principle. Not seating the lower weight firmly in its groove results in an inaccurate reading.

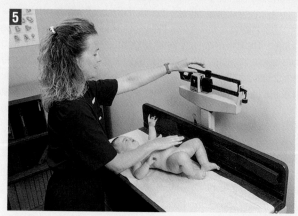

Balance the scale.

PROCEDURE 9-1   Measuring the Weight and Length of an Infant—cont'd

6. Procedural Step. Read the results in pounds and ounces while the infant is lying still. Jot down this value or make a mental note of it. (*Note:* The result on the pictured scale is 15 lb and 2 oz.)

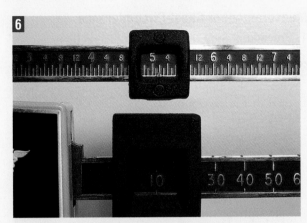

Read the results in pounds and ounces.

7. Procedural Step. Return the balance to its resting position, and lock the scale.

8. Procedural Step. Place the vertex (top) of the infant's head against the headboard at the zero mark. Ask the parent to hold the infant's head in this position.

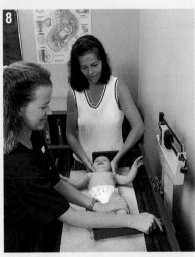

Properly position the infant.

9. Procedural Step. Straighten the infant's knees, and place the soles of his or her feet firmly against the upright footboard (to create a right angle).

10. Procedural Step. Read the infant's length in inches (to the nearest ⅛ inch) from the measure. Jot down this value or make a mental note of it. (*Note:* The result on this scale is 25½ inches.)

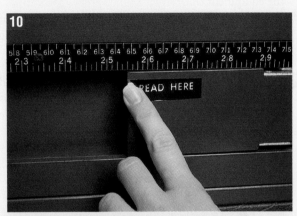

Read the length in inches.

11. Procedural Step. Gently remove the infant from the table, and hand him or her to the parent. Return the headboard and footboard to their resting positions.

12. Procedural Step. Sanitize your hands, and chart the results.

CHARTING EXAMPLE

Date	
8/10/12	9:30 a.m. Wt. 15 lbs. 2 oz. Length 25 ½ in.
	————————————T. Powell, CMA (AAMA)

PROCEDURE 9-1

PROCEDURE 9-2   Measuring Head and Chest Circumference of an Infant

Outcome Measure the head and chest circumference of an infant.

Equipment/Supplies

- Flexible nonstretch tape measure

Measurement of Head Circumference

1. **Procedural Step.** Sanitize your hands, and assemble the equipment.
2. **Procedural Step.** Position the infant. The infant should be placed on his or her back on the examining table. An alternative position is to have the parent hold the infant.
3. **Procedural Step.** Position the tape measure around the infant's head at the greatest circumference. This is usually accomplished by placing the tape slightly above the eyebrows and pinna of the ears and around the occipital prominence at the back of the skull.

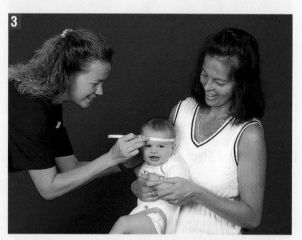

Position the tape measure around the infant's head.

4. **Procedural Step.** Read the results in centimeters (or inches) to the nearest 0.5 cm (or ¼ inch). Jot down this value or make a mental note of it. Sanitize your hands, and chart the results.

CHARTING EXAMPLE

Date	
8/10/12	10:00 a.m. Head circumference: 42.5 cm. ___
	————————————T. Powell, CMA (AAMA)

Measurement of Chest Circumference

1. **Procedural Step.** Position the infant on his or her back on the examining table.
2. **Procedural Step.** Encircle the tape around the infant's chest at the nipple line. It should be snug, but not so tight that it leaves a mark.

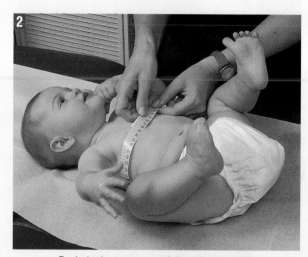

Encircle the tape around the infant's chest.

3. **Procedural Step.** Read the results in centimeters (or inches) to the nearest 0.5 cm (or ¼ inch). Jot down this value or make a mental note of it. Sanitize your hands, and chart the results.

CHARTING EXAMPLE

Date	
8/15/12	10:00 a.m. Chest circumference: 42 cm. ___
	————————————T. Powell, CMA (AAMA)

PROCEDURE 9-3   Calculating Growth Percentiles

Outcome Plot a pediatric growth value on a growth chart.

Equipment/Supplies

* Pediatric growth chart

1. **Procedural Step.** Select the proper growth chart.
2. **Procedural Step.** Locate the child's age in the horizontal column at the bottom of the chart.
3. **Procedural Step.** Locate the growth value in the vertical column under the appropriate category (weight, length or stature, and head circumference).
4. **Procedural Step.** Draw an imaginary vertical line from the child's age mark and an imaginary horizontal line from the child's growth mark. Find the site at which the two lines intersect on the graph, and place a dot on this site.

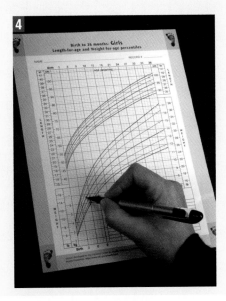

5. **Procedural Step.** To determine the percentile in which the child falls, follow the curved percentile line upward to read the value located on the right side of the chart. Interpolation is needed if the value does not fall exactly on a percentile line. (*Interpolation* means that you must estimate a percentile that falls between a larger and a smaller known percentile.)
6. **Procedural Step.** Chart the results. Include the date and time and each growth percentile.
   Note: The weight (15 lb, 2 oz), length (25½ inches), and head circumference (42.5 cm) of the child in Procedures 9-1 and 9-2 have been plotted on a growth chart. This child is 5 months old. Locate these values on the appropriate growth chart to ensure you obtain the same percentiles.

CHARTING EXAMPLE	
Date	
10/22/12	10:30 a.m. Weight: 55%. Length: 70%.
	Head Circum: 67% ——T. Powell, CMA (AAMA)

Continued

PROCEDURE 9-3   Calculating Growth Percentiles—cont'd

Birth to 36 months: Girls
Length-for-age and Weight-for-age percentiles

NAME _____

RECORD# _____

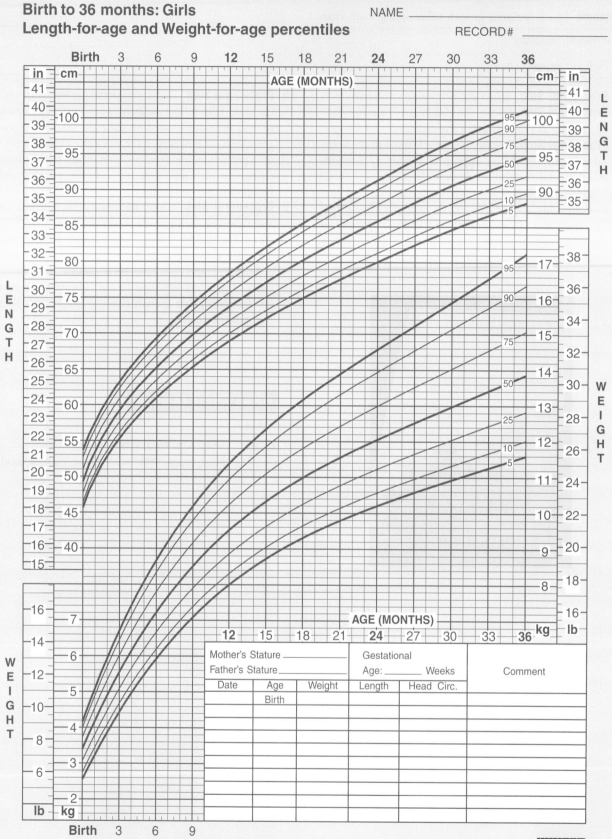

Published May 30, 2000 (modified 4/20/01).
SOURCE: Developed by the National Center for Health Statistics in collaboration with
the National Center for Chronic Disease Prevention and Health Promotion (2000).
http://www.cdc.gov/growthcharts

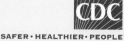

SAFER • HEALTHIER • PEOPLE™

PROCEDURE 9-3   Calculating Growth Percentiles—cont'd

Birth to 36 months: Girls
Head circumference-for-age and
Weight-for-length percentiles

NAME _____

RECORD# _____

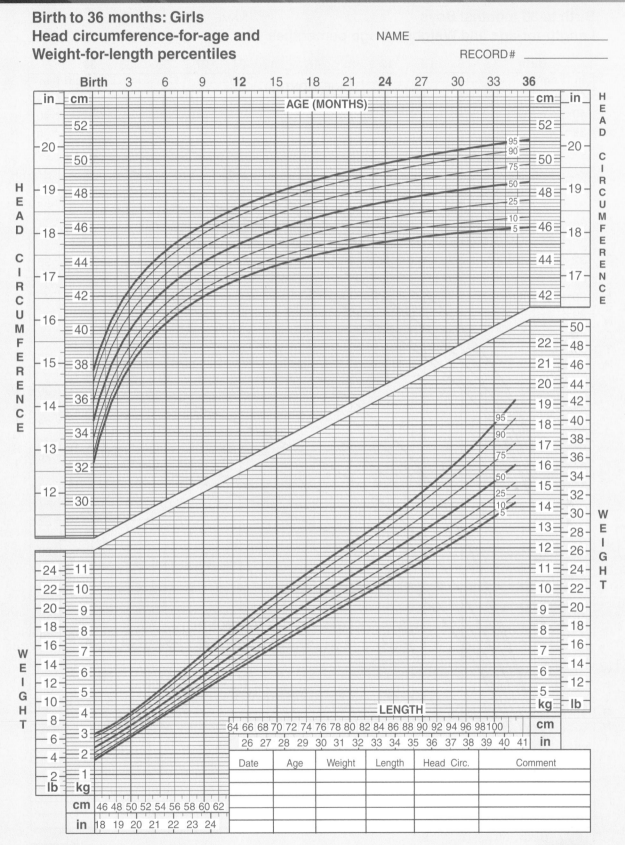

Published May 30, 2000 (modified 10/16/00).
SOURCE: Developed by the National Center for Health Statistics in collaboration with
the National Center for Chronic Disease Prevention and Health Promotion (2000).
http://www.cdc.gov/growthcharts

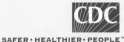

SAFER · HEALTHIER · PEOPLE™

Continued

PROCEDURE 9-3   Calculating Growth Percentiles—cont'd

Birth to 36 months: Boys
Length-for-age and Weight-for-age percentiles

NAME _____

RECORD# _____

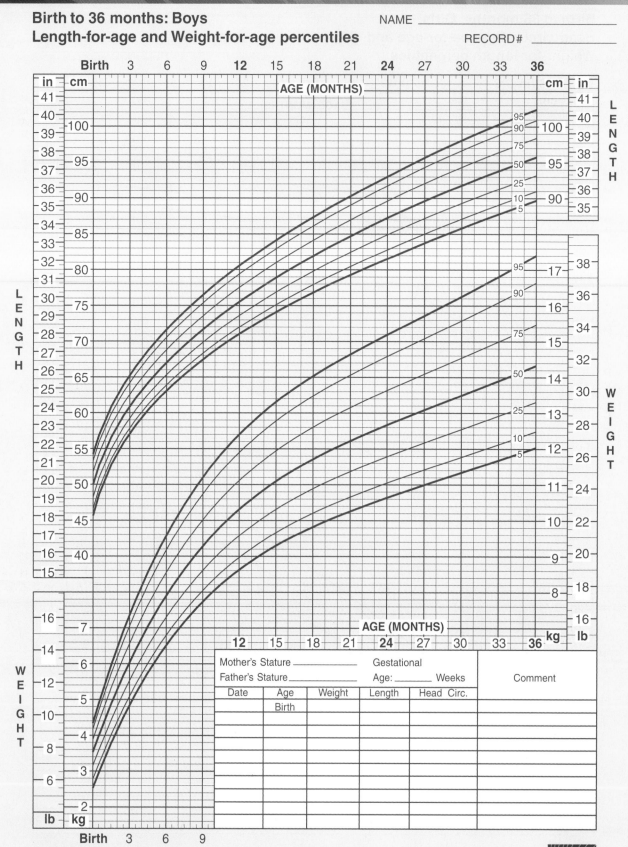

Published May 30, 2000 (modified 4/20/01).

SOURCE: Developed by the National Center for Health Statistics in collaboration with
the National Center for Chronic Disease Prevention and Health Promotion (2000).
http://www.cdc.gov/growthcharts

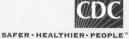

SAFER · HEALTHIER · PEOPLE™

PROCEDURE 9-3   Calculating Growth Percentiles—cont'd

Birth to 36 months: Boys
Head circumference-for-age and
Weight-for-length percentiles

NAME _____

RECORD# _____

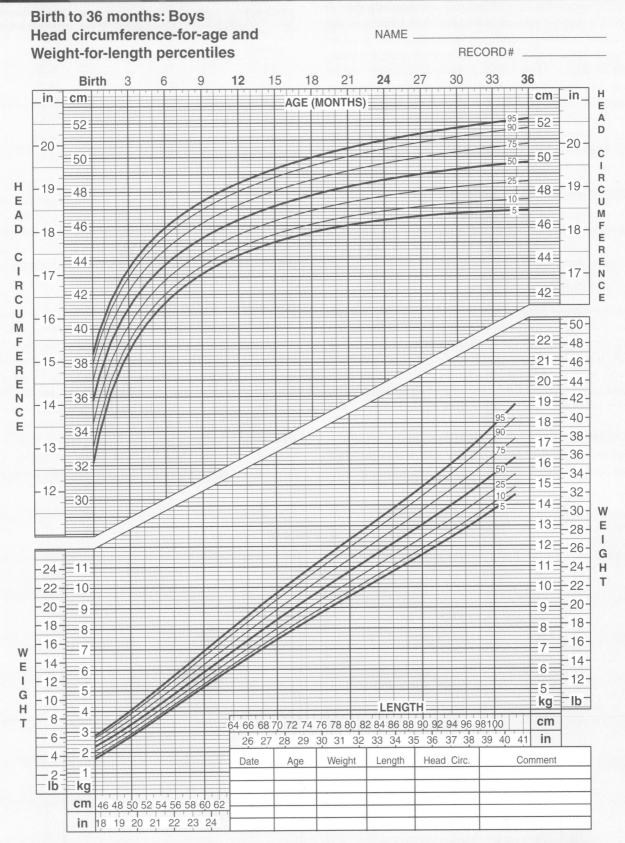

Published May 30, 2000 (modified 10/16/00).
SOURCE: Developed by the National Center for Health Statistics in collaboration with
   the National Center for Chronic Disease Prevention and Health Promotion (2000).
http://www.cdc.gov/growthcharts

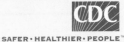

SAFER · HEALTHIER · PEOPLE™

PEDIATRIC BLOOD PRESSURE MEASUREMENT

The American Academy of Pediatrics recommends that all children 3 years old and older have their blood pressure measured annually. Measuring pediatric blood pressure helps to identify children at risk for developing hypertension as adults. High blood pressure in children can be caused by kidney disease and, to a lesser degree, by heart disease. When the condition is treated, the blood pressure usually returns to normal. Overweight children usually have higher blood pressure than children of normal weight. Losing weight through a prescribed diet and regular physical activity often reduces blood pressure in these children.

Special Guidelines for Children

The procedure for measuring blood pressure in children is the same as that for adults and is presented in Chapter 4. Some special pediatric guidelines must be taken into consideration.

Correct Cuff Size

The most important criterion in obtaining an accurate pediatric blood pressure measurement is selecting the correct cuff size. If the cuff is too small, the reading may be falsely high. If the cuff is too large, the reading may be falsely low. Blood pressure cuffs come in a variety of sizes and are measured in centimeters (cm). The size of a cuff refers to its inner inflatable bladder, rather than its cloth cover. Table 9-3 lists the range of cuff sizes commercially available. The name of the cuff (e.g., child, adult) does not imply that it is appropriate for that age. An 8-year-old overweight child may need an adult-sized cuff.

Table 9-3 Acceptable Bladder Dimensions for Arms of Different Sizes

Cuff	Bladder Length, cm	Arm Circumference Range at Midpoint, cm
Newborn	6	Less than 6
Infant	15	6-15
Child	21	16-21
Small adult	24	22-26
Adult	30	27-34
Large adult	38	35-44
Adult thigh	42	45-52

For an accurate blood pressure measurement, the bladder of the cuff should encircle 80% to 100% of the arm. The child's arm circumference should be assessed midpoint between the acromion process (shoulder) and the olecranon process (elbow). Figure 9-5 shows how to determine the correct pediatric cuff size.

Cooperation of the Child

Another important factor to consider when taking pediatric blood pressure is preparing the child for the procedure. It is important to gain the child's cooperation and to ensure that the child is relaxed. Apprehension can cause the blood pressure to be falsely high. To reduce a child's anxiety level, carefully explain the procedure to the child, and, if appropriate, allow him or her to handle the equipment before measuring blood pressure. The blood pressure should be measured after the child has been sitting quietly for 3 to 5 minutes (Figure 9-6).

DETERMINATION OF PROPER CUFF SIZE

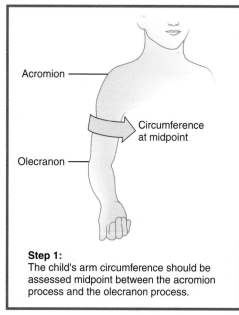

Acromion

Circumference at midpoint

Olecranon

Step 1:
The child's arm circumference should be assessed midpoint between the acromion process and the olecranon process.

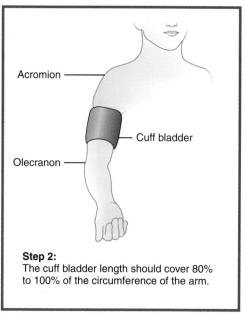

Acromion

Cuff bladder

Olecranon

Step 2:
The cuff bladder length should cover 80% to 100% of the circumference of the arm.

Figure 9-5. Determination of proper blood pressure cuff size.

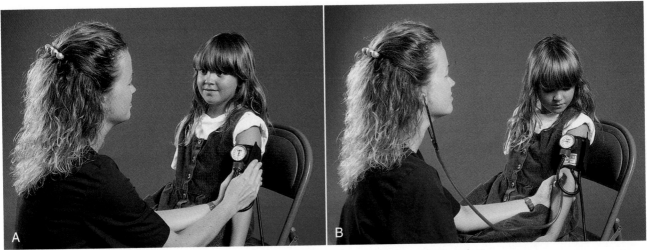

Figure 9-6. Traci measures the blood pressure of a pediatric patient.

What Would You Do? What Would You *Not* Do?

Case Study 2

Wanda Tilley comes to the office with her 10-year-old daughter, Courtney. Courtney has a skin condition on her legs that needs to be evaluated by the physician. Courtney has been obese since she was 4 years old. Mrs. Tilley also is obese and is not too concerned about Courtney's weight. She says that Courtney must have inherited her "fat gene," and there's not much that can be done about it. Courtney's favorite activities are playing video games and reading. She would like to join the community swim team, but she's too embarrassed for anyone to see her in a bathing suit. Courtney says the other kids are always making fun of her at school. She says that they call her "two-ton Tilley" and "double-roll," and they don't want to sit with her at lunch. Courtney wants her mom to home-school her because she's getting to the point where she can't take it anymore. She doesn't want the doctor to examine her because he'll see how fat she is and say bad things about it. ∎

Memories *from* Externship

Traci Powell: I still remember how difficult it was at times as a student. I had been out of high school for more than a year, so I had to get back into the routine of studying. I worried about whether I would do well, whether I would be able to find a good job, and whether I would like medical assisting. Adding to these concerns was the financial burden of putting myself through school. I took advantage of grants and a student loan. Throughout the last 6 months of my education, I also worked full-time as an aide on the midnight shift at a nursing home while attending school full-time during the day. As if that were not enough, my first child was well on her way into this world as I was finishing up the last quarter of my degree. There were so many times that I was tired, frustrated, and broke, but I kept pushing myself to do my best because I knew this was going to be my lifetime career, and I wanted to excel in my profession. My determination paid off. Today I have a great medical assisting position that I love, with an institution that is one of the best employers in the area. ∎

Blood Pressure Classifications

Blood pressure varies depending on the age of the child and his or her height and gender. The National High Blood Pressure Education Program (NHBPEP) prepared a set of tables that physicians use to determine whether a child's blood pressure is higher than the average among children of the same age and height. If a child has a blood pressure that is higher than 90% to 95% of most other children of the same age, height, and gender, the child may have high blood pressure.

The NHBPEP tables (one for boys and one for girls) allow precise classification of blood pressure according to body size, which avoids misclassifying children at the extreme ends of normal growth. A very tall child would not be mistakenly diagnosed as having hypertension, and hypertension would not be missed in a very short child. The NHBPEP tables used by physicians to assist in the diagnosis of hypertension in children can be found at the National Heart, Lung, and Blood Institute website (www.nhlbi.nih.gov/guidelines/hypertension/child_tbl.htm).

Blood pressure varies throughout the day in children as a result of normal fluctuations in physical activity and emotional stress. If a child's blood pressure is elevated, two more readings must be taken at different visits before the physician can make a diagnosis of hypertension.

COLLECTION OF A URINE SPECIMEN

A urinalysis may be performed on a pediatric patient for the following reasons: to screen for the presence of disease as part of a general physical examination, to assist in the diagnosis of a pathologic condition (e.g., urinary tract infection), or to evaluate the effectiveness of therapy. The collection of a urine specimen from a child who exhibits bladder control is performed using the technique outlined in Chapter 16. Collecting a urine specimen from an infant or young child who cannot urinate voluntarily involves the use of a pediatric urine collector. Pediatric urine collectors are designed to be used with both sexes. The urine collector consists of a clear plastic disposable bag containing a hypoallergenic pressure-sensitive adhesive around the opening of the bag. The adhesive firmly attaches the urine collector to the genitalia. Procedure 9-4 outlines the procedure for applying a pediatric urine collector.

PROCEDURE 9-4 Applying a Pediatric Urine Collector

Outcome Apply a pediatric urine collector.

Equipment/Supplies

- Disposable gloves
- Personal antiseptic wipes
- Pediatric urine collector bag
- Urine specimen container and label
- Regular waste container

1. **Procedural Step.** Sanitize your hands.
2. **Procedural Step.** Assemble the equipment.
3. **Procedural Step.** Greet the infant's parent and introduce yourself. Identify the infant and explain the procedure to the parent.
4. **Procedural Step.** Apply gloves. Position the child. The child should be placed on his or her back with the legs spread apart. The medical assistant may need another individual to hold the child's legs apart.
   Principle. This position facilitates cleansing of the genitalia and permits proper application of the urine collector bag.
5. **Procedural Step.** Cleanse the child's genitalia.
   Female: Using a front-to-back motion (pubis to anus), cleanse each side of the meatus with a separate wipe. With a third wipe, cleanse directly down the middle (directly over the urinary meatus). Discard each wipe after cleansing. Allow the area to dry completely.
   Male: If the child is not circumcised, retract the foreskin of the penis. Cleanse the area around the meatus and the urethral opening (meatal orifice) in a manner similar to that used to cleanse the female patient. Use a separate wipe for each swipe. Cleanse the scrotum last, using a fresh wipe. Discard each wipe after cleansing. Allow the area to dry completely.
   Principle. The urinary meatus and surrounding area must be cleansed to prevent contaminants, such as baby powder, fecal material, and microorganisms, from entering the urine specimen, which could affect the test results. A front-to-back motion must be used to prevent drawing microorganisms from the anal area into the area being cleansed. The area must be completely dry to ensure an airtight adhesion of the collection bag to prevent leakage of urine.
6. **Procedural Step.** Remove the paper backing from the urine collector bag. This exposes the hypoallergenic adhesive surface around the opening of the bag. Firmly attach the bag in the following manner:
   Female: Stretch the perineum taut, and firmly place the bottom of the adhesive surface on the infant's perineum. Starting at the perineum and working upward, firmly press the adhesive surface to the skin surrounding the external genitalia, ensuring there is no puckering. The opening of the bag should be directly over the urinary meatus. The excess of the bag should be positioned toward the child's feet.
   Male: Position the bag so that the child's penis and scrotum are projected through the opening of the bag. Starting at the perineum and working upward, firmly press the adhesive surface to the skin surrounding the penis and scrotum, ensuring there is no puckering. The excess of the bag should be positioned toward the child's feet.
   Principle. The adhesive surface of the bag must be attached securely with no puckering to prevent leakage.

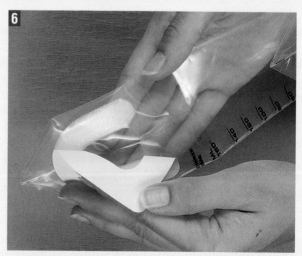

Remove paper backing from the urine collector bag.

PROCEDURE 9-4 Applying a Pediatric Urine Collector—cont'd

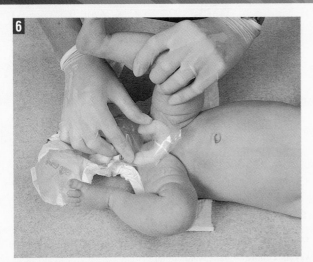

Firmly press the adhesive surface to the skin surrounding the external genitalia.

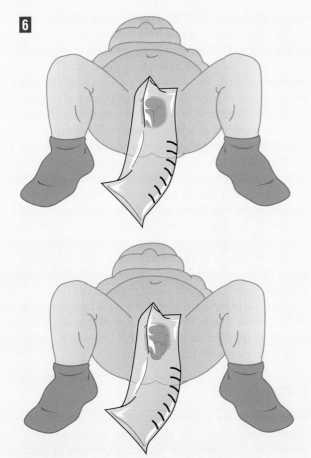

Female: The opening of the bag should be directly over the urinary meatus.
Male: The penis and scrotum are projected through the opening of the bag.

7. **Procedural Step.** Loosely diaper the child. Check the urine collector bag every 15 minutes until a urine specimen is obtained.
   Principle. The diaper helps hold the urine collector bag in place. The bag must be checked frequently. Once the infant has urinated, moisture from the urine may cause the adhesive surface to become loose and leak, especially with an active infant.

8. **Procedural Step.** When the child has voided, gently remove the urine collector bag by holding the bottom of the adhesive surface against the infant's skin and carefully peeling the bag off from the top to the bottom.
   Principle. The bag must be removed gently because pulling the adhesive away too quickly may cause discomfort and irritation of the child's skin.

9. **Procedural Step.** Cleanse the genital area with a personal antiseptic wipe. Rediaper the child.

10. **Procedural Step.** Transfer the urine specimen into a urine specimen container, and tightly apply the lid. Label the container with the child's name and date of birth, the date, the time of collection, and the type of specimen (i.e., urine). Dispose of the collector bag in a regular waste container. (*Note:* The urine collector bag can be used as a urine container to transport the specimen to the laboratory. This is accomplished by folding the adhesive sponge ring in half along its vertical axis and pressing the adhesive surfaces firmly together to ensure a tight seal.)

11. **Procedural Step.** Based on the medical office routine, test the urine specimen, or prepare it for transfer to an outside laboratory; be sure to include a completed laboratory request form. If the specimen cannot be tested or transferred immediately, preserve it by placing it in the refrigerator.
    Principle. Changes occur in a urine specimen that is left sitting out at room temperature, which can lead to inaccurate test results.

12. **Procedural Step.** Remove the gloves, and sanitize your hands.

13. **Procedural Step.** Chart the procedure. Include the date, the time of collection, and the type of specimen (i.e., urine). If the specimen is to be transported to an outside laboratory, indicate this information, including the laboratory tests ordered.

CHARTING EXAMPLE

Date	
8/12/12	10:15 a.m. Urine specimen collected for
	culture. Picked up by Medical Center Lab on
	8/12/12. ————————T. Powell, CMA (AAMA)

PEDIATRIC INJECTIONS

Administering an injection to a child is an important responsibility. The experience a child has with early injections influences the child's attitude toward later ones. If the child is old enough to understand, the procedure should be explained. The medical assistant should be honest and should attempt to gain the child's trust and cooperation. The child should be told the truth about the injection—that it will hurt, but only for a short time. It also is advisable to explain that the medicine will help him or her get better. Another person should be present to assist. The assistant can help position the child and can divert or restrain him or her if necessary. If the child struggles and fights excessively, the medical assistant should delay the injection and consult the physician.

The administration of injections is presented in Chapter 11. Before undertaking the study of pediatric injections, the medical assistant should review this chapter thoroughly, concentrating on the locations of injection sites and the procedures for preparing and administering injections. The same basic technique is used to administer an injection to an adult and a child. Variations in procedure are explained in the following section.

Types of Needles

The gauge and length of the needle used for intramuscular injections vary, depending on the consistency of the medication to be administered and the size of the child. Thick or oily preparations require a larger needle lumen, and the needle must be long enough to reach muscle tissue. A needle length ranging from ⅝ inch to 1 inch is generally used to administer an intramuscular injection to a child, and the gauge of the needle generally ranges between 22 and 25, depending on the viscosity of the medication. The length of the needle used to administer a pediatric subcutaneous injection ranges from ⅜ inch to ½ inch, and the gauge of the needle ranges from 23 to 25.

Intramuscular Injection Sites

Pediatric injection sites vary based on the age of the child. The specific site to be injected is stated in the package insert accompanying the medication. Until the child is walking, the gluteus muscle is small and not well developed, and is covered with a thick layer of fat. An injection in the dorsogluteal site (Figure 9-7) may come dangerously close to the sciatic nerve. The danger is increased if the child is squirming or fighting. Because serious trauma can result from incorrect administration of an injection in this area, the dorsogluteal site should not be used as an injection site for an infant or young child.

The vastus lateralis muscle site is recommended for injections of infants and young children. It is located on the anterior surface of the midlateral thigh, away from major nerves and blood vessels, and it is large enough to accommodate the injected medication (Figure 9-8, *A*). To locate the vastus lateralis site in an infant or young child, divide

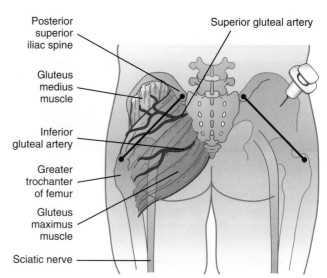

Figure 9-7. Dorsogluteal intramuscular injection site. (Courtesy Wyeth Laboratories, Philadelphia, PA.)

the mid–anterior thigh into thirds. The injection is administered into the middle third of the thigh (Figure 9-8, *B*).

The length of the needle used depends on the overall size of the thigh. It should be long enough to penetrate the muscle belly for proper absorption to occur. A 1-inch needle is often used. To administer the injection, the infant is placed on his or her back. The thigh is grasped to compress the muscle tissue and to stabilize the extremity (Figure 9-9, *A*). The injection is administered as illustrated in Figure 9-9, *B*, by following the procedure outlined in Chapter 11.

The deltoid muscle is shallow and can accommodate only a small amount of medication. In addition, repeated injections at this site are painful. Because the deltoid site is so small in an infant, the deltoid site should not be used to administer an injection until a child is at least 18 months old. To administer the injection, the deltoid muscle mass should be grasped at the injection site and compressed between the thumb and fingers. The needle should be inserted pointing slightly upward toward the shoulder (Figure 9-10).

After the injection is given, the medical assistant or the child's parent should hold the infant and provide comfort and show approval so that the child associates something other than pain with this procedure.

IMMUNIZATIONS

Immunity is the resistance of the body to the effects of harmful agents, such as pathogenic microorganisms and their toxins. The process of becoming immune or rendering an individual immune through the use of a **vaccine** or **toxoid** is known as active, artificial **immunization.** Immunizations build the body's defenses and protect an individual from attack by certain infectious diseases.

Immunizations should be administered to infants and young children during well-child visits according to an immunization schedule (Figure 9-11). The American Acad-

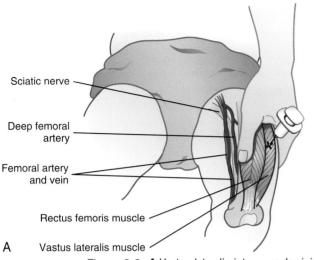

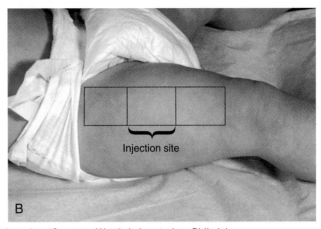

Figure 9-8. **A,** Vastus lateralis intramuscular injection site. (Courtesy Wyeth Laboratories, Philadelphia, PA.) **B,** Location of the vastus lateralis injection site in an infant. Divide the mid-anterior thigh into thirds. The injection is administered into the middle third of the thigh.

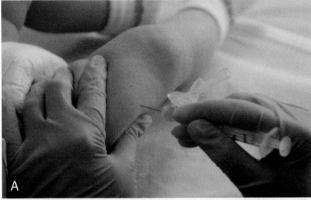

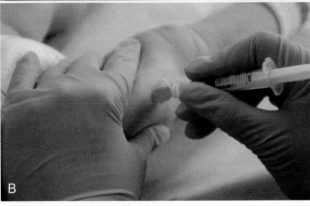

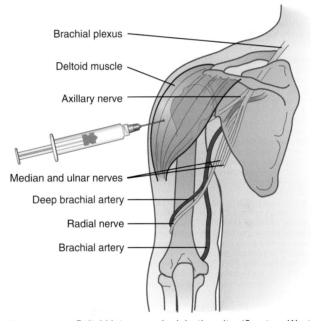

Figure 9-10. Deltoid intramuscular injection site. (Courtesy Wyeth Laboratories, Philadelphia, Penn.)

Figure 9-9. **A,** Compression of the vastus lateralis muscle. **B,** IM injection into the vastus lateralis injection site.

emy of Pediatrics recommends that the schedule outlined in Figure 9-11 should be followed. This schedule is intended as a guide to be used with any modifications needed to meet the requirements of an individual or group.

The medical assistant should be familiar with every immunization that is given, including its use, common side effects, route of administration, dosage, and method of storage. The drug manufacturer includes a package insert with

each vaccine and toxoid that contains valuable information about the drug. Drug references, such as the *Physician's Desk Reference,* also can be used to locate information on immunizations. Immunizations administered to infants and children, along with brand names, routes of administration, and common minor problems, are listed in Table 9-4. Certain immunizations can be administered together in the same injection. A combined immunization is just as effective as the individual immunization and results in fewer injections for the infant or child. For example, diphtheria, tetanus, and pertussis (DTaP), hepatitis B, and polio (DTaP-HepB-IPV) immunizations can be combined together in the same injection. Table 9-5 provides a list of combined immunizations

Recommended Immunization Schedule for Persons Aged 0 Through 6 Years — United States • 2010

For those who fall behind or start late, see the catch-up schedule

Vaccine Age	Birth	1 month	2 months	4 months	6 months	12 months	15 months	18 months	19–23 months	2–3 years	4–6 years
Hepatitis B[1]	HepB	HepB				HepB					
Rotavirus[2]			RV	RV	RV[2]						
Diphtheria, Tetanus, Pertussis[3]			DTaP	DTaP	DTaP	see footnote[3]	DTaP				DTaP
Haemophilus influenzae type b[4]			Hib	Hib	Hib[4]	Hib					
Pneumococcal[5]			PCV	PCV	PCV	PCV				PPSV	
Inactivated Poliovirus[6]			IPV	IPV	IPV						IPV
Influenza[7]					Influenza (Yearly)						
Measles, Mumps, Rubella[8]						MMR		see footnote[8]			MMR
Varicella[9]						Varicella		see footnote[9]			Varicella
Hepatitis A[10]						HepA (2 doses)				HepA Series	
Meningococcal[11]										MCV	

Range of recommended ages for all children except certain high-risk groups

Range of recommended ages for certain high-risk groups

This schedule includes recommendations in effect as of December 15, 2009. Any dose not administered at the recommended age should be administered at a subsequent visit, when indicated and feasible. The use of a combination vaccine generally is preferred over separate injections of its equivalent component vaccines. Considerations should include provider assessment, patient preference, and the potential for adverse events. Providers should consult the relevant Advisory Committee on Immunization Practices statement for detailed recommendations: http://www.cdc.gov/vaccines/pubs/acip-list.htm. Clinically significant adverse events that follow immunization should be reported to the Vaccine Adverse Event Reporting System (VAERS) at http://www.vaers.hhs.gov or by telephone, 800-822-7967.

1. **Hepatitis B vaccine (HepB).** (Minimum age: birth)
   At birth:
   - Administer monovalent HepB to all newborns before hospital discharge.
   - If mother is hepatitis B surface antigen (HBsAg)-positive, administer HepB and 0.5 mL of hepatitis B immune globulin (HBIG) within 12 hours of birth.
   - If mother's HBsAg status is unknown, administer HepB within 12 hours of birth. Determine mother's HBsAg status as soon as possible and, if HBsAg-positive, administer HBIG (no later than age 1 week).
   After the birth dose:
   - The HepB series should be completed with either monovalent HepB or a combination vaccine containing HepB. The second dose should be administered at age 1 or 2 months. Monovalent HepB vaccine should be used for doses administered before age 6 weeks. The final dose should be administered no earlier than age 24 weeks.
   - Infants born to HBsAg-positive mothers should be tested for HBsAg and antibody to HBsAg 1 to 2 months after completion of at least 3 doses of the HepB series, at age 9 through 18 months (generally at the next well-child visit).
   - Administration of 4 doses of HepB to infants is permissible when a combination vaccine containing HepB is administered after the birth dose. The fourth dose should be administered no earlier than age 24 weeks.
2. **Rotavirus vaccine (RV).** (Minimum age: 6 weeks)
   - Administer the first dose at age 6 through 14 weeks (maximum age: 14 weeks 6 days). Vaccination should not be initiated for infants aged 15 weeks 0 days or older.
   - The maximum age for the final dose in the series is 8 months 0 days
   - If Rotarix is administered at ages 2 and 4 months, a dose at 6 months is not indicated.
3. **Diphtheria and tetanus toxoids and acellular pertussis vaccine (DTaP).** (Minimum age: 6 weeks)
   - The fourth dose may be administered as early as age 12 months, provided at least 6 months have elapsed since the third dose.
   - Administer the final dose in the series at age 4 through 6 years.
4. ***Haemophilus influenzae* type b conjugate vaccine (Hib).** (Minimum age: 6 weeks)
   - If PRP-OMP (PedvaxHIB or Comvax [HepB-Hib]) is administered at ages 2 and 4 months, a dose at age 6 months is not indicated.
   - TriHiBit (DTaP/Hib) and Hiberix (PRP-T) should not be used for doses at ages 2, 4, or 6 months for the primary series but can be used as the final dose in children aged 12 months through 4 years. See *MMWR* 1997;46(No. RR-8).
5. **Pneumococcal vaccine.** (Minimum age: 6 weeks for pneumococcal conjugate vaccine [PCV]; 2 years for pneumococcal polysaccharide vaccine [PPSV])
   - PCV is recommended for all children aged younger than 5 years. Administer 1 dose of PCV to all healthy children aged 24 through 59 months who are not completely vaccinated for their age.
   - Administer PPSV 2 or more months after last dose of PCV to children aged 2 years or older with certain underlying medical conditions, including a cochlear implant.

6. **Inactivated poliovirus vaccine (IPV)** (Minimum age: 6 weeks)
   - The final dose in the series should be administered on or after the fourth birthday and at least 6 months following the previous dose.
   - If 4 doses are administered prior to age 4 years a fifth dose should be administered at age 4 through 6 years. See *MMWR* 2009;58(30):829–30.
7. **Influenza vaccine (seasonal).** (Minimum age: 6 months for trivalent inactivated influenza vaccine [TIV]; 2 years for live, attenuated influenza vaccine [LAIV])
   - Administer annually to children aged 6 months through 18 years.
   - For healthy children aged 2 through 6 years (i.e., those who do not have underlying medical conditions that predispose them to influenza complications), either LAIV or TIV may be used, except LAIV should not be given to children aged 2 through 4 years who have had wheezing in the past 12 months.
   - Children receiving TIV should receive 0.25 mL if aged 6 through 35 months or 0.5 mL if aged 3 years or older.
   - Administer 2 doses (separated by at least 4 weeks) to children aged younger than 9 years who are receiving influenza vaccine for the first time or who were vaccinated for the first time during the previous influenza season but only received 1 dose.
   - For recommendations for use of influenza A (H1N1) 2009 monovalent vaccine see *MMWR* 2009;58(No. RR-10).
8. **Measles, mumps, and rubella vaccine (MMR).** (Minimum age: 12 months)
   - Administer the second dose routinely at age 4 through 6 years. However, the second dose may be administered before age 4, provided at least 28 days have elapsed since the first dose.
9. **Varicella vaccine.** (Minimum age: 12 months)
   - Administer the second dose routinely at age 4 through 6 years. However, the second dose may be administered before age 4, provided at least 3 months have elapsed since the first dose.
   - For children aged 12 months through 12 years the minimum interval between doses is 3 months. However, if the second dose was administered at least 28 days after the first dose, it can be accepted as valid.
10. **Hepatitis A vaccine (HepA).** (Minimum age: 12 months)
    - Administer to all children aged 1 year (i.e., aged 12 through 23 months). Administer 2 doses at least 6 months apart.
    - Children not fully vaccinated by age 2 years can be vaccinated at subsequent visits
    - HepA also is recommended for older children who live in areas where vaccination programs target older children, who are at increased risk for infection, or for whom immunity against hepatitis A is desired.
11. **Meningococcal vaccine.** (Minimum age: 2 years for meningococcal conjugate vaccine [MCV4] and for meningococcal polysaccharide vaccine [MPSV4])
    - Administer MCV4 to children aged 2 through 10 years with persistent complement component deficiency, anatomic or functional asplenia, and certain other conditions placing them at high risk.
    - Administer MCV4 to children previously vaccinated with MCV4 or MPSV4 after 3 years if first dose administered at age 2 through 6 years. See *MMWR* 2009; 58:1042–3.

The Recommended Immunization Schedules for Persons Aged 0 through 18 Years are approved by the Advisory Committee on Immunization Practices (http://www.cdc.gov/vaccines/recs/acip), the American Academy of Pediatrics (http://www.aap.org), and the American Academy of Family Physicians (http://www.aafp.org). Department of Health and Human Services • Centers for Disease Control and Prevention

Figure 9-11. Immunization schedule. (From Department of Health and Human Services, Centers for Disease Control and Prevention, United States, 2010.)

Table 9-4 Infant and Childhood Immunizations

Immunization (and Abbreviation)	Brand Names	Route of Administration	Common Minor Problems after Administration
Hep B (hepatitis B vaccine)	Engerix-B Recombivax HB	IM	Mild fever Soreness at injection site
DTaP (Diphtheria and tetanus toxoids and acellular pertussis vaccine)	Acel-Immune Certiva Daptacel Infanrix Tripedia	IM	Fever, irritability, tiredness, poor appetite, and vomiting Redness or swelling at injection site Soreness or tenderness at injection site (occurs 1-3 days after the injection and occurs more often after the 4th or 5th dose in the series than after earlier doses)
Hib (*Haemophilus influenzae* type b vaccine)	ActHIB HibTITER Pedvax HIB	IM	Redness, swelling and warmth at injection site; fever greater than 101°F (38.3°C) (occurs within 1 day after injection; may last 2-3 days)
IPV (inactivated polio vaccine)	IPOL	IM or SC	Soreness at the injection site
PCV (pneumococcal conjugate vaccine)	Prevnar	IM	Redness, swelling, and tenderness at the injection site; fever Irritability and drowsiness Loss of appetite
RV (rotavirus vaccine)	Rotarix RotaShield RotaTeq	Oral	Irritability, temporary diarrhea and vomiting
MMR (measles, mumps, and rubella vaccines)	M-M-R II	SC	Fever, mild rash, swelling of glands in the cheeks or neck (occurs 7-12 days after administration)
Var (varicella) (chickenpox vaccine)	Varivax	SC	Fever, mild rash Soreness or swelling at injection site
Hep A (hepatitis A vaccine)	Havrix Vaqta	IM	Soreness at the injection site Headache, loss of appetite, and tiredness (usually last 1-2 days)
MCV4 (meningococcal vaccine)	Menactra	IM	Pain and redness at injection site Fever (usually lasts 1-2 days)
HPV (human papillomavirus vaccine)	Gardasil	IM	Pain, redness, swelling, or itching at injection site Fever
Influenza vaccine (injection)	Afluria Fluarix FluLaval FluShield Fluvirin Fluzone	IM	Soreness, redness, or swelling at the injection site, fever and malaise Hoarseness; sore, red, or itchy eyes Cough, fever, aches (occur soon after injection and usually last 1-2 days)
Influenza vaccine (nasal spray)	FluMist	IN	Runny nose, nasal congestion or cough Headache, muscle aches, abdominal pain, or occasional vomiting or diarrhea Fever; wheezing

IM, Intramuscular; *IN*, intranasal; *SC*, subcutaneous.

Table 9-5 Infant and Childhood Combination Immunizations

Combined Immunization	Brand Name	Route of Administration
DTaP-HepB-IPV	Pediarix	IM
DTaP-Hib-IPV	Pentacel	IM
DTaP-IPV	Kinrix	IM
DTaP-Hib	TriHIBit	IM
Hib-HepB	Comvax	IM
MMRV	ProQuad	SC

NOTE: See Table 9-4 for the common minor problems that may occur following administration of each individual immunization.
DTaP, Diphtheria, tetanus, and pertussis; *HepB*, hepatitis B; *Hib*, *Haemophilus influenzae* type b; *IM*, intramuscular; *IPV*, inactivated polio vaccine; *MMRV*, measles, mumps, rubella, varicella; *SC*, subcutaneous.

IMMUNIZATION RECORD					
Name					
Birthdate					
Immunization	DATE	DATE	DATE	DATE	DATE
Hep B (Hepatitis B)					
DTaP (Diphtheria, Tetanus, and Pertussis)					
Hib (Haemophilius Influenzae Type b)					
IPV (Inactivated Polio Vaccine)					
PCV (Pneumococcal Conjugate Vaccine)					
RV (Rotavirus vaccine)					
MMR (Measles, Mumps, Rubella)					
Varicella (Chickenpox)					
Hep A (Hepatitis A)					
MCV4 (Meningococcal Vaccine)					
HPV (Human Papillomavirus)					
Influenza					
Tuberculin (Mantoux) RESULT					
Tetanus Booster					
Other					

Figure 9-12. Immunization record card.

administered to infants and children, along with brand names and the routes of administration.

Parents should be provided with an immunization record card (Figure 9-12) at their infant's first well-child visit. They should be instructed to bring this card to every visit so that their child's immunizations can be recorded. Parents should be informed of the possible normal side effects of each immunization and given instructions on how to respond if they occur.

National Childhood Vaccine Injury Act

The National Childhood Vaccine Injury Act (NCVIA), which became effective in 1988, requires that parents be provided with information about the benefits and risks of childhood immunizations. To help medical offices comply with these regulations, the Centers for Disease Control and Prevention developed a set of vaccine information statements. A vaccine information statement (VIS) explains, in lay terminology, the benefits and risks of a vaccine. It also contains information about reporting an adverse reaction, the National Vaccine Injury Compensation Program, and how to get more information about childhood diseases and vaccines. See Figure 9-13 for a DTaP vaccine information statement.

The NCVIA requires that the appropriate VIS be given to the child's parent or guardian each and every time before the child receives a dose of any immunization listed in Table 9-4. The medical assistant must give the parent or guardian enough time to read the VIS and an opportunity to ask questions before the immunization is administered. In addition, the medical assistant must chart the following information in the patient's medical record: the name and publication date of each VIS provided to the parent, and the date the VIS was given to the parent. The publication date of the VIS is located at the bottom left or right corner of the VIS. Vaccine information statements also are available for

pneumococcal polysaccharide, shingles (herpes zoster), rabies, yellow fever, typhoid, Japanese encephalitis, anthrax, and smallpox. Their use is strongly encouraged by the NCVIA, but is not required, because these vaccines are not administered to children on a routine basis.

The NCVIA also requires that the following information be recorded in each patient's medical record or on a permanent office log after administration of the vaccine: the date of administration of the vaccine, the manufacturer and lot number of the vaccine, the signature and title of the health care provider who administered the vaccine, and the name and address of the medical office where the vaccine was administered. Figure 9-14 shows an example of an immunization administrative record that is included in a patient's medical record.

NEWBORN SCREENING TEST

A newborn screening test is performed on an infant to screen for the presence of certain metabolic and endocrine diseases. The diseases that are screened vary by state but typically include phenylketonuria (PKU), biotinidase deficiency, congenital adrenal hyperplasia, maple sugar urine disease, congenital hypothyroidism, galactosemia, homocystinuria, and sickle cell anemia. The most important of these is PKU, which is discussed in greater detail in the following paragraphs.

PKU is a congenital hereditary disease caused by a lack of the enzyme *phenylalanine hydroxylase*. This enzyme is needed to convert phenylalanine, an amino acid, into tyrosine, which is an amino acid needed for normal metabolic functioning. Without this enzyme, phenylalanine accumulates in the blood and, if the accumulation is left untreated, causes mental retardation and other abnormalities, such as tremors and poor muscle coordination. In most cases, on early detection, a special low-phenylalanine diet and close periodic monitoring can prevent adverse effects. Normal development usually occurs if treatment is started before the child reaches 3 to 4 weeks of age. To promote the best development of cognitive abilities, most authorities recommend lifelong dietary restriction of phenylalanine. Although PKU is not a common condition (affecting 1 in every 12,000 births), early diagnosis and treatment lead to a better prognosis.

Phenylalanine can be detected in the blood of an affected infant only after the infant has been receiving breast or formula milk. Infants taking formula can be tested earlier than breastfed infants because formula contains phenylalanine, whereas the "first breast milk," or colostrum, does not. The test results of breastfed infants are usually invalid until the mother begins producing milk.

All states require by law that infants undergo newborn screening. The best time to perform the test is between 1 and 7 days after birth. In most states, the newborn screening test is performed before the infant leaves the hospital. If test results come back indicating abnormal or invalid results, the infant needs to be retested. Most repeat tests are required because of

What Would You Do? What Would You *Not* Do?

Case Study 3

Stacy Jones, a legal secretary, brings her 5-year-old son, Matthew, in for a kindergarten physical. Stacy has read the vaccine information statements for the DTaP, IPV, and MMR immunizations that Matthew will be getting at this visit and has some questions. She wants to know why polio is not given orally anymore. She also wants to know why children are immunized against chickenpox because it is such a harmless disease. She is annoyed because she thinks that children are receiving too many unnecessary injections these days. Matthew is extremely afraid of "shots" and says that no one with a needle is getting anywhere near him. Stacy is protective of Matthew and knows that he will be hard to handle. She wants to know whether this set of immunizations could just be skipped. She says that most of these diseases do not even exist anymore and that she noticed, from reading the vaccine sheets, that there are a lot of possible side effects. ∎

DIPHTHERIA, TETANUS AND PERTUSSIS VACCINE

What You Need to Know

Many Vaccine Information Statements are available in Spanish and other languages. See www.immunize.org/vis.

1. Why get vaccinated?

Diphtheria, tetanus, and pertussis are serious diseases caused by bacteria. Diphtheria and pertussis are spread from person to person. Tetanus enters the body through cuts or wounds.

DIPHTHERIA causes a thick covering in the back of the throat.
• It can lead to breathing problems, paralysis, heart failure, and even death.

TETANUS (Lockjaw) causes painful tightening of the muscles, usually all over the body.
• It can lead to "locking" of the jaw so the victim cannot open his mouth or swallow. Tetanus leads to death in up to 2 out of 10 cases.

PERTUSSIS (Whooping cough) causes coughing spells so bad that it is hard for infants to eat, drink, or breathe. These spells can last for weeks.
• It can lead to pneumonia, seizures (jerking and staring spells), brain damage, and death.

Diphtheria, tetanus, and pertussis vaccine (DTaP) can help prevent these diseases. Most children who are vaccinated with DTaP will be protected throughout childhood. Many more children would get these diseases if we stopped vaccinating.

DTaP is a safer version of an older vaccine called DTP. DTP is no longer used in the United States.

2. Who should get DTaP vaccine and when?

Children should get 5 doses of DTaP vaccine, one dose at each of the following ages:

2 months	15–18 months
4 months	4–6 years
6 months	

DTaP may be given at the same time as other vaccines.

3. Some children should not get DTaP vaccine or should wait

• Children with minor illnesses, such as a cold, may be vaccinated. But children who are moderately or severely ill should wait until they recover before getting DTaP vaccine.

• Any child who had a life-threatening allergic reaction after a dose of DTaP should not get another dose.

• Any child who suffered a brain or nervous system disease within 7 days after a dose of DTaP should not get another dose.

• Talk with your doctor if your child:
 – had a seizure or collapsed after a dose of DTaP,
 – cried non-stop for 3 hours or more after a dose of DTaP,
 – had a fever over 105°F after a dose of DTaP.

Ask your health care provider for more information. Some of these children should not get another dose of pertussis vaccine, but may get a vaccine without pertussis, called **DT**.

4. Older children and adults

DTaP is not licensed for adolescents, adults, or children 7 years of age and older.

But older people still need protection. A vaccine called **Tdap** is similar to DTaP. A single dose of Tdap is recommended for people 11 through 64 years of age. Another vaccine, called **Td**, protects against tetanus and diphtheria, but not pertussis. It is recommended every 10 years. There are separate Vaccine Information Statements for these vaccines.

Diptheria/Tetanus/Pertussis 5/17/2007

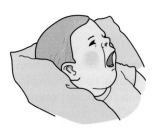

Figure 9-13. Vaccine information statement for diphtheria, tetanus, and pertussis (DTaP). (Courtesy Centers for Disease Control and Prevention, Atlanta, GA.)

5. What are the risks from DTaP vaccine?

Getting diphtheria, tetanus, or pertussis disease is much riskier than getting DTaP vaccine.

However, a vaccine, like any medicine, is capable of causing serious problems, such as severe allergic reactions. The risk of DTaP vaccine causing serious harm, or death, is extremely small.

Mild Problems (Common)
- Fever (up to about 1 child in 4)
- Redness or swelling where the shot was given (up to about 1 child in 4)
- Soreness or tenderness where the shot was given (up to about 1 child in 4).

These problems occur more often after the fourth and fifth doses of the DTaP series than after earlier doses. Sometimes the fourth or fifth dose of DTaP vaccine is followed by swelling of the entire arm or leg in which the shot was given, lasting 1–7 days (up to about 1 child in 30).

Other mild problems include:
- Fussiness (up to about 1 child in 3)
- Tiredness or poor appetite (up to about 1 child in 10)
- Vomiting (up to about 1 child in 50)

These problems generally occur 1–3 days after the shot.

Moderate Problems (Uncommon)
- Seizure (jerking or staring) (about 1 child out of 14,000)
- Non-stop crying, for 3 hours or more (up to about 1 child out of 1,000)
- High fever, over 105°F (about 1 child out of 16,000)

Severe Problems (Very Rare)
- Serious allergic reactions (less than 1 out of a million doses)
- Several other severe problems have been reported after DTaP vaccine. These include:
  – Long-term seizures, coma, or lowered consciousness
  – Permanent brain damage.
  These are so rare it is hard to tell if they are caused by the vaccine.

Controlling fever is especially important for children who have had seizures, for any reason. It is also important if another family member has had seizures. You can reduce fever and pain by giving your child an *aspirin-free* pain reliever when the shot is given, and for the next 24 hours, following the package instructions.

6. What if there is a moderate or severe reaction?

What should I look for?

Any unusual conditions, such as a serious allergic reaction, high fever or unusual behavior. Serious allergic reactions are extremely rare with any vaccine. If one were to occur, it would most likely be within a few minutes to a few hours after the shot. Signs can include difficulty breathing, hoarseness or wheezing, hives, paleness, weakness, a fast heartbeat or dizziness. If a high fever or seizure were to occur, it would usually be within a week after the shot.

What should I do?

- **Call** a doctor, or get the person to a doctor right away.
- **Tell** your doctor what happened, the date and time it happened, and when the vaccination was given.
- **Ask** your doctor, nurse, or health department to report the reaction by filing a Vaccine Adverse Event Reporting System (VAERS) form.

Or you can file this report through the VAERS web site at **www.vaers.hhs.gov**, or by calling **1-800-822-7967**. *VAERS does not provide medical advice.*

7. The National Vaccine Injury Compensation Program

In the rare event that you or your child has a serious reaction to a vaccine, a federal program has been created to help pay for the care of those who have been harmed.

For details about the National Vaccine Injury Compensation Program, call **1-800-338-2382** or visit the program's website at **www.hrsa.gov/vaccinecompensation.**

8. How can I learn more?

- Ask your health care provider. They can give you the vaccine package insert or suggest other sources of information.

- Call your local or state health department's immunization program.

- Contact the Centers for Disease Control and Prevention (CDC):
  – Call **1-800-232-4636 (1-800-CDC-INFO)**
  – Visit the National Immunization Program's website at **www.cdc.gov/vaccines**

U.S. DEPARTMENT OF HEALTH AND HUMAN SERVICES
Centers for Disease Control and Prevention
National Immunization Program

Vaccine Information Statement	
DTaP (5/17/07)	42 U.S.C. § 300aa-26

Figure 9-13, cont'd. Vaccine information statement for diphtheria, tetanus, and pertussis (DTaP). (Courtesy Centers for Disease Control and Prevention, Atlanta, GA.)

IMMUNIZATION ADMINISTRATION RECORD

Name _____
  (first)   (MI)   (last)

DOB _____

Physician _____

Address _____

_____

SITE ABBREVIATIONS:

RVL: Right vastus lateralis
LVL: Left vastus lateralis
RD: Right deltoid
LD: Left deltoid
PO: By mouth
IN: Intranasal

Vaccine	Type of Vaccine[1] (generic abbreviation)	Date Given (mo/day/yr)	Dose	Site	Vaccine		Vaccine Information Statement		Signature and Title of Vaccinator
					Lot #	Mfr.	Date on VIS	Date Given	
Hepatitis B[2] (e.g., HepB, Hib-HepB, DTaP-HepB-IPV) Give IM.									
Diphtheria, Tetanus, Pertussis[2] (e.g., DTaP, DTaP-Hib, DTaP-HepB-IPV, DT, DTaP-Hib-IPV, Tdap, DTaP-IPV, Td) Give IM.									
Haemophilus influenzae **type b[2]** (e.g., Hib, Hib-HepB, DTaP-Hib-IPV, DTaP-Hib) Give IM.									
Polio[2] (e.g., IPV, DTaP-HepB-IPV, DTaP-Hib-IPV, DTaP-IPV) Give IPV SC or IM. Give all others IM.									
Pneumococcal (e.g., PCV, conjugate; PPV, polysaccharide) Give PCV IM. Give PPV SC or IM.									
Rotovirus Give oral.									
Measles, Mumps, Rubella[5] (e.g., MMR, MMRV) Give SC.									
Varicella[5] (e.g., Var, MMRV) Give SC.									
Hepatitis A Give IM									
Meningococcal (e.g., MCV4, MPSV4) Give MCV4 IM and MPSV4 SC.									
Human papillomavirus (e.g., HPV) Give IM									
Influenza[5] (e.g., TIV, inactivated; LAIV, live attenuated) Give TIV IM. Give LAIV IN.									
Other									

1. Record the generic abbreviation for the type of vaccine given (e.g., DTaP-Hib, PCV), *not* the trade name.
2. For combination vaccines, fill in a row for each separate antigen in the combination.

Figure 9-14. Immunization administration record included in a patient's medical record. (Modified from Immunization Action Coalition, St. Paul, Minn.)

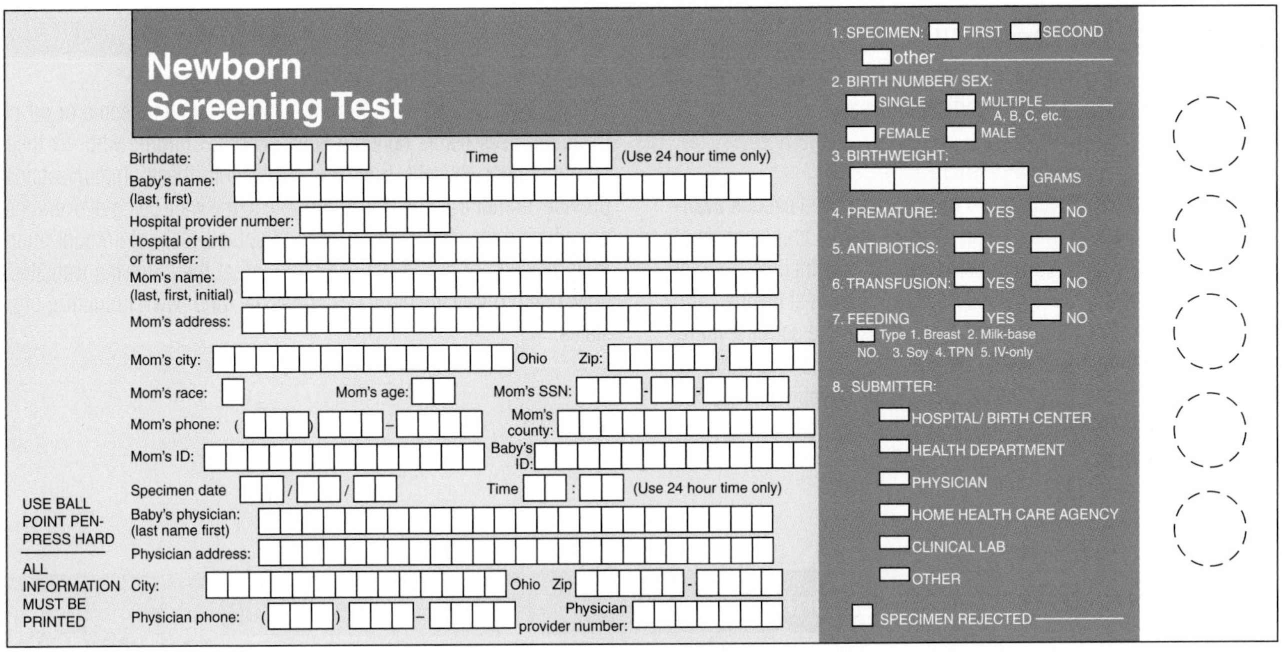
Newborn Screening Test

Birthdate: / / Time : (Use 24 hour time only)
Baby's name: (last, first)
Hospital provider number:
Hospital of birth or transfer:
Mom's name: (last, first, initial)
Mom's address:
Mom's city: Ohio Zip: -
Mom's race: Mom's age: Mom's SSN: - -
Mom's phone: ( ) - Mom's county:
Mom's ID: Baby's ID:
Specimen date / / Time : (Use 24 hour time only)
Baby's physician: (last name first)
Physician address:
City: Ohio Zip -
Physician phone: ( ) - Physician provider number:

USE BALL POINT PEN- PRESS HARD
ALL INFORMATION MUST BE PRINTED

1. SPECIMEN: FIRST SECOND other
2. BIRTH NUMBER/ SEX: SINGLE MULTIPLE A, B, C, etc. FEMALE MALE
3. BIRTHWEIGHT: GRAMS
4. PREMATURE: YES NO
5. ANTIBIOTICS: YES NO
6. TRANSFUSION: YES NO
7. FEEDING YES NO Type 1. Breast 2. Milk-base NO. 3. Soy 4. TPN 5. IV-only
8. SUBMITTER: HOSPITAL/ BIRTH CENTER HEALTH DEPARTMENT PHYSICIAN HOME HEALTH CARE AGENCY CLINICAL LAB OTHER
SPECIMEN REJECTED

Figure 9-15. Newborn screening test card.

invalid test results due to the collection of an inadequate amount of the blood specimen. Newborn screening retesting is often performed in the medical office; therefore the medical assistant needs to acquire the knowledge and technique needed to perform this procedure with skill and accuracy.

The newborn screening test is performed on capillary blood obtained from the fleshy part of the lateral or medial posterior curve of the plantar surface of the infant's heel (Procedure 9-5). The blood specimen is placed on a special filter paper attached to the newborn screening test card (Figure 9-15) and is mailed to an outside laboratory for analysis. The results are ready in a few days. If one of the newborn screening test results is positive, further testing is performed.

PATIENT TEACHING Childhood Immunizations

- Encourage parents to have their children immunized.
- Emphasize to parents the importance of maintaining an immunization record card that documents all of their child's immunizations.
- Provide parents with educational materials on the importance of immunizations.
- Answer questions patients have about childhood immunizations.

What is immunity?

Immunity is the resistance of the body to microorganisms that cause disease. When an individual has an infection, the body responds by producing disease-fighting substances known as *antibodies.* Antibodies usually remain in the body even after the individual has recovered from the disease. This protects the individual from getting that disease again.

How do immunizations prevent disease?

The microorganisms that cause disease or their toxins are weakened or killed and made into vaccines. These vaccines are injected into the body. The body reacts to these vaccines the same way that it responds to the disease itself—by producing antibodies. These antibodies last for a long time, often for life, to defend the body against disease.

What childhood diseases can be prevented through immunization?

The reduction of childhood disease by immunization during the past 40 years has been dramatic. Fourteen diseases can be prevented by routine immunization of children: hepatitis B, diphtheria, tetanus, pertussis (whooping cough), *Haemophilus influenzae* type b infections, polio, measles, mumps, rubella (German measles), chickenpox (varicella), pneumococcal infections (meningitis and blood infections), hepatitis A, rotavirus, and influenza (flu). Except for tetanus, all these diseases are contagious. They can be spread from child to child and from one community to another. When children are not protected against them, serious outbreaks of disease can still occur.

Haven't most of these diseases been eliminated in the United States?

Although most of the vaccine-preventable diseases have been reduced to very low levels in the United States, this is not true worldwide. Some of these diseases are quite prevalent in other countries. An infected traveler can bring these diseases into the United States without knowing it. If Americans were not immunized, these diseases could quickly spread throughout the population and cause an

Continued

PROCEDURE 9-5

epidemic. Only when a disease has been eradicated worldwide is it safe to stop vaccinating for that particular disease.

Do immunizations have side effects?

Vaccines are among the safest and most reliable medications available. Minor side effects may occur, however, after administration of an immunization. They do not last long and may include a slight fever and irritability; redness, swelling, and soreness at the injection site; and a mild rash. Rarely, the effects can be more serious; if any unusual symptoms occur after immunization, it is important to contact the physician immediately. Overall, the benefits of vaccines to prevent childhood diseases are greater than the possible risks for almost all children.

Are immunizations required by law?

Every state has laws requiring immunization against some or all of these diseases before children enter school. Children who get their immunizations benefit from the protection these immunizations provide; immunizations also contribute to the well-being of everyone by reducing the chance for disease to spread. School immunization requirements for each state can be found at the following websites: www.nnii.org/vaccineInfo/index.cfm#state and www.immunize.org/states. ■

PROCEDURE 9-5   Newborn Screening Test

Outcome Collect a capillary blood specimen for a newborn screening test.

Equipment/Supplies

- Disposable gloves
- Infant heel warmer or warm compress
- Antiseptic wipe
- Sterile 2 × 2 gauze pad
- Sterile lancet

- Adhesive bandage
- Newborn screening test card
- Mailing envelope
- Biohazard sharps container

---

1. Procedural Step. Sanitize your hands, and assemble the equipment.

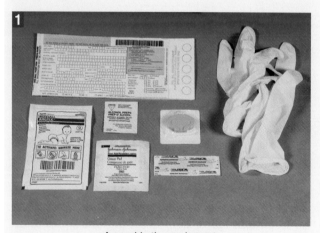

Assemble the equipment.

2. Procedural Step. Greet the infant's parent and introduce yourself. Identify the infant and explain the procedure to the parent.

3. Procedural Step. Complete the information section of the newborn screening card.

4. Procedural Step. Select an appropriate puncture site. The fleshy part of the lateral and medial posterior curves of the plantar surface of the heel can be used.

Principle. The fleshy lateral and medial posterior curves of the heel are used to avoid calcaneal complications such as inflammation of the bone caused by penetrating the bone with the lancet.

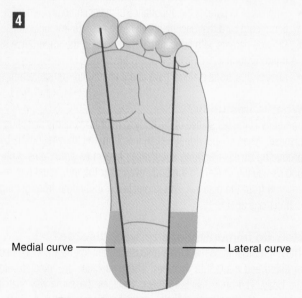

Medial curve ———   ——— Lateral curve

The shading indicates the appropriate area for making the puncture.

Plantar surface of the heel.

PROCEDURE 9-5   Newborn Screening Test—cont'd

5. **Procedural Step.** Warm the puncture site with a commercially available infant heel warmer or a warm compress for approximately 5 minutes.
Principle. Warming the puncture site increases capillary circulation and promotes bleeding.

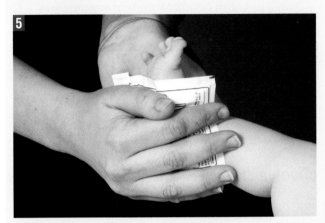

Warm the puncture site.

6. **Procedural Step.** Cleanse the puncture site with an antiseptic wipe, and allow it to air dry. Do not wipe the area with gauze to speed the drying process.
Principle. The site must be allowed to air dry to give the alcohol enough time to destroy microorganisms. If the site is wet, the patient will feel a stinging sensation when the puncture is made.

7. **Procedural Step.** Apply gloves. Grasp the infant's foot around the puncture site, and, without touching the cleansed site, make a puncture with the sterile lancet. The puncture should be made at a right angle to the lines of the skin. Dispose of the lancet in a biohazard sharps container.
Principle. Touching the site after cleansing would contaminate it, and the cleansing process would have to be repeated.

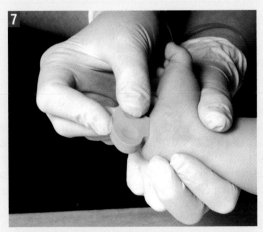

Grasp the infant's foot, and make the puncture.

8. **Procedural Step.** Wipe away the first drop of blood with a gauze pad.
Principle. The first drop of blood is diluted with alcohol and tissue fluid and is not a suitable specimen.

9. **Procedural Step.** Encourage a large drop of blood to form by exerting gentle pressure without excessively squeezing the area. Place one side of the filter paper next to the infant's heel. Touch the drop of blood to the center of the first circle on the test card, and completely fill the first circle with the blood specimen. The proper amount of specimen is obtained when the blood can be observed soaking completely through the filter paper from one side to the other.
Principle. Excessive squeezing would cause dilution of the blood sample with tissue fluid, leading to inaccurate test results.

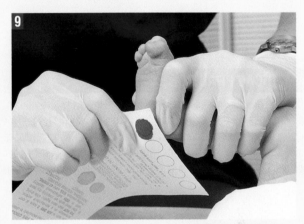

Completely fill the circle with the blood specimen.

10. **Procedural Step.** Repeat Procedure Step 9 until all the circles on the card are completely filled with blood. Be careful not to touch the blood specimens on the card with your gloved hand.
Principle. The circles must be completely filled to ensure enough of a blood sample to perform the test. Most repeat tests are required because of inadequate specimen collection. Touching the blood specimen could lead to inaccurate test results.

11. **Procedural Step.** Hold a piece of gauze over the puncture site, and apply pressure to control the bleeding. Remain with the infant until the bleeding stops. If needed, apply an adhesive bandage.

12. **Procedural Step.** Remove the gloves, and sanitize your hands.

13. **Procedural Step.** Allow the test card to air dry in a horizontal position for at least 3 hours at room temperature on a nonabsorbent surface. Do not allow the wet blood specimen to come in contact with any other surface. Do not expose the test card to heat, moisture, or direct sunlight. Do not place the speci-

Continued

PROCEDURE 9-5

PROCEDURE 9-5   Newborn Screening Test—cont'd

men in a biohazard specimen bag or any other type of plastic bag.

Principle. Placing the test card in a plastic bag interferes with proper drying of the specimen.

14. **Procedural Step.** After the blood is completely dry, place the test card in its protective envelope, and mail it to an outside laboratory for testing within 48 hours.

Principle. The test card should be mailed within 48 hours to ensure accurate test results.

15. **Procedural Step.** Chart the procedure. Include the date and time, the type of procedure, the puncture site location, and information regarding transfer to an outside laboratory.

CHARTING EXAMPLE

Date	
8/15/12	9:30 a.m. Blood specimen collected from ® medial heel. Sent to Newborn Screening Lab on 8/15/12 for newborn screening test.
	—————————— T. Powell, CMA (AAMA)

*e*volve *Check out the Evolve site to access additional interactive activities.*

MEDICAL PRACTICE *and the* LAW

Children are not small adults. They must be treated as individuals, according to their developmental level. Pediatric patients (except for emancipated minors) cannot give written or verbal consent. Make sure a parent or legal guardian is available for consent. A babysitter or grandparent cannot give consent for treatment without written permission from a parent or legal guardian. Similarly, patient information can be given only to a parent or legal guardian.

If your office sees pediatric patients, you have a responsibility to be aware of developmental needs and milestones of children at various ages. This is necessary for accurate developmental assessment. ■

What Would You Do? What Would You *Not* Do? RESPONSES

Case Study 1
Page 323

What Did Traci Do?

❑ Listened patiently to Mrs. Chang and allowed her to vent her frustrations.

❑ Reassured Mrs. Chang that her milk is very nutritious for Christopher. Gave her a brochure on breastfeeding that included information on what to do for sore nipples and engorgement.

❑ Gave Mrs. Chang the names and phone numbers of community resources for nursing mothers.

❑ Told Mrs. Chang that Christopher's weight and length do not fall in the underweight category on his growth chart. Showed her Christopher's growth chart so that she could see that Christopher is progressing normally.

What Did Traci Not Do?

❑ Did not tell Mrs. Chang to cheer up because the colic would eventually go away on its own.

❑ Did not give a personal opinion on whether Mrs. Chang should breastfeed or bottle feed her infant.

What Would You Do?/What Would You *Not* Do? Review Traci's response and place a checkmark next to the information you included in your response. List additional information included in your response.

_____

_____

_____

_____

Case Study 2
Page 337

What Did Traci Do?

❑ Explained to Mrs. Tilley that childhood obesity has doubled in the past 20 years and has become a serious health concern.

❑ Told Mrs. Tilley that she could have a big impact on Courtney's life by preparing healthy meals and eating them with her and by becoming involved in activities with Courtney, such as taking walks.

❑ Spent some time talking with Courtney about her interests and complimented Courtney on her achievements.

What Would You Do? What Would You *Not* Do? RESPONSES—cont'd

❏ Encouraged Courtney to join the swim team. Told her that lots of people do not like to be seen in a bathing suit and encouraged her not to let that stand in her way of doing something she wants to do.

❏ Reassured Courtney that the doctor wants to help her and that he would never say anything bad about her weight.

What Did Traci Not *Do?*

❏ Did not agree with Mrs. Tilley that there is nothing that can be done about Courtney's weight problem.

❏ Did not tell Courtney that she needs to lose weight or she might develop serious health problems such as diabetes.

What Would You Do?/What Would You *Not* Do? Review Traci's response and place a checkmark next to the information you included in your response. List additional information included in your response.

_____

_____

_____

_____

Case Study 3
Page 345

What Did Traci Do?

❏ Explained to Stacy that it is rare, but sometimes a child develops polio from getting the oral polio vaccine. Told her that this does not occur with the injectable polio vaccine.

❏ Explained to Stacy that chickenpox is usually a mild disease, but it can be serious, especially in young infants and adults.

❏ Explained to Stacy that most side effects from vaccines are mild, and that complications from the diseases far outweigh the possible side effects.

❏ Told Stacy that these diseases have been reduced to very low levels in the United States, but they still occur in other countries. Explained that infected travelers can bring these diseases to the United States and infect individuals who are not immunized.

❏ Reminded Stacy that these immunizations are required for Matthew to start kindergarten.

❏ Talked with Matthew on his level about why he needs to be immunized.

❏ Told Matthew that they would play a game so that it wouldn't hurt as much. Taught him to hold up his finger and pretend that it was a birthday candle; when the injection was given, told him to keep blowing out the candle until he was told to stop.

❏ Told Matthew that he could choose a prize from the treasure chest after he had his immunizations.

What Did Traci Not *Do?*

❏ Did not ignore or minimize Stacy's concerns.

❏ Did not tell Stacy that the answers to all her questions are in the vaccine information sheets that she was just given.

❏ Did not tell Stacy it would be all right to skip Matthew's immunizations.

❏ Did not refer to the immunizations as "shots" when talking with Matthew.

❏ Did not tell Matthew that it would not hurt when he gets his immunizations.

What Would You Do?/What Would You *Not* Do? Review Traci's response and place a checkmark next to the information you included in your response. List additional information included in your response.

_____

_____

_____

_____

CERTIFICATION REVIEW

❏ **Pediatrics** is the branch of medicine that deals with the care and development of children and the diagnosis and treatment of diseases in children. A pediatrician is a physician who specializes in pediatrics.

❏ **There are two categories of pediatric office visits:** the well-child visit and the sick-child visit. The purpose of the well-child visit is to receive necessary immunizations and to observe for abnormal conditions associated with the child's stage of development. The purpose of the sick-child visit is to diagnose the condition of a child who is exhibiting the signs and symptoms of disease.

❏ **To evaluate the progress of a child,** the weight, height (or length), and head circumference are measured during each visit and plotted on a growth chart. The child's weight is used to determine nutritional needs and the

proper dosage of a medication to administer to the child. Growth charts provide a means for assessing the child's rate of growth; the physician investigates any significant change or rapid increase or decrease in the child's growth pattern.

❏ **Blood pressure** should be measured in children 3 years old and older to identify children at risk for developing hypertension as adults. To obtain an accurate pediatric blood pressure measurement, the correct cuff size must be used. Blood pressure varies depending on the age of the child and his or her height and gender.

❏ **A urine specimen** may be required from a pediatric patient as part of a general physical examination to assist in the diagnosis of a pathologic condition or to evaluate the effectiveness of therapy. Collecting a urine specimen from an infant or young child who cannot

Continued

CERTIFICATION REVIEW—cont'd

urinate voluntarily requires the use of a pediatric urine collector.

❑ **Administering an injection to a child** uses the same basic technique as that used to administer an injection to an adult. The vastus lateralis muscle is the recommended intramuscular injection site for infants and young children. It is large enough to accommodate the injected medication.

❑ **Immunity** is the resistance of the body to the effects of harmful agents, such as pathogenic microorganisms and their toxins. Immunizations build the body's defenses and protect an individual from attack by certain infectious diseases.

❑ **The National Childhood Vaccine Injury Act** requires that parents be provided with information about the benefits and risks of childhood immunizations through vaccine information sheets (VIS) developed by the Centers for Disease Control and Prevention.

❑ **A newborn screening test** is performed on an infant to screen for the presence of certain metabolic and endocrine diseases. All states require that infants undergo newborn screening. These diseases that are screened vary by state but typically include phenylketonuria (PKU), biotinidase deficiency, congenital adrenal hyperplasia, maple sugar urine disease, congenital hypothyroidism, galactosemia, homocystinuria, and sickle cell anemia. The most important of these is **phenylketonuria (PKU). PKU** is a congenital hereditary disease. If left untreated, PKU can result in mental retardation and other abnormalities. Early diagnosis and treatment can lead to a better prognosis.

TERMINOLOGY REVIEW

Medical Term	Word Parts	Definition
Adolescent		An individual 12 to 18 years old.
Immunity		The resistance of the body to the effects of a harmful agent, such as a pathogenic microorganism and its toxins.
Immunization (active, artificial)		The process of becoming immune or of rendering an individual immune through the use of a vaccine or toxoid.
Infant		A child from birth to 12 months old.
Length (recumbent)		The measurement from the vertex of the head to the heel of the foot in a supine position.
Pediatrician	*pedi/a:* child	A physician who specializes in the care and development of children and the diagnosis and treatment of children's diseases.
Pediatrics	*pedi/a:* child	The branch of medicine that deals with the care and development of children and the diagnosis and treatment of children's diseases.
Preschool child	*pre-:* in front of; before	A child 3 to 6 years old.
School-age child		A child 6 to 12 years old.
Toddler		A child 1 to 3 years old.
Toxoid		A toxin (a poisonous substance produced by a bacterium) that has been treated by heat or chemicals to destroy its harmful properties. It is administered to an individual to prevent an infectious disease by stimulating the production of antibodies in that individual.
Vaccine		A suspension of attenuated (weakened) or killed microorganisms administered to an individual to prevent an infectious disease by stimulating the production of antibodies in that individual.
Vertex		The top of the head.

ON THE WEB

For Information on Child Health:

KidsHealth: www.kidshealth.org

Baby Center: www.babycenter.com

Pediatric on Call: www.pediatriconcall.com

ON THE WEB—cont'd

Kids Source Online: www.kidsource.com

American Academy of Pediatrics: www.aap.org

Child and Youth Health: www.cyh.com

Girl's Health: www.girlshealth.gov

For Information on Childhood Conditions:

Attention-Deficit Hyperactivity Disorder: www.add-adhd.org

Attention Deficit Disorder Association: www.add.org

Cerebral Palsy: www.about-cerebral-palsy.org

American Academy for Cerebral Palsy and Developmental Medicine: www.aacpdm.org

Child Abuse: www.preventchildabuse.org

American Professional Society on the Abuse of Children: www.apsac.org

Cystic Fibrosis: www.cysticfibrosis.com

Cystic Fibrosis Foundation: www.cff.org

Dental Health: Colgate World of Care: www.colgate.com

American Dentistry Association: www.ada.org

The Tooth Fairy Online: www.asis.com/toothfairy

Diabetes: American Diabetes Association: www.diabetes.org

Children with Diabetes: www.childrenwithdiabetes.com

Down Syndrome: downsyndrome.com

National Down Syndrome Society: www.ndss.org

Spina Bifida Association of America: www.sbaa.org

National Sudden and Unexpected Infant/Child Death and Pregnancy Loss Resource Center: www.sidscenter.org

Influenza Information: www.cdc.gov/flu

SIDS Alliance: www.sidsalliance.org

For Information on Immunizations:

Immunization Action Coalition: www.immunize.org

Centers for Disease Control and Prevention: Vaccines and Immunizations: www.cdc.gov/vaccines

American Academy of Pediatrics Childhood Immunization Support Program: www.cispimmunize.org

American Academy of Family Physicians: Recommendations for Immunizations: www.aafp.org

Vaccine Information: www.vaccineinformation.org

The Children's Hospital of Philadelphia Vaccine Education Center: www.chop.edu

Every Child by Two: www.ecbt.org

National Network for Immunization Information: www.immunizationinfo.org

Drug Information Online: www.drugs.com

10

Minor Office Surgery

LEARNING OBJECTIVES	PROCEDURES

Surgical Asepsis

1. State the characteristics of a minor surgical procedure.
2. Identify procedures that require the use of surgical asepsis.
3. Describe the medical assistant's responsibilities during a minor surgical procedure.
4. List the guidelines to follow to maintain surgical asepsis during a sterile procedure.
5. Identify and explain the use and care of instruments commonly used for minor office surgery.

Apply and remove sterile gloves.
Open a sterile package.
Add an article to a sterile field.
Pour a sterile solution.

Wound Healing

1. Explain the differences between a closed and an open wound, and give examples.
2. List and explain the three phases of the healing process.
3. List and describe the different types of wound drainage.
4. List the functions of a dressing.

Change a sterile dressing.

Sutures

1. Explain the method used to measure the diameter of suturing material.
2. Describe the two types of sutures (absorbable and nonabsorbable), and give examples of their uses.
3. Categorize suturing needles according to type of point and shape.

Remove sutures.
Remove surgical staples.
Apply and remove adhesive skin closures.
Set up a tray for each of the following minor surgical procedures:

- Suture insertion
- Sebaceous cyst removal
- Incision and drainage of a localized infection
- Mole removal
- Needle biopsy
- Ingrown toenail removal
- Colposcopy
- Cervical punch biopsy
- Cryosurgery

Medical Office Surgical Procedures

1. Explain the purpose of and procedure for each of the following minor surgical operations: sebaceous cyst removal, incision and drainage of a localized infection, mole removal, needle biopsy, ingrown toenail removal, colposcopy, cervical punch biopsy, and cryosurgery.
2. Explain the principles underlying each step in the minor office surgery procedures.

Assist the physician with minor office surgery.

LEARNING OBJECTIVES

Bandaging

1. State the functions of a bandage, and list the guidelines for applying a bandage.
2. Identify the common types of bandages used in the medical office.
3. Explain the use of a tubular gauze bandage.

PROCEDURES

Apply each of the following bandage turns:
- Circular
- Spiral
- Spiral-reverse
- Figure-eight
- Recurrent

Apply a tubular gauze bandage.

CHAPTER OUTLINE

KEY TERMS

abrasion (ah-BRAY-shun)
abscess (AB-sess)
absorbable suture (ab-SOR-ba-bul SOO-chur)
approximation (ah-PROKS-ih-MAY-shun)
bandage
biopsy (BYE-op-see)
capillary action (KAP-ill-air-ee AK-shun)
colposcope (KOL-poe-skope)
colposcopy (kol-POS-koe-pee)
contaminate (kon-TAM-in-ate)
contusion (kon-TOO-shun)
cryosurgery (KRY-oh-SURJ-er-ee)
exudate (EKS-oo-date)
fibroblast (FYE-broh-blast)
forceps (FORE-seps)
furuncle (FYOOR-un-kul)
hemostasis (hee-moe-STAY-sis)
incision (in-SIH-shun)
infection (in-FEK-shun)
infiltration (in-fill-TRAY-shun)

inflammation (in-flah-MAY-shun)
laceration (lass-ur-AY-shun)
ligate (LIH-gate)
local anesthetic (LOE-kul an-es-STET-ik)
Mayo (MAY-oe) tray
needle biopsy (NEE-dul BYE-op-see)
nonabsorbable suture (non-ab-SOR-ba-bul SOO-chur)
postoperative (post-OP-er-uh-tiv)
preoperative (pree-OP-er-uh-tiv)
puncture (PUNK-shur)
scalpel (SKAL-pul)
scissors
sebaceous cyst (suh-BAY-shus SIST)
serum (SEER-um)
sterile (STARE-ul)
surgery
surgical asepsis (SUR-jih-kul ay-SEP-sis)
sutures (SOO-churz)
swaged (SWAYJD) needle
wound

Introduction to Minor Office Surgery

The term *surgery* is defined as the branch of medicine that deals with operative and manual procedures for correction of deformities and defects, repair of injuries, and diagnosis and treatment of certain diseases. *Minor office surgery* (also known as minor surgery) refers to a surgical procedure that is restricted to the management of minor conditions and injuries that does not require the use of general anesthesia. Minor surgical procedures have the following characteristics:

- Are performed in an ambulatory health care facility, such as a physician's office or clinic
- Can be performed in a short period of time, usually in less than 1 hour
- Require a local anesthetic, a topical anesthetic, or no anesthetic
- Can be performed safely with a minimum of discomfort to the patient
- Do not, under normal circumstances, pose a major risk to life, or function of an organ or body parts

Various types of minor surgical operations are performed in the medical office, such as insertion of sutures, sebaceous cyst removal, incision and drainage of infections, mole removal, needle biopsies, cervical biopsies, and ingrown toe-

nail removal. The physician explains the nature of the surgical procedure and any risks to the patient and offers to answer questions. The medical assistant is responsible for explaining the patient preparation required for the procedure and for obtaining the patient's signature on a written consent to treatment form, which grants the physician permission to perform the surgery (Figure 10-1).

Additional responsibilities of the medical assistant include preparing the treatment room, preparing the patient, preparing the minor surgery tray, assisting the physician during the procedure, administering postoperative care to the patient, and cleaning the treatment room after the procedure.

The treatment room must be spotlessly clean, and the medical assistant should ensure that the physician has adequate lighting for the procedure. The patient is positioned and draped according to the procedure to be performed. The skin is prepared as specified by the physician. Hair around the operative site is a contaminant and may need to be removed by shaving. The skin is cleansed, and an appropriate antiseptic is applied to the area to reduce the number of microorganisms present.

The medical assistant prepares the minor surgery tray using **sterile** technique. The specific instruments and supplies included in each setup vary, depending on the type of

---

(attach label or complete blanks)

First name: _____   Last name: _____

Date of Birth: _____ Month _____ Day _____ Year

Account Number: _____

Procedure Consent Form

I, _____ , hereby consent to have

Dr. _____ perform _____

I have been fully informed of the following by my physician:

1. The nature of my condition.
2. The nature and purpose of the procedure.
3. An explanation of risks involved with the procedure.
4. Alternative treatments or procedures available.
5. The likely results of the procedure.
6. The risks involved with declining or delaying the procedure.

My physician has offered to answer all questions concerning the proposed procedure.

I am aware that the practice of medicine and surgery is not an exact science, and I acknowledge that no guarantees have been made to me about the results of the procedure.

Patient _____   Date _____
(or guardian and relationship)

Witnessed _____   Date _____

Figure 10-1. Consent to treatment form.

surgery to be performed and the physician's preference. The medical assistant must become familiar with the instruments and supplies required for each surgical procedure performed in the medical office.

During the minor surgery, the medical assistant is present to assist the physician as needed and to lend support to the patient. The medical assistant should become completely familiar with the assisting techniques (e.g., swabbing blood from the operative site) required for each surgical procedure performed in the medical office and should learn to anticipate the physician's needs to help the procedure go quickly and smoothly.

After the minor surgery, the medical assistant should remain with the patient as a safety precaution to prevent accidental falls and other injuries and to make sure the patient understands the postoperative instructions. The medical assistant removes and properly cares for all used instruments and supplies and cleans the treatment room in preparation for the next patient.

SURGICAL ASEPSIS

Surgical asepsis, also known as *sterile technique,* refers to practices that keep objects and areas sterile, or free from all living microorganisms and spores. Surgical asepsis protects the patient from pathogenic microorganisms that may enter the body and cause disease. It is always employed under the following circumstances: when caring for broken skin, such as open wounds and suture punctures; when a skin surface is being penetrated, as by a surgical incision for a mole removal or the administration of an injection (the needle must remain sterile); and when a body cavity is entered that is normally sterile, such as during the insertion of a urinary catheter. Sterility of instruments and supplies is achieved through the use of disposable sterile items or by sterilizing reusable articles.

A sterile object that touches any unsterile object is automatically considered contaminated and must not be used. If the medical assistant is in doubt or has a question concerning the sterility of an article, he or she should consider it contaminated and replace it with a sterile article.

Sterility of the hands cannot be attained. Sanitizing the hands renders them medically aseptic and must be performed before and after every surgical procedure using proper technique (see Chapter 2). To prevent contamination of sterile articles, sterile gloves must be worn while picking up or transferring articles during a sterile procedure. Procedure 10-1 describes the procedure for applying and removing sterile gloves.

Specific guidelines must be observed during a sterile procedure to maintain surgical asepsis. See the accompanying box on *Guidelines for Surgical Asepsis.*

INSTRUMENTS USED IN MINOR OFFICE SURGERY

A variety of surgical instruments are used for minor office surgery. Most instruments are made of stainless steel and have either a bright, highly polished finish or a dull finish. The medical assistant should become familiar with the name, use, and proper care of all instruments used in the medical office. Surgical instruments are named by one or more of the following: (1) function (e.g., splinter forceps); (2) design (e.g., mosquito hemostatic forceps); and (3) the individual who developed the instrument (e.g., Kelly hemostatic forceps). The parts of an instrument are illustrated in Figure 10-2; some common instruments are described here and are illustrated in Figure 10-3.

Scalpels

A **scalpel** is a small straight surgical knife consisting of a handle and a thin, sharp steel blade. A scalpel is used to make surgical incisions and can divide tissue with the least possible

---

Guidelines for Surgical Asepsis

1. Take precautions to prevent sterile packages from becoming wet. Wet packages draw microorganisms into the package owing to the capillary action of the liquid, resulting in contamination of the sterile package. If a sterile package that has been prepared at the medical office becomes wet, it must be rewrapped and resterilized; if a disposable sterile package becomes wet, it must be discarded.

2. A 1-inch border around the sterile field is considered contaminated or unsterile because this area may have become contaminated while the sterile field was being set up.

3. Always face the sterile field. If you must turn your back to it or leave the room, a sterile towel must be placed over the sterile field.

4. Hold all sterile articles above waist level. Anything out of sight might become contaminated. The sterile articles also should be held in front of you and should not touch your uniform.

5. To avoid contamination, place all sterile items in the center, not around the edges, of the sterile field.

6. Be careful not to spill water or solutions on the sterile field. The area beneath the field is contaminated, and microorganisms are drawn up onto the field by the capillary action of the liquid, resulting in contamination of the field.

7. Do not talk, cough, or sneeze over a sterile field. Water vapor from the nose, mouth, and lungs is carried outward by the air and contaminates the sterile field.

8. Do not reach over a sterile field. Dust or lint from your clothing may fall onto it, or your unsterile clothing may accidentally touch it.

9. Do not pass soiled dressings over the sterile field.

10. Always acknowledge if you have contaminated the sterile field so that proper steps can be taken to regain sterility.

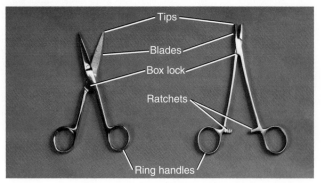

Figure 10-2. Parts of an instrument.

trauma to surrounding structures. Both disposable and reusable scalpels are available. A disposable scalpel consists of a non-slip plastic handle and a permanently attached steel blade that is individually packaged to maintain sterility. Scalpels that are reusable consist of a reusable stainless steel handle to which a disposable steel blade is attached. The blade comes individually packaged in a moisture-proof sterile package.

Scissors

Scissors are cutting instruments that have ring handles and straight (str) or curved (cvd) blades. Both blade tips may be sharp (s/s), both may be blunt (b/b), or one tip may be

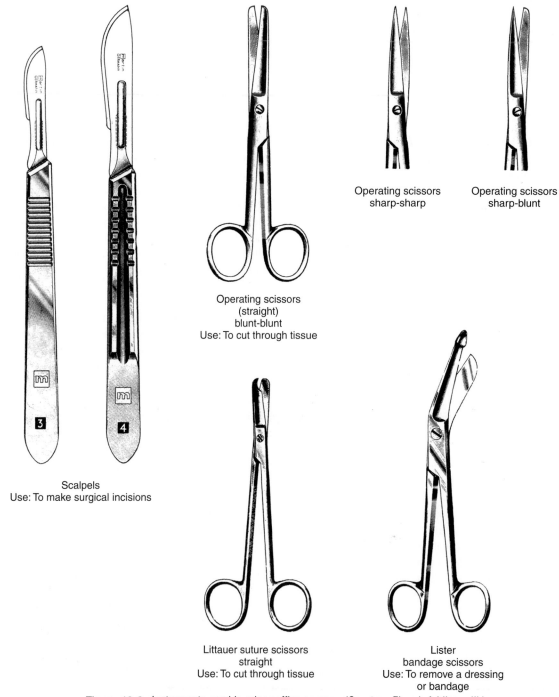

Scalpels
Use: To make surgical incisions

Operating scissors
(straight)
blunt-blunt
Use: To cut through tissue

Operating scissors
sharp-sharp

Operating scissors
sharp-blunt

Littauer suture scissors
straight
Use: To cut through tissue

Lister
bandage scissors
Use: To remove a dressing
or bandage

Figure 10-3. Instruments used in minor office surgery. (Courtesy Elmed, Addison, Ill.)

blunt and the other sharp (b/s). The two parts of a pair of scissors come together at a hinge joint known as a *box lock* (see Figure 10-2). The type of scissors employed depends on the intended use. The various types of scissors are listed and described next.

- *Operating scissors* have straight delicate blades with sharp cutting edges and are used to cut through tissue. They are available with sharp/sharp, blunt/blunt, or blunt/sharp blade tips.

- *Suture scissors* are used to remove sutures. The hook on the tip aids in getting under a suture, and the blunt end prevents puncturing of the tissues.
- *Bandage scissors* are inserted beneath a dressing or bandage to cut it for removal. The flat blunt prow can be inserted beneath a dressing without puncturing the skin.
- *Dissecting scissors* have thick beveled blades with a fine cutting edge used to divide or separate tissue rather than cut it. Dissecting scissors are available with straight or

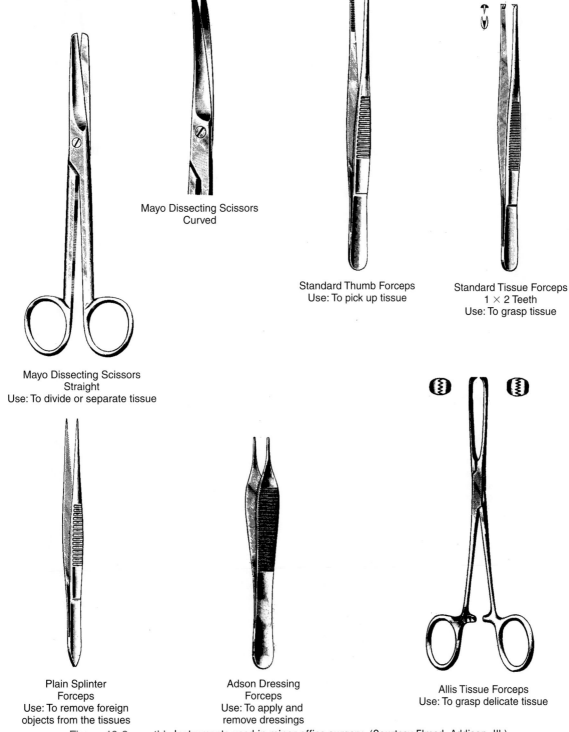

Mayo Dissecting Scissors
Curved

Mayo Dissecting Scissors
Straight
Use: To divide or separate tissue

Standard Thumb Forceps
Use: To pick up tissue

Standard Tissue Forceps
1 × 2 Teeth
Use: To grasp tissue

Plain Splinter
Forceps
Use: To remove foreign
objects from the tissues

Adson Dressing
Forceps
Use: To apply and
remove dressings

Allis Tissue Forceps
Use: To grasp delicate tissue

Figure 10-3, cont'd. Instruments used in minor office surgery. (Courtesy Elmed, Addison, Ill.)

Continued

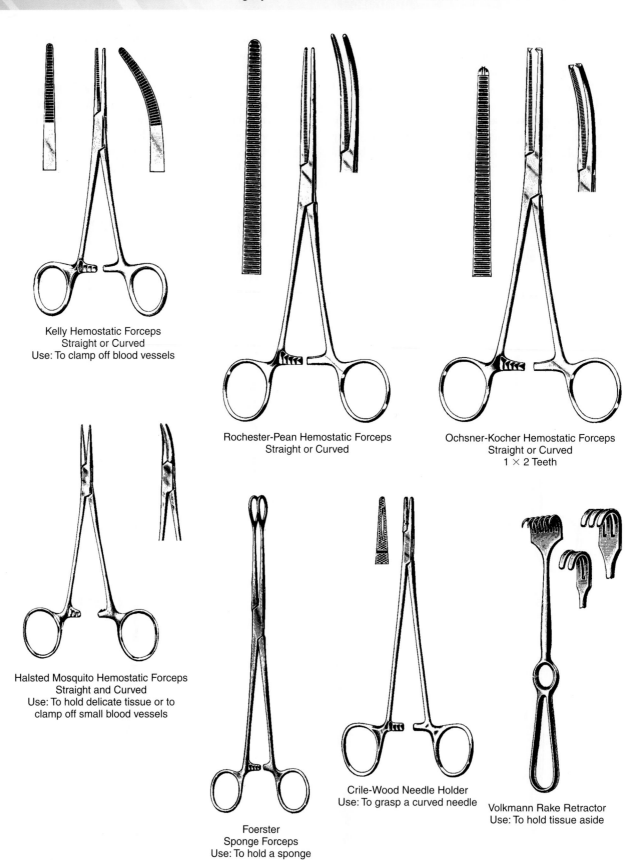

Kelly Hemostatic Forceps
Straight or Curved
Use: To clamp off blood vessels

Rochester-Pean Hemostatic Forceps
Straight or Curved

Ochsner-Kocher Hemostatic Forceps
Straight or Curved
1 × 2 Teeth

Halsted Mosquito Hemostatic Forceps
Straight and Curved
Use: To hold delicate tissue or to
clamp off small blood vessels

Foerster
Sponge Forceps
Use: To hold a sponge

Crile-Wood Needle Holder
Use: To grasp a curved needle

Volkmann Rake Retractor
Use: To hold tissue aside

Figure 10-3, cont'd. Instruments used in minor office surgery. (Courtesy Elmed, Addison, Ill.)

GYNECOLOGIC INSTRUMENTS

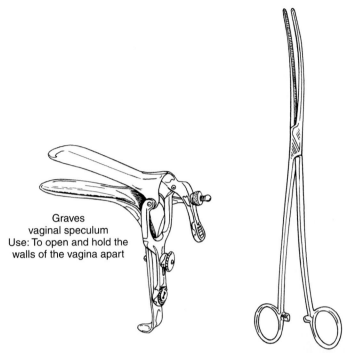

Graves
vaginal speculum
Use: To open and hold the
walls of the vagina apart

Uterine Dressing Forceps
Use: To hold dressings for procedures
involving the vagina, cervix, or uterus

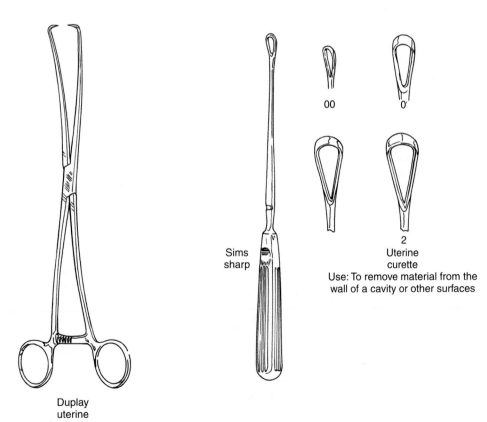

00

0

2
Uterine
curette
Use: To remove material from the
wall of a cavity or other surfaces

Sims
sharp

Duplay
uterine
tenaculum
Use: To grasp and hold the cervix

Figure 10-3, cont'd. Instruments used in minor office surgery. (Courtesy Elmed, Addison, Ill.)

curved blades. Both blade tips of dissecting scissors are blunt.

Forceps

Forceps are instruments for grasping, squeezing, or holding tissue or an item such as sterile gauze. Some forceps have two prongs and a spring handle (e.g., thumb, tissue, splinter, dressing forceps) that provides the proper tension for grasping an object such as tissue, a foreign object, or sterile gauze. Some forceps have serrations (e.g., thumb and hemostatic forceps), which are sawlike teeth that grasp tissue and prevent it from slipping out of the jaws of the instrument. As is shown in Figure 10-3, some varieties have toothed clasps on the handle, known as *ratchets* (see Figure 10-2), to hold the tips securely together and lock them in place (e.g., Allis tissue forceps, hemostatic forceps). The ratchets are designed to allow locked closure of the instrument at two or more positions. The various types of forceps are listed and described next.

- *Thumb forceps* have serrated tips and are used to pick up tissue or to hold tissue between adjacent surfaces.
- *Tissue forceps* have teeth, which are used to grasp tissue and prevent it from slipping. Tissue forceps are identified by the number of apposing teeth on each jaw (e.g., 1×2, 2×3, 3×4). Tissue forceps are sometimes referred to as "rat-toothed" forceps because the pointed projections resemble the teeth of a rat. The teeth should approximate tightly when the instrument is closed.
- *Splinter forceps* have sharp points that are useful in removing foreign objects, such as splinters, from the tissues.
- *Dressing forceps* are used in the application and removal of dressings. They are also used to hold or grasp sterile gauze or sutures during a surgical procedure. Dressing forceps have blunt ends that contain coarse cross-striations used for grasping.
- *Hemostatic forceps* have serrated blades, ratchets, ring handles, and box locks and are available with straight or curved blades. Hemostats are used to clamp off blood vessels and to establish **hemostasis** until the vessels can be closed with sutures. The serrations on a hemostat prevent the blood vessel from slipping out of the jaws of the instrument. The ratchets keep the hemostat tightly shut and locked in place when it is closed. The ring handles allow for a secure grasp of the hemostat and also are used to select the desired ratchet position. The serrated blades should mesh together smoothly when the hemostat is closed; if they spring back open, the instrument is in need of repair. *Mosquito hemostatic forceps* have small, fine tips and are smaller and more delicate than standard Kelly hemostatic forceps. Mosquito hemostatic forceps are used to hold delicate tissue or to clamp off smaller blood vessels, whereas standard hemostatic forceps are used to grasp and compress larger blood vessels.
- *Sponge forceps* have ring handles, ratchets, box locks, and large serrated rings on the blade tips for holding sponges.

A *sponge* is a porous, absorbent pad, such as a 4-inch gauze pad, used to absorb fluids, apply medication, or cleanse an area.

Miscellaneous Instruments

Various miscellaneous instruments used in the medical office are listed and described next.

- *Needle holders* have serrated tips, ring handles, ratchets, and box locks. A needle holder is used to firmly grasp a curved needle for insertion of the needle through the skin flaps of an incision. The serrated tips of a needle holder are designed to hold a curved needle securely without damaging it. A needle holder is sometimes referred to as a "driver" because it functions to "drive" the curved needle through the skin.
- *Retractors* are used to hold tissues aside to improve the exposure of the operative area.

Gynecologic Instruments

Gynecologic surgical procedures are often performed in the medical office; the medical assistant should be familiar with terms related to gynecologic instruments. These are listed and described next.

- A *speculum* is an instrument used to open or distend a body orifice or cavity to permit visual inspection. A vaginal speculum consists of two blades joined at one end, with the lower blade usually a little longer than the upper blade. It is inserted into the vagina and locked into position to open and hold the walls of the vagina apart to allow visual inspection of the vagina and cervix.
- *Uterine dressing forceps* are long slender forceps that have serrated blades, ratchets, and box locks. These forceps are used to hold dressings (such as sterile gauze) for absorbing fluids, applying medication, or cleansing an area of the vagina, cervix, or uterus.
- A *uterine tenaculum* is a hooklike instrument used to grasp and hold the cervix.
- A *curette* is a spoon-shaped instrument used to remove material from the wall of a cavity or other surface.

Care of Surgical Instruments

Surgical instruments are expensive, are delicate yet durable, and last for many years if handled and maintained properly. The care an instrument receives depends to a large degree on the parts making up the instrument (e.g., box lock, ratchet, cutting edge, serrations). The medical assistant works with instruments while setting up a sterile tray, performing certain procedures such as suture removal and sterile dressing change, and cleaning up after minor office surgery and during the sanitization and sterilization process. During each of these procedures, guidelines must be followed to prolong the life span of each instrument and to ensure its proper functioning:

1. Always handle instruments carefully. Dropping an instrument on the floor or throwing an instrument into a basin could damage it.

2. Do not pile instruments in a heap because they become entangled and might be damaged when separated.

3. Keep sharp instruments separate from the rest of the instruments to prevent damaging or dulling the cutting edge. Also, keep delicate instruments, such as lensed instruments, separate to protect them from damage.

4. To prolong the proper functioning of the ratchet, keep instruments with a ratchet in an open position when not in use.

5. Rinse blood and body secretions off an instrument as soon as possible to prevent them from drying and hardening on the instrument.

6. When performing procedures that require surgical instruments, always use the instrument for the purpose for which it was designed. Substituting one type of instrument for another could damage it.

7. Sanitize and sterilize instruments using proper technique.

COMMERCIALLY PREPARED STERILE PACKAGES

Commercially prepared disposable packages are used frequently and may contain one particular article (e.g., sterile dressing) or a complete sterile setup (e.g., one for the removal of sutures). The directions for opening the package are stated on the outside of the package; they should be followed carefully to prevent contamination of the sterile contents. Procedure 10-2 describes opening a sterile package.

One type of commercially prepared package is the peel-apart package (commonly referred to as a *peel-pack*). This type of sterile package has an edge with two flaps that can be pulled apart in the following manner: Grasp each unsterile flap between your bent index finger and extended thumb, and, rolling your hands outward, pull the package apart (Figure 10-4, *A*). The inside of the wrapper and the contents are sterile, and to prevent contamination, they

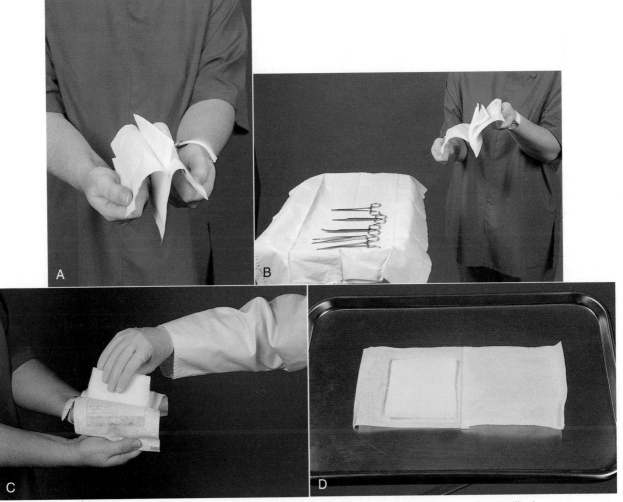

Figure 10-4. Methods for removing the sterile contents of a peel-apart package so that sterility is maintained. **A,** Grasp each flap between a bent index finger and an extended thumb, and roll hands outward to pull apart. **B,** Step back and eject the contents onto the field. **C,** The medical assistant opens the pack, and the physician removes the sterile contents with a gloved hand. **D,** The inside of the peel-apart package can be used as a sterile field.

PROCEDURE 10-1

My Name is Trudy Browning, and I have worked as the office manager of an internal medicine office for the past 7 years. My job includes front and back office duties, including scheduling appointments, transcription, patient calls, patient workups, injections, electrocardiograms, and venipuncture. The most interesting part of my job is dealing with the many different personalities of the patients I come in contact with daily.

A patient who had not been to the clinic for a while came in one day. His graduation from college had been delayed because he had developed a pilonidal cyst that needed to be surgically removed. At onset, these cysts can be very painful and usually require daily cleaning and packing. From my experience with pilonidal cyst care, I knew that 1 to 2 months of treatment are usually required before full recovery is achieved.

The physician and I prepared for the initial treatment and noticed that the surgical site was very large and deep. We knew this treatment would take much longer than usual. Treatment was provided daily for 3 months. Subsequent treatments continued every other day for 2 months. Through our continuous contact, we became good friends with the patient.

Our patient graduated at the end of the spring quarter and moved out of state. He stays in contact with us and is still undergoing treatment. He made a difference in our lives because he always maintained a positive attitude and was very pleasant, making our job easier. We made a difference in his life through the good health care we provided and our continuing friendship. ■

must not be touched with the bare hands. The medical assistant can place the contents of the peel-pack directly on the sterile field by stepping back slightly from the field and gently ejecting or "flipping" the contents onto the center of the sterile field (Figure 10-4, *B*). Stepping back prevents the unsterile outer wrapper and the medical assistant's hands from crossing over the sterile field, which would result in contamination.

The contents of the package also can be removed with a sterile gloved hand. This technique is useful during minor office surgery, when the physician needs additional supplies, such as gauze pads and sutures. The medical assistant opens the sterile package, and the physician removes the sterile contents from the package using a gloved hand (Figure 10-4, *C*). The inside of the package can be used as a sterile field by opening the peel-apart package completely and laying it flat on a clean dry surface (Figure 10-4, *D*).

Once a sterile package has been opened and set up, the medical assistant may need to pour a sterile solution, such as an antiseptic, into a container located on the field. To do so, the steps of surgical asepsis outlined in Procedure 10-3 should be followed.

PROCEDURE 10-1   Applying and Removing Sterile Gloves

Outcome Apply and remove sterile gloves.

The medical assistant must wear sterile gloves to perform a sterile procedure, such as a dressing change, or to assist the physician during minor office surgery. The medical assistant must learn to put on the gloves using the principles of surgical asepsis so as not to contaminate them.

Gloves must be removed in a manner that protects the medical assistant from contaminating the clean hands with pathogens that might be on the outside of the gloves. This is accomplished by not allowing the bare hands to come in contact with the outside of the gloves.

Equipment/Supplies

- Sterile gloves

Applying Sterile Gloves

1. Procedural Step. Remove all rings and put them in a safe place. Wash your hands with an antimicrobial soap.
Principle. Rings may cause the gloves to tear. The warm, moist environment inside gloves provides ideal growing conditions for the multiplication of transient microorganisms on the hands. Washing the hands with an antimicrobial removes these microorganisms and also deposits an antibacterial film on your hands to discourage the growth of bacteria. This prevents the transmission of pathogens.

2. Procedural Step. Choose appropriate-sized gloves; they should not be too small or too large. The gloves should fit snugly but not be too tight.
Principle. If your gloves are too small, they may rip as you apply them or become uncomfortable to wear. If they are too large, you may find it difficult to perform your tasks.

3. Procedural Step. Place the glove package on a clean flat surface. Open the glove package without touching the inside of the wrapper. The tops of the gloves are turned down to form a cuff.

PROCEDURE 10-1   Applying and Removing Sterile Gloves—cont'd

Principle. The hands are not sterile, and the inside of the wrapper is sterile.

4. Procedural Step. Pick up the first glove on the inside of the cuff with the fingers of the opposite hand, being sure not to touch the outside of the glove with your ungloved hand.

Principle. After applying the gloves, the inside of the cuff lies next to your skin and does not remain sterile; therefore it is permissible to pick up the glove by the cuff. The outside of the glove is sterile, and touching it would contaminate it. If a glove becomes contaminated, you must obtain a new pair of gloves and repeat the procedure.

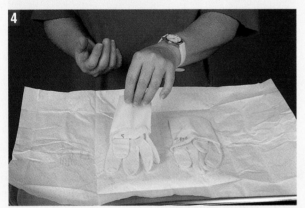

Pick up the first glove on the inside of the cuff.

5. Procedural Step. Step back and pull the glove on. Allow the cuff to remain turned back on itself.

Principle. Stepping back prevents your unsterile hand from passing over the glove still in the glove package, which would contaminate it.

6. Procedural Step. Pick up the second glove by slipping your sterile gloved fingers under its cuff and grasping the opposite side of the cuff with your thumb.

Principle. The cuff is sterile and may be touched by the sterile gloved hand.

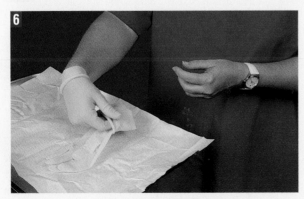

Pick up the second glove.

7. Procedural Step. Remove your thumb from the cuff and pull the glove on. Turn back the cuff.

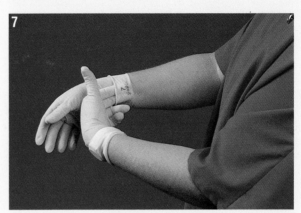

Turn back the cuff.

8. Procedural Step. Turn back the cuff of the first glove by reaching under the cuff with the other gloved hand. Do not allow your sterile gloved hand to come in contact with the inside of the cuff. Adjust the gloves to a comfortable position. Inspect the gloves for tears.

Principle. The area under the folded cuff is sterile and may be touched by the sterile gloved hand. The inside of the cuff has previously been touched by your clean hands and is not sterile. If a tear is present, a new pair of gloves must be applied.

Removing Sterile Gloves

1. Procedural Step. With your gloved left hand, grasp the outside of the right glove 1 to 2 inches from the top. (**NOTE:** It does not matter which glove is removed first—you may start with the left glove if you prefer.)

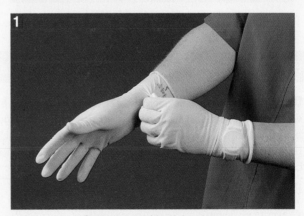

Grasp the outside of the glove.

2. Procedural Step. Slowly pull the right glove off the hand. It turns inside out as it is removed from your hand.

Continued

PROCEDURE 10-1

PROCEDURE 10-2

3. Procedural Step. Pull the right glove free, and scrunch it into a ball with your gloved left hand.

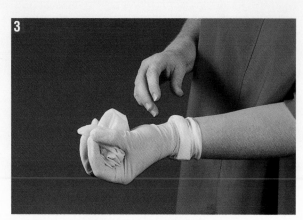

Scrunch the glove into a ball.

4. Procedural Step. Place the index and middle fingers of the right hand on the inside of the left glove. Do not allow your clean hand to touch the outside of the glove.

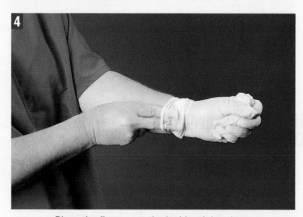

Place the fingers on the inside of the glove.

5. Procedural Step. Pull the second glove off the left hand. It turns inside out as it is removed from your hand, enclosing the balled-up right glove. Discard both gloves in an appropriate waste container. If your gloves are visibly contaminated with blood or other potentially infectious materials, discard them in a biohazard waste container; otherwise, they can be discarded in a regular waste container.

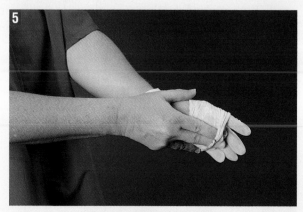

Pull the glove off the hand.

6. Procedural Step. Sanitize your hands thoroughly to remove any microorganisms that may have come in contact with your hands.

---

see DVD

PROCEDURE 10-2   Opening a Sterile Package

Outcome Open a sterile package. A sterile package that has been wrapped after the procedure for wrapping presented in Chapter 3 is opened using the procedure outlined here. The sterile package may be in the form of a commercially prepared disposable package (e.g., sterile dressing change) or a pack that has been assembled and sterilized at the medical office (e.g., sebaceous cyst removal pack); in both cases, the inside of the sterile wrapper serves as the sterile field.

Equipment/Supplies

• Sterile package

1. Procedural Step. Sanitize your hands.
2. Procedural Step. Assemble the equipment.
3. Procedural Step. Check the pack to make sure it is not wet, torn, or opened. These factors cause contamination of the sterile contents and the pack must not

be used. If autoclave tape has been used to close the pack, check to make sure the tape has changed color. **Principle.** Autoclave tape indicates the pack has been through the sterilization process, but it does not verify that the contents of the pack are sterile.

PROCEDURE 10-2   Opening a Sterile Package—cont'd

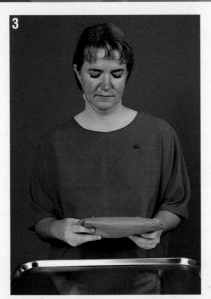

Check the sterilization indicator.

4. Procedural Step. Place the wrapped package on the table so that the top flap of the wrapper opens away from you. Always face the sterile field, and do not talk, laugh, cough, or sneeze over the field. These actions contaminate the sterile field.

5. Procedural Step. Loosen and remove the fastener on the wrapped package, and discard it in a waste container.

6. Procedural Step. Open the first flap away from the body. Handle only the outside of the wrapper.

Principle. The medical assistant should open the sterile package so as not to reach over the sterile contents. Otherwise, dust or lint from unsterile clothing may fall on the contents of the package and cause contamination.

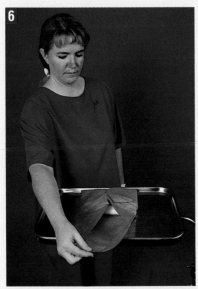

Open the first flap away from the body.

7. Procedural Step. Without crossing over the sterile field, open the left and right flaps.

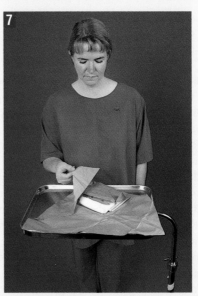

Open the left and right flaps.

8. Procedural Step. Open the flap closest to the body by lifting it toward you. Touch only the outside of the wrapper.

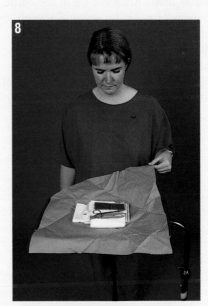

Open the flap closest to the body.

9. Procedural Step. Adjust the sterile wrapper by the corners as needed to make sure it lies in proper position on the tray or table.

10. Procedural Step. Check the sterilization indicator on the inside of the pack to make sure it has changed appropriately. This indicates that the contents of the pack are sterile.

PROCEDURE 10-3   Pouring a Sterile Solution

Outcome Pour a sterile solution.

Equipment/Supplies

- Sterile solution
- Sterile container
- Sterile towel

1. **Procedural Step.** Read the label of the solution to ensure that you have the correct solution.
2. **Procedural Step.** Check the expiration date on the solution. Do not use an outdated solution.
   Principle. Outdated solutions may produce undesirable effects and should be discarded.
3. **Procedural Step.** Check the solution label a second time to make sure you have the correct solution.
4. **Procedural Step.** Place the palm of your hand over the label. Remove the cap by touching only the outside, and place the cap on a flat surface with the open end up. Do not place the cap on the sterile field, as the outside of the cap is contaminated.
   Principle. Palming the label prevents the solution from dripping on the label and obscuring it. Handling the cap by the outside prevents contamination of the inside. Placing the cap with the open end up prevents contamination of the inside of the cap by an unsterile surface.
5. **Procedural Step.** Rinse the lip of the bottle (if it has been previously used) by pouring a small amount of solution into a separate container.
   Principle. Rinsing the lip washes away any microorganisms that may be on it.
6. **Procedural Step.** Pour the proper amount of solution into the sterile container at a height of approximately

6 inches. Do not allow the neck of the bottle to come in contact with the sterile container, and be careful not to splash solution onto the sterile field.
Principle. Pouring from a height of approximately 6 inches reduces splashing and prevents contamination of the sterile container with the outside of the (unsterile) bottle.

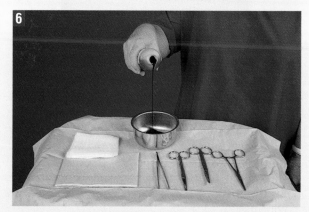

Pour the proper amount of solution.

7. **Procedural Step.** Replace the cap on the container without contaminating it. Check the label a third time to ensure that you have poured the correct solution.

WOUNDS

A **wound** is a break in the continuity of an external or internal surface caused by physical means. Wounds can be accidental or intentional (as when the physician makes an incision during a surgical operation). There are two basic types of wounds: closed and open.

A *closed wound* involves an injury to the underlying tissues of the body without a break in the skin surface or mucous membrane; an example is a contusion, or bruise. A **contusion** results when the tissues under the skin are injured and is often caused by a blunt object. Blood vessels rupture, allowing blood to seep into the tissues, which results in a bluish discoloration of the skin. After several days, the color of the contusion turns greenish yellow as a result of oxidation of blood pigments. Bruising commonly occurs with injuries such as fractures, sprains, strains, and black eyes. *Open wounds* involve a break in the skin surface or mucous membrane that exposes the underlying tissues; ex-

amples include incisions, lacerations, punctures, and abrasions. Figure 10-5 illustrates specific wounds.
- An **incision** is a clean, smooth cut caused by a sharp instrument, such as a knife, razor, or piece of glass. Deep incisions are accompanied by profuse bleeding; in addition, damage to muscles, tendons, and nerves may occur.
- A **laceration** is a wound in which the tissues are torn apart, rather than cut, leaving ragged and irregular edges. Lacerations are caused by dull knives, large objects that have been driven into the skin, and heavy machinery. Deep lacerations result in profuse bleeding, and a scar often results from the jagged tearing of the tissues.
- A **puncture** is a wound made by a sharp-pointed object piercing the skin layers, for example, a nail, splinter, needle, wire, knife, bullet, or animal bite. A puncture wound has a very small external skin opening, and for this reason bleeding is usually minor. A tetanus booster may be administered with this type of wound because

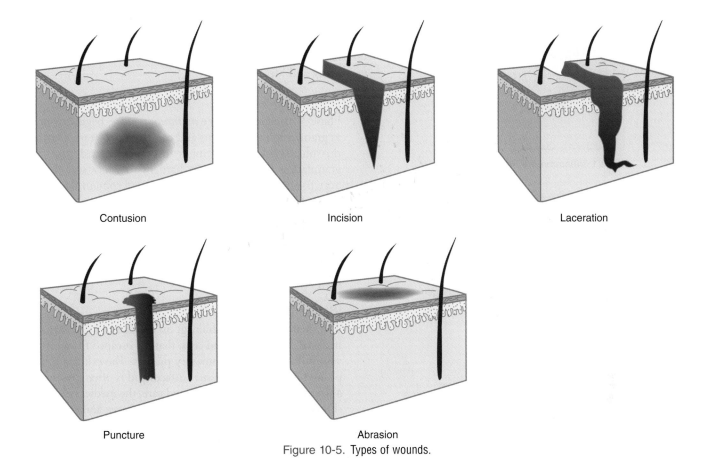

Contusion   Incision   Laceration

Puncture   Abrasion

Figure 10-5. Types of wounds.

the tetanus bacteria grow best in a warm anaerobic environment, such as the one in a puncture.

- An **abrasion** or scrape is a wound in which the outer layers of the skin are scraped or rubbed off, resulting in oozing of blood from ruptured capillaries. Abrasions are often caused by falling on gravel and floors (floor burn). These falls can result in skinned knees and elbows.

Wound Healing

The skin is a protective barrier for the body and is considered its first line of defense. When the surface of the skin has been broken, it is easy for microorganisms to enter and cause **infection.** The body has a natural healing process that works to destroy invading microorganisms and to restore the structure and function of damaged tissues, as is described next.

Phases of Wound Healing

Wound healing occurs in three phases, which are described here and illustrated in Figure 10-6.

Phase 1

Phase 1, also called the *inflammatory phase,* begins as soon as the body is injured. This phase lasts approximately 3 to 4 days. During this phase, a fibrin network forms, resulting

---

PATIENT TEACHING Wound Care

Explain the following to the patient regarding wounds:
- The type of wound that the patient has: incision, laceration, puncture, or abrasion.
- The purpose of suturing the wound: to close the skin and protect against further contamination, to facilitate healing, and to leave a smaller scar.
- If a tetanus toxoid has been administered, explain the purpose of this immunization: to protect against tetanus (lockjaw).
- Teach the patient how to care for the wound, as follows:
  - Keep the dressing clean and dry. If it becomes wet, contact the medical office to schedule a sterile dressing change.
  - Apply an ice bag for swelling (if prescribed by the physician).

- Report immediately any signs that the wound is infected. These signs include the following:
  a. Fever
  b. Persistent or increased pain, swelling, or drainage
  c. Red streaks radiating away from the wound
  d. Increased redness or warmth
- Notify the office if the sutures become loose or break.
- Return as instructed by the physician for the removal of sutures.
- Teach the patient how to apply an ice bag (if prescribed by the physician).
- Give the patient written instructions on wound care to refer to at home.

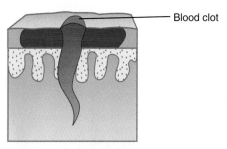

Phase 1: Inflammatory Phase

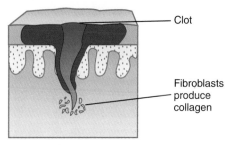

Phase 2: Granulation Phase

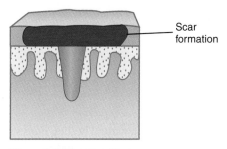

Phase 3: Maturation Phase
Figure 10-6. Phases of wound healing.

in a blood clot that "plugs" up the opening of the wound and stops the flow of blood. The blood clot eventually becomes the scab. The inflammatory process also occurs during this phase. **Inflammation** is the protective response of the body to trauma, such as cuts and abrasions, and to the entrance of foreign matter, such as microorganisms. During inflammation, the blood supply to the wound increases, which brings white blood cells and nutrients to the site to assist in the healing process. The four local signs of inflammation are redness, swelling, pain, and warmth. The purpose of inflammation is to destroy invading microorganisms and to remove damaged tissue debris from the area so that proper healing can occur.

Phase 2

Phase 2 is also called the *granulation phase* and typically lasts 4 to 20 days. During this phase, **fibroblasts** migrate to the wound and begin to synthesize collagen. Collagen is a white protein that provides strength to the wound. As the amount of collagen increases, the wound becomes stronger, and the chance that the wound will open decreases. There also is a growth of new capillaries during this phase to provide the damaged tissue with an abundant supply of blood. As the

capillary network develops, the tissue becomes a translucent red color. This tissue is known as *granulation tissue.* Granulation tissue consists primarily of collagen and is fragile and shiny and bleeds easily.

Phase 3

Phase 3, also known as the *maturation phase,* begins as soon as granulation tissue forms and can last for 2 years. During this phase, collagen continues to be synthesized, and the granulation tissue eventually hardens to white scar tissue. Scar tissue is not true skin and does not contain nerves or have a blood supply.

The medical assistant should always inspect the wound when providing wound care. The wound should be observed for signs of inflammation and the amount of healing that has occurred. This information should be charted in the patient's record.

Wound Drainage

The medical term for drainage is **exudate**. An exudate is material, such as fluid and cells, that has escaped from blood vessels during the inflammatory process. The exudate is deposited in tissue or on tissue surfaces and is often present in a wound. When providing wound care, the medical assistant should always inspect the wound for drainage and chart this information in the patient's record. There are three major types of exudates: serous, sanguineous, and purulent.

- Serous exudate. A serous exudate consists chiefly of **serum,** which is the clear portion of the blood. Serous drainage is clear and watery. An example of a serous exudate is the fluid in a blister from a burn.
- Sanguineous exudate. A sanguineous exudate is red and consists of red blood cells. This type of drainage results when capillaries are damaged, allowing the escape of red blood cells, and is frequently seen in open wounds. A bright-red sanguineous exudate indicates fresh bleeding, and a dark exudate indicates older bleeding.
- Purulent exudate. A purulent exudate contains pus, which consists of leukocytes, dead liquefied tissue debris, and dead and living bacteria. Purulent drainage is usually thick and has an unpleasant odor. It is white in color, but may acquire tinges of pink, green, or yellow depending on the type of infecting organism. The process of pus formation is *suppuration.*

In addition to the exudates just described, mixed types of exudates are often observed in a wound. A *serosanguineous exudate* consists of clear and blood-tinged drainage and is commonly seen in surgical incisions. A *purosanguineous exudate* consists of pus and blood and is often seen in a new wound that is infected.

STERILE DRESSING CHANGE

Surgical asepsis must be maintained when one is caring for and applying a dry sterile dressing (abbreviated as *DSD*) to an open wound. The medical assistant must take care to prevent infection in clean wounds and to decrease infection in wounds already infected. The function of a sterile dressing is to protect the wound from contamination and trauma, to absorb drainage, and to restrict motion, which may interfere with proper wound healing. The size, type, and amount of dressing material used during a sterile dressing change depend on the size and location of the wound and the amount of drainage.

Sterile folded *gauze pads* are used in the medical office for a sterile dressing change. This type of dressing absorbs drainage, but the gauze has a tendency to stick to the wound when the drainage dries. Gauze pads come in a variety of sizes, including 4 × 4, 3 × 3, and 2 × 2; the 4 × 4 size is used most frequently.

Nonadherent pads also are used as a sterile dressing; they have one surface impregnated with agents that prevent the dressing from sticking to the wound. One brand of this type of material is Telfa pads. The nonadherent side, which is shiny, is placed next to the wound. Telfa dressings are often used to cover burned skin. Procedure 10-4 presents the procedure for changing a sterile dressing.

PROCEDURE 10-4 Changing a Sterile Dressing

Outcome Change a sterile dressing.

Equipment/Supplies

- Mayo stand
- Biohazard waste container

Side Table

- Clean disposable gloves
- Antiseptic swabs
- Sterile gloves
- Plastic waste bag
- Surgical tape
- Scissors

Sterile Field

- Sterile dressing
- Sterile thumb forceps

1. **Procedural Step.** Wash your hands with an antimicrobial soap.
2. **Procedural Step.** Assemble the equipment. Set up the nonsterile items on a side table or counter. Position the waterproof waste bag in a location convenient for disposal of contaminated items.

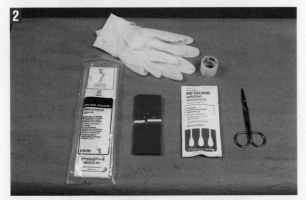

Prepare the side table.

3. **Procedural Step.** Greet the patient and introduce yourself. Identify the patient by full name and date of birth and explain the procedure. Instruct the patient not to move during the procedure. Adjust the light so that it is focused on the dressing.

4. **Procedural Step.** Apply clean gloves. Loosen the tape on the dressing, and pull it toward the wound. Carefully and gently remove the soiled dressing by pulling it upward. Do not touch the inside of the dressing that was next to the open wound. If the dressing is stuck to the wound, it can be loosened by moistening it with a normal saline solution. Place the soiled dressing in the waste bag without allowing the dressing to touch the outside of the bag.

   Principle. Gentle dressing removal avoids unnecessary stress on the wound. Touching the inside of the dressing can transfer an infected discharge to your gloves.

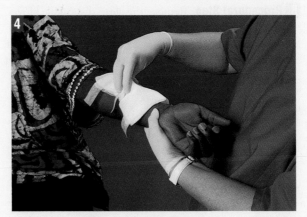

Remove the soiled dressing.

5. **Procedural Step.** Inspect the wound, and observe for the following: amount of healing; presence of inflammation; and presence of drainage, including the amount (scant, moderate, or profuse) and type of drainage.

Continued

PROCEDURE 10-4   Changing a Sterile Dressing—cont'd

Principle. Drainage is classified as serous (containing serum), sanguineous (red and composed of blood), serosanguineous (containing serum and blood), or purulent (containing pus and appearing white with tinges of yellow, pink, or green, depending on the type of infecting microorganism). Purulent drainage is usually thick and has an unpleasant odor.

6. Procedural Step. Open the pouch containing the sterile antiseptic swabs, and place it in a convenient location or hold it in your nondominant hand.

7. Procedural Step. Using the antiseptic swabs, apply the antiseptic to the wound. Apply the antiseptic from the top to the bottom of the wound, working from the center to the outside of the wound. Use a new swab for each motion. Discard each contaminated swab in the waste bag after use.

Principle. The purpose of the antiseptic is to decrease the number of microorganisms in the wound.

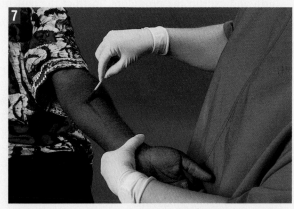

Apply an antiseptic to the wound.

8. Procedural Step. Remove the clean disposable gloves, and discard them in the waste bag without contaminating yourself. Sanitize your hands and prepare the sterile field using surgical asepsis. Items are either

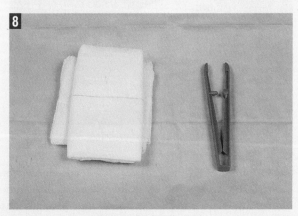

Prepare the sterile field.

placed onto a sterile field or are contained in a pre-packaged setup. Instruct the patient not to talk, laugh, sneeze, or cough over the sterile field.

Principle. Microorganisms are carried in water vapor from the mouth, nose, and lungs, and can be transferred onto the sterile field.

9. Procedural Step. Open a package of sterile gloves, and apply them.

10. Procedural Step. Pick up the sterile dressing with your gloved hand or sterile forceps. Place the sterile dressing over the wound by lightly dropping it in place. Do not move the dressing once you have dropped it into place. Discard the gloves or forceps in the waste bag.

Principle. Dropping the dressing over the wound and not moving it prevent the transfer of microorganisms from the skin to the center of the wound.

11. Procedural Step. Apply hypoallergenic adhesive tape to hold the dressing in place. The tape must be long enough to adhere to the skin, but not so long that it loosens when the patient moves. The strips of tape should be evenly spaced, with strips at each end of the dressing.

12. Procedural Step. Instruct the patient in wound care as follows:

a. Provide the patient with written wound care instructions (see the patient teaching box on wound care in this chapter).

b. Explain the wound care instructions, and ask the patient whether he or she has any questions. Tell the patient to keep the wound clean and dry and to contact the office if signs of infection occur such as excessive swelling, pain, or discharge.

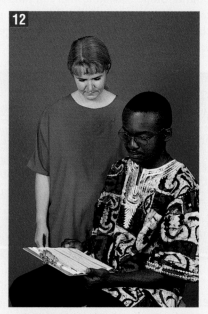

Instruct the patient in wound care.

PROCEDURE 10-4

PROCEDURE 10-4 Changing a Sterile Dressing—cont'd

c. Ask the patient to sign the instruction sheet on the appropriate line.

d. Witness the patient's signature by signing your name in the appropriate space on the form. Include today's date.

e. Before the patient leaves the medical office, make a copy of the instruction sheet. Give a signed copy of the wound care instructions to the patient, and file the original in the patient's medical record.

Principle. The filed copy protects the physician legally in the event that the patient fails to follow the instructions and causes further harm or damage to the wound.

13. **Procedural Step.** Return the equipment. Tightly secure the bag containing the soiled dressing and contaminated articles, and dispose of it in a biohazard waste container.

Principle. Contaminated items must be disposed of properly to prevent the spread of infection.

14. **Procedural Step.** Sanitize your hands.

15. **Procedural Step.** Chart the procedure. Include the date and time, location of the dressing, condition of the wound, type and amount of drainage, care of the wound, and any problems the patient experienced with the wound. Also chart the instructions given to the patient on wound care.

CHARTING EXAMPLE

Date	
9/20/12	10:30 a.m. Dressing changed Ⓛ ant forearm.
	Scant amt of serous drainage noted. Sl redness
	around incision line. Sutures intact and suture
	line in good approximation. Incision cleaned
	Betadine c̄ and DSD applied. No complaints of
	pain or discomfort. Explained wound care.
	Written instructions provided. Signed copy filed
	in chart. To return in 2 days for suture
	removal. ————— T. Browning, CMA (AAMA)

SUTURES

Insertion and removal of **sutures** are commonly performed in the medical office. Sutures may be required to close a surgical incision or to repair an accidental wound. They **approximate**, or bring together, the edges of the wound with surgical stitches and hold them in place until enough healing has taken place so that the wound can withstand ordinary stress and no longer needs support from the sutures. Sutures also protect the wound from further contamination and minimize the amount of scar formation. A **local anesthetic** is necessary to numb the area before the sutures are inserted.

Types of Sutures

Sutures are available in two types: absorbable and nonabsorbable. **Absorbable sutures** are made of a material that is gradually digested and absorbed by the body in a relatively short period of time. The amount of time can range from 7 days to several months, depending on the type of tissue being sutured and the size and type of absorbable suture being used.

Absorbable sutures consist of surgical gut (Surgigut) or synthetic materials, such as polyglycolic acid (Dexon), polyglactin 910 (Vicryl), polydioxanone (PDS II), polyglyconate (Maxon), and poliglecaprone (Monocryl), lactomer

Memories *from* Externship

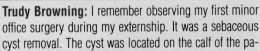

Trudy Browning: I remember observing my first minor office surgery during my externship. It was a sebaceous cyst removal. The cyst was located on the calf of the patient's left leg. I helped in setting up the surgical tray and prepared and draped the site. I tried to explain to the patient what was going to occur to prepare her for the procedure. I think the patient was calmer than I was. The physician entered the room with a medical assistant on hand. Although I was in the room primarily to observe, I helped the physician with his surgical gloves and in numbing the site. I watched the physician make the incision and cut out and remove a large cyst.

Everything was going smoothly until the physician started to suture the wound. I felt like someone had turned the heat up really high; the room seemed to get really hot. I started to feel dizzy. I smiled at the physician and excused myself. He just smiled back at me, and I left the room. I went outside the room and caught my breath. I regained my composure and reentered the room. The physician was still suturing the wound. As I watched him run the needle through the skin and pull the suture tight, it really got to me. I smiled and told the physician that I would wait outside until they were done. After the physician left the room, I went back to help clean up. I felt so stupid. Later that day, the physician looked at me and said: "Got a little warm in there, didn't it?" He just laughed and said that what I did was normal and not to worry about it. He made me feel better about myself. After that incident, I went in alone and helped him with cyst removals, and it didn't bother me at all. ∎

(Polysorb) and Caprosyn (Figure 10-7, *A*). Surgical gut is made from sheep or cow intestine. This type of suturing material is gradually digested by tissue enzymes and is absorbed by the body's tissues 7 to 21 days after insertion, depending on the kind of surgical gut employed. *Plain surgical gut* has a rapid absorption time, whereas *chromic surgical gut* is treated to slow down its rate of absorption in the tissues. Absorbable sutures frequently are used to suture subcutaneous tissue, fascia, intestines, bladder, and peritoneum, and to **ligate,** or tie off, vessels. Because suturing of this type of tissue is generally done during surgery performed by the physician in the hospital with the patient under a general anesthetic, the medical office may not stock absorbable suture material.

Nonabsorbable sutures (Figure 10-7, *B*) are not absorbed by the body and may remain permanently in the body tissues and become encapsulated by fibrous tissue or may be removed (e.g., skin sutures). Nonabsorbable sutures are used to suture skin; this type of suture is used frequently in the medical office. Nonabsorbable sutures are made from materials that are not affected by tissue enzymes. These materials include silk (Sofsilk), nylon (Ethilon), polyester (Ti-Cron, Surgidac), polypropylene (Prolene, Surgipro), polybutester (Novafil and Vascufil), stainless steel, and surgical skin staples.

Suture Size and Packaging

Sutures are measured by their gauge, which refers to the diameter of the suturing material. The sizes range from numbers below 0 (pronounced "aught") to numbers above 0. The diameter of the suture material increases with each number above 0 and decreases with each number below 0. If the size of a particular suture material ranges from 7-0 to 5, available sizes include 7-0, 6-0, 5-0, 4-0, 3-0, 2-0, 0, 1, 2, 3, 4, and 5. Size 7-0 are very fine sutures, and size 5 are very heavy sutures. Size 2-0 (00) sutures have a smaller diameter than size 0 sutures.

Nonabsorbable sutures with a smaller gauge (5-0 to 6-0) are used for suturing incisions in delicate tissue, such as the face and neck, whereas nonabsorbable heavy sutures are used for firmer tissue, such as the chest and abdomen. Finer sutures leave less scar formation and are used when cosmetic results are desired.

Sutures come in a box of individually packaged sutures (Figure 10-8, *A*). The box of sutures is stamped with an expiration date that must be checked each time a suture package is removed from the box. Each individual suture package consists of an outer peel-apart envelope and a sterile inner packet (Figure 10-8, *B*). Packages are labeled according to the type of suture material (e.g., surgical silk),

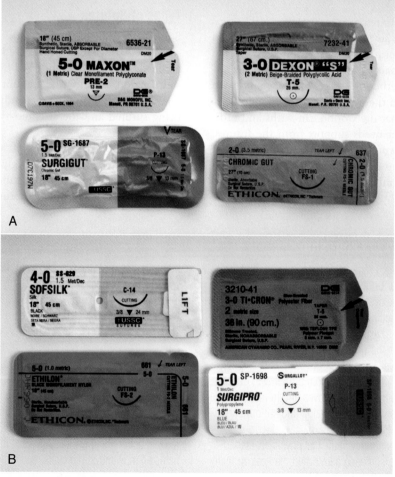

Figure 10-7. Swaged suture packets. **A,** Absorbable sutures. **B,** Nonabsorbable sutures.

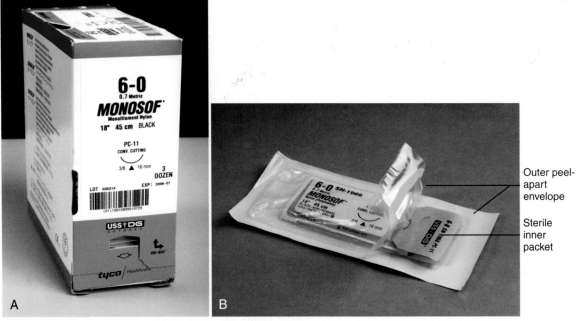

Figure 10-8. **A,** Sutures come in a box of individually packaged sutures. **B,** Each individual suture package consists of an outer peel-apart envelope and a sterile inner packet.

the size (e.g., 4-0), the length of the suturing material (e.g., 18 inches), the date of manufacture, and the expiration date of the suture. The type and size of material used are based on the nature and location of the tissue being sutured and the physician's preference. To repair a laceration of the arm, the physician might use a 4-0 surgical silk suture. The physician informs the medical assistant of the type and size of sutures needed.

Suture Needles

Needles used for suturing are made from stainless steel alloys and are categorized according to their type of point and their shape. A needle with a sharp point is a *cutting needle,* and one with a round point is a *noncutting needle.* Cutting needles (Figure 10-9, *A*) are used for firm tissues such as skin; the sharp point helps push the needle through the tissue. Noncutting or blunt needles are used to penetrate tissues that offer a small amount of resistance, such as the fascia, intestine, liver, spleen, kidneys, subcutaneous tissue, and muscle.

A suture needle may be curved or straight (see Figure 10-9, *A*). *Curved needles* permit the physician to dip in and out of the tissue. A needle holder must be used with a curved needle. A *straight needle* is used when the tissue can be displaced sufficiently to permit the needle to be pushed and pulled through the tissue. Straight needles do not require the use of a needle holder.

Some needles have an eye through which the suture material is inserted; however, most needles are **swaged** (Figure 10-9, *B*). *Swaged* means that the suture and needle are one continuous unit; the needle is permanently attached to the end of the suture. Swaged needles are used frequently because they offer several advantages over eyed needles. One advantage is that the suture material does not slip off the

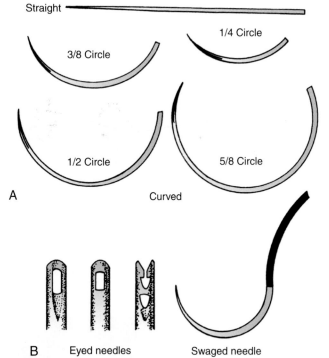

Figure 10-9. Common suture needles. **A,** Needles with a cutting point. **B,** Eyed needles and a swaged needle. (**A** modified from Perspectives on sutures, courtesy Davis & Geck, Danbury, Conn; **B** modified from Nealon TF Jr: Fundamental skills in surgery, ed 4, Philadelphia, 1994, Saunders.)

needle, as might occur with suture material threaded through the eye of a needle. Another advantage is that tissue trauma is reduced because a swaged needle has only a single strand of suture that must be pulled through the tissue compared with a double strand in an eyed needle. The swaged needle can be pulled through the tissue with less resulting trauma. Swaged suture packets are labeled to specify the gauge, type, and length of suture material, the type of needle point (cutting or noncutting), and the needle shape (curved or straight) (see Figure 10-7).

Insertion of Sutures

The medical assistant may be responsible for preparing the suture tray and for assisting the physician during the insertion of the sutures. The physician designates the size and type of suture material and needle required. Because sutures, needles, and suture-needle combinations (swaged needles) are contained in peel-apart packages, they can be added to the sterile field by flipping them onto the sterile field or by placing them there with a sterile gloved hand (Figure 10-10).

Suture Insertion Setup

The items required for a suture insertion setup are listed next.

Items Placed to the Side of the Sterile Field
- Clean disposable gloves
- Antiseptic solution
- Surgical scrub brush

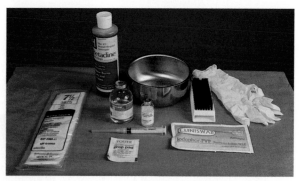

Suture insertion side table.

- Antiseptic swabs
- Sterile gloves
- Local anesthetic
- Antiseptic wipe to cleanse the vial
- Tetanus toxoid with needle and syringe

Items Included on the Sterile Field
- Fenestrated drape
- Syringe and needle for drawing up the local anesthetic
- Hemostatic forceps
- Thumb forceps

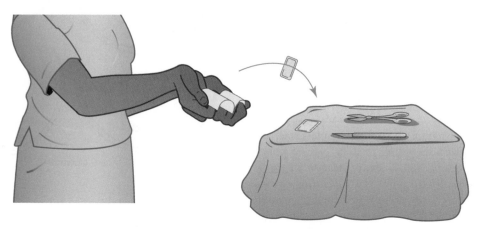

Flipping sutures onto the sterile field.

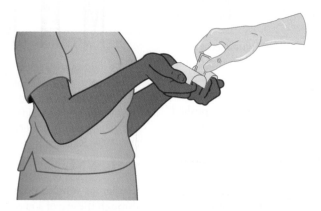

The physician removing the sutures with a sterile gloved hand.
Figure 10-10. Adding sutures to a sterile field.

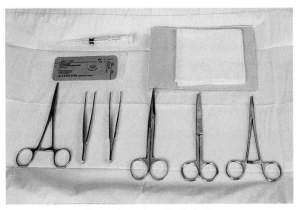

Suture insertion sterile field.

Case Study 1

Kerry Ventura brings her 6-year-old son Cory to the medical office. Cory got a new bike for his birthday and just learned how to ride it without training wheels. While going around a corner, he lost his balance and fell and cut his left knee. The incision is about 1½ inches long. Cory is going to need sutures to approximate the wound. Mrs. Ventura is very upset and blames herself. She says that she should have been watching him more closely. Mrs. Ventura wants to know why Steri-Strips can't be used to close the incision. She says that it would be a lot less painful for Cory than having stitches. When asked to sign the consent to treatment form for Cory, Mrs. Ventura says she does not want to sign the form until her husband has a chance to read it. She says that right now he is in Japan for 2 weeks on a business trip. ■

- Tissue forceps
- Dissecting scissors
- Operating scissors
- Needle holder
- Suture
- Sterile 4 × 4 gauze

Procedure: Suture Insertion

Sutures are inserted as follows:

1. A local anesthetic is used to numb the area.
2. The physician inserts sutures to close a surgical incision or to repair an accidental wound.
3. A sterile dressing may be applied to the operative site.

Postoperative Instructions: Suture Insertion

Postoperative instructions include the following:

1. Keep the dressing clean and dry.
2. Contact the medical office if any signs of infection occur at the incision site, including excessive redness, swelling, discharge, or an increase in pain.
3. Notify the medical office if the sutures become loose or break.

Provide the patient with written instructions on wound care to refer to at home, and instruct the patient when to return for removal of the sutures.

Suture Removal

When the wound has healed such that it no longer needs the support of nonabsorbable suture material, the sutures must be removed. The length of time the sutures remain in place depends on their location and the amount of healing that must occur. Some areas of the body, such as the head and neck, have a good blood supply; the sutures do not need to remain there as long as they do in other areas because this area heals more rapidly.

Sutures must always be left in place long enough for proper healing to occur. The physician determines the length of time, but in general, skin sutures inserted in the face and neck are removed in 3 to 5 days, and sutures in-

serted in other areas, such as the skin of the chest, arms, legs, hands, and feet, are removed in 7 to 14 days.

Surgical Skin Staples

Surgical skin staples are often used to close wounds. Stapling is the fastest method of closure of long skin incisions. In addition, trauma to the tissue is reduced because the tissue does not have to be handled much when the staples are inserted. Surgical staples are stainless steel and are inserted into the skin using a special skin stapler. Skin staplers are available as reusable or disposable devices. The skin stapler holds a cartridge that contains a prescribed number and size of staples (Figure 10-11).

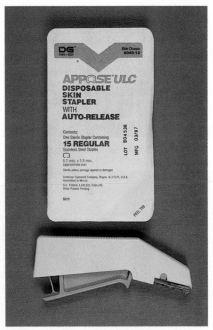

Figure 10-11. Disposable skin stapler.

The physician inserts the staples by gently approximating the tissues with tissue forceps. The skin stapler is held over the site, and the staple is inserted into the skin. Skin stapling produces excellent cosmetic results, and the staples are easy to remove with a specially designed staple remover.

The medical assistant is frequently responsible for removing sutures and staples. This procedure should be done only after the physician has given a written or verbal order to the medical assistant. Procedure 10-5 presents the method used to remove sutures and skin staples.

PROCEDURE 10-5   Removing Sutures and Staples

Outcome Remove sutures and staples.

Equipment/Supplies

- Antiseptic swabs
- Clean disposable gloves
- Sterile 4 × 4 gauze

- Surgical tape
- Mayo stand
- Biohazard waste container

For Suture Removal

- Suture removal kit, which includes the following:
  - Suture scissors
  - Thumb forceps
  - Sterile 4 × 4 gauze

For Staple Removal

- Staple removal kit, which includes:
  - Staple remover
  - Sterile 4 × 4 gauze

1. **Procedural Step.** Wash your hands with an antimicrobial soap. Assemble the equipment.

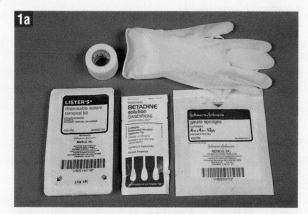

Suture removal setup.

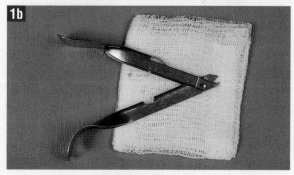

Staple removal setup.

Principle. Washing the hands with an antimicrobial soap removes microorganisms from the hands and also deposits an antimicrobial film on your hands to discourage the growth of bacteria.

2. **Procedural Step.** Greet the patient and introduce yourself. Identify the patient by full name and date of birth and explain the procedure.

3. **Procedural Step.** Position the patient as required to provide good access to the site. Adjust the light so that it is focused on the wound. Verify that the sutures (or staples) are intact and that the incision line is approximated and not gaping. Check that the incision line is not infected. If the incision line is not approximated, or if redness, swelling, or a discharge is present, do not remove the sutures; notify the physician.

Principle. The sutures (or staples) should not be removed unless the incision line is approximated and free from infection.

4. **Procedural Step.** Open the suture or staple removal kit, keeping the contents of the kit sterile. Most kits are opened by peeling back a top cover, which exposes a plastic tray that holds the necessary instruments and supplies.

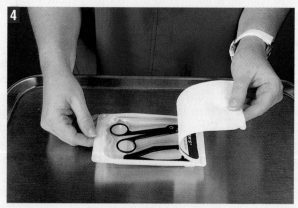

Open the suture removal kit.

PROCEDURE 10-5   Removing Sutures and Staples—cont'd

5. Procedural Step. Apply clean gloves. Cleanse the incision line with an antiseptic swab to destroy microorganisms and to remove any dried exudate encrusted around the sutures or staples. Clean the wound from the top to the bottom, working from the center to the outside of the wound. Use a new swab for each cleansing motion. Allow the skin to dry.

Principle. Dried exudate must be removed to allow unimpeded removal of the sutures or staples.

6. Procedural Step. Remove the sutures or staples. Tell the patient that he or she will feel a pulling or tugging sensation as each suture (or staple) is removed, but that it will not be painful. Count the number of sutures or staples removed. Check the patient's chart to make sure the same number is removed as was inserted by the physician.

To remove sutures:

a. Using the sterile thumb forceps provided in the kit, pick up the knot of the first suture.

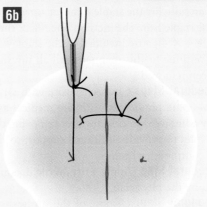

Gently pull the suture out. (Modified from Nealon TF Jr: Fundamental skills in surgery, ed 4, Philadelphia, 1994, Saunders.)

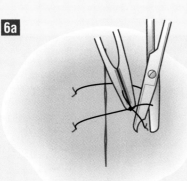

Cut the suture below the knot on the side closest to the skin. (Modified from Nealon TF Jr: Fundamental skills in surgery, ed 4, Philadelphia, 1994, Saunders.)

b. Place the curved tip of the suture scissors under the suture. Using the sterile suture scissors, cut the suture below the knot on the side of the suture closest to the skin. Cut the suture as close to the skin as possible.

c. Using a smooth, continuous motion, gently pull the suture out of the skin. Remove the suture without allowing any portion that was previously outside to be pulled back through the tissue lying beneath the incision line. Place the suture on the 4 × 4 gauze included in the suture kit.

d. Continue in this manner until all the sutures have been removed.

Principle. To prevent infection, the suture must be removed without pulling any portion that has been outside the skin back through the tissue lying beneath the incision line.

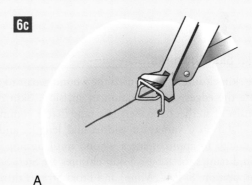

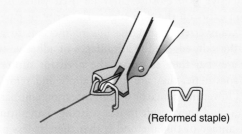

A, Place the bottom jaws of the staple remover under the staple. **B,** Firmly squeeze the staple handles until they are fully closed. (Courtesy Ethicon, Somerville, NJ.)

To remove staples:

a. Gently place the bottom jaws of the staple remover under the staple to be removed.

b. Firmly squeeze the staple handles until they are fully closed.

Continued

PROCEDURE 10-5   Removing Sutures and Staples—cont'd

c. Carefully lift the staple remover upward to remove the staple from the incision line. Place the staple on the 4 × 4 gauze included in the staple kit.

d. Continue in this manner until all the staples have been removed.

7. **Procedural Step.** Cleanse the site with an antiseptic swab. Some physicians want the medical assistant to apply adhesive skin closures after removing the sutures or staples to provide additional support to the wound as it continues to heal.

8. **Procedural Step.** Apply a dry sterile dressing if indicated by the physician.

9. **Procedural Step.** Dispose of the sutures (or staples) and the gauze in a biohazard waste container.

10. **Procedural Step.** Remove the gloves, and sanitize your hands.

11. **Procedural Step.** Chart the procedure. Include the date and time, the status of the sutures (or staples) and incision line, the number of sutures (or staples) removed, the location of the site, care of the wound (i.e., application of an antiseptic or dressing), and the patient's reaction. Chart any instructions given to the patient.

CHARTING EXAMPLE

Date	
9/20/12	10:30 a.m. Sutures intact and incision line in good approximation. No signs of infection. Sutures x6 removed from Ⓡ ant forearm. Incision line cleaned c̄ Betadine and DSD applied. Instructions provided on dressing care. ———————T. Browning, CMA (AAMA)

Adhesive Skin Closures

Adhesive skin closures may be used for wound repair to approximate the edges of a laceration or incision. Skin closures consist of sterile, hypoallergenic tape that is commercially available in a variety of widths and lengths and is strong enough to approximate a wound until healing occurs. Brand names for adhesive skin closures are Steri-Strip (3M Corporation, St Paul, Minn) and Proxi-Strip (Ethicon, Inc., Bridgewater, NJ) (Figure 10-12).

Adhesive skin closures may be used when not much tension exists on the skin edges. The strips of tape are applied transversely across the line of incision to approximate the skin edges. The advantages of adhesive skin closures are that they eliminate the need for sutures and a local anesthetic, they are easy to apply and remove, they have a lower incidence of wound infection compared with sutures, and they result in less scarring than sutures. The disadvantage of this method is that there is less precision in bringing the wound edges together compared with suturing the wound. In addition, adhesive skin closures cannot be used on certain areas of the body where the adhesive has difficulty adhering to the skin. This includes areas that harbor moisture (e.g., palms of the hands, soles of the feet, axillae) and hairy areas of the body (e.g., scalp, a man's chest).

The medical assistant frequently is responsible for applying adhesive skin closures. Procedure 10-6 outlines this

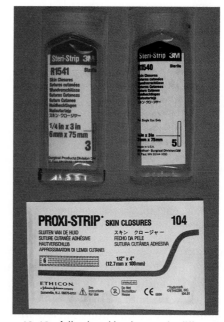

Figure 10-12. Adhesive skin closures in different sizes.

procedure. Approximately 5 to 10 days after application, the skin closures usually loosen and fall off on their own. If they require removal by the medical assistant, the method presented at the end of Procedure 10-6 should be followed.

PROCEDURE 10-6   **Applying and Removing Adhesive Skin Closures**

Outcome Apply and remove adhesive skin closures.

Equipment/Supplies

- Clean disposable gloves
- Sterile gloves
- Antiseptic solution
- Surgical scrub brush
- Antiseptic swabs
- Tincture of benzoin

- Sterile cotton-tipped applicator
- Adhesive skin closure strips
- Sterile 4 × 4 gauze pads
- Surgical tape
- Biohazard waster container

Application of Adhesive Skin Closures

1. Procedural Step. Wash your hands with an antimicrobial soap and assemble the equipment. Check the expiration date on the adhesive skin closures.

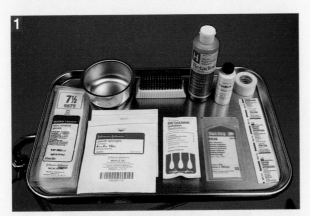

Assemble the equipment.

2. Procedural Step. Greet the patient and introduce yourself.

3. Procedural Step. Identify the patient by full name and date of birth and explain the procedure.

4. Procedural Step. Position the patient as required for application of the strips. Adjust the light so that it is focused on the wound. Apply clean gloves. Inspect the wound for signs of redness, swelling, and drainage. (**NOTE:** Chart this information in the patient's record after completing the procedure.)

5. Procedural Step. Gently scrub the wound using an antiseptic solution (e.g., Betadine solution) and a sterile gauze pad or a surgical scrub brush. Clean at least 3 inches around the wound, removing all debris, skin oil, and exudates. Allow the skin to dry or pat dry with gauze pads. (**NOTE:** Change gloves as needed to maintain cleanliness.)

6. Procedural Step. Apply an antiseptic to the site using antiseptic swabs such as Betadine swabs. Apply the antiseptic from the top to the bottom of the wound, working from the center to the outside of the wound. Use a new swab for each motion. Allow the skin to dry completely.

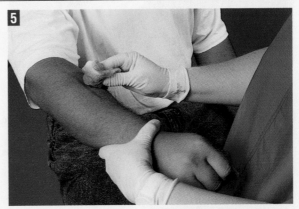

Clean the wound.

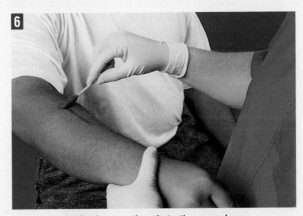

Apply an antiseptic to the wound.

Principle. The antiseptic decreases the number of microorganisms in the wound. The skin must be completely dry to ensure adhesion of the skin closures to the skin.

7. Procedural Step. If dictated by the medical office policy, apply a thin coat of tincture of benzoin to the skin parallel to each side of the wound with a sterile cotton-tipped applicator. Do not allow the tincture of benzoin to touch the wound. Allow the skin to dry. Remove the gloves, and wash your hands with an antimicrobial soap.

Principle. Tincture of benzoin facilitates adhesion of the strips to the skin.

Continued

PROCEDURE 10-6

PROCEDURE 10-6   Applying and Removing Adhesive Skin Closures—cont'd

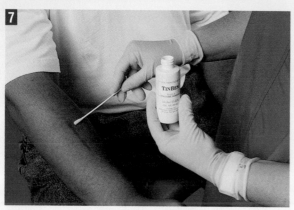

Apply tincture of benzoin.

8. Procedural Step. Open the plastic peel-apart package of strips using sterile technique as follows:

a. Grasp each flap of the package between the thumbs and bent index fingers. Pull the package apart.

b. Peel back the package until it is completely open.

c. Lay the opened package flat on a clean dry surface. The inside of the package serves as the sterile field.

9. Procedural Step. Apply sterile gloves. Fold the card of strips along its perforated tab, and tear off the tab, which exposes the ends of the strips, making them easier to grasp. Peel a strip of tape off the card at a 45-degree angle to the card.

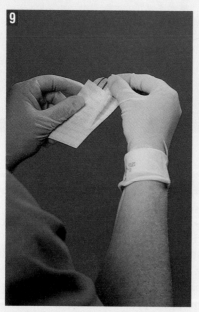

Peel a strip of tape off the card.

10. Procedural Step. Check that the skin surface is dry. Position the first strip over the center of the wound as follows:

a. Secure one end of the strip of tape to the skin on one side of the wound by pressing down firmly on the tape.

b. Stretch the strip transversely across the line of the incision until the edges of the wound are approximated exactly. If necessary, use your gloved hand to assist in bringing the edges of the wound together.

c. Secure the strip on the skin on the other side of the wound by pressing down firmly on the tape.

Principle. Approximating the wound exactly facilitates good healing and minimizes scar formation.

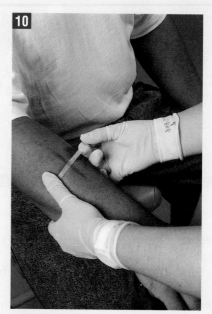

Position the first strip over the center of the wound.

11. Procedural Step. Apply the second strip perpendicular to the wound on one side of the center strip. The space between the strips should be approximately ⅛ inch. Apply a third strip on the other side of the center strip at a ⅛-inch interval. Continue applying the strips at ⅛-inch intervals until the edges of the wound are approximated. If at any time the skin surfaces become moist with perspiration, blood, or serum, wipe the area dry with a sterile gauze pad before applying the next strip.

Principle. Applying the strips in this manner facilitates good approximation of the wound. Spacing the strips at ⅛-inch intervals allows proper drainage of the wound.

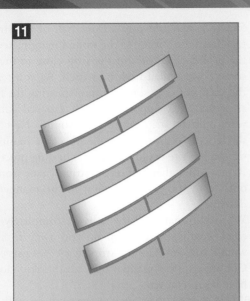

Apply the strips until the edges of the wound are approximated.

12. Procedural Step. Apply two closures approximately ½ inch from the ends of the strips and parallel to the wound (ladder fashion).

Principle. Applying a strip along each edge redistributes the tension and assists in holding the strips firmly in place.

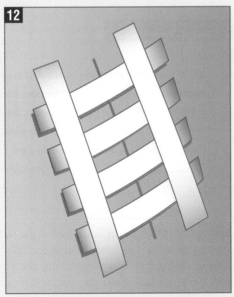

Apply a strip along each edge.

13. Procedural Step. Apply a dry sterile dressing over the strips if indicated by the physician (see Procedure 10-4).

14. Procedural Step. Remove the gloves, and sanitize your hands.

15. Procedural Step. Instruct the patient in wound care as follows:

a. Provide the patient with written wound care instructions (see the patient teaching box on wound care in this chapter).

b. Explain the wound care instructions, and ask the patient whether he or she has any questions.

c. Ask the patient to sign the instruction sheet on the appropriate line.

d. Witness the patient's signature by signing your name in the appropriate space on the form. Include today's date.

e. Before the patient leaves the medical office, make a copy of the instruction sheet. Give a signed copy of the wound care instructions to the patient, and file the original in the patient's medical record.

Principle. An instruction sheet signed by the patient provides legal documentation that wound care instructions were provided to the patient in the event that the patient fails to follow the instructions and causes further harm or damage to the wound.

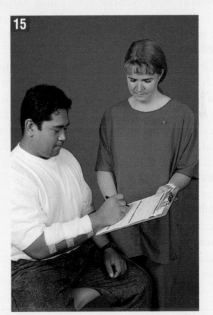

Ask the patient to sign the instruction sheet.

16. Procedural Step. Chart the procedure. Include the date and time, the appearance of the wound, wound preparation, the number of strips applied, the location of the wound, the care of the wound, and the patient's reaction. Chart verbal and written instructions given to the patient concerning wound care.

Continued

PROCEDURE 10-6   Applying and Removing Adhesive Skin Closures—cont'd

PROCEDURE 10-6

CHARTING EXAMPLE

Date	
9/20/12	10:30 a.m. Incision approx 5 cm long located on post Ⓡ forearm. Redness noted on edge of wound. Sl amt of serous drainage noted. Wound scrubbed c̄ Betadine sol and Betadine antiseptic applied. Applied Steri-Strips x4. Incision in good approximation. Applied DSD. Explained wound care. Written instructions provided. Signed copy filed in chart. To return in 5 days for removal of strips. ——————
	—————————T. Browning, CMA (AAMA)

Removal of Adhesive Skin Closures

Adhesive skin closures usually loosen and fall off on their own approximately 5 to 10 days following application. If they require removal, the procedure outlined below should be followed by the medical assistant.

1. **Procedural Step.** Sanitize your hands. Greet the patient and introduce yourself. Identify the patient by full name and date of birth and explain the procedure.
2. **Procedural Step.** Position the patient as required. Adjust the light so that it is focused on the wound. Check that the skin closures are intact and that the incision line is approximated and not gaping. Check that the incision line is not infected. If the incision line is not approximated, or if redness, swelling, or a discharge is present, do not remove the skin closures; notify the physician.
3. **Procedural Step.** Position a 4 × 4 gauze pad in a convenient location. Apply clean gloves.
4. **Procedural Step.** Remove the skin closures as follows:
   a. Gently grasp one end of a strip of tape with the dominant hand.
   b. Stabilize the skin with one finger of the nondominant hand.

c. Slowly loosen and peel off one half of the strip of tape from the outside to the wound margin, keeping the peeled-off section of the strip close to the skin surface and pulled back over itself. As you remove the strip from the skin, continue moving the finger as necessary to support the newly exposed skin. Always pull the strip toward the wound. Never pull the strip away from the wound because tension on the wound site could disrupt the healing process.
   d. Remove the other half of the strip of tape from the outside to the wound margin in the manner just described.
   e. When both halves of the strip are completely loosened, gently lift the strip up and away from the wound surface. Place the strip on a 4 × 4 gauze pad.
   f. Continue in this manner until all the skin closures have been removed.
5. **Procedural Step.** Cleanse the site with an antiseptic swab. Apply a dry sterile dressing if indicated by the physician (see Procedure 10-4).
6. **Procedural Step.** Dispose of the strips and gauze in a biohazard waste container. Remove the gloves, and sanitize your hands.
7. **Procedural Step.** Chart the procedure. Include the date and time, the status of the skin closures, the number of skin closures removed, the location of the site, the care of the wound, and the patient's reaction. Chart any instructions given to the patient.

CHARTING EXAMPLE

Date	
9/25/12	10:30 a.m. Skin closures intact and in good approximation. No signs of infection. Strips x 4 removed from Ⓡ post forearm. Incision line cleaned c̄ Betadine and DSD applied. Instructions provided on dressing care.
	—————————T. Browning, CMA (AAMA)

ASSISTING WITH MINOR OFFICE SURGERY
Tray Setup

Assisting with minor office surgery requires a thorough knowledge of the instruments and supplies for each tray setup and the type of assistance required by the physician during the surgery. The medical assistant must be able to work quickly and efficiently and to anticipate the physician's needs.

The instruments and supplies for the surgery must be set on a sterile field. Many offices maintain index cards indicating the appropriate instruments and supplies for each minor office surgery tray setup. The card also may include information regarding the type of skin preparation, the position of the patient, the physician's glove size, the type of suture material, preoperative instructions, and postoperative instructions. The index cards are generally kept in a file box and are filed alphabetically by the type of surgery. The medical assistant should pull the card before setting up for the minor office surgery and use it as a guide to ensure that all required articles are placed on the sterile field. The medical assistant may set up the sterile tray before or after preparing the patient's skin. The sterile tray setup must not become contaminated. If the medical assistant must turn away from the sterile tray or leave the room after setting up, a sterile towel must be placed over the tray to maintain sterility.

Methods Used to Set Up a Sterile Tray

A common method used to set up a sterile tray is to use prepackaged sterile setups wrapped in disposable sterilization paper or muslin that are prepared by the medical office through autoclave sterilization (see Procedure 10-2). These setups are labeled according to use (e.g., suture pack, cyst removal pack) and contain most of the instruments and supplies required for the minor office surgery indicated on the label. The medical assistant opens the wrapped package on a flat surface, such as a **Mayo tray.** A Mayo tray is a broad, flat metal tray placed on a stand that can be used to hold sterile instruments and supplies; the inside of the wrapped package is sterile and serves as the sterile field. Several additional articles not contained in the prepackaged setup (e.g., an antiseptic, sterile 4 × 4 gauze pads, disposable syringes and needles, sutures) may need to be added to the sterile field when the package is opened. If an antiseptic solution is poured into a basin on the sterile field, this is performed according to Procedure 10-3. Items in peel-apart packages are added by flipping them onto the sterile field or by placing them on the field using a sterile gloved hand.

Another method used to set up a sterile tray is to place all necessary articles on the sterile field by flipping them onto the sterile field from peel-apart packages. With this method, the sterile field is prepared by placing a sterile towel over a tray such as a Mayo tray or another flat surface. The sterile towel must be handled by the corners only so as not to contaminate it. It must not be fanned through the air, but instead must be laid down gently and slowly to prevent airborne contamination.

Side Table

Some articles required for minor office surgery are not placed on the sterile field but are set on an adjacent table or counter. These articles, such as a surgical scrub brush, are not sterile and must not be placed on the sterile field. The local anesthetic, which is a sterile solution, is in a vial that is not sterile and must *not* be placed on the sterile field. The physician needs to apply gloves to perform the surgery. Although the gloves are sterile, the outside wrapper is not; the package of gloves must not be placed on the sterile field. In addition, it is easier for the physician to apply gloves from a side table or counter. To facilitate applying the gloves, the medical assistant opens the outside wrapper for the physician.

Skin Preparation

The patient's skin must be prepared before the minor office surgery because the skin contains an abundance of microorganisms. If these microorganisms were to enter the body through the operative site, a wound infection could develop. It is impossible to sterilize skin because chemical

agents required to kill all living microorganisms are too strong to be placed on the skin surfaces. The operative site and an area surrounding it must be cleaned and prepared in such a way as to remove as many microorganisms as possible to reduce the risk of surgical wound contamination.

Shaving the Site

Hair supports the growth of microorganisms, and the physician may want the medical assistant to shave the skin at and around the operative site. Shave preparation trays are commercially available and include several gauze sponges, a measured amount of antiseptic soap, a container for soapy water, and a disposable safety razor. The skin should be pulled taut as it is shaved, and the medical assistant must be careful to prevent nicks. When all the hair has been removed, the shaved area should be rinsed and dried thoroughly.

Cleansing the Site

The operative site must be cleaned with an antiseptic solution such as povidone-iodine (Betadine Surgical Scrub) or chlorhexidine gluconate (Hibiclens) (Figure 10-13). The medical assistant should scrub the operative area with a surgical scrub brush using a firm circular motion, moving from the inside outward. The area is rinsed using gauze pads saturated with water and is blotted dry with sterile gauze.

Antiseptic Application

When the patient's skin has been shaved (if required) and cleansed, an antiseptic is applied to the operative area, followed by the application of a sterile drape. The antiseptic decreases the number of microorganisms on the patient's skin; a common antiseptic is Betadine. A disposable sterile *fenestrated drape* (Figure 10-14) is the type of drape most commonly used. It has an opening that is placed directly over the operative site. A fenestrated drape covers a wide area of skin around the operative area, leaving only the operative site

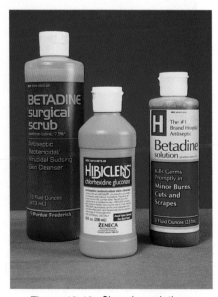

Figure 10-13. Cleansing solutions.

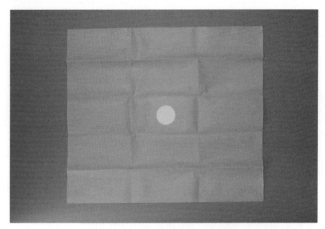

Figure 10-14. Fenestrated drape.

exposed. This provides a sterile area around the operative site and decreases contamination of the patient's surgical wound.

Local Anesthetic

Minor office surgeries often require the use of a local anesthetic; the local anesthetic most frequently used in the medical office is lidocaine hydrochloride (Xylocaine). The physician injects the local anesthetic into the tissue surrounding the operative site, a process termed *infiltration*, to produce a loss of sensation in that area and prevent the patient from feeling pain during the surgery. When first injected into the tissues, lidocaine causes the patient to experience a brief burning or stinging sensation at the injection site. The local anesthetic begins working in 5 to 15 minutes and has a duration of action of 1 to 3 hours, depending on the type of anesthetic.

Some physicians prefer to use a local anesthetic containing *epinephrine.* Epinephrine is a vasoconstrictor that pro-

longs the local effect of the anesthetic and decreases the rate of systemic absorption of the local anesthetic. It accomplishes this by constricting blood vessels at the operative site. The physician informs the medical assistant of the type, strength, and amount of local anesthetic needed for the minor office surgery. Xylocaine is available in 0.5%, 1%, 1.5%, and 2% solutions. The physician may order 1 ml of Xylocaine 2% with epinephrine to suture a laceration of the forearm.

Preparing the Anesthetic

The local anesthetic is drawn up into the syringe according to the procedure presented in Chapter 11. The vial must first be cleansed using an antiseptic wipe. The correct amount of anesthetic solution is withdrawn into the syringe. This may be performed by the medical assistant or the physician. The medical assistant withdraws the anesthetic into the syringe and hands it to the physician, who has not yet applied sterile gloves. The physician injects the anesthetic into the patient's tissues and then applies sterile gloves to begin the surgery.

The physician may prefer to draw the anesthetic solution into the syringe after he or she has applied sterile gloves. The medical assistant should first show the label of the vial to the physician and should then hold the vial securely while the physician withdraws the medication (Figure 10-15). The medical assistant must hold the vial because the outside of the vial is medically aseptic and cannot be touched by the physician's sterile gloved hand.

If the medical assistant prepares the anesthetic injection, the needle and syringe are not placed on the sterile field, but are assembled off to the side. If the physician withdraws the anesthetic, the needle and syringe are placed on the sterile field.

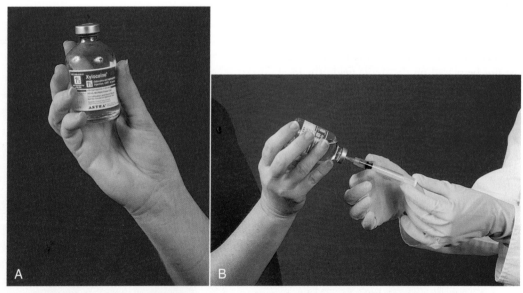

Figure 10-15. Drawing up the local anesthetic. **A,** Trudy holds up the vial so that the physician can verify the name and strength of the local anesthetic. **B,** Trudy holds the vial securely while the physician withdraws the medication.

Assisting the Physician

The type of assistance required by the physician during minor office surgery is based on the type of surgery and the physician's preference. Some physicians want the medical assistant to apply sterile gloves and assist directly by handing instruments and supplies from the sterile field. An instrument should be handed to the physician in a firm, confident manner so that the instrument does not slip out of the physician's hand and drop on the floor. The instrument should be placed in the physician's hand in its functional position, that is, the position in which it is to be used (Figure 10-16). If the instrument is handed correctly, the physician should not have to reposition the instrument to use it.

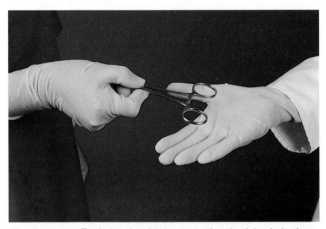

Figure 10-16. Trudy hands a hemostat to the physician in its functional position.

The medical assistant is responsible for adding any instruments or supplies to the sterile field that the physician requires after the surgery has begun, such as another hemostat, additional 4 × 4 gauze pads, and sutures. This is generally accomplished using peel-apart packages and by either flipping the contents onto the sterile field or by holding the package open and allowing the physician to remove the contents with a gloved hand. In assisting with minor office surgery, it is essential to know all steps in the procedure, so that the physician's needs are anticipated, and the surgery proceeds smoothly and efficiently.

The physician may obtain a tissue specimen that is sent to the laboratory for histologic examination. The specimen must be placed in an appropriate-sized container with a preservative. The medical assistant is responsible for labeling the specimen container. An unlabeled specimen is a cause for rejection of the specimen by an outside laboratory. Two *unique identifiers* should be used to label the specimen. A unique identifier is information that clearly identifies a specific patient, such as the patient's name and date of birth. A specimen can be labeled by attaching a computerized bar code label to the specimen. A specimen can also be labeled by hand-writing the information on the label, which should include the patient's name and date of birth, the date and time of collection, the medical assistant's initials, and any other information required by the laboratory, such as the source of the specimen. The information should be printed legibly, and the medical assistant should be certain that the information is accurate to avoid a mix-up of specimens. The medical assistant also must complete a laboratory requisition to accompany the specimen; this is known as a *biopsy requisition* (Figure 10-17).

DIAGNOSTIC PATHOLOGY ASSOCIATES, INC

HISTOPATHOLOGY/CYTOPATHOLOGY REQUISITION

BILL TO: ☐ ACCOUNT ☐ MEDICARE ☐ BLUE SHIELD ☐ PATIENT ☐ MEDICAID ☐ OTHER	PATIENT NAME (LAST, FIRST, MIDDLE INITIAL)		PATIENT ID	ROOM NO.

SEX	BIRTHDATE / /	DATE COLLECTED	TIME COLLECTED A.M. P.M.	REQUESTING PHYSICIAN	SPECIAL INSTRUCTIONS

RESPONSIBLE PARTY NAME	RESPONSIBLE PARTY ADDRESS	CITY, STATE, ZIP

PHONE	MEDICAID ID NUMBER	MEDICARE HIC NUMBER	INSURANCE COMPANY NAME

INSURANCE COMPANY ADDRESS	GROUP NUMBER	CONTRACT NUMBER	COVERAGE CODE	PATIENT/INSURED RELATIONSHIP ☐ SELF ☐ SPOUSE ☐ DEPEND.

PATIENT AUTHORIZATION: I AUTHORIZE THE RELEASE OF ANY MEDICAL INFORMATION NECESSARY TO PROCESS A CLAIM. I PERMIT A COPY OF THIS AUTHORIZATION TO BE USED IN PLACE OF THE ORIGINAL AND REQUEST PAYMENT OF ANY MEDICAL INSURANCE BENEFITS EITHER TO ME OR TO THE PARTY WHO ACCEPTS ASSIGNMENT.	SIGNED X_____	DATE _____

TISSUE EXAM: ☐ GROSS & MICROSCOPIC ☐ GROSS ONLY SPECIMEN TYPE: ☐ BIOPSY ☐ SCRAPING ☐ BRUSHING ☐ WASHING ☐ FLUIDS ☐ FINE NEEDLE ☐ OTHER _____ _____	SOURCE OF SPECIMEN: ☐ PHONE REPORT (NEXT WORKING DAY) COPIES TO:_____	CLINICAL DIAGNOSIS: PATIENT HISTORY:

Figure 10-17. Biopsy requisition. (Courtesy Diagnostic Pathology Associates, Columbus, OH.)

Case Study 2

Abbey Mendy is having a sebaceous cyst removed from her neck. She wants to know why the antiseptic applied to her neck is orange, and whether it is going to stain her skin permanently. During the procedure, Abbey reaches her hand up to adjust her hair and accidentally touches the physician's gloved hand. After the procedure, a sterile dressing is applied to her neck, and she is given an appoint-

ment to return to have her sutures removed. Abbey becomes alarmed when she is told that the cyst will be sent to the laboratory for a biopsy. She wants to know whether the physician is not telling her everything about her condition, and is concerned that maybe he thinks she has cancer. Abbey asks if her neighbor can take out her sutures. She says that he has worked as a veterinary assistant for the past 8 years and has lots of experience in removing stitches. ■

Highlight on the History of Surgery

Primitive Surgery

Surgery evolved from very primitive beginnings. The first record of a surgical operation dates back to 350,000 BC. Primitive humans believed that headaches were caused by demons that had gained entrance to the head and were unable to get out. To release the demons, a hole was chiseled through the patient's skull with a sharp flint. Early operating instruments consisted of sharpened flints and crude hammers. Sharpened animal teeth were used for bloodletting and drainage of abscesses. Ancient records show that suturing materials consisted of dried gut, dried tendon, strips of hide, horsehair, and fibers from tree bark. To help form a clot, bleeding wounds were covered with materials such as rabbit fur, shredded tree bark, egg yolk, and cobwebs.

Early 1800s

In the early 1800s, surgical instruments were still almost nonexistent. Kitchen knives and penknives doubled as scalpels, and table forks were used as retractors. Physicians would use household pincushions to hold their suturing needles. The same sponges were used for every patient to wipe away blood and other secretions. Because of these conditions, the most trivial operations were likely to be followed by infection, and death occurred in half of all surgical operations. Joseph Lister, an English surgeon, was one of the first individuals to advocate the use of antiseptics during surgery. Lister insisted on the use of antiseptics on the hands of his surgical team, instruments, wounds, and dressings. Many surgeons ridiculed Lister's ideas, but in 1879 his antiseptic principles were, at long last, formally adopted by the medical profession. Today, Lister is known as the father of modern surgery.

Mid-1800s

Anesthetic agents, such as ether and chloroform, were discovered in the mid-1800s. Before this time, various methods were used to subdue and restrain patients during surgery, such as having the patient consume alcohol before the operation and strapping the patient to the operating table. With the advent of anesthetics, new surgical procedures never before considered possible came into existence. This resulted in new demands for surgical instruments and the necessity for smaller and more delicate instruments.

Late 1800s and Early 1900s

The late 1800s and early 1900s saw dramatic advances in surgical operations and techniques. The most notable include the invention of the steam sterilizer, which permitted sterilization of surgical instruments and supplies; the use of surgical gowns, caps, masks, and gloves during surgery; the monitoring of a patient's condition while under anesthesia; the development of stainless steel, which provided a superior material for manufacturing surgical instruments; and the establishment of standards for manufacturing and packaging sutures. Other discoveries important to surgery during this time included the discovery of x-rays by Wilhelm Röntgen; the discovery of penicillin by Alexander Fleming; the discovery by William Halsted that cocaine could be used as a local anesthetic; and the development of endoscopic instruments, such as the laryngoscope, bronchoscope, and sigmoidoscope, for viewing internal structures of the body.

Breakthroughs in surgical technology established through the ages laid the foundation for present-day complex surgical procedures, such as laser surgery, open-heart surgery, and microsurgery. It is incredible to think that it all started with a sharpened flint! ■

When the minor office surgery is completed, the physician may want the medical assistant to place a dry sterile dressing over the surgical wound to protect it from contamination or injury or to absorb drainage. The medical assistant also is responsible for assisting the patient and cleaning the examining room.

Procedure 10-7 describes the medical assistant's responsibilities while assisting with minor office surgery. Specific instruments and supplies required for the minor office surgery depend on the type of surgery being performed and

the physician's preference. Knowing the name and function of the surgical instruments shown in Figure 10-3 enables the medical assistant to set up for each type of minor surgery performed in the medical office. If the medical office uses prepackaged sterile setups, the medical assistant should have already assembled the instruments and supplies in the package during the sanitization and sterilization process; however, the instruments and supplies should be checked after the pack is opened to ensure that all the sterile articles are included.

PROCEDURE 10-7   Assisting with Minor Office Surgery

Outcome Set up a surgical tray, and assist with minor office surgery.

Equipment/Supplies

- Mayo stand
- Instruments and supplies for the type of surgery to be performed
- Biohazard waste container

Preparing the Tray

1. **Procedural Step.** Determine the type of minor office surgery to be performed. The physician instructs the medical assistant as to the type of surgery and provides any additional information needed to set up for the surgery, such as the type of local anesthetic and sutures to be used. If the medical office maintains a minor office surgery filing system, pull the file card that indicates the instruments and supplies required for the type of surgery to be performed.

2. **Procedural Step.** Prepare the examining room. Make sure the room is clean and well lighted.

3. **Procedural Step.** Sanitize your hands.

4. **Procedural Step.** Set up nonsterile articles on a side table or counter. If a specimen container is included in the setup, perform one of the following (based on the medical office policy):

   a. Attach a computer-generated bar code label to the specimen container *or*

   b. Clearly label the tubes and containers with the patient's name and date of birth, the date, your initials, and any other information required by the laboratory, such as the source of the specimen.

   Principle. Articles that are not sterile cannot be placed on the sterile field because they would contaminate it. Two unique identifiers should be used when labeling the specimen (e.g., patient's name and date of birth).

5. **Procedural Step.** Wash your hands with an antimicrobial soap and set up the minor office surgery tray on a clean, dry, flat surface, using the principles of surgical asepsis. The sterile tray can be set up as follows:

   Prepackaged setup:

   a. Select the appropriate package from the supply shelf, and place it on a Mayo tray or other flat surface

   b. Open the prepackaged setup using the inside of the wrapper as the sterile field. Check the sterilization indicator to make sure the contents of the pack are sterile.

   c. Add other articles to the sterile field that are needed for the surgery but not contained in the sterile package, such as 4 × 4 gauze, sutures, and a fenestrated drape. If sutures are required for the setup, make sure to check the expiration date of the sutures.

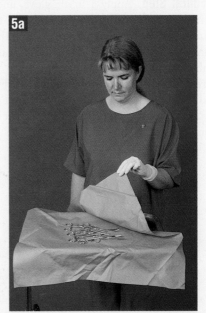

Open the sterile pack using the inside of the wrapper as the sterile field.

Transferring articles to a sterile field:

a. Pick up the folded sterile towel by two corner ends and allow it to unfold; make sure it does not touch an unsterile surface.

b. Lay the sterile towel down gently and slowly over the Mayo tray, making sure it does not brush against an unsterile surface such as your uniform. Do not allow your arms to pass over the towel as

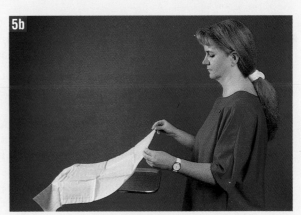

Lay the sterile towel down gently and slowly.

Continued

PROCEDURE 10-7   Assisting with Minor Office Surgery—cont'd

you lay it down because this would result in contamination of the sterile field.

c. Transfer instruments and supplies to the sterile field from wrapped or peel-apart packages.

Principle. The principles of surgical asepsis must be followed to prevent contamination of the sterile field.

6. Procedural Step. Apply a sterile glove, and arrange the articles neatly on the sterile field. Do not allow one article to lie on top of another. Check that all the instruments and supplies required for the surgery are available on the sterile field.

Principle. Instruments and supplies can be located quickly and efficiently on a neat and orderly sterile field. Sterile gloves must be used to prevent contamination of the sterile articles.

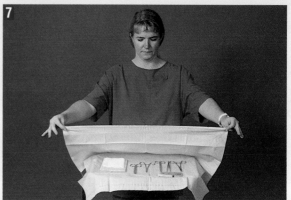

Cover the tray setup with a sterile towel.

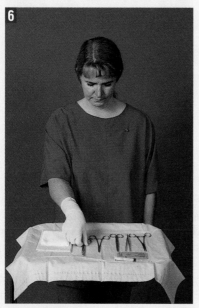

Arrange the articles neatly on the sterile field.

7. Procedural Step. Cover the tray setup with a sterile towel by picking up the towel by two corner ends and placing it gently and slowly over the setup. Do not allow your arms to pass over the sterile field as you lay it down.

Principle. The towel prevents the sterile tray from becoming contaminated. The towel must be picked up by the corner ends to prevent contaminating it and should be moved slowly and not fanned through the air to prevent airborne contamination. Passing the arms over the sterile field results in contamination of the field.

Preparing the Patient

8. Procedural Step. Greet the patient and introduce yourself. Identify the patient by full name and date of birth. Explain the procedure, and prepare the patient for the minor office surgery as outlined below:

a. Try to allay the patient's fear or anxiety.

b. Ask the patient whether he or she needs to void before the surgery.

c. Provide instructions to the patient about any clothing that must be removed and putting on an examination gown, if required. Enough clothing must be removed to expose the operative area completely and to avoid getting the antiseptic or blood on the patient's clothing.

d. Instruct the patient not to move during the procedure and not to talk, laugh, sneeze, or cough over the sterile field.

Principle. Minor office surgery is often a frightening experience for the patient, and reassurance should be offered to reduce apprehension. The amount of clothing that must be removed depends on the type of minor office surgery being performed. By moving, the patient may accidentally contaminate the sterile field or touch the operative site. Microorganisms are carried in water vapor from the mouth, nose, and lungs and can be transferred onto the sterile field.

9. Procedural Step. Position the patient. The position is determined by the type of minor office surgery to be performed. The patient is positioned in such a way as to provide the best possible exposure and accessibility to the operative site. **NOTE:** If a difficult position must be maintained, such as the knee-chest position, the patient should not be positioned until the physician is ready to begin the minor office surgery.

10. Procedural Step. Adjust the light so that it is focused on the operative site.

PROCEDURE 10-7 Assisting with Minor Office Surgery—cont'd

11. Procedural Step. Prepare the patient's skin by performing the following:
a. Apply clean disposable gloves.
b. If hair is present, the skin at and around the operative site may need to be shaved. The skin should be pulled taut as it is shaved. The area is rinsed and dried thoroughly.
c. Cleanse the patient's skin with an antiseptic solution and a surgical scrub brush using a firm, circular motion and moving from the inside outward. Do not return to an area just cleansed. The area is rinsed using gauze pads saturated with water and blotted dry with a sterile gauze pad.
d. Apply an antiseptic to the site using antiseptic swabs such as Betadine. Allow the skin to dry. Alternatively, the physician may place a fenestrated drape over the operative site and then apply the antiseptic.
e. Remove the gloves, and sanitize your hands.

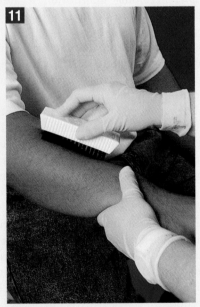

Cleanse the patient's skin with an antiseptic solution.

12. Procedural Step. Verify that everything is prepared for the minor office surgery, and inform the physician that the patient is ready.

Assisting the Physician

13. Procedural Step. Assist the physician as required during the minor office surgery, following the principles of surgical asepsis. The physician drapes the patient, injects the local anesthetic, and performs the surgery.

The responsibilities of the medical assistant may include the following:
a. Uncover the sterile tray setup by picking up the sterile towel covering it. The towel should be picked up by two corner ends and removed slowly and gently without allowing the arms to pass over the sterile field.
b. Open the outer glove wrapper for the physician to facilitate the application of sterile gloves.
c. Withdraw the local anesthetic into a syringe and hand it to the physician, or hold the vial while the physician withdraws the local anesthetic. If lidocaine (Xylocaine) is used, the physician or medical assistant should inform the patient to expect a brief burning or stinging sensation as it is injected into the tissues.
d. Adjust the light as needed by the physician for good visualization of the operative site.
e. Restrain patients such as children.
f. Relax and reassure the patient during the minor office surgery.
g. Hand instruments and supplies to the physician. (Sterile gloves are required.)
h. Keep the sterile field neat and orderly. (Sterile gloves are required.)
i. Hold a basin in which the physician can deposit soiled instruments and supplies, such as hemostats and gauze sponges. (Clean gloves are required.)

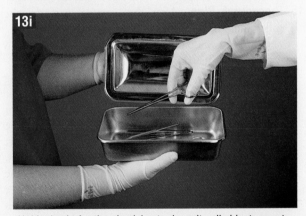

Hold a basin for the physician to deposit soiled instruments.

j. Retract tissue from an area to allow the physician the best access to and visibility of the operative site. (Sterile gloves are required.)
k. Sponge blood from the operative site. (Sterile gloves are required.)
l. Add instruments and supplies to the sterile field as required by the physician.
m. Hold the specimen container to accept a tissue specimen received from the physician. (Clean

Continued

PROCEDURE 10-7   Assisting with Minor Office Surgery—cont'd

gloves are required.) Do not touch the inside of the container because it is sterile. After the physician inserts the specimen, replace the container lid and close it tightly.

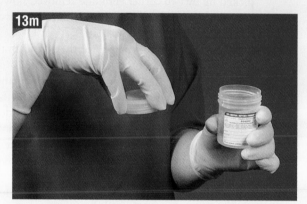

Hold the container to accept a tissue specimen.

n. After the physician has inserted a suture, cut the ends of the suture material approximately ⅛ inch above the knot of the suture (sterile gloves are required).

14. **Procedural Step.** Apply a sterile dressing to the surgical wound, if ordered by the physician (see Procedure 10-4).

Principle. The sterile dressing protects the wound from contamination and injury and absorbs drainage.

15. **Procedural Step.** After the surgery, perform the following:

a. Stay with the patient as a safety precaution and to assist and instruct the patient.

b. Ensure that postoperative instructions regarding any type of medical care to be administered at home are understood. If the patient has a wound or if sutures have been inserted, he or she should be told to keep the area clean and dry and to report any signs of infection, such as excessive redness, swelling, discharge, or increased pain. Provide the patient with written wound care instructions (see the patient teaching box on wound care in this chapter). Ask the patient if he or she has any questions. Have the patient sign the instruction sheet. Witness the patient's signature. Before the patient leaves the office, make a copy of the instruction sheet. Give a copy to the patient and file the original in the patient's chart.

c. Relay information regarding the return visit for postoperative care, such as the removal of sutures or a dressing change.

d. Help the patient off the table to prevent falls.

e. Instruct the patient to get dressed, offering assistance if needed.

f. Any instructions or information given must be charted in the patient's medical record.

Principle. The patient (especially an elderly one) may become dizzy after the minor office surgery and may fall when getting off the examining table. The filed copy protects the physician legally, in the event that the patient fails to follow instructions and causes harm or damage to the operative site.

16. **Procedural Step.** If a specimen was collected, it must be transferred to the laboratory in a tightly closed, properly labeled specimen container. Prepare the specimen for transport. Complete a biopsy request form to accompany the specimen. Place the specimen container in a biohazard specimen bag and seal it. Insert the biopsy request in the outer pocket of the bag and tuck the requisition under the flap. Place the bag in the appropriate location for pickup by the laboratory. Record information in the patient's chart, including the date the specimen was picked up or sent to the laboratory and the name of the laboratory.

Principle. Recording information regarding transport of the specimen documents that the specimen was sent to the laboratory.

17. **Procedural Step.** Clean the examining room. Handle the instruments carefully so as not to damage them. Be especially careful with sharp instruments to prevent cutting yourself. Blood and body secretions should be rinsed off the instruments immediately to prevent them from drying and hardening. The instruments must be sanitized and sterilized when it is convenient to do so; follow the procedures presented in Chapter 3. Discard disposable articles contaminated with blood or other potentially infectious materials in a biohazard waste container.

Principle. Surgical instruments are expensive and must be handled carefully to prolong their life span. Hardened blood and secretions on an instrument are difficult to remove. Disposable articles must be discarded in an appropriate manner to prevent the spread of infection.

CHARTING EXAMPLE	
Date	
9/25/12	2:00 p.m. Applied DSD to Ⓡ post forearm. Instructed patient on suture care. Written instructions provided. Signed copy filed in chart. To return in 5 days for removal of sutures. Sebaceous cyst specimen sent to Medical Center Laboratory for biopsy on 9/25/12. ———T. Browning, CMA (AAMA)

MEDICAL OFFICE SURGICAL PROCEDURES

The most common surgical procedures performed in the medical office are presented on the following pages. A discussion of the procedure and the items required for each tray setup are included. The medical assistant should take into account, however, that the instruments and supplies may vary slightly from those listed here, based on the physician's preference.

Sebaceous Cyst Removal

A **sebaceous cyst** (also known as an epidermal cyst) is a thin, closed sac or capsule located just under the surface of the skin. A sebaceous cyst forms when the outlet of a sebaceous (oil) gland becomes obstructed. The cyst contains *sebum,* which is made up of secretions from the sebaceous gland. The built-up secretion of sebum causes swelling, and the lining of the cyst consists of the stretched sebaceous gland. A sebaceous cyst is usually white or yellow in appearance and varies in size from less than ¼ inch (0.6 cm) in diameter to nearly 2 inches (5 cm) in diameter. It is usually a movable, dome-shaped mass with a smooth surface that is filled with a thick, fatty-white, cheesy material that has a foul odor. This type of cyst can occur anywhere on the body except on the palms of the hands and the soles of the feet—these areas do not contain sebaceous glands. Sebaceous cysts tend to occur most frequently on the scalp, face (Figure 10-18), ears, neck, back, and genital area.

A sebaceous cyst is usually slow-growing, painless, and nontender and may disappear on its own. A sebaceous cyst usually does not require surgical removal unless it becomes infected. An infected cyst is painful, tender, red, and swollen and may have a grayish-white, foul-smelling discharge. Because it is difficult to remove an infected sebaceous cyst, the physician usually drains the cyst and allows it to heal and then performs the cyst excision at a later time. Other reasons for removing a sebaceous cyst include cosmetic concerns and the need to reduce discomfort from a cyst that is located in a body area that is easily irritated, such as the armpit.

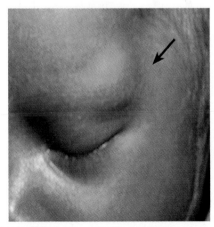

Figure 10-18. Sebaceous cyst. (From Weston, Lane, Morelli: In Sanders MJ: Mosby's paramedic textbook, ed 3, St Louis, 2007, Mosby.)

Surgical excision of a sebaceous cyst is a simple procedure that involves complete removal of the sac wall and its contents. Most sebaceous cysts are benign and are not usually biopsied unless they have an unusual appearance that may indicate a more serious problem. The side tray setup presented below includes the items needed for a tissue biopsy (specimen container and laboratory request form); however, these items would not be placed on the tray if the physician determines that a biopsy of the sebaceous cyst is not warranted.

Sebaceous Cyst Setup

The items required for a sebaceous cyst setup are listed.

Items Placed to the Side of the Sterile Field
- Clean disposable gloves
- Antiseptic solution
- Surgical scrub brush
- Antiseptic swabs
- Sterile gloves
- Local anesthetic
- Antiseptic wipe to cleanse the vial
- Specimen container with preservative and label
- Laboratory request form
- Surgical tape

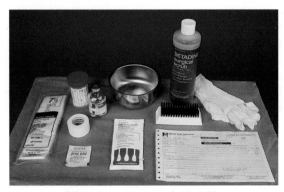

Sebaceous cyst removal side table.

Items Included on the Sterile Field
- Fenestrated drape
- Needle and syringe for drawing up the local anesthetic
- Scalpel and blade
- Dissecting scissors
- Hemostatic forceps
- Tissue forceps
- Thumb forceps
- Operating scissors
- Needle holder
- Sutures
- Sterile 4 × 4 gauze

Procedure: Sebaceous Cyst Removal

A sebaceous cyst is removed as follows:
1. A local anesthetic is used to numb the area.
2. The physician makes an incision using either a single cut down the center or an oval cut on both sides of the cyst.

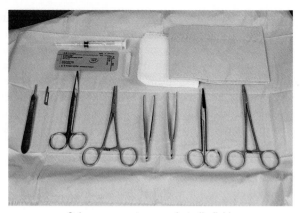

Sebaceous cyst removal sterile field.

The physician then removes the cyst and sutures the surgical incision (Figure 10-19).

3. If the cyst is to be biopsied, it is placed in a specimen container with a preservative and sent to the laboratory for examination by a pathologist.
4. A sterile dressing is applied to the operative site.

Postoperative Instructions: Sebaceous Cyst Removal

Postoperative instructions include the following:

1. Keep the dressing clean and dry.
2. Report any signs that the wound is infected, which include fever, increased pain, swelling, redness, warmth, and discharge.
3. Notify the medical office if the sutures become loose or break.

Provide the patient with written instructions on wound care to refer to at home, and instruct the patient when to return for removal of the sutures.

Surgical Incision and Drainage of Localized Infections

An **abscess** is a collection of pus in a cavity surrounded by inflamed tissue (Figure 10-20, *A*). It is caused by a pathogen that invades the tissues, usually via a break in the skin. An abscess serves as a defense mechanism of the body to keep an infection localized by walling off the microorganisms, preventing them from spreading through the body (Figure 10-20, *B*). A **furuncle,** also known as a *boil,* is a localized staphylococcal infection that originates deep within a hair follicle (Figure 10-21). Furuncles produce pain and itching. The skin initially becomes red and then turns white and necrotic over the top of the furuncle. Erythema and induration usually surround it.

Incision and Drainage Setup

The items required for an incision and drainage cyst setup are listed.

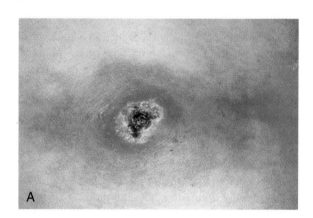

A

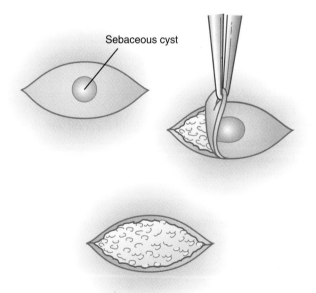

Sebaceous cyst

Figure 10-19. Sebaceous cyst removal. The physician makes an incision, removes the cyst, and sutures the surgical incision. (From Nealon TF Jr: Fundamental skills in surgery, ed 4, Philadelphia, 1994, Saunders.)

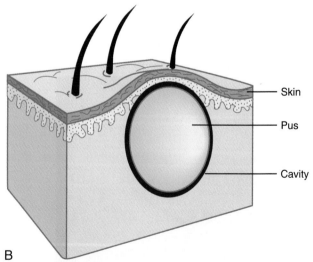

Skin

Pus

Cavity

B

Figure 10-20. **A,** Staphylococcus skin abscess. **B,** An abscess is a collection of pus in a cavity surrounded by inflamed tissue. (**A** from Braverman IM: Skin signs of systemic disease, ed 3, Philadelphia, 1998, WB Saunders. **B** from Nealon TF Jr: Fundamental skills in surgery, ed 4, Philadelphia, 1994, Saunders.)

ED: Made no change to credit lin
OK? Instructions were confusing

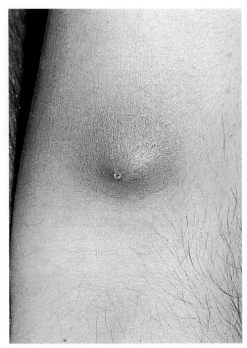

Figure 10-21. Furuncle resulting from a *Staphylococcus aureus* infection. (From LaFleur Brooks M: Exploring medical language: a student-directed approach, ed 7, St Louis, 2009, Mosby.)

Items Placed to the Side of the Sterile Field
- Clean disposable gloves
- Antiseptic solution
- Surgical scrub brush
- Antiseptic swabs
- Sterile gloves
- Local anesthetic
- Antiseptic wipe to cleanse the vial
- Iodoform gauze packing material
- Rubber Penrose drain
- Surgical tape

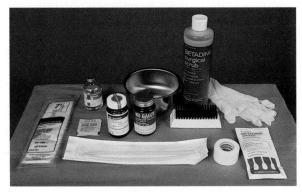

Incision and drainage side table.

Items Included on the Sterile Field
- Fenestrated drape
- Needle or syringe for drawing up the local anesthetic
- Scalpel and blade

- Dissecting scissors
- Hemostatic forceps
- Tissue forceps
- Thumb forceps
- Operating scissors
- Sterile 4 × 4 gauze

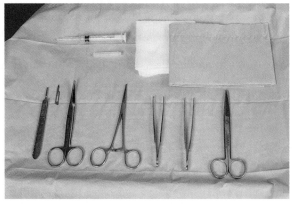

Incision and drainage sterile field.

Procedure: Incision and Drainage
Localized infections, such as abscesses, furuncles, and infected sebaceous cysts, that do not rupture and drain naturally may need to be incised and drained by the physician as follows:
1. A local anesthetic is generally used for the procedure.
2. A scalpel is used to make the incision. The physician then allows the pus to drain out using gauze to absorb pus and blood. Either gauze packing or a rubber Penrose drain is inserted into the wound to keep the edges of the tissues apart; this facilitates drainage of the exudate. The exudate contains pathogenic microorganisms; the medical assistant should be careful to avoid contact with the exudate while assisting with the minor surgery.
3. A sterile dressing of several thicknesses is applied over the operative site to absorb the drainage.

Postoperative Instructions: Incision and Drainage
Postoperative instructions include the following:
1. Keep the dressing clean and dry.
2. Report any signs that the wound is infected, which include fever, increased pain, swelling, redness, warmth, and discharge.

Provide the patient with written instructions on wound care to refer to at home, and instruct the patient when to return for removal of the gauze packing or Penrose drain.

Mole Removal

A mole (also known as a *nevus*) is a small growth on the human skin. An individual may be born with moles, which are known as *congenital nevi*, but may develop moles over time known as *acquired nevi*. According to the American Academy of Dermatology, the majority of moles appear during the first 20 years of an individual's life. Moles can occur anywhere on the skin, and between 10 and 40 moles on the body is considered normal. Large numbers of moles can be concentrated on the back, chest, and arms. Most moles are benign and exhibit the following characteristics:

- Usually range in color from brown to nearly black in color but can be a pinkish flesh color to dark blue or even black. Dark-colored moles consist of a cluster of melanocytes. Melanocytes produce the pigment *melanin,* which is responsible for the dark color of moles.
- Shape is usually round or oval and may be smooth or rough.
- Size is usually smaller than a pencil eraser but can range from barely visible to quite a large area.
- May form a raised area on the skin or may be flat
- May sometimes have hairs growing out of them

The most common types of moles are skin tags, flat moles, and raised moles. *Skin tags* or *acrochordon* are small, painless, benign growths that project from the skin from a small narrow stalk known as a *peduncle.* They are flesh colored or slightly darker, often appear in groups, and range from 1 mm to 5 mm in size (Figure 10-22). Skin tags occur most often during and after middle age in adults who are overweight or have diabetes. Skin tags are most frequently found in body areas where the skin creases, such as the eyelids, neck, armpits, upper chest, and groin. Occasionally, a skin tag becomes irritated as the result of shaving or rubbing from clothing or jewelry.

A *flat mole* is any dark spot or irregularity in the skin. A *raised mole,* as the name implies, extends above the skin. It can be a variety of colors and runs deeper than flat moles (Figure 10-23).

Although most moles are benign, some moles may be precancerous and are known as *dysplastic nevi* (Figure 10-24). Dysplastic nevi are usually larger than normal moles and have an irregular coloration and shape. The center of dysplastic nevi may be raised and darkened. According to the National Cancer Institute, dysplastic nevi are more likely than ordinary moles to develop into malignant melanoma. Because of this, dysplastic nevi are often biopsied or removed and biopsied to determine whether they are malignant.

Melanoma is a very serious type of skin cancer that can sometimes develop within a mole. Melanoma is most apt to

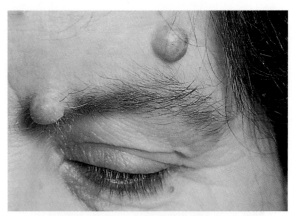

Figure 10-23. Raised moles. (From Forbes CD: Color atlas and text of clinical medicine, ed 3, St Louis, 2003, Mosby.)

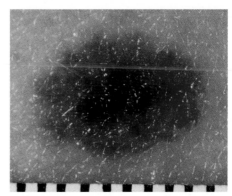

Figure 10-24. Dysplastic nevi. (From Goldman L: Cecil medicine, ed 23, Philadelphia, 2008, Saunders.)

be found on the upper backs of men and on the lower legs of women. Studies show that excessive sun exposure, especially severe blistering sunburns early in life, increase the risk of developing certain melanomas. If discovered early, it may be possible to completely remove the melanoma and reduce the spread of skin cancer. Left untreated, melanoma can be fatal.

Any moles exhibiting the following characteristics common to melanoma (Figure 10-25) should be evaluated by a physician:

- Asymmetric: one half of the mole is different from the other half.
- Irregular border: the edges of the mole are notched, uneven, or blurred rather than round or distinct.
- Color varies from one area of the mole to another: various shades of tan, brown, and black (and sometimes white, red, or blue) are present.
- Diameter is larger than ¼ inch (6 mm), which is about the diammeter of a pencil eraser.
- Other signs: the mole is painful or tender, itches, bleeds, oozes, or has a scaly appearance.

Moles are removed for a variety of reasons, which include the following: cosmetic to improve an individual's appearance, to reduce irritation and discomfort from a mole that is rubbing against clothing or that is in the way when shaving. A more serious reason for removing a mole is that the mole

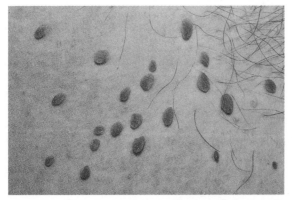

Figure 10-22. Skin tags. (From White GM, Cox NH: Diseases of the skin: a color atlas and text, ed 2, St Louis, 2006, Mosby.)

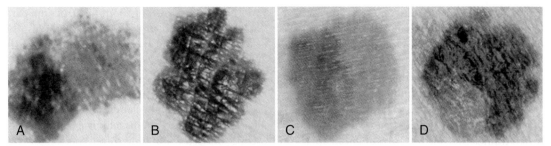

Figure 10-25. The ABCDs of melanoma. A: Asymmetry (one half unlike the other half). B: Border (edges of mole are notched, uneven, or blurred). C: Color varied from one area to another; shades of tan, brown, and black, and sometimes white, red, or blue. D: Diameter larger than ¼ inch or 6 mm (diameter of a pencil eraser). (From Christensen BL: Adult health nursing, ed 5, St Louis, 2006, Mosby.)

is suspected of being precancerous (dysplastic nevus) or cancerous (melanoma). Several methods may be used for mole removal. The most common methods include shave excision, surgical excision, and laser surgery. The method used depends on the type of mole being removed, including its size, shape and color, and location. In some cases, a biopsy of the mole is taken before the mole is removed to determine whether the mole is benign or malignant.

Mole Shave Excision Setup

The items required for a shave excision setup are listed.

Items Placed to Side of the Sterile Field

- Clean disposable gloves
- Antiseptic solution
- Surgical scrub brush
- Container with water
- Sterile 4 × 4 gauze
- Antiseptic swabs
- Sterile gloves
- Local anesthetic
- Antiseptic wipe to cleanse the vial
- Electrocautery instrument
- Specimen container with preservative and label
- Laboratory request form

Items Placed on the Sterile Field

- Fenestrated drape
- Needle and syringe for drawing up the local anesthetic
- Scalpel and blade
- Sterile 4 × 4 gauze

Procedure: Mole Shave Excision

A shave excision is most commonly used to remove protruding moles. It can also be used to remove skin tags. This procedure is not used to remove dysplastic nevi because it might leave mole cells beneath the surface of the skin, which could cause the mole to grow back again. Sutures are not generally required for a shave excision. After the numbing effect of the anesthetic wears off, the area will be tender and sore. As healing occurs, a scab forms, which usually falls off within 1 to 2 weeks, leaving a red mark. As healing progresses, a flat, white mark usu-

ally remains in the place of the mole, which is approximately the same size as the mole. Over time, it fades to a barely visible scar. A mole is removed using the shave excision procedure as follows:

1. The physician numbs the area with a local anesthetic.
2. The physician uses a scalpel to shave off the protruding part of the mole until the area is flush with the level of the surrounding skin.
3. The physician may use an electrocautery instrument to destroy the tissue below the surface of the mole and to control bleeding.
4. A topical antibiotic is applied to the area.
5. A sterile dressing is applied to the operative site.
6. The mole shavings may be placed in a specimen container with a preservative and sent to the laboratory for examination by a pathologist.

Surgical Mole Excision Setup

The items required for a surgical excision setup are listed.

Items Placed to Side of the Sterile Field

- Clean disposable gloves
- Antiseptic solution
- Surgical scrub brush
- Container with water
- Sterile 4 × 4 gauze
- Antiseptic swabs
- Sterile gloves
- Local anesthetic
- Antiseptic wipe to cleanse the vial
- Electrocautery instrument
- Specimen container with preservative and label
- Laboratory request form

Items Placed on the Sterile Field

- Fenestrated drape
- Needle and syringe for drawing up the local anesthetic
- Scalpel and blade
- Tissue forceps
- Operating scissors
- Needle holder
- Sutures
- Sterile 4 × 4 gauze

Procedure: Surgical Mole Excision

The surgical excision procedure is often used when the physician suspects that a mole is precancerous or cancerous. A scalpel is used to remove the entire mole, as well as a border of surrounding skin and tissue underlying the mole, to remove all the mole cells. A scar commonly forms after this procedure; however, it usually fades over time. A mole is removed using the surgical excision procedure as follows:

1. The physician numbs the area with a local anesthetic.
2. The physician uses a scalpel to cut an oval border surrounding the mole and removes the mole with tissue forceps.
3. The physician may use an electrocautery instrument to control bleeding.
4. The physician inserts sutures to close the surgical incision.
5. A sterile dressing is applied to the operative site.
6. The mole is placed in a specimen container with a preservative and is sent to the laboratory for examination by a pathologist.

Postoperative Instructions: Shave Excision and Surgical Excision

Postoperative instructions for both a shave excision and a surgical excision of a mole include the following:

1. Keep the dressing clean and dry.
2. Report any signs that the wound is infected, which include fever, increased pain, swelling, redness, warmth, and discharge.
3. If sutures have been inserted, notify the medical office if they become loose or break.
4. To reduce scarring, protect the area from the ultraviolet (UV) rays of the sun by staying out of the sun or using a good sunscreen with a sun protection factor (SPF) of 15 or higher.

Provide the patient with written instructions on wound care to refer to at home. If sutures have been inserted, instruct the patient when to return for removal of the sutures.

Laser Mole Surgery

Laser surgery is used to remove small or flat moles that are brown or black in color. This procedure involves the use of a laser beam of light, which evaporates the mole tissue. The laser beam also seals off blood vessels, which avoids the need for sutures. Because the laser light cannot penetrate deeply enough, this method generally is not used on raised moles, deep moles, large moles, or dysplastic nevi.

Removing a mole with a laser reduces the amount of tissue destruction in the surrounding tissue, which minimizes scarring. This procedure does not require a local anesthetic. No pain is involved during the procedure; the patient feels only a mild tingling when the laser pulses. A scab forms, which usually falls off within 1 to 2 weeks. Once the scab falls off, the area is usually reddish, and it may take several weeks before normal skin color returns. Repeated treatments (one to three) may be required before the mole is completely removed.

The medical assistant should instruct the patient to keep the area clean and dry. The area should also be protected from the UV rays of the sun by staying out of the sun or by using a good sunscreen with an SPF of 15 or higher.

Needle Biopsy

A **biopsy** is the removal and examination of tissue from the living body. The tissue usually is examined under a microscope. Biopsies are most often performed to determine whether a tumor is malignant or benign; however, a biopsy also may be used as a diagnostic aid for other conditions, such as infections. A **needle biopsy** is a type of biopsy in which tissue from deep within the body is obtained by the insertion of a biopsy needle through the skin. A biopsy needle consists of an outer needle for making the puncture and a forked inner needle for obtaining the tissue specimen (Figure 10-26, *A*). The inner needle detaches tissue from a part of the body and brings it to the surface through its lumen (Figure 10-26, *B*). The advantage of a needle biopsy is that a sample of tissue can be obtained that might otherwise require a major surgical operation.

Needle Biopsy Setup

The items required for a needle biopsy are listed.

Items Placed to the Side of the Sterile Field

- Clean disposable gloves
- Antiseptic solution
- Surgical scrub brush
- Antiseptic swabs
- Sterile gloves
- Local anesthetic
- Antiseptic wipe to cleanse the vial
- Specimen container with preservative and label
- Laboratory request form
- Surgical tape

Items Included on the Sterile Field

- Fenestrated drape
- Needle and syringe for drawing up the local anesthetic
- Biopsy needle
- Sterile 4 × 4 gauze

Procedure: Needle Biopsy

1. The procedure is performed with the patient under a local anesthetic, and because an incision is not required, the patient does not have to undergo the discomfort and inconvenience of an operative recovery.
2. The tissue specimen is placed in a container with a preservative and is sent to the laboratory for examination by a pathologist.
3. A small dressing, placed over the needle puncture site, is usually sufficient to protect the operative site and promote healing.
4. After the procedure, the patient should be observed for any evidence of complications related to the procedure.

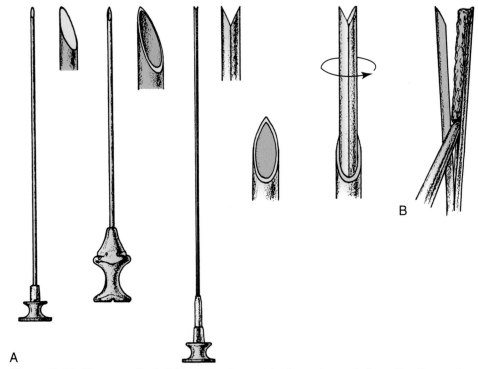

A

B

Figure 10-26. Biopsy needle. **A,** A biopsy needle consists of an outer needle for making the puncture and a forked inner needle for obtaining the specimen. **B,** The inner needle detaches tissue from a part of the body and brings it to the surface through its lumen. (Modified from Nealon TF Jr: Fundamental skills in surgery, ed 4, Philadelphia, 1994, Saunders.)

Postoperative Instructions: Needle Biopsy

1. A bruise typically occurs at the biopsy site and will gradually disappear within several weeks.
2. Keep the dressing clean and dry.
3. Rest and avoid strenuous activity and heavy lifting for 2 days following the procedure.
4. Report any signs that the wound is infected, which include fever, increased pain, swelling, redness, warmth, and discharge.

Ingrown Toenail Removal

An ingrown toenail occurs when the edge of the toenail grows deeply into the nail groove and penetrates the surrounding skin, resulting in pain and discomfort to the patient (Figure 10-27, *A*). An ingrown nail can occur in both the nails of the hands and feet; however, it is most apt to occur in the toenails. External pressure, such as from tight shoes, or from trauma, improper nail trimming, or infection, can cause an ingrown toenail. The protruding nail acts as a foreign body, usually resulting in secondary infection and inflammation. In mild cases, this condition is treated by inserting a small piece of cotton packing under the toenail to raise the nail edge away from the tissue of the nail groove (Figure 10-27, *B*). In severe and recurring cases, part of the nail must be surgically removed (Figure 10-27, *C* and *D*). Severe cases cause pain, swelling,

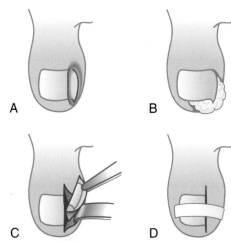

A   B

C   D

Figure 10-27. Ingrown toenail. **A,** The edge of the toenail grows deeply into the nail groove. **B,** In mild cases, treatment consists of inserting a small piece of cotton packing under the toenail. **C,** In severe and recurring cases, a wedge of the nail is surgically removed. **D,** A strip of surgical tape is applied over the area. (From Nealon TF Jr: Fundamental skills in surgery, ed 4, Philadelphia, 1994, Saunders.)

redness, and drainage (Figure 10-28). The toenail removal procedure relieves pain by decreasing nail pressure on the soft tissues.

Ingrown Toenail Removal Setup

The items required for removal of an ingrown toenail are listed.

Items Placed to the Side of the Sterile Field
- Clean disposable gloves
- Antiseptic solution
- Surgical scrub brush
- Antiseptic swabs
- Sterile gloves
- Local anesthetic
- Antiseptic wipe to cleanse the vial
- Antibiotic ointment
- Surgical tape

Items Included on the Sterile Field
- Fenestrated drape
- Needle and syringe for drawing up the local anesthetic
- Surgical toenail scissors
- Hemostatic forceps
- Operating scissors
- Sterile 4 × 4 gauze

Procedure: Ingrown Toenail

An ingrown toenail is removed as follows:
1. Before the surgical procedure is performed, the affected foot must be soaked in tepid water containing an antibacterial skin solution for 10 to 15 minutes to soften the nail plate and decrease the possibility of bacterial infection.
2. The patient is placed in a reclining position with the foot adequately supported, and the toe is shaved to remove hair, which would act as a contaminant.
3. An antiseptic is applied to the affected toe, which is then numbed using a local anesthetic.
4. Using surgical toenail scissors, the physician surgically removes a wedge of the nail (see Figure 10-27, *C*).

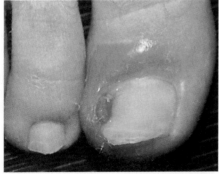

Figure 10-28. Ingrown toenail. (From Seidel HM: Mosby's guide to physical examination, ed 6, St Louis, 2006, Mosby.)

5. An antibiotic ointment is applied to the area.
6. A sterile gauze dressing or a strip of surgical tape is applied over the area to protect the operative site and to promote healing (see Figure 10-27, *D*).

Postoperative Instructions: Ingrown Toenail

Postoperative instructions include the following:
1. Elevate the foot for 24 hours following the procedure.
2. Keep the area clean and dry.
3. Cleanse the toe daily with warm water and gently dry the area.
4. Apply an antibiotic ointment daily until the wound has completely healed.
5. Wear loose-fitting shoes for 2 weeks following the procedure.
6. Avoid strenuous exercise for 2 weeks following the procedure.
7. Contact the medical office if any signs of infection occur, which include increasing pain, redness, swelling, and drainage from the toe.

Provide the patient with written instructions on wound care to refer to at home, and instruct the patient on the importance of wearing properly fitting shoes and on the proper procedure for nail trimming. The nail should be cut straight across with the corners of the nail protruding from the end of the toe.

Colposcopy

Colposcopy is the visual examination of the vagina and cervix by means of a lighted instrument with a binocular magnifying lens, known as a **colposcope** (Figure 10-29). The purpose of colposcopy is to examine the vagina and cervix to detect areas of abnormal tissue growth that may not be visible with the naked eye (Figure 10-30). Colposcopy is performed following abnormal Pap test results and to evaluate a vaginal or cervical lesion observed during a pelvic examination. The primary goal of colposcopy is to prevent cervical cancer by detecting precancerous lesions early and treating them.

Blood cells make it more difficult for the physician to observe the cervix; therefore, a colposcopy is usually performed 1 week after the end of the menstrual period. To prepare for the procedure, the patient should be told not to douche; use tampons, vaginal medications, or spermicides; or have intercourse for 24 hours before the examination. The lens of the colposcope is positioned approximately 12 inches (30 cm) from the opening of the vagina. The lens magnifies tissue, facilitating the inspection of cervical cells and the obtaining of a biopsy specimen. For a routine colposcopic examination, a magnification ranging from 6× to 15× is generally used. The colposcope may be placed on an adjustable stand or attached to the side of the examining table and swung out before use.

Colposcopy Setup

The items required for colposcopy are listed.

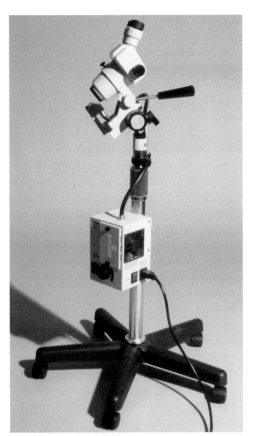

Figure 10-29. A colposcope. (From Apgar BS, Brotzman GL, Spitzer M: Colposcopy: principles and practice—an integrated textbook and atlas, Philadelphia, 2002, Saunders.)

Items Placed to the Side of the Sterile Field
- Colposcope
- Sterile gloves
- Normal saline
- Acetic acid (3%)
- Lugol's iodine solution

Items Included on the Sterile Field
- Vaginal speculum
- Long, sterile, cotton-tipped applicators
- Uterine tenaculum
- Uterine dressing forceps

Procedure: Colposcopy

Colposcopy is performed as follows:

1. The patient is assisted into a lithotomy position and is prepared as for a pelvic examination.
2. The physician inserts a vaginal speculum into the vagina.
3. A long, cotton-tipped applicator moistened with saline is used to wipe the cervix to remove the mucous film that normally covers it. The saline also provides better visualization of the cervical epithelium because dry cervical epithelium is not transparent and does not allow satisfactory viewing of the vascular pattern of the cervix.
4. The colposcope is focused on the cervix, and the physician inspects the saline-moistened cervix.
5. The cervix is swabbed with acetic acid, using a long, cotton-tipped applicator. The acetic acid dissolves cervical mucus and other secretions. It also causes abnormal tissue to turn white, which allows easier visualization of abnormal areas of the cervix.
6. The cervical epithelium also may be stained with Lugol's iodine solution using a long, cotton-tipped applicator. This provides another means to identify unhealthy epithelium. The healthy epithelium of the cervix contains glycogen, which is able to absorb the iodine, causing the epithelium to stain a dark brown color. Conversely, abnormal epithelium, such as would constitute a malignancy, does not contain glycogen and is unable to absorb the iodine.
7. If an abnormal area is observed, the physician obtains a cervical biopsy specimen using punch biopsy forceps, which is described next.

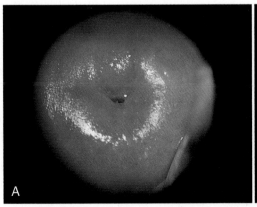
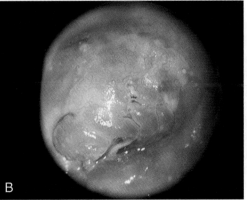

Figure 10-30. **A,** Normal cervix. **B,** Abnormal cervix. (From Damjanov I: Pathology for the health-related professions, ed 3, St Louis, 2006, Saunders.)

Cervical Punch Biopsy

A cervical biopsy is performed in combination with colposcopy to remove a cervical tissue specimen for examination by a pathologist. The purpose of the biopsy is to detect the presence of cervical dysplasia or cancer of the cervix. *Cervical dysplasia* is an abnormal growth of cells on the surface of the cervix that are precancerous. *Precancerous* means that abnormal cells have the potential to develop into cancer in the future. Cervical dysplasia can range from mild, to moderate, to severe. A cervical punch biopsy can also be used to diagnose polyps on the cervix and genital warts. Genital warts may indicate infection with human papillomavirus (HPV), which is a risk factor for developing cervical cancer. Performing a cervical punch biopsy helps the physician determine the type of abnormal tissue present on the cervix, so that the physician can determine the best form of treatment for the patient's condition.

Cervical biopsies are most frequently performed following abnormal Pap test results. Although an abnormal Pap test result is a cause for concern, the majority of abnormal Pap tests are not caused by cervical cancer, but rather by a vaginal infection. To prevent inaccurate test results, the cervical biopsy is usually performed 1 week after the end of the menstrual period, when the cervix is the least vascular. To prepare for the procedure, the patient should be told not to douche; use tampons, vaginal medications, or spermicides; or have intercourse for 24 hours before the procedure to prevent inaccurate test results.

Cervical Punch Biopsy Setup

The items required for a cervical punch biopsy are listed.

Items Placed to the Side of the Sterile Field
- Colposcope
- Sterile gloves
- Lugol's iodine solution
- Monsel's solution
- Specimen container with preservative and label
- Laboratory request form
- Sanitary pad

What Would You Do? What Would You *Not* Do?

Case Study 3

Sadira Wisal has been referred to the office by her family physician for a colposcopy. Her last Pap test came back as abnormal, and a repeat Pap test 3 months later also was abnormal. While having her vital signs taken, Sadira bursts into tears. She tearfully explains that she's afraid that she has cancer, and that no one at her regular physician's office told her what to expect from this procedure. Sadira does not understand why she has to have this procedure done, and she does not know what the physician will be doing during the procedure. She says that she feels stupid, but she does not even know what a cervix is. Sadira also worries that the procedure will affect her ability to have children. ■

Items Included on the Sterile Field
- Vaginal speculum
- Long, sterile, cotton-tipped applicators
- Cervical punch biopsy forceps
- Uterine dressing forceps
- Uterine tenaculum
- Sterile 4 × 4 gauze

Procedure: Cervical Punch Biopsy

A cervical punch biopsy is performed as follows:

1. The patient is positioned and draped in a lithotomy position. An anesthetic is not needed because the cervix has few pain receptors. The patient may experience no discomfort during the procedure or a certain amount of discomfort ranging from mild to moderate in intensity. Some patients experience mild cramping and pinching when the specimen is being removed from the cervix.
2. The physician inserts a vaginal speculum into the vagina for proper visualization of the cervix.
3. The cervix is wiped with saline and then swabbed with ascetic acid.
4. To assist in obtaining the specimen, the physician may stain the cervix with Lugol's iodine solution.
5. The colposcope is focused on the cervix, and the physician inspects the cervix.
6. Using cervical biopsy punch forceps, the physician obtains several tissue specimens (Figure 10-31, *A*) from the abnormal cervical epithelium (Figure 10-31, *B*). The patient may feel a pinching sensation and mild cramps each time a specimen is removed from the cervix.
7. The specimen is placed in a container with a preservative and is sent to the laboratory for examination by a pathologist.
8. If bleeding occurs, the physician controls it with gauze packing, a hemostatic solution (e.g., Monsel's solution), or electrocautery.
9. The patient is given a sanitary pad at the office after the procedure to absorb any discharge.

Postoperative Instructions: Cervical Punch Biopsy

Postoperative instructions include the following:

1. A minimum amount of cramping and bleeding may follow the procedure and last up to 1 week. Contact the medical office if the bleeding lasts longer than 2 weeks.
2. If Monsel's solution is used to control bleeding, a thick, dark-colored vaginal discharge may occur following the procedure and may last for several days.
3. Do not douche, use tampons, or have intercourse for 1 week following the procedure to allow proper healing of the cervix to take place.
4. Contact the medical office if any of the following occurs: bleeding that is heavier than normal menstrual bleeding, a foul-smelling vaginal discharge, fever, or lower abdominal pain.

Provide the patient with written instructions to refer to at home. An appointment is scheduled approximately 1 week

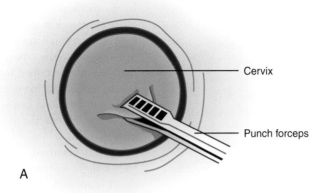

A

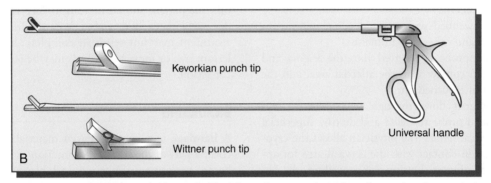

B

Figure 10-31. Cervical punch biopsy. **A,** Obtaining a tissue specimen from the cervix using cervical biopsy punch forceps. **B,** Cervical biopsy punch forceps. (Courtesy Elmed, Addison, Ill.)

following the procedure to make sure that healing is taking place and to discuss the biopsy results.

Cryosurgery

Cervical Cryosurgery

Cervical **cryosurgery,** also known as *cryotherapy,* uses freezing temperatures to treat certain gynecologic conditions. Cryosurgery is most often performed as a treatment for cervical dysplasia to destroy abnormal cervical cells that show changes that may lead to cancer. Cryosurgery is done only after a colposcopy confirms the presence of cervical dysplasia. Cryosurgery is also used for the treatment of chronic cervicitis, which is inflammation of the cervix.

Cervical cryosurgery can be performed without an anesthetic, although occasionally a mild analgesic is necessary immediately afterward. The cryosurgery unit consists of a long metal cryoprobe attached to a cooling-agent tank (Figure 10-32). The principal cooling agents are liquid nitrogen and compressed nitrogen gas. The cryoprobe is inserted into the vagina and placed firmly in contact with the abnormal area. The cooling agent flows through the cryoprobe, freezing the cervical tissue to $-20°$ C. This causes the abnormal cells to die and slough off so that the cervical covering can eventually be replaced with new, healthy epithelial tissue. Regeneration of cervical tissue occurs within approximately 4 to 6 weeks after the procedure. Following

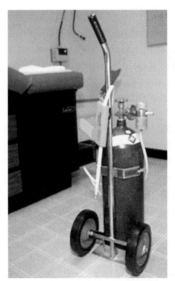

Figure 10-32. Cryosurgery unit. (From Zakus S: Clinical skills for medical assistants, ed 4, Philadelphia, 2001, Saunders.)

cryosurgery, the patient will be required to have a Pap test every 3 to 6 months for a period of time determined by the physician.

Cryosurgery Setup

The items required for cryosurgery are listed.

Items Placed to the Side of the Sterile Field
- Cryosurgery unit
- Sanitary pads

Items Included on the Sterile Field
- Vaginal speculum
- Acid-saline solution
- Long, cotton-tipped applicators

Procedure: Cervical Cryosurgery

Cryosurgery is performed as follows:
1. The patient is draped and assisted into the lithotomy position.
2. The physician inserts a vaginal speculum for proper visualization of the cervix.
3. The cervix is swabbed with an acid-saline solution to remove mucus and other contaminants.
4. The metal cryoprobe is inserted into the vagina and placed firmly in contact with the affected area, and the cryosurgery unit is turned on.
5. The cooling agent flows through the cryoprobe and causes the metal probe to freeze and destroy superficial abnormal cervical tissue. The physician allows the cryoprobe to come in contact with the cervical area for approximately 3 minutes. During the procedure, the patient may experience some pain resembling menstrual cramping.
6. The cryoprobe is removed for 3 to 5 minutes to permit the cervical tissue to return to its normal temperature. The freezing procedure is then repeated for an additional 3 minutes.
7. When the procedure has been completed, the medical assistant should assist the patient as necessary and observe her for signs of discomfort or vertigo.
8. The patient is given a sanitary pad at the office after the procedure to absorb any discharge.

Postoperative Instructions: Cervical Cryosurgery

Postoperative instructions include the following:
1. Normal activities can be resumed the day following the cryosurgery.
2. On the first postoperative day, a clear, watery vaginal discharge occurs, which lasts for 2 to 4 weeks. The discharge is caused by the shedding of the dead cervical tissue and gradually diminishes as the healing progresses.
3. Use sanitary pads (rather than tampons) to absorb the watery discharge.
4. Do not douche, use tampons, or have intercourse for 2 to 3 weeks following the procedure to allow proper healing of the cervix to take place.
5. Contact the medical office if any of the following occurs: bleeding that is heavier than normal menstrual bleeding, a foul-smelling vaginal discharge, fever, or lower abdominal pain.

Provide the patient with written instructions to refer to at home. The patient must schedule a return visit 6 weeks after the procedure to ensure that proper healing has occurred.

Skin Lesions

In the medical office, cryosurgery also may be used to remove benign skin lesions, such as common warts and skin tags. Only a small amount of cooling agent is required for skin lesions, so the cryosurgery unit is considerably smaller than the one described for cervical cryosurgery. Most physicians use liquid nitrogen contained in a small, pressurized, stainless steel canister with an attached probe. The physician applies the liquid nitrogen to the skin lesion until it turns white, which indicates that freezing of the tissue has occurred. During the procedure, the patient feels a slight burning or stinging sensation as the cooling agent is applied. After cryosurgery, a blister develops and dries to a scab in 1 week to 10 days and eventually sloughs off. The patient should be told to keep the area clean and dry until the scab has sloughed off. In some cases, the treatment may not result in complete destruction of the lesion; two or more treatments may be required to remove the lesion.

BANDAGING

A **bandage** is a strip of woven material used to wrap or cover a part of the body. The function of the bandage may be to apply pressure to control bleeding, to protect a wound from contamination, to hold a dressing in place, or to protect, support, or immobilize an injured part of the body.

Guidelines for Application

The bandage should be applied so that it feels comfortable to the patient, and it must be fastened securely with metal clips or adhesive tape. Guidelines for applying a bandage are as follows:
1. Observe the principles of medical asepsis during the application of a bandage.
2. Ensure that the area to which a bandage is applied is clean and dry.
3. Do not apply a bandage directly over an open wound. To prevent contamination of the wound, apply first a sterile dressing and then the bandage. The bandage should extend at least 2 inches (5 cm) beyond the edge of the dressing,
4. To prevent irritation, do not allow the skin surfaces of two body parts (e.g., two fingers) to touch. In addition, the patient's perspiration provides a moist environment that encourages the growth of microorganisms. A piece of gauze should be inserted between the two body parts.
5. Ensure that joints and prominent parts of bones are padded to prevent the bandage from rubbing the skin and causing irritation.
6. Bandage the body part in its normal position with joints slightly flexed to avoid muscle strain.
7. Apply the bandage from the distal to the proximal part of the body to aid the venous return of blood to the heart.

8. As you apply the bandage, ask the patient whether it feels comfortable. The bandage should fit snugly enough that it does not fall off, but not so tightly that it impedes circulation.

9. If possible, leave the fingers and toes exposed when bandaging an extremity. This provides the opportunity to check them for signs of impairment in circulation. Signs indicating that the bandage is too tight include coldness, pallor, numbness, cyanosis of the nail beds, swelling, pain, and tingling sensations. If any of these signs occurs, loosen the bandage immediately.

10. If a bandage roll is dropped during the procedure, obtain a new bandage and begin again.

Types of Bandages

Three basic types of bandages are used in the medical office. A *roller bandage* is a long strip of soft material wound on itself to form a roll. It ranges from ½ to 6 inches (1.3 to 15.2 cm) wide and from 2 to 5 yards (1.83 to 4.57 m) long. The width used depends on the part being bandaged. Roller bandages usually are made of sterilized gauze. Gauze is porous and lightweight, molds easily to a body part, and is relatively inexpensive and easily disposed of. Because it is made of loosely woven cotton, however, it may slip and fray

easily. *Kling gauze* is a special type of gauze that stretches; this allows it to cling, and, as a result, it molds and conforms better to the body part than does regular gauze.

Elastic bandages are made of woven cotton that contains elastic fibers. One brand name of elastic bandages is the Ace bandage. Although elastic bandages are expensive, they can be washed and used again. The medical assistant must be extremely careful when applying an elastic bandage because it is easy to apply it too tightly and impede circulation. Elastic adhesive bandages also may be used; these have an adhesive backing to provide a secure fit.

Bandage Turns

Five basic bandage turns are used, alone or in combination. The type of turn used depends on which body part is to be bandaged, and whether the bandage is used for support or immobilization or for holding a dressing in place.

The *circular turn* is applied to a part of uniform width, such as toes, fingers, or the head. Each turn completely overlaps the previous turn. Two circular turns are used to anchor a bandage at the beginning and end of a spiral, spiral-reverse, figure-eight, or recurrent turn (Figure 10-33).

The *spiral turn* is applied to a part of uniform circumference, such as the fingers, arms, legs, chest, or abdomen.

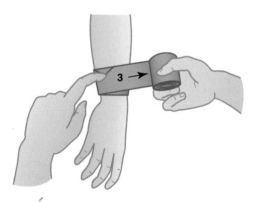

1. Place the end of the roller bandage on a slant.

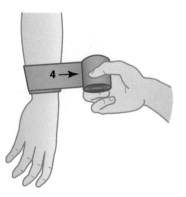

2. Encircle the part while allowing the corner of the bandage to extend.

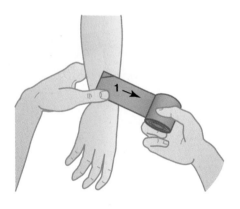

3. Turn down the corner of the bandage.

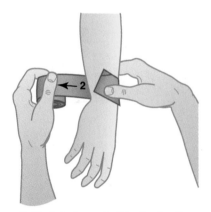

4. Make another circular turn around the part.

Figure 10-33. Procedure for anchoring a bandage.

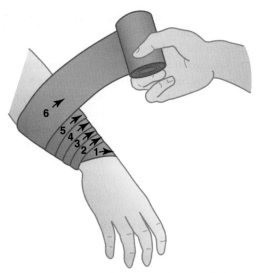

Figure 10-34. Procedure for making the spiral turn.

Each spiral turn is carried upward at a slight angle and should overlap the previous turn by one-half to two-thirds the width of the bandage (Figure 10-34).

The *spiral-reverse turn* is useful for bandaging a part that varies in width, such as the forearm or lower leg. Reversing each spiral turn allows for a smoother fit and prevents gaping caused by variation in the contour of the limb. The thumb is used to make the reverse halfway through each spiral turn. The bandage is directed downward and folded on itself while it is kept parallel to the lower edge of the previous turn. Each turn should overlap the previous one by two-thirds the width of the bandage. The reverse turn is used as often as necessary to provide a uniform fit (Figure 10-35).

The *figure-eight turn* generally is used to hold a dressing in place or to support and immobilize an injured joint, such as the ankle, knee, elbow, or wrist. The figure-eight turn consists of slanting turns that alternately ascend and descend around the part and cross over one another in the middle, resembling the figure eight. Each turn overlaps the previous one by two-thirds the width of the bandage (Figure 10-36).

The *recurrent turn* is a series of back-and-forth turns used to bandage the tips of fingers or toes, the stump of an amputated extremity, or the head. The bandage is anchored by using two circular turns and is passed back and forth over the tip of the part to be bandaged, first on one side and then on the other side of the first center turn. Each turn should overlap the previous turn by two-thirds the width of the bandage (Figure 10-37).

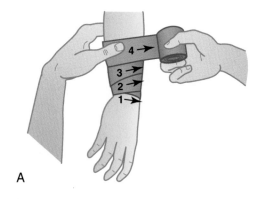

A

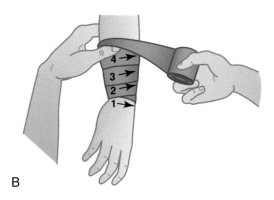

B

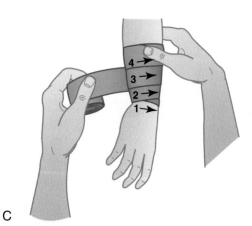

C

Figure 10-35. Procedure for making the spiral-reverse turn. **A,** Encircle the part while keeping the bandage at a slant. **B,** Reverse the spiral turn using the thumb or index finger, and direct the bandage downward to fold it on itself. **C,** Keep the bandage parallel to the lower edge of the previous turn.

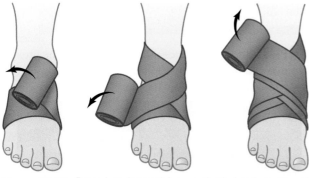

Figure 10-36. Procedure for applying an elastic bandage around the ankle using a figure-eight turn. (From Leake MJ: A manual of simple nursing procedures, Philadelphia, 1971, Saunders.)

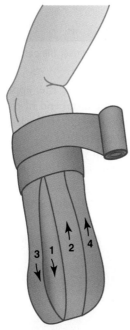

Figure 10-37. Procedure for using the recurrent turn to bandage the end of a stump.

Tubular Gauze Bandages

A tubular gauze bandage consists of seamless elasticized gauze fabric dispensed in a roll. It is used to cover round body parts, such as fingers, toes, arms, and legs, and fits like a sleeve. This type of bandage is easier to apply than a roller bandage and it adheres more securely to the body part. Tubular gauze is not sterile and should not be applied over open wounds; however, it can be applied over a sterile dressing to hold it in place. The gauze is available in varying widths; selection of the width is based on the body part to be bandaged. Table 10-1 lists tubular gauze widths and the body parts each size can be used to bandage.

The gauze is applied by means of a plastic or metal frame–like applicator, which comes in different sizes. The applicator must be larger than the part to be bandaged to allow the gauze to slide easily over the body part. To assist in selecting the proper gauze width, each applicator is marked with a size that corresponds to the size on the tubular gauze bandage box. Procedure 10-8 outlines the method for applying a tubular gauze bandage to a finger.

PROCEDURE 10-8

Table 10-1	Tubular Gauze Bandage Widths and Recommended Application Sites
Width, inches	**Recommended Application Sites**
$\frac{5}{8}$	Fingers and toes of infants Small fingers and toes of adults
1	Hands and feet of infants Fingers and toes of adults Over bulky dressings
$1\frac{1}{2}$	Arms and legs of infants Arms and feet of children Small hands, arms, and feet of adults
$2\frac{5}{8}$	Legs, thighs, and heads of children Arms and lower legs of adults Small thighs and small heads of adults
$3\frac{5}{8}$	Legs, thighs, lower legs, shoulders, arms, and heads of adults Trunks of infants
5	Large heads and small trunks of adults
7	Trunks of adults

PROCEDURE 10-8   Applying a Tubular Gauze Bandage

Outcome Apply a tubular gauze bandage.

Equipment/Supplies

- Applicator
- Roll of tubular gauze
- Adhesive tape
- Bandage scissors

Continued

PROCEDURE 10-8   Applying a Tubular Gauze Bandage—cont'd

1. **Procedural Step.** Sanitize your hands. Greet the patient by full name and date of birth and introduce yourself. Identify the patient and explain the procedure.

2. **Procedural Step.** Assemble the equipment. The applicator selected should be larger than the part to be bandaged. The proper gauze width must be used to ensure a secure fit.
   Principle. The applicator should be larger than the body part to allow the gauze to slide easily over the body part.

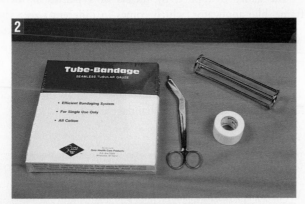

Assemble the equipment.

3. **Procedural Step.** Place the gauze bandage on the applicator as follows:
   a. Pull a sufficient length of gauze from the dispensing box roll.
   b. Spread apart the open end of the gauze, using your fingers.
   c. Slide the gauze over one end of the applicator. Continue loading the applicator by gathering enough gauze on the applicator to complete the bandage.
   d. Cut the roll of gauze near the opening of the box.

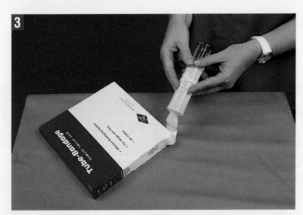

Slide the gauze over one end of the applicator.

4. **Procedural Step.** Place the applicator over the proximal end of the patient's finger.

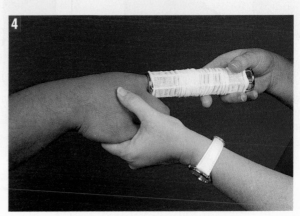

Place the applicator over the patient's finger.

5. **Procedural Step.** Move the applicator from the proximal end to the distal end of the patient's finger, while leaving the bandage on the length of the finger. The bandage should be held in place at the base of the patient's fingers with your fingers.
   Principle. The bandage should be held in place to prevent it from sliding, which would not ensure complete coverage of the affected part.

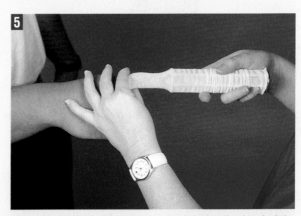

Move the applicator from the proximal to the distal end of the patient's finger.

6. **Procedural Step.** Pull the applicator 1 to 2 inches past the end of the patient's finger. Continue to hold the bandage in place with your fingers.
   Principle. The bandage must extend beyond the length of the patient's finger to secure it at the distal end.

7. **Procedural Step.** Rotate the applicator one full turn to anchor the bandage.
   Principle. Anchoring the bandage holds it securely in place.

PROCEDURE 10-8   Applying a Tubular Gauze Bandage—cont'd

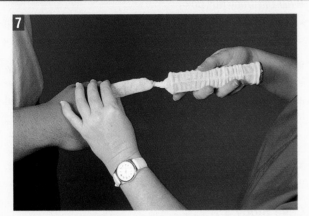

Rotate the applicator one full turn.

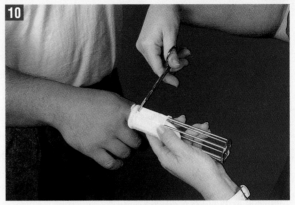

Cut unused gauze from the applicator.

8. **Procedural Step.** Move the applicator forward again toward the proximal end of the patient's finger.
   Principle. Moving the applicator forward applies a second layer of bandaging material to the patient's finger.

9. **Procedural Step.** Move the applicator forward approximately 1 inch past the original starting point of the bandage, and anchor it using another rotating motion.
   Principle. Anchoring the bandage holds it securely in place.

10. **Procedural Step.** Repeat this procedure for the number of layers desired. Finish the last layer at the proximal end. Cut unused gauze from the applicator, and remove the applicator.

11. **Procedural Step.** Apply adhesive tape at the base of the finger to secure the bandage.

12. **Procedural Step.** Sanitize your hands, and record the procedure. Include the date and time and location of the bandage application and any instructions given to the patient.

CHARTING EXAMPLE

Date	
9/30/12	10:00 a.m. Tubular gauze bandage applied
	to ®̃ index finger. Explained bandage care.
	—————————— T. Browning, CMA (AAMA)

evolve *Check out the Evolve site to access additional interactive activities.*

MEDICAL PRACTICE *and the* LAW

Surgical procedures are invasive and painful, and they have the potential for harmful complications and subsequent lawsuits. Before having a surgical procedure performed, the patient must sign a consent to treatment form. It is the medical assistant's responsibility to witness the patient's signature, but it is the physician's responsibility to inform the patient of the procedure to be performed and its risks, alternative procedures, and benefits. The physician may delegate some or all of these tasks to the medical assistant, but *do not* accept this responsibility. Patients cannot sign for themselves if they are minors or if they are impaired by drugs or disease, such as Alzheimer's disease. In these cases, consent must be obtained from the legal guardian or next of kin. Before asking a patient to sign a consent to treatment form, ask whether he or she has any questions. If so, make sure the information is given before the consent is signed. Make sure you know what procedures in your office require informed consent.

During the procedure, your duty is to assist the physician and maintain surgical asepsis. If this is broken, you must inform the physician and remedy the situation. There is no such thing as "almost sterile."

After the surgical procedure, the medical assistant must give the patient home care instructions. Home care must be performed exactly to ensure proper healing. Instructions should be given verbally, demonstrated, and given in writing. Written instructions must be in the correct language and at the patient's reading level. Pictures included with the written instructions can clarify difficult points. Many offices purchase preprinted instructions for common surgical procedures. Make sure the signs of infection are listed on these sheets, along with instructions to call the physician if they occur, or if any other problems or questions arise. ■

What Would You Do? What Would You *Not* Do? RESPONSES

Case Study 1
Page 379

What Did Trudy Do?

❏ Tried to calm and reassure Mrs. Ventura. Told her that children at this age are prone to accidents and that she should not blame herself.

❏ Told Mrs. Ventura that Cory's wound could not be held together effectively with Steri-Strips. Explained that sutures would help the wound heal better.

❏ Told Mrs. Ventura that the doctor could not perform the procedure unless she signs the consent form. Explained that Cory's wound should be sutured as soon as possible to prevent infection and to minimize scarring.

❏ Asked Mrs. Ventura whether she would like to talk with the doctor again about any questions she has about the procedure before signing the form.

What Did Trudy Not Do?

❏ Did not prepare Cory for the suture insertion procedure until Mrs. Ventura signed the consent to treatment form.

What Would You Do?/What Would You *Not* Do? Review Trudy's response and place a checkmark next to the information you included in your response. List additional information you included in your response.

_____
_____
_____
_____

Case Study 2
Page 390

What Did Trudy Do?

❏ Explained to Abbey that the antiseptic contains iodine, which appears orange when it is applied to the skin. Assured her that the iodine would not stain her skin permanently and that it would wear off in a few days.

❏ Calmly and discreetly opened a new pair of sterile gloves so that the physician could reapply sterile gloves. Reminded Abbey not to move during the procedure.

❏ Told Abbey that all tissues removed from patients are routinely sent to the laboratory for a biopsy. Reassured her that the doctor has told her everything he knows about her condition.

❏ Made it clear to Abbey that her neighbor is not permitted to remove her sutures. Stressed to her that the doctor needs to check her incision before the sutures are removed to ensure that proper healing has occurred.

What Did Trudy Not Do?

❏ Did not scold Abbey for contaminating the physician's sterile gloved hand.

What Would You Do?/What Would You *Not* Do? Review Trudy's response and place a checkmark next to the information you included in your response. List additional information you included in your response.

_____
_____
_____
_____

Case Study 3
Page 404

What Did Trudy Do?

❏ Listened empathetically to Sadira, and tried to calm and reassure her.

❏ Spent some time going over the colposcopy procedure and what to expect.

❏ Answered as many of Sadira's questions as possible. Reassured her that a lot of people do not know what a cervix is, and that she was asking some very good questions.

❏ Asked the physician to spend some time talking with Sadira before the procedure to answer the questions that Trudy was not qualified to answer.

❏ Ensured that Sadira understood all of the information about the procedure before asking her to sign a consent to treatment form.

What Did Trudy Not Do?

❏ Did not tell Sadira that her family physician and staff should have spent some time explaining the procedure to her so that she did not have to worry so much.

❏ Did not tell Sadira that she does not have cancer.

What Would You Do?/What Would You *Not* Do? Review Trudy's response and place a checkmark next to the information you included in your response. List additional information you included in your response.

_____
_____
_____
_____

- **Surgical asepsis** refers to practices that keep objects and areas sterile or free of all living microorganisms. It is always employed when caring for broken skin, when a skin surface is being penetrated, and when a body cavity that is normally sterile is entered.

- **During a sterile procedure, specific guidelines** must be followed. Do not allow sterile packages to become wet. A 1-inch border around the sterile field is considered contaminated. Always face the sterile field. Hold all sterile articles above waist level. All sterile items should be placed in the center of the sterile field. Do not spill water or solutions on the sterile field. Do not talk, cough, or sneeze over a sterile field. Do not reach over a sterile field. Do not pass soiled dressings over a sterile field. Always acknowledge if you have contaminated the sterile field.

- **A wound** is a break in the continuity of an external or internal surface caused by physical means. The two basic types of wounds are closed and open. A closed wound involves an injury to the underlying tissue without a break in the skin surface, such as a contusion. An open wound involves a break in the skin surface that exposes the underlying tissues; examples include incisions, lacerations, punctures, and abrasions.

- **The body has a natural healing process** that works to destroy invading microorganisms and to restore the structure and function of the damaged tissue. Wound healing occurs in three phases: inflammatory phase, granulation phase, and maturation phase.

- **The function of a sterile dressing** is to protect a wound from contamination and trauma, to absorb drainage, and to restrict motion, which may interfere with proper wound healing.

- **Sutures** are available in two types: absorbable and nonabsorbable. Absorbable sutures consist of surgical gut or synthetic materials that are gradually digested by tissue enzymes and absorbed by the body's tissues. Nonabsorbable sutures are not absorbed by the body and either remain permanently in the body tissues or are removed. They are made from silk, cotton, linen, nylon, braided polyester, polypropylene, polybutester, stainless steel, and surgical skin staples.

- **Needles for suturing** are categorized as cutting needles (having a sharp point) or noncutting needles (having a round or blunt point). Cutting needles are used for skin, and noncutting needles are used to penetrate tissues that offer a small amount of resistance, such as the viscera, subcutaneous tissue, muscle, and peritoneum. A swaged needle is one in which the suture and needle are one continuous unit.

- **Surgical skin staples** are often used to close wounds. Stapling is the fastest method of closing long skin incisions. In addition, trauma to the tissue is reduced because the tissue does not have to be handled much when inserting the staples.

- **Adhesive skin closures** may be used for wound repair to approximate the edges of a laceration or incision. They are used when not much tension exists on the skin edges. Advantages of adhesive skin closures are that they eliminate the need for skin sutures and a local anesthetic, they are easy to apply and remove, and they result in less scarring than skin sutures.

- **The instruments and supplies for a minor office surgery** depend on the surgery to be performed. Many offices maintain index cards that indicate the appropriate instruments and supplies for each minor office surgery tray setup.

- **The patient's skin must be prepared** before the minor office surgery because the skin contains an abundance of microorganisms. Skin preparation involves shaving the site, scrubbing the site with an antiseptic cleansing solution, and applying an antiseptic.

- **The use of a local anesthetic,** such as Xylocaine, is often required for minor office surgery. Xylocaine with epinephrine prolongs the local effect of the anesthetic and decreases the rate of systemic absorption by constricting blood vessels at the operative site.

- **A sebaceous cyst** is a thin, closed sac or capsule that contains secretions from a sebaceous, or oil, gland. It forms when the outlet of the gland becomes obstructed. A sebaceous cyst is usually painless and nontender and may disappear on its own A sebaceous cyst usually does not require surgical removal unless it becomes infected. Other reasons for removing a sebaceous cyst include cosmetic concerns and to reduce discomfort from a cyst that is located in a body area that is easily irritated, such as the armpit.

- **An abscess** is a collection of pus in a cavity surrounded by inflamed tissue. An abscess serves as a defense mechanism of the body to keep an infection localized by walling off the microorganisms, preventing them from spreading through the body. A furuncle (boil) is a localized staphylococcal infection that originates deep within a hair follicle.

- **A mole** (also known as a nevus) is a small growth on human skin. The most common types of moles are skin tags, flat moles, and raised moles. Moles are removed for a variety of reasons, which include the following: cosmetic to improve an individual's appearance, to reduce irritation and discomfort from a mole that is rubbing against clothing or that is in the way when shaving. A more serious reason for removing a mole is that the mole is suspected of being precancerous (dysplastic nevus) or cancerous (melanoma).The most common methods for mole removal include shave excision, surgical excision, and laser surgery.

Continued

CERTIFICATION REVIEW—cont'd

❏ **A biopsy** is the removal and examination of tissue from the living body. It is most often performed to determine whether a tumor is malignant or benign. A needle biopsy is a type of biopsy in which tissue from deep within the body is obtained by the insertion of a biopsy needle through the skin. The advantage of a needle biopsy is that a sample of tissue can be obtained that might otherwise require a major surgical operation.

❏ **An ingrown toenail** occurs when the edge of the toenail grows deeply into the nail groove and penetrates the surrounding skin, resulting in pain and discomfort to the patient. The protruding nail acts as a foreign body, usually resulting in secondary infection and inflammation. Severe cases cause pain, swelling, redness, and drainage. The toenail removal procedure relieves pain by decreasing nail pressure on the soft tissues.

❏ **Colposcopy** is the visual examination of the vagina and cervix by means of a colposcope, a lighted instrument with a binocular magnifying lens. The purpose of colposcopy is to examine the vagina and cervix to determine areas of abnormal tissue growth. Colposcopy is performed following an abnormal cytology report from a Pap test, to evaluate a vaginal or cervical lesion observed during a pelvic examination. The primary goal of colposcopy is to prevent cervical cancer by detecting precancerous lesions early and treating them.

❏ **A cervical punch biopsy** is usually performed in combination with colposcopy to remove a cervical tissue specimen for examination by a pathologist. The purpose of the biopsy is to detect the presence of cervical dysplasia or cancer of the cervix. Cervical biopsies are often performed following an abnormal Pap test result.

❏ **Cervical cryosurgery** is most often performed as a treatment for cervical dysplasia to destroy abnormal cervical cells that show changes that may lead to cancer. Cryosurgery is also used for the treatment of chronic cervicitis, which is inflammation of the cervix. A cooling agent is applied to the infected area, which causes the cells to die and slough off so that the cervical covering can eventually be replaced with new, healthy epithelial tissue.

❏ **A bandage** is a strip of woven material used to wrap or cover a part of the body. The function of the bandage may be to apply pressure to control bleeding, to protect a wound from contamination, to hold a dressing in place, or to protect, support, or immobilize an injured part of the body.

TERMINOLOGY REVIEW

Medical Term	Word Parts	Definition
Abrasion		A wound in which the outer layers of the skin are damaged; a scrape.
Abscess		A collection of pus in a cavity surrounded by inflamed tissue.
Absorbable suture		Suture material that is gradually digested and absorbed by the body.
Approximation		The process of bringing two parts, such as tissue, together through the use of sutures or other means.
Bandage		A strip of woven material used to wrap or cover a part of the body.
Biopsy	*bi/o:* life *-opsy:* to view	The surgical removal and examination of tissue from the living body. Biopsies are generally performed to determine whether a tumor is benign or malignant.
Capillary action		The action that causes liquid to rise along a wick, a tube, or a gauze dressing.
Colposcope	*colp/o:* vagina *-scope:* instrument used for visual examination	A lighted instrument with a binocular magnifying lens used to examine the vagina and cervix.
Colposcopy	*colp/o:* vagina *-scopy:* visual examination	The visual examination of the vagina and cervix using a colposcope.
Contaminate		As it relates to sterile technique, to cause a sterile object or surface to become unsterile.
Contusion		An injury to the tissues under the skin that causes blood vessels to rupture, allowing blood to seep into the tissues; a bruise.

☺ TERMINOLOGY REVIEW—cont'd

Medical Term	Word Parts	Definition
Cryosurgery	*cry/o:* cold	The therapeutic use of freezing temperatures to destroy abnormal tissue.
Exudate		A discharge produced by the body's tissues.
Fibroblast	*fibr/o:* fibrous tissue *blast:* developing cell	An immature cell from which connective tissue can develop.
Forceps		A two-pronged instrument for grasping and squeezing.
Furuncle		A localized staphylococcal infection that originates deep within a hair follicle. Also known as a *boil.*
Hemostasis	*hem/o:* blood *stasis:* control, stop	The arrest of bleeding by natural or artificial means.
Incision		A clean cut caused by a cutting instrument.
Infection		The condition in which the body, or part of it, is invaded by a pathogen.
Infiltration		The process by which a substance passes into and is deposited within the substance of a cell, tissue, or organ.
Inflammation		A protective response of the body to trauma and the entrance of foreign matter. The purpose of inflammation is to destroy invading microorganisms and to remove damaged tissue debris from the area so that proper healing can occur.
Laceration		A wound in which the tissues are torn apart, leaving ragged and irregular edges.
Ligate		To tie off and close a structure such as a severed blood vessel.
Local anesthetic		A drug that produces a loss of feeling and an inability to perceive pain in only a specific part of the body.
Mayo tray		A broad, flat metal tray placed on a stand and used to hold sterile instruments and supplies when it has been covered with a sterile towel.
Needle biopsy	*bi/o:* life *-opsy:* to view	A type of biopsy in which tissue from deep within the body is obtained by the insertion of a biopsy needle through the skin.
Nonabsorbable suture		Suture material that is not absorbed by the body and either remains permanently in the body tissue and becomes encapsulated by fibrous tissue or is removed.
Postoperative	*post-:* after	After a surgical operation.
Preoperative	*pre-:* before	Preceding a surgical operation.
Puncture		A wound made by a sharp-pointed object piercing the skin.
Scalpel		A surgical knife used to divide tissues.
Scissors		A cutting instrument.
Sebaceous cyst		A thin, closed sac or capsule that contains fatty secretions from a sebaceous gland.
Serum		The clear, straw-colored part of the blood that remains after the solid elements have been separated out of it.
Sterile		Free of all living microorganisms and bacterial spores.
Surgery		The branch of medicine that deals with operative and manual procedures for correction of deformities and defects, repair of injuries, and diagnosis and treatment of certain diseases.
Surgical asepsis	*a:* without or absence of *-sepsis:* infection	Practices that keep objects and areas sterile or free from microorganisms.
Sutures		Material used to approximate tissues with surgical stitches.
Swaged needle		A needle with suturing material permanently attached to its end.
Wound		A break in the continuity of an external or internal surface caused by physical means.

ON THE WEB

For Information on Surgery and Emergency Medicine:

American College of Surgeons: www.facs.org

American Red Cross: www.redcross.org

Ethicon Incorporated: www.ethicon.com

Federal Emergency Management Agency: www.fema.gov

11

Administration of Medication and Intravenous Therapy

LEARNING OBJECTIVES	PROCEDURES
Introduction to the Administration of Medication	
1. Explain the difference between administering, prescribing, and dispensing medication.	Research a drug using the *Physician's Desk Reference* (PDR).
2. State the common routes for administering medication.	Interpret a drug package insert
3. List and describe the six sections of the PDR.	Calculate drug dosage.
4. List and describe the categories of information in a drug package insert.	Complete a prescription form.
5. Describe the Food and Drug Administration's responsibilities with respect to drugs.	Complete a medication record form.
6. List and define the four names of drugs.	
7. Classify drugs according to preparation.	
8. Classify drugs according to the action they have on the body.	
9. List the guidelines for writing metric and apothecary notations.	
10. List and describe the five schedules for controlled drugs.	
11. List and explain the parts of a prescription.	
12. Describe the functions performed by an electronic medical record (EMR) prescription program.	
13. Explain the purpose of a medication record.	
14. Describe the factors that affect the action of drugs in the body.	
15. List and describe the possible adverse effects of medication.	
16. List the guidelines for preparing and administering medication.	
Oral Administration	
1. Explain why the oral route is most frequently used to administer medication.	Prepare and administer oral medications.
2. State where the absorption of most oral medications occurs.	
Parenteral Administration	
1. State the advantages and disadvantages of the parenteral route of administration.	Reconstitute a powdered drug for parenteral administration.
2. Identify the parts of a needle and syringe and explain their functions.	Withdraw medication from a vial.
3. State the ranges of gauge and length of needles for each of the following injections: intradermal, subcutaneous, and intramuscular.	Withdraw medication from an ampule. Locate appropriate subcutaneous injection sites.
4. State the purpose of safety-engineered syringes.	Administer a subcutaneous injection.
5. Describe the dispensing units available for injectable medications.	Locate each of the following intramuscular injection sites: dorsogluteal, deltoid, vastus lateralis, and ventrogluteal.
6. State which tissue layers of the body are used for intradermal, subcutaneous, and intramuscular injections.	Administer an intramuscular injection.
7. List the medications commonly administered through each of the following routes: intradermal subcutaneous, and intramuscular.	Administer an injection using the Z-track method. Administer an intradermal injection.
8. Explain the reason for administering medication with the Z-track method.	

Tuberculin Testing

1. Explain the difference between active and latent tuberculosis.
2. Explain the purpose of tuberculin skin testing.
3. Identify the categories of individuals who should have a tuberculin test.
4. Explain the significance of a positive reaction to a tuberculin test.
5. List the diagnostic procedures that might be performed following a positive tuberculin test.
6. State the guidelines that should be followed when administering and reading a Mantoux test.
7. State the advantages of the tuberculosis blood test.

Allergy Testing

1. Define an allergy, and name common allergens.
2. Explain what occurs during an allergic reaction.
3. List the guidelines for direct skin allergy testing.
4. State the purpose of each of the following types of allergy tests: patch testing, skin-prick testing, intradermal skin testing, and in vitro blood testing.

Intravenous Therapy

1. Explain the advantages of outpatient intravenous (IV) therapy.
2. Identify the role of the entry-level medical assistant in IV therapy.
3. State the indications for outpatient IV therapy.
4. Describe how medication is administered through each of the following methods: direct IV injection, intermittent IV administration, and continuous IV administration.
5. Identify when each of the following medications may be administered intravenously in an outpatient setting: antibiotics, chemotherapy, monoclonal antibodies, and analgesics.
6. State when each of the following may be administered intravenously in an outpatient setting: fluids and electrolytes, nutritional supplements, and blood products.

Administer a Mantoux test, and read the test results.
Complete a tuberculosis test record card.

Perform allergy skin testing.

Introduction to the Administration of Medication
Administering, Prescribing, and Dispensing Medication
Legal Aspects
Routes of Administration
Drug References
Food and Drug Administration
Drug Nomenclature
Classification of Drugs Based on Preparation
  Liquid Preparations
  Solid Preparations
Classification of Drugs Based on Action
Systems of Measurement for Medication
  Metric System
  Apothecary System
  Household System
Converting Units of Measurement
Controlled Drugs
Prescription
  Parts of a Prescription
  Generic Prescribing
  Completing a Prescription Form
  EMR Prescription Program

Medication Record
Factors Affecting Drug Action
  Therapeutic Effect
  Undesirable Effects of Drugs
Guidelines for Preparation and Administration of Medication
Oral Administration
Parenteral Administration
  Parts of a Needle and Syringe
  Safety-Engineered Syringes
  Preparation of Parenteral Medication
  Storage
  Reconstitution of Powdered Drugs
  Subcutaneous Injections
  Intramuscular Injections
  Intradermal Injections
Tuberculin Skin Testing
  Tuberculosis
  Purpose of Tuberculin Testing
  Tuberculin Skin Test Reactions
  Tuberculin Skin Testing Methods
  Mantoux Test

KEY TERMS

adverse reaction (AD-vers ree-AK-shun)
allergen (AL-er-jen)
allergy (AL-er-jee)
ampule (AM-pyool)
anaphylactic reaction (an-uh-ful-AK-tik ree-AK-shun)
autoimmune disease
chemotherapy
controlled drug
conversion (kon-VER-shun)
cubic centimeter (KYOO-bik SEN-tih-mee-ter)
DEA number
dose
drug
enteral nutrition
gauge (GAYJ)
hemophilia
immune globulin
induration (in-dur-AY-shun)
infusion

inhalation (in-hal-AY-shun)
inscription (in-SKRIP-shun)
intradermal injection (in-tra-DER-mal in-JEK-shun)
intramuscular (in-tra-MUS-kyoo-lar) injection
intravenous (in-tra-VEE-nus) (IV) therapy
oral (OR-ul) administration
parenteral (par-EN-ter-al)
pharmacology (far-ma-KOL-oh-jee)
prescription
signatura (sig-na-CHUR-ah)
subcutaneous (sub-kyoo-TAY-nee-us) injection
sublingual (sub-LIN-gwal) administration
subscription (sub-SKRIP-shun)
superscription (soo-per-SKRIP-shun)
topical (TOP-ih-kul) administration
transfusion
vial (VIE-ul)
wheal (WEE-ul)

Introduction to the Administration of Medication

Pharmacology is the study of drugs and includes the preparation, use, and action of drugs in the body. A **drug** is a chemical that is used for the treatment, prevention, or diagnosis of disease. Most drugs are produced synthetically, but they also can be obtained from other sources, such as animals, plants, and minerals.

ADMINISTERING, PRESCRIBING, AND DISPENSING MEDICATION

Medication may be administered, prescribed, or dispensed in the medical office. Medication that is *administered* is actually given to a patient at the office. Medication is *pre-scribed* when a physician provides a patient with a handwritten or computer-generated prescription for a drug to be filled at a pharmacy. Prescriptions also can be telephoned or faxed to the pharmacy by the physician, depending on the preference of the patient. *Dispensed* medication is given to a patient at the office to be taken at home, for example, the physician gives a patient drug samples to take home.

LEGAL ASPECTS

An important responsibility of the medical assistant is the administration of medication. (One should check the laws of the state to ensure that it is legally permissible for the medical assistant to administer medication.) The medical assistant should administer medication only under the direction of the physician. In all states, it is unlawful to administer medication in the medical office without the consent of the physician.

ROUTES OF ADMINISTRATION

[handwritten: Know Routes & what they mean]

[handwritten: under tounge]

Common routes of administration of medication are oral, sublingual, inhalation, rectal, vaginal, topical, intradermal, subcutaneous (SC), intramuscular (IM), and intravenous (IV). The route of administration depends on the type of drug being given, the dosage form, the intended action, and the rapidity of response desired. The route by which medication is most commonly administered in the medical office is the parenteral route. **Parenteral** refers to sites outside the gastrointestinal tract; this term is most commonly used to refer to the administration of medication by injection.

DRUG REFERENCES

The medical assistant is obligated to become familiar with the drugs that are most frequently used in his or her office. It is essential to know their indications, adverse reactions, routes of administration, dosage, and storage. With each drug (including drug samples and injectable medications), the manufacturer includes a *package insert* (PI), which contains valuable information regarding the drug. In addition, many drug references are available. The *Physician's Desk Reference* (PDR) is frequently used in the medical office. The PDR contains information on most major prescription pharmaceutical products available in the United States. The drug information in the PDR consists of the actual drug package insert. Figure 11-1 provides guidelines for using the PDR. These guidelines not only assist in learning how to use the PDR, but they also provide the necessary information for understanding how to interpret drug package inserts. Drug information is also available on the Internet on certain recognized websites; many of these sites are listed at the end of the chapter under the section entitled *On the Web: For Information on Pharmacology.*

FOOD AND DRUG ADMINISTRATION

The U.S. Food and Drug Administration (FDA) is a federal agency in the Department of Health and Human Services. The FDA is responsible for determining whether new food products, drugs, vaccines, medical devices, cosmetics, and other products are safe before they are released for human use.

The FDA determines the safety and effectiveness of prescription and nonprescription (over-the-counter [OTC]) drugs. Pharmaceutical manufacturers are required to submit new drug applications to the FDA for review and approval before products can be released for human use.

The FDA also is responsible for determining whether a medication will be available with or without a prescription. Medications that require a prescription have been determined by the FDA to be safe and effective when used under the guidance of a physician. Prescription medication labels must bear the following statement: *Caution: Federal law prohibits dispensing without a prescription.*

Nonprescription medications are drugs that the FDA determines to be safe and effective for use without physician supervision. Nonprescription medications have a low incidence of adverse reactions when the consumer follows the directions and warnings on the label. Examples of nonprescription medications include mild pain relievers, topical antibiotics, topical corticosteroids, cold medications, and laxatives.

DRUG NOMENCLATURE

[handwritten: know these]

Each drug has four names: chemical, generic, official, and brand (also known as *trade*) names.

1. **Chemical name.** The chemical name provides a precise description of the drug's chemical composition; pharmaceutical manufacturers and pharmacists are most concerned with the chemical makeup of a drug.
2. **Generic name.** The generic name is assigned by the pharmaceutical manufacturer who develops the drug, before it receives official approval by the FDA. The generic name is often a shortened derivative of the chemical name.
3. **Official name.** The official name is the name under which the drug is listed in official publications, such as the *United States Pharmacopeia* (USP) and the *National Formulary* (NF). Official publications set specific standards to regulate the strength, purity, packaging, safety, labeling, and dosage form of each drug. The generic name is frequently used for the official name.
4. **Brand name.** The brand name is the name under which a pharmaceutical manufacturer markets a drug. Because a drug may be manufactured by more than one pharmaceutical company, it may have several brand names. The generic name of a common analgesic is acetaminophen; brand names for this drug include Tylenol, Tempra, Datril, Exdol, Panadol, and Liquiprin.

The medical assistant should be familiar with the generic and brand names of medications commonly prescribed and administered in the medical office.

What Would You Do? What Would You *Not* Do?

Case Study 1

Carol Okasinski, 56 years old, is a new patient. She was a patient of another physician in the community; however, his receptionist was often rude to her, and she decided not to go there anymore. Mrs. Okasinski is obese and has hypertension, type 2 diabetes, osteoarthritis in her hands and knees, and problems with depression. While filling in the health history form, she says she cannot fill in the names of the medications she is taking. She is on a lot of medications prescribed by her previous physician. She says she could not get the childproof pill containers open because of the arthritis in her hands, so she had her husband throw away the childproof containers and transfer each medication into an easy-to-open plastic container. She knows when to take her medications, but she does not know the names of them or why she is taking them. She has brought in a bag with all her medications in their plastic containers. ∎

GUIDELINES FOR USING THE PHYSICIAN'S DESK REFERENCE

The *Physician's Desk Reference* (PDR) is published anually by the Medical Economics Company with the cooperation of the pharmaceutical manufacturers whose products are included in it. This reference includes essential information on most major prescription pharmaceutical products available in the United States. The PDR is divided into sections, which are described below.

SECTION 1: MANUFACTURER'S INDEX

The Manufacturer's Index lists pharmaceutical manufacturers in alphabetical order along with a list of drugs that are manufactured by each company. This index provides all of the necessary information, should the manufacturer need to be contacted regarding a particular drug.

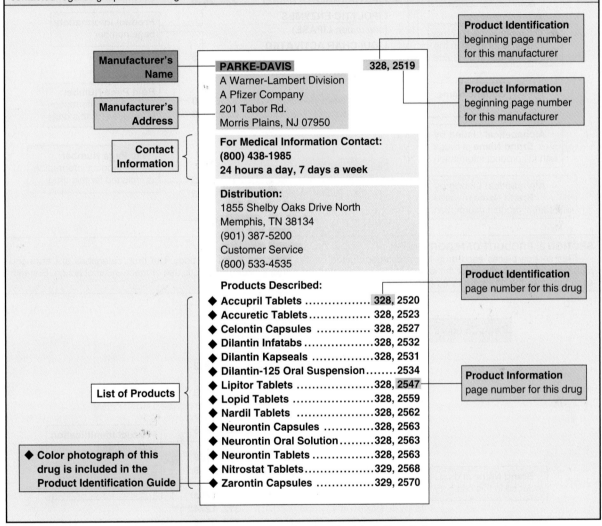

Figure 11-1. Guidelines for using the *Physician's Desk Reference.*

Continued

SECTION 2: BRAND AND GENERIC NAME INDEX
This section consists of an alphabetical listing of the drugs included in the PDR by both generic and brand names. This section allows for the quick and easy location of drug information.

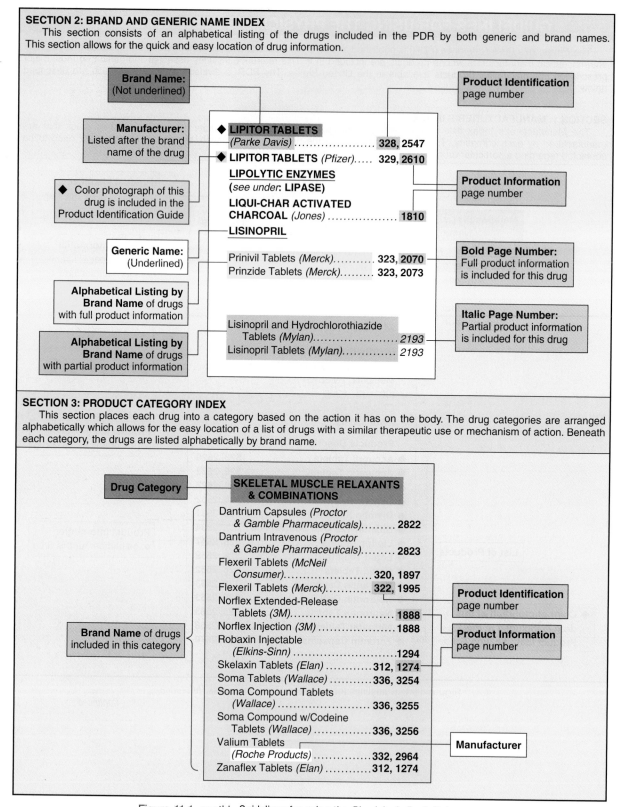

SECTION 3: PRODUCT CATEGORY INDEX
This section places each drug into a category based on the action it has on the body. The drug categories are arranged alphabetically which allows for the easy location of a list of drugs with a similar therapeutic use or mechanism of action. Beneath each category, the drugs are listed alphabetically by brand name.

Figure 11-1, cont'd. Guidelines for using the *Physician's Desk Reference.*

SECTION 4: PRODUCT IDENTIFICATION GUIDE

This section provides a full-color (actual size) photograph of the tablets and capsules included in the PDR.
The drugs are arranged alphabetically by manufacturer. A variety of other dosage forms are also illustrated, but are shown in less than actual size (e.g., inhalers, injectable drugs in vials). This section provides valuable assistance in identifying a drug.

SECTION 5: PRODUCT INFORMATION

This index makes up the main section of the PDR and contains product information on approximately 3000 drug products. The drugs are arranged alphabetically by manufacturer; under the manufacturer, the drugs are listed alphabetically by brand name. The information included in this section consists of the actual drug package inserts. The following information is included for each medication:

DESCRIPTION: This category consists of a general description of the drug and includes the following information: brand name (with pronunciation), generic name, drug category, dosage form (e.g., tablets, capsules), route of administration, chemical name and structural formula, and the inactive ingredients contained in the drug. This category also indicates if the product requires a prescription (Rx) or if it is available over-the-counter (OTC). The symbol C and a Roman numeral appearing next to the drug indicates that it is a scheduled drug and that a prescription written for this drug requires the physician's DEA number.

CLINICAL PHARMACOLOGY: This category describes how the drug functions in the body to produce its therapeutic effect. Also included is an analysis of the absorption, distribution, metabolism, and excretion of the drug after it enters the body.

INDICATIONS AND USAGE: This category presents a list of the conditions that the drug has been formally approved to treat by the U.S. Food and Drug Administration (FDA).

CONTRAINDICATIONS: This category includes situations in which the drug should not be used because the risk of using the drug in these situations outweighs any possible benefit. Contraindications include administration of the drug to patients known to have a hypersensitivity (allergy) to it and use of the drug in patients who have a substantial risk of being harmed by it because of their particular age, sex, concurrent use of another drug, disease state, or condition (e.g., pregnancy).

WARNINGS: This category describes serious adverse reactions and potential safety hazards that may occasionally occur with the use of the drug and what should be done if they occur.

PRECAUTIONS: This category includes information regarding any special care that needs to be taken by the physician for the safe and effective use of the drug. Information typically presented in this category includes:

- **General Precautions:** Lists any disease states or situations that may require special consideration when the drug is being taken.
- **Information for Patients:** Includes information that should be relayed to the patient to ensure safe and effective use of the drug.
- **Laboratory Tests:** Indicates the laboratory tests that may be helpful in following the patient's response to the drug or in identifying possible adverse reactions to the drug.
- **Drug Interactions:** Lists any known interactions of this drug with other drugs that can affect the proper functioning of the drug.
- **Laboratory Test Interactions:** Includes any laboratory tests that may be affected when taking the medication.
- **Pregnancy:** Indicates the pregnancy category of the drug.

ADVERSE REACTIONS: This category describes the unintended and undesirable effects that may occur with the use of the drug. Some adverse reactions are harmless and therefore often tolerated by the patient in order to obtain the therapeutic effect of the drug. Other adverse reactions may be harmful to the patient and warrant discontinuing the medication.

OVERDOSAGE: This category describes symptoms associated with an overdosage of the drug, as well as the complications that can occur and the treatment to institute for an overdosage.

DOSAGE AND ADMINISTRATION: This category lists the recommended adult dosage, the usual dosage range of the drug, and the route of administration (e.g., by mouth, sublingual, IM). Also included is information about the intervals recommended between doses, the usual duration of treatment, and any modification of dosage needed for special groups such as children, the elderly, and patients with renal or hepatic disease.

HOW SUPPLIED: This category indicates the dosage forms that are available (e.g., 20-mg tablets), the units in which the dosage form is available (e.g., bottles of 100; 5-ml multiple-dose vial), information to help identify the dosage form (shape and color), and the handling and storage conditions for the drug.

Figure 11-1, cont'd. Guidelines for using the *Physician's Desk Reference.*

CLASSIFICATION OF DRUGS BASED ON PREPARATION

Drugs are available in two basic forms: liquid and solid. A medication may be available in both these forms (liquid and solid), which permits it to be administered to different types of patients. A liquid preparation of an antibiotic is administered to young children, and the solid preparation (e.g., tablets) of the same medication is administered to older children and adults. The following list includes the common categories of drugs based on preparation.

Liquid Preparations

Elixir   A drug that is dissolved in a solution of alcohol and water. Elixirs are sweetened and flavored and are taken orally. *Example:* Dimetapp elixir.

Emulsion   A mixture of fats or oils in water. *Example:* Durezol ophthalmic emulsion

Liniment   A drug combined with oil, soap, alcohol, or water. Liniments are applied externally, using friction, to produce a feeling of heat or warmth. *Example:* Heet liniment.

Lotion   An aqueous preparation that contains suspended ingredients. Lotions are used to treat external skin conditions. They work to soothe, protect, and moisten the skin and to destroy harmful bacteria. *Example:* Caladryl lotion.

Solution   A liquid preparation that contains one or more completely dissolved substances. The dissolved substance is known as the solute, and the liquid in which it is dissolved is known as the solvent. Most drugs administered parenterally (by injection) consist of solutions. *Example:* Depo-Provera injectable solution.

Spirit   A drug combined with an alcoholic solution that is volatile (a substance that is volatile evaporates readily). *Example:* Aromatic spirit of ammonia.

Spray   A fine stream of medicated vapor, usually used to treat nose and throat conditions. *Example:* Dristan nasal spray.

Suspension   A drug that contains solid insoluble drug particles in a liquid; the preparation must be shaken before administration. *Example:* Amoxicillin oral suspension.

Suspension aerosol   A pressurized form in which solid aerosol or liquid drug particles are suspended in a gas to be dispensed in a cloud or mist. *Example:* Proventil inhalation aerosol.

Syrup   A drug dissolved in a solution of sugar, water, and sometimes a flavoring to disguise an unpleasant taste. *Example:* Robitussin cough syrup.

Tincture   A drug dissolved in a solution of alcohol or alcohol and water. *Example:* Tincture of iodine.

Solid Preparations

Tablet   A powdered drug that has been pressed into a disc. Some tablets are scored, that is, they are marked with an indentation so that they can be broken into halves or quarters for proper dosage. *Example:* Tylenol tablets.

Chewable tablet   A powdered drug that has been flavored and pressed into a disc. Chewable tablets are often used for antacids, antiflatulents, and children's medications. *Example:* Pepto-Bismol chewable tablets.

Sublingual tablet   A powdered drug that has been pressed into a disc and is designed to dissolve under the tongue, which permits its rapid absorption into the bloodstream. *Example:* Nitroglycerin sublingual tablets (Nitrostat).

Enteric-coated tablet   A tablet coated with a substance that prevents it from dissolving until it reaches the intestines. The coating protects the drug from being destroyed by gastric juices and prevents it from irritating the stomach lining. To prevent the active ingredients from being released prematurely in the stomach, enteric-coated tablets must not be crushed or chewed. *Example:* Ecotrin enteric-coated aspirin.

Capsule   A drug contained in a gelatin capsule that is water-soluble and functions to prevent the patient from tasting the drug. *Example:* Benadryl capsules.

Sustained-release capsule   A capsule that contains granules that dissolve at different rates to provide a gradual and continuous release of medication. This reduces the number of doses that must be administered. (Sustained-release medication also comes in other preparations, such as tablets and caplets.) *Example:* Sudafed 12-hour sustained-release capsules.

Caplet   A drug contained in an oblong tablet with a smooth coating to make swallowing easier. *Example:* Advil caplets.

Lozenge   A drug contained in a candy-like base. Lozenges are circular and are designed to dissolve on the tongue. *Example:* Chloraseptic throat lozenges.

Cream   A drug combined in a base that is generally nongreasy, resulting in a semisolid preparation. Creams are applied externally to the skin. *Example:* Hydrocortisone topical cream.

Ointment   A drug with an oil base, resulting in a semisolid preparation. Ointments are applied externally to the skin and are usually greasy. *Example:* Cortisporin topical ointment.

Suppository   A drug mixed with a firm base, such as cocoa butter, that is designed to melt at body temperature. A suppository is shaped into a cylinder or a cone for easy insertion into a body cavity, such as the rectum or vagina. *Example:* Preparation H suppositories.

Transdermal patch   A patch with an adhesive backing, which contains a drug, that is applied to the skin. The drug enters the circulation after being absorbed through the skin. *Example:* Nitroglycerin patches (Nitro-Dur).

CLASSIFICATION OF DRUGS BASED ON ACTION

Drugs also can be classified according to the action they have on the body. The medical assistant should know in which category a particular drug belongs and its primary uses and major therapeutic effects. Table 11-1 contains classifications based on action and examples of drugs that

Table 11-1 Classification of Drugs Based on Action

Drug Category	Primary Use and Major Therapeutic Effects	COMMONLY PRESCRIBED DRUGS	
		Generic	Brand
Analgesics (Opioid)	**Used** to manage moderate to severe pain **Work** by altering perception of and response to painful stimuli **Vicodin** 500/5 mg **Darvocet-N** 50/325 mg 100/650 mg	codeine/APAP fentanyl hydrocodone/APAP hydrocodone/ASA hydrocodone/ibuprofen meperidine oxycodone oxycodone/APAP oxycodone/ASA propoxyphene propoxyphene N/APAP tramadol	▶Tylenol w/ Codeine (III) Actiq ▶Vicodin (III) Lortab/ASA (III) ▶Vicoprofen (III) Demerol (II) ▶OxyContin (II) ▶Percocet (II) Percodan (II) Darvon (IV) ▶Darvocet-N (IV) ▶Ultram
Analgesics (Barbiturate)	**Used** to manage moderate to severe pain of tension headaches **Work** by relieving pain and relaxing muscle contractions	butalbital/APAP/caffeine butalbital/ASA/caffeine	▶Fioricet (III) Fiorinal (III)
Analgesics/Antipyretics	**Used** to manage mild to moderate pain and to reduce fever **Work** by relieving pain and reducing fever **Naprosyn** 250 mg 375 mg 500 mg	acetaminophen aspirin **NSAID** diclofenac ibuprofen naproxen	Tylenol* Bayer* Ecotrin* Voltaren Advil* ▶Motrin* Aleve* ▶Anaprox ▶Naprosyn
Anesthetics (Local)	**Used** to produce local anesthesia through loss of feeling to a body part **Work** by preventing initiation and conduction of normal nerve impulses in body part	lidocaine dibucaine	Xylocaine Nupercainal ointment*
Antacids	**Used** to treat heartburn, hyperacidity, indigestion, and gastro-esophageal reflux disease, and to promote healing of ulcers **Work** by neutralizing gastric acid to relieve gastric pain and irritation	aluminum hydroxide/ magnesium hydroxide calcium carbonate sodium bicarbonate/ASA	Maalox* Mylanta* Tums* Alka-Seltzer*
Anti-Alzheimer's Agents	**Used** to treat mild to moderate dementia associated with Alzheimer's disease **Work** by elevating acetylcholine concentration in the cerebral cortex	donepezil memantine rivastigmine	▶Aricept ▶Namenda Exelon
Antianemics	**Iron Supplements** **Used** to prevent or cure iron-deficiency anemia **Work** by increasing amount of iron in body **Vitamin B$_{12}$ Injections** **Used** to treat pernicious anemia **Work** by increasing amount of vitamin B$_{12}$ in body **Folic Acid Supplements** **Used** to promote normal fetal development **Work** by stimulating production of red blood cells, white blood cells, and platelets	ferrous sulfate iron dextran Cyanocobalamin folic acid	Feosol* DexFerrum InFed Cobex Cyanoject ▶Folvite

*Available OTC (over-the-counter).
▶Top-200 most prescribed drugs.
(II): schedule II drug, (III): schedule III drug, (IV): schedule IV drug.

Continued

Table 11-1 Classification of Drugs Based on Action—cont'd

		COMMONLY PRESCRIBED DRUGS	
Drug Category	Primary Use and Major Therapeutic Effects	Generic	Brand
Antianginals	*Used* to relieve or prevent angina attacks *Work* by increasing blood supply to myocardial tissue **Imdur** 60 mg **Nitrostat** 0.3 mg 0.4 mg 0.6 mg	*Nitrates* isosorbide dinitrate isosorbide mononitrate nitroglycerin *Beta Blockers* atenolol propranolol metoprolol *Calcium Channel Blockers* amlodipine bepridil diltiazem nifedipine verapamil	Sorbitrate ▶Imdur Nitro-Bid Nitro-Dur Nitrostat Tenormin Inderal ▶Toprol-XL ▶Norvasc Vascor Cardizem Dilacor XR Adalat Procardia-XL ▶Calan Isoptin Verelan
Antianxiety Agents	*Used* to treat anxiety *Work* at many levels in central nervous system to produce anxiolytic (anxiety-relieving) effect **Xanax** 0.25 mg 0.5 mg 1 mg 2 mg	alprazolam buspirone chlordiazepoxide diazepam lorazepam	▶Xanax (IV) BuSpar Librium (IV) ▶Valium (IV) ▶Ativan (IV)
Anticholinergics	*Used* to decrease preoperatively oral and respiratory secretions *Work* by blocking effects of acetylcholine in autonomic nervous system	atropine	Atro-Pen
Anticoagulants	*Used* to prevent and treat venous thrombosis, pulmonary embolism, and myocardial infarction by preventing clot extension and formation *Work* by delaying or preventing blood coagulation **Coumadin** 1 mg 2 mg	heparin enoxaparin warfarin	 ▶Lovenox ▶Coumadin
Anticonvulsants	*Used* to prevent or relieve seizures *Work* by decreasing incidence and severity of seizures **Neurontin** 100 mg 300 mg 400 mg	carbamazepine clonazepam divalproex gabapentin lamotrigine phenytoin pregabalin topiramate	Tegretol ▶Klonopin (IV) ▶Depakote ▶Neurontin ▶Lamictal ▶Dilantin ▶Lyrica ▶Topamax

*Available OTC (over-the-counter).
▶Top-200 most prescribed drugs.
(II): schedule II drug, (III): schedule III drug, (IV): schedule IV drug.

Table 11-1 Classification of Drugs Based on Action—cont'd

Drug Category	Primary Use and Major Therapeutic Effects	Generic (Commonly Prescribed Drugs)	Brand
Antidepressants	**Used** to prevent, cure, or alleviate depression, and to treat anxiety disorders (panic attacks) and obsessive-convulsive disorder **Work** by inhibiting reuptake of neurotransmitters in the central nervous system	**Selective Serotonin Reuptake Inhibitors (SSRIs)** citalopram escitalopram fluoxetine fluvoxamine paroxetine sertraline	▶Celexa ▶Lexapro ▶Prozac Luvox ▶Paxil ▶Zoloft
	Prozac 10 mg 20 mg **Wellbutrin-SR** 100 mg 150 mg	**Serotonin-Norepinephrine Reuptake Inhibitors (SNRIs)** desvenlafaxine duloxetine venlafaxine	Pristiq ▶Cymbalta ▶Effexor XR
		Miscellaneous amitriptyline bupropion mirtazapine nefazodone trazodone	▶Elavil ▶Wellbutrin-SR ▶Remeron Serzone ▶Desyrel
Antidiabetics	**Oral Hypoglycemics** **Used** to manage non–insulin-dependent type 2 diabetes mellitus **Work** by stimulating release of insulin from pancreas and increasing sensitivity to insulin	glimepiride glipizide glyburide metformin pioglitazone rosiglitazone	▶Amaryl ▶Glucotrol XL ▶Micronase ▶Glucophage ▶Actos ▶Avandia
	Insulins **Used** to manage diabetes mellitus **Work** by reducing blood glucose levels	regular insulin NPH insulin NPH/regular insulin insulin glargine insulin lispro	Humulin R* Novolin R* Humulin N* Novolin N* Humulin 70/30* Novolin 70/30* ▶Lantus Humalog
	Amaryl 2 mg 4 mg **Glucotrol XL** 5 mg 10 mg		
Antidiarrheals	**Used** to control and relieve diarrhea **Work** by inhibiting peristalsis, reducing fecal volume, and preventing loss of fluids and electrolytes **Lomotil** 2.5/0.025 mg	bismuth subsalicylate diphenoxylate/atropine kaolin/pectin loperamide	Pepto-Bismol* Lomotil (V) Kaopectate* Imodium*

Continued

Table 11-1 Classification of Drugs Based on Action—cont'd

Drug Category	Primary Use and Major Therapeutic Effects	COMMONLY PRESCRIBED DRUGS	
		Generic	Brand
Antidysrhythmics	**Used** to control or prevent cardiac dysrhythmias **Work** by decreasing myocardial excitability and slowing conduction velocity **Inderal** 10 mg 20 mg 40 mg 60 mg 80 mg	metoprolol procainamide propranolol	▶Lopressor ▶Toprol XL Pronestyl Inderal
Antiemetics	**Used** to prevent or relieve nausea and vomiting **Work** by depressing chemoreceptor trigger zone in central nervous system to inhibit nausea and vomiting	dronabinol ondansetron prochlorperazine promethazine meclizine	Marinol (III) Zofran Compazine ▶Phenergan Bonine*
Antiflatulents	**Used** to relieve discomfort of excess gas and bloating in gastrointestinal tract **Work** by causing coalescence of gas bubbles in intestinal tract	simethicone	Gas-X* Mylanta Gas*
Antifungals	**Used** to treat fungal infections **Work** by killing or inhibiting growth of susceptible fungi **Diflucan** 50 mg 100 mg 200 mg	amphotericin B clotrimazole fluconazole itraconazole ketoconazole miconazole nystatin terbinafine	Fungizone Gyne-Lotrimin* ▶Diflucan Sporanox Nizoral Monistat* Mycostatin* ▶Lamisil
Antigout Agents	**Used** to prevent attacks of gout **Work** by inhibiting production of uric acid **Zyloprim** 100 mg 300 mg	allopurinol colchicine	▶Zyloprim Colchicine tablets
Antihelmintics	**Used** to treat worm infections (pinworms, roundworms, hookworms) **Work** by destroying worms	mebendazole	Vermox
Antihistamines	**Used** to relieve symptoms associated with allergies (increased sneezing; rhinorrhea; itchy eyes, nose, and throat) **Work** by blocking effects of histamine at histamine receptor sites **Allegra** 60 mg 180 mg	brompheniramine cetirizine chlorpheniramine desloratadine diphenhydramine fexofenadine/ pseudoephedrine levocetirizine loratadine promethazine	Dimetane* ▶Zyrtec* Chlor-Trimetron* Teldrin* ▶Clarinex Benadryl* ▶Allegra Xyzal ▶Claritin* ▶Phenergan

*Available OTC (over-the-counter).
▶Top-200 most prescribed drugs.
(II): schedule II drug, (III): schedule III drug, (IV): schedule IV drug.

Table 11-1 Classification of Drugs Based on Action—cont'd

		COMMONLY PRESCRIBED DRUGS	
Drug Category	**Primary Use and Major Therapeutic Effects**	**Generic**	**Brand**
Antihypertensives	*Used* to manage hypertension *Work* by causing systemic vasodilation to reduce blood pressure	**Angiotensin-Converting Enzyme (ACE) Inhibitors**	
	Accupril	benazepril	Lotensin
	5 mg	captopril	Capoten
	10 mg	enalapril	▶Vasotec
	20 mg	lisinopril	▶Prinivil
	40 mg	quinapril	▶Accupril
		ramipril	▶Altace
	Cozaar		
	25 mg	**Peripherally Acting Adrenergic Blockers**	
	50 mg	clonidine	▶Catapres
		doxazosin	Cardura
	Toprol XL	prazosin	Minipress
	50 mg		
	100 mg	**Angiotensin II Receptor Antagonists**	
	200 mg	candesartan	Atacand
		irbesartan	▶Avapro
	Cardizem	losartan	▶Cozaar
	30 mg	olmesartan	▶Benicar
	60 mg	telmisartan	Micardis
	90 mg	valsartan	▶Diovan
	120 mg		
		Beta-Blockers	
		atenolol	▶Tenormin
		carvedilol	▶Coreg
		metoprolol	▶Lopressor
			▶Toprol XL
		propranolol	Inderal
		sotalol	Betaspace
		Calcium Channel Blockers	
		amlodipine	▶Norvasc
		diltiazem	▶Cardizem
		felodipine	Plendil
		Vasodilators	
		hydralazine	Apresoline
		Miscellaneous	
		amlodipine/atorvastatin	Caudet
		amlodipine/benazepril	▶Lotrel
		bisoprolol/ hydrochlorothiazide	Ziac
		irbesartan/ hydrochlorothiazide	▶Avalide
		losartan/ hydrochlorothiazide	▶Hyzaar
		olmesartan/ hydrochlorothiazide	▶Benicar HCT
		triamterene/ hydrochlorothiazide	▶Maxzide
		valsartan/ hydrochlorothiazide	Diovan HCT

Continued

Table 11-1 Classification of Drugs Based on Action—cont'd

Drug Category	Primary Use and Major Therapeutic Effects	Generic	Brand
Antiimpotence Agents	**Used** to treat erectile dysfunction **Work** by promoting increased blood flow to penis	sildenafil	▶Viagra
		tadalafil	▶Cialis
	Viagra	vardenafil	Levitra
	25 mg 50 mg 100 mg		
Antiinfectives	**Used** to treat infections **Work** by killing or inhibiting growth of bacteria	**Penicillins**	
	Amoxil	amoxicillin	▶Amoxil
			▶Trimox
	125 mg 250 mg	amoxicillin/clavulanate	▶Augmentin
	250 mg	ampicillin	Omnipen
		benzathine penicillin	Bicillin
	500 mg	penicillin V	▶Veetids
		procaine penicillin	Wycillin
	Zithromax	**Macrolides**	
		azithromycin	▶Zithromax
	250 mg	clarithromycin	Biaxin
	250 mg	erythromycin	Ery-Tab
		Cephalosporins	
		cefaclor	Ceclor
		cefdinir	▶Omnicef
		cefprozil	▶Cefzil
		ceftriaxone	Rocephin
		cefuroxime	Ceftin
		cephalexin	▶Keflex
	Keflex	**Fluoroquinolones**	
	250 mg 500 mg	ciprofloxacin	▶Cipro
		levofloxacin	▶Levaquin
		moxifloxacin	Avelox
	Cipro	ofloxacin	Floxin
	250 mg 500 mg	**Tetracyclines**	
		doxycycline	Doryx
			▶Vibramycin
	750 mg	minocycline	Arestin
		tetracycline	Achromycin
			Sumycin
	Macrobid	**Aminoglycosides**	
		gentamicin	Garamycin
	100 mg	kanamycin	Kantrex
		neomycin	Neobiotic
		tobramycin	Nebcin
		Sulfonamides	
		sulfamethoxazole	Gantanol
		trimethoprim/ sulfamethoxazole	▶Bactrim
		Miscellaneous	
		Clindamycin	Cleocin
		chloramphenicol	Chloromycetin
		nitrofurantoin	▶Macrobid
			Macrodantin
		vancomycin	Vancocin

*Available OTC (over-the-counter).
▶Top-200 most prescribed drugs.
(II): schedule II drug, (III): schedule III drug, (IV): schedule IV drug.

Table 11-1 Classification of Drugs Based on Action—cont'd

Drug Category	Primary Use and Major Therapeutic Effects	COMMONLY PRESCRIBED DRUGS	
		Generic	Brand
Antiinflammatory Agents	**Used** to relieve signs and symptoms of osteoarthritis and rheumatoid arthritis in adults **Work** by decreasing pain and inflammation **Celebrex** 100 mg 200 mg	aspirin celecoxib etodolac ibuprofen indomethacin meloxicam nabumetone naproxen piroxicam valdecoxib	Bayer* Ecotrin* ►Celebrex Lodine Advil* Motrin* Indocin ►Mobic ►Relafen Aleve* Anaprox Naprosyn Feldene Bextra
Antimanics	**Used** to treat bipolar affective disorders **Work** by altering cation transport in nerves and muscles **Eskalith** **Eskalith CR** 300 mg 450 mg	lithium	Eskalith Eskalith CR
Antimigraines	**Used** in acute treatment of migraine attacks **Work** by causing vasoconstriction in large intracranial arteries	sumatriptan	►Imitrex
Antineoplastics	**Used** to treat tumors **Work** by preventing development, growth, or proliferation of malignant cells	cyclophosphamide methotrexate	Cytoxan Mexate Folex
Anti-Parkinson's Agents	**Used** to treat symptoms of Parkinson's disease **Work** by restoring balance between acetylcholine and dopamine in central nervous system **Sinemet** 10/100 mg 25/100 mg 50/200 mg 25/250 mg	carbidopa/levodopa ropinirole	Sinemet Requip

Continued

Table 11-1 Classification of Drugs Based on Action—cont'd

Drug Category	Primary Use and Major Therapeutic Effects	COMMONLY PRESCRIBED DRUGS	
		Generic	Brand
Antiprotozoals	*Used* to treat protozoal infections *Work* by destroying protozoa	Metronidazole	Flagyl

Flagyl

250 mg 500 mg FLAG 375 m / 375 mg

| Antipsychotics | *Used* to treat psychotic disorders
Work by blocking dopamine and serotonin receptors in central nervous system | haloperidol
aripiprazole
olanzapine
risperidone
quetiapine | Haldol
▶Abilify
▶Zyprexa
▶Risperdal
▶Seroquel |

Risperdal

1 mg 2 mg 3 mg 4 mg

| Antiretrovirals | *Used* to manage human immunodeficiency virus (HIV) infections and to reduce maternal-fetal transmission of HIV
Work by inhibiting replication of retroviruses | efavirenz
emtricitabine
lamivudine
ritonavir
tenofovir
zidovudine | Sustiva
Emtriva
Epivir
Norvir
Viread
Retrovir |

Retrovir

100 mg

Antispasmodics	*Used* to control hypermotility in irritable bowel syndrome, spastic colitis, spastic bladder, and pylorospasm *Work* by preventing or relieving spasms of gastrointestinal or genitourinary tract	dicyclomine hyoscyamine	Bentyl Levsin
Antituberculars	*Used* to treat tuberculosis *Work* by killing or inhibiting growth of mycobacteria	isoniazid rifampin	INH Rifadin
Antitussives	*Used* in prevention or relief of coughs caused by minor viral upper respiratory infections or inhaled irritants *Work* by suppressing cough reflex by direct effect on cough center in central nervous system	benzonatate chlorpheniramine/ hydrocodone dextromethorphan guaifenesin/codeine	Tessalon Tussionex (III) Robitussin DM* Robitussin A-C (V)
Antiulcers	*Used* to manage ulcers, gastroesophageal reflux disease, heartburn, indigestion, and gastric hyperacidity *Work* by preventing accumulation of acid in stomach	***Proton Pump Inhibitors*** esomeprazole lansoprazole omeprazole pantoprazole rabeprazole	 ▶Nexium ▶Prevacid ▶Prilosec* ▶Protonix ▶AcipHex

Prevacid

15 mg 30 mg

| | | ***H_2-Receptor Antagonists***
cimetidine
famotidine
ranitidine |
Tagamet*
▶Pepcid AC*
▶Zantac* |
| Antivirals | *Used* to manage herpes infections
Work by inhibiting viral replication | acyclovir
famciclovir
valacyclovir | ▶Zovirax
Famvir
▶Valtrex |

Valtrex

500 mg 1 g

*Available OTC (over-the-counter).
▶Top-200 most prescribed drugs.
(II): schedule II drug, (III): schedule III drug, (IV): schedule IV drug.

Table 11-1 Classification of Drugs Based on Action—cont'd

Drug Category	Primary Use and Major Therapeutic Effects	COMMONLY PRESCRIBED DRUGS	
		Generic	Brand
Bone Resorption Inhibitors	**Used** to treat and prevent osteoporosis **Work** by inhibiting resorption of bone **Fosamax** 5 mg 10 mg 40 mg	alendronate ibandronate raloxifene risedronate	▶Fosamax Boniva ▶Evista ▶Actonel
Bronchodilators	**Used** to manage reversible airway obstruction caused by asthma or chronic obstructive pulmonary disease **Work** by relaxing smooth muscle of respiratory tract resulting in bronchodilation **Singulair** 4 mg 5 mg 10 mg	albuterol fluticasone/salmeterol formoterol ipratropium/albuterol levalbuterol montelukast salmeterol theophylline tiotropium	▶Proventil ▶Advair Diskus Foradil ▶Combivent Xopenex ▶Singulair Serevent Bronkodyl ▶Spiriva
Cardiac Glycosides	**Used** to treat congestive heart failure and cardiac arrhythmias **Work** by increasing strength and force of myocardial contractions and slowing heart rate **Lanoxicaps** 0.1 mg	digitoxin digoxin	Crystodigin ▶Digitek Lanoxicaps ▶Lanoxin
Central Nervous System Stimulants	**Used** to treat narcolepsy and manage attention-deficit/hyperactivity disorder **Work** by increasing level of catecholamines in central nervous system **Adderall (II)** 5 mg 10 mg 20 mg 30 mg	atomoxetine dextroamphetamine dextroamphetamine saccharate and sulfate lisdexamfetamine methylphenidate	▶Strattera Dexedrine (II) ▶Adderall (II) Vyvanse (II) ▶Ritalin (II) ▶Concerta (II)

Continued

Table 11-1 Classification of Drugs Based on Action—cont'd

Drug Category	Primary Use and Major Therapeutic Effects	COMMONLY PRESCRIBED DRUGS	
		Generic	Brand

Contraceptives (Hormonal)	**Used** to prevent pregnancy and to regulate menstrual cycle
	Work by inhibiting ovulation
	
	Ortho-Novum
	
	7/7/7
	
	1/35
		Oral Contraceptives
		ethinyl estradiol/
		  drospirenone
		ethinyl estradiol/
		  levonorgestrel
		ethinyl estradiol/
		  norethindrone
		
		ethinyl estradiol/
		  norgestimate
			▶Yasmin
			Yaz
			Alesse
			Levien
			Kariva
			▶Ortho-Novum
			▶Loestrin Fe
			▶Ortho Tri-Cyclen
			Tri-Sprintec

		Injectable Contraceptives medroxyprogesterone	▶Depo-Provera
		Transdermal Contraceptives ethinyl estradiol/ norelgestromin	▶Ortho Evra
		Vaginal Ring Contraceptives ethinyl estradiol/ etonogestrel	NuvaRing
Corticosteroids	**Systemic Corticosteroids** **Used** to treat inflammation, allergies, asthma, and autoimmune disorders and as replacement therapy in adrenal insufficiency **Work** by suppressing inflammation and modifying normal immune response	cortisone fluticasone hydrocortisone methylprednisolone triamcinolone	Cortone ▶Flovent Cortef Medrol Depo-Medrol Aristocort
	Nasal Corticosteroids **Used** to treat chronic nasal inflammatory conditions (e.g., allergic rhinitis) **Work** by suppressing inflammation and reducing hypersecretions of respiratory tract	fluticasone mometasone prednisone triamcinolone	▶Flonase ▶Nasonex ▶Deltasone ▶Nasacort
Decongestants	**Used** to decrease nasal congestion **Work** by producing vasoconstriction in respiratory tract mucosa	oxymetazoline phenylephrine pseudoephedrine	Afrin* Dristan* Neo-Synephrine* Sudafed*
Diuretics	**Used** to manage hypertension, edema in congestive heart failure, and renal disease **Work** by removing excess fluid from the body by increasing urine output **Lasix** 20 mg 40 mg 80 mg	**Loop Diuretics** bumetanide furosemide **Thiazide Diuretics** chlorthalidone hydrochlorothiazide **Potassium-Sparing Diuretics** spironolactone triamterene	Bumex ▶Lasix Hygroton ▶Microzide Aldactone Dyrenium

*Available OTC (over-the-counter).
▶Top-200 most prescribed drugs.
(II): schedule II drug, (III): schedule III drug, (IV): schedule IV drug.

Table 11-1 Classification of Drugs Based on Action—cont'd

Drug Category	Primary Use and Major Therapeutic Effects	COMMONLY PRESCRIBED DRUGS	
		Generic	Brand
Electrolyte Replacements	*Used* to treat or prevent electrolyte depletion *Work* by replacing electrolytes in body **Klor-Con** KLOR-CON 8 — 600 mg KLOR-CON 10 — 750 mg	*Potassium Supplements* potassium chloride	▶K-Dur ▶Klor-Con
Emetics	*Used* to treat poisoning *Work* by inducing vomiting	syrup of ipecac	
Expectorants	*Used* to manage coughs by expelling mucus *Work* by decreasing viscosity of bronchial secretions to promote clearance of mucus from respiratory tract	guaifenesin	Robitussin* Mucinex* Naldecon*
Hormone Replacements	*Used* to treat moderate to severe vasomotor symptoms of menopause *Work* by restoring hormonal balance **Premarin** PREMARIN 0.3 — 0.3 mg PREMARIN 0.625 — 0.625 mg PREMARIN 0.3 — 0.9 mg PREMARIN 1.25 — 1.25 mg PREMARIN 2.5 — 2.5 mg	conjugated estrogens conjugated estrogen/ progesterone estradiol/norethindrone	▶Premarin ▶Prempro Activella
Immunizations	*Used* to prevent (vaccine-preventable) diseases *Work* by stimulating body to produce antibodies	diphtheria, tetanus toxoids, and acellular pertussis vaccine	Acel-Imune Certiva Daptacel Infanrix Tripedia
		Haemophilus b conjugate vaccine	ActHIB HibTITER
		hepatitis A vaccine	Havrix Vaqta
		hepatitis B vaccine	Engerix-B Recombivax HB
		human papillomavirus vaccine	Gardasil
		inactivated polio vaccine	IPOL
		influenza virus vaccine types A and B	Afluria FluShield Fluzone FluMist
		measles, mumps, and rubella vaccine	M-M-R II
		meningococcal conjugate vaccine	Menactra
		pneumococcal conjugate vaccine	Prevnar Pneumovax II
		rotavirus	Rotarix RotaShield
		rubella vaccine	Meruvax II
		varicella vaccine	Varivax

Continued

Table 11-1 Classification of Drugs Based on Action—cont'd

Drug Category	Primary Use and Major Therapeutic Effects	COMMONLY PRESCRIBED DRUGS	
		Generic	Brand
Immunosuppressants	**Used** to treat severe rheumatoid arthritis and to prevent and treat rejection of transplanted organs **Work** by inhibiting body's normal immune response	cyclosporine methotrexate	Sandimmune Neoral Rheumatrex
Laxatives	**Used** to relieve constipation **Work** by promoting defecation of normal, soft stool	bisacodyl docusate phenolphthalein psyllium	Dulcolax* Colace* Phenolax* Metamucil*
Lipid-Lowering Agents	**Used** to lower cholesterol to reduce risk of myocardial infarction and stroke **Work** by inhibiting enzyme needed to synthesize cholesterol in body **Lipitor** PD 155 10 **10 mg** **20 mg** S P 712 **40 mg**	atorvastatin ezetimibe ezetimibe/simvastatin fenofibrate fluvastatin gemfibrozil lovastatin pravastatin rosuvastatin simvastatin	▶Lipitor ▶Zetia ▶Vytorin ▶Tricor Lescol Lopid ▶Mevacor ▶Pravachol ▶Crestor ▶Zocor
Muscle Relaxants (Skeletal)	**Used** to treat acute painful musculoskeletal conditions **Work** by relaxing skeletal muscles **Flexeril** MSD 931 **10 mg**	baclofen carisoprodol cyclobenzaprine metaxalone methocarbamol tizanidine	▶Lioresal ▶Soma ▶Flexeril Skelaxin Robaxin ▶Zanaflex
Ophthalmic Antiinfectives	**Used** to treat eye infections **Work** by destroying bacteria	dexamethasone/ tobramycin moxifloxacin polymyxin/bacitracin polymyxin/neomycin polymyxin/trimethoprim tobramycin	TobraDex Vigamox Polysporin Neosporin Polytrim Tobrex
Otic Preparations	**Used** to treat ear conditions ***Antiinfectives*** **Work** by relieving ear pain ***Antiinfectives*** **Work** by treating otitis externa ***Cerumenolytics*** **Work** by softening cerumen	 benzocaine neomycin/polymyxin/ hydrocortisone ofloxacin carbamide peroxide	 Auralgan Cortisporin Otic Floxin Otic Debrox*
Platelet Inhibitors	**Used** to reduce incidence of myocardial infarction and stroke **Work** by interfering with ability of platelets to adhere to each other	clopidogrel Salicylates	▶Plavix Aspirin*
Sedatives and Hypnotics	**Used** for short-term treatment of insomnia **Work** by promoting sleep by central nervous system depression **Ambien** 5401 5421 **5 mg** **10 mg**	eszopiclone flurazepam hydroxyzine phenobarbital temazepam zolpidem	▶Lunesta (IV) Dalmane (IV) Atarax Vistaril Luminal (IV) ▶Restoril (IV) ▶Ambien (IV)

*Available OTC (over-the-counter).
▶Top-200 most prescribed drugs.
(II): schedule II drug, (III): schedule III drug, (IV): schedule IV drug.

Table 11-1 Classification of Drugs Based on Action—cont'd

Drug Category	Primary Use and Major Therapeutic Effects	COMMONLY PRESCRIBED DRUGS	
		Generic	Brand
Smoking Deterrents	***Used*** to manage nicotine withdrawal to cease cigarette smoking ***Work*** by providing nicotine during controlled withdrawal from cigarette smoking	bupropion nicotine varenicline	Zyban Nicorette Gum* Nicotrol Inhaler Nicoderm Patch* Commit Lozenges* Chantix
Thrombolytic Agents	***Used*** for acute management of coronary thrombosis (myocardial infarction) ***Work*** by dissolving existing clots	alteplase anistreplase reteplase streptokinase	Activase Eminase Retavase Streptase
Thyroid Preparations	***Thyroid Hormones*** ***Used*** as replacement or substitute therapy for diminished or absent thyroid functioning of many causes ***Work*** by increasing basal metabolic rate	levothyroxine	▶Levoxyl ▶Synthroid
	Levoxyl 0.05 mg		
	Antithyroid Agents ***Used*** to treat hyperthyroidism ***Work*** by inhibiting thyroid hormone synthesis, reducing basal metabolic rate	methimazole	Tapazole
Urinary Tract–Antispasmodics	***Used*** to treat overactive bladder function ***Work*** by inhibiting bladder contractions	oxybutynin tolterodine	Ditropan ▶Detrol
Vasopressors	***Used*** to treat severe allergic reactions and cardiac arrest ***Work*** by increasing blood pressure and cardiac output and by dilating bronchi	epinephrine	Adrenalin EpiPen
Weight Control Agents	***Used*** to manage obesity		
	Appetite Suppressants ***Work*** by suppressing appetite center in central nervous system	diethylpropion phentermine sibutramine orlistat	Tenuate (IV) Fastin (IV) Meridia (IV) Xenical Ali*
	Meridia 5 mg 10 mg 15 mg		
	Lipase Inhibitors ***Work*** by inhibiting action of lipase to decrease absorption of dietary fats		

are commonly administered and prescribed in the medical office.

SYSTEMS OF MEASUREMENT FOR MEDICATION

Three systems of measurement are used in the United States for prescribing, administering, and dispensing medication: the metric system, the apothecary system, and the household system. The metric system is the most common system used to measure medication because it provides a more exact measurement and is easier to use. Some physicians oc-casionally use the apothecary system; the medical assistant should be familiar with this system. The third system of measurement, the household system, is the least accurate and generally is used only when a patient takes liquid medication at home.

Systems of measurement have units of weight, volume, and length. *Weight* refers to the heaviness of an item, and *volume* refers to the amount of space occupied by a substance. *Length* is a unit of linear measurement of the distance from one point to another. Although length is not used to administer medication, it is used in other aspects of the medical office. The head circumference of infants is measured in centimeters (cm), a metric unit of linear measurement.

To prepare and administer medication properly and to avoid medication errors, the medical assistant must have a thorough knowledge of the specific units of measurement for these three systems and must be able to convert within each and from one system to another. A basic discussion of the metric, apothecary, and household systems is presented next. A more thorough study of these systems, including conversion of units and dose calculation, is included in Chapter 11 of the Study Guide.

Metric System

The metric system was developed in France in the latter part of the 18th century in an effort to simplify measurement. Most European countries are required by law to use this system for the measurement of weight, volume, and length. Overall, the metric system is used for most scientific and medical measurements. Pharmaceutical companies use the metric system to measure and label medications.

The metric system employs a uniform decimal scale based on units of 10, making it very flexible and logical. The basic metric units of measurement are the gram, liter, and meter. The *gram* is a unit of weight used to measure solids, the *liter* is a unit of volume used to measure liquids, and the *meter* is a linear unit used to measure length or distance. The metric units used most often in the administration of medication in the medical office are the milligram, gram, milliliter, and cubic centimeter. Because a **cubic centimeter (cc)** is the amount of space occupied by 1 milliliter (ml), these two units can be used interchangeably (i.e., 1 ml = 1 cc).

Prefixes added to the words *gram, liter,* and *meter* designate smaller or larger units of measurement in the metric system. The same prefixes are used with all three units. For example, *milli-* is used as follows: *milli*gram, *milli*liter, and *milli*meter. A prefix changes the value of the basic unit of measurement by the same amount. The prefix *milli-* describes a unit that is $\frac{1}{1000}$ of the basic unit: 1 gram is equal to 1000 milligrams, 1 liter is equal to 1000 milliliters, and 1 meter is equal to 1000 millimeters. The box *Metric Notation Guidelines* lists the metric units of measurement and equivalent values in different units. Specific guidelines are used in the medical notation of metric units and doses, which also are presented in the box. To read prescriptions and medication orders, to record medication administration, and, most important, to avoid medication errors, the medical assistant must be familiar with and be able to follow these guidelines.

Apothecary System

The apothecary system is older and less accurate than the metric system. It was brought to the United States from England during the 18th century. Pharmacists used this system during the colonial period to compound and measure medications. This system is gradually being phased out

for measurement of medication in favor of the metric system. Until that process is completed, however, the medical assistant must be familiar with this system and be able to use it to administer medication.

The basic unit of weight in the apothecary system is the *grain,* derived from the weight of a large grain of wheat, which was used to balance the material being weighed. The next largest unit of measurement is the *scruple;* however, this unit is not used to administer medication. The remaining units, in order of increasing weight, are *dram, ounce,* and *pound.* The pound is not generally used in the administration of medication. The medical assistant should note, however, that in the apothecary system the pound is equal to 12 ounces, in contrast to the more familiar *avoirdupois* pound used to measure body weight, which is equal to 16 ounces.

Measures of liquid volume in the apothecary system correlate closely with measures of dry weight in the same system. The smallest unit of measurement is the *minim,* meaning "the least." A minim is approximately equivalent to a volume of water that weighs 1 grain. A minim glass or a syringe calibrated in minims must be used to measure with this unit. The remaining units of liquid volume in the apothecary system, in order of increasing volume, are *fluid dram, fluid ounce, pint, quart,* and *gallon.* The basic unit of linear measurement is the *inch,* followed by *foot, yard,* and *mile.* Most Americans are familiar with apothecary units of measurement because of their use in everyday life. For example, milk is available in pints, quarts, and gallons, and height is measured in feet and inches.

The box *Apothecary Notation Guidelines* lists the units of measurement in the apothecary system and equivalent values in different units. It also includes guidelines for the medical notation of apothecary units.

Household System

The household system is more complicated and less accurate for administering liquid medication than either the metric or the apothecary system. Nevertheless, most individuals are familiar with this system because of its frequent use in the United States. This system of measurement may be the only one the patient can understand and safely use to take liquid medication at home. Most patients are more comfortable measuring medication in drops and teaspoons than in minims and milliliters. In addition, the patient is more likely to have household measuring devices on hand than to have metric measuring devices. If a precise measurement is needed, however, the metric system must be used, and the medical assistant should instruct the patient in the use of the metric measuring device.

Volume is the only household unit of measurement used to administer medication. The basic unit of liquid volume in the household system is the *drop (gtt),* which is approximately equal to 0.6 ml in the metric system and 1 minim in the apothecary system. These units cannot be considered exact equivalents because the size of the drop varies based on temperature, the viscosity of the liquid, and the size of

Metric Notation Guidelines

Follow these guidelines when using the metric notation of measurement and dosage.

1. The units of metric measurement are written using the following abbreviations:

    Weight

    microgram: mcg or μg

    milligram: mg

    gram: g

    kilogram: kg

    Volume

    milliliter: ml

    liter: L

2. Do not use a period with the abbreviations for metric units because it might be mistaken for another letter or symbol.

    Correct: mg

    ml

    Incorrect: mg.

    ml.

3. Use Arabic numerals (e.g., 1, 2, 3, 4) to express the quantity of the dose.

    Correct: 4 mg

    Incorrect: $\overline{\text{iv}}$ mg

4. Place the numeral that expresses the quantity of the dose in front of the abbreviation. To make it easier to read, leave a (single) space between the quantity and the abbreviation.

    Correct: 5 ml

    Incorrect: ml 5

    5ml

5. Write a fraction of a dose as a decimal.

    Correct: 0.5 g

    Incorrect: ½ g

6. If the dose is a fraction of a unit, place a zero before the decimal point as a means of focusing on the fractional dose. This reduces the possibility of misreading the dose as a whole number.

    Correct: 0.5 g (this reduces the possibility of not seeing the decimal point and reading the dose as 5 grams)

    Incorrect: .5 g

7. Do not place a decimal point and a zero after a whole number. The decimal point may be overlooked, resulting in a 10-fold overdose error.

    Correct: 1 ml (this reduces the possibility of not seeing the decimal point and reading the dose as 10 ml)

    Incorrect: 1.0 ml

Metric System: Conversion of Equivalent Values

Weight

1000 micrograms = 1 milligram

1000 milligrams = 1 gram

1000 grams = 1 kilogram

Volume

1000 milliliters = 1 liter

1000 liters = 1 kiloliter

1 milliliter = 1 cubic centimeter

---

the dropper. The remaining units, in order of increasing volume, are *teaspoon, tablespoon, ounce (fluid ounce), cup,* and *glass.* Table 11-2 lists the units of liquid volume measurement in the household system and equivalent values in different units.

Table 11-2 Household System: Conversion of Common Values	
Abbreviations	
drop:	gtt
teaspoon:	tsp
tablespoon:	T
ounce:	oz
cup:	c
Volume	
60 gtt =	1 tsp
3 tsp =	1 T
6 tsp =	1 oz
2 T =	1 oz
6 oz =	1 teacup
8 oz =	1 glass

CONVERTING UNITS OF MEASUREMENT

Changing from one unit of measurement to another is known as **conversion.** Conversion is required when medication is ordered in a unit of measurement that differs from the medication's label. The dose quantity must be mathematically translated or converted to the unit of measurement of the medication on hand. If the physician orders 5 grams of an oral solid medication, and the medication label expresses the drug strength in milligrams, the medical assistant would need to convert the grams into milligrams to know how much medication to administer. Converting units of measurement can be classified into the following categories: (1) conversion of units within a measurement system, and (2) conversion of units from one measurement system to another.

Converting units within a measurement system allows a quantity to be expressed in two different but equal units of measurement within *one* system. An example of converting units of weight within the metric system is as follows: 1 gram is equal to 1000 milligrams. Converting from one measurement system to another allows a quantity written in one measurement system to be expressed in an equivalent unit of measurement in *another* system. An example of a

Apothecary Notation Guidelines

Follow these guidelines when using the medical notation of apothecary units and dosage.

1. The units of apothecary measurement are usually written with abbreviations and symbols as follows:

   Weight

   grain: gr

   dram: dr or ℨ

   ounce: oz or ℥

   Volume

   minim: ♏

   fluid dram: fℨ; fluid ounce: f℥

   pint: pt

   quart: qt

   gallon: gal

2. When writing symbols and abbreviations to express apothecary units, use lowercase roman numerals to express the dose quantity.

   Correct: ℥ vi̇ (6 ounces)

   Incorrect: ℥6

3. Place the roman numeral expressing dose quantity after the symbol or abbreviation.

   Correct: ℨ ii̇ (2 drams)

                gr v (5 grains)

   Incorrect: ii ℨ

               v gr

4. A line may be placed over the roman numerals. Dots are placed above the line for emphasis as a safeguard against error.

   Correct: f ℨ iii̇ (3 fluid drams)

   Incorrect: f ℨ III

5. Write ss to designate one half of a dose, and place it after the apothecary symbol or abbreviation.

   Correct: gr ss

   Incorrect: gr ½

6. Write fractions (other than ½) in Arabic numerals, and place them after the apothecary symbol or abbreviation.

   Correct: gr ¼

   Incorrect: gr 0.25; ¼ gr

   Note: If abbreviations and symbols are not used to express apothecary units of measurement, Arabic numerals must be used to express dose quantity and are placed before the unit of measurement. *Example:* ¼ grain.

Apothecary System: Conversion of Equivalent Values

Weight

60 grains = 1 dram

8 drams = 1 ounce

12 ounces = 1 pound

Volume

60 minims = 1 fluid dram

8 fluid drams = 1 fluid ounce

16 fluid ounces = 1 pint

2 pints = 1 quart

4 quarts = 1 gallon

---

conversion from the apothecary system to the metric system is as follows: 1 grain (apothecary system) is equivalent to 60 milligrams (metric system).

Conversion requires the use of a conversion table to indicate the equivalent values of various units of measurement. Conversion tables of equivalent values in these three measurement systems are included in this chapter:

Metric conversion—*Metric Notation Guidelines* box

Apothecary conversion—*Apothecary Notation Guidelines* box

Household conversion—Table 11-2

Tables used to convert from one system to another consist of approximate rather than exact equivalents, and a 10% error usually occurs in making these conversions. Conversion tables used to convert from one system to another are presented in Table 11-3.

The medical assistant must be careful when using conversion tables to avoid errors in interpolation. The numbers on conversion tables are small and close together; it is easy to misread the chart from one column to the other. To reduce this possibility, a straightedge, such as a ruler, should be used when reading a conversion table.

CONTROLLED DRUGS

By means of federal and state legislation, restrictions are placed on drugs that have potential for abuse. These drugs are known as **controlled drugs.** They are classified into five categories, called *schedules,* which are based on their abuse potential. Table 11-4 lists, describes, and provides examples of the schedules for controlled drugs.

To administer, prescribe, or dispense controlled drugs, the physician must register every year with the Drug Enforcement Administration (DEA). The physician is assigned a registration number known as the **DEA number.** Every time a prescription for a controlled drug is written, the physician must put his or her DEA number in the appropriate space on the prescription blank.

PRESCRIPTION

A **prescription** is a physician's order authorizing the dispensing of a drug by a pharmacist. Prescriptions can be authorized in different forms, including hand-written, computer-generated, and telephoned or faxed to a pharmacy.

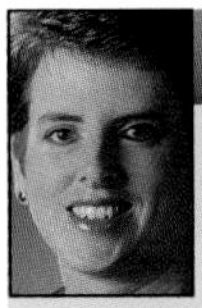

My Name is Theresa Cline, and I work for four physicians in a family practice medical office. I have worked there ever since I graduated from college with an associate's degree in medical assisting. One experience that I will never forget taught our entire office staff a valuable lesson. It involved a woman who came to our office because she had lacerated her wrist while using a butcher knife. After the wound was sutured, I gave her a tetanus injection because she was past due for one. Shortly thereafter, she became very nauseated and dizzy, and I made her lie down on the examining table. She asked me to get her a cold drink of water, and I left the room to do so. Apparently, while I was gone, she must have tried to sit up or turn over because she rolled off the table and struck the back of her head on the floor. She sustained a laceration to her scalp, which also had to be sutured. Owing to her persistent symptoms of severe nausea, vomiting, and headache, it was decided that she should be admitted to the hospital for neurologic observation and x-ray studies.

The vital lesson that this experience taught everyone in our office was that you must never leave a patient alone, not even for a minute to get something, if there is the slightest indication that he or she is not feeling perfectly fine. Another staff member should be called to obtain whatever is needed. From that point on, this has been our office policy and procedure. ■

Abbreviations and symbols are usually used to write a prescription. They also are used to record medication information in the patient's chart. Common abbreviations used in the medical office for writing prescriptions are included in Table 11-5.

The medical assistant should ensure that all prescription pads are kept in a safe place and out of reach of individuals who may want to obtain drugs illegally. The stock supply of prescription pads should be locked in a drawer.

Parts of a Prescription

A prescription is a hand-written (Figure 11-2) or computer-generated document that includes directions to the pharmacist for filling the prescription and instructions to the patient for taking the medication. The specific information that the prescription must include follows:

- **Date.** A pharmacist cannot fill a prescription unless the date the prescription was issued is indicated on the prescription. The reason for this is that a prescription expires after a certain length of time. In most states, a prescription for a drug (with the exception of controlled drugs) expires 1 year from the date of issue. After this time, the prescription (or any refills left on the prescription) cannot be filled.
- **Physician's name, address, telephone number, and fax number.** This information is preprinted on prescription forms that are hand-written and automatically printed on forms that are computer generated. This information identifies the physician issuing the prescription and pro-

Table 11-3 Conversion Charts for Systems of Measurement

CONVERSION CHART FOR METRIC AND APOTHECARY SYSTEMS (COMMON APPROXIMATE EQUIVALENTS)					
Metric System to Apothecary System			**Apothecary System to Metric System**		
Weight			**Weight**		
60 mg	=	1 gr	15 gr	=	1000 mg (1 g)
1 g	=	15 gr	10 gr	=	600 mg
29 g	=	1 dr	7½ gr	=	500 mg
30 g	=	1 oz	5 gr	=	300 mg
1 kg	=	2.2 lb	3 gr	=	200 mg
			1½ gr		100 mg
Volume			**Volume**		
0.06 ml	=	1 ♏	1 gr	=	60 mg
1 ml (cc)	=	15 ♏	¾ gr	=	50 mg
4 ml	=	1 ℨ	½ gr	=	30 mg
30 ml	=	1 ℥	¼ gr	=	15 mg
500 ml	=	1 pt	⅙ gr	=	10 mg
1000 ml (1 L)	=	1 qt	⅛ gr	=	8 mg
			1/12 gr	=	5 mg
			1/15 gr	=	4 mg
			1/20 gr	=	3 mg
			1/30 gr	=	2 mg
			1/40 gr	=	1.5 mg
			1/50 gr	=	1.2 mg
			1/60 gr	=	1 mg
			1/100 gr	=	0.6 mg
			1/120 gr	=	0.5 mg
			1/150 gr	=	0.4 mg
			1/200 gr	=	0.3 mg
			1/300 gr	=	0.2 mg
			1/600 gr	=	0.1 mg

EQUIVALENCES IN HOUSEHOLD, APOTHECARY, AND METRIC UNITS (VOLUME)		
Household	**Apothecary**	**Metric**
1 gtt	= 1 ♏	= 0.06 ml
15 gtt	= 15 ♏	= 1 ml (1 cc)
1 tsp	= ⅙ ℥	= 5 (4) ml*
1 T	= ½ ℥	= 15 ml
2 T	= 1 ℥	= 30 ml
1 oz	= 1 ℥	= 30 ml
1 teacup	= 6 ℥	= 180 ml
1 glass	= 8 ℥	= 240 ml

*The American standard teaspoon is accepted as 5 ml; however, 4 ml can be used as the equivalent to provide a more accurate conversion.

Table 11-4 Classification of Controlled Drugs

Classification	Description and Prescription Regulations	EXAMPLES	
		Generic	Brand
Schedule I	High potential for abuse Currently no accepted medical use in treatment in the United States There is a lack of accepted safety for use of the drug under medical supervision Use may lead to severe physical or psychological dependence May be used for research with appropriate limitations Not available for prescribing	GHB heroin LSD marijuana MDMA (Ecstasy) mescaline methaqualone (Quaalude) psilocybin	
Schedule II	High potential for abuse Currently accepted medical use in treatment in the United States or a currently accepted medical use with severe restrictions Abuse may lead to severe psychological or physical dependence Prescription must be in writing in indelible ink or typed Emergency telephone order permitted only for immediate amount needed to treat patient; written prescription must be provided to pharmacist within 7 days No refills allowed Manufacturer's label marked C-II	**Analgesics** cocaine codeine fentanyl hydrocodone hydromorphone meperidine methadone morphine oxycodone oxycodone/APAP oxycodone/ASA **Central Nervous System Stimulants** dextroamphetamine lisdexamfetamine methylphenidate methamphetamine **Sedatives/Hypnotics** amobarbital glutethimide pentobarbital secobarbital	 Duragesic Dilaudid Demerol Dolophine Roxanol OxyContin Percocet Percodan Adderall Vyvanese Ritalin, Concerta Desoxyn Amytal Doriden Nembutal Seconal
Schedule III	Less potential for abuse than drugs in Schedules I and II Currently accepted medical use in treatment in the United States Abuse may lead to moderate or low physical dependence or high psychological dependence Telephone and fax orders permitted If authorized by physician, prescription can be refilled five times within 6 months from issue date Prescription expires 6 months from issue date Manufacturer's label marked C-III	**Anabolic Steroids** oxandrolone oxymetholone **Analgesics** buprenorphine butalbital compound codeine combined with nonopioid analgesic hydrocodone combined with nonopioid analgesic **Central Nervous System Stimulant** benzphetamine **Male Hormone** testosterone **Sedative/Hypnotic** butabarbital	 Anavar Anapolon Buprenex Fioricet, Fiorinal Tylenol w/ codeine, Empirin w/ codeine Vicodin, Lortab, Lorcet, Tussionex, Vicoprofen Didrex Depotest, Delatestryl Butisol

Table 11-4 Classification of Controlled Drugs—cont'd

Classification	Description and Prescription Regulations	EXAMPLES	
		Generic	Brand
Schedule IV	Lower potential for abuse than drugs in Schedule III Currently accepted medical use in treatment in the United States Abuse may lead to limited physical or psychological dependence Telephone and fax orders permitted If authorized by physician, prescription can be refilled five times within 6 months of issue date Prescription expires 6 months from issue date Manufacturer's label marked C-IV	**Analgesics** butorphanol pentazocine propoxyphene **Antianxiety Agents** alprazolam chlordiazepoxide diazepam halazepam lorazepam meprobamate oxazepam **Anticonvulsant** clonazepam **Central Nervous System Stimulants** modafinil pemoline **Sedatives/Hypnotics** chloral hydrate eszopiclone ethchlorvynol flurazepam midazolam phenobarbital temazepam triazolam zaleplon zolpidem **Weight Control Agents** diethylpropion phentermine sibutramine	Stadol Talwin Darvon, Darvocet-N Xanax Librium Valium Paxipam Ativan Equanil Serax Klonopin Provigil Cylert Noctec Lunesta Placidyl Dalmane Versed Luminal Restoril Halcion Sonata Ambien Tenuate Fastin Meridia

Schedule V	Low potential for abuse
	Accepted medical use in United States
	Abuse may lead to limited physical or psychological dependence
	Telephone and fax orders permitted
	Prescribing policies determined by state and local regulations. In most states:
	  Number of refills determined by physician
	  Prescription expires 1 year from issue date
	  Some are available without prescription to patients older than 18 years of age (with proper identification)
	Manufacturer's label marked C-V
		Cough suppressants with small amounts of codeine
		Antidiarrheals containing paregoric
		diphenoxylate/atropine
			Robitussin A-C, Cheracol syrup
			Parepectolin, Kapectolin PG
			
			Lomotil

Table 11-5 Common Abbreviations and Symbols Used in Medication Documentation

Abbreviation or Symbol	Meaning	Abbreviation or Symbol	Meaning
$\overline{aa}$	of each	OS	left eye
ac	before meals	OTC	over-the-counter
AD	right ear	OU	in each eye
ad lib	as desired	$\overline{3}$ or oz	ounce
aq	water	$\overline{p}$	after
admin	administer, administration	pc	after meals
AM or a.m.	morning	Pt or pt	patient
APAP	acetaminophen	per	by
AS	left ear	PM or p.m.	evening
ASA	aspirin	po or PO	by mouth
AU	in each ear	prn	as needed
bid	twice a day	qAM	every morning
$\overline{c}$	with	qd	every day
cap(s)	capsule(s)	qh	every hour
cc	cubic centimeter	q (2, 3, 4) h	every (2, 3, 4) hours
DAW	dispense as written	qid	four times a day
dil	dilute	qod	every other day
3 or dr	dram	qs	of sufficient quantity
elix	elixir	Rx	take
g	gram	$\overline{s}$	without
gr	grain	SC or SQ	subcutaneous
gtt(s)	drop(s)	SL	sublingual
h or hr	hour	sol	solution
hs	at bedtime	ss	one half
ID	intradermal	STAT	immediately
IM	intramuscular	T	tablespoon
IN	inhalation	tab(s)	tablet(s)
IV	intravenous	tid	three times a day
kg	kilogram	tsp	teaspoon
L	liter	#	number
liq	liquid	×	times
m	minim	Ø	no, none
med(s)	medication(s)	$\dot{\imath}$	one
mg	milligram	$\dot{\imath\imath}$	two
min	minute	$\dot{\imath\imath\imath}$	three
ml	milliliter	$\dot{\imath v}$	four
NPO	nothing by mouth	$\overline{v}$	five
OD	right eye		

vides the necessary information should the pharmacist have a question and need to contact the medical office.

- **Patient's name and address.** This information is important for insurance billing and for properly dispensing the medication.
- **Patient's age.** The patient's age is important to the pharmacist when he or she double checks the physician's order to ensure that the proper dose is being dispensed. The most common errors in dosage occur among children and the elderly, who may not require the standard dose of a drug because these age groups metabolize drugs differently. The patient's age also allows the pharmacist to double check that the drug is age appropriate for the patient. For example, *ciprofloxacin* (e.g., Cipro) should not be taken by children and adolescents because this antibiotic can damage cartilage in individuals younger than 18 years old.
- **Superscription.** The superscription consists of the symbol *Rx.* This symbol comes from the Latin word *recipe* and means "take."

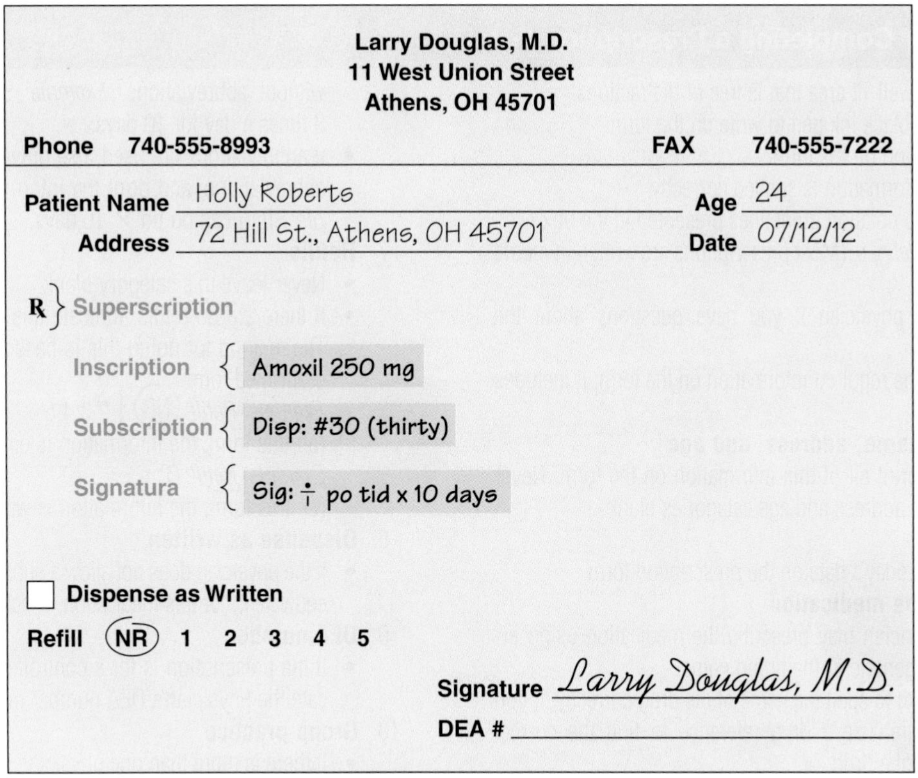
Larry Douglas, M.D.
11 West Union Street
Athens, OH 45701

Phone 740-555-8993 FAX 740-555-7222

Patient Name Holly Roberts Age 24
Address 72 Hill St., Athens, OH 45701 Date 07/12/12

℞ } Superscription

Inscription { Amoxil 250 mg

Subscription { Disp: #30 (thirty)

Signatura { Sig: ī po tid x 10 days

☐ Dispense as Written

Refill (NR) 1 2 3 4 5

Signature Larry Douglas, M.D.
DEA #

Figure 11-2. Example of a hand-written prescription.

- **Inscription.** The inscription states the name of the drug and the dose (e.g., Amoxil 250 mg). Most drugs are available in various doses; it is important that the correct dose be prescribed. For example, Amoxil comes in the following doses: 125 mg, 250 mg, and 500 mg.
- **Subscription.** The subscription gives directions to the pharmacist. At present, it is generally used to designate the number of doses to be dispensed. To prevent a prescription from being altered illegally, it is recommended that numbers and letters be used to indicate the quantity to be dispensed (e.g., #30 [thirty]).
- **Signatura.** The signatura (abbreviated *Sig.*) is a Latin term that means "write" or "label" and indicates the information to be included on the medication label. It consists of directions to the patient for taking the medication. The name of the medication also is included on the label so that the patient can identify the medication.
- **Refill.** This part of the prescription indicates the number of times the prescription may be refilled.
- **Physician's signature.** A prescription cannot be filled unless it is signed by the physician.
- **DEA number.** The number assigned to the physician by the Drug Enforcement Administration must appear on the prescription for a controlled drug. See Table 11-4 for examples of controlled drugs.

Generic Prescribing

Generic prescribing means that the physician writes the prescription using the generic rather than the brand name of the drug. Because many pharmaceutical manufacturers may produce the same generic drug and sell it under different brand names, price competition often results. If the physician prescribes a drug using its generic name, the pharmacist is permitted to fill it with the drug that offers the best savings to the patient. In addition, most states allow the pharmacist the option of filling the prescription with a chemically equivalent generic drug, even if the drug has been prescribed by brand name. If the physician wants the prescription to be filled with a specific brand of drug, instructions must be indicated on the prescription form, such as "Dispense as Written (DAW)," or words of a similar meaning (see Figure 11-2).

Completing a Prescription Form

The physician is responsible for having accurate and pertinent information on the prescription form. If delegated by the physician, a prescription form can be completed by the medical assistant and signed by the physician. The physician must review the prescription thoroughly before signing it to ensure all of the information is correct. If the medical assistant is delegated this responsibility, he or she must carefully follow the important guidelines presented in the box *Guidelines for Completing a Prescription Form.*

EMR Prescription Program

Electronic medical record (EMR) software includes a prescription program, which greatly reduces the amount of time needed to prescribe and refill medication. The prescription program generates and prints a prescription(s) on a regular sheet of 8½ × 11-inch paper, which is then signed

Guidelines for Completing a Prescription Form

- Work in a quiet, well-lit area that is free of distractions.
- Use an indelible black ink pen to write on the form.
- Print all information on the form.
- Ensure that all information is spelled correctly.
- Review the metric notation guidelines presented in the box *Metric Notation Guidelines*. (Most prescriptions are written in metric units.)
- Always ask the physician if you have questions about the prescription.
- Complete all of the required information on the form; it includes the following:

  1. **Patient's name, address, and age**
     - Clearly print all of this information on the form. Never leave the address and age categories blank.
  2. **Date**
     - Indicate today's date on the prescription form.
  3. **Name of the medication**
     - The physician may prescribe the medication using either the generic or the brand name.
     - Make sure to spell the name of the drug correctly. If you are unsure, use a drug reference to find the correct spelling of a drug.
  4. **Medication dosage**
     - Never leave a decimal point "naked." If the dosage is a fraction of a unit, a zero must be placed before the decimal point as a means of focusing on the fractional dose. This reduces the possibility of misreading the dose as a whole number. *Example:* 0.5 ml (*not* .5 ml).
     - Never place a decimal point and a zero after a whole number because the decimal point may be overlooked, resulting in a 10-fold overdose error. *Example:* 5 mg (*not* 5.0 mg).
  5. **Quantity to dispense**
     - Use numbers and letters to indicate the quantity to be dispensed. *Example:* Disp: #30 (thirty).
     - Ensure that the quantity is correct. The number of prescribed pills should match the duration of treatment. *Example:* If the patient has been prescribed 3 tablets a day for 7 days, the quantity should be written as follows: Disp: #21 (twenty-one).
  6. **Directions for taking the medication**
     - Clearly indicate the directions for taking the medication. Many authorities recommend writing the directions

without abbreviations. *Example:* Sig: Take 1 capsule 3 times a day for 10 days.
- If abbreviations are used, use only commonly accepted abbreviations, and print the information clearly. *Example:* Sig: ī cap po tid × 10 days.

  7. **Refills**
     - Never leave this category blank.
     - If there are no refills, indicate this clearly on the form. The method for doing this is based on the setup of the preprinted form.
       Example: Refill: (NR) 1 2 3 4 5
       (on this form, the information is circled)
       Example: Refill: Ø
       (on this form, the information is written in)
  8. **Dispense as written**
     - If the physician does not allow a substitution (e.g., generic equivalent) for this medication, check this category.
  9. **DEA number**
     - If the prescription is for a controlled drug, clearly indicate the physician's DEA number on the form.
  10. **Group practice**
      - If there is more than one physician in the practice, circle (or check) the name of the physician prescribing the medication. This avoids confusion if the pharmacist cannot read the physician's signature.
        Example:
        James Ortman, MD, (Mark Rothstein, MD), Richard Bontrager, MD
      - Give the prescription to the physician to review and sign.
      - Document the prescription order in the patient's medication record if directed by the physician. Some offices use multiple-copy prescription pads. In this case, file the copy of the prescription in the patient's medical record.
      - Give the prescription to the patient. Provide the patient with guidelines for taking the medication (see patient teaching box on prescription medications).
      - Ask the patient whether he or she has any questions about the medication.

by the physician and given to the patient (Figure 11-3). The program can also transmit the prescription electronically (by e-fax or e-mail) to the patient's pharmacy. Both of these features eliminate the need for the pharmacist to decipher the physician's handwriting.

To use an EMR prescription program, the physician first selects the medication. The program displays a list of available dosage strengths and preparation forms (e.g., tablets, oral solution, parenteral solution, suppository) for that medication. The physician highlights the dosage strength and preparation desired and enters the information into the computer. Next, the physician selects additional information related to the prescription, such as dosage frequency and number of refills using fill-in boxes, drop-down lists,

PRESCRIPTION: (Give to the pharmacist)	PRESCRIPTION: (Give to the pharmacist)
Huntington Clinic 701 Concord Ave Lexington, KY 48710 614-871-0033 Doctor: John Blauser, MD For: Danielle Travis Age: 28 DOB: 08/08/84 Date: 10/27/2012 Address: 101 Coventry Lane Lexington, KY 48710 Rx: Amoxil (Generic - amoxicillin) (Dose/unit - 250 mg) (Form - Caps) (Disp - #30) (Frequency - One three times daily for 10 days) (Route - By mouth) (Refills-0). Dr: _____ *John Blauser, MD* _____	Huntington Clinic 701 Concord Ave Lexington, KY 48710 614-871-0033 Doctor: John Blauser, MD For: Danielle Travis Age: 28 DOB: 08/08/84 Date: 10/27/2012 Address: 101 Coventry Lane Lexington, KY 48710 Rx: Tylenol-3 (Generic - Acetaminophen/Codeine) (Dose/unit - 1 to 2) (Form - Tabs) (Disp - #15)(fifteen) (Frequency - Every 4 hours as needed for moderate to severe pain) (Route - By mouth) (Refills-0). Dr: _____ *John Blauser, MD* _____

Figure 11-3. Example of a computer-generated prescription.

PATIENT TEACHING   Prescription Medications

To avoid adverse reactions, teach patients the proper guidelines for taking prescription medication. These guidelines are as follows:

Know the names of all your prescription and nonprescription medications. Know the generic and brand names of each of your medications. Nonprescription drugs are known as *over-the-counter* (OTC) drugs; they are drugs that can be purchased without a prescription. Vitamin supplements and herbal products are considered OTC drugs.

Know why you are taking each medication. It is important to know the desired therapeutic outcome, dosage, frequency and time of administration, and common side effects of each medication, and guidelines ("do's and dont's") to follow when taking the medication. Never take your medication in the dark or without your reading glasses (if needed for close vision).

Take your medication exactly as prescribed, at the right times and in the right amounts. The medication may not work properly if it is not taken as directed. If the dose is too small, the drug may not produce its intended therapeutic effect; exceeding the recommended dosage could result in a toxic effect. Make sure you know what to do if you are late in taking a dose or miss a dose of your medication. It is also important to know if any other medication or food interferes with your medication and should be avoided.

Inform the physician if new symptoms or adverse effects develop when you are taking the medication. The physician may need to change your dosage or prescribe a different medication. There are usually alternative medications that the physician can prescribe to treat your condition.

Take the medication for the prescribed duration of time, even after you begin to feel better. If you do not complete the entire course of drug therapy, your condition may recur. Not taking all of a prescribed antibiotic may cause an infection to return, and it may be worse than the first infection.

Tell the physician if you decide not to take your medication. Otherwise, the physician may think your medication is not working. Not taking a medication prescribed by the physician could be serious because this may allow your condition to worsen.

Do not take additional medications, including OTC medications, without checking with the physician. All drugs, including OTC medications, are designed to have an effect on the body. Some combinations of drugs cause serious reactions. In some cases, one drug cancels the effects of another and prevents it from working.

Never take a medication that was prescribed for someone else. Physicians prescribe medication based on an individual's age, weight, sex, and condition. Taking a medication prescribed for someone else can have serious results.

Keep all medications in their original containers to avoid taking the wrong medication by mistake. Store your medications in their original containers from the pharmacy. Basic information about your medication is on the original container. Medications that are not clearly marked may be taken inadvertently by the wrong person.

Store your medications in a safe place, away from the reach of children. If you have young children, make sure your

Continued

medication is dispensed in containers with child-resistant safety closures. After taking your medication, make sure that the cap of the container is closed tightly. Accidental drug poisoning in children is a common and preventable problem. Also, do not take your medication in front of young children because they may want to mimic your behavior.

Store medications in a cool, dry place or as stated on the label. Do not store capsules or tablets in the bathroom or

kitchen because heat or moisture may cause the medication to break down.

Discard unused portions of prescription medications and outdated OTC medications. Medications should be discarded by flushing them down the toilet. Medications that are past their expiration dates may produce adverse effects in the body.

---

and check-boxes. The program automatically checks the prescription against any drug allergies the patient may have. It also checks for potential interactions with other medications being taken by the patient. Once the physician has entered the prescription into the computer, the medication is recorded in the patient's medication record. The prescription is then printed out, signed by the physician, and given to the patient or sent electronically to the pharmacy. The prescription program usually provides access to extensive and current product information on all FDA-approved medications.

The EMR prescription program usually has the capability to compare the prescription against the *formulary* or list of drugs covered by the patient's insurance plan. If the prescription is not in the patient's formulary, the physician is advised of alternate drugs that are covered by the patient's insurance plan.

The EMR prescription program also has the capability to quickly refill a prescription and print a list of medications being taken by the patient. The patient can use this list to keep track of the medication he or she is taking (Figure 11-4).

MEDICATION RECORD

A medication record form (Figure 11-5) includes detailed information about each medication, so that the physician can tell at a glance what medications and how much the patient is taking. Both prescription medication and over-the-counter (OTC) medication, including vitamin supplements and herbal products, must be recorded in the medication record.

The medication record is part of the patient's medical record. The medical assistant is often responsible for documenting medication information in the medication record. Care must be taken to ensure the information is correct and clearly stated.

In a paper-based patient record (PPR), the medical office may use a preprinted form to record the medication that a patient is taking. With an EMR, the medical assistant enters this information into a digital form on the screen of the monitor using free-text entry, drop-down lists, and check-boxes.

A medication record typically includes the following information:

- Patient's name and date of birth
- Any drug allergies
- Date the medication was prescribed (Rx) or date the patient started taking the medication (OTC)
- Name and dose of the medication
- Frequency of administration of the medication
- Route of administration
- Prescription or OTC medication category
- Refills (Rx medication only)
- Date the patient stopped taking the medication

What Would You Do? What Would You *Not* Do?

Case Study 2

Linda Cardwell calls the medical office. Her daughter Rachel, 9 years old, was seen in the office 10 days ago. Rachel was diagnosed with strep throat, and the physician ordered Amoxil 250 mg tid × 7 days. Mrs. Cardwell says that after 3 days of taking the medication, Rachel was much better, so she stopped giving her the Amoxil because it was causing her to have diarrhea. Mrs. Cardwell says that her 12-year-old son started feeling achy all over and she gave him the Amoxil for 2 days, and it seemed to help. She also says that her husband started complaining of sinus problems, so she also gave him the Amoxil for 2 days. Mrs. Cardwell says that now Rachel's throat is hurting again, and she has a fever. She wants to know whether Rachel has developed another case of strep throat. Mrs. Cardwell says she does not know what to do because she does not have any Amoxil left to give Rachel. ■

FACTORS AFFECTING DRUG ACTION
Therapeutic Effect

Each drug has an intended therapeutic effect—the reason the patient takes the medication. Certain factors affect the therapeutic action of drugs in the body, causing patients to respond differently to the same drug. Because of this, the drug therapy may need to be adjusted to meet these variations, which include the following.

Huntington Clinic
701 Concord Ave
Lexington, KY 48710
614-871-0033

Patient: Clare Andrews
    352 Pinewood Dr.
    Lexington, KY 48710

Age/DOB: 12/25/1970
EMRN: 7016780

Medication List

Medication	Refills	Start
Abilify 15 mg tablet	0	24Sep2011
TAKE 1 TABLET DAILY		
Acetaminophen-Codeine #3 300-30 mg tablet	0	23Sep2012
TAKE 1 TABLET EVERY 6 TO 8 HOURS AS NEEDED FOR PAIN		
Clonazepam 1 mg tablet	0	24Sep2011
TAKE 1 TABLET EVERY 8 HOURS PRN		
Etodolac CR 500 mg tablet extended release 24 hour	0	21Sep2011
1-2 TABLETS PO ONCE DAILY WITH FOOD		
Fish Oil 1000 mg capsule	11	7Apr2011
TAKE 1 CAPSULE DAILY		
Flovent HFA 44 mcg/act aerosol	3	6Jan2011
INHALE 2 PUFFS TWICE DAILY		
Fluticasone Propionate 50 mcg/act suspension	3	9Sep2011
USE 2 SPRAYS IN EACH NOSTRIL ONCE DAILY		
Lamictal 200 mg tablet	0	24Sep2011
TAKE 2 TABLETS DAILY		
Omeprazole 20 mg capsule delayed release	11	24Sep2011
TAKE 1 TABLET DAILY		
Pamine 2.5 mg tablet	0	6Jan2011
TAKE 1 TABLET 3 TIMES DAILY		
Proventil HFA 108 (90 base) mcg/act aerosol solution	3	21Jul2012
INHALE 1-2 PUFFS EVERY 4-6 HOURS AS NEEDED AND AS DIRECTED		
Tramadol HCl 50 mg tablet	0	29Apr2011
TAKE 1 TABLET EVERY 6 HOURS		
Voltaren 1% gel	6	24Sep2011
APPLY 2 GRAMS TOPICALLY 4 TIMES DAILY		
WelChol 625 mg tablet	11	29Apr2012
TAKE 3 TABLETS TWICE DAILY WITH MEALS		

Figure 11-4. Example of a computer-generated patient medication list.

Age

Children and the elderly tend to respond more strongly to drugs than young and middle-aged adults. The physician may calculate smaller doses for very young and geriatric patients.

Route of Administration

Medications administered by different routes are absorbed at different rates. Drugs administered orally are absorbed slowly because they must be digested first. Parenterally administered drugs are absorbed more quickly than orally administered drugs because they are injected directly into the body.

Size

A patient's body size has an effect on drug action. A thin individual may require a smaller quantity of a drug, and an obese individual may require more.

Time of Administration

A drug administered through the oral route is absorbed more rapidly when the stomach is empty than when it contains food. A drug may not produce the desired effect or may be absorbed too slowly if it is taken when food is present. Some drugs irritate the stomach's lining, however, and must be taken with food. The drug package insert or a drug reference should always be consulted to determine when a drug should be taken.

Tolerance

A patient taking a certain drug over a period of time may develop a tolerance to it. This means that the same dose of a drug no longer produces the desired effect after prolonged administration. The physician should be notified to determine whether a change of drug or dosage is needed.

MEDICATION RECORD

Patient ___John Walsh___

Birthdate ___6/10/49___

ALLERGY
Ø

DATE	MEDICATION AND DOSAGE	FREQUENCY	RX	OTC	REFILLS		STOP
2/18/11	Cipro 250 mg	ī q 12 h po x 10 days	X				2/28/11
6/10/11	Prevacid 15 mg	ī qd po	X				7/10/11
6/10/11	Lipitor 10 mg	ī qd po	X		1/6/12		
6/10/11	Prozac 20 mg	ī qd po	X		1/6/12		
12/3/11	Tobrex Ophthalmic Solution	ī gtt q3h OD	X				12/10/11
2/5/12	Echinacea	ī qd po		X			
3/15/12	Nitrostat 0.4 mg	ī prn pain SL Rep q 5 min prn pain, not to exceed 3 tabs	X				
3/15/12	Inderal 40 mg	ī bid po	X				
3/15/12	St. Joseph's ASA Enteric Coated 81 mg	ī qd po		X			

Figure 11-5. Example of a medication record.

Memories *from* Externship

Theresa Cline: I can clearly remember the first time I gave an injection at my externship site. I was worried that I would forget how to give an injection and look bad in front of my externship supervisor and the patient. What made things worse is that the patient was a woman with very thin arms. I was giving her a flu shot, and I was so scared that the needle would hit her bone even though I was only using a 1-inch needle. When I walked into the room, my supervisor told the woman that I was a student and asked her if it was all right if I gave her the flu injection. The woman laughed and said, "Well, I guess so." That made me feel even more nervous. The patient then asked if it was my first shot. I told her "yes" and she said, "Just don't hurt me." When it came time to give the injection, everything that I had ever learned about injections came back to me. I gave the injection, and the woman told me I did a good job and that she didn't even feel it. That made me feel so good! My supervisor said, "If you can give a shot to her, you can give a shot to anyone." Every injection after that was a "piece of cake." I've learned just to take a deep breath before each difficult situation encountered in the office, and everything will work out. ∎

Undesirable Effects of Drugs

A drug may cause undesirable effects, which may occur immediately or may be delayed hours or even days after administration of the medication.

Adverse Reactions

Most drugs produce unintended and undesirable effects known as **adverse reactions.** Adverse reactions are secondary effects that occur along with the therapeutic effect of the drug. Some adverse reactions, referred to as *side effects,* are harmless and are often tolerated by the patient to obtain the therapeutic effect of the drug. Most patients are willing to tolerate the dry mouth and drowsiness that may accompany an antihistamine to obtain its therapeutic effect. Other adverse reactions, such as a decrease in blood pressure or an allergic reaction, can be harmful to the patient and warrant discontinuing the medication.

Drug Interactions

When certain medications are used at the same time, drug interactions may produce undesirable effects. The medical assistant should inquire about other medications the patient is taking and record this information in the patient's chart for review by the physician.

Allergic Drug Reaction

The patient may exhibit an allergic reaction to a drug. The reaction is usually mild and takes the form of a rash, rhinitis, or pruritus. Occasionally, a patient has a severe allergic reaction that occurs suddenly and immediately. This is known as an **anaphylactic reaction.**

An anaphylactic reaction is the least common but the most serious type of allergic reaction. Symptoms begin with sneezing, urticaria (hives), itching, erythema, angioedema, and disorientation. Erythema is reddening of the skin caused by dilation of superficial blood vessels in the skin. Angioedema is a localized urticaria of the deeper tissues of the body. If not treated, the symptoms of anaphylaxis quickly increase in severity and progress to dyspnea, cyanosis, and shock. Blood pressure decreases, and the pulse becomes weak and thready. Convulsions, loss of consciousness, and death may occur if treatment is not initiated promptly.

To prevent an anaphylactic reaction to a drug or to reduce its danger, the medical assistant should stay with the patient after administration of the medication. The medical assistant should be especially alert for signs of an anaphylactic reaction after administering allergy skin tests or a penicillin or allergy injection. If a reaction occurs, the physician should be notified immediately so that he or she can begin treatment immediately. Treatment generally consists of one or more injections of epinephrine, depending on the severity of the reaction. Epinephrine goes to work immediately to reverse the life-threatening symptoms of anaphylaxis. When the patient is stabilized, he or she is usually given an injection of an antihistamine. The antihistamine takes longer to begin working but helps alleviate urticaria, itching, angioedema, and erythema. The medical assistant must ensure that an ample supply of epinephrine is on hand at all times. Many offices maintain emergency crash carts for this purpose.

Idiosyncratic Reaction

An idiosyncratic reaction is an abnormal or peculiar response to a drug that is unexplained and unpredictable. Elderly patients are most prone to idiosyncratic reactions to drugs and should be monitored closely when they are taking a new medication.

GUIDELINES FOR PREPARATION AND ADMINISTRATION OF MEDICATION

To prevent medication errors, the medical assistant should follow these guidelines when preparing and administering any drug:

1. Work in a quiet, well-lit atmosphere that is free of distractions.
2. Always ask if you have a question about the medication order.
3. Know the drug to be given.
4. Select the proper drug. Check the label of the medication three times—as it is taken from its storage location, before preparing the medication, and after preparing the medication. Do not use a drug if the label is missing or is difficult to read.
5. Do not use a drug if the color has changed, if a precipitate has formed, or if it has an unusual odor.
6. Check the expiration date before preparing the drug for administration.
7. Prepare the proper dose of the drug. The term **dose** refers to the quantity of a drug to be administered at one time. Each medication has a dose range, or range of quantities of the drug that can produce therapeutic effects. It is important to administer the exact dose of the drug. A dose that is too small would not produce a therapeutic effect, and a dose that is too large could be harmful or even fatal to the patient.
8. Correctly identify the patient so that the drug is administered to the intended patient. When medication is administered, the patient should be identified by his or her full name and date of birth.
9. Before administering the medication, check the patient's records or question the patient to ensure that he or she is not allergic to the medication.
10. If you are giving an injection, determine the appropriate route and site at which to administer the injection; the route and site are dictated by the type of injection being given. An allergy injection is given through the SC route, and an antibiotic injection is given through the IM route. The site must be free from abrasions, lesions, bruises, and edema.
11. Use the proper technique to administer the medication.
12. Stay with the patient after administering the medication.
13. Document information properly in the patient's medical record immediately after administering the drug. Include the date and time, the name of the medication, the lot number (if required), the dose given, the route of administration, the site of administration, and any unusual observations or patient reactions. Sign the recording with your name and credentials. If you administer a medication that contains a fraction of a unit, place a 0 before the decimal point (e.g., 0.5 mg, not .5 mg) so that the dosage is not misread as 5 mg. A decimal point and a zero should never be placed after a whole number. The decimal point may be overlooked and misread, resulting in a 10-fold overdose error (e.g., 20 mg, not 20.0 mg).
14. Always follow the seven "rights" of preparing and administering medication in the medical office:
    Right drug
    Right dose
    Right time
    Right patient
    Right route
    Right technique
    Right documentation

ORAL ADMINISTRATION

The oral route is the most convenient and most used method of administering medication. **Oral administration** means that the drug is given by mouth in either a solid form (e.g., tablet, capsule) or a liquid form (e.g., suspension, syrup). Absorption of most oral medications occurs in the small intestine, although some may be absorbed in the mouth and stomach.

Many patients find it easier to swallow a tablet or a capsule with a glass of water. Water should not be offered after the patient has received a cough syrup, however, because the water would dilute the medication's beneficial effects. Unless the patient has a malabsorption problem or is unable to swallow, the oral route is considered the safest and most desirable route for administering medication. Procedure 11-1 outlines the procedure for the administration of oral medications.

PROCEDURE 11-1   Administering Oral Medication

Outcome Administer oral solid and liquid medications.

Equipment/Supplies

- Medication ordered by the physician
- Medicine cup
- Medication tray

---

1. **Procedural Step.** Sanitize your hands.
2. **Procedural Step.** Assemble the equipment.
3. **Procedural Step.** Work in a quiet, well-lit atmosphere.
   Principle. Good lighting aids the medical assistant in reading the medication label.
4. **Procedural Step.** Select the correct medication from the shelf. Compare the medication with the physician's instructions. Check the drug label three times—while removing the medication from storage, while preparing the medication, and after preparing the medication. Check the expiration date.
   Principle. If the medication is outdated, consult the physician because it may produce undesirable effects for which the medical assistant could be held responsi-

ble. To prevent a drug error, the medication should be carefully compared with the physician's instructions.
5. **Procedural Step.** Calculate the correct dose to be given, if necessary.
6. **Procedural Step.** Remove the bottle cap, touching the outside of the lid only.
   Principle. Touching the inside of the lid contaminates it.
7. **Procedural Step.** Check the drug label again, and pour the medication.
   a. *Solid Medications.* Pour the correct number of capsules or tablets into the bottle cap. Transfer the medication to a medicine cup, being careful not to touch the inside of the cup.
      Principle. Pouring the medication into the lid prevents contamination of the medication and lid.
   b. *Liquid Medications.* Place the lid of the bottle on a flat surface with the open end facing up. Palm the surface of the label.
   c. With the opposite hand, place the thumbnail at the proper calibration on the medicine cup, and

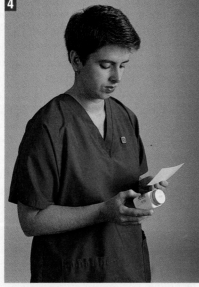

Compare the medication with the physician's instructions.

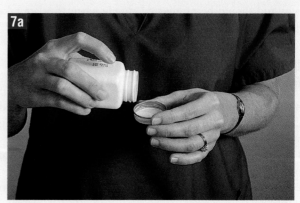

Pour the correct number of capsules or tablets into the bottle cap.

PROCEDURE 11-1 Administering Oral Medication—cont'd

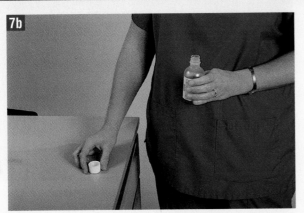

Place the lid of the bottle on a flat surface with the open end facing up.

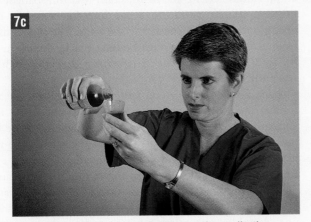

Hold the cup at eye level, and pour the medication.

hold the cup at eye level. Pour the medication, and read the dose at the lowest level of the meniscus. (The meniscus is the curved surface of the liquid in a container. When a liquid is poured into a medicine cup, capillary action causes the liquid in contact with the cup to be drawn upward, resulting in a curved surface in the middle.)

Principle. Placing the bottle cap with the open end up prevents contamination of the inside of the cap. Palming the medication label prevents the medication from dripping on the label and obscuring it.

8. **Procedural Step.** Replace the bottle cap, and check the drug label a third time to ensure it is the correct medication. Return the medication to its storage location.

9. **Procedural Step.** Greet the patient and introduce yourself. Identify the patient by full name and date of birth and explain the procedure. Explain the purpose of administering the medication.

Principle. It is crucial that no error be made in patient identity.

10. **Procedural Step.** Hand the medicine cup containing the medication to the patient, along with a glass of water. (If the medication is a cough syrup, do not offer water.)

Principle. Water helps the patient swallow the medication.

11. **Procedural Step.** Remain with the patient until the medication is swallowed. If the patient experiences any unusual reaction, notify the physician.

12. **Procedural Step.** Sanitize your hands.

13. **Procedural Step.** Chart the procedure. Include the date and time, the name of the medication, the dosage given, the route of administration, and any significant observations or patient reactions. The Latin abbreviation *po,* which means "by mouth," can be used to indicate the route of administration.

CHARTING EXAMPLE	
Date	
2/12/12	9:30 a.m. Acetaminophen, 650 mg, po.
	———————— T. Cline, CMA (AAMA)

PARENTERAL ADMINISTRATION

The parenteral route of drug administration has several advantages. Medications given subcutaneously, intramuscularly, and intravenously are absorbed more rapidly and completely than medications given orally. In some cases, the parenteral route is the only way a drug can be given (e.g., insulin, most immunizations). If the patient is unconscious or has a gastric disturbance, such as nausea or vomiting, the parenteral route may be used to administer medication. If state laws permit, the medical assistant is usually responsible for administering SC, IM, and intradermal injections. IV medications are sometimes administered in the medical office and are discussed in greater detail later in the section on IV therapy.

The parenteral route also has disadvantages, such as pain and the possibility of infection as a result of breaking the skin. The medical assistant can minimize pain by inserting and withdrawing the needle quickly and smoothly and by withdrawing the needle at the same angle as for insertion. If injections are given repeatedly (e.g., allergy injections), the site should be rotated to prevent the overuse of one site, which may cause irritation and tissue damage. Rotating sites also allows for better absorption of the drug.

When recording the administration of a medication in the patient's chart, the medical assistant must include the site of injection (e.g., right upper arm, left dorsogluteal). This assists in proper site rotation for patients who receive repeated injections. In addition, the information provides a reference point should a problem arise with the injection site.

Medical asepsis must be used when parenteral medications are administered. In addition, the needle and the inside of the syringe must remain sterile. These practices reduce the danger of microorganisms entering the patient's body during the administration of medication. The medical assistant must follow the Occupational Safety and Health Administration (OSHA) standard when administering medication as a means of protecting himself or herself from bloodborne pathogens (see Chapter 2). Procedure 11-2 describes how to prepare an injection.

Parts of a Needle and Syringe

Needle

The needle consists of several parts (Figure 11-6). The *hub* of the needle fits onto the top of the syringe. The *shaft* is inserted into the body tissue. The opening in the shaft of the needle, known as the *lumen,* is continuous with the needle hub. Medication flows from the syringe and through the lumen of the needle. The *point* of the needle is located at the end of the needle shaft. The point is sharp so that it can penetrate body tissues easily. The top of the needle is slanted and is called the *bevel.* The bevel is designed to make a narrow, slitlike opening in the skin. This narrow opening closes quickly when the needle is removed to prevent leakage of medication, and it heals quickly.

The length of the needle ranges between ⅜ and 3 inches; the length used is based on the type of injection being given and the size of the patient. Refer to Figure 11-7 for examples of various needle lengths. Administering an IM injection to an obese adult requires a longer needle to reach the

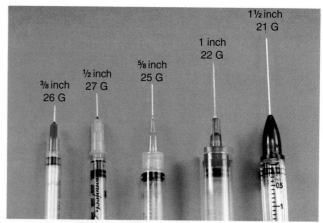

Figure 11-7. Needle lengths and gauges.

muscle tissue than would be required for a normal-size adult. Administering an IM injection to a thin patient requires a shorter needle to avoid inserting a needle too deeply and possibly penetrating the bone. The needle used to give an IM injection must be longer than the one used for an SC injection so that it penetrates deeply enough to reach the muscle tissue.

Each needle has a certain **gauge;** needle gauges for administering medication range between 18 G and 27 G. The gauge of a needle is determined by the diameter of the lumen: As the size of the gauge increases, the diameter of the lumen decreases (see Figure 11-7). A needle with a gauge of 23 has a smaller lumen diameter than a needle with a gauge of 21. Thick or oily preparations must be given with a large lumen because they are too thick to pass through a smaller one. A needle with a larger lumen makes a larger needle track in the tissues. To reduce pain and tissue damage, a needle with the smallest gauge appropriate for the solution and route of administration is always chosen.

Syringe

The syringe is used for inserting fluids into the body. It is made of plastic and must be disposed of after one use. The syringe with an attached needle is packaged in a cellophane wrapper or a rigid plastic container. Information regarding the syringe's capacity and the needle's length and gauge is printed on the wrapper of the syringe and needle (Figure 11-8). Syringes and needles also are available in separate packages. In this case, the medical assistant must attach a needle to the syringe before drawing medication into the syringe.

The parts of a syringe are the barrel, flange, and plunger (see Figure 11-6). The *barrel* of the syringe holds the medication and contains calibrated markings to measure the proper amount of medication. Most syringes are calibrated in milliliters (ml) (or cubic centimeters [cc])—the unit of measurement used most often to administer parenteral medication. The medical assistant should become familiar with reading the graduated scales on syringes. At the end of the barrel is a rim known as the *flange,* which helps in in-

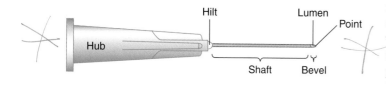

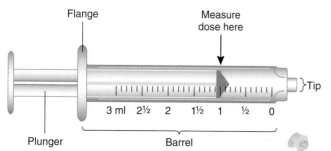

Figure 11-6. Diagram of a needle and a 3-ml syringe, with parts identified.

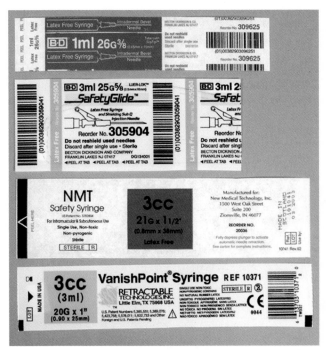

Figure 11-8. Examples of syringe and needle packages labeled according to contents.

jecting the medication. The flange also prevents the syringe from rolling when it is placed on a flat surface. The *plunger* is a movable cylinder that slides back and forth in the barrel. It is used to draw medication into the syringe when an injection is prepared and to push medication out of the syringe when an injection is administered.

Various types of syringes are available to administer injections. The choice is based on the type of injection

being given (e.g., tuberculin skin test, allergy injection, antibiotic injection) and the amount of medication being administered. The types of syringes used most often in the medical office include hypodermic, insulin, and tuberculin (Figure 11-9).

Hypodermic syringes are available in 2-, 2.5-, 3-, and 5-ml sizes and are calibrated in milliliters (or cubic centimeters). They are commonly used to administer IM injections.

The *insulin syringe* is designed especially for the administration of an insulin injection, and the barrel is calibrated in units. The most common type is the U-100 syringe, which is calibrated into 100 units in increments of 2.

Tuberculin syringes are employed to administer a small dose of medication, such as when administering a tuberculin skin test. The tuberculin syringe has a capacity of 1 ml, and the calibrations are divided into tenths (0.10) and hundredths (0.01) of a milliliter.

Syringes also are available with capacities of 10, 20, 30, 50, and 60 ml; however, they are not used for administering medication, but rather for medical treatments, such as irrigating wounds and draining fluid from cysts.

Safety-Engineered Syringes

The Occupational Safety and Health Administration (OSHA) stipulates requirements to reduce needlestick and other sharps injuries among health care workers. As was discussed in Chapter 2, employers are required to evaluate and implement commercially available safer medical devices that reduce occupational exposure to the lowest extent feasible.

Safer medical devices include safety-engineered syringes. *Safety-engineered syringes* incorporate a built-in safety feature to reduce the risk of a needlestick injury. Figure 11-10

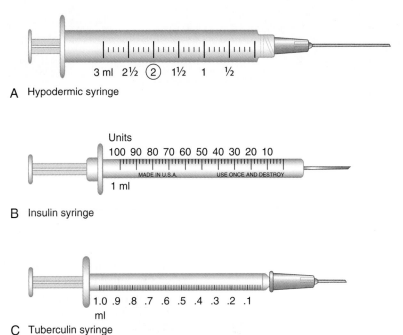

A   Hypodermic syringe

B   Insulin syringe

C   Tuberculin syringe

Figure 11-9. Various syringes used to administer injections. **A**, Hypodermic. **B**, Insulin (U-100). **C**, Tuberculin.

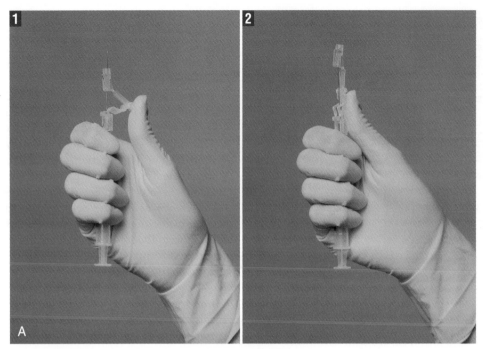

A. Hinged-Shield Syringe (Becton-Dickinson Safety Glide Syringe)
1. After administering the injection, push the lever of the hinged shield forward.
2. Continue pushing until the needle tip is fully covered by the shield, then discard the syringe in a biohazard sharps container.

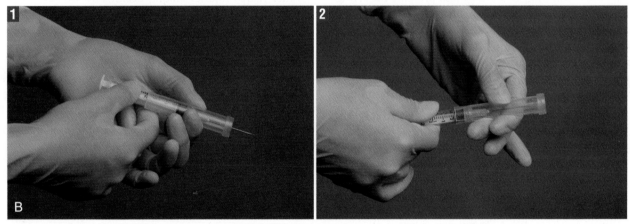

B. Sliding-Shield Syringe (Monoject Safety Syringe)
1. After administering the injection, extend the sliding shield forward fully until a click is heard.
2. Lock the shield by twisting it in either direction until a click is heard. Discard the syringe in a biohazard sharps container.

Figure 11-10. Safety-engineered syringes.

illustrates types of safety-engineered syringes and the methods for using them.

Preparation of Parenteral Medication

Medication used for injections is available in various types of dispensing units—vials, ampules, and prefilled syringes and cartridges.

Vials

A **vial** is a closed glass container with a rubber stopper; a soft metal or plastic cap protects the rubber stopper and must be removed the first time the medication is used. An injectable medication may be available in a single-dose vial, a multiple-dose vial, or both (Figure 11-11). A vial is labeled with specific information as illustrated in Figure 11-12.

Before the medication can be withdrawn, some vials require mixing (e.g., reconstituting a powdered drug, mixing a vial that separates on standing). Vials that require mixing should be rolled between the hands rather than shaken because shaking would cause the medication to foam, creating air bubbles that may enter the syringe when the medication is withdrawn.

To remove medication from a vial, an amount of air exactly equal to the amount of liquid to be removed is in-

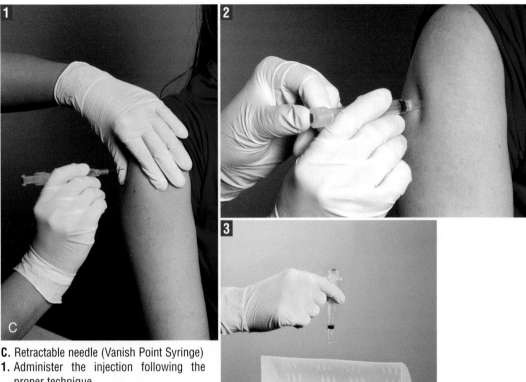

C. Retractable needle (Vanish Point Syringe)
1. Administer the injection following the proper technique.
2. After administering the medication, continue depressing the plunger with the thumb. Use firm pressure past the point of initial resistance. This action delivers the full dose of medication to the patient and activates the needle retraction device, causing the needle to retract automatically from the patient's skin and into the barrel of the syringe.
3. Discard the syringe in a biohazard sharps container.

Figure 11-10, cont'd. Safety-engineered syringes.

jected into the vial. The air should be inserted above the fluid level to avoid creating bubbles in the medication. If air is not injected first, a partial vacuum is created, and it is difficult to remove the medication. During the withdrawal of medication, the needle opening should be inserted below the fluid level to prevent the entrance of air bubbles. Air bubbles can be removed by tapping the barrel of the syringe with the fingertips. If the bubbles are allowed to remain, they take up space that the medication should occupy, which would prevent the patient from receiving the full dose of medication.

Ampules

An **ampule** is a small, sealed glass container that holds a single dose of medication (see Figure 11-11). An ampule has a constriction in the stem, known as the *neck,* which helps in opening it. Before opening, the medical assistant must ensure that there is no medication in the stem by tap-

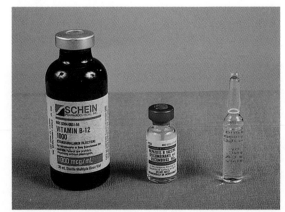

Figure 11-11. The multiple-dose vial *(left)* and the single-dose vial *(middle)* consist of a closed glass container with a rubber stopper. The ampule *(right)* consists of a small, sealed glass container that holds a single dose of medication.

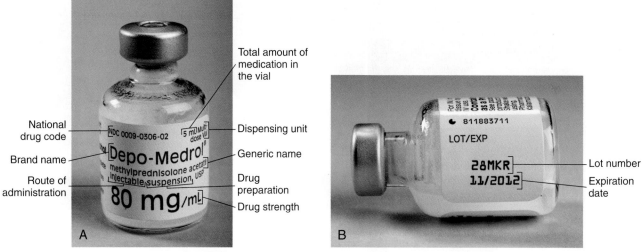

National drug code

Brand name

Route of administration

Total amount of medication in the vial

Dispensing unit

Generic name

Drug preparation

Drug strength

Lot number

Expiration date

Figure 11-12. Information included on the label of a medication vial.

ping it lightly. A colored ring around the neck indicates where the ampule is prescored for easy opening. The ampule is opened by holding it firmly with gauze and breaking off the stem with a strong steady pressure.

A hazard with medication in ampules is the possibility of small glass particles getting into the ampule as the stem is broken off. When the medication is withdrawn into the syringe, the glass particles also might be withdrawn. To prevent this problem, a needle with a filter should be used that filters out small glass particles (Figure 11-13).

The needle opening is inserted into the base of the ampule below the fluid level to withdraw medication. To prevent contamination, the needle should not be permitted to touch the outside of the ampule. Air should never be injected into the ampule because it could force out some of the medication.

Prefilled Syringes

Some drugs come in *prefilled disposable syringes.* Using this type of dispensing unit does not require drawing up the medication. The name of the drug, the dose, and the expiration date are printed on the syringe. (Figure 11-14).

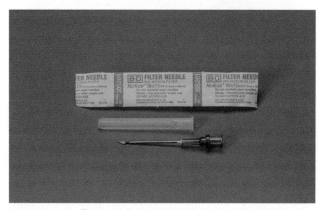

Figure 11-13. Filter needle used to withdraw medication from an ampule.

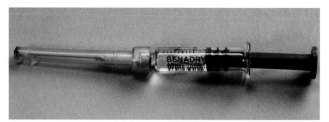

Figure 11-14. A prefilled disposable syringe of medication.

Storage

The medical assistant should always read the drug package insert to determine the proper method for storing each parenteral medication because improper storage may alter the effectiveness of the medication.

Reconstitution of Powdered Drugs

Some parenteral medications are stable for only a short time in liquid form; these medications are prepared and stored in powdered form and require the addition of a liquid before administration. The process of adding a liquid to a powdered drug is known as *reconstitution.* The liquid used to reconstitute a powdered drug is known as the *diluent* and usually consists of sterile water or normal saline. The powdered drug is contained in a single-dose or multiple-dose vial and is accompanied by specific instructions for reconstitution. An example of a parenteral medication that requires reconstitution is the measles, mumps, and rubella (MMR) immunization (Figure 11-15). The procedure for reconstituting powdered drugs is outlined in Procedure 11-3.

Subcutaneous Injections

A **subcutaneous injection** is made into the subcutaneous tissue, which consists of adipose (fat) tissue and is located just under the skin (Figure 11-16). Subcutaneous tissue is located all over the body; however, certain sites are more commonly used because they are located where bones and

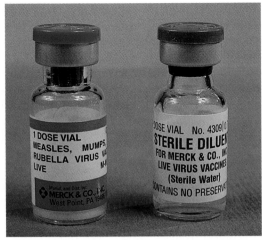

Figure 11-15. The measles, mumps, and rubella (MMR) vaccine is a parenteral medication that requires reconstitution before administration. The vial on the left contains the medication in powdered form, and the vial on the right contains the sterile diluent.

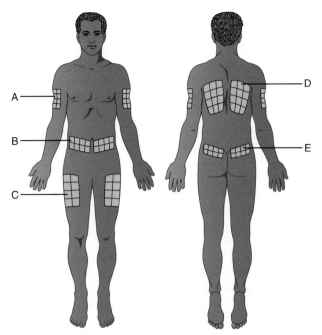

Figure 11-17. Common sites for subcutaneous injections. **A,** Upper outer arm. **B,** Lower abdomen. **C,** Upper outer thigh. **D,** Upper back. **E,** Flank region.

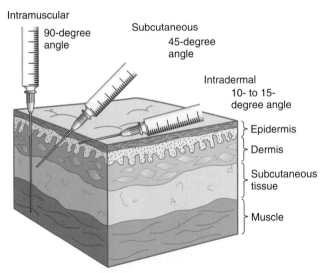

Figure 11-16. Angle of insertion for intradermal, subcutaneous, and intramuscular injections.

blood vessels are not near the surface of the skin. These sites include the upper lateral part of the arms, the anterior thigh, the upper back, and the abdomen (Figure 11-17). Absorption of medication from an SC injection occurs mainly through capillaries, resulting in a slower absorption rate than with IM injections. To ensure proper absorption, tissue that is grossly adipose, hardened, inflamed, or edematous should not be used as an injection site.

The needle length varies from ½ to ⅝ inch, and the gauge ranges from 23 G to 25 G. Elderly and dehydrated patients tend to have less SC tissue, and obese patients have more. The length of the needle should be adjusted accordingly to ensure the medication is administered into the subcutaneous tissue and not into muscle tissue.

Subcutaneous tissue is sensitive to irritating solutions and large volumes of medications; therefore, drugs given subcutaneously must be isotonic, nonirritating, nonviscous, and water-soluble. The amount of medication injected through the SC route should not exceed 1 ml. More than this amount results in pressure on sensory nerve endings, causing discomfort and pain.

Medications commonly administered through the SC route include epinephrine, insulin, and allergy injections. Patients who receive allergy injections must wait in the medical office for 15 to 20 minutes after the injection to be observed for an allergic reaction. Procedure 11-4 outlines the administration of a subcutaneous injection.

Intramuscular Injections

Intramuscular injections are made into the muscular layer of the body, which lies below the skin and subcutaneous layers (see Figure 11-16). The amount of medication that can be injected into muscle tissue is more than the amount that can be injected into subcutaneous tissue. An amount of up to 3 ml can be injected into the gluteal or vastus lateralis muscles, although older and very thin adults are able to tolerate only 2 ml or less in these sites.

Absorption is more rapid by this route than by the SC route because there are more blood vessels in muscle tissue. Medication that is irritating to subcutaneous tissue is often given intramuscularly because there are fewer nerve endings in deep muscle tissue. Most parenteral medications administered in the medical office are given through the IM route; examples include immunizations, antibiotics, injectable contraceptives, vitamin B$_{12}$, and corticosteroids.

The needle for an adult must be long enough to reach muscle tissue and varies in length from 1 to 3 inches. A 1½-inch needle is typically used for an average-sized adult, whereas a 1-inch needle is often used for a thin adult or a child, and a needle of 2 to 3 inches may be needed for an obese adult. The gauge of the needle used ranges from 18 G to 23 G, depending on the viscosity of the medication. Procedure 11-5 outlines the technique for the administration of an IM injection.

Intramuscular Injection Sites

The sites chosen for IM injections are away from large nerves and blood vessels. The medical assistant should practice locating these sites to become familiar with them. The area should always be fully exposed to permit clear visualization of the injection site.

Dorsogluteal Site

The dorsogluteal site is often used to administer IM injections in the medical office. In adults and children older than 3 years of age, the gluteal muscles are well developed and can absorb a large amount of medication. The patient should lie on the abdomen with the toes pointed inward, which aids in relaxation of the gluteal muscles. The medication is injected into the upper outer quadrant of the gluteal area. This site is located by palpating the greater trochanter and the posterior superior iliac spine. An imaginary line is then drawn between these two points, and the injection is administered above and outside of this area (Figure 11-18, *A*). The dorsogluteal site can also be located by dividing the buttocks into quadrants. The site is located in the upper outer quadrant approximately 2 to 3 inches below the iliac crest. The medical assistant must be *extremely* careful to maintain the proper boundary lines to avoid injection into the sciatic nerve or the superior gluteal artery (see Figure 11-18, *A*).

Deltoid Site

The deltoid area is easily accessible and can be used when the patient is sitting or lying down. This site is small because major nerves and blood vessels surround it, and large

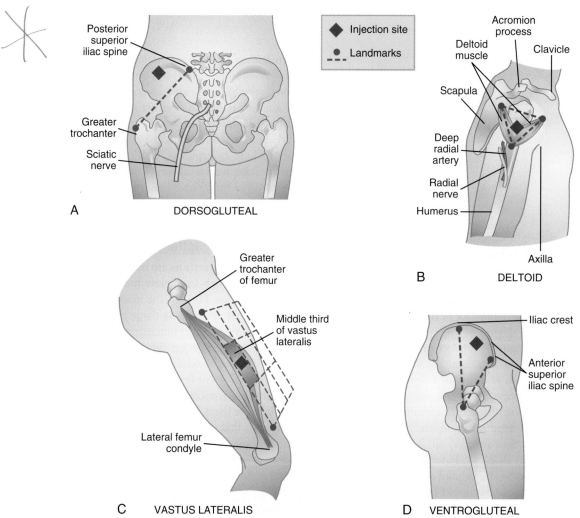

Figure 11-18. Sites of intramuscular injections. **A,** Dorsogluteal muscle. **B,** Deltoid muscle. **C,** Vastus lateralis. **D,** Ventrogluteal muscle. (From Leahy JM, Kizilay PE: Foundations of nursing practice: a nursing process approach, Philadelphia, 1988, Saunders.)

amounts of medication (no more than 1 ml) and repeated injections should not be given in this area. The medication is injected into the deltoid muscle.

The medical assistant should ensure that the entire arm is exposed by having the patient's sleeve completely pulled up or by removing the sleeve from the arm if it cannot be pulled up. A tight sleeve constricts the arm and causes unnecessary bleeding from the puncture site.

The deltoid site is located by palpating the lower edge of the acromion process, which forms the base of a triangle in line with the midpoint of the lateral side of the arm, opposite the axilla (Figure 11-18, B). This site also may be located by placing four fingers horizontally across the deltoid muscle with the top finger along the acromion process. The injection site is located two to three fingerwidths below the acromion process, which is about 1 to 2 inches below the acromion process (Figure 11-19).

Vastus Lateralis Site

The vastus lateralis is used because it is not near major nerves and blood vessels and is a relatively thick muscle (Figure 11-18, C). This site is particularly desirable for infants and children younger than 3 years old whose gluteal muscles are not yet well developed. The area is bounded by the midanterior thigh on the front of the leg and the midlateral thigh on the side. The proximal boundary is a hand's breadth below the greater trochanter, and the distal boundary is a hand's breadth above the knee. It is easier to give an injection in the vastus lateralis if the patient is lying down, but a sitting position also can be used.

Ventrogluteal Site

The ventrogluteal site is growing in acceptability as an IM injection site because the subcutaneous layer is relatively small and the muscle layer is thick. The site is located away from major nerves and blood vessels. Through palpation, the greater trochanter of the femur, the anterior superior iliac spine, and the iliac crest can be located. If the injection is being made into the patient's left side, the palm of the right hand is placed on the greater trochanter, and the index finger is placed on the anterior superior iliac spine. The middle finger is spread posteriorly as far as possible away from the index finger, to touch the iliac crest. The hand position is reversed if the injection is being made into the patient's right side. The triangle formed by the fingers is the area into which the injection is given. An injection into the ventrogluteal site can be administered when the patient is lying prone or on one side (Figure 11-18, D).

Z-Track Method

Medications that are irritating to subcutaneous and skin tissue or that discolor the skin must be given intramuscularly using the Z-track method; one medication that is administered by this method is iron dextran (Imferon). The dorsogluteal, ventrogluteal, and vastus lateralis sites all can be used as areas to administer a Z-track injection.

The Z-track method is similar to the IM injection procedure except that the skin and subcutaneous tissue at the injection site are pulled to the side before the needle is inserted. This causes a zigzag path through the tissues when the needle is removed and the skin is released. The zigzag path prevents the medication from reaching the subcutaneous layer or skin surface by sealing off the needle track (Figure 11-20). The procedure for administering medication using the Z-track method is outlined in Procedure 11-6.

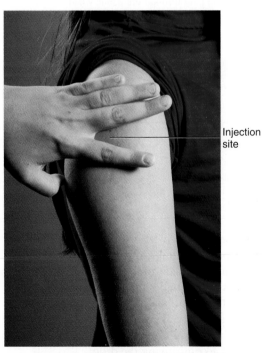

Injection site

Figure 11-19. Location of the deltoid site.

What Would You Do? What Would You *Not* Do?

Case Study 3

Danielle Roush, 16 years old, has come to the office with her mother. Danielle is complaining of a painful sore throat, fever, and severe aching in both of her ears. The physician diagnoses her with strep throat and otitis media, and prescribes a parenteral antibiotic to be given deep IM. Danielle says that she's a basketball player and on the varsity team at her high school. She says that she is always too embarrassed to change or take a shower in front of the other girls because she's so skinny. Danielle would like to have the injection in her arm because it would be too embarrassing to have it in the buttocks. ∎

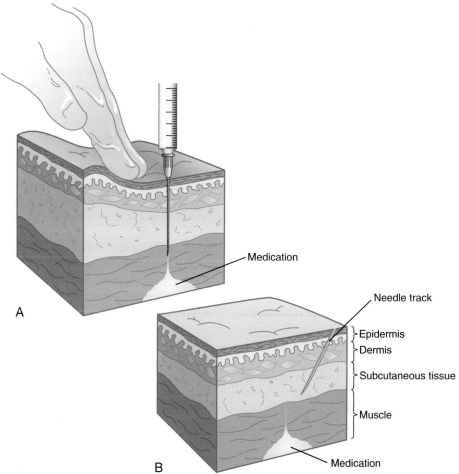

Figure 11-20. Z-track intramuscular injection method. **A,** The skin and subcutaneous tissue are pulled to the side before the needle is inserted. **B,** This causes a zigzag path through the tissue when the skin is released, which seals off the needle track.

PROCEDURE 11-2   Preparing an Injection

Outcome Prepare an injection from an ampule and a vial.

Equipment/Supplies

- Medication ordered by the physician
- Appropriate needle and syringe
- Antiseptic wipe
- Medication tray

1. Procedural Step. Sanitize your hands.

2. Procedural Step. Assemble the equipment.

3. Procedural Step. Work in a quiet and well-lit atmosphere.
Principle. Good lighting aids the medical assistant in reading the medication label.

4. Procedural Step. Select the proper medication. Compare the medication with the physician's instructions. Check the drug label three times—while removing the medication from storage, before withdrawing the medication into the syringe, and after preparing the medication. Check the expiration date.

Principle. The medication should be carefully identified to prevent administration of the wrong medication. Outdated medication should not be used because it could produce undesirable effects.

5. Procedural Step. Calculate the correct dose to be given, if necessary. If you have any questions regarding the administration of the medication, check the package insert accompanying the drug.

6. Procedural Step. Open the syringe and the needle package. If necessary, assemble the needle and syringe.
Principle. Disposable needles and syringes may come already assembled together in a package or in separate

PROCEDURE 11-2   Preparing an Injection—cont'd

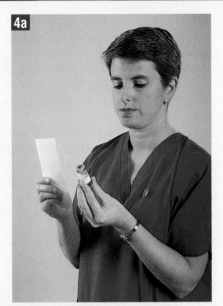

Compare the medication with the physician's instructions.

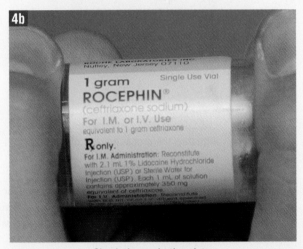

Check the expiration date.

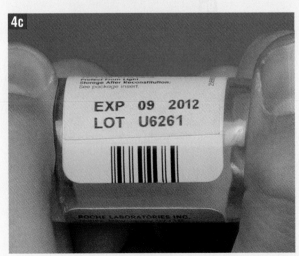

Check the drug label three times.

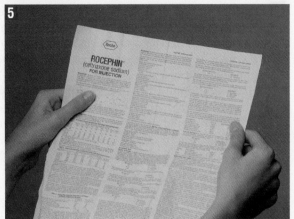

Check the package insert.

packages that require assembly of the needle and syringe.

7. **Procedural Step.** Check to ensure that the needle is attached firmly to the syringe by loosening the guard on the needle, grasping the needle at the hub, and tightening it. Break the seal on the syringe by moving the plunger back and forth several times.

8. **Procedural Step.** Check the drug label again to ensure it is the correct medication. If required, mix the medication by rolling the vial between your hands to obtain a uniform suspension of the medication.

9. **Procedural Step.** Withdraw the medication following these steps.

Withdrawing Medication From a Vial

a. **Procedural Step.** Remove the soft metal or plastic cap protecting the rubber stopper of an unused vial to expose the rubber stopper. Open the antiseptic; wipe and cleanse the rubber stopper and allow it to dry.

Principle. Cleansing the top of the vial removes dust and bacteria. The alcohol must be allowed to dry to prevent it from adhering to the needle and mixing with the medication.

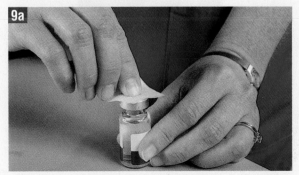

Cleanse the rubber stopper.

Continued

PROCEDURE 11-2   Preparing an Injection—cont'd

b. Procedural Step. Place the vial in an upright position on a flat surface. Remove the needle guard. Pull back on the plunger to draw an amount of air into the syringe equal to the amount of medication to be withdrawn from the vial.

Principle. Air must be injected into the vial first to prevent the formation of a partial vacuum in the vial, which would make it difficult to remove medication.

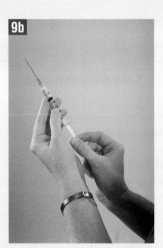

Draw air into the syringe.

c. Procedural Step. With the vial on a flat surface, use moderate pressure on the barrel of the syringe to insert the needle through the center of the rubber stopper at a 90-degree angle. Continue to apply pressure until the needle reaches the empty space between the stopper and fluid level. Be careful not to bend the needle. Push down on the plunger to inject the air into the vial, keeping the needle opening above the fluid level. (*Note:* If you are using a

retractable safety syringe, do not push too hard on the plunger to avoid activating the retracting mechanism prematurely.)

Principle. The center of the rubber stopper is thinner and easier to penetrate. The air must be inserted above the fluid level to avoid creating air bubbles in the medication.

d. Procedural Step. Invert the vial while holding onto the syringe and plunger. Hold the syringe at eye level, and withdraw the proper amount of medication. Keep the needle opening below the fluid level.

Principle. The needle opening must be below the fluid level to prevent the entrance of air bubbles into the syringe.

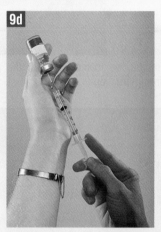

Withdraw the proper amount of medication.

e. Procedural Step. Remove any air bubbles in the syringe by holding the syringe in a vertical position and tapping the barrel carefully with the fingertips until they disappear.

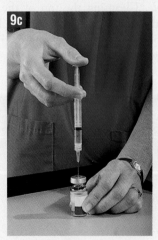

Inject air into the vial.

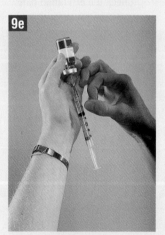

Tap the barrel with the fingertips to remove air bubbles.

PROCEDURE 11-2   Preparing an Injection—cont'd

Principle. Tapping the barrel too forcefully could cause the needle to bend. Air bubbles take up space the medication should occupy, preventing the patient from getting the proper dose of medication.

f. **Procedural Step.** Remove any air remaining at the top of the syringe by slowly pushing the plunger forward and allowing the air to flow back into the vial.

g. **Procedural Step.** Carefully remove the needle from the rubber stopper, and replace the needle guard. (*Note:* After drawing up the medication, some facilities require that the needle used to draw up the medication be removed from the syringe and replaced with a new sterile needle. This is because the point of the needle may not be as sharp after it has been inserted into rubber stopper of the medication vial. The medical assistant should follow the policy set forth by his or her medical office.)
Principle. The needle must remain sterile. The needle guard prevents the needle from becoming contaminated.

h. **Procedural Step.** Check the drug label for the third time, and return the medication to its proper storage location.

Withdrawing Medication From an Ampule

a. **Procedural Step.** Remove the needle (and needle guard) from the syringe, and attach a filter needle (and needle guard).

b. **Procedural Step.** Open the antiseptic wipe, and cleanse the neck of the ampule.
Principle. Cleansing the neck of the ampule removes dust and bacteria.

c. **Procedural Step.** Tap the stem of the ampule lightly to remove any medication in the neck of the ampule.

d. **Procedural Step.** Check the medication label a second time and place a piece of gauze around the neck of the ampule. Hold the base of the ampule between the first two fingers and the thumb of one hand. Hold the neck of the vial between the first two fingers and the thumb of the other hand. Apply a strong steady pressure with the thumbs, and break off the stem by snapping it quickly and firmly away from the body. Discard the stem and gauze in a biohazard sharps container.

e. **Procedural Step.** Place the ampule on a flat surface. Remove the needle guard. Insert the filter needle opening below the fluid level.
Principle. The filter needle prevents glass particles from being withdrawn into the syringe.

f. **Procedural Step.** Withdraw the proper amount of medication by pulling back on the plunger. Keep the needle opening below the fluid level to prevent the entrance of air bubbles into the syringe. Tilt the

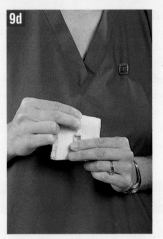

Snap off the stem away from the body.

ampule as needed to keep the needle opening immersed in the fluid.

Note: There is another method that can be used to remove medication from an ampule. Choose the method that is easiest for you. To perform this method, invert the ampule, making sure to keep the needle opening below the fluid level. Withdraw the proper amount of medication by pulling back on the plunger. Move the needle downward as necessary to keep the needle opening immersed in the fluid.
Principle. Air bubbles take up space the medication should occupy, resulting in an inaccurate measurement of medication.

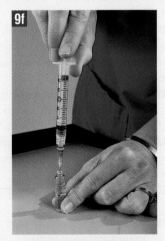

Withdraw the medication.

g. **Procedural Step.** Remove the needle from the ampule, and replace the needle guard. Check the drug label for the third time, and dispose of the glass ampule in a biohazard sharps container.

Continued

PROCEDURE 11-2   Preparing an Injection—cont'd

h. **Procedural Step.** Remove the filter needle (and guard) from the syringe, and discard it in a biohazard sharps container. Reapply the needle (and guard) for administering the medication.

i. **Procedural Step.** If air bubbles are in the syringe, remove the needle guard, hold the syringe in a vertical position, and tap the barrel with the fingertips until the bubbles disappear. Remove the air at the top of the syringe by slowly pushing the plunger forward. If the syringe contains excess fluid, hold the syringe vertically over a sink with the needle tip up and slanted toward the sink. Slowly eject the excess fluid into the sink. Replace the needle guard.

PROCEDURE 11-3   Reconstituting Powdered Drugs

Outcome Reconstitute a powdered drug for parenteral administration.

Equipment/Supplies

- Medication ordered by the physician
- Appropriate needle and syringe
- Antiseptic wipe
- Medication tray

1. **Procedural Step.** Follow steps 1 through 8 of Procedure 11-2.

2. **Procedural Step.** From the vial of the powdered drug, withdraw an amount of air equal to the amount of liquid to be injected into the vial.
   Principle. Removing air from the powdered drug vial allows room for injection of the diluent.

3. **Procedural Step.** Inject the air removed from the powdered drug vial into the vial of diluent.
   Principle. Air must be injected into the vial to prevent formation of a partial vacuum in the vial, which would make it difficult to remove the diluent.

4. **Procedural Step.** Invert the diluent vial, and withdraw the proper amount of liquid into the syringe. Remove air bubbles from the syringe, and carefully remove the needle from the vial.

5. **Procedural Step.** Insert the needle into the powdered drug vial, and inject the diluent into the vial. Remove the needle from the vial, and replace the needle guard.

6. **Procedural Step.** Roll the vial between the hands to mix the powdered drug and liquid (unless indicated otherwise by the drug package insert).
   Principle. Shaking the vial may cause air bubbles to form.

7. **Procedural Step.** Label multiple-dose vials with the date of preparation and your initials.

8. **Procedural Step.** Administer the injection.

9. **Procedural Step.** Store multiple-dose vials as indicated by the manufacturer's instructions. Because reconstituted drugs are stable for a short time, carefully check the date of preparation on the multiple-dose vial before administering it again.

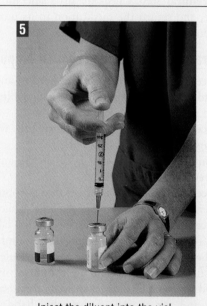

Inject the diluent into the vial.

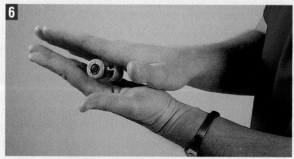

Roll the vial between the hands.

PROCEDURE 11-4 Administering a Subcutaneous Injection

Outcome Administer a subcutaneous injection.

Equipment/Supplies

- Medication ordered by the physician
- Appropriate needle and syringe
- Antiseptic wipe
- Sterile 2 × 2 gauze pad
- Disposable gloves
- Biohazard sharps container

1. **Procedural Step.** Sanitize your hands, and prepare the injection (see Procedure 11-2).

2. **Procedural Step.** Greet the patient and introduce yourself. Identify the patient by full name and date of birth. Explain the procedure and the purpose of the injection.
Principle. It is crucial that no error be made in patient identity. An apprehensive patient may need reassurance.

3. **Procedural Step.** Select an appropriate injection site. The upper arm, thigh, back, and abdomen are recommended sites for a subcutaneous injection. See Figure 11-17.
Principle. The entire area should be exposed to ensure a safe and comfortable injection.

4. **Procedural Step.** Prepare the injection site. Cleanse the area with an antiseptic wipe. Using a circular motion, start with the injection site, and move outward. Do not touch the site after cleansing it.
Principle. Using a circular motion carries contaminants away from the injection site. Touching the site after cleansing contaminates it, and the cleansing process needs to be repeated.

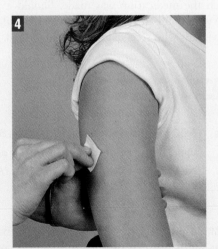

Cleanse the area with an antiseptic wipe.

5. **Procedural Step.** Allow the area to dry completely.
Principle. If the area is not permitted to dry, the antiseptic may enter the tissues when the skin is pierced, resulting in irritation and patient discomfort.

6. **Procedural Step.** Apply gloves, and remove the needle guard. Position your nondominant hand on the area surrounding the injection site. The skin may be held taut, or the area surrounding the injection site may be grasped and held in a cushion fashion.
Principle. Gloves provide a barrier against bloodborne pathogens. In normal adults, the needle enters the subcutaneous tissue when the skin is held taut. Grasping the area around the injection site is recommended for a thin or dehydrated patient. This ensures that the subcutaneous tissue, and not muscle tissue, is entered.

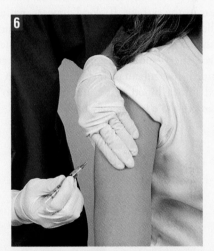

Grasp the area surrounding the injection site.

7. **Procedural Step.** Hold the barrel of the syringe between your thumb and index finger. Insert the needle quickly and smoothly at a 45-degree or 90-degree angle, depending on the length of the needle. With a ½-inch needle, a 90-degree angle should be used; with a ⅝-inch needle, a 45-degree angle should be used. Insert the needle to the hub.
Principle. Inserting the needle quickly and smoothly minimizes tissue trauma and pain. Needle length determines the angle of insertion to ensure placement of the medication in subcutaneous tissue.

8. **Procedural Step.** Remove your hand from the skin.
Principle. Medication injected into compressed tissue causes pressure against nerve fibers and is uncomfortable for the patient.

Continued

PROCEDURE 11-4

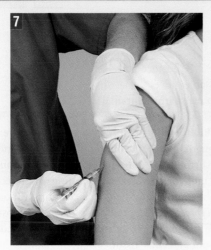

Insert the needle at a 45-degree angle.

9. Procedural Step. Hold the syringe steady and pull back gently on the plunger to determine whether the needle is in a blood vessel, in which case blood would appear in the syringe. If blood appears, withdraw the needle, prepare a new injection, and begin again.
Principle. Moving the syringe after the needle has entered the tissue causes patient discomfort. Drugs intended for subcutaneous administration but injected into a blood vessel are absorbed too quickly, and undesirable results may occur.

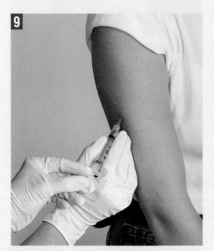

Pull back gently to determine whether the needle is in a blood vessel.

10. Procedural Step. Inject the medication slowly and steadily by depressing the plunger. If you are using a retractable safety syringe, activate it at this time following the steps outlined in Figure 11-10, *C*, and continue to step 12.
Principle. Rapid injection creates pressure and destroys tissue, both of which are uncomfortable for the patient.

11. Procedural Step. Place the antiseptic wipe or a gauze pad gently over the injection site and quickly remove the needle, keeping it at the same angle as for insertion.
Principle. Withdrawing the needle quickly and at the same angle as for insertion reduces patient discomfort. The antiseptic wipe or gauze pad placed over the injection site helps prevent tissue movement as the needle is withdrawn, reducing patient discomfort. Using a gauze pad prevents a stinging sensation from the alcohol.

12. Procedural Step. Apply gentle pressure to the injection site with the antiseptic wipe or gauze pad. If you are using a safety syringe with a shield, activate the safety feature at this time following the steps outlined in Figure 11-10.
Principle. Gentle pressure helps distribute the medication so that it is completely absorbed. Avoid vigorous massaging because this could damage underlying tissue.

13. Procedural Step. Properly dispose of the needle and syringe in a biohazard sharps container.
Principle. Proper disposal is required by the Occupational Safety and Health Administration (OSHA) standard to prevent accidental needlestick injuries.

14. Procedural Step. Remove gloves, and sanitize your hands.

15. Procedural Step. Chart the procedure. Include the date and time, the name of the medication, the lot number (if required), the dosage given, the route of administration, the injection site used, and any significant observations or patient reactions.
Principle. The lot number indicates the batch in which the medication was made. Should a problem arise with that batch, the drug can be recalled, and the individuals who received it can be identified.

CHARTING EXAMPLE

Date	
2/17/12	3:30 p.m. Ragweed allergy inj, 0.20 cc, SC Ⓡ
	upper arm. Arm checked 15 min. after admin.
	No reaction noted. ——T. Cline, CMA (AAMA)

16. Procedural Step. Stay with the patient to ensure that he or she is not experiencing any unusual reactions. (*Note:* If an allergy injection has been given, the patient should remain at the medical office for 15 to 20 minutes to ensure that an allergic reaction does not occur.) Check the patient's arm after the waiting period, and observe for induration and redness. If the patient experiences such a reaction, notify the physician immediately.

PROCEDURE 11-5 Administering an Intramuscular Injection

Outcome Administer an intramuscular injection.

Equipment/Supplies

- Medication ordered by the physician
- Appropriate needle and syringe
- Antiseptic wipe
- Sterile 2 × 2 gauze pad
- Disposable gloves
- Biohazard sharps container

1. **Procedural Step.** Sanitize your hands, and prepare the injection (see Procedure 11-2).

2. **Procedural Step.** Greet the patient and introduce yourself. Identify the patient by his/her full name and date of birth. Explain the procedure and purpose of the injection.
   Principle. Make sure that you administer the medication to the right patient. Explain the purpose of the injection. Assistance may be needed for restraining infants and children.

3. **Procedural Step.** Select an appropriate intramuscular (IM) injection site. See Figure 11-18 for the recommended IM injection sites. Remove the patient's clothing as necessary to ensure the entire area is exposed.
   Principle. Major nerves and blood vessels may lie in close proximity to the intramuscular injection sites. The medical assistant should develop skill and accuracy in locating the proper sites.

4. **Procedural Step.** Prepare the injection site. Cleanse the area with an antiseptic wipe. Using a circular motion, start with the injection site and move outward. Do not touch the site after cleansing it.
   Principle. Using a circular motion carries contaminants away from the injection site. Touching the site after cleansing contaminates it, and the cleansing process needs to be repeated.

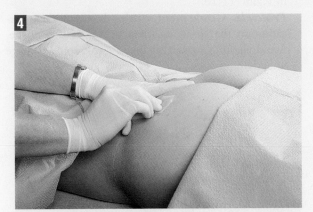

Cleanse the site with an antiseptic wipe.

5. **Procedural Step.** Allow the area to dry completely.
   Principle. If the area is not permitted to dry, the antiseptic may enter the tissues when the skin is pierced, resulting in irritation and patient discomfort.

6. **Procedural Step.** Apply gloves, and remove the needle guard. Using the thumb and first two fingers of the nondominant hand, stretch the skin taut over the injection site.
   Principle. Gloves provide a barrier against bloodborne pathogens. Stretching the skin taut permits easier insertion of the needle and helps ensure that the needle enters muscle tissue.

7. **Procedural Step.** Hold the barrel of the syringe like a dart, and insert the needle quickly and smoothly at a 90-degree angle to the patient's skin with a firm motion. Insert the needle to the hub.

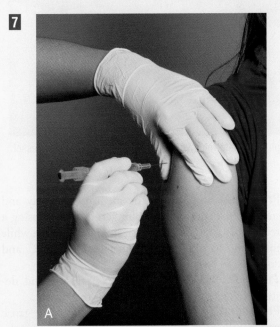

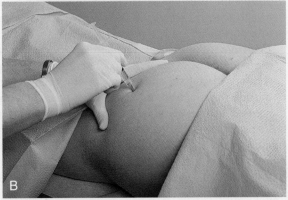

Insert the needle at a 90-degree angle.

Continued

PROCEDURE 11-5   Administering an Intramuscular Injection—cont'd

Principle. The needle is inserted at a 90-degree angle and to the hub to ensure that it reaches muscle tissue. Inserting the needle quickly and smoothly minimizes tissue trauma and pain.

8. Procedural Step. Hold the syringe steady, and pull back gently on the plunger to determine whether the needle is in a blood vessel. If blood appears, withdraw the needle, prepare a new injection, and begin again.

Principle. Moving the syringe after the needle has penetrated the tissue causes patient discomfort. If drugs intended for intramuscular administration are injected into a blood vessel, the result is faster absorption of the medication. This may produce undesirable results.

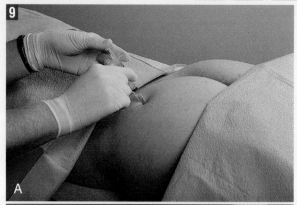

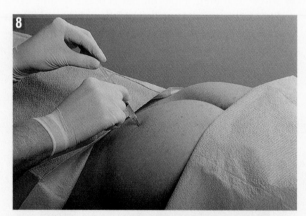

Aspirate to determine whether the needle is in a blood vessel.

9. Procedural Step. Inject the medication slowly and steadily by depressing the plunger. If you are using a retractable safety syringe, activate it at this time while following the steps outlined in Figure 11-10, *C*, and continue to step 11.

Principle. Rapid injection creates pressure and destroys tissue, causing discomfort for the patient.

10. Procedural Step. Place the antiseptic wipe or gauze pad gently over the injection site and remove the needle quickly, keeping it at the same angle as for insertion.

Principle. Withdrawing the needle quickly and at the same angle as for insertion reduces patient discomfort. Placing the antiseptic wipe or gauze pad over the injection site helps prevent tissue movement as the needle is withdrawn, also reducing patient discomfort. Using a gauze pad prevents a stinging sensation from the alcohol.

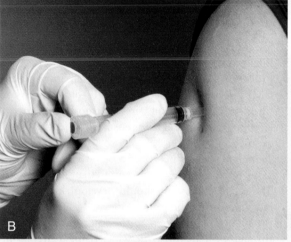

A-B, Inject the medication slowly and steadily.

11. Procedural Step. Apply gentle pressure to the injection site with an antiseptic wipe or gauze pad. If you are using a safety syringe with a shield, activate the safety feature at this time following the steps outlined in Figure 11-10.

Principle. Gentle pressure helps distribute the medication so that it is absorbed by the muscle tissue. Avoid vigorous massaging because this could damage underlying tissues.

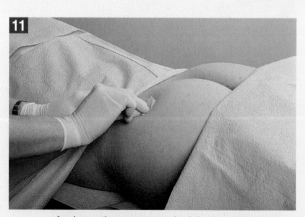

Apply gentle pressure to the injection site.

PROCEDURE 11-5   Administering an Intramuscular Injection—cont'd

12. Procedural Step. Properly dispose of the needle and syringe in a biohazard sharps container.
Principle. Proper disposal is required by the OSHA standard to prevent accidental needlestick injuries.

13. Procedural Step. Remove the gloves, and sanitize your hands.

14. Procedural Step. Chart the procedure. Include the date and time, the name of the medication, the lot number (if required), the dosage given, the route of administration, the injection site used, and any significant observations or patient reactions.
Principle. The lot number indicates the batch in which the medication was made. Should a problem arise with that batch, the drug can be recalled, and individuals who received it can be identified.

CHARTING EXAMPLE

Date	
2/20/12	9:30 a.m. Rocephin (Lot #: U6261) Admin 1 gram, IM, (L) dorsogluteal. Tolerated injection well.
	—————————————————— T. Cline, CMA (AAMA)

15. Procedural Step. Stay with the patient to ensure he or she is not experiencing any unusual reactions. If the patient experiences an unusual reaction, notify the physician immediately.

PROCEDURE 11-6   Z-Track Intramuscular Injection Technique

Outcome Administer an intramuscular injection using the Z-track method.

Equipment/Supplies

- Medication ordered by the physician
- Appropriate needle and syringe
- Antiseptic wipe

- Disposable gloves
- Biohazard sharps container

1. Procedural Step. Follow steps 1 through 5 of Procedure 11-5.

2. Procedural Step. Apply gloves, and remove the needle guard. With the nondominant hand, pull the skin away laterally from the injection site approximately 1 to 1½ inches.

3. Procedural Step. Insert the needle quickly and smoothly at a 90-degree angle.

4. Procedural Step. Aspirate to determine whether the needle is in a blood vessel. If blood appears, withdraw the needle and discard the needle and syringe. Prepare another injection and begin again.

5. Procedural Step. Inject the medication slowly and steadily.

6. Procedural Step. After injecting the medication, wait 10 seconds before withdrawing the needle to allow initial absorption of the medication.

7. Procedural Step. Withdraw the needle quickly, keeping it at the same angle as for insertion.

8. Procedural Step. Release the traction on the skin to seal off the needle track; doing so prevents the medication from reaching the subcutaneous tissue and skin surface.

9. Procedural Step. Do not apply pressure to the site because this could cause the medication to seep out.

10. Procedural Step. If you are using a safety syringe with a shield, activate the safety feature at this time following the steps outlined in Figure 11-10.

11. Procedural Step. Properly dispose of the needle and syringe in a biohazard sharps container.

12. Procedural Step. Remove your gloves, and sanitize your hands.

13. Procedural Step. Chart the procedure. Include the date and time, the name of the medication, the lot number (if required), the dosage given, the route of administration, the injection site used, and any significant observations or patient reactions.

CHARTING EXAMPLE

Date	
2/20/12	10:30 a.m. Iron dextran (Lot #: 1445) Admin 100 mg, IM, Z-track into (R) dorsogluteal. No complaints of discomfort. —————————
	—————————————— T. Cline, CMA (AAMA)

14. Procedural Step. Stay with the patient to ensure he or she is not experiencing any unusual reactions. If the patient experiences an unusual reaction, notify the physician immediately.

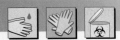

Intradermal Injections

An **intradermal injection** is given into the dermal layer of the skin, at an angle almost parallel to the skin (see Figure 11-16). Absorption is slow; only a small amount of medication may be injected (0.01 to 0.2 ml). The sites most often used for an intradermal injection are areas where the skin is thin, such as the anterior forearm and the middle of the back. The upper arm also is used to administer an intradermal injection.

The needle used is short, usually ⅜ to ⅝ inch long, and the lumen has a small diameter, usually 25 G to 27 G. A tuberculin syringe is often used for administering the injection. The capacity of the syringe is small (1 ml), and the calibrations are divided into tenths and hundredths of a milliliter. The fine calibrations allow a very small amount of medication to be administered, which is required with an intradermal injection. Procedure 11-7 outlines the technique for the administration of an intradermal injection.

The most frequent use of intradermal injections is to administer a skin test, such as an allergy test or a tuberculin test. The medication for the appropriate test is placed into the skin layers, and a small, raised area known as a **wheal** is produced at the injection site, owing to distention of the skin (Figure 11-21). At a time dictated by the type of test being administered, the results are read and interpreted. Most allergy tests can be read and interpreted at the medical office a short time (usually 15 to 20 minutes) after administration of the test, whereas tuberculin testing requires 48 hours before the results can be read.

The skin testing medication interacts with the body tissues; if no reaction occurs, the wheal disappears within a short time, and the only visible sign left is the puncture site. If a reaction to the skin test occurs, induration results, indicating a positive reaction. Erythema also may be present at the test site; however, for most skin tests, the extent of induration is the only criterion used to assess a positive reaction.

TUBERCULIN SKIN TESTING
Tuberculosis

Tuberculosis (TB) is an infectious bacterial disease that can occur in almost any part of the body but usually attacks the lungs. Tuberculosis affecting the lungs is known as *pulmonary tuberculosis,* whereas tuberculosis occurring in other parts of the body is known as *extrapulmonary tuberculosis* and is most apt to occur in the brain, spine, kidneys, bones, and joints. The name of the bacterium that causes tuberculosis is *Mycobacterium tuberculosis,* which is a rod-shaped bacterium. Shortly (within weeks) after infection, a small percentage of individuals infected with the TB bacteria develop active pulmonary tuberculosis. In these individuals, the TB bacteria are able to overcome the body's defense system. This is most apt to occur in young children and individuals with a weakened immune system. The TB bacteria then begin to multiply and attack the body, resulting in the destruction of tissue.

Symptoms of active pulmonary tuberculosis include a chronic cough lasting 3 weeks or longer that produces a mucopurulent sputum, occasional hemoptysis (coughing up blood), and chest pain. Systemic symptoms include fatigue, loss of appetite, weakness, unexplained weight loss, chills, low-grade fever, and sweating at night. If active tuberculosis is left untreated, it can result in serious complications such as permanent lung damage and even death.

Most people (90%) infected with the TB bacterium do not develop the active disease because their body defenses protect them. Body defenses may be able to destroy the TB bacteria immediately after they enter the body and completely clear them from the body. If this is not possible, the TB bacteria are engulfed by white blood cells known as macrophages. The body then builds a fibrous wall of tissue around these macrophages (infected with TB bacteria) to encapsulate them. Some of the TB bacteria may remain alive inside the capsule in a dormant or inactive state. During this time, the individual experiences no symptoms and

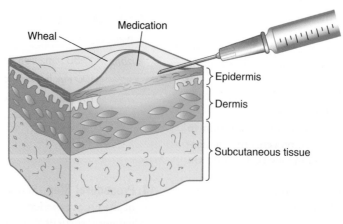

Figure 11-21. Intradermal injections are used to administer skin tests. Enough medication must be deposited in the skin layers to form a wheal.

cannot spread the disease to others. Individuals are said to have a latent tuberculosis infection (LTBI) and the only sign indicating that they have been infected with tuberculosis is a positive reaction to a TB test.

Individuals with latent tuberculosis may go on to develop active tuberculosis. This occurs in approximately 10% of individuals with LTBI. About half of these individuals develop active tuberculosis within 2 years after the initial infection, and the other half develop tuberculosis many years, even decades, after becoming infected. The TB bacteria break out of the capsule and cause the symptoms of active tuberculosis (described previously). The development of LTBI into active tuberculosis is most apt to occur when the body's immune system is weakened, such as during a serious illness, or in patients who have an immune disorder such as human immunodeficiency virus (HIV) infection. The difference between active tuberculosis and latent tuberculosis is outlined in Table 11-6.

Purpose of Tuberculin Skin Testing

The purpose of tuberculin skin testing (TST) is to identify individuals who are infected with *M. tuberculosis*. TST is recommended for individuals who are at higher risk for TB exposure or infection, or at higher risk for progressing from latent tuberculosis to active tuberculosis. Examples include individuals who have close day-to-day contact with someone with active tuberculosis, individuals who have immigrated from a country with a high incidence of TB, and individuals who work or reside in facilities or institutions with people who are at high risk for TB (e.g., hospitals and other health care facilities, correctional facilities, and nursing homes). Tuberculin skin testing may also be required as a prerequisite for employment, college entrance, entrance into the military service, and so on. A positive reaction to a tuberculin skin test occurs 2 to 10 weeks after an individual is infected with tuberculosis. Because of this, a patient recently infected with TB bacteria may show a false-negative test result and should be retested 10 weeks later.

The medical assistant is responsible for administering the tuberculin test and for reading the test results. Although tuberculin skin testing is relatively easy to perform, the procedure must be followed exactly to ensure accurate results. A patient with a tuberculous infection may fail to react to the test if it is not performed correctly.

Tuberculin Skin Test Reactions

The substance used in the skin test is tuberculin, which consists of a purified protein derivative (PPD) extracted from a culture of *M. tuberculosis* (the causative agent of tuberculosis), to test for sensitivity to the TB organism. The tuberculin PPD solution contains no live tuberculosis organisms and is completely harmless, making it safe to administer to people of all ages.

When introduced into the skin of an individual with an active or latent case of tuberculosis, tuberculin causes localized thickening of the skin, resulting in induration. **Induration,** which indicates a positive reaction, is an abnormally raised hardened area with clearly defined margins caused by an accumulation of small, sensitized lymphocytes (a type of white blood cell) that occurs in the area in which the tuberculin was injected into the skin (Figure 11-22). Tuberculin skin test reactions are based on the amount of induration

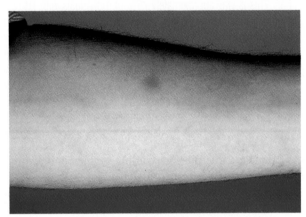

Figure 11-22. Positive tuberculin skin test. (From Nairn R: Immunology for medical students, ed 2, Philadelphia, 2007, Mosby.)

Table 11-6 Differences Between Active TB and Latent TB		
Characteristics	**Active TB**	**Latent TB**
Symptoms	Patient usually feels sick and has symptoms of TB such as cough, fever, and weight loss.	Patient feels fine and has no symptoms.
TB bacterial status	Active TB bacteria are present in the body.	TB bacteria are present in the body that are alive but inactive.
TB test results	Patient usually has a positive TST or QFT-G blood test result.	Patient usually has a positive TST or QFT-G blood test result.
Diagnostic tests	Patient may have an abnormal chest x-ray and a positive sputum test.	Patient has a normal chest x-ray and a negative sputum test.
Ability to infect others	Patient is infectious and may spread the disease to others.	Patient is not infectious and cannot spread the TB to others.
Treatment	Patient needs treatment for active TB.	Physician may consider treatment for latent TB to prevent active TB disease.

QFT, QuantiFERON–TB Gold; *TB,* tuberculosis; *TST,* tuberculin skin testing.

Highlight on Tuberculosis

Despite advances in treatment, tuberculosis remains a primary cause of illness and death worldwide, especially in Africa and Asia. According to the World Health Organization (WHO), approximately two billion people—making up one third of the world's population—are infected with the tuberculosis (TB) bacterium. Worldwide, eight million people become ill each year with tuberculosis, and an estimated two million people die from this disease annually. New infection occurs at a rate of one per second. Factors that contribute to the high prevalence of tuberculosis include the human immunodeficiency virus (HIV) epidemic and the increase in drug-resistant strains of TB bacteria.

In the United States, new cases of tuberculosis have been declining steadily from more than 26,000 new cases in 1992 to fewer than 13,000 new cases in 2008. This is the lowest rate recorded in the United States since national reporting began in 1953. However, an estimated 9 to 14 million Americans have latent tuberculosis infection, and about 10% of them will develop tuberculosis at some point in their lives.

What part of the body becomes infected?

Although any part of the body can be infected, the TB organism prefers body tissues with high oxygen concentrations, such as the lungs. This is why approximately 75% of individuals with TB have pulmonary tuberculosis. When another part of the body is affected, the condition is known as extrapulmonary tuberculosis. Symptoms of extrapulmonary tuberculosis depend on the part of the body that is affected. For example, TB occurring in the spine may cause back pain, collapsed vertebrae, and leg paralysis; TB occurring in the kidneys may cause kidney damage and blood in the urine; TB occurring in the joints may cause arthritis-like symptoms.

Is TB contagious?

Pulmonary tuberculosis is contagious, whereas extrapulmonary tuberculosis is not contagious. Pulmonary tuberculosis is transmitted through the air by droplet infection. Droplet infection is an infection caused by inhaling pathogens (such as TB bacteria) from an infected individual. The TB bacteria are suspended on a fine spray of moisture droplets expelled from the upper respiratory tract of an individual with active pulmonary tuberculosis during talking, coughing, or sneezing; one sneeze can release as many as 40,000 moisture droplets. Fortunately, pulmonary tuberculosis is not highly contagious, and frequent or prolonged contact with an infected individual is usually required before the disease develops. This is because the natural defense mechanisms in the upper respiratory tract prevent most inhaled TB bacteria from reaching the lungs.

Who is at risk for TB?

Individuals at greatest risk for developing tuberculosis once they are infected with *Mycobacterium tuberculosis* include infants and young children, whose immune systems are not fully developed; the elderly, whose immune systems are diminished; and individuals with conditions that weaken the immune system such as diabetes mellitus, malnutrition, and prolonged corticosteroid drug therapy. Individuals with HIV infection are at very high risk for developing tuberculosis. Infection with HIV suppresses the immune system, making it difficult for the body to defend itself from TB infection or progression of latent tuberculosis infection (LTBI) to active TB. Because of this, tuberculosis is one of the leading causes of death among people with HIV infection. There has also been an increase in crowded living environments conducive to the transmission of tuberculosis, which include long-term care facilities such as nurs-

---

present and are interpreted according to the manufacturer's instructions that accompany the test.

A positive reaction to a tuberculin skin test indicates the presence of a tuberculous infection; however, it does not differentiate between active and latent forms of the infection. Therefore, a positive reaction warrants additional diagnostic procedures before the physician can make a final diagnosis. Other procedures used to detect an active tuberculous infection include chest x-ray and microbiologic examination and culture of the patient's sputum for TB bacteria.

Tuberculin Skin Testing Methods

Two methods are available for tuberculin skin testing: the Mantoux test and the Tine multiple puncture test. The Mantoux test is the most common method used for tuberculin skin testing. The Mantoux test is administered using an intradermal needle and syringe. The Mantoux test is considered a more specific and accurate test because a known amount of tuberculin is used to perform the test.

The Tine multiple puncture test uses a sterile plastic unit containing four stainless-steel tines for puncturing the skin. The tines are approximately 2 mm long and are impregnated with tuberculin. The patient is inoculated intradermally to a

depth of 1 to 2 mm by pressing the disc onto the skin, causing the tuberculin on the tines to be deposited into the skin layers. The amount of tuberculin injected into the patient's skin cannot be precisely controlled with the Tine mulitple puncture test; therefore, it is rarely used anymore. Because of this, this unit will focus on the Mantoux test.

Mantoux Test

The Mantoux test is named after Charles Mantoux, the French physician who developed the test. The Mantoux test is administered through an intradermal injection using a tuberculin syringe with a capacity of 1.0 ml and a short (⅜ to ½ inch) needle with a gauge of 26 to 27. The standard injected dose is 0.1 ml of tuberculin PPD solution containing 5 TU (tuberculin units). Brand names for Mantoux tests include Tubersol and Aplisol. Once opened, a vial of tuberculin PPD solution expires after 30 days and must be discarded. This is because oxidation and degradation of tuberculin reduce its potency, which can lead to inaccurate test results. The medical assistant should write the expiration date on the vial upon opening. Before withdrawing tuberculin from the vial, the medical assistant should check both the manufacturer's expiration date and

Highlight on Tuberculosis—cont'd

ing homes, drug rehabilitation centers, correctional facilities, and homeless shelters.

Why is the Mantoux test the preferred method of skin testing?

The tuberculin skin test is used to identify individuals infected with the TB bacteria and who have active or latent tuberculosis. Early identification of individuals with active infectious tuberculosis leads to early treatment and prevents the spread of TB. Most authorities believe that the Mantoux tuberculin test method is more specific and accurate than the Tine multiple puncture test. This is because the Mantoux test uses a known amount of tuberculin (0.1 ml of PPD), compared with the tine test, in which the tuberculin cannot be as precisely controlled. Because of this, the Tine test is rarely used anymore.

How is TB treated?

Fortunately, active tuberculosis can be treated if it is diagnosed early. Antibiotics have been available since the 1940s to cure tuberculosis and thereby help prevent its spread. The two most powerful antibiotics used to treat tuberculosis are isoniazid and rifampin. Unless antibiotic drug resistance occurs, most patients are able to leave the hospital shortly after beginning drug therapy. Discharge, however, does not mean that the patient is cured. Compared with most other infectious diseases, treatment for tuberculosis is lengthy, typically lasting 6 months to 1 year. After 2 to 4 weeks of drug therapy, the active disease is no longer contagious and the patient can resume a normal lifestyle. If the patient does not comply with the drug therapy regimen, however, some of the TB bacteria will survive and the patient will be at risk for recurrence of the disease

and the development of drug-resistant TB strains. Many physicians recommend treating individuals with LTBI to prevent it from developing into active tuberculosis later in life.

Is there a vaccine for tuberculosis?

The bacille Calmette-Guérin (BCG) vaccine is used to prevent or reduce the severity of tuberculosis. It was named for Calmette and Guérin, the French scientists who developed it in 1906. The BCG vaccine is not widely used in the United States because of the low risk of TB infection in this country. It is often administered to infants and young children in other countries where there is a high incidence of tuberculosis. The BCG vaccine does not usually protect adults from developing pulmonary tuberculosis and does not provide lifelong immunity to tuberculosis. BCG vaccination may also cause an individual to have a false-positive test result on a tuberculin skin test. Research is currently being conducted to develop a TB vaccine that is more effective than the BCG vaccine.

Is TB a reportable disease?

Tuberculosis is a reportable disease; therefore, physicians must notify the local health department of cases of tuberculosis. The physician is also required to keep public health officials informed of the patient's compliance with the drug therapy regimen. To help prevent the spread of tuberculosis, public health officials conduct investigations to locate people who may have been infected by individuals known to have TB. ∎

---

the 30-day expiration date marked by the medical assistant on the vial.

It is important to properly store the tuberculin PPD solution because it can be adversely affected by exposure to light and heat. The vial should be stored in the dark as much as possible; exposure to bright light should be avoided because this can diminish the potency of the PPD solution. A vial that has been exposed to light for an extended period of time should be discarded. The vial must be stored in the refrigerator at a temperature between 35° F to 46° F (2° C to 8° C). The vial should be returned to its refrigerated storage area as soon as possible after the proper dosage is drawn up into a syringe.

It is important that the medical assistant draw up the proper amount of tuberculin PPD solution. Injecting too much of the solution might elicit a reaction not caused by a tuberculous infection, and injecting too little of the solution results in insufficient solution being injected into the skin to elicit a reaction. This will invalidate the test because if no reaction occurs, it cannot be accepted as a negative reaction.

The medical assistant must make sure to inject the tuberculin solution into the superficial skin layers to form

a tense, pale, raised area known as a **wheal.** If the injection is made into the subcutaneous layer, a wheal will not form and the test will yield a false-negative result, whereas a too-shallow injection may cause leakage of the tuberculin solution onto the skin. In either case, the medical assistant must repeat the test at a site at least 2 inches (5 cm) away.

The medical assistant should not apply pressure to the site after injecting the tuberculin PPD solution because the solution is not intended to be absorbed into the tissues. In addition, applying pressure may cause leakage of the solution through the needle puncture site. The wheal will disappear on its own within a few minutes and should not be covered with an adhesive bandage.

Guidelines for Administering a Mantoux Test

1. Use the anterior forearm, approximately 4 inches (10 cm) below the bend in the elbow, as the site of administration of the test. Avoid the following areas because they make the test harder to perform and interfere with good visualization and palpation of test reactions:
   - Hairy areas of the skin
   - Areas with visible veins

- Scar tissue
- Red or swollen areas
- Bruised areas
- Areas with lesions, dermatitis, or other skin irritations
- Muscle ridges

2. Cleanse the skin thoroughly with an antiseptic wipe and allow it to dry completely before administering the test.

3. Be sure to inject the tuberculin slowly into the superficial layers of the skin. If the injection is performed correctly, a wheal should appear that is approximately 6 to 10 mm (⅜ inch) in diameter. If blood appears at the puncture site once the test has been administered, this is not significant and will not interfere with the test. The blood can be removed by gently blotting the area with a gauze pad, making sure not to apply pressure.

4. Once the test has been administered, the results must be read within 48 to 72 hours.

Guidelines for Reading Mantoux Test Results

1. The test results must be read in good lighting within 48 to 72 hours.

2. Use both inspection and palpation to read the test results. Induration may not always be visible and therefore must be assessed through palpation.

3. If induration is present, rub your fingertip lightly from the area of normal skin (without induration) to the indurated area to assess its size. The diameter of induration must be assessed and measured transversely to the long axis of the forearm (left to right, not up and down). Measure the widest diameter of induration in millimeters using a flexible millimeter ruler. (*Note:* If you have difficulty locating the edges of the induration, the following technique will help. Take a ballpoint pen and place the tip of it on normal skin adjacent to the induration at a 45-degree angle. Then push the pen toward the indurated area. The pen will make an ink line on the normal skin and then will stop at the edge of the induration. Repeat this technique on the opposite side of the induration.

4. The extent of induration present is the only criterion used to determine a positive reaction (Figure 11-23). If erythema is present without induration, the results are interpreted as negative.

5. Record all reactions in millimeters to the nearest millimeter. If no induration is present, the results should be recorded as 0 mm. Results should never be recorded as positive or negative.

6. The interpretation of the test results depends on:
   a. Measurement (in mm) of the induration
   b. The individual's risk of being infected with tuberculosis (e.g., close contact with an individual with active TB increases the risk of being infected)
   c. The individual's risk of progression to disease if infected (e.g., HIV-infected individuals are more apt to progress from LTBI to active TB)

7. Mantoux tuberculin test results are interpreted according to the guidelines presented in Table 11-7. The procedure

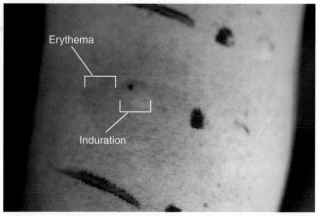

Figure 11-23. Positive tuberculin skin test showing induration and erythema. Induration is the only criterion used to determine a positive reaction. (From Abbas AK: Basic immunology: functions and disorders of the immune system, ed 3, Philadelphia, 2004, Saunders.)

for administering and reading a Mantoux test is presented in Procedure 11-7.

Two-Step Tuberculin Skin Test

The two-step tuberculin test is recommended by the Centers for Disease Control (CDC) for the initial baseline testing of adults who are required to undergo periodic tuberculin skin testing. For example, most health care workers are required to have an initial tuberculin skin test when hired and then a yearly test thereafter. Upon employment, the initial tuberculin skin test should consist of a baseline two-step test.

To understand the purpose of a two-step tuberculin skin test, it is first necessary to understand what can sometimes occur in individuals who were infected with tuberculosis many years ago. Over a period of years, the ability of the immune system of an individual with a previous TB infection to react to the tuberculin solution may gradually diminish. When a tuberculin skin test is administered to such an individual, the body does not react at all or only weakly reacts, resulting in a false-negative test result. For example, a 42-year-old individual who was infected with tuberculosis during childhood may have a negative test result to an initial tuberculin skin test.

Administering a tuberculin skin test to an individual with a previous TB infection causes stimulation or "boosting" of the patient's immune system that takes place over several days following administration of the test. Basically, the first test "jogs the memory" of the immune system to recognize and react to the tuberculin. If another test is administered following the first test, there is often a strong reaction to the tuberculin, resulting in a positive test result. This boosted reaction is caused by an old TB infection and should not be interpreted as a newly acquired infection. Misinterpretation could result in an unnecessary investigation to identify the source of the infection and unnecessary treatment of individuals. Although the booster effect can occur in an individual in any age group, it is most apt to

Table 11-7 Interpretation of the Tuberculin Mantoux Skin Test*

Interpretation of the Mantoux skin test results is based on the individual's risk of being infected with tuberculosis and the risk of progression to disease if infected. Individuals with impaired immunity are more likely to have a weaker response to a tuberculin skin test. Because of this, there are three cut-off points for identifying a positive reaction to a Mantoux test.

Positive Reaction

An induration of 5 mm or more is classified as positive in individuals with the following high-risk factors for developing TB:
1. Individuals infected with HIV
2. Individuals who have had recent close contact with individuals who have active TB
3. Individuals who have fibrotic changes on a chest radiograph consistent with previously healed TB
4. Individuals who have had organ transplants
5. Individuals on immunosuppressive drug therapy (e.g., prolonged high-dose corticosteroid therapy, TNF/alpha-antagonist drug therapy [Remicade, Enbrel, Humira])

Negative Reaction

An induration of 4 mm or less

Positive Reaction

An induration of 10 mm or more is classified as positive in individuals who do not meet the above criteria but who have other risk factors for TB, including the following:
1. Individuals who inject illegal drugs
2. Individuals with the following conditions that weaken the immune system: diabetes mellitus, chronic renal failure, being 10% or more below ideal body weight, silicosis, gastrectomy, jejunoileal bypass, certain hematologic disorders such as leukemias and lymphomas, carcinoma of the head, neck, or lungs
3. Residents and employees of the following high-risk congregate settings: hospitals and other health care facilities, correctional facilities, nursing homes, homeless shelters, drug rehabilitation centers, residential facilities for patients with AIDS
4. Recent immigrants from countries with a high incidence of TB (Asia, Africa, the Caribbean, Latin America, Eastern Europe, and Russia)
5. Children younger than 4 years of age
6. Infants, children, and adolescents exposed to adults at high risk for developing TB
7. Mycobacteriology laboratory personnel

Negative Reaction

An induration of 9 mm or less

Positive Reaction

An induration of 15 mm or more is classified as positive in individuals at low risk for developing TB, including the following:
Individuals with no known risk factors for TB

Negative Reaction

An induration of 14 mm or less

*The cut-off point may sometimes vary from state-to-state from those presented in this table.
AIDS, Acquired immunodeficiency syndrome; *HIV,* human immunodeficiency virus; *TB,* tuberculosis; *TNF,* tumor necrosis factor.

occur in older individuals who were infected with tuberculosis at a younger age.

To perform a two-step tuberculin test, the medical assistant administers the Mantoux test and instructs the patient to return to have the test read within 48 to 72 hours as outlined in Procedure 11-7. If the test result is positive, the individual is considered infected with TB bacteria, and further skin testing is not warranted. If the test result is negative, a second test is performed 1 to 3 weeks after the first test. If the second test result is negative, the patient is classified as noninfected, and a positive reaction later on to a subsequent test is likely to represent a new infection. If the second test result is positive, this is most likely caused by a boosted reaction indicating the patient was previously infected with *M. tuberculosis.* Refer to Figure 11-24 for a diagram to assist in interpreting two-step tuberculin skin testing.

When periodic TB testing is required, the two-step tuberculin skin test needs to be completed only *once.* The initial test (consisting of two tests) indicates the true baseline reading of the individual's tuberculosis status. Any subsequent tuberculin skin test performed on a periodic basis (after a two-step test) needs to consist of only one skin test.

Tuberculosis Blood Test

The QuantiFERON–TB Gold (QFT-G) test is a new blood test used to identify individuals who are infected with *M. tuberculosis* (the causative agent of tuberculosis). As with the tuberculin skin test, the QFT-G test cannot differentiate between active and latent forms of the infection. Therefore, a positive result warrants additional diagnostic procedures, such as a chest x-ray and microbiologic examination and culture of the patient's sputum, before the physician can make a diagnosis.

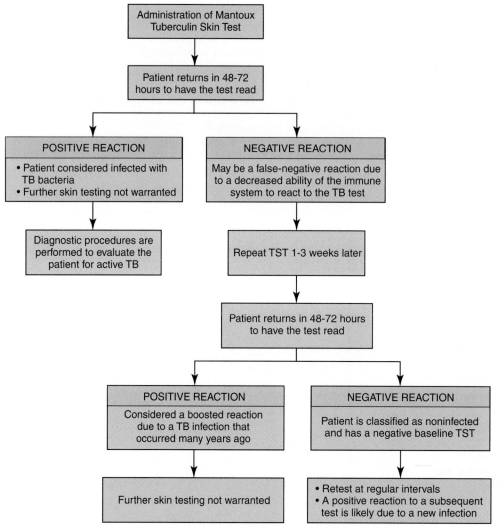

Figure 11-24. Interpretation of the two-step Mantoux tuberculin skin test.

The QFT-G test was approved for use in the United States by the Food and Drug Administration (FDA) in 2005. The CDC recently came out with guidelines indicating that the QFT-G test can be used in all situations in which the Mantoux tuberculin skin test is currently being used. A number of laboratories across the United States perform QFT-G blood testing for tuberculosis.

If the blood specimen for the QFT-G test is drawn in the medical office, several guidelines must be followed to ensure accurate test results. The blood specimen must be drawn into several evacuated tubes containing heparin; the blood drawing tubes are often provided by the laboratory performing the test. The blood specimen must be stored at room temperature and transported to the laboratory within 12 hours for processing.

Once the blood specimen reaches the laboratory, it is incubated overnight for 16 to 24 hours. The QFT-G test works by measuring the immune response of an individual. When the body is infected with *M. tuberculosis,* certain lymphocytes (a type of white blood cell) in the blood become sensitized and release a substance known as interferon

gamma (IFN-gamma). The test measures the amount of IFN-gamma released by the sensitized lymphoctyes in the patient's blood specimen. The patient is likely to be infected with *Mycobacterium* infection if he or she registers an IFN-gamma level above the positive cut-off value. On the other hand, if the patient is not infected with *M. tuberculosis,* his or her blood will not contain sensitized lymphocytes and there will not be a release of IFN-gamma. In this case, the test result is recorded as negative, indicating that the patient is unlikely to be infected with *M. tuberculosis.*

QFT-G test results are interpreted as follows:

Positive: Individuals who test positive are likely to be infected with *M. tuberculosis* and should be evaluated further for latent TB or active TB.

Negative: Healthy adults who test negative are unlikely to have a *M. tuberculosis* infection and usually do not require further evaluation.

Indeterminate: An indeterminate result indicates that the *M. tuberculosis* infection status cannot be determined because of factors that invalidate the test results. These factors include the following: improper handling and storage of the blood specimen, a delay of longer than 12 hours in transporting the specimen to the laboratory, and the inability of the patient's blood to respond to the test because of a severely weakened immune system, such as in a patient undergoing chemotherapy. If a test result is indeterminate, the QFT-G test should be repeated using a fresh blood specimen.

The QFT-G test offers several advantages over the Mantoux tuberculin skin test (TST), which include the following:

1. The patient needs to visit the office only one time to have his or her blood drawn. This alleviates the problem that sometimes occurs with patients undergoing the TST, in which a patient does not return for the second visit to have the results read.

2. The results are available within 24 hours compared with the 48 to 72 hours required for a TST.

3. The QFT-G test is an objective evaluation, whereas the TST is a subjective evaluation. If the TST test is not measured correctly, inaccurate test results may occur.

4. The QFT-G test is not affected by the booster effect, which can occur with TST, thus eliminating the need for two-step tuberculin skin testing.

5. The QFT-G test provides a positive or negative test result, and risk factors do not have to be taken into consideration when positive reactions are interpreted, as is required with the TST.

6. An individual who has been vaccinated for tuberculosis with the bacillus Calmette-Guérin (BCG) vaccine does not show a false-negative result on the QFT-G test, as can occur with a TST.

A disadvantage of the QFT-G test is that the patient's blood specimen must be delivered within 12 hours to the laboratory performing the test. This is because the lymphocytes in the blood specimen begin to die after this time period has passed.

ALLERGY TESTING

Allergy

An **allergy** is an abnormal hypersensitivity of the immune system of the body to substances that are ordinarily harmless; these substances are known as **allergens.** Allergens enter the body by being inhaled, by being swallowed, by being injected, or by contact with the skin. Almost any substance in the environment can be an allergen. Some common allergens are plant pollens, mold, house dust, animal dander, latex, dyes, soaps, detergents, cosmetics, certain foods and medications, and venom from insect stings.

The exact cause of allergies is not fully understood. In many cases, the tendency to develop allergies seems to be inherited because children of allergic parents tend to exhibit more allergic symptoms than children of nonallergic parents. Although allergies can develop at any age, children are more apt to develop allergies than are older individuals.

Allergic Reaction

The immune system of an individual with allergies interprets certain allergens (e.g., pollen, mold, house dust) as invaders. The first time the allergen enters the body of an allergic individual, it stimulates the body to produce antibodies to that allergen. These antibodies are usually of a type known as *immunoglobulin (Ig)E antibodies.* After the initial sensitization, allergic antibodies combine with the allergen in the body, resulting in an allergen-antibody reaction. When such a reaction occurs, histamine is released in significant amounts, causing allergic symptoms (e.g., sneezing, watery eyes, runny nose). Allergen-antibody reactions may involve any system of the body; however, they most frequently affect the respiratory and integumentary systems. Allergic symptoms can range from mild to very severe, as is the case with the potentially fatal anaphylactic reaction.

Depending on the allergen and the body system affected, allergies appear in different forms in an individual and commonly include allergic rhinitis, asthma, urticaria, contact dermatitis, eczema, and food allergies. Symptoms exhibited by an allergic individual depend on an individual's form of allergy. Table 11-8 lists the common clinical forms of allergies and symptoms of allergies.

Diagnosis and Treatment

The best way to prevent allergic symptoms is to identify and avoid the offending allergen or allergens. The first and most important step in this process is the completion of a careful and detailed medical history by the physician. Of particular importance to the diagnosis of an allergy are the patient's home and work environments, diet, and living habits. The physician also performs a thorough physical examination to detect conditions resulting from allergies, such as nasal polyps, wheezing, skin rashes, and urticaria.

When the medical history and physical examination have been completed, the physician may order diagnostic tests. Allergy testing is performed to confirm information obtained through the medical history and physical examination. The allergy tests ordered most often are direct skin testing and in vitro blood testing, which are described in greater detail in the following section. The general treatment of allergies includes avoiding the allergen(s) (if possible); alleviating the symptoms through drug therapy such as antihistamines, decongestants, bronchodilators, and inhaled steroids; and decreasing the sensitivity of the body to the allergen by the administration of allergy injections, or desensitization injections (known as immunotherapy).

Types of Allergy Tests

The purpose of allergy testing is to determine the specific substances or allergens that are causing the patient's allergic symptoms. The two main categories of allergy tests are direct skin tests and the in vitro blood test. The medical assistant is often responsible for performing direct skin testing in the medical office. The in vitro blood test is performed

Table 11-8 Clinical Forms of Allergies

Hay fever (seasonal allergic rhinitis)	Caused by allergy to mold or the pollen of trees, grasses, or weeds. The term *hay fever* is misleading because hay fever is not caused by hay, and it does not result in fever. English physicians first used the term *hay fever* in the early 1800s when treating patients with allergies to grass pollens. Symptoms of hay fever and the common cold are almost identical: episodes of sneezing, itching, and watery eyes; runny and stuffy nose; and burning sensation of the palate and throat. Hay fever is seasonal, occurring when there is pollen in the air. Depending on geographic location, hay fever may occur in spring, summer, or fall, and last until first frost.
Perennial allergic rhinitis	Inflammation of mucous membranes of the nose caused by allergies. Symptoms include nasal congestion, sneezing, and runny nose. With perennial rhinitis, the nasal mucosa is inflamed year-round. This type of allergic rhinitis is commonly caused by allergens that are always present in the environment, such as house dust and animal dander.
Allergic asthma	Condition characterized by coughing, chest tightness, shortness of breath, and wheezing. During an asthma attack, the bronchiole tubes constrict and become clogged with mucus, which accounts for many of the symptoms of allergic asthma. Asthma can occur at any age but is more common in children and young adults and, if not treated, can lead to serious complications such as permanent lung damage. It is frequently, but not always, associated with a family history of allergy. Any common allergen, such as house dust, pollens, mold, or animal dander, may trigger an allergic asthma attack.
Urticaria	Urticaria, or hives, is an outbreak on the skin of welts of varying sizes that are redder or paler than surrounding skin and are accompanied by intense itching. When swellings are large and invade deeper tissues, the condition is known as *angioedema*. Hives may develop on the face or lips or even internally. Allergies to food or drugs (especially penicillin and aspirin) and insect bites often cause hives, but they also may result from underlying disease or occur after exercise. In many cases the exact causes of urticaria cannot be determined. 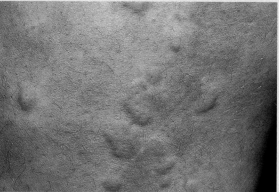 (From Forbes CD: Color atlas and text of clinical medicine, ed 3, Philadelphia, 2002, Mosby.)
Contact dermatitis	Rash caused by direct contact of the skin with an allergen, such as cosmetics, perfumes, deodorants, latex, plastics, certain plants, and clothing treated with certain preservatives or dyes. Symptoms include swelling, blistering, oozing, and scaling. Rash usually occurs only on the areas of the body that have been in contact with the allergen. The most common causes of contact dermatitis are poison ivy, poison oak, and sumac. 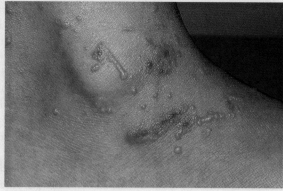 (From Forbes CD: Color atlas and text of clinical medicine, ed 3, Philadelphia, 2002, Mosby.)

Table 11-8 Clinical Forms of Allergies—cont'd	
Eczema	Noncontagious rash accompanied by redness, itching, vesicles, oozing, crusting, and scaling. Eczema is a common allergic reaction in children, but it also may occur in adults, usually in a more severe form. A rash commonly appears on the face, neck, and folds of the elbows and knees. Eczema frequently is associated with allergies, and substances to which a person is allergic may aggravate it. Foods may be important factors, particularly milk, fish, or eggs. Allergens that are inhaled, such as dust and pollen, rarely cause eczema. 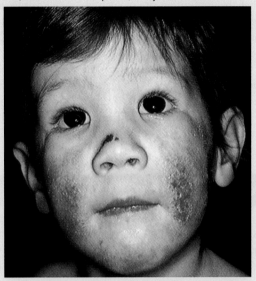 (From Leifer G: Introduction to maternity and pediatric nursing, ed 5, St Louis, 2009, Saunders.)
Food allergy	An immune system reaction that occurs soon after eating a food to which an individual is allergic. The most common symptoms that occur when a patient has a food allergy are urticaria (hives), asthma symptoms (such as wheezing and shortness of breath), gastrointestinal symptoms (such as nausea, vomiting, diarrhea, abdominal pain), and swelling of the lips, face, tongue, or throat. The most common foods that cause allergies are milk, soy, eggs, peanuts, tree nuts (e.g., walnuts), fish, shellfish, and wheat. The primary treatment for a food allergy involves avoidance of the food. If the individual has a severe allergy to a food, such as peanuts, consuming the food can cause an anaphylactic reaction, which can be life threatening. Treatment involves the immediate injection of epinephrine.

on a blood specimen by an outside laboratory. The medical assistant may be responsible for performing a venipuncture to obtain the blood specimen.

Direct Skin Testing

Direct skin testing involves applying extracts of common allergens to the skin and observing the body's reaction to them. The extract is applied either topically to the skin (patch testing) or into the superficial skin layers (skin-prick testing and intradermal testing). The advantage of direct skin testing is that test results are obtained immediately. This in vivo administration of allergens has the potential, however, to cause adverse reactions, the least common but most serious being an anaphylactic reaction. The medical assistant should have a thorough knowledge of the symptoms of an anaphylactic reaction and should alert the physician immediately if the patient begins to exhibit them.

Regardless of the specific type of direct skin test used (patch, skin-prick, or intradermal), some general guidelines should be followed:

1. Instruct the patient to discontinue the use of antihistamines for 3 days before the skin testing. Antihistamines block the response of histamine, which may suppress skin

testing reactions and lead to false-negative test results. Certain medications decrease the immune response of the body to skin testing, which could cause a false-negative test result. These medications include tricyclic antidepressants, corticosteroids, theophylline, beta-blockers, angiotensin-converting enzyme (ACE) inhibitors, and nifedipine. If the patient is taking any of these medications, the physician must determine if it is possible to take the patient off of the medication. If it is not feasible, the physician may order in vitro allergy blood testing, which is not affected by medication.

2. Verify that the area of application is free from hair, scar tissue, and dermatitis to permit good visualization and palpation of test reactions. Recommended sites include the anterior forearm, the upper arm, and the middle of the back. The back is usually used for patch and skin-prick testing, and the upper arm and forearm are typically used for intradermal skin testing.

3. Cleanse the area of application thoroughly with an antiseptic wipe, and allow it to dry completely.

4. Wear gloves when the allergy testing involves puncture of the skin, which includes skin-prick testing and intradermal skin testing. Gloves protect the medical assistant

from exposure to bloodborne pathogens, as required by the OSHA standard.

5. Space the allergen extracts at least 1 inch apart to provide enough surface area for a sizable reaction. If not enough surface area is available, large adjacent reactions may run together, making it difficult to read test results.

6. Label the test sites so that the application site of each allergen extract can be identified later when reading results.

7. Closely observe the patient after the procedure for a systemic reaction to the skin testing. The patient should remain at the office for at least 30 minutes following the procedure for observation.

8. Make the patient aware that the skin testing may cause a mild allergic reaction, such as a runny nose, sneezing, and mild wheezing 8 to 24 hours after skin-prick and intradermal skin testing. Instruct the patient to contact the physician immediately if a more severe reaction than this occurs, such as difficulty in breathing, dizziness, or swelling of the face, lips, or mouth.

Quality Control

Positive and negative controls should be performed with each skin testing procedure to ensure reliable and valid test results. Controls are performed at the same time and in the same way that the allergy skin testing is performed.

Negative Control: To perform a negative skin test control, a substance that should not cause a reaction in a normal person is inserted into the patient's superficial skin layers. The negative control usually consists of normal saline. Some patients have a condition known as *dermo-*

Highlight on Allergens

House Dust

There are many components in house dust to which an individual may be allergic; the most significant of these is the house dust mite. Dust mites thrive in warm humid conditions and feed on scales shed from human skin; they are often found in mattresses, carpets, stuffed animals, and upholstered furniture. An individual who is allergic to house dust reacts to the waste products of these dust mites.

There is no shortage of food for the dust mite because one person sheds up to 1 g of scales per day, which is enough to feed thousands of mites for months. *Dermatophagoides pteronyssinus* and *Dermatophagoides farinae* are the most common house dust mites and are present in varying numbers in virtually every home. Mites occur in greatest numbers in bedding, particularly in mattresses; there may be 5000 mites in each gram of dust from a mattress. Sufferers often notice that symptoms become much worse when the bedding is disturbed and allergenic material becomes airborne. Practices that eliminate dust also reduce the number of dust mites in a household.

Insect Stings

It is estimated that 1 of every 125 Americans is allergic to the venom from insect stings. Approximately 40 people in the United States die each year from a severe allergic reaction to insect venom. The incidence of deaths is low because most people know they need to obtain medical attention immediately if an allergic reaction begins.

Almost all insects whose venom can cause allergic reactions belong to the group Hymenoptera, which includes honeybees and bumblebees, wasps, yellow jackets, and hornets. When a honeybee stings, its stinger remains embedded in the victim's skin, causing the bee to die as it tries to tear itself away. Wasps, yellow jackets, and hornets are more aggressive than bees and can sting repeatedly. Hornets are the most aggressive of the group and may sting even when not provoked. Yellow jackets are close behind in aggressiveness, but wasps usually sting only if someone interferes with them near their nest.

If an insect sting does not cause an allergic reaction within 30 minutes, chances are excellent that no problem will occur. A normal reaction to an insect sting includes localized pain, redness, swelling, and itching lasting 1 to 2 days. Any generalized reaction not arising directly from the area of the sting is almost certain to be an anaphylactic reaction, which begins with such symptoms as sneezing, urticaria, itching, angioedema, erythema, and disorientation and progresses to difficulty in breathing, dizziness, faintness, and loss of consciousness. Medical care should be sought immediately because most fatalities occur within 2 hours following the sting. Because time is a factor, individuals who are known to have a severe allergy to insect stings are provided with an anaphylactic emergency treatment kit that contains epinephrine in a prefilled syringe and oral antihistamines. They can carry the kit with them so that treatment for a severe allergic reaction can be started as soon as possible.

Penicillin

Penicillin is a common cause of allergic drug reactions. Approximately 2% to 5% of individuals are allergic to penicillin. The reaction may be mild and completely overlooked or confused with the symptoms of the disease being treated with penicillin, or it can be more serious and take the form of severe dermatitis or an anaphylactic reaction. Death as a result of a severe anaphylactic reaction is rare, occurring in only 0.01% of patients being treated with penicillin.

Penicillin was discovered in 1929 by Sir Alexander Fleming, but it was not used as a therapeutic drug until 1940. By 1944, it was evident that some of the side effects of penicillin were allergic reactions; the first recorded death as a result of an anaphylactic reaction to penicillin occurred in 1945.

Oral administration of penicillin is safer than a penicillin injection because it has a lower frequency of severe allergic reactions. There have been only six reported deaths from oral administration of penicillin.

Approximately 95% of serious reactions occur within 1 hour after a penicillin injection. The best preventive measure is to keep the patient under direct observation for at least 30 minutes after administration of the injection. ■

graphism, which causes them to have a reaction just from the irritating effect of a needle pricking their skin. Running a negative control ensures that positive skin test reactions are truly positive and are not due to another factor, such as dermographism.

Positive Control: To perform a positive control, a substance that should cause a reaction in a nonallergenic patient is inserted into the patient's superficial skin layers. The substance used for the positive control is histamine. The positive control should produce a reaction that consists of at least 3 mm of induration surrounded by erythema. Patients who are taking an antihistamine or who have a depressed immune system due to a disease or immunosuppressive medication may have a false-negative reaction to a skin test. Running a positive control ensures that negative skin test reactions are truly negative and are not just due to another factor, as in a patient who has taken an antihistamine.

Types of Direct Skin Tests

Patch Testing

Patch testing is primarily used to identify allergens that cause contact dermatitis. Patch testing involves the topical application of each allergen to the skin, using a "patch." A patch consists of a small piece of gauze or filter paper impregnated with the allergen, which is applied to the skin and taped in place with hypoallergenic tape (Figure 11-25). Allergens commonly applied include plants, topical drugs, latex, resins, metals, cosmetics, dyes, and chemicals. The patient should be instructed to leave the patches in place, keep them dry, and return to the medical office in 48 hours to have the results read. When the patient returns to the office, the patches are carefully removed, and the results are read 20 minutes later. The delayed reading time allows lessening of redness that may occur from the tape removal.

Test results are recorded as positive or negative. Positive reactions cause a small area of contact dermatitis characterized by itching, erythema, induration, and vesiculation (Figure 11-26). In strongly positive responses, the reaction may extend beyond the margins of the patch. Positive results are graded further on a quantitative 1+ to 3+ scoring system according to the type of reaction (Table 11-9).

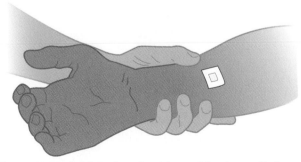

Figure 11-25. Patch testing. A patch consists of a small piece of gauze or filter paper impregnated with the allergen, which is applied to the skin and taped in place.

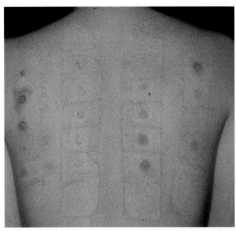

Figure 11-26. Patch test showing positive results. (From Shiland BJ: Mastering healthcare terminology, ed 3, St Louis, 2010, Mosby.)

Table 11-9 Guidelines for Recording Direct Skin Test Results	
Patch Test	
—	No reaction
+1	Presence of erythema and edema, possibly papules
+2	Presence of erythema, edema, and vesicles, possibly papules
+3	Erythema, vesicles, and severe edema
Skin-Prick Testing and Intradermal Testing	
—	No reaction
±1	Induration 1 mm or less
+1	Induration greater than 1 mm and up to 5 mm in diameter
+2	Induration greater than 5 mm and up to 10 mm in diameter
+3	Induration greater than 10 mm and up to 15 mm in diameter
+4	Induration greater than 15 mm in diameter

Skin-Prick Testing

Skin-prick testing usually is performed to diagnose allergies to common allergens, particularly those that are inhaled, such as house dust, pollens, and molds. It is also used to test for food allergies; the most common foods that cause allergies are milk, soy, eggs, peanuts, tree nuts (e.g., walnuts), fish, shellfish, and wheat.

Skin-prick testing involves the application of numerous allergen extracts to the skin, followed by the pricking of each with a sterile needle or another sharp instrument (Figure 11-27). The number of allergen extracts applied during one office visit usually ranges between 20 and 30. Pricking the skin deposits the allergens in the outer layers of the skin to allow each to react with the body tissues.

The following guidelines should be followed for skin-prick testing: The extracts should be placed on the skin in rows in a specific pattern. This, along with labeling the test sites with a felt-tipped pen, tracks the location of each extract. Only a single drop of extract should be placed on the skin; more than this amount may cause the extracts to dif-

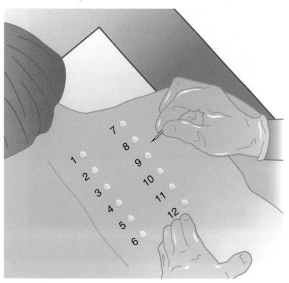

Figure 11-27. Skin-prick testing. Skin-prick testing involves the application of numerous allergen extracts to the skin, followed by the pricking of each with a sterile needle.

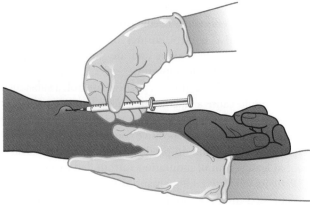

Figure 11-28. Intradermal skin testing. Intradermal testing involves the injection of a small amount of allergen extract into the superficial skin layers through the intradermal route of administration.

fuse and run together. A sterile needle should be passed through the drop, and the point should lightly lift the top layer of skin without causing bleeding. It is important to wipe the needle dry with a sterile swab between pricks to prevent one extract from mixing with the next, leading to inaccurate test results.

The maximum reaction is usually seen in 15 to 20 minutes. During this time, the test sites should be left uncovered, and the patient should be instructed not to touch them. These areas should not be wiped because this removes the allergen extract, resulting in false-negative results. The results are read (after 15 to 20 minutes) using a millimeter ruler.

An area of induration surrounded by redness and itching characterizes a positive reaction. Positive results are recorded by measuring the size of the induration in millimeters and converting it to a numeric scale based on the extent of the induration (see Table 11-9). Any redness should be ignored. See Figure 11-28 for an illustration of skin test results. If a negative or only a mild reaction occurs and the

physician still suspects the presence of an allergy, the physician may order intradermal skin testing.

Intradermal Skin Testing

Intradermal skin testing is similar to skin-prick testing but it is more sensitive. The number of skin tests performed during one office visit ranges from 5 to 30. Because there is a greater chance of adverse allergic reactions to intradermal skin testing, the physician often starts with skin-prick testing in individuals who are suspected of being highly allergic as determined by the medical history and results of the physical examination.

Intradermal skin testing involves the injection of a small amount (0.02 to 0.05 ml) of allergen extract into the superficial skin layers through the intradermal route of administration (see Figure 11-28). A tuberculin syringe is used to administer the test, and the allergen extract is injected until a wheal forms (see Procedure 11-7). After 15 to 20 minutes, the test sites are observed for reactions. Positive reactions are characterized by an area of induration surrounded by redness and itching. As with skin-prick testing, positive results are recorded by measuring the size of the induration in millimeters and converting it to a numeric scale based on the amount of induration present (Figure 11-29; see Table 11-9).

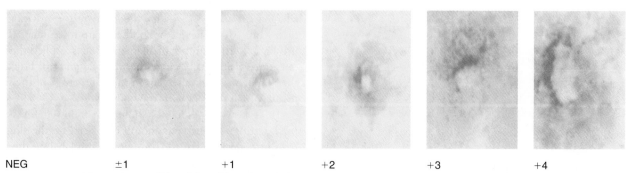

NEG   ±1   +1   +2   +3   +4

Figure 11-29. Skin-prick and intradermal skin test results. (Copyright and courtesy Hollister-Stier, Spokane, Wash.)

In Vitro Allergy Blood Testing

An in vitro allergy blood test measures the amount of IgE antibodies in the blood that respond to common allergens. Examples of in vitro blood tests include enzyme-linked immunosorbent assay (ELISA), the radioallergosorbent test (RAST), and ImmunoCAP. To perform the test, a sample of the patient's blood is sent to an outside laboratory, where it is exposed to allergens suspected of causing an allergic reaction in that patient. A detection device is used to measure the level of IgE antibodies that respond to each allergen being tested, and the results are reported as a numeric value. An elevated level of IgE antibodies responding to an allergen indicates the patient is allergic to that allergen.

Advantages of the in vitro blood test over direct skin testing are as follows: The results are not affected by medication (e.g., antihistamines); there is no danger of adverse allergic reactions because the test is performed in vitro,

meaning outside the body; and in vitro blood testing can be performed on patients who have skin eruptions and are unable to undergo direct skin testing because of the lack of an intact skin surface area. In vitro blood testing is expensive, however, and does not provide immediate test results, which are available with direct skin testing. Blood testing is often used to test for allergies when it is not possible to perform skin testing. These situations include the following:

1. The physician does not want the patient to be taken off of a medication that interferes with skin test results.
2. The physician suspects that skin testing could result in an anaphylactic reaction in that patient.
3. The patient suffers from a severe skin condition such as widespread dermatitis.
4. The skin testing may be difficult to perform, as in a child younger than 4 years of age.

 PROCEDURE 11-7   Administering an Intradermal Injection

Outcome Administer an intradermal injection and read the test results.

Equipment/Supplies:

- Skin test solution ordered by the physician
- Appropriate needle and syringe
- Antiseptic wipe
- Sterile 2 × 2 gauze pad

- Disposable gloves
- Millimeter ruler
- TB skin test record card
- Biohazard sharps container

---

1. **Procedural Step.** Sanitize your hands and prepare the injection (see Procedure 11-2).
2. **Procedural Step.** Greet the patient and introduce yourself. Identify the patient by full name and date of birth. Explain the procedure and purpose of the injection.
   Principle. It is crucial that no error be made in patient identity. Explain the purpose of the injection to reassure an apprehensive patient.
3. **Procedural Step.** Select an appropriate injection site. The anterior forearm and the middle of the back are recommended sites for an intradermal injection. If using the anterior forearm, position the arm on a firm surface with the palm facing upward.
   Principle. The entire area should be exposed to ensure a safe and comfortable injection.
4. **Procedural Step.** Prepare the injection site. Cleanse the area with an antiseptic wipe. Using a circular motion, start with the injection site and move outward. Do not touch the site after cleansing it.
   Principle. Using a circular motion will carry material away from the injection site. Touching the site after cleansing will contaminate it, and the cleansing process will need to be repeated.
5. **Procedural Step.** Allow the area to dry completely.
   Principle. If the area is not permitted to dry, the

antiseptic may enter the tissue when the skin is pierced, resulting in irritation and patient discomfort. In addition, the antiseptic may cause a reaction that could be mistaken for a positive test response.

6. **Procedural Step.** Apply gloves, and remove the needle guard. With the nondominant hand, stretch the skin taut at the proposed site of administration. Insert the needle at a 10- to 15-degree angle (almost parallel to the skin), with the bevel upward. The needle should be inserted about ⅛ inch until the bevel of the needle

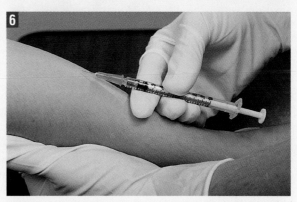

Insert the needle at a 10- to 15-degree angle with the bevel upward.

Continued

PROCEDURE 11-7   Administering an Intradermal Injection—cont'd

just penetrates the skin. Slight resistance may be felt as the needle is inserted. No aspiration is needed.

Principle. Gloves provide a barrier against blood-borne pathogens. Stretching the patient's skin taut will permit easier insertion of the needle. The needle should be inserted at an angle almost parallel to the skin, to ensure penetration within the dermal layer of the skin. The needle must be inserted with the bevel facing up to allow proper wheal formation. If the needle is inserted with the bevel facing down, the skin test solution will be absorbed into the underlying subcutaneous tissue, and a wheal will not form.

7. **Procedural Step.** Release the stretched skin. Hold the syringe steady, and inject the skin test solution slowly and steadily by depressing the plunger until a firm, tense, pale wheal forms (approximately 6 to 10 mm in diameter). Expect to feel a certain amount of resistance as you inject the solution; this helps in indicating that the needle is properly located in the superficial skin layers rather than in the deeper subcutaneous tissue. If a wheal does not form, the test must be repeated at another site that is at least two inches (5 cm) from the first site. If you are using a retractable safety syringe, activate it at this time following the steps outlined in Figure 11-10, *C,* and continue to Step 9.

Principle. Moving the syringe once the needle has entered the skin causes patient discomfort. Test results are considered reliable only if a wheal forms.

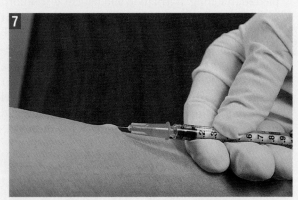

Inject the medication to form a wheal.

8. Procedural Step. Place the antiseptic wipe or gauze pad gently over the injection site and remove the needle quickly and at the same angle as for insertion.

Principle. Withdrawing the needle quickly and at the angle of insertion reduces patient discomfort. The antiseptic wipe or gauze pad placed over the injection site helps prevent tissue movement as the needle is withdrawn, also reducing patient discomfort.

9. Procedural Step. Do not apply pressure to the injection site. If blood appears at the injection site, blot the site lightly with a gauze pad. If you are using a safety syringe with a shield, activate the safety feature at this time following the steps outlined in Figure 11-10.

Principle. Applying pressure may cause leakage of the testing solution through the needle puncture site, resulting in inaccurate test results.

10. **Procedural Step.** Properly dispose of the needle and syringe in a biohazard sharps container.

Principle. Proper disposal of the needle and syringe is required by the Occupational Safety and Health Administration (OSHA) Standard to prevent accidental needlestick injuries.

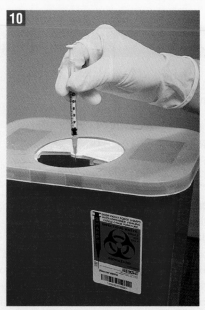

Properly dispose of the needle and syringe.

11. Procedural Step. Remove gloves and sanitize your hands.

12. Procedural Step. Stay with the patient to make sure that he or she is not experiencing any unusual reactions. The medical assistant should be especially careful and alert for any sign of a patient reaction when administering allergy skin tests. If the patient experiences an unusual reaction, notify the physician immediately.

13. Procedural Step. Perform one of the following, based on the type of skin test being administered.

Allergy Skin Tests

a. Read the test results within 20 to 30 minutes, using inspection and palpation at the site of the in-

PROCEDURE 11-7 **Administering an Intradermal Injection—cont'd**

jection to assess the presence of and to determine the amount of induration. Interpret the skin test results according to the information outlined in Table 11-9.

b. Chart the procedure. Include the date and time, the injection site used, the names of the skin tests, the skin test results, and any significant observations or patient reactions.

CHARTING EXAMPLE

Date	
2/15/12	Allergy skin tests, ID, Ⓡ ant forearm.
	Results: House dust +2
	Cat dander +4
	Dog dander –
	Ragweed +4
	Mixed fungi +3
	—————————— T. Cline, CMA (AAMA)

Mantoux Tuberculin Skin Test

a. Inform the patient of the date and time to return to the medical office to have the results read. Results must be read within 48 to 72 hours after the test has been administered. Stress the importance of returning to the office to have the results read, even if the test site does not exhibit a reaction. Failure to return warrants having to repeat the test.

b. Chart the procedure. Include the date and time, the name of the tuberculin purified protein derivative (PPD) solution, the dosage given, the manufacturer and lot number, the route of administration, the injection site used, and any significant observations or patient reactions. The lot number indicates the batch in which the tuberculin solution was made. Should a problem arise with that

CHARTING EXAMPLE

Date	
2/15/12	10:00 a.m. Tubersol Mantoux test 5 TU,
	0.10 ml, ID. Connaught Laboratories,
	Lot #: C0832AA. Admin Ⓡ ant forearm.
	Pt to return on 2/17/12 to have results
	read. —————— T. Cline, CMA (AAMA)

batch, the tuberculin solution can be recalled and the individuals who received it can be identified.

c. Instruct the patient in the care of the test site as follows:
- Continue your normal daily personal hygiene activities.
- Do not cover the test site with an adhesive bandage.
- Avoid the use of ointments, lotions, and sunscreens.
- Mild itching, swelling, or irritation may normally occur at the test site.
- Do not touch, scratch, press on, or rub the test site. This could alter the test results. If the test site itches, apply a cold compress to the area.
- Pat the arm dry after washing it. Do not rub it dry.

Reading Mantoux Test Results

Equipment/Supplies

- Millimeter ruler
- Disposable gloves
- Tuberculin test record card

1. **Procedural Step.** Greet the patient and introduce yourself. Identify the patient by full name and date of birth and explain the procedure.
2. **Procedural Step.** Work in a quiet well-lit atmosphere. Check the patient's chart to determine which arm was used to administer the test.
3. **Procedural Step.** Sanitize your hands and apply gloves.
4. **Procedural Step.** Position the patient's arm on a firm surface with the arm flexed at the elbow.
5. **Procedural Step.** Locate the application site. The result should be read transversely to the long axis of the forearm, meaning "across" the forearm.
6. **Procedural Step.** Gently rub your fingertip over the test site and lightly palpate for the presence of induration. If induration is present, the area should be lightly rubbed from the area of normal skin (without induration) to the indurated area to assess the size of the area of induration. If the margins of induration are irregular, assess the widest diameter of induration across the forearm.

Principle. Induration is the only criterion used in determining a positive reaction. If erythema is present without induration, the results are interpreted as negative.

7. **Procedural Step.** Measure the diameter of the induration with a flexible millimeter ruler (supplied by the manufacturer).

Continued

PROCEDURE 11-7   Administering an Intradermal Injection—cont'd

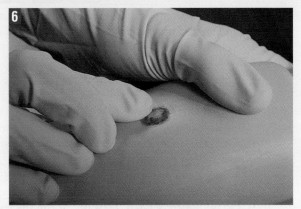

Lightly palpate for induration.

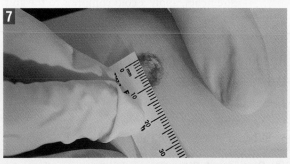

Measure the induration.

8. Procedural Step. Remove gloves and sanitize your hands.

9. Procedural Step. Chart the results. Include the date and time, the name of the test (Mantoux), and the test results (recorded in millimeters). If no induration is present, 0 mm should be recorded. The results of the

CHARTING EXAMPLE

Date	
2/17/12	3:00 p.m. Tubersol Mantoux test: 9 mm.
	Pt provided c̄ TB record card. Scheduled
	for TB retesting on 2/28/12. ————————
	——————————— T. Cline, CMA (AAMA)

Mantoux test are interpreted according to the guidelines outlined in Table 11-7.

10. Procedural Step. Complete a tuberculin test record card and give it to the patient.

Principle. The record card provides the patient with a permanent record of the test results.

10

TUBERCULOSIS TEST RECORD

Name	Date Admin: 2/15/12
Carrie Fee	Date Read: 2/17/12
MANTOUX TEST	**RESULT**
Tubersol, 5 TU	_9_ mm

Logan Family Practice
401 St. George St.
St. Augustine, FL 32084
(904) 555-3933

Performed by _T. Cline_, **CMA** (AAMA)

INTRAVENOUS THERAPY

Intravenous (IV) therapy is the administration of a liquid agent directly into a patient's vein, where it is distributed throughout the body by way of the circulatory system (Figure 11-30). The veins most commonly used for IV therapy are the peripheral veins of the arm and hand. The liquid agent may consist of basic fluids, medication, nutrients, blood, or blood products. When fluids, medications, or nutrients are administered through the IV route, the technique is called an **infusion.** When whole blood or blood products are administered through the IV route, the procedure is called a **transfusion.**

Most IV therapy occurs in a hospital setting on both an inpatient and an outpatient basis. IV therapy also is administered in outpatient ambulatory settings, such as medical offices and clinics, urgent care centers, ambulatory infusion clinics, and the patient's home (Figure 11-31).

Advantages of Outpatient Intravenous Therapy

Administration of IV therapy in an outpatient setting is growing in acceptance by patients and the medical community. Outpatient IV therapy is more convenient for the patient and reduces medical costs through earlier discharge from the hospital or avoidance of hospitalization altogether.

Earlier Hospital Discharge

When a hospitalized patient is receiving IV therapy and requires continued therapy, it is not always necessary or cost effective to keep the patient in the hospital. If the patient is medically stable, he or she may no longer need the careful observation and daily nursing care provided by a hospital. By receiving IV therapy in an outpatient setting, the patient can be discharged earlier. Most patients, particularly children, are more comfortable in their home environment, which often contributes to faster healing. An example of

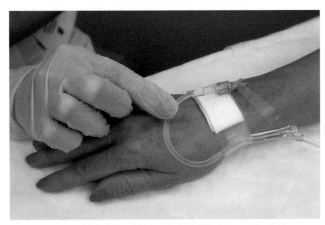

Figure 11-30. IV therapy. (From Potter PA, Perry AG: Basic nursing: essentials for practice, ed 5, St Louis, 2002, Mosby.)

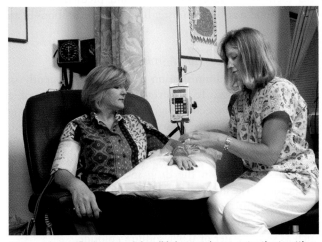

Figure 11-31. Patient receiving IV therapy in an outpatient setting. (Photo by Margaret Hartshorn: Courtesy of the Arizona Arthritis Center [www.arthritis.arizona.edu].)

this is a hospitalized patient with an infection who still needs IV antibiotic therapy but no longer needs to be hospitalized, and receives the therapy at an infusion clinic.

Avoidance of Hospitalization

Outpatient IV therapy provides an alternative to patients with an acute or chronic illness that requires IV therapy. Patients who do not require hospitalization for their condition are able to obtain their IV therapy in an outpatient setting. This allows patients the option of being able to continue their daily routine without major interruptions and provides them with greater independence and control over their condition. An example of this is a patient with rheumatoid arthritis who needs IV infliximab (Remicade) therapy and receives that therapy at the rheumatology medical office.

Medical Office–Based Intravenous Therapy

Some medical offices provide outpatient IV therapy. Outpatient IV therapy may be provided in an oncology office for the administration of IV chemotherapy. With the advent of

newer rheumatology medications that must be given intravenously, some rheumatology offices have started to provide this service. There are distinct advantages to medical office–based IV therapy. It allows the physician to provide closer monitoring of a patient's response to the IV therapy and any adverse reactions exhibited by the patient. These benefits have prompted more physicians to consider office-based IV therapy.

Based on the potential future growth of IV therapy in the medical office and the current growth of other IV outpatient settings, such as infusion clinics and the patient's home, there is a need for medical assistants to acquire some basic knowledge in IV therapy. The medical assistant is often responsible for scheduling IV therapy and providing the patient with IV therapy instructions and information, such as the length of time required for the therapy. In addition, patients may have questions that the medical assistant may need to answer (or refer to the proper individual for answering) regarding their outpatient IV therapy. The entry-level medical assistant should be familiar with the basic theory of outpatient IV therapy, which is presented here.

Advanced IV theory and initiating, maintaining, and discontinuing IV therapy are not entry-level medical assisting competencies and are not addressed in this text. Certain requirements must be met before the medical assistant can perform IV therapy in the medical office. The medical assistant first should check the laws of his or her state to determine whether it is legally permissible for the medical assistant to perform this procedure. The medical assistant must acquire the proper training (theory and skills) by completing a recognized IV therapy training program, including supervised clinical practice. Although the IV procedure can appear simple when performed by an expert, it is a difficult skill that requires considerable practice to perfect.

Indications for Outpatient Intravenous Therapy

Outpatient IV therapy has been shown to be a safe and effective alternative to inpatient IV therapy for the treatment of certain conditions. Before prescribing outpatient IV therapy, the physician assesses the need for the therapy by determining whether the following criteria are met: The patient's condition warrants the use of IV therapy, no alternative routes are feasible or appropriate to deliver the therapy, and the patient does not need to be hospitalized to receive the IV therapy. After determining the need for outpatient IV therapy, the physician prescribes the appropriate medication or fluid and treatment plan, orders laboratory tests to monitor the patient's progress, and assesses the patient after the IV therapy.

Scheduling the IV Therapy

If the patient receives the IV therapy at an outpatient site other than the medical office (e.g., an infusion clinic), the medical assistant may be responsible for scheduling the necessary services and providing the patient with IV therapy instructions, such as the length of time required for the therapy, any dietary restrictions, whether to wear loose-fitting comfortable clothing, and whether someone needs to transport the patient to and from the appointment.

Medical Office Guidelines

Medical offices that provide IV therapy on-site usually set up a special room to deliver the therapy, which often includes a lounge chair to provide for patient comfort during the therapy. With office-based IV therapy, the entry-level medical assistant is responsible for scheduling the IV therapy and providing the patient with the IV therapy instructions listed previously. The medical office employs an IV practitioner, such as a nurse or a specially trained medical assistant, to initiate, maintain, and discontinue the IV therapy. This practitioner must be completely familiar with all aspects of the IV therapy, including indications and uses, actions, dose and rate of infusion, incompatibilities, contraindications and precautions, antidote, and adverse effects. During the IV therapy, the practitioner must monitor carefully the patient's response to the therapy and be alert for adverse or allergic reactions. After the therapy is completed, the IV practitioner provides the patient with follow-up instructions, such as information on normal side effects that may occur when the patient returns home and any adverse reactions that need to be reported to the medical office.

Administration of IV Therapy

IV therapy may be administered in an outpatient setting for a variety of reasons. These include the following, which are discussed in greater detail in the next section:
- Administration of IV medication
- Replacement of fluids and electrolytes
- Administration of nutritional supplements
- Administration of blood products
- Emergency administration of IV medication and fluids

Administration of Intravenous Medication

IV medication administration is the process of delivering medication directly into a patient's vein. The IV route provides a rapid and effective method for administering medication to a patient. It also provides more accurate dosing than other routes because the medication enters the body directly from the circulatory system. This allows the medication to bypass barriers to drug absorption, such as the digestive tract (from oral administration) or muscle tissue (from IM administration), which makes it easier to control the actual amount of drug delivered to the body.

Medication may have to be administered through the IV route, as opposed to other, less invasive routes such as oral administration, for many reasons, including the following:
- A rapid systemic response to the medication is desired.
- Therapeutic blood levels of the medication need to be maintained.
- The medication is destroyed by stomach acids, digestive enzymes, or both.
- The medication cannot be absorbed into the body through the gastrointestinal tract.

- The medication is toxic and could damage the lining of the gastrointestinal tract.
- The medication is painful or irritating when given by other parenteral routes (IM or SC injection).

Intravenous Administration Methods

IV medication can be administered by three methods: direct IV injection, intermittent IV administration, and continuous IV administration.

Direct Intravenous Injection

The direct IV injection method (known as an *IV push*) involves the administration of the medication as a single dose into the vein over a short time, usually less than 10 minutes. It is usually administered through a vascular access device that is already in place. Medication administered through this method produces immediate and predictable results and is a good way to administer lifesaving medications in an emergency.

Intermittent Intravenous Administration

Intermittent IV administration is employed frequently in outpatient settings. It involves the administration of a medication over a specific length of time (termed the *rate of infusion*) and at specified intervals. Before it is administered, the medication first must be diluted in a moderate amount of an IV fluid (25 to 250 ml). The amount and type of IV fluid are indicated in the drug insert accompanying the medication. The intermittent IV administration of ceftriaxone (Rocephin) (an antibiotic) requires that it first be reconstituted and then diluted in 50 to 100 ml of an IV fluid, such as sterile water or 0.9% sodium chloride.

The rate of infusion for administering an IV medication intermittently depends on the medication being administered and typically ranges from 15 minutes to several hours. This information also is specified in the drug insert accompanying the medication. The recommended rate for the intermittent infusion of ceftriaxone is 15 to 30 minutes. The recommended rate of infusion for IV infliximab is at least 2 hours.

The interval of time between doses is determined by the physician and depends on the medication being administered and the patient's condition. The physician may prescribe the following outpatient treatment plan for a patient with Lyme disease: IV ceftriaxone intermittently once a day for 14 days. In this instance, the interval of time between doses is 24 hours, or 1 day.

Continuous Intravenous Administration

Continuous IV administration, also known as an *IV drip*, is most often used in a hospital or home setting. It involves the infusion of medication over a continuous period of time (4 to 24 hours). Continuous IV administration is used to maintain a constant therapeutic blood level of the medication. The medication is diluted in a large quantity (250 to 1000 ml) of an IV fluid (Figure 11-32), such as 0.9% sodium chloride (normal saline) or 5% dextrose in water

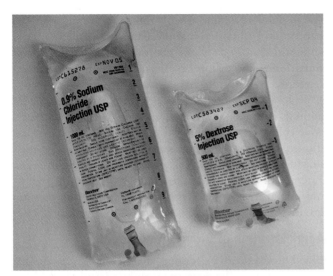

Figure 11-32. IV fluid bags.

(D5W). Because of the time required for continuous administration, this method of administration generally is not used to administer IV medications in the medical office.

Intravenous Medications Administered in an Outpatient Setting

Medications that are most commonly administered intravenously in an outpatient setting are listed next, along with the conditions each is used to treat.

Antibiotics

The physician may prescribe IV antibiotic therapy to treat a serious infection to prevent the infection from spreading and to avoid the development of serious complications. The IV route allows the antibiotic to achieve high blood concentrations quickly, permitting it to go to work on the infection immediately.

Examples of infections for which the physician may prescribe IV antibiotic therapy in an outpatient setting include osteomyelitis, cellulitis endocarditis, bacterial meningitis, Lyme disease, bacterial pneumonia, bacterial septicemia, pyelonephritis, pelvic inflammatory disease, acquired immunodeficiency syndrome (AIDS)-related infections, severe urinary tract infections, and nonhealing wound infections.

Chemotherapy

Chemotherapy is broadly defined as the use of chemicals to treat disease. More specifically, chemotherapy refers to the use of antineoplastic medications to treat different types of cancer. In most cases, chemotherapy works by interfering with the ability of cancer cells to grow or reproduce. The IV route is commonly used to administer chemotherapy because most antineoplastic medications are toxic and irritating and must be delivered to the body through a vein. These types of medications cause pain and trauma to the tissues if administered by other parenteral routes (i.e., IM or SC).

IV chemotherapy may take only a few minutes or several hours to administer and may be given on a daily, weekly, or monthly basis. The frequency and length of the chemotherapy treatment depend on the type of cancer being treated, the medications that are being administered, and the patient's overall health and ability to tolerate the medications. IV chemotherapy is often administered in an outpatient setting, such as a medical oncology office or an infusion clinic.

Monoclonal Antibodies

One use of monoclonal antibodies is to treat inflammatory diseases; infliximab (Remicade) is a monoclonal antibody. Individuals with certain inflammatory diseases have too much of a normally occurring protein (tumor necrosis factor [TNF]) in their bodies. TNF causes inflammation in the body, but in too large amounts, it attacks healthy tissues. Infliximab works by binding with TNF and blocking its action, reducing the inflammatory response of the body. In doing so, however, infliximab also lowers the ability of the body to fight infection.

IV infliximab therapy is often administered in an outpatient setting for treatment of the following conditions: Crohn's disease, rheumatoid arthritis, ulcerative colitis, ankylosing spondylitis, and psoriatic arthritis. Infliximab works to reduce the symptoms of the patient's condition and to initiate and maintain remission of the disorder. However, infliximab has some undesirable side effects and is very expensive. Because of this, it is administered only when patients with these conditions have had an inadequate response to conventional therapy.

Analgesics

When a patient is not able to manage pain using oral pain medication, the physician may prescribe a narcotic pain medication administered through the IV route. Conditions for which the physician may prescribe IV analgesic therapy in an outpatient setting include migraine headache, cancer-related pain, and the pain associated with AIDS conditions.

Some patients receive IV narcotic analgesics at home through the use of an ambulatory IV pump (Figure 11-33) that is controlled by the patient. This type of IV analgesic therapy is known as *patient-controlled analgesia* (PCA). When the patient experiences pain, he or she presses a button attached to the PCA pump. The PCA pump is programmed to deliver a predetermined dose of the narcotic analgesic intravenously to the patient to relieve the pain. The pump is preset to prevent overmedication, and it includes a locking device for security of the medication.

Replacement of Fluids and Electrolytes

To remain healthy, the body must maintain an adequate fluid and electrolyte balance. This balance can be altered by a variety of conditions. Conditions that may cause a depletion of fluids and electrolytes include vomiting and diarrhea, excessive perspiration (from fever or hot weather), and starvation. If an individual experiences an excessive loss of fluids or electrolytes, they must be replaced as soon as possible to prevent dehydration. Infants and children are especially vulnerable to dehydration.

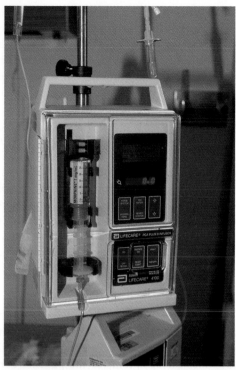

Figure 11-33. Patient-controlled anesthesia pump. (From Elkin MK, Perry AG, Potter PA: Nursing interventions and clinical skills, ed 3, St Louis, 2004, Mosby.)

The best way to replace fluids and electrolytes is through oral consumption; however, this may not always be possible, such as when the patient is experiencing excessive vomiting. In these instances, IV fluid therapy may be prescribed. The physician determines the specific IV fluid and amount of fluid to treat the patient's condition using the following information:

- Patient's diagnosis (e.g., prolonged diarrhea)
- Other coexisting medical conditions
- Length of the current illness
- Patient's body size and weight
- Physician's findings from the physical examination
- Laboratory test results

Examples of IV fluids commonly used to replace fluids and electrolytes include 0.9% sodium chloride and Ringer's solution. IV fluids are administered by continuous administration in the following outpatient settings: urgent care centers, infusion clinics, and the patient's home. Because of the length of time required for continuous administration, the medical office does not typically administer IV fluids and electrolytes except in an emergency situation (see later).

Administration of Nutritional Supplements

IV therapy can be used to administer nutritional supplements to patients in an outpatient setting who are unable to eat or have conditions causing poor absorption of nutrients from the gastrointestinal tract. IV nutritional therapy provides the nutrients necessary for basic health maintenance

and to promote healing. The IV route is used only when the patient has a condition that prevents use of other routes of administration, such as the oral or enteral routes. **Enteral nutrition** is the delivery of nutrients through a tube inserted into the gastrointestinal tract.

Examples of specific conditions that may require the IV administration of nutritional supplements include ulcerative colitis, Crohn's disease, short bowel syndrome, celiac disease, pancreatitis, esophageal cancer, AIDS-related malnutrition, and malnutrition related to an eating disorder. Parenteral IV nutrition is often administered in the following outpatient settings: infusion clinics and the patient's home.

Administration of Blood Products

Blood products can be administered to a patient in an outpatient setting. The most frequently administered blood products are discussed next.

Immune Globulin

Immune globulin consists of antibodies that must be given through the IV route of administration. Immune globulin is obtained from pooled human plasma that has been tested and found to be safe and free of bloodborne pathogens, such as HIV and the hepatitis viruses.

Intravenous immune globulin (IVIG) therapy is used to treat patients with immune deficiencies who are unable to produce their own antibodies, such as chronic inflammatory demyelinating polyneuropathy. It also is used in the treatment of a variety of autoimmune diseases, such as multiple sclerosis, myasthenia gravis, and lupus erythematosus. An **autoimmune disease** is a condition in which, for some unknown reason, the body's immune system attacks the body's own cells.

The IVIG dose is based on the patient's weight, and the medication is infused slowly over many hours. The number and frequency of treatments depend on the patient's condition. Patients who cannot produce their own antibodies usually receive an IVIG treatment once a month, whereas patients with autoimmune diseases may require a treatment to boost their immune system only when there is a flare-up of their condition.

Hemophilia Factors

Hemophilia is an inherited bleeding disorder characterized by deficiency of a clotting factor needed for proper coagulation of the blood. Without this factor, a hemophiliac may bleed spontaneously or after trauma to any tissues or organs of the body. The most common sites of bleeds are joints and muscles. The missing blood clotting factor must periodically be administered intravenously to an individual with hemophilia. If treatment is delayed, this can lead to irreversible damage to the affected tissues and even death. Many patients with hemophilia receive their intravenous clotting factors at home, making it more convenient and easier for them to manage their condition.

Emergency Administration of Intravenous Medication and Fluids

Having the capability to initiate an IV line is important in an emergency situation. It provides an access route for the IV administration of lifesaving medications and fluids. Emergency situations sometimes arise in the medical office. While waiting for emergency medical services to transport the patient to the hospital, an IV line may be established to administer medication and fluids to the patient as soon as possible. Situations occurring in the medical office that may benefit from establishing IV access include myocardial infarction, stroke, anaphylactic reaction, diabetic emergencies, and heat-related injuries such as heatstroke.

⊖volve *Check out the Evolve site to access additional interactive activities.*

MEDICAL PRACTICE *and the* LAW

Medications have the potential to do great good and great harm. Many lawsuits are medication related, so the medical assistant has a tremendous responsibility to follow all procedures to avoid doing harm.

Many patients are prescribed multiple medications from various physicians. When performing a medication evaluation, ask the patient to bring in all medications he or she is currently taking. Include over-the-counter medications such as aspirin, vitamins, and herbal products.

When administering medications, first check a current medication reference to determine potential adverse effects. See the *Physician's Desk Reference* or package insert for this information. This information also may be available on a computer program. Next check for patient allergies. Check the chart, then ask the patient about allergies before administering the medication. Be sure the patient knows why the drug is being given, its name, and common side effects. Watch the patient take the drug if given orally. If given parenterally, use proper technique to prevent injury. Follow the seven "rights" of medication administration, and check the medication label three times before administering any medication. This all may seem cumbersome, but if any steps are omitted and the patient has a serious adverse reaction, you could be held liable.

Controlled drugs have specific laws that regulate their ordering, storing, and dispensing. Failure to adhere to these regulations could cause the physician to lose his or her license. Be aware of drug-seeking behaviors of patients and physical symptoms of addiction. You also have a duty to be aware of coworkers' behavior and to report to the physician any individual who appears chemically impaired or whom you suspect of diverting medications for personal use. ∎

What Would You Do? What Would You *Not* Do? RESPONSES

Case Study 1
Page 420

What Did Theresa Do?

❑ Asked Mrs. Okasinski what pharmacy she uses. Called the pharmacy and asked them to fax a copy of her medications to the medical office. Used the information from the pharmacy and the Product Identification section of the PDR to identify Mrs. Okasinski's medications.

❑ Wrote the names of her medications in her chart for the physician to review.

❑ Explained to Mrs. Okasinski that when she has her prescriptions filled, she should request nonchildproof containers so that she will be able to use the original containers, which have the name and prescription information on them. This will make it easier to tell her medications apart.

❑ After the physician was finished with Mrs. Okasinski, made a list of all the medications she would be taking based on the physician's order. Went over each medication with Mrs. Okasinski, and gave her a copy of the medication list to keep as a reference.

What Did Theresa Not Do?

❑ Did not criticize Mrs. Okasinski for taking her medications out of their original containers.

What Would You Do?/What Would You *Not* Do? Review Theresa's response and place a checkmark next to the information you included in your response. List additional information you included in your response.

_____

_____

_____

Case Study 2
Page 448

What Did Theresa Do?

❑ Explained to Mrs. Cardwell that for the infection to be completely eliminated from Rachel's body, she needed to be given all of the medication.

❑ Stressed to Mrs. Cardwell that medication prescribed to one person should never be given to someone else because it might cause him or her to have a bad reaction.

❑ Explained to Mrs. Cardwell that if side effects of medication ever occur, it is important to call the medical office for information on what to do.

❑ Told Mrs. Cardwell that Rachel needs to be seen by the doctor again and scheduled an appointment for her. Asked if any other family members needed an appointment with the doctor.

Continued

What Did Theresa Not *Do?*

❑ Did not tell Mrs. Cardwell that she should have known better than to give Rachel's antibiotic to the other family members.

What Would You Do?/What Would You *Not* Do? Review Theresa's response and place a checkmark next to the information you included in your response. List additional information you included in your response.

_____
_____
_____
_____

Case Study 3
Page 461

What Did Theresa Do?

❑ Explained to Danielle that if the injection were given in her arm, it would not be absorbed very well and she might not get better.

❑ Explained to Danielle that injections are given to patients every day at the office and that Danielle does not need to be embarrassed.

❑ Told Danielle that she would be draped extra well and that it would only take a minute to give the injection.

What Did Theresa Not *Do?*

❑ Did not disregard Danielle's concerns.
❑ Did not give the injection in the deltoid.

What Would You Do?/What Would You *Not* Do? Review Theresa's response and place a checkmark next to the information you included in your response. List additional information you included in your response.

_____
_____
_____
_____

CERTIFICATION REVIEW

❑ **Pharmacology** is the study of drugs and includes the preparation, use, and action of drugs in the body. Medication that is *administered* is given to the patient at the office. Medication is *prescribed* when a physician provides the patient with a written prescription for a drug to be filled at a pharmacy. *Dispensed* medication is either given or sold to the patient at the office to be taken at home. Common routes of administration of medication are oral, sublingual, inhalation, rectal, vaginal, topical, intradermal, subcutaneous, intramuscular, and intravenous.

❑ **Drug package inserts** are included with each drug manufactured by a pharmaceutical company. The *Physician's Desk Reference* is a drug reference frequently used in the medical office to research information on prescription drugs. The U. S. Food and Drug Administration is responsible for determining the safety and effectiveness of drugs for human use.

❑ **Each drug has four names.** The chemical name of a drug provides a precise description of a drug's chemical composition. The generic name is assigned by the pharmaceutical manufacturer who first develops the drug. The official name is the name under which the drug is listed in official publications. The brand name is the name under which a pharmaceutical manufacturer markets a drug.

❑ **Three systems of measurement** are used in the United States for prescribing and administering medication: the metric system, the apothecary system, and the household system. The metric system is the most common system used to administer, prescribe, and dispense

medication because it is more exact and easier to use. Conversion is required when medication is ordered in one unit of measurement, and the medication label expresses the drug strength in a different unit.

❑ **Controlled drugs** are drugs that have potential for abuse. They are classified into five categories based on their abuse potential. To prescribe or dispense controlled drugs, the physician must register each year with the Drug Enforcement Agency (DEA). The physician is assigned a DEA number that must appear on the prescription of every controlled drug that he or she writes.

❑ **A prescription** is a physician's order authorizing the dispensing of a drug by a pharmacist. The prescription includes directions to the pharmacist for filling the prescription and instructions to the patient for taking the medication. Prescriptions can be authorized in different forms, including hand-written, computer-generated, and telephoned or faxed to a pharmacy.

❑ **The therapeutic effect** of a drug is its desired effect. Factors that affect the therapeutic action of drugs include age of the patient, route of administration, body size, time of administration, and tolerance to the drug.

❑ **Most drugs produce adverse reactions.** They may be harmless and tolerated to obtain the therapeutic effect of the drug. Some adverse reactions are harmful to some patients and warrant discontinuing the medication.

❑ **A patient can have an allergic reaction** to a drug after administration. The reaction is usually mild and may take the form of a rash, rhinitis, or pruritus. Occasionally, a severe allergic reaction occurs suddenly and immediately. This reaction is known as an *anaphylactic reaction.*

❏ **The seven "rights"** of preparing and administering medication in the medical office include the right drug, right dose, right time, right patient, right route, right technique, and right documentation.

❏ **The oral route** is the most convenient and most widely used method of administering medication. Absorption of most oral medication occurs in the small intestine, although some may be absorbed in the mouth and stomach.

❏ **The parenteral routes** of administration include subcutaneous, intramuscular, and intravenous. With parenteral administration, medications are absorbed more rapidly and completely. In some cases, such as when a patient is unconscious, the parenteral route is the only way a drug can be given.

❏ **A syringe** is used to insert fluids into the body. Various types of syringes are available to administer injections. The types used most often in the medical office are hypodermic, insulin, and tuberculin. Each needle has a certain gauge, which refers to the diameter of the lumen. As the size of the gauge increases, the diameter of the lumen decreases. Thick or oily preparations must be given with a large lumen because they are too thick to pass through a smaller one. The length of the needle ranges between $3/8$ inch and 3 inches; the length used is based on the type of injection being given and the size of the patient. Safety-engineered syringes incorporate a built-in safety feature to reduce the risk of a needlestick injury.

❏ **The most common dispensing units** for injectable medications include vials, ampules, and prefilled disposable syringes or cartridges that hold a single dose of medication.

❏ **A subcutaneous injection** is made into the subcutaneous tissue, which consists of adipose tissue. The needle length varies from $1/2$ to $5/8$ inch, and the gauge ranges from 23 G to 25 G. The amount of medication injected subcutaneously should not exceed 1 ml. More than this amount causes pain and discomfort to the patient.

❏ **Intramuscular injections** are made into the muscular layer of the body. An amount of up to 3 ml may be given intramuscularly. The length of the needle varies from 1 to 3 inches depending on the size of the patient, and the gauge ranges from 18 G to 23 G depending on the viscosity of the medication. Intramuscular injection sites include the following: dorsogluteal, deltoid, vastus lateralis, and ventrogluteal.

❏ **An intradermal injection** is given into the dermal layer of the skin. The size of the needle ranges from $3/8$ to $5/8$ inch, and the lumen ranges from 25 G to 27 G. The most frequent use of intradermal injections is to administer a skin test such as an allergy test or a tuberculin test (Mantoux test).

❏ **Tuberculosis** is an infectious bacterial disease that can occur in almost any part of the body but usually attacks the lungs. Tuberculosis affecting the lungs is known as pulmonary tuberculosis, whereas tuberculosis occurring in other parts of the body is known as extrapulmonary tuberculosis. The purpose of tuberculin testing is to detect the presence of a tuberculin infection. A positive reaction to a tuberculin test indicates the presence of a tuberculous infection; however, it does not differentiate between the active and latent forms of the infection. A positive reaction warrants additional diagnostic procedures before a final diagnosis can be made.

❏ **Allergy skin testing** determines the specific allergens that are causing the patient's allergic symptoms. Direct skin testing involves applying extracts of common allergens to the skin and observing the body's reaction to them. Direct skin testing includes patch testing, skin-prick testing, and intradermal skin testing. In vitro allergy blood testing is performed by an outside laboratory on a blood specimen and measures the amount of immunoglobulin (Ig)E antibodies in the blood that respond to common allergens. Examples of in vitro allergy blood tests include enzyme-linked immunosorbent assay (ELISA), radioallergosorbent testing (RAST), and ImmunoCAP.

❏ **Intravenous (IV) therapy** is the administration of a liquid agent directly into a patient's vein, where it is distributed throughout the body via the circulatory system. The veins most commonly used for IV therapy are the peripheral veins of the arm and hand. The liquid agent may consist of basic IV fluids, medication, nutrients, blood, or blood products. When IV fluids, medications, or nutrients are administered through the intravenous route, the technique is called an *infusion.* When whole blood or blood products are administered through the intravenous route, the procedure is called a *transfusion.*

❏ **IV therapy may be administered** in an outpatient setting for the following: administration of medication, replacement of fluids and electrolytes, administration of nutritional supplements, administration of blood products, and emergency administration of IV medication and IV fluids.

❏ **IV medication administration** is the process of delivering medication directly into a patient's vein. The IV route provides a rapid and effective method for administering medication to a patient. It also provides more accurate dosing than other routes because the medication enters the body directly from the circulatory system.

❏ **The direct IV injection method** (known as an *IV push*) involves the administration of the medication as a single

Continued

CERTIFICATION REVIEW—cont'd

dose into the vein over a short period of time, usually less than 10 minutes. It is usually administered through a vascular access device that is already in place. Medication administered through this method produces immediate and predictable results, and this method is a good way to administer lifesaving medications in an emergency.

❏ **Intermittent IV medication administration** is frequently employed in outpatient settings. It involves the IV administration of a medication over a specific length of time (termed the *rate of infusion*) and at specified intervals. Before being administered, the medica-

tion must first be diluted in a moderate amount of an IV fluid (25 to 250 ml).

❏ **Continuous IV administration,** also known as an *IV drip,* is most often used in a hospital or home setting. It involves the infusion of medication over a continuous period of time (4 to 24 hours). Continuous IV administration is used to maintain a constant therapeutic blood level of a medication. The medication is diluted in a large quantity (250 to 1000 ml) of an IV fluid (see Figure 11-28), such as 0.9% sodium chloride (known as *normal saline*) or 5% dextrose in water (known as *D5W*).

TERMINOLOGY REVIEW

Medical Term	Word Parts	Definition
Adverse reaction		An unintended and undesirable effect produced by a drug.
Allergen		A substance that is capable of causing an allergic reaction.
Allergy		An abnormal hypersensitivity of the body to substances that are ordinarily harmless.
Ampule		A small sealed glass container that holds a single dose of medication.
Anaphylactic reaction		A serious allergic reaction that requires immediate treatment.
Autoimmune disease	*auto-:* self	A condition in which the body's immune system produces antibodies that attack the body's own cells. The cause is unknown.
Chemotherapy	*chem/o-:* chemical *-therapy:* treatment	The use of chemicals to treat disease. Chemotherapy is most often used to refer to the treatment of cancer using antineoplastic medications.
Controlled drug		A drug that has restrictions placed on it by the federal government because of its potential for abuse.
Conversion		Changing from one system of measurement to another.
Cubic centimeter		The amount of space occupied by 1 milliliter (1 ml = 1 cc).
DEA number		A registration number assigned to physicians by the Drug Enforcement Administration for prescribing or dispensing controlled drugs.
Dose		The quantity of a drug to be administered at one time.
Drug		A chemical used for the treatment, prevention, or diagnosis of disease.
Enteral nutrition	*enter/o-:* intestines *-al:* pertaining to	The delivery of nutrients through a tube inserted into the gastrointestinal tract.
Gauge		The diameter of the lumen of a needle used to administer medication.
Hemophilia	*hem/o-:* blood *-philia:* love	An inherited bleeding disorder caused by a deficiency of a clotting factor needed for proper coagulation of the blood.
Immune globulin		A blood product consisting of pooled human plasma containing antibodies.
Induration		An abnormally raised, hardened area of the skin with clearly defined margins.
Infusion		The administration of fluids, medications, or nutrients into a vein.
Inhalation administration		The administration of medication by way of air or other vapor being drawn into the lungs.
Inscription		The part of a prescription that indicates the name of the drug and the drug dosage.

TERMINOLOGY REVIEW—cont'd

Medical Term	Word Parts	Definition
Intradermal injection	*intra-:* within *derm/o:* skin *-al:* pertaining to	Introduction of medication into the dermal layer of the skin.
Intramuscular injection	*intra-:* within *muscul/o:* muscle *-ar:* pertaining to	Introduction of medication into the muscular layer of the body.
Intravenous (IV) therapy	*intra-:* within *ven/o:* vein *-ous:* pertaining to	The administration of a liquid agent directly into a patient's vein, where it is distributed throughout the body by way of the circulatory system.
Oral administration		Administration of medication by mouth.
Parenteral		Administration of medication by injection.
Pharmacology	*pharmac/o-:* drugs *-ology:* study of	The study of drugs.
Prescription		A physician's order authorizing the dispensing of a drug by a pharmacist.
Signatura		The part of a prescription that indicates the information to print on the medication label.
Subcutaneous injection	*sub-:* under, below *cutane/o:* skin *-ous:* pertaining to	Introduction of medication beneath the skin, into the subcutaneous or fatty layer of the body.
Sublingual administration	*sub-:* under, below *lingu/o:* tongue *-al:* pertaining to	Administration of medication by placing it under the tongue, where it dissolves and is absorbed through the mucous membrane.
Subscription	*sub-:* under, below	The part of the prescription that gives directions to the pharmacist and usually designates the number of doses to be dispensed.
Superscription	*super-:* over, above	The part of a prescription consisting of the symbol Rx (from the Latin word recipe, meaning "take").
Topical administration		Application of a drug to a particular spot, usually for a local action.
Transfusion	*trans-:* through, across	The administration of whole blood or blood products through the intravenous route.
Vial		A closed glass container with a rubber stopper that holds medication.
Wheal		A tense, pale, raised area of the skin.

ON THE WEB

For Information on Pharmacology:

Food and Drug Administration: www.fda.gov

Drug Enforcement Administration: www.usdoj.gov/dea

RxList: The Internet Drug Index: www.rxlist.com

Drug Topics: www.drugtopics.com

Medline Plus: www.medlineplus.gov

Health Square: www.healthsquare.com

For Information on Alcohol and Drug Abuse:

Alcoholics Anonymous (AA): www.aa.org

National Institute on Alcohol Abuse and Alcoholism (NIAAA): www.niaaa.nih.gov

Continued

ON THE WEB—cont'd

National Council on Alcoholism and Drug Dependence (NCADD): www.ncadd.org

National Institute on Drug Abuse: www.nida.nih.gov

National Clearinghouse for Alcohol and Drug Information: http://ncadi.samhsa.gov

Substance Abuse and Mental Health Services Administration: www.samhsa.gov

Partnership for a Drug Free America: www.drugfree.org

Institute for a Drug-Free Workplace: www.drugfreeworkplace.org

Al-Anon/Alateen: www.al-anon.alateen.org

Mothers Against Drunk Driving (MADD): www.madd.org

For Information on Tuberculosis:

American Lung Association: www.lungusa.org

American Thoracic Society: www.thoracic.org

National Center for TB Prevention: www.cdc.gov/nchstp/tb

For Information on Allergies:

American Academy of Allergy, Asthma, and Immunology: www.aaaai.org

National Institute of Allergy and Infectious Diseases (NIAID): www3.niaid.nih.gov

Asthma and Allergy Foundation of America: www.aafa.org

12

Cardiopulmonary Procedures

Electrocardiography

1. Trace the path of the blood through the heart, starting with the right atrium.
2. Describe the heart's conduction system.
3. State the purpose of electrocardiography.
4. Identify each of the following components of the ECG cycle:
   - P wave
   - QRS complex
   - T wave
   - P-R segment
   - ST segment
   - P-R interval
   - Q-T interval
   - Baseline following the T wave
5. State the purpose of the standardization mark.
6. State the functions of the electrodes, amplifier, and galvanometer.
7. List the 12 leads that are included in an ECG.
8. Describe the function served by each of the following:
   - Three-channel recording
   - Teletransmission
   - Interpretive electrocardiography
   - EMR connectivity
9. Identify each of the following types of artifact, and state its causes:
   - Muscle
   - Wandering baseline
   - 60-cycle interference
   - Interrupted baseline

Record a 12-lead, three-channel ECG.

Holter Monitor Electrocardiography

1. List the reasons for applying a Holter monitor.
2. State the guidelines for wearing a Holter monitor.
3. Explain the use of the patient diary in Holter monitor electrocardiography.

Instruct a patient in the guidelines for wearing a Holter monitor.
Apply a Holter monitor.

Cardiac Dysrhythmias

1. Identify each of the following cardiac dysrhythmias, and explain its causes:
   - Premature atrial contraction
   - Paroxysmal atrial tachycardia
   - Atrial flutter
   - Atrial fibrillation
   - Premature ventricular contraction
   - Ventricular tachycardia
   - Ventricular fibrillation

Identify cardiac dysrhythmias on a 12-lead ECG.

Pulmonary Function Testing

1. List the different pulmonary function tests.
2. List indications for performing spirometry testing.
3. Describe each of the following: FVC, FEV_1, and FEV_1/FVC ratio.
4. Explain the difference between predicted values and measured values.
5. Describe patient preparation for spirometry.
6. Explain how to calibrate a spirometer.
7. Explain the purpose of post-bronchodilator spirometry.

Perform a spirometry test.

Peak Flow Measurement

1. Identify the symptoms of an asthma attack.
2. List examples of asthma triggers.
3. Explain the difference between long-term control and quick-relief asthma medications.
4. Describe the purpose of a peak flow meter.
5. State the purpose of peak flow measurements.

Measure a patient's peak flow rate.

Home Oxygen Therapy

1. Explain why oxygen is needed by the body.
2. Describe what occurs when the body cannot maintain an adequate blood oxygen level.
3. Identify the conditions that may require home oxygen therapy.
4. List and describe the information that is included on a prescription for home oxygen therapy.
5. List and describe the three common types of oxygen delivery systems along with the advantages and disadvantages of each.
6. List and describe the two types of devices used to administer home oxygen therapy.
7. State the usage and safety guidelines that should be followed by a patient on home oxygen therapy.

CHAPTER OUTLINE

Introduction to Electrocardiography
Structure of the Heart
Conduction System of the Heart
Cardiac Cycle
   Waves
   Baseline, Segments, and Intervals
Electrocardiograph Paper
Standardization of the Electrocardiograph
Electrocardiograph Leads
   Electrodes
   Bipolar Leads
   Augmented Leads
   Chest Leads
Paper Speed
Patient Preparation
Maintenance of the Electrocardiograph
Electrocardiographic Capabilities
   Three-Channel Recording Capability
   Teletransmission
   Interpretive Electrocardiograph
   EMR Connectivity
Artifacts
   Muscle Artifact
   Wandering Baseline Artifact

   60-Cycle Interference Artifact
   Interrupted Baseline Artifact
Holter Monitor Electrocardiography
   Purpose
   Digital Holter Monitor
   Patient Preparation
   Electrode Placement
   Patient Diary
   Event Marker
   Evaluating Results
   Maintenance of the Holter Monitor
Cardiac Dysrhythmias
   Premature Atrial Contraction
   Paroxysmal Atrial Tachycardia
   Atrial Flutter
   Atrial Fibrillation
   Premature Ventricular Contraction
   Ventricular Tachycardia
   Ventricular Fibrillation
Pulmonary Function Tests
   Spirometry
   Post-Bronchodilator Spirometry

KEY TERMS

amplitude (AM-pli-tood)
artifact (AR-tih-fakt)
atherosclerosis (ath-roe-skler-OH-sus)
baseline
cardiac cycle
dysrhythmia (dis-RITH-mee-ah)
ECG cycle
electrocardiogram (ee-LEK-troe-KAR-dee-oh-gram) (ECG)
electrocardiograph (ee-LEK-troe-KAR-dee-oh-graf)
electrode (ee-LEK-trode)
electrolyte (ee-LEK-troe-lite)
flow rate

hypoxemia
hypoxia
interval (IN-ter-val)
ischemia (is-KEEM-ee-ah)
normal sinus rhythm
oxygen therapy
peak flow rate
segment
spirometer (spih-ROM-ih-ter)
spirometry (spih-ROM-ih-tree)
wheezing

Introduction to Electrocardiography

The **electrocardiograph** is an instrument used to record the electrical activity of the heart. The **electrocardiogram (ECG)** is the graphic representation of this activity. The ECG exhibits the amount of electrical activity produced by the heart and the time required for the impulse to travel through the heart.

Cardiovascular disorders can cause abnormal changes to occur on the ECG. Because of this, electrocardiography is used for the following purposes:

- To evaluate the following symptoms: chest pain, shortness of breath, dizziness, or heart palpitations
- To detect an abnormality in the heart's rate or rhythm (**dysrhythmia**)
- To detect the presence of impaired blood flow to the heart muscle (**cardiac ischemia**)
- To help diagnose damage to the heart caused by a myocardial infarction
- To determine the presence of hypertrophy (enlargement) of the heart
- To detect inflammation of the heart muscle (**myocarditis**) or the lining of the heart (**pericarditis**)
- To assess the effect on the heart of digitalis and other cardiac drugs
- To determine the presence of electrolyte disturbances
- To assess the progress of rheumatic fever
- To detect congenital heart defects

- Performed before surgery to assess cardiac risk during surgery
- As part of a complete physical examination

A 12-lead resting ECG cannot detect all cardiovascular disorders nor can it always detect impending heart disease such as a myocardial infarction. An ECG is taken with the patient in a resting state and records only about 10 seconds of the heart's electrical activity. If a patient has a dysrhythmia that occurs intermittently, the abnormal heartbeat may not occur during this brief time period. A patient who experiences angina pectoris does not typically have symptoms while in a resting state (see *Patient Teaching: Angina Pectoris*), and an ECG run on such a patient may appear normal. Because of this, an ECG must be used in combination with the patient's symptoms, health history, physical examination, and other diagnostic and laboratory tests to obtain a complete assessment of cardiac functioning.

The medical assistant is frequently responsible for recording ECGs in the medical office. The medical assistant must acquire knowledge, and skill must be acquired in the following aspects of electrocardiography: preparation of the patient, operation of the electrocardiograph, identification and elimination of artifacts, and care and maintenance of the electrocardiograph.

Electrocardiographs are available in single-channel and three-channel recording formats. Because most medical offices use a three-channel ECG, the information in this chapter focuses on the three-channel electrocardiograph (Figure 12-1).

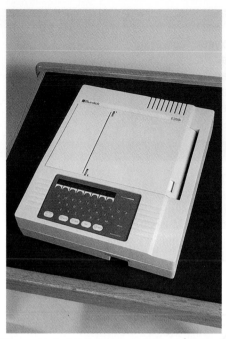

Figure 12-1. A three-channel electrocardiograph.

STRUCTURE OF THE HEART

The human heart consists of four chambers. The right and left atria are the small upper chambers of the heart, and the right and left ventricles are the large lower chambers (Figure 12-2). Blood enters the right atrium from two large veins—

the superior vena cava and the inferior vena cava—which bring it back from its circulation through the body. The blood entering the right atrium is deoxygenated, meaning it contains very little oxygen and is high in carbon dioxide.

From the right atrium, the blood enters the right ventricle. It is pumped from here to the lungs by way of the pulmonary artery. The blood picks up oxygen in the lungs in exchange for carbon dioxide and returns to the left atrium of the heart through the pulmonary veins. From the left atrium, the blood enters the left ventricle. This is the most muscular and powerful chamber of the heart and serves to pump blood to the entire body. Blood exits from the left ventricle through the aorta, which distributes it to all parts of the body to nourish the tissues with oxygen and nutrients. The coronary arteries consist of two small arteries that branch off the aorta and innervate the heart (Figure 12-3). These arteries have numerous branches, which supply the heart itself with oxygen and nutrients.

CONDUCTION SYSTEM OF THE HEART

The *sinoatrial (SA) node* is located in the upper portion of the right atrium, just below the opening of the superior vena cava. It consists of a knot of modified myocardial cells that have the ability to send out an electrical impulse without an external nerve stimulus. In this way, the SA node initiates and regulates the heartbeat and is often referred to as the "pacemaker" of the heart. In a normal individual, the SA node generates electrical impulses at a rate of 60 to 100 times per minute.

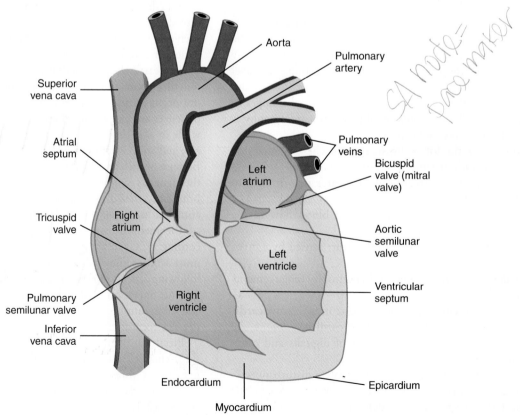

SA node = pacemaker

Figure 12-2. Diagram of the heart.

Putting It All into Practice

My Name is Janet Canterbury, and I work in the medical laboratory of an internal medicine office. I also run electrocardiograms, apply and remove Holter monitors, perform pulmonary function tests, and assist with cardiac stress testing.

One of my most rewarding experiences was when a young woman came into the office with severe chest pain. I immediately helped her back to an examining room. I ran an electrocardiogram, as ordered by the physician. After the physician read the electrocardiogram, he indicated the results did not look good and that the patient would have to be transported to the hospital. I went into the patient's room to comfort her. She asked me if she was going to have to go to the hospital. I replied, "Possibly." She immediately said, "No!" Then I began to explain to her how important it was to have more tests to make sure she would be alright. She finally agreed to go. After being taken to the hospital by an ambulance, she was later transferred to another hospital for a heart catheterization. A few weeks passed, and she came into the office. She hugged me and thanked me for possibly saving my life. It felt so good that I could help make a difference in a patient's life. ∎

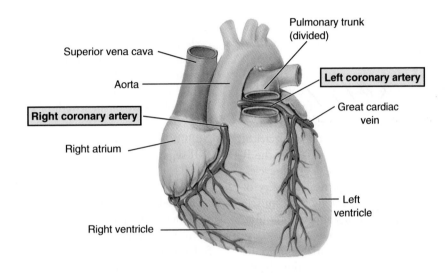

ANTERIOR

Figure 12-3. Coronary arteries. (From Applegate EJ: The anatomy and physiology of the learning system, ed 3, St Louis, 2006, Saunders.)

Each electrical impulse discharged by the SA node is distributed to the right and left atria and causes them to contract. This contraction forces blood through the open cuspid valves and into the ventricles. The impulse is picked up by the *atrioventricular (AV) node,* another knot of modified myocardial cells located at the base of the right atrium. The AV node delays the impulse momentarily to allow for complete contraction of the atria and filling of the ventricles with blood from the atria. The AV node then transmits the electrical impulse to the *bundle of His.* The bundle of His divides into right and left branches known as the *bundle branches,* which relay the impulse to the *Purkinje fibers.* The Purkinje fibers distribute the impulse evenly to the right and left ventricles, causing them to contract; this forces blood out of the right ventricle and into the pulmonary artery and out of the left ventricle into the aorta. Ejection of blood into the aorta causes the blood pressure and pulse to be produced. The entire heart then relaxes momentarily. The SA node initiates a new impulse, and the cycle repeats (Figure 12-4).

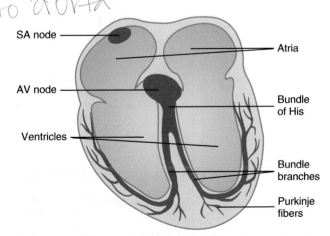

Figure 12-4. Diagram of the heart, identifying the structures involved with the conduction of an electrical impulse through the heart.

CARDIAC CYCLE

The **cardiac cycle** represents one complete heartbeat. It consists of the contraction of the atria, the contraction of the ventricles, and the relaxation of the entire heart (as described previously). The electrocardiograph records the electrical activity that causes these events in the cardiac cycle. The **ECG cycle** is the graphic representation of the cardiac cycle (Figure 12-5).

Waves

The normal ECG cycle consists of a P wave; the Q, R, and S waves (known as the *QRS complex*); and a T wave. The ECG cycle is recorded from left to right, beginning with the P wave.

P wave   The P wave represents the electrical activity associated with the contraction of the atria, or *atrial depolarization.*

QRS complex   The QRS complex represents the electrical activity associated with the contraction of the ventricles, or *ventricular depolarization,* and consists of the Q wave, the R wave, and the S wave. The ventricles are larger than the atria and therefore require a stronger electrical stimulus to depolarize the ventricles. That is why the R wave is taller than the P wave on the ECG graph cycle.

T wave   The T wave represents the electrical recovery of the ventricles, or *ventricular repolarization.* The muscle cells are recovering in preparation for another impulse. (*Note:* Electrical recovery, known as *atrial repolarization,* occurs following the P wave. This repolarization occurs at the same time as ventricular depolarization [QRS complex]. Because of this, atrial repolarization is masked

or hidden by the QRS complex and does not appear as a separate wave on the ECG cycle.)

U wave   Occasionally, a U wave follows a T wave. It is a small wave that is associated in some as yet undefined way with repolarization of the Purkinje fibers or repolarization of the papillary muscles of the heart.

Baseline, Segments, and Intervals

The flat, horizontal line that separates the various waves is known as the **baseline.** Following the U wave, the heart is at rest or *polarized.* Because no electrical activity is occurring in the heart during this time, the electrocardiograph does not have anything to record, which is why the baseline is flat.

The waves deflect either upward (positive deflection) or downward (negative deflection) from the baseline. The ECG cycle between the P wave and the T wave is divided into segments and intervals for the purpose of interpretation and analysis of the ECG by the physician. A **segment** is the portion of the ECG between two waves, and an **interval** is the length of a wave or the length of a wave with a segment.

Segments

P-R segment   The P-R segment represents the time interval from the end of the atrial depolarization to the beginning of the ventricular depolarization. It is the time needed for the impulse to be delayed at the AV node and then travel through the bundle of His and Purkinje fibers to the ventricles.

S-T segment   The S-T segment represents the time interval from the end of the ventricular depolarization to the beginning of repolarization of the ventricles.

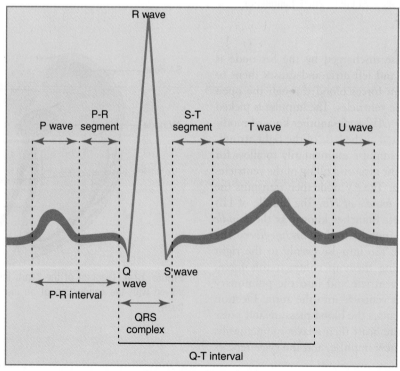

Figure 12-5. ECG cycle.

Intervals

P-R interval   The P-R interval represents the time interval from the beginning of the atrial depolarization to the beginning of the ventricular depolarization.

Q-T interval   The Q-T interval is the time interval from the beginning of the ventricular depolarization to the end of repolarization of the ventricles.

Baseline   The baseline after the T wave (or U wave, if present) represents the period when the entire heart returns to its resting, or polarized, state.

ELECTROCARDIOGRAPH PAPER

Electrocardiograph paper is divided into two sets of squares for the accurate and convenient manual measurement of the waves, intervals, and segments (Figure 12-6). Each small square is 1 mm high and 1 mm wide. Each large square (made up of 25 small squares) is 5 mm high and 5 mm wide. By manually measuring the various waves, intervals, and segments of the ECG graph cycle with ECG calipers or an ECG ruler, the physician is able to determine whether the electrical activity of the heart falls within normal limits. Heart disease can trigger abnormal changes in the ECG cycle, causing the results to fall outside of normal limits. For example, cardiac ischemia (often due to coronary artery disease) can cause a depressed S-T segment and an inverted T wave. A myocardial infarction can cause a larger than normal Q wave and an elevated S-T segment.

Electrocardiograph paper contains a thermosensitive coating. A black or red graph is printed on top of this coating. The electrocardiograph uses a thermal print head to produce the ECG tracing. The print head has the ability to generate heat in a prescribed pattern. When the thermosensitive paper comes in contact with the heated print head, the coating turns black in the areas where it is heated, producing the ECG tracing. In addition to being heat-sensitive, ECG paper is pressure sensitive and should be handled carefully to avoid making impressions that would interfere with proper reading of the ECG.

STANDARDIZATION OF THE ELECTROCARDIOGRAPH

The electrocardiograph machine must be standardized, or calibrated, when an ECG is recorded. This is a quality control measure that ensures an accurate and reliable recording. It also means that an ECG run on one electrocardiograph compares in accuracy with a recording run on another machine. An ECG run on a properly calibrated electrocardiograph results in an accurate and reliable representation of the electrical activity of the patient's heart.

By international agreement, 1 millivolt (mV) of electricity should cause the stylus to move 10 mm high in **amplitude** (10 small squares). During the recording, the machine allows 1 mV to enter the electrocardiograph machine, which should result in an upward deflection of 10 mm. The marking that occurs on the ECG paper is known as a *standardization mark* (Figure 12-7). The width of the mark made by the machine is approximately 2 mm (two small squares). A three-channel electrocardiograph automatically records standardization marks on the ECG; a standardiza-

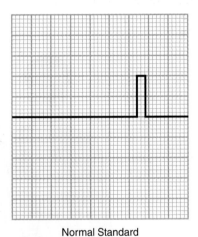

Normal Standard
Standardization mark is
10 mm high

Figure 12-7. Standardization mark.

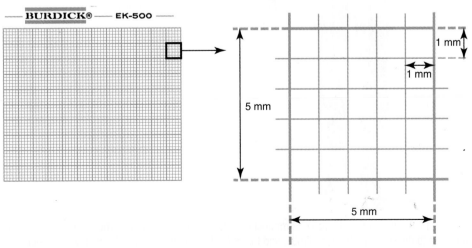

Figure 12-6. Diagram of ECG paper with a section enlarged to indicate the sizes of the large and small squares.

tion mark is recorded at the beginning and end of each of the ECG strips included in the three-channel recording (see Figure 12-12). If the standardization mark is more or less than 10 mm in amplitude, it must be adjusted; otherwise, the ECG recording may not be accurate. The manufacturer's operating manual must be consulted for proper adjustment information. An electrocardiograph must never be adjusted without use of the operating manual.

ELECTROCARDIOGRAPH LEADS

The standard ECG consists of 12 leads. A *lead* is a tracing of the electrical activity of the heart between two electrodes. Each lead provides an electrical "photograph" of the heart's activity from a different angle. Together, the 12 leads, or "photographs," facilitate a thorough interpretation of the heart's activity.

The electrical impulses given off by the heart are picked up by **electrodes** and conducted into the machine through lead wires. Electrodes are composed of a substance that is a good conductor of electricity. The electrical impulses given off by the heart are very small (0.0001 to 0.003 volt). To produce a readable ECG, they must be made larger, or amplified, by a device known as an *amplifier*, located within the electrocardiograph. The amplified voltages are changed into mechanical motion by the *galvanometer* and recorded on the electrocardiograph paper by a thermal print head (Figure 12-8).

Ten lead wires are attached to the patient and are used to take the 12 electrical "photographs" of the heart. There are four limb lead wires: the right arm lead wire (RA), the left arm lead wire (LA), the right leg lead wire (RL), and the left leg lead wire (LL). The right leg lead wire is known as the *ground*. It is not used for the actual recording, but serves as an electrical reference point. The chest lead wires are abbreviated with a "V" and use six chest lead wires.

Electrodes

Disposable electrodes are used to record a resting 12-lead electrocardiogram. The electrode contains a thin layer of a metallic substance; this metallic substance is a good conductor of electricity. The electrode is square in shape and has a tab extending from one end (Figure 12-9, *A*). The tab allows for the firm attachment of an alligator clip (Figure 12-9, *B*).

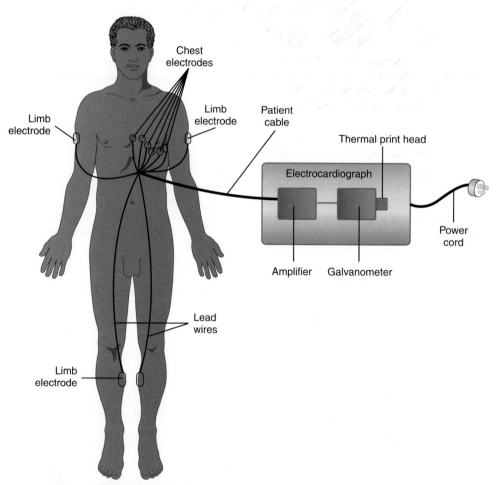

Figure 12-8. Diagram of the basic components of the electrocardiograph. The limb electrodes are attached to the fleshy parts of the limbs, and the lead wires are arranged to follow body contour. The patient cable is not dangling, and the power cord points away from the electrocardiograph.

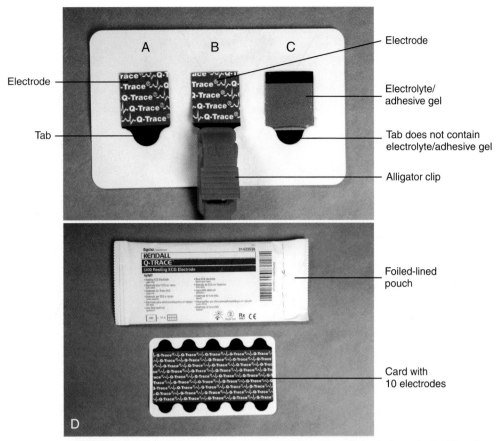

Figure 12-9. Resting 12-lead ECG electrodes. **A,** Disposable resting 12-lead electrode. **B,** The tab allows for attachment of the alligator clip. **C,** The back of the electrode contains an electrolyte gel combined with an adhesive. **D,** Disposable 12-lead electrodes are packaged in a foil-lined pouch and come on a card that contains 10 electrodes.

The back of the electrode contains an electrolyte gel combined with an adhesive (Figure 12-9, *C*). An **electrolyte** is a substance that facilitates the transmission of the heart's electrical impulse. Skin is a poor conductor of electricity; therefore, an electrolyte must be used when recording an ECG. The adhesive allows for firm adherence of the electrode to the patient's skin. There is no adhesive on the tab of the electrode to allow for attachment of the alligator clip. The electrode is applied to the skin and held in place with its adhesive backing; it is thrown away after use.

Disposable 12-lead electrodes come on a card containing 10 electrodes (Figure 12-9, *D*). A foil-lined pouch is used to hold ten cards of electrodes (or 100 electrodes per pouch). The foil-lined pouch preserves moisture to prevent the electrolyte from drying out.

Each electrode pouch (and the box containing the pouches) is stamped with an expiration date. The medical assistant must always check the expiration date of the electrodes before applying them. The electrolyte gel on outdated electrodes may be dried out; a dried out electrolyte is unable to transmit a good ECG signal.

Electrodes are sensitive to environmental conditions and must be stored properly to prevent electrolyte drying. Electrodes should be stored in a cool area (less than 75° F or 24° C) away from sources of heat. When an electrode pouch is opened, the medical assistant should seal the pouch by folding over the end of it and then place the pouch (containing the remaining electrode cards) in a zip-lock plastic bag to preserve moisture.

Bipolar Leads

The first three leads of the 12-lead ECG are the bipolar leads; they are leads I, II, and III. The bipolar leads use two of the limb electrodes to record the heart's electrical activity. Lead I records the electrical current traveling between the right arm and the left arm, lead II records the electrical current traveling between the right arm and the left leg, and lead III records the electrical current traveling between the left arm and the left leg (Figure 12-10).

Lead II shows the heart's rhythm more clearly than the other leads. Because of this, the physician often requests a *rhythm strip*, which is a longer recording (approximately 12 inches) of lead II (see Figure 12-12).

Augmented Leads

The next three leads are the augmented leads: aVR (augmented voltage—right arm), aVL (augmented voltage—left arm), and aVF (augmented voltage—left leg or foot). Lead

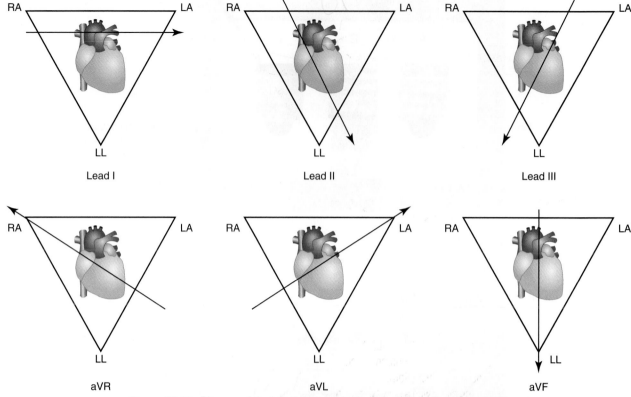

Figure 12-10. Diagram of the heart's voltage for leads I, II, III, aVR, aVL, and aVF.

Highlight on Cardiac Stress Testing

Description

A cardiac stress test (also known as an *exercise tolerance test* or *exercise ECG*) is a diagnostic procedure used to evaluate the cardiovascular health of individuals with known heart disease and individuals at high risk for developing heart disease, particularly coronary artery disease (CAD). Cardiac stress testing is usually performed in a hospital under the direction of a cardiologist and a cardiac technician so that emergency equipment and trained personnel are available to deal with any unusual situations that might arise. (**NOTE:** A *nuclear cardiac stress test* is a type of stress test that employs the use of a radioactive material injected through an IV and is described in Chapter 14.)

Purpose

The purpose of cardiac stress testing is as follows:

1. To evaluate symptoms of ischemic heart disease that cannot be assessed by a resting electrocardiogram. Ischemic heart disease occurs as a result of inadequate blood supply to the myocardium, which is most commonly caused by atherosclerosis. **Atherosclerosis** is a condition in which fibrous plaques of fatty deposits and cholesterol build up on the inner walls of arteries. This causes narrowing and partial blockage of the lumen of these arteries, along with hardening of the arterial wall. Atherosclerosis in the coronary arteries is called *coronary artery disease (CAD)*. During rest, the myocardium supplied by the partially blocked artery may receive an adequate blood supply. If the individual exercises, however, the artery may not be able to supply enough blood to the myocardium, resulting in myocardial ischemia. Myocardial ischemia can cause chest discomfort and certain abnormal changes on the ECG (see *Patient Teaching: Angina Pectoris*).

2. To assist in evaluating symptoms indicating the presence of cardiac dysrhythmias.

3. To assess the effectiveness of cardiac drug therapy.

4. To follow the course of rehabilitation after a myocardial infarction or a cardiac surgical procedure, such as a coronary bypass operation or a coronary stent placement.

5. To determine an individual's fitness level for a strenuous exercise program, such as jogging.

Patient Preparation

Patient preparation for a cardiac stress test includes the following:

1. Refrain from smoking for 4 hours before the test.

2. Avoid strenuous physical activities for 8 to 12 hours before the test.

3. Do not consume alcohol or food and beverages containing caffeine for 12 hours before the test. These substances may interfere with obtaining accurate results.

Highlight on Cardiac Stress Testing—cont'd

4. Do not eat or drink anything except water for 4 hours before the test. This reduces the likelihood of nausea that may accompany strenuous activity after a meal.
5. Certain cardiac medications may need to be discontinued 1 to 2 days before the test; this determination is made by the physician.
6. Wear loose, comfortable clothing and sports shoes suitable for exercising.

How the Test Works

- Cardiac stress testing involves the continuous electrocardiographic monitoring of an individual during physical exercise. During exercise, the body's need for oxygen places added demands or "stress" on the heart, making it work harder. A cardiac stress test evaluates the response of the heart to maximum or near-maximum exertion.
- A resting 12-lead ECG is usually performed before a cardiac stress test, and the results of the resting ECG are compared with the results of the cardiac stress test.
- The stress test is accomplished by having the patient use a treadmill while connected to an electrocardiograph machine through lead wires and electrodes (see illustration).
- The intensity of the physical exertion starts with a slow "warm-up" walk on the treadmill. The speed and incline of the treadmill are gradually increased every 3 minutes until the patient's target heart rate is reached. During this time, the ECG is continuously displayed on a computer screen. The patient's blood pressure, heart rate, and physical symptoms are also monitored during the test.
- If the signs and symptoms of cardiac ischemia appear, the test is stopped. These symptoms include severe dyspnea, chest discomfort or pain, pallor, weakness, and dizziness. The test is also stopped if the ECG shows abnormal changes, if a serious, irregular heartbeat occurs, or if there is an abnormal change in blood pressure.
- Once the exercising is complete, the patient's blood pressure, heart rate, and ECG are monitored until they return to normal.

Interpretation of Results

The patient's response to the cardiac stress test is used to determine normal or abnormal results. A normal response is a gradual increase in the patient's blood pressure as physical exertion increases, whereas an abnormal response is a sudden increase or decrease in the patient's blood pressure. The electrocardiogram of a normal individual undergoing exercise exhibits a shortened P-R interval and a compressed QRS complex. An abnormal tracing indicative of myocardial ischemia results in a depressed S-T segment and an inverted T wave. An abnormal cardiac stress test usually warrants further testing, such as coronary angiography, to assess the extent and severity of the heart disease. ■

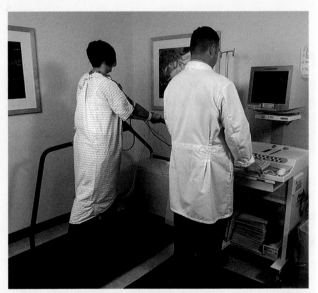

Cardiac treadmill stress test. (From deWit SC: Medical-surgical nursing: concepts and practice, St Louis, 2008, Saunders.)

---

aVR records the electrical current traveling between the right arm electrode and a central point between the left arm and left leg. Lead aVL records the electrical current traveling between the left arm electrode and a central point between the right arm and left leg. Lead aVF records the electrical current traveling between the left leg electrode and a central point between the right and left arms. Leads I, II, III, aVR, aVL, and aVF provide an electrical "photograph" of the heart's activity from side to side and from the top to the bottom of the heart (see Figure 12-9).

Chest Leads

The last six leads are the chest, or precordial, leads: V_1, V_2, V_3, V_4, V_5, and V_6. These leads record the heart's voltage from front to back. The electrical current traveling through the heart is recorded from a central point "inside" the heart to a point on the chest wall where the electrode is placed. These points correspond to the chest electrode placement sites. Figure 12-11 shows the proper location of the electrodes for the six chest leads. To ensure an accurate and reliable recording, the medical assistant must be able to locate these electrode placement sites accurately (by palpating the patient's chest). For example, if V_1 and V_2 are placed in the third intercostal spaces (instead of the fourth intercostal spaces), changes can occur to the P and T waves, which can falsely indicate heart disease. When first learning to locate the electrode sites for each chest lead, it helps to mark their locations on the patient's chest with a felt-tipped pen.

What Would You Do? What Would You *Not* Do?

Case Study 1

Camilla Rossi is 22 years old and works at a Waffle House during the day and goes to business school at night. She comes to the office because she has been experiencing some heart problems. Over the past month, she has had three episodes of tachycardia, palpitations, trouble breathing, and profuse sweating. She is really scared that she has heart disease. Her grandfather just died from a heart attack, and she is afraid she will die next. The physician orders an ECG, but Camilla is reluctant to have the procedure. She is embarrassed about having to disrobe from the waist up, and she is worried that she will get shocked by all the wires coming out of the machine. She says that she does not have health insurance, and she does not know how she would pay for such a fancy test. She wants to know whether there is a less expensive way to find out what is wrong with her. ■

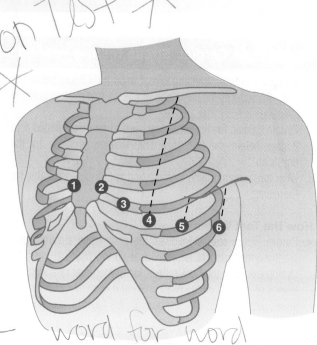

Figure 12-11. Recommended positions for ECG chest electrodes:
1. V_1, fourth intercostal space at right margin of sternum
2. V_2, fourth intercostal space at left margin of sternum
3. V_3, midway between positions 2 and 4
4. V_4, fifth intercostal space at junction of left midclavicular line
5. V_5, at horizontal level of position 4 at left anterior axillary line
6. V_6, at horizontal level of position 4 at left midaxillary line

PAPER SPEED

Normally, the ECG is recorded with the paper moving at a speed of 25 mm/sec. Occasionally, the ECG cycles are close together, making the recording difficult to read. The medical assistant can change the paper speed to 50 mm/sec to spread out the cycles. To alert the physician to the change, the medical assistant must make a notation of it on the recording.

PATIENT PREPARATION

Minimal preparation is required for an ECG. The medical assistant should instruct the patient in the following guidelines, which facilitate placement of the electrodes and ensure good adhesion of the electrodes to the patient's skin.

1. Do not apply body lotion, oil, or powder on the day of the test. This may make it more difficult to apply the electrodes.
2. Wear comfortable clothing and a shirt or blouse that can be removed easily.
3. Women should not wear full-length hosiery, such as panty hose or tights.

MAINTENANCE OF THE ELECTROCARDIOGRAPH

Electrocardiographs require periodic maintenance. The casing of the electrocardiograph should be cleaned frequently with a soft cloth, slightly dampened with a mild detergent, to remove dust and dirt. Commercial solvents and abrasives should not be used because they can damage the finish of the casing.

The patient's cables, lead wires, and power cord should be cleaned periodically with a cloth moistened with a disinfectant cleaner. The cables should never be immersed in the cleaning solution because this could damage them.

Inspect the cables frequently for cracks or fraying, and replace them if needed. Check the metal tip of each lead wire for adhesive/electrolyte gel residue, which can interfere with the transmission of a good ECG signal from the electrode. Remove any residue with an alcohol wipe using pressure and friction.

The reusable alligator clips should be cleaned thoroughly with an alcohol wipe after patient use. Check the alligator clips periodically to make sure they fit snugly on the metal tip of each lead wire.

ELECTROCARDIOGRAPHIC CAPABILITIES

Electrocardiographs have a variety of capabilities that permit specific recording and transmittal options.

Three-Channel Recording Capability

An electrocardiograph with a three-channel recording capability can record the electrical activity of the heart through three leads simultaneously. This is in contrast to a single-channel electrocardiograph, which records only one lead at a time. The advantage of a three-channel electrocardiograph is that an ECG can be produced in less time than would be required if each lead were recorded separately.

The leads that are recorded simultaneously are leads I, II, and III; followed by aVR, aVL, and aVF; followed by V_1,

V₂, and V₃; followed by V₄, V₅, and V₆. Each lead is automatically labeled by the electrocardiograph with its appropriate abbreviation.

Recording three leads at one time requires three-channel recording paper, which is designed in a standard 8½ × 11-inch format. This size printout fits easily into a paper-based medical record (PPR). Most three-channel electrocardiographs have a *copy capability* that quickly produces a duplicate copy of an ECG that has just been recorded. Some three-channel electrocardiographs have a memory storage capability in which a specified number of ECGs can be stored in the machine for later retrieval. In this way, an ECG that has been misplaced can be retrieved from the electrocardiograph's memory and printed out again. Figure 12-12 is an example of a three-channel ECG recording that also includes a rhythm strip. Procedure 12-1 describes how to run a 12-lead three-channel ECG.

Teletransmission

An electrocardiograph with teletransmission capabilities can transmit a recording performed at the medical office electronically (by telfax, modem, Ethernet, or wirelessly) to an ECG data interpretation site. The recording is interpreted by a cardiologist (often along with a computer analysis) at the interpretation site, and the ECG recording, along with its interpretation, is electronically transmitted to the sending office the same day. Patient information (e.g., age, sex, height, weight, medications) must be relayed to the ECG site to assist in the interpretation. This information is entered into the electrocardiograph by the medical assistant (using a keyboard) and is transmitted automatically with the ECG recording.

Interpretive Electrocardiograph

An electrocardiograph with interpretive capabilities has a built-in computer program that analyzes the recording as it is being run. Interpretive electrocardiographs provide immediate information on the heart's activity, leading to earlier diagnosis and treatment. Patient data are used in the interpretation of the ECG and must be entered into the electrocardiograph using a keyboard before running the recording. The data generally required are the patient's age, sex, height, weight, and medications, which are presented at the top of the recording. The computer analysis of the ECG

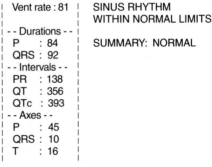

```
Name : Jane Doe
ID   : 34
Date : 04/06/73      Time : 11:37
Age  : 20            Sex  : Female
Hgt  : 64 IN         Wgt  : 130 LBS
Med1 :
Med2 :
Ccl1 :
Ccl2 :
Cmnt :
```

```
| Vent rate : 81  |    SINUS RHYTHM
|                 |    WITHIN NORMAL LIMITS
|- - Durations - -|
| P   : 84        |    SUMMARY: NORMAL
| QRS : 92        |
|- - Intervals - -|
| PR  : 138       |
| QT  : 356       |
| QTc : 393       |
|- - Axes - -     |
| P   : 45        |
| QRS : 10        |
| T   : 16        |
```

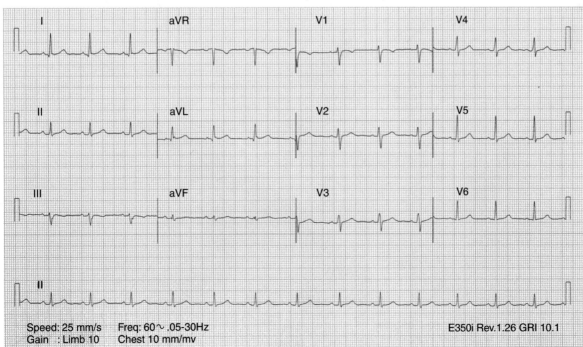

Speed: 25 mm/s   Freq: 60〜 .05-30Hz   E350i Rev.1.26 GRI 10.1
Gain : Limb 10   Chest 10 mm/mv

Figure 12-12. A three-channel ECG with a rhythm strip.

is also printed at the top of the recording, along with the reason for each interpretation (Figure 12-13). The results are reviewed and interpreted further by the physician before a diagnosis is made and treatment is initiated.

EMR Connectivity

EMR (electronic medical record) connectivity allows the electrocardiograph machine to be linked with the office's computer system, either wirelessly or through a USB port. This enables a digital image of the recording to be sent from the electrocardiograph machine to the computer. EMR software can display the digital image of the ECG on the screen of the computer. The software also analyzes the ECG and displays this information along with the reason for each interpretation. If needed, a copy of the ECG report can be printed out on a regular sheet of paper using an ink-jet or laser printer. The ECG report is reviewed and interpreted further by the physician before a diagnosis is made and treatment is initiated. The ECG report is then stored electronically in the patient's EMR.

ARTIFACTS

The medical assistant is responsible for producing a clear and concise ECG recording that can be read and interpreted by both a computer and the physician. Structures sometimes appear in the recording that are not natural and interfere with the normal appearance of the ECG cycles. They are known as **artifacts** and represent additional electrical activity that is picked up by the electrocardiograph. The presence of artifacts affects the quality of the recording, making it difficult to manually measure the ECG cycles. Artifacts can also sometimes cause a false-positive result on an ECG that is analyzed by a computer. The medical assistant should be able to identify artifacts and correct them. There are several types of artifacts; the most common are muscle, wandering baseline, and 60-cycle interference (also known as AC artifacts).

In some circumstances, as when individuals have trouble holding still or in buildings with older electrical systems, normal methods to eliminate muscle and 60-cycle interference artifacts may be unsuccessful. Electrocardiographs

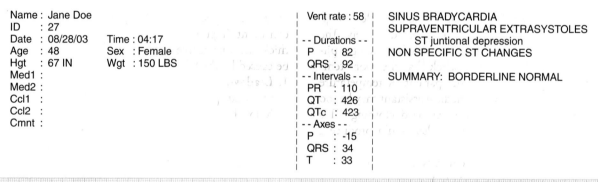

```
Name : Jane Doe
ID   : 27
Date : 08/28/03      Time : 04:17
Age  : 48            Sex  : Female
Hgt  : 67 IN         Wgt  : 150 LBS
Med1 :
Med2 :
Ccl1 :
Ccl2 :
Cmnt :
```

```
Vent rate : 58
- - Durations - -
P    : 82
QRS  : 92
- - Intervals - -
PR   : 110
QT   : 426
QTc  : 423
- - Axes - -
P    : -15
QRS  : 34
T    : 33
```

SINUS BRADYCARDIA
SUPRAVENTRICULAR EXTRASYSTOLES
  ST juntional depression
NON SPECIFIC ST CHANGES

SUMMARY: BORDERLINE NORMAL

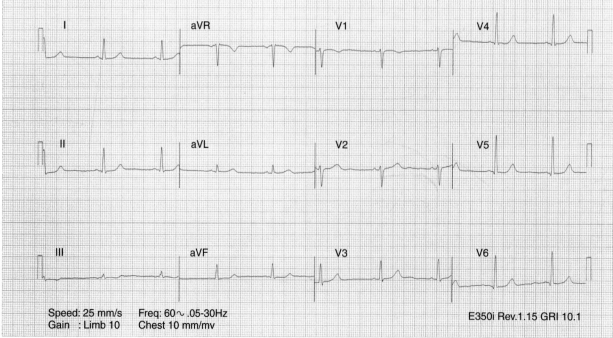

Speed: 25 mm/s   Freq: 60∿ .05-30Hz   E350i Rev.1.15 GRI 10.1
Gain : Limb 10   Chest 10 mm/mv

Figure 12-13. An ECG recording that has been analyzed by an interpretive electrocardiograph. The computer analysis is printed at the top of the recording, along with the reason for each interpretation.

have an artifact filter that can reduce artifacts when all else fails. Because the *artifact filter* also affects the diagnostic accuracy of the ECG, it should be used as little as possible.

If the medical assistant is unable to correct an artifact, the physician should be consulted. It is possible that the machine is broken. If an electrocardiograph service technician has to be contacted, the medical assistant should have the following information available to aid the service technician in locating the problem:

1. What already has been done to locate and correct the problem
2. Leads in which the artifact occurs
3. A sample of the artifact recorded by the machine

Muscle Artifact

A muscle artifact (Figure 12-14, *A*) can be identified by its fuzzy, irregular baseline. There are two types of muscle artifacts: those caused by involuntary muscle movement (somatic tremor) and those caused by voluntary muscle movement. Muscle artifacts may be caused by the following:

1. **An apprehensive patient.** To reduce the patient's apprehension and relax muscles, explain the procedure and reassure the patient that having an ECG recorded is a painless procedure.
2. **Patient discomfort.** Ensure that the table is wide enough to support the patient's arms and legs adequately. The patient can be made more comfortable by placing a pillow under his or her head. Check that the room temperature is comfortable for the patient. A temperature that is warm enough for the medical assistant may be too cold for the patient who has removed clothing. This could result in shivering, which also would produce a muscle artifact on the ECG.
3. **Patient movement.** The patient must be instructed to lie still and not talk during the recording.
4. **A physical condition.** Several nervous system disorders, such as Parkinson's disease, prevent relaxation, and the patient trembles continually. For these individuals, it is difficult to obtain an ECG that is free of artifacts. The artifacts can be reduced, however, by asking the patient to place his or her hands under the buttocks with the palms facing downward.

Wandering Baseline Artifact

A wandering baseline artifact (Figure 12-14, *B*) can be caused by the following:

1. **Loose electrodes.** The medical assistant should ensure that the electrodes are attached firmly to the patient's skin. A loose electrode results in poor transmission of the electrical impulse from the patient's skin to the electrode. If an electrode pulls loose, it can be reattached with hypoallergenic tape or replaced with a new electrode. The alligator clips should be attached firmly to the tabs of the electrodes. To prevent pulling of the lead wires on the electrodes, the patient cable should be well supported on the table or the patient's abdomen and should not be allowed to dangle. Pulling on the electrodes can cause the electrodes to pull away from the patient's skin.

2. **Dried-out electrolyte.** If the electrolyte gel on an electrode is dried out, the medical assistant must replace it with a new electrode. Always check the expiration date stamped on the electrode pouch (or box) to make sure the electrodes are within their expiration date.
3. **Body creams, oils, or lotions** on the skin in the area where the electrode is applied. This prevents good adhesion of the electrodes to the patient's skin. The medical assistant should remove these by rubbing with alcohol, using friction.
4. **Excessive movement of the chest wall during respiration.** The medical assistant should encourage the patient to relax and breathe more calmly, using the diaphragm rather than expanding the chest.

60-Cycle Interference Artifact

A 60-cycle interference artifact (also known as an AC artifact) is caused by electrical interference. Electric current can "leak" or spread out from the power used by electrical appliances in the room in which the ECG is being run. This current may be picked up by the patient and carried into the electrocardiograph, where it would show up on the ECG recording as a 60-cycle interference artifact. This type of artifact appears as small, straight, spiked lines that are consistent (Figure 12-14, *C*), causing the baseline to be thick and unreadable. A 60-cycle interference artifact can be caused by the following:

1. **Lead wires not following body contour.** Dangling lead wires can pick up electric current. Arrange the wires to follow body contour and to lie flat.
2. **Other electrical equipment in the room.** Lamps, autoclaves, electrically powered examining tables, or other electrical equipment that is plugged in may be leaking electric current. Unplug all nearby electrical equipment. (*Note:* Jewelry and watches do not interfere with the recording, therefore it is not necessary for the patient to remove these items unless they interfere with proper placement of the electrodes.)
3. **Wiring in the walls, ceilings, or floors.** Try moving the patient table away from the walls.
4. **Improper grounding of the electrocardiograph.** The machine is automatically grounded when it is plugged in. Check the three-pronged plug of the ECG machine to make sure the prongs are not loose or damaged. Ensure that the plug is securely in the wall outlet. The right leg electrode is not used for recording the leads, but it picks up electric current that has "leaked" onto the patient and carries it into the electrocardiograph. The electric current is carried away by the machine's grounding system.

Interrupted Baseline Artifact

Occasionally, an interrupted baseline (Figure 12-14, *D*) occurs that may be caused by the metal tip of a lead wire becoming detached or by a frayed or broken patient cable. If the latter is the case, a new patient cable should be ordered from the manufacturer.

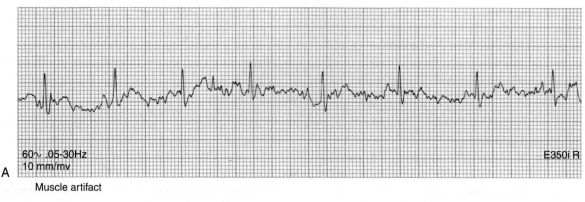

60∼ .05-30Hz
10 mm/mv

E350i R

A

Muscle artifact

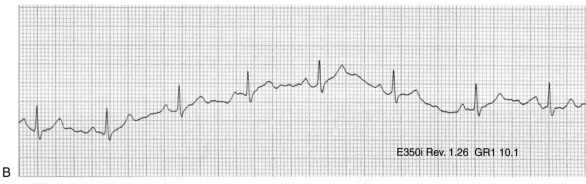

E350i Rev. 1.26 GR1 10.1

B

Wandering baseline

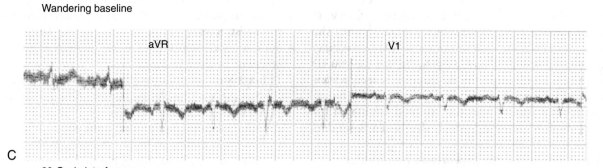

aVR

V1

C

60-Cycle interference

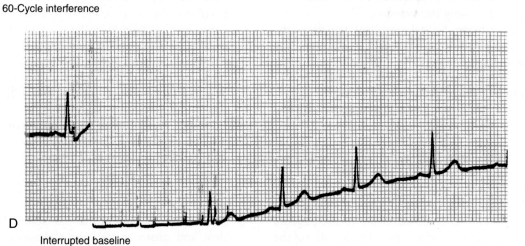

D

Interrupted baseline

Figure 12-14. **A-D,** Examples of ECG artifacts. (**D** from Long BW: Radiography essentials for limited practice, ed 3, St Louis, 2010, Saunders.)

PROCEDURE 12-1   Running a 12-Lead, Three-Channel Electrocardiogram

Outcome Record a 12-lead electrocardiogram.

Equipment/Supplies

- Three-channel electrocardiograph
- Disposable electrodes
- ECG paper

1. Procedural Step. Work in a quiet, relaxing atmosphere away from sources of electrical interference.

2. Procedural Step. Sanitize your hands, and assemble the equipment. Check the expiration date of the electrodes. Greet the patient and introduce yourself. Identify the patient by full name and date of birth.

Principle. The electrolyte gel on outdated electrodes may be dried out, which can cause artifacts on the ECG.

3. Procedural Step. Help the patient relax by explaining the procedure. Tell the patient that having an ECG recording is painless. Explain that he or she must lie still, breathe normally, and not talk while the ECG is being recorded so that an accurate ECG can be obtained.

Principle. Explaining the procedure helps reassure apprehensive patients. The patient should be mentally and physically relaxed for an accurate ECG recording; an apprehensive or moving patient produces muscle artifacts. Heavy breathing or sighing can cause a wandering baseline artifact.

4. Procedural Step. Prepare the patient. Ask him or her to remove clothing from the waist up. The lower legs also must be uncovered. Provide a female patient with a gown, and instruct her to put it on with the opening in front. Assist the patient into a supine position on the table. The table should support the arms and legs adequately so that they do not dangle. Properly drape the patient to prevent exposure and to provide warmth. A pillow can be used to support the patient's head.

Principle. The chest, upper arms, and lower legs must be uncovered to allow proper placement of the electrodes. The patient should be kept warm, and the arms and legs should not be allowed to dangle; otherwise, muscle artifacts could result.

5. Procedural Step. Position the electrocardiograph so that the power cord points away from the patient and does not pass under the table. It is usually easier for the medical assistant to work on the left side of the patient.

Principle. Proper positioning of the electrocardiograph reduces 60-cycle interference artifacts.

6. Procedural Step. Prepare the patient's skin for application of the disposable electrodes. If the patient has sweaty or oily skin or has used lotion, rub the area to which the electrode will be applied with alcohol, and allow it to dry. If the patient's chest is hairy, dry shave it at each electrode site before applying the electrode.

Principle. The patient's skin must be dry and free of oil and body hair so that the adhesive backing of the electrodes sticks to the patient's skin and stays on during the procedure.

7. Procedural Step. Remove a card containing 10 electrodes from its foil-lined pouch and reseal the pouch. Apply the limb electrodes. Firmly apply the adhesive backing of the electrodes to the fleshy part of each of the four limbs (upper arms and lower legs). The electrode tabs should point toward the center of the body. The tabs of the arm electrodes should point downward, and the tabs of the leg electrodes should point upward. The adhesive backing of the electrode allows it to adhere firmly to the patient's skin.

Principle. The pouch should be resealed to preserve moisture and prevent the electrolyte on the remaining electrodes from drying out. The electrodes must be

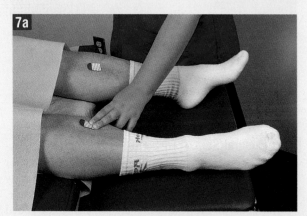

Apply the leg electrodes.

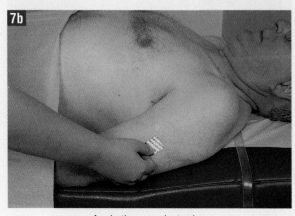

Apply the arm electrodes.

Continued

PROCEDURE 12-1   Running a 12-Lead, Three-Channel Electrocardiogram—cont'd

firmly attached to permit good transmission of the electrical impulse from the patient's skin to the electrode. Loose electrodes can cause artifacts to occur on the recording, making it difficult to analyze the recording. The tabs of the electrodes should be positioned toward the center of the body to provide a more stable connection when the lead wire is attached to the electrode and to prevent the lead wires from pulling onto the electrodes and causing artifacts.

8. Procedural Step. Apply the chest electrodes. Properly locate each electrode placement site using palpation, and apply the electrode with the tab pointing downward. Continue until all six of the chest electrodes have been applied.

Principle. Positioning the tabs of the electrodes downward prevents the lead wires from pulling and causing artifacts.

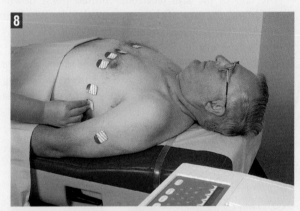

Apply the chest electrodes.

9. Procedural Step. Connect the lead wires to the electrodes. This is accomplished by inserting an alligator clip onto the metal tip of each lead wire. Next, firmly attach an alligator clip to the tab of each electrode. The ends of the lead wires are usually color-coded

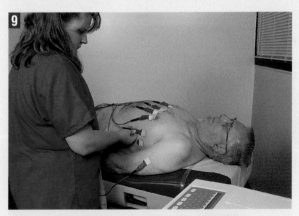

Connect the lead wires to the electrodes.

(e.g., red for the arms and green for the legs) and identified with abbreviations to help the medical assistant connect the proper lead to each electrode. Arrange the lead wires to follow body contour.

Principle. The lead wires must be attached correctly to ensure an accurate and reliable ECG. Arranging the lead wires to follow body contour reduces the possibility of 60-cycle interference artifacts.

10. Procedural Step. Plug the patient cable into the machine. The cable should be supported on the table or on the patient's abdomen to prevent pulling of the lead wires on the electrodes.

Principle. Pulling of the lead wires on the electrodes can cause the electrodes to pull away from the skin, resulting in artifacts.

11. Procedural Step. Turn on the electrocardiograph. Enter patient data using the soft-touch keypad. Always use your fingertips to enter the data. Pencils and other sharp objects can damage the keyboard. As the data are entered, they are displayed on the LCD screen. Patient data to be entered generally include the patient's name, a patient identification number, age, sex, height, weight, and medications.

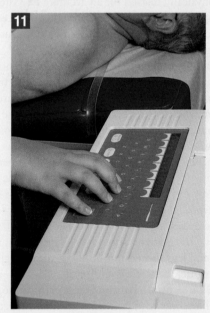

Enter patient data.

12. Procedural Step. Remind the patient to lie still, breathe normally, and not talk. Press the AUTO (automatic) button, and run the recording. The machine automatically inserts a standardization mark at the beginning of each ECG strip, followed by the recording of the 12-lead ECG in a three-channel format. Another standardization mark is inserted at the end of each ECG strip.

PROCEDURE 12-1 Running a 12-Lead, Three-Channel Electrocardiogram—cont'd

(*Note:* With most three-channel electrocardiographs, the machine checks for a clear ECG signal after the AUTO button is pressed. If the signal is "noisy," this may indicate that an electrode does not have a good connection with the patient's skin. The machine usually indicates which electrode is causing the problem [e.g., "V₆ noisy"]. Apply firm pressure to the electrode causing the problem. If this does not correct the problem, replace the electrode with a new one and/or place a piece of nonallergenic tape over the electrode.)

13. Procedural Step. After the ECG has been recorded:

a. Check the printout to ensure the standardization mark is 10 mm high. If it is more or less than 10 mm, adjust the standardization mark according

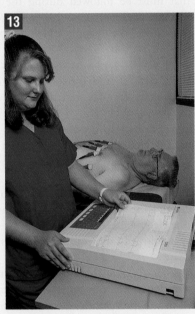

Check the standardization mark.

to the manufacturer's instructions, and run another ECG.

b. Check the direction of the R wave in lead I. If your patient's limb leads are attached correctly, the R wave on lead I should have a positive deflection. If it has a negative deflection, the limb leads are not attached correctly. Reattach the limb leads properly and run another recording.

c. Observe the recording for artifacts. If an artifact is present, determine the cause of the artifact, correct the problem, and run another ECG.

14. Procedural Step. Inform the patient that you are finished and he or she can now talk or move. Turn the machine off. Disconnect the lead wires. Remove and discard the electrodes.

15. Procedural Step. Assist the patient in stepping down from the table.

16. Procedural Step. Sanitize your hands. Chart the procedure. Include the date and time and the name of the procedure (12-lead ECG). Place the recording in the patient's medical record, and put the record in the appropriate place to be reviewed by the physician.

CHARTING EXAMPLE	
Date	
6/12/12	10:30 a.m. Completed a 12-lead ECG.
	Recording to physician for review. ————
	———————— J. Canterbury, CMA (AAMA)

17. Procedural Step. Return all equipment to its proper storage place.

HOLTER MONITOR ELECTROCARDIOGRAPHY

A Holter monitor is a portable ambulatory monitoring system for the continuous recording of the electrical activity of the heart for 24 hours or longer (Figure 12-15). The monitor is named for Dr. Norman Holter, an American biophysicist who invented this cardiac monitoring device. The original Holter monitor consisted of a large pack of equipment worn on the patient's back.

A Holter monitor is also known as an ambulatory electrocardiographic monitor (AEM). The purpose of a Holter monitor is to detect cardiac abnormalities that occur while the patient is engaged in his or her normal daily routine. Because of this, the Holter system is designed so that the patient is able to maintain his or her usual daily activities with minimal inconvenience while being monitored.

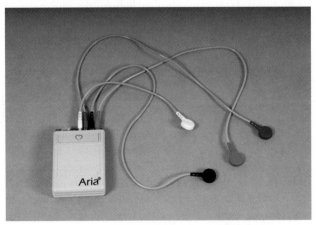

Figure 12-15. Digital Holter monitor.

A Holter monitor is similar to a resting 12-lead ECG in that the electrical impulses given off by the heart are picked up by electrodes and transmitted through lead wires to a recording device. It is different from a resting 12-lead ECG in that only about 10 seconds of the heart's activity are recorded with a 12-lead ECG, whereas a Holter monitor records the heartbeat continuously for an extended period of time. This allows the Holter monitor to pick up cardiac abnormalities that do not occur during the brief recording period of a resting 12-lead ECG.

Purpose

Holter monitor electrocardiography is an important noninvasive procedure used to diagnose cardiac rate, rhythm, and conduction abnormalities. Specifically, it is most frequently used for the following purposes:

- To assess the rate and rhythm of the heart during daily activities
- To evaluate patients with unexplained chest pain, dizziness, or syncope (fainting)
- To discover intermittent cardiac dysrhythmias not picked up on a routine resting 12-lead ECG. A resting ECG records only between 40 and 50 heartbeats, whereas a Holter monitor records approximately 100,000 heartbeats in a 24-hour period.
- To detect myocardial ischemia
- To assess the effectiveness of antidysrhythmic medications (e.g., digitalis, antianginal medications)
- To assess the effectiveness of a pacemaker

Digital Holter Monitor

Holter monitors are available in two formats. The newer format consists of a digital monitor that uses either an external (removable) or an internal (nonremovable) memory card to document the heart's activity (see Figure 12-15). The older type of Holter monitor consists of a magnetic tape monitor that uses a cassette tape to record the activity of the heart. Because most facilities have phased out magnetic tape monitors, the remainder of this unit will focus on the digital monitor.

A digital Holter monitor is lightweight and battery-powered. The monitor can be clipped onto a belt around the patient's waist. It can also be held in a protective pouch, which is hung around the patient's neck with a strap known as a *lanyard*. Digital monitors can continuously record the electrical activity of the heart for 24 hours, 48 hours, or 72 hours. Most physicians order a 24-hour recording, but they may occasionally order a 48- or 72-hour recording when the heart's activity needs to be recorded for a longer period of time. Throughout the monitoring period, the system continuously records the electrical activity of the heart and stores it on the memory card. The monitor may have a small LCD screen that displays the date and time along with the remaining recording time. The Holter monitor automatically stops recording after the monitoring period has been completed.

Some physicians have Holter monitors in their medical offices. The medical assistant is responsible for preparing the

Memories *from* Externship

Janet Canterbury: During my externship, I was at an office where electrocardiograms were one of the many procedures that were performed. For my first electrocardiogram, the patient was a man who had a lot of hair on his chest, and I would need to shave the electrode placement sites on his chest. I was very nervous, but the procedure went well. When the electrocardiogram was run, he told me that I did a wonderful job and that it did not hurt at all to have his chest shaved. I realized then that it was not so bad after all. That patient made me feel so good about what I do and helped me feel confident in the procedures I had ahead of me. ■

patient, applying and removing the monitor, and instructing the patient in patient preparation requirements and the guidelines that must be followed during the monitoring period (see the box *Holter Monitor Patient Guidelines*). Procedure 12-2 describes how to apply a Holter monitor.

Patient Preparation

The medical assistant should instruct the patient in the preparation required for the test, which includes the following:

1. Take a shower or bath before coming to the medical office to have the Holter monitor applied. You will not be able to shower or bathe again until the monitor is removed.
2. Do not apply body lotion, oil, or powder to your chest before or during the test. This may make it more difficult to apply the electrodes.
3. Take your usual medications unless the physician specifies otherwise.
4. Wear loose, comfortable clothing with a shirt or blouse that buttons down the front for easier application of the electrodes and to prevent the electrodes from rubbing against clothing and becoming loose.

Electrode Placement

The purpose of the electrodes is to pick up the electrical impulses given off by the heart. The impulses are then transmitted through the lead wires and patient cable to the monitor. A special type of electrode is used with the Holter monitor. It usually consists of foam and is round or rectangular in shape with an electrode plate and a snap for attaching a lead wire. The electrode has an adhesive backing and a central sponge pad that contains an electrolyte gel (Figure 12-16). This type of electrode is disposable and must be discarded after use.

The newer Holter monitors are three-channel recording systems. This means that the monitor can record three leads at one time. Depending on the brand and model of monitor, a three-channel monitor uses between four and seven electrodes that are placed at various locations on the patient's chest. Information on the number of electrodes and their locations is diagrammed in an electrode placement chart included in the operating manual that accompanies

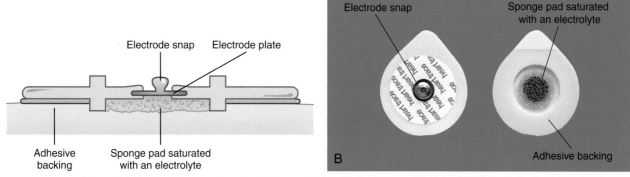

Figure 12-16. **A,** Diagram of an electrode used with a Holter monitor. **B,** Holter monitor electrode (front and back).

Holter Monitor Patient Guidelines

Most routine activities can be performed while wearing a Holter monitor, except those that can damage the monitor or cause artifacts on the recording. Artifacts affect the quality of the recording and can lead to false-positive results on ECG recordings analyzed by a computer. The following guidelines must be relayed to the patient to ensure an accurate and reliable electrocardiographic recording:

1. Participate in your normal everyday activities during the monitoring period. The purpose of Holter monitoring is to determine how your heart functions during your usual daily activities. Avoid engaging in activities, however, that cause excessive sweating (such as vigorous physical exercise), which might cause the electrodes to become loose or fall off.
2. Do not shower, bathe, or swim while wearing the monitor because water can damage the monitor and loosen the electrodes. A sponge bath can be taken if needed.
3. Check periodically to make sure the monitor indicator light is still on and that all the electrodes and lead wires are still attached to the chest.
4. Do not touch or move the electrodes or lead wires during the monitoring period to prevent artifacts from appearing in the recording.
5. If a lead wire detaches from an electrode, snap it back onto the electrode as soon as possible, and record this information in the patient diary.
6. If an electrode comes loose, press down around the edges of the electrode and apply tape to the electrode to restore the contact. Record this information in the patient diary. Contact the medical office if an electrode comes off and cannot be replaced.
7. Do not handle the monitor or take it out of its pouch.
8. Do not use an electric blanket, hair dryer, electric shaver, heating pad, microwave oven, or electric toothbrush while wearing the monitor. Other items and areas to avoid during the testing period include magnets, metal detectors, and areas with high-voltage electrical wires. These items or areas can cause electrical interference artifacts, which may affect the quality of the recording.

9. Record your activities and emotional states in the patient diary. With each entry, note the time that the activity or emotional state occurred.
   The following activities should be recorded:
   - Physical exercise associated with daily activities (e.g., walking, housework, gardening, employment-related activities)
   - Walking up or down stairs
   - Periods of inactivity (e.g., sitting in a chair, lying on a couch)
   - Driving
   - Smoking
   - Urination
   - Bowel movements
   - Meals (including alcohol and caffeinated beverages)
   - Sexual intercourse
   - Medications consumed
   - Sleep periods (including naps)
   The following are examples of emotional states that should be recorded:
   - Anger
   - Excitement
   - Anxiety
   - Fear
   - Laughter
10. Record the physical symptoms experienced during each activity. If you do not experience anything abnormal during an activity, leave that symptom space blank. Following are examples of physical symptoms that should be recorded:
    - Shortness of breath
    - Chest pain
    - Neck, arm, or face pain
    - Heart palpitations
    - Nausea
    - Dizziness
    - Faintness

the Holter monitor. To reduce artifacts during the recording period, these electrodes are typically placed over bone, such as on the sternum or ribs. The medical assistant should make sure the electrodes are properly placed to ensure an accurate recording. When first learning to place these elec-

trodes, it may help to mark their locations on the patient's chest with a felt-tipped pen.

The monitor's effectiveness should be checked after hooking up the patient to ensure that a clear signal is being relayed from the electrodes to the monitor. This check is performed by accessing the *Lead Status* screen on the LCD display screen located on the monitor. The quality of the ECG signal for each lead is displayed on the screen. The ECG signal should be clear and strong. If the signal is "noisy," this may indicate that an electrode does not have a good connection with the patient's skin. The medical assistant should apply gentle pressure to each electrode to improve contact with the patient's skin. If a problem still exists, the monitor may be malfunctioning and in need of repair.

Patient Diary

An important aspect of the Holter monitor procedure is the completion of a diary by the patient (Figure 12-17). All activities and emotional states must be documented during the monitoring period, along with the time of their occurrence. In addition, any physical symptoms experienced by the patient during the activity must be indicated next to each activity. A dysrhythmia or ECG change recorded by the Holter monitor can then be compared with the information in the patient's diary. This allows the physician to correlate patient activities, emotional states, and symptoms with cardiac activity to determine if a certain activity triggers an ECG abnormality.

Event Marker

Some Holter monitor models have an *event marker* button, which is used along with the patient diary for patient evaluation. When the event marker button is pressed, a beep may sound as an audible feedback. The patient should be told to depress the button momentarily when experiencing a symptom and then record the time and nature of the symptom in the Holter diary. Depressing the button places an electronic signal on the recording. This signal highlights the specific portion of the recording where the symptom occurred. When the patient data are analyzed by a computer, the time of the event along with an *ECG event strip* will be included in the ECG report.

Evaluating Results

At the end of the monitoring period, the Holter monitor system is removed from the patient. The information on the memory card is then uploaded to a computer. Specialized ECG software performs calculations on the data and prepares an ECG summary report of the monitoring period, which is then displayed on the screen of the computer.

The computer-generated ECG report summarizes information about the patient's heart rate and rhythm and any abnormalities that occurred during the monitoring period. The report also includes selected samples of the patient's cardiac activity, including patient event strips and any abnormal cardiac activity exhibited by the patient, such as dysrhythmias. The results of the ECG summary report are reviewed and interpreted further by the physician. The physician also reviews the patient's diary to determine if there is a correlation between any of the patient's activities, emotional states, or symptoms and ECG abnormalities. The ECG report can be printed out on regular sheets of paper using an ink-jet or laser printer and stored in a PPR (patient-based paper record). It can also be stored electronically in the patient's EMR (electronic medical record).

PATIENT DIARY		
TIME	ACTIVITY	SYMPTOM
AM PM	*Start recording*	
8:30 AM	Ate breakfast Smoked cigarette	
9:15 AM	Driving freeway	Chest pounding
10:35 AM	Argued with boss	Chest pain
10:45 AM	Took medication	
12:30 PM	Ate lunch	
1:15 PM	Walked up two flights of stairs	Stomach burning Pain in left arm

Page 1

PATIENT DIARY		
TIME	ACTIVITY	SYMPTOM

Page 2

Figure 12-17. Holter monitor patient diary.

Maintenance of the Holter Monitor

At the end of each recording period, the battery should be removed from the monitor and discarded. Leaving a battery in the monitor could result in corrosion of the battery, which could damage the monitor. The casing of the monitor should be cleaned frequently, using a soft cloth moistened with a mild disinfectant to remove dust and dirt. Commercial solvents and abrasives should not be used because they can damage the finish of the casing. The patient cable and lead wires should be cleaned periodically with a cloth moistened with a mild disinfectant. The cable and lead wires should never be immersed in the cleaning solution because this could damage them. The snap of each lead wire should be cleaned with alcohol and a small brush to eliminate any trace of gel remaining after the use of disposable electrodes. The monitor should be stored in a dry, dust-free area.

PROCEDURE 12-2 Applying a Holter Monitor

Outcome Apply a Holter monitor.

Equipment/Supplies

- Holter monitor (with an internal memory card)
- Battery
- Disposable pouch and lanyard or a belt clip
- Disposable electrodes
- Razor

- Antiseptic wipes
- Gauze pads
- Abrasive pad
- Nonallergenic tape
- Patient diary

---

1. Procedural Step. Assemble the equipment.

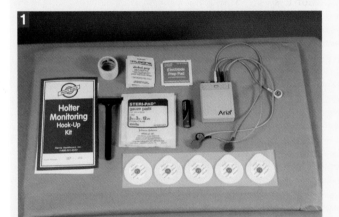

Assemble the equipment.

2. Procedural Step. Prepare the equipment. Install a new high-quality alkaline battery according to the markings on the battery holder to ensure correct battery polarity. Check the expiration date on the electrodes.
Principle. A new battery must be installed each time the monitor is used to ensure sufficient power throughout the monitoring period. The electrolyte on outdated electrodes may be dried out, which can cause artifacts on the ECG.

3. Procedural Step. Connect the Holter monitor to the computer using a docking station or a computer cable connected to a USB port. Enter patient demographic data into the computer. Patient data to be entered generally include the patient's name and date of birth

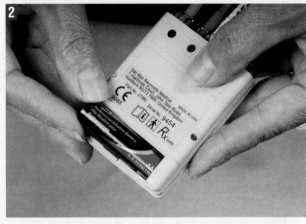

Insert the battery.

and a patient identification number. Download this information to the Holter monitor.
Principle. The data are used to identify the recording. They are also used in computer-assisted interpretation of the ECG.

4. Procedural Step. Sanitize your hands. Greet the patient and introduce yourself.

5. Procedural Step. Identify the patient by full name and date of birth, and explain the procedure. Tell the patient that the Holter monitor will record the heartbeat without interfering with his or her daily activities. Tell the patient that, because of its small size, the monitor will be fairly inconspicuous. Instruct the patient in the guidelines for wearing a Holter monitor (see the *Holter Monitor Patient Guidelines* box). Emphasize to the patient that is it important to maintain daily activities during the monitoring period.

Continued

PROCEDURE 12-2   Applying a Holter Monitor—cont'd

Principle. The patient must follow the guidelines carefully to ensure an accurate recording.

6. **Procedural Step.** Prepare the patient by asking him or her to remove clothing from the waist up.

Principle. Clothing must be removed for placement of the chest electrodes.

7. **Procedural Step.** Place the patient in a sitting position.

8. **Procedural Step.** Locate the chest electrode sites by following the electrode placement diagram included in the operating manual.

Prepare an area of skin slightly larger than an electrode at each placement site as follows:

a. If the patient's chest is hairy, dry shave it at each electrode site.

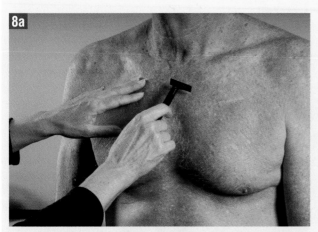

Shave the chest.

b. Rub the skin with an alcohol wipe to remove any dirt, perspiration, or body oils that might be on the skin. Allow the area to dry completely.

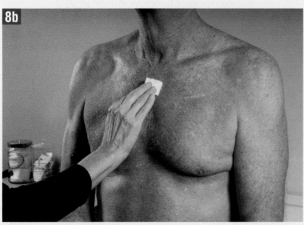

Rub the skin with an alcohol wipe.

c. Slightly abrade the skin with a gauze pad or an abrasive pad until the skin is reddened. This is accomplished by rubbing the skin lightly with six or seven small circular motions. On a patient with normal skin, use about the same pressure used to file the fingernails with a fingernail file. Use less pressure on geriatric patients and patients with sensitive skin or poor skin condition.

Principle. Shaving the chest improves the adherence of the electrodes and makes them easier to remove. The placement sites should be rubbed with a skin abrasive to remove dry, dead skin, which improves adherence of the electrodes and increases conductivity of the electrical signal from the skin surface to the electrode.

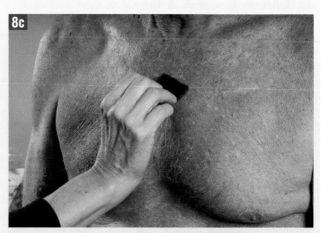

Slightly abrade the skin with a skin abrader.

9. **Procedural Step.** Attach a color-coded lead wire to the snap of each electrode.

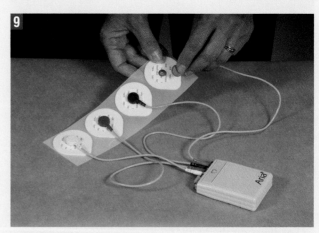

Snap the color-coded lead wires onto the electrodes.

10. **Procedural Step.** Apply the chest electrodes as follows: Determine the first electrode to be applied by looking at the color-coded chest electrode placement

PROCEDURE 12-2   Applying a Holter Monitor—cont'd

chart. Grasp the first electrode by the colored lead wire snap cover, and remove the electrode from its protective backing. Avoid touching the adhesive to prevent loss of its stickiness. Check that the electrolyte gel is moist. If it is dry, obtain a new electrode.
Principle. The ends of the lead wires are color-coded for proper placement of each lead. The electrolyte gel should be moist to ensure good conduction of electrical impulses.

11. Procedural Step. Apply the electrode (with attached lead wire) to the first chest electrode site. Ensure a firm seal by running your finger around the outer edge of the electrode with a firm pressure until it is firmly attached to the skin. Do not press down in the middle of the electrode.
Principle. The electrodes must be firmly attached to permit good transmission of the electrical impulse from the patient's skin to the electrode. Loose electrodes can cause artifacts on the recording, making it difficult to analyze the recording. Pressing down on the middle of the electrode may cause some of the electrolyte gel to be forced out from under the electrode, interfering with good conduction of the electrical signal from the patient's heart.

are transmitted through the lead wires and the patient cable to the monitor.

13. Procedural Step. Plug the patient cable into the monitor, and turn on the monitor. Check the ECG signal quality by accessing the *Lead Status* screen on the LCD display screen located on the monitor. The quality of the ECG signal for each lead is displayed on the screen. The ECG signal should be clear and strong. If the signal is "noisy," this may indicate that an electrode does not have a good connection with the patient's skin. Apply gentle pressure to each electrode to improve contact with the patient's skin.
Principle. A clear signal ensures an accurate and reliable ECG recording.

14. Procedural Step. Place a strip of nonallergenic tape over each electrode and cover of the lead wire.
Principle. Applying tape prevents the lead wire from detaching from the electrode.

15. Procedural Step. Check to make sure the date and time displayed on the screen of the monitor are accurate, and start the monitor.

16. Procedural Step. Place the disposable lanyard and pouch around the patient's neck, and insert the monitor into the pouch.

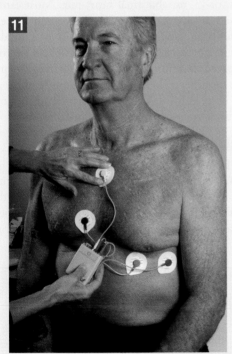
Ensure a firm seal of each electrode.

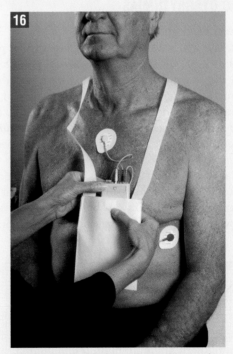
Insert the monitor into a disposable pouch.

12. Procedural Step. Repeat steps 10 and 11 until all the chest electrodes have been applied.
Principle. The electrodes pick up and conduct the electrical impulses given off by the heart. The impulses

17. Procedural Step. Tell the patient to redress while being careful not to pull on the lead wires.

18. Procedural Step. Complete the patient information section of the patient diary, and record the starting time

Continued

PROCEDURE 12-2   Applying a Holter Monitor—cont'd

in the patient diary. Give the diary to the patient, and provide him or her with instructions on completing it. ***Principle.*** The beginning time must be recorded for later correlation of the patient diary with cardiac activity. The patient diary is used to correlate patient symptoms with cardiac activity.

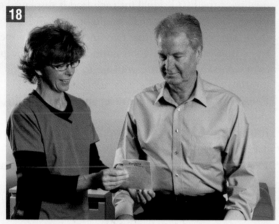

Provide the patient with instructions on completion of the diary.

19. Procedural Step. Instruct the patient when to return for removal of the monitor. Remind the patient not to forget to bring the diary.

20. Procedural Step. Sanitize your hands, and chart the procedure in the patient's medical record. Include the date and time, the name of the procedure (application of a Holter monitor), and the beginning time. Also chart instructions given to the patient.

CHARTING EXAMPLE

Date	
6/15/12	2:00 p.m. Applied Holter monitor.
	Starting time: 2:15 p.m. Instructed pt on
	recording data in diary. To return on
	6/16/12 at 2:30 p.m. for removal of
	monitor————D. Arnold, CMA (AAMA)

CARDIAC DYSRHYTHMIAS

The normal ECG graph cycle consists of a P wave, a QRS complex, and a T wave, which repeat in a regular pattern (see Figure 12-5). The term **normal sinus rhythm** refers to an ECG that is within normal limits. This means that the waves, intervals, segments, and cardiac rate fall within the normal range. The normal heart rate ranges from 60 to 100 beats per minute. A rate slower than 60 beats per minute is *sinus bradycardia,* and a rate faster than 100 beats per minute is *sinus tachycardia.*

Cardiac **dysrhythmia** is the term used to describe abnormal electrical activity in the heart causing an irregular heartbeat. Cardiac dysrhythmias can be classified into one of the following categories: (1) extra beats, (2) an abnormal

rhythm, or (3) an abnormal heart rate. Most cardiac dysrhythmias are harmless; however, some can be serious or even life-threatening. The medical assistant should be able to recognize basic cardiac dysrhythmias on an electrocardiographic recording for the purpose of alerting the physician of their presence. The dysrhythmias the medical assistant should be able to identify are presented next, along with brief descriptions and significant clinical aspects.

Premature Atrial Contraction

Description

A premature atrial contraction (PAC) is characterized by a beat that comes before the next normal beat is due. The most distinguishing feature is that the P wave of the premature beat has a different shape from the P wave of the nor-

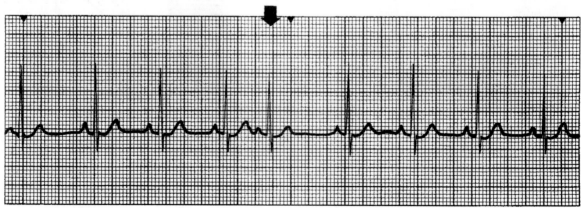

Premature atrial contraction. (From Huang S et al: Coronary care nursing, Philadelphia, 1989, Saunders.)

mal beat. The premature atrial contraction has a normal QRS complex and a normal T wave, similar to the other ECG graph cycles.

Clinical Significance

Premature atrial contractions are common in healthy individuals and are often associated with the intake of stimulants, such as caffeine and tobacco. They also can be associated with more serious atrial dysrhythmias and structural heart disease.

Paroxysmal Atrial Tachycardia

Description

Paroxysmal atrial tachycardia (PAT) is an abrupt episode of tachycardia with a constant heart rate that usually falls between 150 and 250 beats per minute. Paroxysmal atrial tachycardia is characterized by a rhythm that has a sudden onset and termination. The sudden increase in rate occurs in short bursts and lasts only a few seconds, after which the rate returns to what it was before the paroxysmal atrial tachycardia occurred. Because of the increase in heart rate, the ECG graph cycles are very close together. With paroxysmal atrial tachycardia, the patient experiences a sudden pounding or fluttering of the chest associated with weakness, breathlessness, and acute apprehension. Occasionally, the patient experiences syncope.

Clinical Significance

Paroxysmal atrial tachycardia is one of the most common rhythm disorders, often occurring in healthy patients with no underlying heart disease and young adults with normal hearts. It also can occur in individuals with organic heart disease.

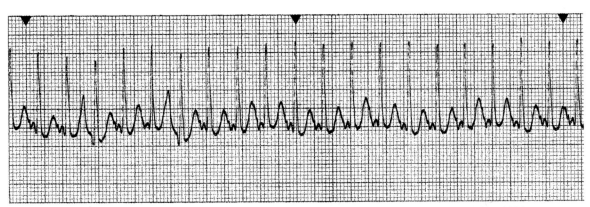

Paroxysmal atrial tachycardia. (From Huang S et al: Coronary care nursing, Philadelphia, 1989, Saunders.)

PATIENT TEACHING   Angina Pectoris

Answer questions the patient has about angina pectoris.

What is angina pectoris?

Angina pectoris is a symptom, or a set of symptoms, rather than a disease. Its name is a Latin term that means "pain in the chest." Angina pectoris occurs when the muscle tissue of the heart does not receive enough oxygenated blood, resulting in discomfort or pain under the sternum.

What causes angina pectoris?

For most patients, the cause of angina is atherosclerosis. *Atherosclerosis* is a condition in which fibrous plaques of fatty deposits and cholesterol build up on the inner walls of the arteries. This causes narrowing and partial blockage of the lumen of these arteries, along with hardening of the arterial wall. Atherosclerosis in the coronary arteries is called coronary artery disease (CAD). CAD results in a reduction in oxygenated blood flow to the heart muscle. Despite the narrowing, enough oxygen may still reach the heart muscle for normal needs. More oxygen is needed, however, when situations occur that increase the workload of the heart, such as physical activity, emotional stress, a heavy meal, and exposure to cold weather. If the coronary arteries cannot deliver enough oxygen

to the heart muscle during these times of increased need, angina pectoris results.

What happens during an angina episode?

Individuals experience angina in different ways, including the following: severe indigestion, tightness or burning, heaviness, ache, and squeezing or crushing pressure in the center of the chest. Other symptoms that may occur with an angina episode include shortness of breath, sweating, nausea, weakness, fatigue, heart palpitations, and dizziness. The chest discomfort that occurs with an angina episode varies greatly. It can feel only mildly uncomfortable, or it may be intense and accompanied by a feeling of suffocation and doom. Pain is usually felt beneath the sternum and may radiate to the neck, throat, jaw, left shoulder, arm, or back. In most cases, the pain lasts no longer than a few minutes and is relieved by resting. Severe and prolonged anginal pain generally suggests a myocardial infarction (heart attack) caused by complete blockage of the coronary arteries and requires immediate medical attention.

What tests might be ordered by the physician?

For patients who exhibit angina pectoris, the physician may order one or more of the following: a 12-lead electrocardiogram, chest

Continued

x-ray, blood tests, and a cardiac stress test. These tests assist in detecting coronary artery narrowing and blockage. To determine the exact location and extent of blockage, a more specific test, known as *coronary angiography,* may be performed.

What type of treatment might be prescribed by the physician?

The goal of treating angina is to reduce the workload of the heart and increase the oxygen supply to the heart. This is accomplished by resting when an angina attack occurs. In addition, the physician often prescribes medications, the most common one being nitroglycerin. Nitroglycerin is usually taken sublingually. It works by reducing the workload of the heart and increasing the oxygen supply

to the heart by dilating the coronary arteries. Nitroglycerin also can be administered through patches worn on the skin or an ointment rubbed into the skin.

To help prevent more serious heart disease from developing, the physician generally recommends lifestyle changes, such as a diet low in cholesterol and saturated fat, weight reduction, controlling high blood pressure, smoking cessation, exercise, and stress reduction. For patients with severe blockage of the coronary arteries, balloon angioplasty with coronary stent placement or coronary artery bypass surgery may be recommended.

Provide the patient with educational materials on angina pectoris and coronary artery disease. ▪

Atrial Flutter

Description

Atrial flutter is a rapid, regular fluttering of the atrium in which the heart rate falls between 250 and 350 beats per minute. More than one P wave precedes each QRS complex, and the P waves appear as saw-toothed spikes between the QRS complexes. The number of waves can range from just one extra P wave to eight falling in rapid succession, but all have the same size and shape. The QRS complexes of an atrial flutter configuration are normal; however, the T wave is usually lost in the P waves.

Clinical Significance

Atrial flutter rarely occurs in healthy individuals. It is found in patients with underlying heart disease. Atrial flutter is not specific to any particular heart disease; it can occur in patients with mitral valve disease, coronary artery disease, acute myocardial infarction, chronic lung disease, hypertensive heart disease, and pulmonary emboli, and in patients who have undergone cardiac surgery.

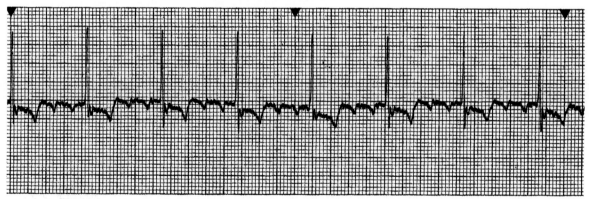

Atrial flutter. (From Johnson R, Swartz MH: A simplified approach to electrocardiography, Philadelphia, 1986, Saunders.)

Atrial Fibrillation

Description

Atrial fibrillation is characterized by an ECG in which the P waves have no definite pattern or shape. The P waves appear as irregular wavy undulations between the QRS complexes. The QRS complexes in atrial fibrillation are normal but do not have a definite pattern. It is difficult to measure accurately the atrial rate because the P waves are not discernible; however, the atria are contracting between 400 and 500 times per minute. The ventricular rate may be rapid (150 to 180 beats per minute) or relatively normal.

Clinical Significance

Atrial fibrillation is a common dysrhythmia that can occur in healthy individuals and in patients with a variety of cardiac diseases. In healthy individuals, it can be initiated by emotional stress, excessive alcohol consumption, and vomiting. In individuals younger than 50 years old, the common causes of atrial fibrillation are congenital heart disease and rheumatic heart disease with mitral valve involvement. In individuals older than 50, atrial fibrillation is caused by diseases capable of producing **ischemia** or hypertrophy of the atria, such as coronary artery disease, mitral valve disease, and hypertensive heart disease.

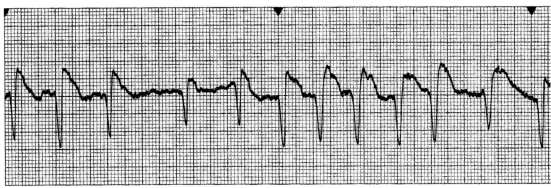

Atrial fibrillation. (From Huang S et al: Coronary care nursing, Philadelphia, 1989, Saunders.)

Premature Ventricular Contraction

Description

Premature ventricular contractions (PVCs) are among the most common rhythm disturbances seen on an ECG. The PVC is characterized by a beat that comes early in the cycle, is not preceded by a P wave, has a wide and distorted QRS complex, and has a T wave opposite in direction to the R wave of the QRS complex. Because of the unusual configuration of the QRS complex, the premature ventricular contraction easily stands out from the normal ECG graph cycles. The baseline distance after the PVC is usually longer than the normal distance between the other cycles. In other words, the premature ventricular contraction is followed by a pause before the next normal beat.

Clinical Significance

Premature ventricular contractions are seen in normal individuals in all age groups and are caused by anxiety, smoking, caffeine, alcohol, and certain medications (e.g., epinephrine, isoproterenol, aminophylline). PVCs can occur with virtually any type of heart disease but are seen most often in patients with hypertensive heart disease, ischemic heart disease, lung disease with hypoxia, and digitalis toxicity. PVCs also are common in individuals with mitral valve prolapse.

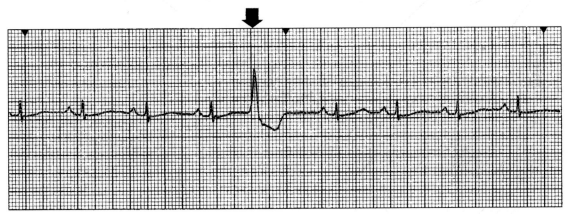

Premature ventricular contraction. (From Huang S et al: Coronary care nursing, Philadelphia, 1989, Saunders.)

Ventricular Tachycardia

Description

Ventricular tachycardia consists of a series of three or more consecutive premature ventricular contractions that occur at a rate of 150 to 250 per minute. The tachycardia may occur paroxysmally and last only a short time, or it may persist for a long time. The QRS complexes are bizarre and widened, and no P waves are present. Sustained ventricular tachycardia is a life-threatening dysrhythmia because the rapid ventricular rate prevents adequate filling time for the heart, leading to reduced cardiac output that often degenerates into ventricular fibrillation and cardiac arrest.

Clinical Significance

Ventricular tachycardia is usually seen in patients with acute or chronic heart disease. Runs of ventricular tachycardia indicate coronary artery disease. Ventricular tachycardia also occurs as a complication of a myocardial infarction.

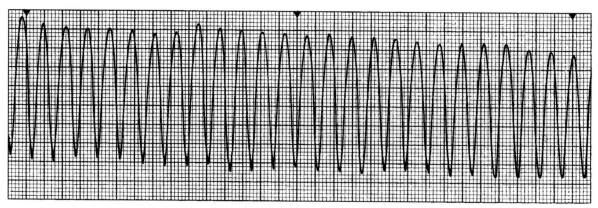

Ventricular tachycardia. (From Huang S et al: Coronary care nursing, Philadelphia, 1989, Saunders.)

Ventricular Fibrillation

Description

Ventricular fibrillation (V-fib) is the most serious dysrhythmia. With this type of dysrhythmia, the ventricles do not beat in a coordinated manner, but instead they twitch or fibrillate. Because of this, virtually no blood is ejected into the systemic circulation. On an ECG, ventricular fibrillation is characterized by irregular, chaotic undulations of the baseline. There are no recognizable P waves, QRS complexes, or T waves in the irregular line of jagged spikes. Because the ventricles are twitching irregularly, there is no effective ventricular pumping action, resulting in no circulation. Ventricular fibrillation is a serious dysrhythmia that must be treated immediately because it can lead to sudden death.

Clinical Significance

The most common cause of ventricular fibrillation is an acute myocardial infarction. It also can occur in patients with organic heart disease and cardiac dysrhythmias. It may be preceded by a dysrhythmia such as premature ventricular contractions or ventricular tachycardia, or it may occur spontaneously.

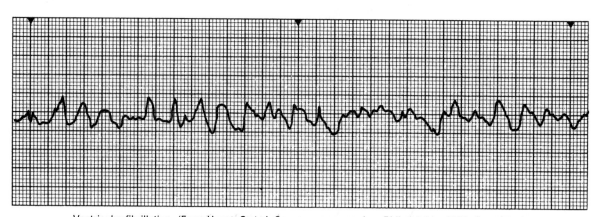

Ventricular fibrillation. (From Huang S et al: Coronary care nursing, Philadelphia, 1989, Saunders.)

PULMONARY FUNCTION TESTS

The purpose of a pulmonary function test (PFT) is to assess lung functioning, assisting in the detection and evaluation of pulmonary disease. Pulmonary function tests include spirometry, lung volumes, diffusion capacity, arterial blood gas studies, pulse oximetry, and cardiopulmonary exercise tests. The most frequently performed pulmonary function test is spirometry, which is described in detail in the next section. Procedure 12-3 outlines how to use a spirometer.

Spirometry

Spirometry is a simple, noninvasive screening test that is often performed in the medical office. A computerized electronic instrument known as a **spirometer** is used to conduct the test. A spirometer measures how much air is pushed out of the lungs and how fast it is pushed out. The spirometry report is printed out as a table and graph. Spirometry is considered a screening test, and abnormal test results require that the patient undergo additional pulmonary function tests and possibly a computed tomography scan before a diagnosis can be made. Indications for performing spirometry include the following:

1. Patients who exhibit symptoms of lung dysfunction such as dyspnea
2. Individuals at high risk for lung disease because of smoking or exposure to environmental pollutants such as coal dust, asbestos, and exhaust fumes
3. Patients with lung disease, such as asthma, chronic bronchitis, and emphysema
4. Patients who are to undergo surgery (to assess probable lung performance during an operation)
5. Patients who need to be evaluated for lung disability or impairment for a compensation program (e.g., coal miners)

Spirometry Test Results

The results obtained from spirometry testing provide numerous measurements that help the physician assess lung functioning. The most important parameters are described next.

Forced Vital Capacity

Forced vital capacity (FVC) is the maximum volume of air (measured in liters) that can be expired when the patient exhales as forcefully and rapidly as possible and for as long as possible. Forced vital capacity is obtained by having the patient perform a breathing maneuver. The patient is instructed to take a deep breath until the lungs are completely full. Following this, the patient is told to blow all the air out of the lungs and into the mouthpiece as hard and as fast as possible until no more air can be expelled. To be considered an adequate test, the patient must forcibly blow out all the air from the lungs and continue smooth, continuous exhaling for at least 6 seconds. To be considered a valid test, a minimum of three acceptable efforts must be obtained.

What Would You Do? What Would You *Not* Do?

Case Study 2

Joel Matthews, 48 years old, is at the office for a biannual checkup. Joel had a mild heart attack 2 years ago. Since then, he has completely changed his life. He's become a vegetarian and practices yoga every morning before going to work. After he gets home, he jogs 10 miles. He also lifts weights every other day and takes herbal vitamin supplements. Since his heart attack, he has lost 40 lb and says that he has never felt better. The only thing he cannot seem to do is give up smoking. He started smoking when he was 17 years old and has cut back from 2 packs to 1 pack a day. He keeps trying to stop but says that he has been smoking so long that it might not be possible. Besides, with all the other healthy stuff he is doing, he thinks it probably cancels out the bad effect of the cigarettes. Joel is very concerned that if he does stop smoking, he will gain back all of the weight that it took him so long to lose. ■

Some patients have difficulty performing the FVC breathing maneuver because they have a physical impairment or poor motivation, or they do not understand the instructions. The medical assistant should be patient and work with these individuals to help them perform the maneuver. If patients are unable to perform the maneuver after eight attempts, however, testing should be discontinued. At this point, fatigue may affect the accuracy of the results, and additional efforts are not recommended.

Forced Expiratory Volume after 1 Second

Forced expiratory volume after 1 second (FEV_1) is the volume of air (in liters) that is forcefully exhaled during the first second of the FVC breathing maneuver. The spirometer automatically determines this parameter from the FVC maneuver.

FEV_1/FVC Ratio

In patients with healthy lungs, 70% to 75% of the air exhaled (FVC) is exhaled in the first second (FEV_1) of the breathing maneuver. This comparison is known as the *FEV_1/FVC ratio,* and it is expressed as a percentage. A patient with healthy lungs may have a FEV_1/FVC ratio of 85%. This means that 85% of the exhaled air was exhaled during the first second of the breathing maneuver.

In patients with chronic obstructive pulmonary disease, the FEV_1/FVC ratio is less than 70% to 75%. These patients are unable to move most of their exhaled air out of the lungs during the first second because of an obstruction to the airflow, such as inflammation or damaged lung tissue. Based on the FEV_1/FVC ratio, the obstruction is characterized as mild (61% to 69%), moderate (45% to 60%), or severe (less than 45%). Figure 12-18 shows a graph of spirometry parameters in a patient with healthy lungs and in a patient with obstructive pulmonary disease.

Evaluation of Results

To evaluate the spirometry test results fully, certain demographic factors must be taken into consideration, including the patient's age, sex, weight, and height. These demographic factors are used to calculate the *predicted values,* which is what the results should be for a patient with healthy lungs. When the test is run, the physician compares the patient's *measured values* with the predicted values. For example, the FVC predicted value is 6 liters, and the FVC measured value is 4 liters. This means that the patient should have been able to exhale 6 liters of air (based on age, sex, weight, and height), but he or she was able to exhale only 4 liters of air.

The computerized spirometer automatically calculates predicted values using demographic information entered into the machine by the medical assistant. The predicted values and the measured values are printed on the spirometry report. Figure 12-19 shows an example of these results. Comparing the measured values with the predicted values assists the physician in detecting the presence of pulmonary disease.

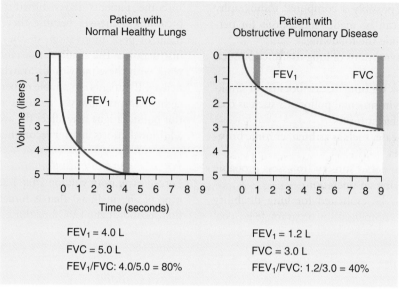

Figure 12-18. Spirometry parameters.

Parameter	Predicted Values	Measured Values
FVC	6.00 liters	4.00 liters
FEV$_1$	5.00 liters	2.00 liters
FEV$_1$/FVC	83%	50%

Figure 12-19. Predicted values compared with measured values. This individual exhibits a moderate airflow obstruction.

Patient Preparation

Patient preparation is essential to obtain accurate test results. To prepare for the test, the patient should be instructed to do the following:

1. Do not eat a heavy meal for 8 hours before the test. (The patient must exert the diaphragm muscles, and a full stomach may interfere with this action.)
2. Stop smoking at least 8 hours before the test.
3. Do not take bronchodilators for 4 hours before the test.
4. Do not engage in strenuous activity for 4 hours before the test.
5. Wear loose, nonrestrictive clothing to keep the chest area as free as possible, which makes it easier to perform the breathing maneuver.

Calibration of the Spirometer

To ensure accurate and valid test results, the spirometer should be calibrated each day that the machine is used. Calibration is performed by injecting a known quantity of air into the spirometer. A large 3-liter spirometry syringe is used to inject 3 liters of air into the machine. The output should read 3 L, and the reading should not vary by more than 3%. If the machine is not properly calibrated, the medical assistant should consult the operating manual and adjust the machine as required.

Post-Bronchodilator Spirometry

If the results of the spirometry test indicate a possible obstruction, the physician usually orders a post-bronchodilator spirometry test. This test is performed by having the patient inhale a bronchodilator and running a spirometry test approximately 10 to 15 minutes later. The purpose of this test is to inform the physician as to how treatment would work in patients whose airways are obstructed. If the FVC or FEV$_1$ parameter increases by at least 15%, the result is reported as positive for bronchodilator responsiveness. This means that the obstruction may be reversible or partially reversible through the use of medication.

What Would You Do? What Would You *Not* Do?

Case Study 3

Walter Conrad, 62 years old, comes to the office because he has been getting short of breath when he goes up and down stairs. He has worked in the coal mines his whole life and has just retired. The physician orders a pulmonary function test. Walter tries to breathe like he is supposed to during the test, but he cannot do it, and he is getting dizzy from trying so hard. He also is having problems with the nose clips. He says they pinch his nose, and he feels like he is being smothered. After four attempts, he puts down the spirometer in frustration and wants to know if he can come back some other time. He says that he is thinking his symptoms are not that bad after all, and maybe he will just wait and see what happens and will come back if they get worse. ■

Highlight on Smoking and Chronic Obstructive Pulmonary Disease

COPD Defined

Chronic obstructive pulmonary disease (COPD) is a chronic airway obstruction that results from emphysema or chronic bronchitis or a combination of these conditions. COPD is a chronic, debilitating, irreversible, and sometimes fatal disease.

More than 12 million Americans have been diagnosed with COPD; however, it is estimated that an additional 12 million Americans have the disease and remain undiagnosed. Smoking tobacco is the primary cause of COPD. In the United States, approximately 80% to 90% of deaths due to COPD are caused by smoking. According to the American Lung Association, COPD is the fourth leading cause of death in the United States, behind heart disease, cancer, and stroke. COPD claims the lives of more than 120,000 Americans each year.

Emphysema

Emphysema is most often seen in older individuals with a long history of smoking. Emphysema due to smoking is caused by irreversible damage to the alveoli in the lungs from toxins present in cigarette smoke (see illustration). As alveoli continue to be damaged, the lungs are able to transfer less and less oxygen to the bloodstream. In addition, air becomes trapped in the damaged alveoli, making it difficult to remove during exhalation. Because of this, the primary symptom of emphysema is shortness of breath. Other symptoms include chronic cough, tiredness, and limited exercise tolerance. More than 3 million people in the United States have been diagnosed with emphysema; of these, 52% are men and 48% are women. The reason is not yet understood, but fortunately only 10% to 15% of long-term smokers develop emphysema.

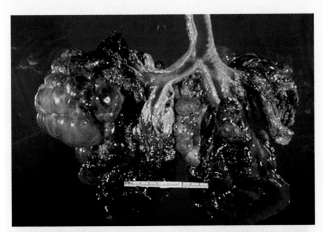

Emphysema caused by smoking. (From Little JW: Dental management of the medically compromised patient, ed 7, St Louis, 2008, Mosby. Courtesy R.N. McLay, J.H. Harrison, C.D. Fermin, H. Johnson, Tulane Gross Pathology Tutorial. Last modified July 15, 1997, Tulane University School of Medicine. Available at: http://www.som.tulane.edu/classware/pathology/medical_pathology/mcpath. Accessed August 22, 2006.)

Chronic Bronchitis

Chronic bronchitis is an inflammation of the lining of the bronchiole tubes that causes swelling and excess production of mucus. Swelling and excess mucus narrow the bronchiole tubes and restrict airflow into and out of the lungs. Symptoms include chronic cough, shortness of breath, and coughing up of mucus. To be classified as chronic bronchitis, the symptoms must last 3 or more months out of the year for at least 2 years. As the disease progresses, the lips and skin may exhibit cyanosis resulting from lack of oxygen in the blood. Chronic bronchitis is most often caused by long-term irritation of the bronchial tubes due to cigarette smoking; other causes include air pollution and exposure to dust or toxic gases in the workplace (e.g., coal mines). Chronic bronchitis often precedes or accompanies emphysema. It is estimated that 12 million Americans have chronic bronchitis. This condition affects individuals of all ages but has a higher incidence in individuals over 45 years of age. Women are more than twice as likely to be diagnosed with chronic bronchitis than men.

Symptoms of COPD

Damage to the lungs caused by COPD occurs gradually over many years. In fact, more than 90% of patients who have COPD are over the age of 45 at the time of their diagnosis. Because there are no early symptoms, many people do not know they have COPD. By the time an individual experiences symptoms, it is usually a sign that irreversible lung damage has already occurred. The first symptoms of COPD include mild shortness of breath on exertion and occasional coughing. The disease slowly becomes more pronounced with severe episodes of dyspnea and coughing even after modest activity. As the disease progresses, the heart also can be affected and shortness of breath is present all the time, even while sitting quietly. At this point, the individual's quality of life is greatly diminished. When the lungs and the heart are no longer able to deliver oxygen to the body's tissues, death occurs.

Treatment for COPD

The best treatment for COPD caused by smoking is for the patient to stop smoking. Continued smoking makes the COPD worse; quitting smoking slows the disease process. There are programs, support groups, and stop-smoking aids (e.g., nicotine patch, Zyban) to help individuals quit smoking. Other forms of treatment depend on the patient's condition and degree of lung impairment and may include the following:

1. Bronchodilators to relax and widen the bronchial tubes to increase airflow. They may be inhaled as aerosol sprays or taken orally.
2. Expectorants to thin the mucus so that it is easier to expel.
3. Antibiotics to treat infections that could interfere further with breathing and lung function.
4. Corticosteroids to reduce inflammation in the airways.
5. Breathing exercises to strengthen the muscles used to breathe.
6. Maintaining overall good health habits, which include proper nutrition, adequate sleep, and regular exercise.
7. Oxygen therapy for patients with low blood oxygen to help with shortness of breath, allowing them to be more active.
8. Special measures include avoiding extremes (heat and cold) of temperature, getting an annual influenza immunization, avoiding individuals with respiratory infection, and reducing exposure to air pollution.
9. Lung transplantation surgery is being performed on some patients who are in the later stages of COPD.

PROCEDURE 12-3   Spirometry Testing

Outcome Perform a spirometry test.

Equipment/Supplies

- Spirometer
- Disposable tubing
- Disposable mouthpiece

- Disposable nose clips
- Waste container

1. **Procedural Step.** Sanitize your hands. Assemble and prepare the equipment. Calibrate the spirometer according to the manufacturer's instructions. Apply a disposable mouthpiece to the mouthpiece holder, which is attached to the spirometer by a cable.
   Principle. Calibration of the spirometer ensures accurate and valid test results.

2. **Procedural Step.** Greet the patient and introduce yourself. Identify the patient and explain the procedure. Tell the patient that he or she will be wearing nose clips and performing a breathing maneuver several times to see how well his or her lungs are functioning. Ask the patient whether he or she prepared properly for the procedure.

3. **Procedural Step.** Prepare the patient. Have the patient remove any heavy or constricting clothing, such as a jacket or a sweater. Also, ask the patient to loosen tight clothing, such as a necktie or a tight collar. If the patient is chewing gum, ask him or her to discard it in a waste container.
   Principle. Heavy outer clothing, tight clothing, or gum may make it difficult for the patient to perform the breathing maneuvers.

4. **Procedural Step.** Measure the patient's weight and height precisely.
   Principle. Precise weight and height measurements are required for the accurate calculation of predicted values.

5. **Procedural Step.** Have the patient sit near the machine. The patient should be seated to prevent dizziness or possible fainting during the procedure. Enter the following data into the computer database of the spirometer: patient's age, sex, weight, and height, and any other information required, such as the patient's identification number and whether the patient smokes.
   Principle. Demographic data need to be entered for the computer to calculate the predicted values.

6. **Procedural Step.** Instruct the patient in the breathing maneuver. The following procedure should be described and demonstrated to the patient:
   a. Relax and take the deepest breath possible until your lungs are completely filled with air.
   b. Place the mouthpiece in your mouth, and seal your lips tightly around it.
   c. Blow out as hard as you can and for as long as possible until your lungs are completely empty. Do

not block the opening of the mouthpiece with your tongue.
   d. Remove the mouthpiece from your mouth.
   Principle. The lips must be tightly sealed around the mouthpiece so that all of the air leaving the mouth enters the mouthpiece.

7. **Procedural Step.** Tell the patient you will repeat the instructions during the test. Encourage the patient to remain calm during the procedure. Gently apply nose clips to the patient's nose. Hand the mouthpiece to the patient, and tell him or her to hold it close to the mouth.
   Principle. Fear or anxiety can make the results less reliable. Nose clips prevent air from escaping from the nostrils and ensure that all breathing is done through the mouth.

8. **Procedural Step.** Begin the test. When the patient is ready, press the start button on the spirometer. Actively coach the patient as follows:
   a. "Now relax and take in a big breath—in—in—in—more—keep inhaling."
   b. "Put the mouthpiece in your mouth and blow hard. Keep going—keep going—keep going—more—more—more—you're almost there—a little more. That's good. You can stop now."
   c. "Take out the mouthpiece and rest for a while. You did a great job."
   Principle. Coaching the patient helps to obtain accurate test results.

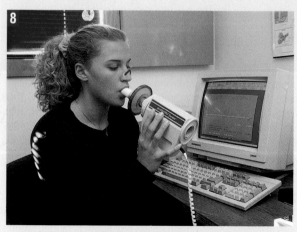

Instruct the patient to blow into the mouthpiece.

PROCEDURE 12-3   Spirometry Testing—cont'd

9. Procedural Step. If the patient does not perform the breathing maneuver correctly, inform him or her of what modifications are needed for the next effort. Continue until three acceptable efforts have been obtained.
Principle. Three acceptable efforts must be obtained to ensure valid test results.

10. Procedural Step. Gently remove the nose clips from the patient's nose. Remove the mouthpiece from the mouthpiece holder. Dispose of the mouthpiece and nose clips in a regular waste container.

11. Procedural Step. Allow the patient to remain seated for a few minutes.
Principle. The patient may feel light-headed after the procedure.

12. Procedural Step. Sanitize your hands. Print the report, and label it with the patient's name, the date, and your initials. Chart the procedure. Include the

CHARTING EXAMPLE

Date	
6/20/12	9:00 a.m. Spirometry test run. Obtained
	3 acceptable efforts. Pt stated she was
	tired following the test. Report to
	physician for review. —————
	————— J. Canterbury, CMA (AAMA)

date, the time, the name of the procedure, and the patient's reaction. Place the spirometry report in the patient's medical record, and put the record in the appropriate place for review by the physician.

13. Procedural Step. Clean the spirometer according to the manufacturer's instructions.

PEAK FLOW MEASUREMENT

Asthma

Asthma is a chronic lung disease that affects the small airways of the lungs. The trachea divides into the right and left primary bronchi. After the primary bronchi enter the lungs, they branch into smaller bronchi (known as secondary and tertiary bronchi) and then into even smaller passages known as bronchioles (Figure 12-20). The bronchioles continue to branch and finally lead into microscopic alveolar ducts, which terminate in clusters of tiny air sacs known as alveoli. Asthma affects the smaller bronchi (secondary and tertiary bronchi) and the bronchioles of the lungs.

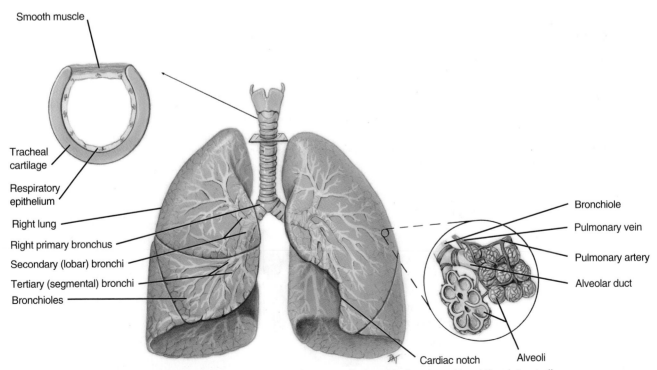

Figure 12-20. The primary bronchi divide into secondary and tertiary bronchi and then into smaller passages known as *bronchioles*. (From Applegate EJ: The anatomy and physiology of the learning system, ed 3, St Louis, 2006, Saunders.)

Asthma can occur at any age but is more common in children and young adults. Asthma affects boys more frequently before puberty and girls more frequently after puberty. In the United States, there are approximately 20 million individuals with asthma; of these, 6 million are children. Each year, more than 4000 deaths result from asthma.

Asthma is characterized by chronic inflammation of the small airways of the lungs and recurrent attacks of coughing, chest tightness, shortness of breath, and wheezing. **Wheezing** is a continuous, high-pitched, whistling, musical sound heard particularly during exhalation and sometimes during inhalation. In most patients, an asthma attack is followed by a symptom-free period. Asthma can be controlled by recognizing the warning signs and symptoms of an attack and treating them when they first occur. Failure to treat asthma can lead to serious complications, such as permanent lung damage.

The exact cause of asthma is not known. It is thought to be caused by a combination of factors, including genetics, certain childhood respiratory infections, and contact with allergens or exposure to certain viral infections in infancy or early childhood.

Asthma Attack

An asthma attack is also known as an asthma flare-up or an asthma episode. Asthma attacks are highly individualized. Depending on the patient, asthma attacks vary in frequency and severity and may come on suddenly or gradually. An asthma attack may last for only 10 to 15 minutes or it may last for hours or even days.

In a normal individual, the airways to the lungs are fully open, allowing air to move easily into and out of the lungs. In a patient with asthma, the airways are always inflamed and hypersensitive to certain stimuli that do not affect the airways of normal individuals. These stimuli are known as asthma triggers because they can "trigger" an asthma attack.

Asthma triggers vary from one patient to another and may also vary from one season to the next. Examples of common allergens that may trigger an asthma attack include house dust, pollens, molds, animal danders, and cockroaches. Asthma attacks can also be triggered by environmental irritants, activities, or events, including air pollutants, tobacco smoke, chemical fumes (e.g., perfume, paint, gasoline), vigorous physical exercise, upper respiratory viral infections, exposure to cold, and emotional stress. It is sometimes difficult to determine what specific triggers cause a patient's asthma attack.

When the inflamed airways of a patient with asthma are stimulated by a trigger, a series of reactions occur that affect the bronchial tubes. The bronchial tubes begin to constrict and swell, causing the patient to experience asthma symptoms. Sometimes the symptoms are mild and go away, either on their own, or with minimal treatment with medication. At other times, the symptoms become worse, leading to a full-blown asthma attack. During a severe asthma attack, the bronchial tubes continue to constrict and swell and become clogged with mucus (Figure 12-21). This results in less air moving into and out of the lungs, which leads to a decrease in the amount of oxygen available to the body. The narrowed bronchial tubes and decreased oxygen supply cause the patient to experience coughing, chest tightness, shortness of breath, and wheezing. It is important to treat symptoms when they first begin to occur to prevent them from getting worse and causing a severe asthma attack, which may require emergency care.

Diagnosis and Treatment

The physician diagnoses asthma through a careful and detailed medical history. Of particular importance to the diagnosis of asthma are the patient's symptoms, family history of asthma, home and work environment, and living habits. The physician also performs a thorough physical examination to detect symptoms resulting from asthma, such as wheezing. When the medical history and physical examination have been completed, the physician usually orders laboratory and diagnostic tests, which may include pulmonary function tests (such as spirometry), allergy testing, and arterial blood gas studies.

Although asthma is a chronic disease with no cure, most patients with asthma are able to lead a normal life through proper management and treatment. The general treatment of asthma includes identifying and avoiding asthma triggers (if possible) and preventing and alleviating the symptoms through drug therapy. Two general categories of medication

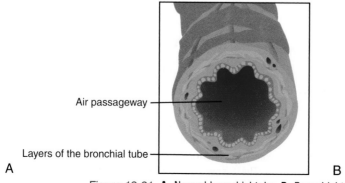
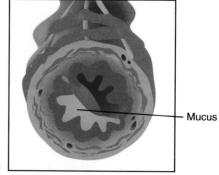

Air passageway

Layers of the bronchial tube

Mucus

A   B

Figure 12-21. **A,** Normal bronchial tube. **B,** Bronchial tube during an asthma attack.

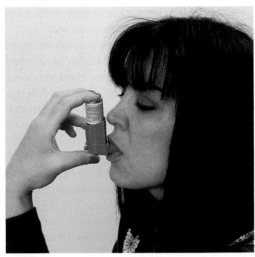

Figure 12-22. An inhaler is often used to deliver asthma medication to the bronchial tubes of the lungs. (From Potter PA: Basic nursing: essentials for practice, ed 6, St Louis, 2007, Mosby.)

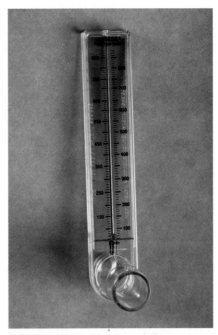

Figure 12-23. Manual peak flow meter.

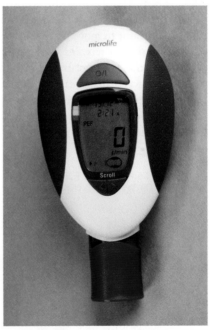

Figure 12-24. Digital peak flow meter.

are prescribed for asthma: long-term control medication and quick-relief medication.

Long-term control medication helps relieve bronchial inflammation and prevents symptoms from occurring. Control medication helps the patient have fewer and milder asthma attacks and is typically taken every day. Corticosteroids are an example of a control medication; brand names include Flovent, Azmacort, Vanceril, and AeroBid. Other examples of long-term control medication include Singulair, Accolate, Serevent, Alupent, and Advair.

Quick-relief medication (also called *rescue medication*) opens the airways quickly by dilating the bronchial tubes. It is taken when the patient is experiencing symptoms to prevent or control an asthma attack. Fast-acting bronchodilators are an example of quick-relief medication; brand names include Proventil, Ventolin, and Xopenex.

Many asthma medications are delivered through an *inhaler* (Figure 12-22), which allows the medication to go directly to the lungs. Quick-relief medications can be used in a breathing machine known as a *nebulizer* to treat an asthma attack at home. Other asthma medications are administered orally; however, they take longer to work because they first have to travel through the digestive and circulatory systems before reaching the lungs.

Peak Flow Meter

A peak flow meter is a portable, handheld manual or digital device used to measure a breathing maneuver performed by the patient. *A manual peak flow meter* consists of a plastic tube with a sliding indicator that manually moves along a scale of numbers when the patient performs the breathing maneuver (Figure 12-23). A *digital peak flow meter* automatically measures the breathing maneuver and displays the measurement digitally on a screen (Figure 12-24). Because the manual meter is currently used most often, the remainder of this unit will focus on the manual peak flow meter.

A peak flow meter is used to measure how quickly air flows out of the lungs when the patient exhales forcefully. Peak flow meters are frequently used by patients with asthma and are recommended for patients with moderate to severe asthma. The measurements obtained from a peak flow meter are not as accurate as those obtained by spirometry; however, a peak flow meter can be used easily by a patient at home.

Peak flow measurements provide patients with important information such as when to take their medication and how severe an asthma attack is. Several different brands of peak flow meters are available, and peak flow measurements between brands may vary. Because of this, a patient who purchases more than one meter should always buy the same brand to provide consistency between measurements.

Peak flow meters can be purchased over-the-counter and are available in two ranges: a low range and a full range. The *low-range meter* has a range from zero to 300 and is used by young children and some older patients. The *full-range meter* has a range from zero to 800 and is used by older children, teenagers, and adults (Figure 12-25). An adult has much larger bronchial tubes than a child and needs the wider range.

Peak Flow Rate

The **peak flow rate** (PFR) is the maximum volume of air measured in liters per minute (L/min) that can be exhaled when the patient blows into a peak flow meter as forcefully and as rapidly as possible. The PFR is obtained by having the patient perform a breathing maneuver.

The patient is instructed to take a deep breath until the lungs are completely full. Following this, the patient is told to blow all the air out of the lungs and into the mouthpiece of the peak flow meter as hard and as fast as possible. When the patient blows into the peak flow meter, his or her breath causes the sliding indicator to move up the scale of the meter. The indicator stops and remains at the patient's peak flow rate. To obtain the most accurate PFR, the patient should perform three acceptable breathing maneuvers, and then record the highest of the three measurements. The three measurements should be about the same to show that an acceptable breathing maneuver was performed each

time. This is especially important to note when parents are evaluating a child's peak flow measurement.

The medical assistant is often responsible for instructing a newly diagnosed asthma patient in the procedure for using a peak flow meter. In addition, the medical assistant may be responsible for obtaining the peak flow rate of a patient with asthma at the medical office. The procedure for measuring peak flow rate is outlined in Procedure 12-4.

Schedule of Use

A peak flow meter should be used on a regular schedule by patients with moderate to severe asthma to determine how well their asthma is being controlled. The physician determines each patient's schedule based on the severity and frequency of asthma symptoms. Most physicians recommend that the patient use a peak flow meter at least once a day, preferably in the morning before taking asthma medication. A peak flow measurement should also be obtained when the patient is having symptoms. If the patient has a more severe form of asthma, the physician may want the patient to use a peak flow meter twice a day—in the morning and in the evening.

Peak flow measurements are usually recorded on a peak flow chart (Figure 12-26), which allows the patient and the physician to track changes in the patient's lung function over a period of time. A peak flow chart consists of graph paper with a range of peak flow numbers (usually from 50 to 800 L/min) listed in a vertical column on the left side of the graph paper. The patient indicates the date and time at the top of the chart. After obtaining a peak flow measurement, the patient places a dot across from the peak flow number in the appropriate column. A sample peak flow

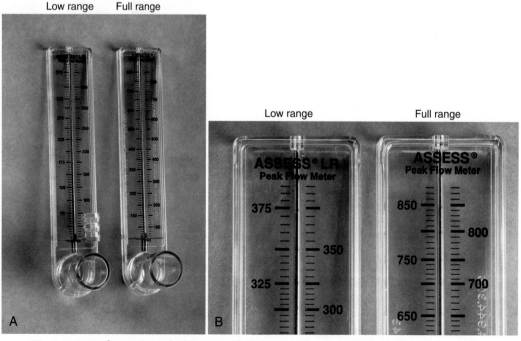

Figure 12-25. Comparison of a low-range (**A, B:** *left*) and full-range (**A, B:** *right*) peak flow meter.

PEAK FLOW CHART

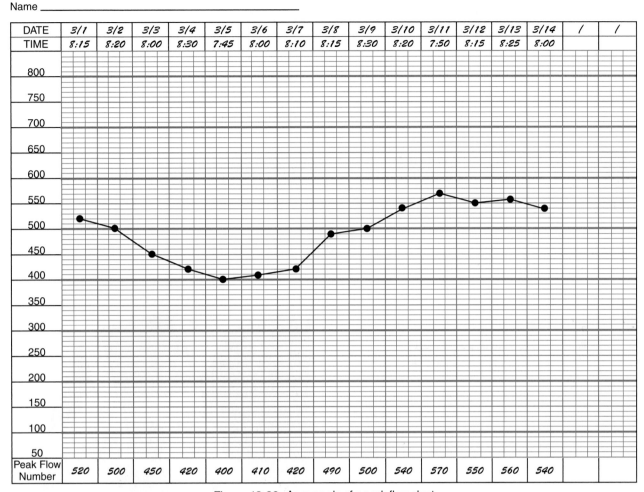

Name _____

DATE	3/1	3/2	3/3	3/4	3/5	3/6	3/7	3/8	3/9	3/10	3/11	3/12	3/13	3/14	/	/
TIME	8:15	8:20	8:00	8:30	7:45	8:00	8:10	8:15	8:30	8:20	7:50	8:15	8:25	8:00		
Peak Flow Number	520	500	450	420	400	410	420	490	500	540	570	550	560	540		

Figure 12-26. An example of a peak flow chart.

chart usually accompanies a peak flow meter and can be photocopied for ongoing use.

Purpose of Peak Flow Measurements

Peak flow measurements allow physicians and patients to monitor changes in the patient's airflow to determine how well the patient's asthma is being controlled. A high number usually means that air is moving easily out of the patient's lungs. A low number usually means that the airways are narrowed and air cannot move easily through them, resulting in a decrease in oxygen available to the body.

Peak flow measurements are used for the following:

1. *Monitor how well the asthma is being controlled.* Peak flow measurements assist the physician in determining how well a patient's asthma is being controlled and in knowing what medications to prescribe to keep the patient's asthma in control.

2. *Change or adjust medication.* Peak flow measurements help to determine if a patient's daily medications need to be adjusted or changed. If the patient is doing well as

indicated by high peak flow measurements, the physician may be able to lower the dosage of the patient's medication or discontinue certain medications altogether.

3. *Recognize early changes before symptoms occur.* Peak flow measurements may show changes before the patient feels them. A patient's PFR may drop hours or even days before asthma symptoms occur. For example, the patient may feel fine, but when a peak flow measurement is taken, the reading is slightly decreased. By taking medication before symptoms occur, it may be possible to stop the attack quickly to avoid a severe asthma attack.

4. *Determine the severity of an asthma episode.* When the patient is having symptoms or an asthma attack, the PFR can be used to determine the severity of the symptoms or the severity of the attack. This allows the patient to decide when to use quick-relief medication and, if necessary, when to seek emergency care. It also allows the patient to determine his or her response to treatment during an asthma attack by measuring PFR before and after taking quick-relief medication.

5. *Assist in identifying asthma triggers.* Asthma triggers can sometimes be identified by measuring the PFR before and after exposure to a trigger suspected of causing the asthma.

Care and Maintenance

It is important to instruct the patient in the proper care of the (manual) peak flow meter because dirt collecting on the meter may result in inaccurate measurements. The meter is cleaned by washing it weekly with warm soapy water and then rinsing it thoroughly with warm water. Excess water should be removed by gently shaking the meter. The meter should then be allowed to air-dry completely before it is used. Many peak flow meters can be cleaned by placing them in the dishwasher on the top shelf; check the manufacturer's instructions for this information. The peak flow meter should be inspected periodically for damage such as cracks, which could cause air to leak out of the meter, leading to inaccurate readings. With proper care, a peak flow meter should last 2 to 3 years.

 PROCEDURE 12-4   Measuring Peak Flow Rate

Outcome   Measure a patient's peak flow rate.

Equipment/Supplies

- Peak flow meter
- Disposable mouthpiece
- Waste container

---

1. Procedural Step. Sanitize the hands. Assemble and prepare the equipment. Move the sliding indicator on the peak flow meter to the bottom of the numbered scale. Apply a disposable mouthpiece to the mouthpiece holder.
Principle. Not placing the marker at the bottom of the numbered scale leads to inaccurate test results. The disposable mouthpiece prevents the spread of microorganisms from one patient to another.

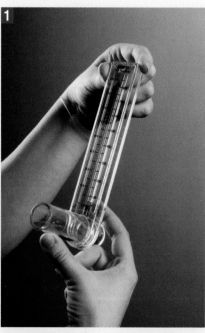

Move indicator to bottom of scale.

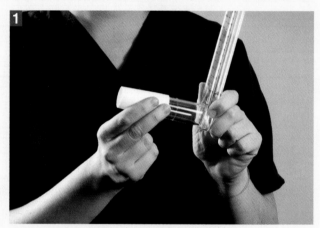

Apply a disposable mouthpiece.

2. **Procedural Step.** Greet the patient and introduce yourself. Identify the patient and explain the procedure. Tell the patient that he or she will be performing a breathing maneuver several times to see how well his or her lungs are functioning.
3. **Procedural Step.** Prepare the patient. Have the patient remove any heavy or constricting clothing, such as a jacket or a sweater. Also, ask the patient to loosen tight clothing, such as a necktie or a tight collar. If the patient is chewing gum, ask him or her to discard it in a waste container.
   Principle. Heavy outer clothing, tight clothing, or gum may make it difficult for the patient to perform the breathing maneuver.
4. **Procedural Step.** Instruct the patient in the breathing maneuver. The following procedure should be described and demonstrated to the patient.
   a. Relax and take the deepest breath possible until your lungs are completely filled with air.

PROCEDURE 12-4   Measuring Peak Flow Rate—cont'd

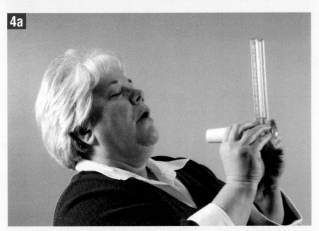

The patient takes a deep breath.

b. Place the mouthpiece in your mouth, and seal your lips tightly around it.

c. Blow out as hard and fast as you can until your lungs are completely empty. Try to move the marker as high as you can on the numbered scale. Do not block the opening of the mouthpiece with your tongue.

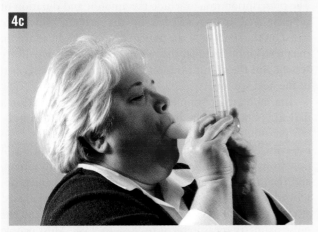

The patient blows out hard and fast.

d. Remove the mouthpiece from your mouth.

Principle. The lips must be tightly sealed around the mouthpiece so that all of the air leaving the mouth enters the mouthpiece. The force of the air coming out of the patient's lungs causes the marker to move upward on the scale. The reading depends on how hard the patient blows out the air in his or her lungs.

5. **Procedural Step.** Tell the patient you will repeat the instructions during the test. Encourage the patient to remain calm during the procedure.

Principle. Fear or anxiety can make the results less reliable.

6. **Procedural Step.** Place a new disposable mouthpiece on the peak flow meter, and slide the marker to the

bottom of the numbered scale. Hand the peak flow meter to the patient.

7. **Procedural Step.** Instruct the patient to stand up straight and look straight ahead.

8. **Procedural Step.** Begin the test. Actively coach the patient…
   a. "Now relax and take in a big breath—in—in—in—"
   b. "Put the mouthpiece in your mouth and blow hard."
   c. "Take out the mouthpiece and rest for a while. You did a great job."

9. **Procedural Step.** Note the number where the indicator stopped on the scale of the peak flow meter. Jot down the number on a piece of paper.

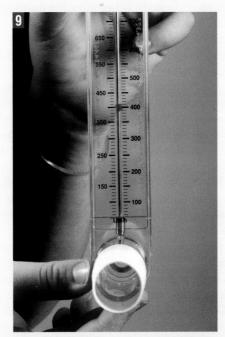

Note where the indicator stopped on the scale.

10. **Procedural Step.** If the patient coughs or does not perform the breathing maneuver correctly, do not write down the number. Inform the patient of what modifications are needed for the next effort.

11. **Procedural Step.** Continue until three acceptable efforts have been obtained. Make sure to slide the marker to the bottom of the scale before each measurement.

Principle. Three acceptable efforts must be obtained to ensure valid test results. If the patient performs the breathing maneuver correctly, the numbers from the three tests should be about the same.

12. **Procedural Step.** Take the peak flow meter from the patient, and remove the mouthpiece from the mouthpiece holder. Dispose of the mouthpiece in a regular waste container.

Continued

PROCEDURE 12-4   Measuring Peak Flow Rate—cont'd

13. **Procedural Step.** Sanitize your hands. Note the highest of the three peak flow measurements. (Do not calculate an average.) Chart the procedure. Include the date, the time, the name of the procedure, and the highest peak flow expiratory reading.

14. **Procedural Step.** Clean the peak flow meter by washing it in warm soapy water, rinsing it thoroughly, and allowing it to dry completely.

CHARTING EXAMPLE	
Date	
6/21/12	10:30 a.m. PFR: 400 L/min. Pt stated she was tired following the test. ———— ————————— D. Brown, CMA (AAMA)

HOME OXYGEN THERAPY

Oxygen is a colorless, odorless, and tasteless gas that is vital to the human body. Oxygen is transported by the blood to various tissues of the body. When it reaches the tissues, oxygen is taken into the cells, where it combines with glucose to produce energy. Energy is necessary to the body for carrying out all metabolic processes that sustain life such as breathing and beating of the heart.

When the lungs cannot deliver enough oxygen to the body, there is a reduction in the amount of oxygen in the blood, resulting in hypoxemia. **Hypoxemia** is defined as a decrease in the oxygen saturation of the blood. Hypoxemia, in turn, leads to **hypoxia,** which is a reduction in the oxygen supply to the tissues of the body. Failure to maintain an adequate blood oxygen level can result in progressive deterioration of the patient, beginning with the death of cells and, if prolonged, organ failure and eventually body system failure and death.

There are certain conditions, such as severe chronic obstructive pulmonary disease (COPD), that reduce the amount of oxygen in the body, resulting in hypoxemia. In these cases, the physician may write a prescription for home oxygen therapy. **Oxygen therapy** is the administration of supplemental oxygen at concentrations greater than room air to treat or prevent hypoxemia. Oxygen therapy increases the oxygen supply to the lungs, which, in turn, raises blood oxygen to normal levels and increases the availability of oxygen to the tissues. Oxygen therapy helps to alleviate the effects of low oxygen levels such as shortness of breath and fatigue and helps the patient have a better quality of life and live longer.

Home oxygen therapy is most commonly prescribed for patients with severe COPD caused by smoking. Other common causes of hypoxemia that may require home oxygen therapy include asthma, occupational lung disease, lung cancer, cystic fibrosis, and congestive heart failure.

Oxygen Prescription

The physician determines a patient's need for oxygen therapy through clinical observation of the patient and by measuring the oxygen level of the patient's blood. Clinical signs of hypoxemia include cyanosis, dyspnea, tachypnea, tachycardia, and anxiety. The oxygen level of the blood is typically measured by arterial blood gas (ABG) analysis and through pulse oximetry. A normal individual should have an ABG analysis of 75 to 100 mm Hg and a pulse oximetry reading above 94%. An ABG analysis less than or equal to 55 mg Hg and a pulse oximetry reading less than or equal to 88% warrants the use of supplemental oxygen. The goal of oxygen therapy is to maintain a blood oxygen level of 65 mm Hg (as measured through ABG analysis) and 90% to 93% (as measured through pulse oximetry).

Once the need for supplemental oxygen has been determined, the physician must write a prescription for oxygen therapy that is filled by a home medical supply company. The prescription must include the amount and duration of supplemental oxygen needed by the patient, which are based on the severity of the patient's condition. In addition, the prescription includes the recommended oxygen delivery system and the administration device, which are described in the next section.

The amount of supplemental oxygen prescribed for a patient is known as the **flow rate,** which is measured in liters per minute (L/min). For example, if a patient has been prescribed 2 L/min, each minute, 2 liters of oxygen will flow from the patient's oxygen delivery system into tubing, and then into the patient's upper airway. As previously described, the flow rate prescribed by the physician is targeted at raising the patient's ABG analysis to 65 mm Hg and the pulse oximetry measurement to 90% to 93%. Most people with COPD start out with a flow rate of 1 to 2 liters per minute. As their COPD worsens over time, the flow rate might increase to 3 to 6 L/min.

The duration of oxygen therapy refers to the number of hours per day oxygen therapy is administered and, depending on the patient's lung function, can vary from a few hours a day up to 15 or more hours per day. Some patients need oxygen only when sleeping or exercising, whereas other patients with more severe hypoxemia may require continuous oxygen therapy. *Continuous oxygen therapy* refers to the use of oxygen for more than 15 hours a day.

Once oxygen therapy is initiated, periodic assessment of the patient's blood oxygen level is required. This assessment is necessary to make sure that the patient still requires oxygen therapy, and that the amount and duration of oxygen are adequate to meet the patient's oxygen needs.

Oxygen Delivery Systems

There are three common delivery systems for providing supplemental oxygen to a patient: compressed oxygen gas, liquid oxygen, and an oxygen concentrator. The type of delivery system prescribed by the physician is based on the patient's condition, the patient's personal preference, the ease of equipment use, and cost. Each of these delivery systems can be used alone or in combination with another system to meet the oxygen needs of the patient. These systems are described in greater detail below.

Compressed Oxygen Gas

Compressed oxygen gas is oxygen gas compressed under high pressure and then stored in a container referred to as a *cylinder* or *tank*. Compressed oxygen cylinders vary in size from very large stationary cylinders to small portable cylinders that can be carried around (Figure 12-27, *A*). A large

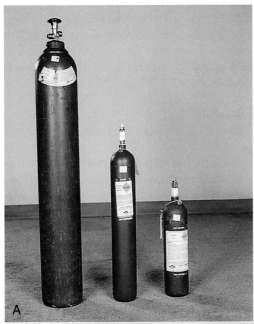

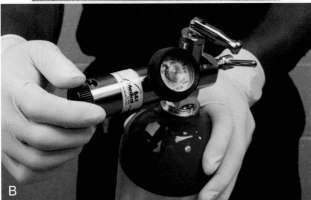

Figure 12-27. **A,** Compressed oxygen cylinders. **B,** Oxygen cylinder with regulator and flow meter attached. (**A** from Henry MC: EMT prehospital care, ed 4, St Louis, 2009, Mosby. **B** from Aehlert B: Paramedic practice today: above and beyond, 2-volume set, St Louis, 2009, Mosby.)

cylinder of compressed oxygen is used at home by the patient. A small cylinder is placed in a carrying device such as a shoulder bag and is used when the patient goes outside the home.

The cylinder is equipped with a regulator and a flow meter that control the flow rate of the oxygen (Figure 12-27, *B*). The flow of oxygen out of the cylinder is constant. To conserve oxygen and avoid waste, an oxygen-conserving device may be attached to the system. An oxygen-conserving device releases the oxygen gas only when the patient inhales and cuts off the release of oxygen when the patient exhales. Advantages and disadvantages of compressed oxygen gas include the following:

Advantage
- Compressed oxygen gas is less expensive than liquid oxygen.

Disadvantages
- The oxygen cylinders must be refilled frequently.
- A compressed oxygen gas cylinder cannot be taken on a commercial airliner.

Liquid Oxygen

When oxygen gas is subjected to an extremely cold temperature, it changes from a gas to a very cold liquid. The liquid oxygen is stored in an insulated tank with a lining similar to a thermos. Oxygen in a liquid form takes up much less space than compressed oxygen gas, for example, 1 liter of liquid oxygen is equal to 860 liters of compressed oxygen gas. Because of this, a container of liquid oxygen lasts four times longer than compressed oxygen gas of the same weight.

A liquid oxygen system consists of a large stationary tank that serves as the primary reservoir of oxygen (Figure 12-28). A small portable tank weighing between 5 and 13 pounds is filled from the large primary tank for use outside the home

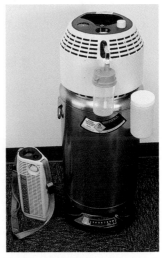

Figure 12-28. Liquid oxygen tank (stationary tank and portable tank). (From Perry AG: Clinical nursing skills and techniques, ed 7, St Louis, 2010, Saunders.)

(see Figure 12-28). The portable tank can be hung over the shoulder or pulled on a roller cart. When liquid oxygen is released from its tank, it changes into a gas and the patient breathes it in, similar to breathing in compressed oxygen gas. Advantages and disadvantages of liquid oxygen include the following.

Advantage

- Because it takes up less space and is easier to transport than compressed oxygen gas, liquid oxygen is often preferred by individuals who want to maintain an active life.

Disadvantages

- Liquid oxygen is more expensive than compressed oxygen gas.
- The contents of a liquid oxygen tank evaporate, making it necessary to have the tank refilled often.
- A liquid oxygen portable tank cannot be taken on a commercial airliner.

Oxygen Concentrator

An oxygen concentrator is an electrically powered device that weighs about 35 pounds and is about the size of a large suitcase (Figure 12-29, *A*). It works by separating oxygen out of the air, concentrating it, and then storing it for use by the patient. The oxygen concentrator is equipped with a built-in flow meter, which allows the prescribed flow rate to be set.

Small, portable, battery-powered oxygen concentrator systems weighing about 10 pounds have recently been developed (Figure 12-29, *B*). They can provide a patient with oxygen for about 8 hours when used at a flow rate of 2 L/min. For many patients, portable oxygen concentrators have replaced the need to use liquid oxygen or compressed gas cylinders for mobility. Advantages and disadvantages of oxygen concentrators include the following:

Advantages

- Oxygen concentrators do not need to be resupplied with oxygen from a home medical supply company.
- Oxygen concentrators are less expensive and safer than oxygen cylinders.
- Portable oxygen concentrators that are battery powered offer the patient even greater freedom and mobility than other oxygen delivery systems.
- Some portable oxygen concentrators have been approved by the Federal Aviation Administration (FAA) for use on commercial airlines.

Disadvantage

- Because oxygen concentrators use electricity, if the power goes out, the patient must have a compressed oxygen gas cylinder for use as a backup.

Oxygen Administration Devices

A device must be used to administer the oxygen to the upper airway of the patient from the delivery system. The device used depends on the expected duration of therapy and the personal preference and needs of the patient. The most commonly used devices to administer home oxygen therapy are a nasal cannula and a face mask, which are described in greater detail below.

Nasal Cannula

A nasal cannula is the most frequently used device for administering home oxygen therapy. A nasal cannula consists of soft plastic tubing with a two-pronged device that is inserted into the patient's nose (Figure 12-30, *A*). The tubing of the prongs loops over the patient's ears and is secured under the chin (Figure 12-30, *B*). The tubing connects to the delivery system (i.e., compressed oxygen cylinder, liquid oxygen, or oxygen concentrator). The primary advantage of

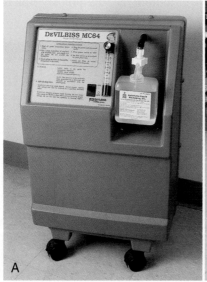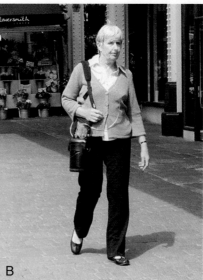

Figure 12-29. **A,** Stationary oxygen concentrator. **B,** Portable oxygen concentrator. (**A** from Sorrentino S: Mosby's textbook for long-term care nursing assistants, ed 5, St Louis, 2006, Mosby. **B** from Perry AG: Clinical nursing skills and techniques, ed 7, St Louis, 2010, Saunders.)

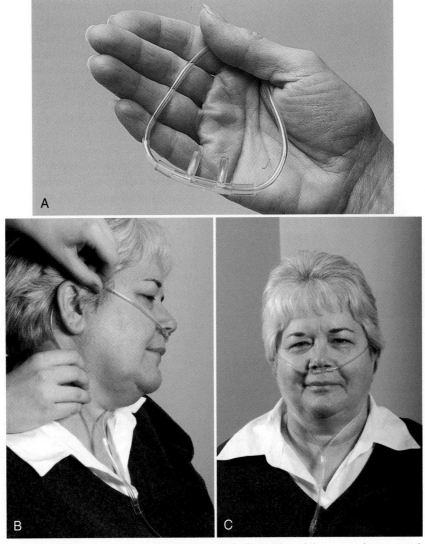

Figure 12-30. **A,** Nasal cannula showing prongs. **B-C,** The tubing of the prongs loops over the patient's ears and is secured under the chin. (**A** from Potter P: Canadian fundamentals of nursing, ed 4, Canada, 2010, Mosby.)

a nasal cannula is that it does not interfere with the patient's ability to talk, eat, or drink.

The concentration of oxygen inhaled by the patient depends on the flow rate prescribed by the physician. A nasal cannula can deliver oxygen at a flow rate between 0.25 and 6 L/min. If the flow rate is greater than 4 L/min, it can dry out the patient's nasal passages. To prevent this from occurring, a humidifier should be used to provide moisture for a flow rate above 4 L/min.

The cannula should be washed once or twice a week using liquid soap and water, rinsed thoroughly, and allowed to air-dry. The cannula should be replaced with a new cannula every 2 to 4 weeks.

Face Mask

A face mask consists of plastic and fits over the patient's nose and mouth. A face mask strap is then tightened around the patient's head to ensure a secure fit (Figure 12-31). Oxygen tubing is used to connect the face mask to the oxygen delivery system. A face mask is not used as frequently as a nasal cannula to administer oxygen because it is bulky and must be removed for eating or drinking and to communicate effectively.

A face mask is often used for patients who need a high flow of oxygen. It can deliver oxygen to the patient at a flow rate between 5 and 15 L/min. Wearing a nasal cannula for an extended period of time can cause irritation of the nose. Because of this, the patient might prefer to wear a nasal cannula during the day and a face mask at night to reduce the irritation that may occur from a nasal cannula. A face mask is also preferred by the patient if he or she has nasal congestion from a cold.

The face mask should be washed once or twice a week using liquid soap and water, then rinsed thoroughly and dried. The face mask should be replaced with a new one every 2 to 4 weeks, or sooner if it becomes cracked or discolored.

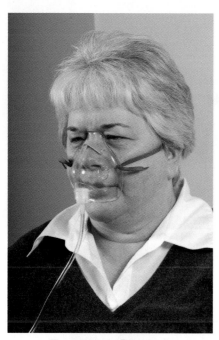

Figure 12-31. Face mask.

Oxygen Guidelines

The home medical supply company that provides the patient with the oxygen equipment gives the patient specific instructions on safe use, care, and maintenance of the equipment. Listed below are general usage and safety guidelines that should be followed by the patient.

Usage

1. Contact the physician if any of the symptoms of a low blood oxygen level occur, which include frequent headaches, anxiety, cyanosis of the lips or fingernails, drowsiness, confusion, restlessness, and slow, shallow, difficult, or irregular breathing.
2. Keep the oxygen delivery system clean and free from dust.
3. Do not change the oxygen flow rate unless directed to do so by the physician.
4. Do not use alcohol or take any other sedating drugs, as these substances will slow the breathing rate.
5. Order more oxygen from a home medical company in a timely manner.
6. To prevent the cheeks or skin behind the ears from becoming irritated from the tubing, tuck some gauze under the tubing. If you have persistent redness under your nose, contact the physician.
7. Oxygen therapy dries out the inside of the patient's nose and mouth. Use water-based lubricants (e.g., K-Y Jelly) on the lips or nostrils to relieve the drying effect. Do not use oil-based products such as petroleum jelly.
8. Do not use more than 40 to 50 feet of tubing with the oxygen delivery system to avoid bending or twisting of tubing to ensure unobstructed oxygen flow.
9. People are not allowed to bring compressed oxygen cylinders or liquid oxygen tanks on board an airplane. Many airlines will provide oxygen if notified 48 to 72 hours in advance.

Safety

Oxygen is a safe gas as long as it is used properly. Oxygen itself is not flammable, nor will it explode; however, it greatly increases the combustion rate of a fire. If something catches fire, oxygen will make the flame hotter and cause it to burn faster and more vigorously. The result is that a fire involving oxygen can appear explosive-like.

1. Store oxygen in a clean, dry, well-ventilated room. If kept in a closed area such as a closet, the small amount of oxygen gas that is continually vented from these units can accumulate in a confined space and become a fire hazard.
2. Compressed oxygen cylinders and liquid oxygen tanks must remain upright at all times. Secure oxygen cylinders and tanks to a fixed object, or place in a stand.
3. Never smoke while using oxygen. Do not allow smoking in the room where the oxygen is kept. Post "No Smoking: Oxygen in Use" signs where oxygen is kept.
4. Keep the oxygen supply at least 6 to 8 feet away from open flames such as gas stoves, lighted fireplaces, and candles.
5. Keep the oxygen supply at least 6 to 8 feet away from intense heat such as radiators, furnaces, and space heaters.
6. Keep the oxygen supply away from flammable products such as cleaning fluid, paint thinner, and aerosol sprays.
7. Do not lubricate oxygen equipment with oil or grease, as these substances are flammable.
8. Be sure to have functioning smoke detectors in the home.
9. Buy a fire extinguisher, and be familiar with how to use it.

evolve *Check out the Evolve site to access additional interactive activities.*

What Would You Do? What Would You *Not* Do? RESPONSES

Case Study 1
Page 510

What Did Janet Do?
- ❑ Tried to reduce Camilla's fears by talking with her calmly and quietly.
- ❑ Explained to Camilla that an ECG is the best screening test available to check for heart problems.
- ❑ Reassured Camilla that she would be draped during the procedure and that she would be exposed as little as possible.
- ❑ Told Camilla that the wires may look a little scary, but there is no chance of being shocked by them. Explained that she won't feel anything when the test is being run.
- ❑ Told Camilla that she could talk with the billing clerk about setting up a payment plan for the test. Provided her with information about community resources that might help her pay for the test.

What Did Janet Not *Do?*
- ❑ Did not tell Camilla that she was too young to have heart problems.
- ❑ Did not tell Camilla that she needed to act more mature about being tested.

What Would You Do?/What Would You *Not* Do? Review Janet's response and place a checkmark next to the information you included in your response. List additional information you included in your response.

_____

_____

_____

_____

Case Study 2
Page 529

What Did Janet Do?
- ❑ Commended Joel on his weight loss and positive lifestyle changes.
- ❑ Shared a positive story with Joel about a patient who stopped smoking and did not gain weight.
- ❑ Asked Joel whether he would like any of the latest information on smoking cessation.

What Did Janet Not *Do?*
- ❑ Did not agree that Joel's positive lifestyle changes would counteract the bad effects of smoking.

- ❑ Did not lecture Joel on the dangers of smoking because if he has been smoking since age 17 and has been trying to quit, he already knows what they are.

What Would You Do?/What Would You *Not* Do? Review Janet's response and place a checkmark next to the information you included in your response. List additional information you included in your response.

_____

_____

_____

_____

Case Study 3
Page 530

What Did Janet Do?
- ❑ Removed the nose clips and empathized with Mr. Conrad that the test is hard to do and that the nose clips do fit very snugly.
- ❑ Explained to Mr. Conrad that it is normal to feel dizzy and that it is only temporary.
- ❑ Allowed Mr. Conrad to rest for a while. Tried to relax and calm him by talking with him about his family and interests.
- ❑ Talked to Mr. Conrad about the importance of performing the test. Told him that detecting a problem early would help him get the treatment he needs as soon as possible so that his condition will not get worse.
- ❑ Asked Mr. Conrad whether he would try the test one more time.

What Did Janet Not *Do?*
- ❑ Did not criticize Mr. Conrad for not being able to perform the test.
- ❑ Did not force Mr. Conrad to stay if he did not want to, but scheduled another pulmonary function test for him before he left the office.

What Would You Do?/What Would You *Not* Do? Review Janet's response and place a checkmark next to the information you included in your response. List additional information you included in your response.

_____

_____

_____

_____

CERTIFICATION REVIEW

- ❑ **The electrocardiograph** records the heart's electrical activity. An electrocardiogram (ECG) is the graphic representation of this activity.
- ❑ **The heart consists of four chambers:** the right and left atria and the right and left ventricles. The SA node consists of a knot of modified myocardial cells that have the ability to send out an electrical impulse, which initiates and regulates the heartbeat. The AV node delays the impulse momentarily to give the ventricles a chance to fill with blood. The impulse is transmitted to

Continued

CERTIFICATION REVIEW—cont'd

the bundle of His, and the Purkinje fibers distribute the impulse evenly to the right and left ventricles, causing them to contract.

❑ **The cardiac cycle** represents one complete heartbeat. It consists of the contraction of the atria, the contraction of the ventricles, and the relaxation of the entire heart. The electrocardiograph records the electrical activity that causes these events in the cardiac cycle.

❑ **The ECG cycle** consists of a P wave, a QRS complex, and a T wave. The P wave represents the contraction of the atria, the QRS complex represents the contraction of the ventricles, and the T wave represents the electrical recovery of the ventricles.

❑ **The electrocardiograph must be standardized** when recording an ECG. This ensures an accurate and reliable recording. A normal standardization mark should be 10 mm high. If it is more or less than this, the electrocardiograph machine must be adjusted.

❑ **The standard ECG consists of 12 leads.** Each lead records the heart's activity from a different angle. The 12 leads are I, II, III, aVR, aVL, aVF, V_1, V_2, V_3, V_4, V_5, and V_6.

❑ **The electrical impulses** given off by the heart are picked up by electrodes and conducted into the machine through lead wires. An electrolyte assists in transmission of the heart's electrical impulses. An electrolyte consists of a chemical substance that promotes conduction of an electrical current.

❑ **An electrocardiograph** with a three-channel recording capability can record three leads simultaneously. An electrocardiograph with telephone transmission capabilities can transmit a recording over a telephone line to an ECG data interpretation site. An electrocardiograph with interpretive capabilities has a built-in computer program that analyzes the recording as it is being run.

❑ **Artifacts** represent additional electrical activity that is picked up by the electrocardiograph. A muscle artifact has a fuzzy, irregular baseline and is caused by voluntary and involuntary muscle movement. A wandering baseline artifact can be caused by electrodes that are too loose and by body creams, oils, or lotions on the skin. An alternating current artifact is caused by electrical interference and is characterized by small, straight spiked lines on the ECG. An interrupted baseline is caused by the metal tip of a lead wire becoming detached or by a broken patient cable.

❑ **Holter monitor electrocardiography** monitors and records the cardiac activity of a patient for 24 hours. It is used to evaluate patients with unexplained syncope, to discover intermittent cardiac dysrhythmias, and to assess the effectiveness of antiarrhythmic medications.

❑ **Normal sinus rhythm** refers to an ECG that is within normal limits. Cardiac abnormalities known as *dysrhythmias* include extra beats, an abnormal rhythm, and an abnormal heart rate. Cardiac dysrhythmias include atrial premature contraction, paroxysmal atrial tachycardia, atrial flutter, atrial fibrillation, premature ventricular contraction, ventricular tachycardia, and ventricular fibrillation.

❑ **The purpose of a pulmonary function test** is to assess lung functioning, assisting in the detection and evaluation of pulmonary disease. The most frequently performed pulmonary function test is spirometry; an instrument known as a *spirometer* is used to conduct the test. A spirometer measures how much air is pushed out of the lungs and how fast that occurs.

❑ **The most important parameters obtained from spirometry testing** are FVC, FEV_1, and the FEV_1/FVC ratio. The measured values are compared with the predicted values to detect the presence of pulmonary disease. To obtain accurate spirometry test results, it is essential that the following be performed: proper patient preparation, proper calibration of the spirometry machine, and correct performance of the breathing maneuver. Post-bronchodilator spirometry assists the physician in determining how treatment would work for patients with obstructive lung disease.

❑ **A peak flow meter** is used to measure how quickly air flows out of the lungs when the patient exhales forcefully. Peak flow meters are frequently used by patients with asthma. The peak flow rate (PFR) is the maximum volume of air measured in liters per minute that can be exhaled when the patient blows into a peak flow meter as forcefully and as rapidly as possible. A peak flow meter should be used on a regular schedule by patients with moderate to severe asthma to determine how well their asthma is being controlled.

❑ **Oxygen therapy** is the administration of supplemental oxygen at concentrations greater than room air to treat or prevent hypoxemia. Home oxygen therapy is most commonly prescribed for patients with severe COPD caused by smoking. Other common causes of hypoxemia that may require home oxygen therapy include asthma, occupational lung disease, lung cancer, cystic fibrosis, and congestive heart failure. The physician determines a patient's need for oxygen therapy through clinical observation of the patient and by measuring the oxygen level of the patient's blood. There are three common delivery systems for providing supplemental oxygen to a patient: compressed oxygen gas, liquid oxygen, and an oxygen concentrator. The most commonly used devices to administer home oxygen therapy are a nasal cannula and a face mask.

⟳ TERMINOLOGY REVIEW

Medical Term	Word Parts	Definition
Amplitude		Refers to amount, extent, size, abundance, or fullness.
Artifact		Additional electrical activity picked up by the electrocardiograph that interferes with the normal appearance of the ECG cycles.
Atherosclerosis	*ather/o-:* yellowish, fatty plaque *-sclerosis:* hardening of	Buildup of fibrous plaques of fatty deposits and cholesterol on the inner walls of an artery that causes narrowing, obstruction, and hardening of the artery.
Baseline		The flat horizontal line that separates the various waves of the ECG cycle.
Cardiac cycle	*cardi/o:* heart	One complete heartbeat.
Dysrhythmia	*dys-:* difficult, painful, abnormal *rhythm:* rhythm *-ia:* condition of diseased or abnormal state	An irregular heart rate or rhythm; also termed *arrhythmia.*
ECG cycle		The graphic representation of a heartbeat.
Electrocardiogram (ECG)	*electr/o-:* electrical, electrical activity *cardi/o:* heart *-gram:* record of	The graphic representation of the electrical activity of the heart.
Electrocardiograph	*electr/o-:* electrical, electrical activity *cardi/o:* heart *-graph:* instrument used to record	The instrument used to record the electrical activity of the heart.
Electrode	*electr/o-:* electrical, electrical activity	A conductor of electricity, which is used to promote contact between the body and the electrocardiograph.
Electrolyte	*electr/o-:* electrical, electrical activity	A chemical substance that promotes conduction of an electrical current.
Flow rate		The number of liters of oxygen per minute that come out of an oxygen delivery system.
Hypoxemia	*hypo-:* below, deficient *ox/i:* oxygen *-emia:* blood condition	A decrease in the oxygen saturation of the blood.
Hypoxia	*hypo-:* below, deficient *ox/i:* oxygen *-ia:* condition of diseased or abnormal state	A reduction in the oxygen supply to the tissues of the body.
Interval		The length of a wave or the length of a wave with a segment.
Ischemia	*isch/o-:* deficiency, blockage *-emia:* blood condition	Deficiency of blood in a body part.
Normal sinus rhythm		Refers to an ECG that is within normal limits.
Oxygen therapy		The administration of supplemental oxygen at concentrations greater than room air to treat or prevent hypoxemia
Peak flow rate		The maximum volume of air that can be exhaled when the patient blows into a peak flow meter as forcefully and as rapidly as possible.
Segment		The portion of the ECG between two waves.
Spirometer	*spir/o-:* breathe, breathing *-meter:* instrument used to measure	An instrument for measuring air taken into and expelled from the lungs.
Spirometry	*spir/o-:* breathe, breathing *-metry:* measurement	Measurement of an individual's breathing capacity by means of a spirometer.
Wheezing		A continuous, high-pitched whistling musical sound heard particularly during exhalation and sometimes during inhalation.

ON THE WEB

For Information on Heart Disease:

American Heart Association: www.americanheart.org

National Heart, Lung, and Blood Institute: www.nhlbi.nih.gov

American Association of Cardiovascular and Pulmonary Rehabilitation: www.aacvpr.org

My Heart Central: www.healthcentral.com/heart-disease

Cardiology Channel: www.cardiologychannel.com

American College of Cardiology: www.acc.org

The National Coalition for Women with Heart Disease: www.womenheart.org

For Information on Lung Disease:

American Lung Association: www.lungusa.org

Pulmonary Channel: www.pulmonarychannel.com

Lung Cancer Online: www.lungcanceronline.org

American Association for Respiratory Care: www.aarc.org

Emphysema: emphysema.org

For Information on Smoking Cessation:

Quit Net: www.quitnet.com

Smoking Cessation: www.smoking-cessation.org

National Center for Tobacco-free Kids: www.tobaccofreekids.org

Why Quit.com: www.whyquit.com

Quit Smoking Now: www.smokefree.gov

The Quit Smoking Company: www.quitsmoking.com

13

Colon Procedures and Male Reproductive Health

LEARNING OBJECTIVES

Fecal Occult Blood Testing

1. Explain the purpose of a fecal occult blood test.

2. Describe the patient preparation for fecal occult blood testing (guaiac slide method).
3. Explain the purpose of each type of preparation for fecal occult blood testing (guaiac slide method).

Sigmoidoscopy

1. Explain the purpose of a digital rectal examination before a sigmoidoscopic examination.
2. Explain the purpose of a sigmoidoscopy.
3. Describe the patient preparation for a sigmoidoscopy.

Colonoscopy

1. Explain the purpose of a colonoscopy.

2. List the conditions that can be detected and assessed during a colonoscopy.
3. Describe the patient preparation for a colonoscopy.

Male Reproductive Health

1. List the symptoms of prostate cancer.
2. Explain the purpose of the digital rectal examination (DRE).
3. Explain the purpose of the prostate-specific antigen (PSA) test.
4. State the risk factors for testicular cancer.

5. Describe the TSE schedule.

PROCEDURES

Instruct a patient in the preparation and procedure for a fecal occult blood test (guaiac slide test).
Develop a fecal occult blood test.

Instruct a patient in the preparation required for a sigmoidoscopy.
Assist the physician with sigmoidoscopy.

Instruct a patient in the preparation required for a colonoscopy.

Assist the physician with a digital rectal examination.
Instruct a patient in the preparation for a PSA test.

Teach a patient how to perform a testicular self-examination (TSE).

CHAPTER OUTLINE

Introduction to Colon Procedures
Structure of the Large Intestine
Blood in the Stool
Fecal Occult Blood Test
  Guaiac Slide Test
  Quality Control

Other Types of Stool Tests
  Fecal Immunochemical Test
  Fecal DNA Test
Sigmoidoscopy
  Purpose
  Patient Preparation for Sigmoidoscopy

KEY TERMS

biopsy (BIE-op-see)
colonoscope (KOL-un-oh-skope)
colonoscopy (KOL-un-OS-koe-pee)
endoscope (EN-doe-skope)
insufflate (IN-suf-flate)

melena (ma-LEE-na)
occult (ah-KULT) blood
peroxidase (per-OKS-ih-dase)
sigmoidoscope (sig-MOYD-oh-skope)
sigmoidoscopy (sig-moyd-OS-koe-pee)

Introduction to Colon Procedures

Colon procedures are performed in the medical office or clinic and include the fecal occult blood test (FOBT), sigmoidoscopy, and sometimes colonoscopy, which are presented in this chapter. The FOBT is a screening test used to detect blood in the stool for the early detection of colorectal cancer. Stool specimens must be collected by the patient at home. Some patients initially may be reluctant to comply with the FOBT patient preparation requirements and collection of the stool specimens. The medical assistant can help by explaining the purpose of the test to the patient. If the patient understands the benefits to be derived from the test, he or she is more likely to participate as required.

Medical assistants are often responsible for explaining to a patient the preparation required for a sigmoidoscopy and colonoscopy. The medical assistant should make sure the patient thoroughly understands the instructions. If the patient does not prepare properly, the procedure must be cancelled, which requires the patient to go through the preparation procedure again. The medical assistant assists the physician during a sigmoidoscopy, and he or she should have a thorough knowledge of the responsibilities accompanying this procedure.

STRUCTURE OF THE LARGE INTESTINE

The medical assistant should be familiar with the structure of the large intestine. The large intestine is divided into three parts, which include the *cecum, colon, and rectum* (Figure 13-1). The *cecum* is the first part of the large intestine. It consists of a blind pouch to which the appendix is attached.

The cecum leads into the ascending colon and joins with the *ileum,* which is the last part of the small intestine.

The colon makes up most of the large intestine. It averages 60 inches in length and is divided into four sections, which include the *ascending colon,* the *transverse colon,* the *descending colon,* and the *sigmoid colon.* The sigmoid colon is identified by its S-shaped curve and connects the descending colon with the rectum. The *rectum* is located between the colon and the anus. The anus contains sphincter muscles and opens to the outside as a means of expelling waste from the body.

The primary functions of the large intestine include absorption of water and preparation of fecal material for elimination. Mucus is secreted from glands embedded in the intestinal wall (mucosa) of the large intestine. The mucus binds the fecal material together and protects the wall of the large intestine from the irritating effects of substances moving through it.

BLOOD IN THE STOOL

Blood in the stool can indicate a number of gastrointestinal conditions, including hemorrhoids, diverticulitis, polyps, colitis, upper gastrointestinal ulcers, and colorectal cancer. Some of these conditions (e.g., hemorrhoids) produce visible red blood on the outside of the stool, making it easy to detect. Blood entering the stool in an amount of 50 ml or greater from conditions affecting the upper gastrointestinal tract (e.g., peptic ulcers) causes the stool to exhibit **melena**, meaning it is black and tarlike. The dark color is a result of oxidation of the iron in the blood (heme) by intestinal and bacterial enzymes. If a minute quantity of blood is present, however, it is not possible to detect it with the unaided eye.

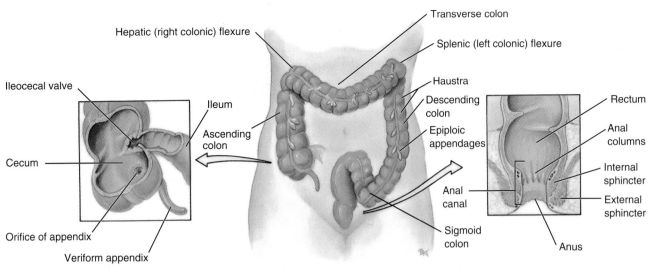

Figure 13-1. Large intestine. (From Applegate E: The anatomy and physiology learning system, ed 3, St Louis, 2006, Saunders.)

This hidden, or nonvisible, blood is termed **occult blood**, and its presence can be determined by testing the stool for blood.

Colorectal cancer is one of the most common forms of cancer in individuals older than the age of 50 years (see *Highlight on Colorectal Cancer*). During the early asymptomatic stages, almost all lesions (e.g., benign and malignant tumors) of the colon and rectum bleed a small amount on an intermittent basis, and this is usually in the form of occult blood. Discovery of occult blood in the stool does not mean that a patient has colorectal cancer. It does, however, warrant further diagnostic procedures, such as a colonoscopy, to determine if colorectal cancer is present. Early diagnosis and treatment of colorectal cancer increase the patient's survival rate. In most cases, when more pronounced symptoms of colorectal cancer start to appear (e.g., visible bleeding from the rectum, a change in bowel habits, abdominal pain), the cancer has reached an advanced stage.

FECAL OCCULT BLOOD TEST

Guaiac Slide Test

Routine screening of stool specimens for occult blood is frequently performed in the medical office. The guaiac slide test is a chemical test used to screen for fecal occult blood and is discussed in detail in this chapter. This test is commercially available with the brand names of Hemoccult, ColoScreen (Figure 13-2), and Seracult.

Fecal blood loss greater than 5 ml per day results in a positive reaction on a guaiac slide test. Individuals normally may lose up to 3 ml per day of blood in the feces, owing to minor insignificant abrasions of the nasopharynx and gastrointestinal tract, such as from brushing the teeth. To allow for normal blood loss, the guaiac slide test does not show a positive reaction until the blood in the stool reaches a level of 5 ml (or more) per day.

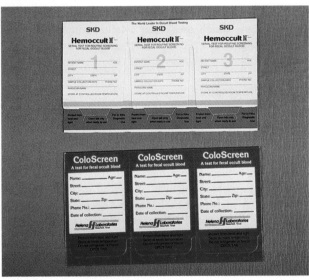

Figure 13-2. Examples of fecal occult blood testing kits. Hemoccult *(top)* and ColoScreen *(bottom)*.

The guaiac slide test is a simple and inexpensive method to screen for the presence of fecal occult blood; however, care must be taken to reduce the occurrence of false-positive and false-negative test results. This test is designed to assess the presence of blood in stool specimens collected from three bowel movements on three different days. The purpose of using three specimens is to provide for the detection of blood from gastrointestinal lesions that exhibit intermittent bleeding, meaning they do not bleed every day. The patient must collect the three specimens at home and return the prepared slides to the medical office for developing. The medical assistant is responsible for providing the patient with instructions on patient preparation and collection and proper care and storage of the slides until they are returned to the medical office.

Purpose

The primary use of the guaiac slide test is to screen for the presence of occult blood caused by colorectal cancer. Other conditions that can cause blood in the stool include the following:

- Hemorrhoids
- Anal fissures
- Colorectal polyps
- Diverticulitis
- Peptic ulcers
- Ulcerative colitis
- Gastroesophageal reflux disease (GERD)
- Crohn's disease

A positive test result on the guaiac slide test indicates only the presence of blood in the stool; the source and cause of the bleeding must still be determined. This means that additional diagnostic procedures must be performed before the physician can make a final diagnosis. These procedures may include colonoscopy, sigmoidoscopy, a double-contrast barium enema radiographic study, computed tomography (CT) colonography, and a newer procedure known as *capsule endoscopy*, which uses a tiny wireless camera (that the patient swallows as a pill) to take photographs of the digestive tract.

Patient Preparation

Patient preparation for a guaiac slide test plays an important role in ensuring accurate test results. The patient must follow a special diet, beginning 3 days before the test, and must continue the diet until all three slides have been prepared. The patient is placed on a high-fiber, meat-free diet. Meat contains animal blood, which could lead to a false-positive test result. A high-fiber diet is used because it encourages bleeding from lesions that may bleed only occasionally. In addition, fiber adds bulk, which promotes bowel elimination and ensures adequate specimen collection.

Certain medications irritate the gastrointestinal tract, which may result in a small amount of bleeding, and thus could result in a false-positive result on the guaiac slide test. Medications that should be avoided include ibuprofen (Motrin, Advil), naproxen (Aleve), and more than one adult aspirin per day. In addition, an iron supplement may cause a false-positive result, and a vitamin C supplement (greater than 250 mg per day) can cause a false-negative result. All of these substances should be discontinued before testing. Table 13-1 lists the specific patient preparation requirements for fecal occult blood testing using the guaiac slide test.

Quality Control

Quality control methods must be employed with the guaiac slide test to ensure reliable and valid results. It is important to properly store the box containing the guaiac slides and developing solution. Adverse storage conditions can result in deterioration of the developing solution and the active reagents impregnated on the filter paper of the slides, leading to inaccurate test results. The box must be stored at a room temperature between 59° F (15° C) and 86° F (30° C). The contents of the box must be protected from heat, sunlight, and strong fluorescent light. In addition, the box should not be stored in close proximity to volatile chemicals such as ammonia, bleach, bromine, iodine, and disinfectant cleaners. If stored properly, the slides and developer will remain effective until the expiration date that is stamped on the side of the box, each slide itself, and the container of developing solution.

A quality control procedure must be performed *after* the patient's test has been developed, read, and interpreted. This ensures that the test results are accurate and valid. The Hemoccult slide test contains an on-slide performance monitor that consists of positive and negative monitor areas. This monitor is located on the developing side of the filter paper under the back flap of the cardboard slide. The positive

Table 13-1 Patient Preparation for the Fecal Occult Guaiac Slide Test

Dietary and Medication Guidelines:
Beginning 3 days before obtaining the first stool specimen, the patient should follow certain diet and medication modifications. These modifications should be followed until all three slides have been prepared.

Meats	Eat no red or rare meat (beef and lamb) or liver. Small amounts of well-cooked pork, poultry, and fish are permitted. Red meat contains animal blood that could cause a false-positive test result.
Vegetables	Eat moderate amounts of raw and cooked vegetables. Especially advised are lettuce, spinach, corn, and celery. Do not consume horseradish, turnips, broccoli, cauliflower, and radishes. These foods contain peroxidase, which sometimes can cause a false-positive test result.
Fruits	Eat moderate amounts of apples, bananas, oranges, peaches, pears, and plums. Avoid vitamin C in excess of 250 mg a day from citrus fruits and juices. Do not consume melons, because they contain peroxidase.
Miscellaneous High-Fiber Foods	Eat moderate amounts of whole-wheat bread, bran cereal, and popcorn. Foods high in fiber provide roughage to promote bowel elimination and encourage bleeding from "silent" lesions that bleed only occasionally.
Medications	Do not take medications or vitamin supplements that contain iron or vitamin C in excess of 250 mg for 3 days before and during the collection period. In addition, based on the patient's medication therapy, the physician may stipulate additional medication restrictions. Certain medications cause irritation of the gastrointestinal tract, which may result in a small amount of bleeding. Nonsteroidal anti-inflammatory drugs (NSAIDs) and more than one adult aspirin a day should be avoided for at least 7 days before and continuing through the test period. Examples of NSAIDs include ibuprofen (Advil, Motrin) and naproxen (Aleve). Acetaminophen (Tylenol) can be taken as needed.
Special Guidelines	Inform the physician, and do not consume any of the food items listed previously if you know, from past experience, that they cause you severe gastrointestinal discomfort or serious diarrhea. Ensure that the diet modifications have been followed for 3 days before collecting the first stool specimen. Do not initiate the test during a menstrual period or in the first 3 days after a menstrual period. The test should not be conducted when blood is visible in the stool or urine, such as from bleeding from hemorrhoids or a urinary tract infection. These conditions would result in false-positive test results. Store the slides with the flaps in a closed position at room temperature, and protect them from heat, sunlight, and fluorescent light. The slides must also be stored away from volatile chemicals such as ammonia, bleach, and other household cleaners. Improper storage can result in deterioration of the active reagents on the slides, leading to inaccurate test results.

monitor area contains a control chemical that has been impregnated into the filter paper during the manufacturing process.

The medical assistant should apply 1 drop of the developing solution between the positive and negative performance monitor areas on each of the three slides. The results must be read within 10 seconds after application of the developer. If the slides and developer are functioning properly, the positive area turns blue, whereas the negative area shows no color change. Failure of the expected control results to occur indicates an error, and the test results are not considered valid; possible causes include the use of outdated slides or developing solution; an error in technique; and subjection of the slides to heat, sunlight, strong fluorescent light, or volatile chemicals. Procedure 13-1 outlines the medical assistant's responsibilities related to fecal occult blood testing using the Hemoccult guaiac slide test. Procedure 13-2 describes the development of a Hemoccult slide test.

What Would You Do? What Would You *Not* Do?

Case Study 1
Beatrice Bernard is 52 years old and has come to the office for a physical examination. The physician wants Mrs. Bernard to perform a Hemoccult test. After being told the purpose of the test and how to prepare for it, Mrs. Bernard expresses some concerns. She does not like the idea of what she has to do to perform the test because it does not seem sanitary to her. She also thinks it will be a lot of work to prepare for the test. She has red meat for dinner at least four times a week, and she does not understand why she has to eliminate it from her meals. She says she takes a baby aspirin every day for "heart health" and would prefer not to stop taking it. Mrs. Bernard says that she has always taken very good care of herself, and she has never had problems with her colon. She also says no history of colon cancer has been reported in her family. Mrs. Bernard is too embarrassed to talk about this topic with the physician. She says she may just throw the test away when she gets home. ■

Highlight on Colorectal Cancer

Incidence

Colorectal cancer is used to describe both cancer of the colon and cancer of the rectum. Based on what area is affected, these cancers are often referred to separately as colon cancer (see illustration below) and rectal cancer. Colorectal cancer is the third leading cause of cancer-related deaths in the United States for both men and women.

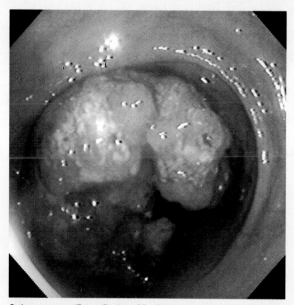

Colon cancer. (From Forbes CD: Color atlas and text of clinical medicine, ed 3, Philadelphia, 2003, Mosby.)

According to the American Cancer Society, every year approximately 150,000 people are diagnosed with colorectal cancer, and approximately 50,000 people die every year from this disease. As the U.S. population of baby boomers ages, these numbers may increase.

Risk Factors

The following factors increase the risk of developing colorectal cancer:

- *Age.* The risk of colorectal cancer increases significantly after 50 years of age and reaches a peak from ages 60 to 75 years. More than 90% of individuals diagnosed with colorectal cancer are older than 50 years of age.
- *Colorectal polyps.* A colorectal *polyp* is a grapelike growth that protrudes from the inner lining (mucosa) of the colon or rectum (see Figure 13-6). Individuals with large polyps or numerous polyps are particularly at risk for colorectal cancer. Most cases of colorectal cancer arise from *adenomatous* polyps that gradually become malignant over many years. Colorectal polyps are fairly common in individuals older than 50 years of age. Approximately 1 in 20 colorectal polyps can become cancerous if not removed.
- *Personal history of colorectal cancer.* Individuals who have been diagnosed previously with colorectal cancer are at higher risk for developing it in other parts of the colon and rectum, even if it was completely removed.
- History of inflammatory bowel disease of long duration, such as ulcerative colitis and Crohn's disease
- Strong family history of colorectal cancer

OTHER TYPES OF STOOL TESTS

Two types of newer tests are now available to screen for colorectal cancer. They include the fecal immunochemical test and the fecal DNA test.

Fecal Immunochemical Test

The fecal immunochemical test (FIT) is a fecal occult blood test that uses antibodies to detect blood in the stool. Examples of brand names for this test are Hemoccult ICT and QuickVue iFOB (Figure 13-3). The stool specimen for an FIT is collected by the patient at home in a similar manner to the guaiac slide test. Although the FIT is more expensive than the guaiac slide test, it is more sensitive to the presence of lower gastrointestinal (GI) bleeding than is the guaiac test. This test is not affected by drugs or food and therefore does not require medication or dietary restrictions. In addition, FIT has fewer false-positive test results than the guaiac slide test. When a fecal occult blood test is positive, the patient must undergo a colonoscopy. Reducing the number of false-positive test results, in turn, reduces the number of unnecessary colonoscopies that are performed.

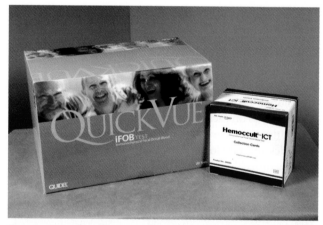

Figure 13-3. Fecal immunochemical tests: QuickVue iFOB *(left)* Hemoccult ICT *(right)*.

Fecal DNA Test

A fecal DNA test (PreGen Plus) was recently developed, and its advantages and disadvantages are still being investigated. This test uses DNA technology to detect abnormal

Highlight on Colorectal Cancer—cont'd

- Known family history of hereditary colorectal cancer syndromes such as familial adenomatous polyposis (FAP) or hereditary nonpolyposis colon cancer (HNPCC)
- Other factors that have been associated with a higher incidence of colorectal cancer include smoking; heavy alcohol consumption; obesity; a diet high in fat, red meat, and processed meats (e.g., hot dogs, luncheon meats); low intake of fresh fruits and vegetables; and physical inactivity.

Symptoms

No or very few symptoms occur during the early stages of colorectal cancer. If colorectal cancer is detected and treated while the patient is still asymptomatic, the patient has a 90% chance of 5-year survival. By comparison, the 5-year survival rate for patients in whom colorectal cancer is diagnosed after symptoms appear is only 40%, and the 5-year survival rate when the cancer has spread to distant organs (metastasized) such as the liver or lungs is only 11%.

Symptoms that occur when colorectal cancer is more developed include the following:
- Bleeding from the rectum
- Blood in the stool
- A change in the shape of the stool (e.g., stools that are narrower than usual)
- A change in bowel habits (e.g., diarrhea, constipation)
- General abdominal discomfort (e.g., aches, pains, cramps)
- Unexplained weight loss
- Constant fatigue

Recommendations for Early Detection

For the early prevention and detection of colorectal cancer, the American Cancer Society recommends that all adults 50 years old and older who are at average risk for colorectal cancer be screened using one of the screening tests listed below. Tests that detect both polyps and cancer are preferred over those tests that detect just cancer. Individuals with risk factors for colorectal cancer should be screened at an earlier age and with greater frequency. For example, an individual who has a family history of colorectal cancer should begin colorectal cancer screening at 40 years of age.

Tests that detect both polyps and cancer include the following:
- Sigmoidoscopy: every 5 years*
- Colonoscopy: every 10 years
- Double-contrast barium enema: every 5 years*
- CT colonography (virtual colonoscopy): every 5 years*

Tests that detect cancer only include these:
- Fecal occult blood test: every year*
- Fecal immunochemical test: every year*
- Fecal DNA test: interval uncertain*

Cause

The cause of colorectal cancer is unknown, but studies have shown a higher incidence of this disease in countries, such as the United States, whose populations have a diet that is high in meat and animal fat and low in fiber. This finding is supported by the fact that in countries such as Japan, in which the diet is high in fiber and low in fat, the incidence of colorectal cancer is much lower. ∎

*Colonoscopy should be performed if test results are positive.

cells that are shed into the stool from cancerous growths or colorectal polyps. The fecal DNA test is much more expensive than other forms of stool testing. No special preparation is needed for this test. The patient is required to collect an entire stool sample in a special container. The container and an ice pack are then placed in a shipping box and mailed to a laboratory within 24 hours after collection. When a fecal DNA test is positive, the patient must undergo a colonoscopy.

PROCEDURE 13-1 Fecal Occult Blood Testing: Guaiac Slide Test

Outcome Instruct a patient in specimen collection for a Hemoccult guaiac slide test.

Equipment/Supplies

- Hemoccult slide testing kit

1. Procedural Step. Obtain a Hemoccult testing kit. Check the expiration date on the slides.
Principle. Outdated slides can lead to inaccurate test results.

2. Procedural Step. Greet the patient and introduce yourself. Identify the patient and explain the purpose of the test. Tell the patient that the test should not be conducted during a menstrual period or when hemorrhoids are bleeding or a urinary tract infection is present.
Principle. Bleeding from other (identifiable) sources causes a false-positive test result.

3. Procedural Step. Instruct the patient in proper preparation for the test. See the box *Highlight on Colorectal Cancer* for the specific guidelines the patient should follow. Tell the patient to begin the diet

Continued

PROCEDURE 13-1   Fecal Occult Blood Testing: Guaiac Slide Test—cont'd

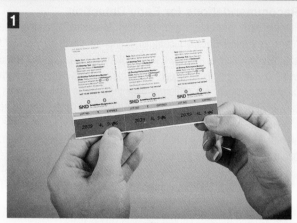

Check the expiration date.

modifications 3 days before collecting the first stool specimen. Encourage the patient to adhere to the diet modifications.

Principle. The diet modifications may discourage patient compliance. The medical assistant should reinforce the importance of adhering to the diet requirements. Improper patient preparation can lead to inaccurate test results.

4. Procedural Step. Provide the patient with the Hemoccult testing kit. The kit consists of three identical cardboard slides attached to one another; each slide contains two squares, labeled "A" and "B." Three wooden applicator sticks and written instructions also are included in the testing kit.

Principle. Three slides are provided so that three stool specimens can be collected. The two squares in

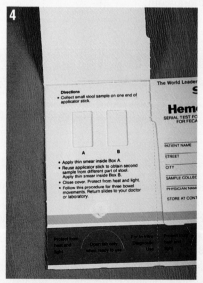

Each slide contains two squares labeled "A" and "B."

each slide (A and B) contain filter paper impregnated with guaiac, a chemical necessary for detection of blood in the stool.

5. Procedural Step. Instruct the patient on completion of the information required on the front flap of each card. This includes the patient's name, address, phone number, and age and the date of the specimen collection. A ballpoint pen should be used to write this information.

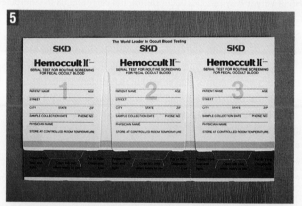

Instruct the patient on how to complete the information section on the slides.

6. Procedural Step. Provide instructions on proper care and storage of the slides. Make it clear that the slides must be stored (with the flaps in a closed position) at room temperature and protected from heat, sunlight, strong fluorescent light, and volatile chemicals.

Principle. Adverse storage conditions can result in deterioration of the active reagents impregnated on the filter paper, leading to inaccurate test results.

7. Procedural Step. Instruct the patient on initiation of the test by telling him or her to begin the diet modifications and then to collect a stool specimen from the first bowel movement after the 3-day preparatory period.

8. Procedural Step. Instruct the patient on proper collection of the stool specimen:

a. Fill in the sample collection date on the front flap of the first cardboard slide.

b. Use a clean, dry container to collect the stool sample. The sample must be collected before it comes in contact with toilet bowl water. Allow the stool to fall into the collection container.

c. Use one of the wooden applicators to obtain a specimen from one part of the stool sample.

d. Open the front flap of the first cardboard slide (located on the left in the series of three).

e. Spread a very thin smear of the specimen over the filter paper in the square labeled "A."

PROCEDURE 13-1   Fecal Occult Blood Testing: Guaiac Slide Test—cont'd

f. Using the same wooden applicator, obtain another specimen from a different area of the stool.

g. Spread a thin smear of the specimen over the filter paper in the square labeled "B."

h. Close the front flap of the cardboard slide.

i. Discard the wooden applicator in a waste container. Do not flush it down the toilet.

j. Place the slides in a regular paper envelope to air-dry overnight.

Principle. Two squares are included in each slide to allow specimen collection from different parts of the stool because occult blood is not always uniformly distributed throughout the stool. Thick specimens prevent adequate light penetration through the filter paper, making it difficult to interpret the test results.

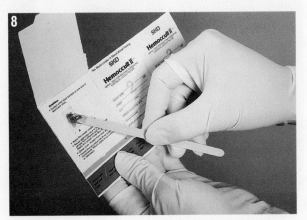

Spread a thin smear of the specimen over the filter paper.

9. **Procedural Step.** Instruct the patient to continue the testing period on 3 different days until all three specimens have been obtained as follows.

a. Repeat Procedural Step 8 after the second bowel movement the next day. If you do not have a bowel movement on the next day, then collect the specimen on the following day. The specimens should be collected on 3 different days. Use the cardboard slide located in the middle of the series of three.

b. Repeat Procedural Step 8 after the third bowel movement, using the cardboard slide located to the right in the series of three.

c. Allow the completed slides to air-dry overnight in the paper envelope.

10. **Procedural Step.** Instruct the patient to place the cardboard slides in the envelope lined with foil, seal carefully, and return them as soon as possible to the medical office. Emphasize to the patient that only the foil-lined envelope can be used to mail the slides; a standard envelope cannot be used. Inform the patient that the slides must be returned no later than 14 days after the first specimen is collected.

Principle. Standard paper envelopes are not approved by U.S. postal regulations for mailing fecal occult blood testing slides. Slides should not be developed after 14 days, as the test results may not be accurate.

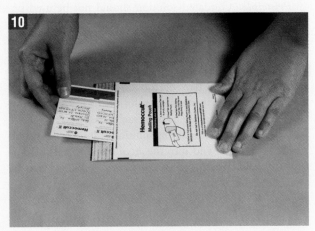

Place the cardboard slides in the envelope.

11. **Procedural Step.** Give the patient an opportunity to ask questions; ensure that the patient understands the instructions for patient preparation and collection of the stool specimen and for storage of the slides.

Principle. Improper patient preparation and poor collection technique can lead to inaccurate test results.

12. **Procedural Step.** Record in the patient's chart. Include the date and documentation that the Hemoccult test and instructions were given to the patient.

Note: The ColoScreen and Seracult guaiac slide tests use a procedure similar to that of the Hemoccult test.

PROCEDURE 13-1

PROCEDURE 13-2   Developing the Hemoccult Slide Test

Outcome Develop a Hemoccult slide test.

Equipment/Supplies

- Disposable gloves
- Prepared cardboard slides
- Hemoccult developing solution
- Waste container

1. Procedural Step. Assemble the equipment. Check the expiration date on the developing solution bottle. The developing solution contains hydrogen peroxide and must be stored away from heat and light. It must be tightly capped when not in use.

Principle. Outdated solution should not be used because it can lead to inaccurate test results. The solution should be stored properly because it is flammable and evaporates easily.

2. Procedural Step. Sanitize your hands and apply gloves. Open the back flap of the cardboard slides. Apply 2 drops of the developing solution to the guaiac test paper underlying the back of each smear.

Principle. The developing solution is absorbed through the filter paper and into the stool specimen. This solution could irritate the skin and eyes; if contact occurs, immediately rinse the area with water.

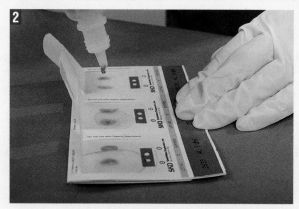

Apply 2 drops of developing solution.

3. Procedural Step. Read the results within 60 seconds. Fecal blood loss greater than 5 ml per day results in a positive reaction, which is indicated by any trace of blue on or at the edge of the fecal smear. If no detectable color change occurs, the result is considered negative.

Principle. In the presence of hydrogen peroxide, the heme compound in hemoglobin oxidizes guaiac, causing it to turn blue within 60 seconds after the developer is added. The reading time is important because the color reaction may fade after 2 to 4 minutes.

4. Procedural Step. Perform the quality control procedure as follows:

a. Apply 1 drop of developing solution between the positive and negative control performance indicators on each of the three slides.

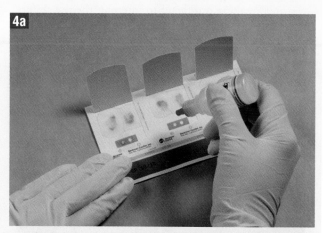

Apply 1 drop of developing solution to the control area.

b. Read the results within 10 seconds.

c. The positive area should turn blue and the negative area should show no color change. Failure of the expected control results to occur indicates an error and that the test results are invalid.

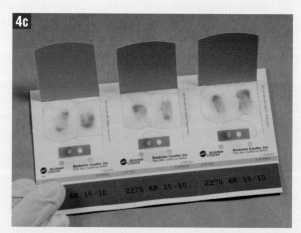

The positive area should turn blue, and the negative area should show no color change.

PROCEDURE 13-2 Developing the Hemoccult Slide Test—cont'd

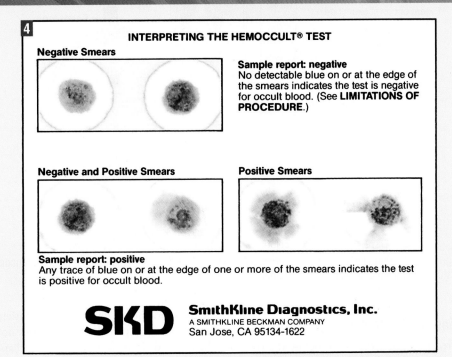

INTERPRETING THE HEMOCCULT® TEST

Negative Smears

Sample report: negative
No detectable blue on or at the edge of the smears indicates the test is negative for occult blood. (See **LIMITATIONS OF PROCEDURE**.)

Negative and Positive Smears

Positive Smears

Sample report: positive
Any trace of blue on or at the edge of one or more of the smears indicates the test is positive for occult blood.

SKD **SmithKline Diagnostics, Inc.**
A SMITHKLINE BECKMAN COMPANY
San Jose, CA 95134-1622

Principle. The quality control procedure must be performed after developing, reading, and interpreting the slides. Quality control procedures ensure the accuracy and reliability of the test results.

5. **Procedural Step.** Properly dispose of the Hemoccult slides in a regular waste container.

Principle. Fecal material is not considered regulated medical waste and can be discarded in a regular waste container.

6. **Procedural Step.** Remove gloves and sanitize your hands. Chart the results. Include the date and time, the brand name of the test (Hemoccult), and the test results for each slide (recorded as positive or negative).

CHARTING EXAMPLE	
Date	
9/08/12	9:00 a.m. Pt provided with a Hemoccult test and instructions for the procedure.
	———————————— M. Baer, CMA (AAMA)
9/14/12	10:30 a.m. Hemoccult test:
	Slide 1: Negative
	Slide 2: Negative
	Slide 3: Negative
	———————————— M. Baer, CMA (AAMA)

SIGMOIDOSCOPY

Sigmoidoscopy is the visual examination of the mucosa of the rectum and the lower third of the colon using a flexible fiberoptic **sigmoidoscope** (Figure 13-4). Before a patient undergoes a sigmoidoscopy, the physician explains the nature of the procedure and any risks to the patient and offers to answer questions. The medical assistant is responsible for obtaining the patient's signature on a written consent to treatment form, which grants the physician permission to perform the procedure.

Purpose

Sigmoidoscopy may be performed following a positive fecal occult blood test to determine the source and cause of the bleeding. It is also performed to evaluate patient symptoms related to the colon such as lower abdominal pain, diarrhea, or constipation. Conditions that can be detected and assessed during a sigmoidoscopy include lesions (benign or malignant tumors), polyps, hemorrhoids, fissures, infection, and inflammation. It is especially valuable as a diagnostic procedure for detecting inflammatory bowel disease such as ulcerative colitis and Crohn's disease.

A sigmoidoscopy has certain limitations. Because a sigmoidoscopy reaches only the lower third of the colon, the physician may not be able to determine the cause of the patient's symptoms or bleeding. In this situation, the physician may order a colonoscopy to be performed at a later date. If the sigmoidoscopy detects the presence of a precancerous polyp or colorectal cancer, a colonoscopy must be performed for means of detecting additional polyps or cancer that may be present in the rest of the colon.

PROCEDURE 13-2

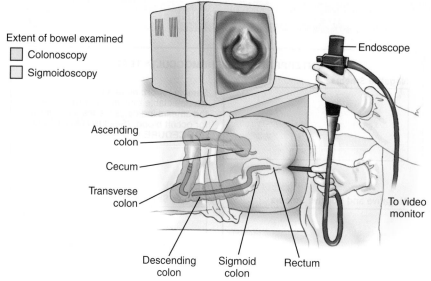

Figure 13-4. Sigmoidoscopy and colonoscopy. (From Lafleur Brooks M: Exploring medical language: A student-directed approach, ed 7, St Louis, 2009, Mosby.)

Patient Preparation for Sigmoidoscopy

The patient is required to prepare the colon before the sigmoidoscopy. The lower third of the colon must be flushed out completely, so that it is empty and free of fecal material; this is known as a *partial bowel prep* because only a portion of the colon needs to be prepared. Bowel preparation is one of the most important parts of the sigmoidoscopy. Fecal material can interfere with good visualization of the wall of the colon, making it difficult for the physician to detect abnormalities.

The medical assistant is responsible for providing the patient with instructions on preparing the colon. The medi-

cal assistant should encourage the patient to follow the instructions exactly. If the patient does not prepare properly, the sigmoidoscopy is usually cancelled and must be rescheduled, which requires the patient to go through the bowel preparation procedure again. The patient preparation instructions may vary slightly from one facility to another. General patient preparation recommendations for a sigmoidoscopy are outlined in Table 13-2.

Digital Rectal Examination

A digital examination of the anal canal and rectum is performed before a sigmoidoscopy. Using a well-lubricated, gloved index finger, the physician palpates the rectum for

Table 13-2 Patient Preparation for Sigmoidoscopy	
It is important to follow the patient preparation requirements as carefully as possible to ensure accurate results. The following preparation is required for a sigmoidoscopy:	
Beginning 5 days before the procedure	Discontinue taking iron, aspirin, and aspirin products. Iron can alter the color of the wall of the colon, and aspirin may cause bleeding if a polyp is removed from the colon.
Beginning 2 days before the procedure	Discontinue taking nonsteroidal anti-inflammatory drugs such as ibuprofen and naproxen to minimize the risk of bleeding if a polyp is removed.
Medication restrictions	The physician will advise the patient of any other medication restrictions that need to be followed.
The day before the procedure and continuing until your examination is completed	a. Do not consume any solid food or milk products. b. Consume only gelatin (Jell-O) or popsicles (except purple or red, which could be mistaken for blood in the colon). c. Drink only clear liquids (water, apple juice, sport drinks [e.g., Gatorade], soft drinks, clear broth). Do not drink alcohol. d. Coffee or tea is permitted with no milk or cream.
The evening before the procedure	a. Drink the following laxative between 5 and 7 PM: one 10-ounce bottle of magnesium citrate. b. Continue drinking plenty of clear liquids throughout the evening.
The day of the procedure	a. You may continue drinking clear liquids until 4 hours before the procedure. b. Two hours before the examination: Insert one Fleet's enema rectally by following the package instructions. One hour before the procedure: Insert another Fleet's enema.

the presence of tenderness, hemorrhoids, polyps, and tumors. Any palpable abnormality is viewed directly when the endoscope is inserted. An **endoscope** is an instrument (e.g., sigmoidoscope, colonoscope) that consists of a tube and an optical system that is used for direct visual inspection of organs or cavities. The digital examination also helps relax the sphincter muscles of the anus and prepares the patient for the insertion of the endoscope.

Sigmoidoscope

A flexible fiberoptic sigmoidoscope consists of a control head and a long flexible insertion tube attached to a light source (Figure 13-5). The insertion tube is ½ inch (1.3 cm) in diameter and 24 inches (60 cm) long, which allows the physician to view approximately one third of the colon, which includes the rectum and sigmoid colon.

The sigmoidoscope is composed of extremely thin fibers of bendable glass that transmit light and images of the colon back to the physician. The image, magnified ten times by the fiberoptic system, is viewed by the physician through the eye lens located in the handle of the sigmoidoscope. Alternatively, the sigmoidoscope may have a videocamera attached to the distal end of the flexible insertion tube, which permits the physician to view images of the colon and rectum on a display screen (see Figure 13-4).

Procedure

When the sigmoidoscopy is performed, the patient is placed on his or her left side in the Sims position. The distal end of the sigmoidoscope is lubricated and inserted into the anus and rectum and then slowly advanced into the colon until it reaches the sigmoid colon. A small amount of air is usually blown, or **insufflated**, into the colon through tub-

ing attached to the air control valve located on the head of the sigmoidoscope. The function of the air is to distend the lumen of the colon for better visualization. In addition, suction equipment can be used to remove secretions, such as mucus, blood, and liquid feces, which interfere with proper visualization of the intestinal mucosa. The physician then slowly withdraws the sigmoidoscope while carefully observing the mucosa of the colon for abnormalities.

If the physician discovers an abnormal lesion during the examination, a long thin instrument is passed through the lumen of the insertion tube to remove a specimen for **biopsy**. In addition, if a suspicious-looking polyp is discovered, the physician may remove it (polypectomy) or take a biopsy of it for analysis by the laboratory. Removal of a precancerous polyp prevents it from developing into colon cancer in the future (see *Highlight on Colorectal Cancer*). Procedure 13-3 outlines the medical assistant's role during a sigmoidoscopy.

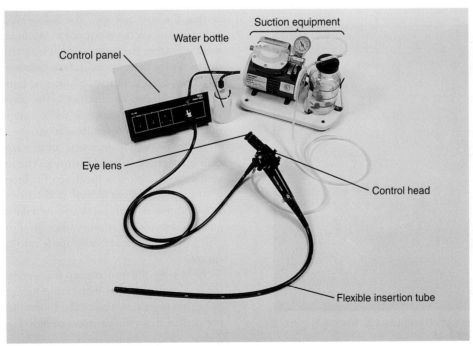

Figure 13-5. Flexible fiberoptic sigmoidoscope.

COLONOSCOPY

A **colonoscopy** is the visual examination of the mucosa of the rectum and the entire length of the colon (sigmoid colon, descending colon, transverse colon, and ascending colon) using a flexible fiberoptic **colonoscope**. A colonoscope is basically a sigmoidoscope but with a longer insertion tube. The colonoscope has a videocamera attached to the distal end of the flexible insertion tube. The camera transmits images of the colon to a video screen for viewing by the physician (see Figure 13-4).

Before a patient undergoes a colonoscopy, the physician explains the nature of the procedure and any risks to the patient and offers to answer questions. The medical assistant may be responsible for obtaining the patient's signature on a written consent to treatment form, which grants the physician permission to perform the procedure.

Purpose

Colonoscopy is often performed following a positive fecal occult blood test to determine the source and cause of the bleeding. It is also performed to evaluate patient symptoms related to the colon such as lower abdominal pain. Colonoscopy is considered the "gold standard" for assessing abnormalities of the colon. Conditions that can be detected and assessed during a colonoscopy include the following:

- Lesions of the colon or rectum (e.g., benign or malignant growths)
- Colorectal polyps (Figure 13-6)
- Hemorrhoids
- Fissures
- Infection and inflammation

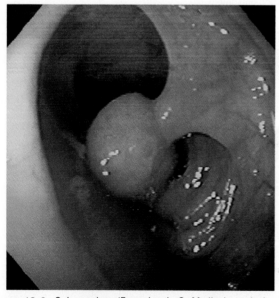

Figure 13-6. Colon polyp. (From Lewis S: Medical-surgical nursing, ed 7, St Louis, 2007, Mosby.)

Colonoscopy is particularly valuable for the early detection of symptomatic and asymptomatic colorectal cancer. Early detection of colorectal cancer leads to early diagnosis and treatment, which increases the chance of survival for patients with this disease.

Patient Preparation for Colonoscopy

A colonoscopy is usually performed in a hospital on an outpatient basis or in a large medical clinic. The rectum and the entire colon must be flushed out completely so that it is empty and free of fecal material; this is known as a *full bowel prep*. This is one of the most important parts of the colonoscopy. Fecal material can interfere with good visualization of the wall of the colon, making it difficult for the physician to detect abnormalities.

The medical assistant may be responsible for providing the patient with instructions on preparing the colon. The patient should be encouraged to follow the instructions exactly. If the patient does not prepare properly, the colonoscopy is usually cancelled and must be rescheduled, which requires the patient to go through the bowel preparation procedure again. The patient preparation instructions may vary from one facility to another. General patient preparation recommendations for a colonoscopy are outlined in Table 13-3, along with patient instructions following the procedure.

Procedure

A sedative is administered intravenously before the colonoscopy. The sedative causes the patient to become relaxed, sleepy, and less aware of what is taking place. Some patients do not remember the procedure at all afterward.

The procedure itself is similar to a sigmoidoscopy. The patient is placed on his or her left side in Sims position. The physician performs a digital rectal examination before inserting the colonoscope. The colonoscope is advanced all the way through the entire colon (approximately 4 to 5 feet) until it reaches the cecum. Air is inserted into the colon to distend it for better visualization. Suction is used to remove secretions such as mucus, blood, and liquid feces that interfere with proper visualization. The physician then slowly withdraws the colonoscope while carefully observing the mucosa of the colon for abnormalities.

If the physician discovers an abnormal lesion, a long thin instrument is passed through the lumen of the insertion tube to remove a specimen for biopsy. In addition, if a suspicious-looking polyp is discovered, the physician may remove it (polypectomy) or take a biopsy of it for analysis by the laboratory. Removal of a precancerous polyp prevents it from developing into colon cancer in the future.

Following the procedure, the patient may experience some bloating, abdominal cramping, and flatulence. If a polyp has been removed or if a biopsy has been performed, the patient may exhibit traces of blood in the stool for 1 to 2 days.

Table 13-3 Patient Preparation for Colonoscopy

It is important to follow the patient preparation requirements as carefully as possible to ensure accurate results. The following preparation is required for a colonoscopy:

Beginning 5 days before the procedure	Discontinue taking iron, aspirin, and aspirin products. Iron can alter the color of the wall of the colon, and aspirin may cause bleeding if a polyp is removed from the colon.
Beginning 2 days before the procedure	Discontinue taking nonsteroidal anti-inflammatory drugs such as ibuprofen and naproxen to minimize the risk of bleeding if a polyp is removed.
Medication restrictions	The physician will advise the patient of any other medication restrictions that need to be followed.
Beginning 1 day before the procedure and continuing until your examination is completed	a. Do not consume any solid food or milk products. b. Consume only gelatin (Jell-O) or popsicles (except purple or red, which could be mistaken for blood in the colon). c. Drink only clear liquids (water, apple juice, sport drinks [e.g., Gatorade], soft drinks, clear broth). Do not drink alcohol. d. Coffee or tea is permitted with no milk or cream.
Bowel preparation	Take a laxative on the afternoon (between 2 PM and 4 PM) before the procedure. The laxative is often in a powdered form (e.g., Colyte) and comes in a package that is attached to a plastic gallon container. Read the package instructions for preparing the laxative solution. The gallon container is filled with drinking water and mixed with the powdered laxative. After preparing the laxative solution, store it in the refrigerator. Most patients find it easier to drink the solution if it is chilled. a. Begin the bowel preparation by drinking one 8-ounce glass of the liquid laxative solution every 10 to 15 minutes until 2 quarts (eight 8-ounce glasses) have been consumed. It is best to drink the solution quickly rather than slowly sipping it. b. After drinking the first few glasses, you may experience nausea and a bloated feeling. This is temporary and will disappear once you start having bowel movements. If this occurs, you can slow down the drinking process or stop for 30 minutes and then resume drinking the solution every 15 minutes. c. Your first bowel movement should occur approximately 1 hour after you begin drinking the solution. You will need to have a bowel movement about 10 to 15 times. If your bowel movement is clear to pale yellow in color after drinking the first 2 quarts of the solution, you can stop drinking the solution. If your stool is not clear, continue drinking the solution every 15 minutes until your bowel movement is clear.
After midnight on the night before the examination	a. Do not eat or drink anything, including water. b. If medications need to be taken (as approved by the physician), take them with only a sip of water.
Transportation	Arrange to have someone drive you home following the procedure. You will be sedated during the procedure and cannot drive yourself, nor can you use public transportation.
Following the procedure	You may experience some bloating, abdominal cramping, and flatulence. If you had a polyp removed or a biopsy taken, it is normal to experience traces of blood in the stool for 1 to 2 days. Contact the office if you experience significant rectal bleeding, faintness, dizziness, shortness of breath, or heart palpitations.

PROCEDURE 13-3   Assisting With a Sigmoidoscopy

Outcome Assist with a sigmoidoscopy.

Equipment/Supplies

- Flexible sigmoidoscope
- Disposable gloves
- Water-soluble lubricant
- Drape
- Biopsy forceps

- Sterile specimen container with a preservative
- 4 × 4 gauze squares
- Tissue
- Waste container

1. Procedural Step. Sanitize your hands.

2. Procedural Step. Assemble the equipment. Check that the light source on the sigmoidoscope is working.

3. Procedural Step. Greet the patient and introduce yourself. Identify the patient by full name and date of birth. Ask the patient whether he or she has prepared

Continued

PROCEDURE 13-3 *(side tab)*

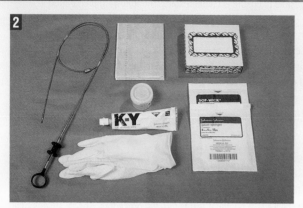

Assemble the equipment.

properly for the procedure. Explain the sigmoidoscopy procedure to the patient.

Principle. The patient must prepare properly to allow the physician to visualize the mucosa of the colon. Explaining the procedure helps reduce patient apprehension.

4. **Procedural Step.** Ask the patient whether he or she needs to empty the bladder before the examination. If a urine specimen is needed, the medical assistant requests that the patient void into a specimen container.

Principle. An empty bladder makes the examination easier and more comfortable for the patient.

5. **Procedural Step.** Instruct and prepare the patient for the examination. Ask him or her to remove all clothing from the waist down and to put on an examining gown with the opening in back.

6. **Procedural Step.** Assist the patient onto the examining table. Place the patient on his or her left side in the Sims position.

Principle. The Sims position is recommended for sigmoidoscopy.

7. **Procedural Step.** Properly drape the patient so that only the anus is exposed. Some medical offices use fenestrated drapes with the circular opening placed over the anus.

Principle. Draping the patient reduces exposure and provides warmth.

8. **Procedural Step.** Reassure the patient, and help him or her relax the muscles of the anus and rectum by breathing slowly and deeply through the mouth. As the sigmoidoscope is inserted, the patient feels some pressure and the urge to defecate. This pressure is caused by the insertion of the sigmoidoscope, and the patient should be reassured that although it is uncomfortable, it will last only a short time.

9. **Procedural Step.** Assist the physician as required during the examination. The medical assistant may be responsible for the following:
   a. Lubricating the physician's gloved index finger for the digital examination.
   b. Placing lubricant on the distal end of the sigmoidoscope before insertion into the rectum. The sigmoidoscope should be well lubricated to facilitate insertion.

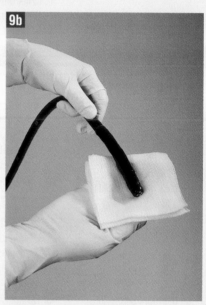

Place lubricant on the sigmoidoscope.

   c. Assisting with the suction equipment as required.
   d. Assisting with the collection of a biopsy specimen of a lesion or polyp by handing the biopsy forceps to the physician and holding the container to accept the specimen. Do not touch the inside of the container because it is sterile. After the physician inserts the specimen, replace the container lid and close it tightly.

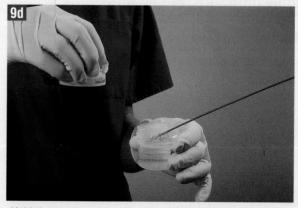

Hold the specimen container to accept the biopsy specimen.

PROCEDURE 13-3   Assisting With a Sigmoidoscopy—cont'd

10. **Procedural Step.** When the examination is completed, the medical assistant should apply gloves and clean the patient's anal region of any excess lubricant, using tissue wipes. Discard the tissues in the regular waste container.

11. **Procedural Step.** Remove gloves and sanitize your hands. Assist the patient off the examining table. Instruct him or her to get dressed.

12. **Procedural Step.** If a biopsy specimen was taken, prepare the specimen for transportation to the laboratory. Label the container with the patient's name and date of birth, date, and source of the specimen. Complete a biopsy request form to accompany the specimen. Place the specimen container in a biohazard specimen bag, and seal the bag. Insert the biopsy requisition into the outside pocket of the bag, and tuck the top of the requisition under the flap. Place the bag

in the appropriate location for pickup by the laboratory. Chart the transport of the specimen to an outside laboratory.

13. **Procedural Step.** Clean the examining room in preparation for the next patient. The sigmoidoscope should be sanitized and disinfected with a high-level disinfectant according to the manufacturer's recommendations.

CHARTING EXAMPLE	
Date	
8/15/12	11:00 a.m. Biopsy specimen transported to Medical Center Laboratory for pathology. ———————— M. Baer, CMA (AAMA)

Introduction to Male Reproductive Health

Two important areas related to male reproductive health are prostate screening and testicular self-examination. Preventive examinations and tests can assist in the detection of prostate and testicular cancers. Both of these areas are described in the following section.

PROSTATE CANCER

According to the American Cancer Society, prostate cancer is the second most common cause of cancer deaths in men, lung cancer being the most common. Every year, approximately 200,000 men are diagnosed with prostate cancer, and approximately 27,000 die from this disease. The incidence of prostate cancer increases after age 50. Prostate cancer is found more often in African American men and men with a family history of prostate cancer.

The prostate gland surrounds the urethra and is located just below the bladder and in front of the rectum (Figure 13-7). It is approximately the size and shape of a walnut, and its function is to secrete fluid that transports sperm.

In the early stages, prostate cancer often causes no symptoms. Symptoms that occur when the cancer is more developed include the following:

- Difficulty in urinating
- Weak or interrupted urinary flow
- Pain or burning during urination
- Frequent urination, especially at night
- Blood in the urine
- Pain in the lower back, pelvis, or upper thighs

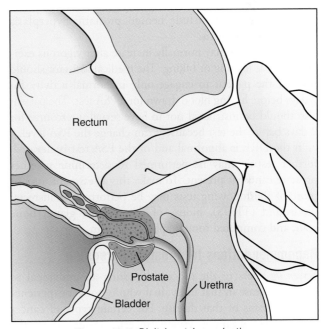

Figure 13-7. Digital rectal examination.

PROSTATE CANCER SCREENING

The primary screening tests for prostate cancer are the digital rectal examination (DRE) and the prostate-specific antigen (PSA) test.

Digital Rectal Examination

The digital rectal examination (DRE) is a quick and simple procedure that causes only momentary discomfort. During the examination, the physician inserts a lubricated gloved finger into the patient's rectum. Because the prostate gland is located in front of the rectum, the physician is able to palpate the surface of the prostate gland through the rectal wall (see Figure 13-7). The physician palpates the gland to determine whether it is enlarged or has an abnormal consistency. Normally, the prostate gland should feel soft, whereas malignant tissue is firm and hard. The sensitivity of the DRE is limited, however, because the physician can palpate only the posterior and lateral aspects of the prostate gland.

Prostate-Specific Antigen Test

The prostate-specific antigen (PSA) test is a screening test that measures the amount of PSA in the blood. PSA is a protein normally produced by the cells of the membrane that covers the prostate gland. The normal range for PSA is 0 to 4 ng/ml of blood. The PSA level may become elevated in men who have a benign or malignant growth in the prostate. A PSA level of 4 to 10 ng/ml is considered slightly elevated; levels between 10 and 20 ng/ml are considered moderately elevated; and a value greater than 20 ng/ml is considered highly elevated. The higher the PSA level, the more likely that cancer is present. Other conditions (other than prostate cancer) that can cause an elevated PSA level include benign prostatic hyperplasia (BPH) and prostatitis.

The PSA level may normally increase after vigorous exercise, such as jogging or biking. The medical assistant should instruct the patient to engage only in normal activity for 2 days before having blood drawn for a PSA test. The patient also should be instructed not to have sexual intercourse for 2 days before the test because it can change the PSA level.

If the DRE is abnormal and/or the PSA test is elevated, further testing may be performed to determine whether prostate cancer is present. To make this assessment, one or more of the following tests may be performed: transrectal ultrasound (TRUS), biopsy of the prostate gland, bone scan, and computed tomography (CT) scan.

Recommendations for Prostate Screening

Screening refers to the process of testing an individual to detect a disease in that individual who is not yet experiencing symptoms of that disease. For certain types of cancer (e.g., colorectal cancer, cervical cancer), screening allows the cancer to be discovered early, when it is more treatable, which increases the patient's survival rate.

The DRE and PSA screening tests for prostate cancer have certain limitations. Abnormal results from both of these tests do not necessarily indicate that cancer is present. In addition, normal results from these tests do not mean that cancer is *not* present. An elevated PSA test may lead to a biopsy and the detection of cancer in an individual, which can pose a dilemma. Many prostate cancers are slow growing and do not result in the death of an individual, particularly if the man is older or in poor health. Because it is sometimes difficult to determine the aggressiveness of the cancer, these individuals may still be treated with surgery or radiation, which can seriously affect a man's quality of life.

The American Cancer Society (ACS) believes that available evidence does not currently support routine testing for prostate cancer. The ACS recommends that health care providers discuss the potential benefits and limitations of prostate screening with men older than 50 years of age. Following this discussion, the PSA test and the DRE should be offered annually to men 50 years and older who are at average risk for prostate cancer and have at least a 10-year life expectancy. Those men who indicate a preference for testing should be tested. The ACS recommendation provides men with knowledge of the advantages and disadvantages of early detection and treatment of prostate cancer, which then allows them to share in the decision of whether or not to be tested.

TESTICULAR SELF-EXAMINATION

The purpose of testicular self-examination (TSE) is early detection of testicular cancer. In the past 40 years, testicular cancer among young Caucasian men has more than

---

TESTICULAR SELF-EXAMINATION

1
Take a warm bath or shower.

2
Stand in front of a mirror. Look for any swelling of the skin of the scrotum.

3
Place the index and middle fingers of both hands on the underside of one testicle and the thumbs on top of the testicle.

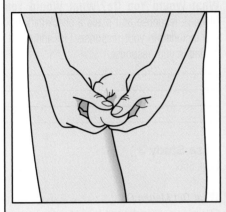

4
Apply a small amount of pressure and gently roll the testicle between the thumb and fingers of both hands, feeling for lumps, swelling, or any change in the size, shape, or consistency of the testicle. A normal testicle should feel smooth, egg-shaped and rather firm. It is also normal for one testicle to be larger or hang lower than the other testicle.

5
Find the epididymis so that you do not confuse it with a lump. The epididymis is a soft tubular cord, located behind the testicle, that functions in storing and carrying sperm.
(Note: Tenderness in the area of the epididymis is considered normal.)

6
Repeat the examination outlined above on the other testicle.

7
Report any of the following abnormalities to the physician: any unusual lump, a feeling of heaviness in the scrotum, a dull ache in the lower abdomen or groin, enlargement of one of the testicles, tenderness or pain in a testicle, or any change in the way the testicle feels.

Figure 13-8. Testicular self-examination.

---

doubled. Although testicular cancer can develop at any age, it is most common in males 15 to 34 years old. If detected early, it has a very high cure rate. Most cases of testicular cancer are detected by men themselves, either by accident or when performing a TSE. Certain risk factors increase a man's chance of getting testicular cancer, including the following:

- History of cryptorchidism (undescended testicles)
- Family history of testicular cancer
- Cancer of the other testicle
- Caucasian race (testicular cancer is five times more common in Caucasian men than in African American men)

TSE should be performed monthly, starting at 15 years of age. A good idea is for the patient to choose an easy-to-remember date each month, such as the first day of the month. The best time to perform the examination is after taking a warm bath or shower. Heat allows the scrotal skin to relax and become soft, making it easier to palpate the underlying testicular tissues.

The most common sign of testicular cancer is a small, hard, painless lump (about the size of a pea) located on the front or side of the testicle. Any abnormality of the testicles should be reported to the physician immediately. It does not mean that the patient has cancer, however; the physician must make that determination. Figure 13-8 outlines the procedure for a TSE.

evolve *Check out the Evolve site to access additional interactive activities.*

MEDICAL PRACTICE *and the* LAW

Colon procedures can be embarrassing for the patient. Many colon procedures can be diagnostic for cancer. This combination makes these procedures very stressful for the patient. Professionalism, compassion, and a caring attitude can alleviate many fears. Many invasive procedures require written informed consent.

While assisting with a sigmoidoscopy, assist the patient and maintain proper positioning as comfortably as possible. Be aware of the patient's condition, and inform the physician if the patient is not tolerating the procedure well.

Malpractice
Malpractice laws require a minimal level of care and of doing good, or beneficence. Malpractice is a type of negligence, which is a tort, or wrong. Torts can be done intentionally or accidentally (negligently) and can be caused by something that was done or by something that was omitted. ∎

What Would You Do? What Would You *Not* Do? RESPONSES

Case Study 1
Page 553

What Did Megan Do?

❏ Relayed to Mrs. Bernard that this is not the most fun test to perform, but that if colon cancer is detected early, the cure rate is very high.

❏ Explained to Mrs. Bernard that colon cancer increases after age 50, and that an individual can develop colon cancer without a family history of it.

❏ Told Mrs. Bernard that during the early stages of colon cancer, no symptoms occur, so it is possible to feel fine but still have a problem.

❏ Explained to Mrs. Bernard in greater detail the reason for not eating red meat or taking aspirin during the testing period.

❏ Told Mrs. Bernard that disposable gloves could be given to her to take home to wear when she collected the specimens.

❏ Explained to Mrs. Bernard that the physician talks with patients every day about these types of things, and it is important to talk with him about all aspects of her health so that she receives the best care possible.

❏ Told Mrs. Bernard that the office would call her in 3 days to see whether she has any questions or is having any problems with the test.

What Did Megan Not Do?

❏ Did not tell Mrs. Bernard that she is getting older and needs to be more concerned about performing health screening tests.

What Would You Do?/What Would You *Not* Do? Review Megan's response and place a checkmark next to the information you included in your response. List additional information you included in your response.

_____
_____
_____
_____

Case Study 2
Page 561

What Did Megan Do?

❏ Told Dr. Mitchell that the physician cannot perform a sigmoidoscopy unless the colon has been properly prepared.

❏ Explained that the colon needs to be cleaned out, so the physician can see the wall of the colon to check for abnormalities.

❏ Went over the preparation instructions with Dr. Mitchell again and gave him another instruction sheet to take home.

❏ Rescheduled his appointment and told him that he would be called the day before the examination to be reminded of his appointment and to see whether he has any questions regarding the preparation.

What Did Megan Not Do?

❏ Told Dr. Mitchell that an entire office hour had been scheduled for his examination and that other patients could have been seen during this time.

What Would You Do?/What Would You *Not* Do? Review Megan's response and place a checkmark next to the information you included in your response. List additional information you included in your response.

_____
_____
_____

Case Study 3
Page 566

What Did Megan Do?

❏ Listened patiently and tried to reassure and calm Mr. Bota. Told him that physicians do not yet know what causes prostate cancer.

❏ Explained that the PSA test is a screening test and that he should not jump to conclusions about the results.

❏ Told Mr. Bota that the physician would talk with him about his test results in a short while.

❏ Commended Mr. Bota on his healthy lifestyle habits and encouraged him to continue with them.

❏ Gave Mr. Bota some brochures on male reproductive health to read while he waited to be seen by the physician.

What Did Megan Not Do?

❏ Did not tell Mr. Bota that there was nothing to worry about.

What Would You Do?/What Would You *Not* Do? Review Megan's response and place a checkmark next to the information you included in your response. List additional information you included in your response.

_____
_____
_____
_____

CERTIFICATION REVIEW

- ❑ **Blood in the stool** may indicate many gastrointestinal conditions, including hemorrhoids, diverticulosis, polyps, colitis, upper gastrointestinal ulcers, and colorectal cancer. Hidden, or nonvisible, blood in the stool is termed occult blood, and its presence can be determined through fecal occult blood testing.

- ❑ **Fecal occult blood testing** is routinely performed in the medical office using the guaiac slide test (e.g., Hemoccult, ColoScreen, Seracult). Patient preparation for the test is important to ensure accurate test results. A positive test result warrants further diagnostic procedures, such as colonoscopy, sigmoidoscopy, a double-contrast barium enema radiographic study, and CT colonography.

- ❑ **Sigmoidoscopy** is the visual examination of the mucosa of the rectum and sigmoid colon using a flexible fiberoptic sigmoidoscope. Sigmoidoscopy may be performed to detect the presence of lesions, polyps, hemorrhoids, fissures, infection, and inflammation. It is especially valuable in the early detection of colorectal cancer.

- ❑ **Colonoscopy** is the visual examination of the mucosa of the rectum and the entire length of the colon using a flexible fiberoptic colonoscope. The colonoscope has a videocamera attached to the distal end of the insertion tube, which transmits images of the colon to a video screen for viewing by the physician. A colonoscopy is usually performed following a positive fecal occult blood test to determine the source and cause of the bleeding. It is also performed to evaluate patient symptoms related to the colon.

- ❑ **A digital rectal examination** is performed by the physician before the sigmoidoscopy to palpate the rectum for tenderness, hemorrhoids, polyps, or tumors. The digital examination also helps relax the sphincter muscles of the anus for insertion of the sigmoidoscope.

- ❑ **The prostate gland** surrounds the urethra and secretes fluid that transports sperm. The primary screening tests for prostate cancer are the digital rectal examination (DRE) and the prostate-specific antigen (PSA) test. If the test results indicate the possibility of cancer, further testing may be done, which may include one or more of the following: transrectal ultrasound (TRUS), biopsy of the prostate gland, bone scan, and CT scan.

- ❑ **The purpose of the testicular self-examination (TSE)** is to detect testicular cancer early. Testicular cancer is most common between 15 and 34 years of age. The TSE should be performed monthly beginning at age 15. Any abnormality should be reported to the physician immediately.

TERMINOLOGY REVIEW

Medical Term	Word Parts	Definition
Biopsy	*bi/o-:* life *-opsy:* to view	The surgical removal and examination of tissue from the living body. Biopsies generally are performed to determine whether a tumor is benign or malignant.
Colonoscopy	*colon/o-:* colon *-scopy:* visual examination	The visualization of the rectum and the entire colon using a colonoscope
Colonoscope	*colon/o-:* colon *-scope:* instrument used for visual examination	An endoscope that is specially designed for passage through the anus to permit visualization of the rectum and the entire length of the colon
Endoscope	*endo-:* within *-scope:* instrument used for visual examination	An instrument that consists of a tube and an optical system that is used for direct visual inspection of organs or cavities
Insufflate		To blow a powder, vapor, or gas (e.g., air) into a body cavity
Melena		The darkening of the stool caused by the presence of blood in an amount of 50 ml or greater
Occult blood		Blood in such a small amount that it is not detectable by the unaided eye
Peroxidase	*-oxia:* oxygen *-ase:* enzyme	(As it pertains to the guaiac slide test) A substance that is able to transfer oxygen from hydrogen peroxide to oxidize guaiac, causing the guaiac to turn blue
Sigmoidoscope	*sigmoid/o-:* sigmoid (colon) *-scope:* instrument used for visual examination	An endoscope that is specially designed for passage through the anus to permit visualization of the rectum and sigmoid colon
Sigmoidoscopy	*sigmoid/o-:* sigmoid (colon) *-scopy:* visual examination	The visual examination of the rectum and sigmoid colon using a sigmoidoscope

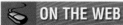
ON THE WEB

For Information on Colorectal Cancer:

American Cancer Society: www.cancer.org

National Cancer Institute: www.cancer.gov

Prevent Cancer Foundation: www.preventcancer.org

Colon Cancer Alliance: www.ccalliance.org

Oncology Channel: www.oncologychannel.com

For Information on Prostate Cancer:

Prostate Health: www.prostatehealth.com

Prostate Information: www.prostateinfo.com

Prostate.com: www.prostate.com

Prostate Cancer Foundation: www.prostatecancerfoundation.org

Prostatitis Foundation: www.prostatitis.org

Male Health: www.malehealthcenter.com

14

Radiology and Diagnostic Imaging

LEARNING OBJECTIVES

Radiology

1. State the function of radiographs in medicine.
2. Explain the importance of proper patient preparation for a radiographic examination.
3. Explain the function of a contrast medium.
4. Describe the purpose of a fluoroscope.
5. Describe each of the following positions used for radiographic examinations:
   - Anteroposterior
   - Posteroanterior
   - Right and left lateral
   - Supine
   - Prone
6. Explain the purpose of each of the following types of radiographic examinations:
   - Mammography
   - Bone density scan
   - Upper gastrointestinal radiography
   - Lower gastrointestinal radiography
   - Intravenous pyelography

Diagnostic Imaging

1. Explain the purpose of each of the following diagnostic imaging procedures:
   - Ultrasonography
   - Computed tomography
   - Magnetic resonance imaging
   - Nuclear medicine
2. Explain how nuclear medicine is used to produce an image of a body part or organ.
3. State the guidelines that may be required for nuclear medicine.

Digital Radiology

1. Explain the advantages of digital radiology.

PROCEDURES

Instruct a patient in the proper preparation necessary for each of the following types of radiographic examinations:
   - Mammography
   - Bone density scan
   - Upper gastrointestinal radiography
   - Lower gastrointestinal radiography
   - Intravenous pyelography

Instruct a patient on the purpose and advance preparation for each of the following diagnostic imaging procedures:
   - Ultrasonography
   - Computed tomography
   - Magnetic resonance imaging
   - Nuclear medicine

KEY TERMS

contrast medium
echocardiogram (EK-oh-KAR-dee-oh-gram)
enema (EN-em-ah)
fluoroscope (FLOOR-oh-skope)
fluoroscopy (floor-OS-koe-pee)
radiograph (RAY-dee-oh-graf)
radiography (ray-dee-OG-rah-fee)

radiologist (ray-dee-AH-lah-jist)
radiology (ray-dee-AH-lah-jee)
radiolucent (ray-dee-oh-LOO-sent)
radiopaque (ray-dee-oh-PAYK)
sonogram (SON-oh-gram)
ultrasonography (ul-trah-son-AH-grah-fee)

Introduction to Radiology

Radiology is the branch of medicine that deals with the use of radiation and other imaging techniques (such as ultrasound, computed tomography [CT] scans, magnetic resonance imaging [MRI], and nuclear medicine) in the diagnosis and treatment of disease. A **radiologist** is a physician who specializes in the diagnosis and treatment of disease using radiation and other imaging techniques.

Wilhelm Konrad Röntgen, a German physicist, discovered x-rays on November 8, 1895, while working with a cathode ray tube. He noticed that these rays could pass through solid materials, such as paper, wood, and human skin. Because he did not know what they were, he named them *x-rays*. The rays have since been renamed *roentgen rays* after their discoverer; however, they are better known as "x-rays."

X-rays are high-energy electromagnetic waves that are invisible and have a short wavelength that enables them to penetrate solid materials. X-rays are used to visualize internal structures and serve as a diagnostic aid in determining the presence of disease. They are especially useful for detecting abnormal conditions associated with the skeletal system such as fractures. X-rays also are used therapeutically in the treatment of disease conditions, such as malignant neoplasms.

X-rays can be taken using the conventional film method or digitally with the use of a computer. The conventional film method is described in this section, and the digital method is described later in this chapter. When conventional radiographs are taken, radiographic film is loaded into a device known as an *x-ray cassette*. The cassette is placed behind the part being examined, and a shadow or image of the internal body structure photographed is produced on the film. After the x-ray has been taken, the film must be processed. A radiologic technician takes the cassette into a dark room and develops the image using an x-ray processor. **Radiograph** is the term for the permanent record of the picture produced on the radiographic film.

An orthopedic medical office may have its own radiograph machine, but more often radiographs are taken in a hospital by radiology personnel or large medical clinic. Some radiographs, such as a chest x-ray, require no advance preparation, whereas others, such as a lower gastrointestinal (GI) study, require a great deal of special preparation. Medical assistants are usually responsible for patient instruction in the type of preparation necessary for a particular radiographic examination and for ensuring that the patient understands the importance of the preparation. If the patient does not prepare properly, the radiograph may be of poor quality, and the procedure may need to be rescheduled. This section provides an introduction to the study of radiographs, with a focus on the patient preparation necessary for common radiographs.

CONTRAST MEDIA

Radiography relies on differences in density between various body structures to produce shadows of varying intensity on the radiographic film. There is a difference in density between bone and flesh (bone is denser than flesh). Bone absorbs more x-rays and does not allow them to reach the radiographic film. This leaves that part of the film unexposed and causes white areas to appear on the processed film. If the x-rays penetrate an organ or structure, a black area appears on the film. Because the lungs contain air, x-rays are able to penetrate them easily. As a result, the lungs appear black on the processed film. The ribs absorb the x-rays and appear as white shadows on the film (Figure 14-1). A structure, such as lung tissue, that permits the passage of x-rays is **radiolucent.** A structure, such as bone, that obstructs the passage of x-rays and causes an image to be cast on the film is **radiopaque.**

In many cases, the natural densities of two adjacent organs or structures are similar. In this instance, a **contrast medium** (also known as a contrast agent) must be used to make a particular structure visible on the radiograph. Contrast media are usually radiopaque chemical compounds that cause the body tissue or organ to absorb more radiation. This absorption provides a contrast in density between the tissue or organ and the surrounding area. The tissue or organ becomes visible and appears white on the processed radiograph. Substances used as contrast media must be able to be ingested or injected into the body tissues or organs without causing harm to the patient. Contrast media are administered to the patient through various routes. Some are administered orally; others are injected into a vein or are delivered through an IV line or an enema.

Barium sulfate and inorganic iodine compounds are commonly used radiopaque contrast media. Barium sulfate is a chalky compound that is water-insoluble and does not allow penetration by x-rays. It is frequently used for examination of the GI tract because barium is not absorbed into the body through the GI tract and does not alter its normal function. Iodine salts are radiopaque and are combined

What Would You Do? What Would You *Not* Do?

Case Study 1

Jose Ramirez is a 7-year-old boy with episodes of unexplained abdominal pain and vomiting during the past 6 months. The medical office has scheduled an upper GI radiographic study at the local hospital. Mrs. Ramirez wants to know how best to prepare Jose for the procedure, so that he will not be so afraid of the x-ray room and equipment. She asks what she can do so that he will drink the barium solution. She says he will not drink milk, and if the barium tastes anything like milk, it will be hard to get him to drink the barium. Mrs. Ramirez wants to know whether Jose can hold his favorite toy (a Tonka truck) during the procedure to comfort him. She also wants to know whether the barium solution has any side effects. ■

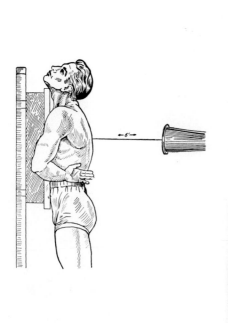
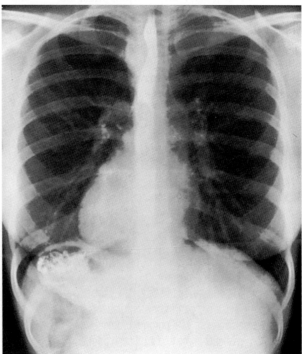

Figure 14-1. Posteroanterior view of the chest. Position of patient and radiograph. (From Meschan I: Synopsis of radiologic anatomy with computed tomography, Philadelphia, 1980, Saunders.)

with other compounds for radiographic examination of structures such as the urinary tract and blood vessels. Iodine contrast media consist of clear liquids and are usually injected. Iodine sometimes may produce an allergic reaction, and before administration, patients should be asked whether they have an allergy to iodine. Patients with known allergies may be given an iodine sensitivity test as a precautionary measure.

FLUOROSCOPY

A **fluoroscope** is an instrument used to view internal organs and structures of the body directly on a display screen. Examination of a patient with a fluoroscope is known as **fluoroscopy.** A radiopaque medium is often used with fluoroscopy to outline various parts of the body. The patient is positioned between the radiographic tube and a fluorescent screen composed of zinc cadmium sulfide crystals. When the x-rays pass through the body and strike the crystals, visible light is emitted so that the radiologist can view (on a screen) the action of body organs or structures, such as the stomach and intestines. During fluoroscopy, the radiologist can take radiographs that permit the study of the structure in detail and serve as a permanent record.

POSITIONING THE PATIENT

The position of the patient is determined by the purpose of the examination and the area examined. The patient is generally positioned so that several different views can be taken to provide a complete three-dimensional picture of the part examined. Articles such as jewelry and hairpins must be removed so the image on the radiograph is not obscured. To prevent blurring of the image on the film, patients must maintain the position in which they are placed and not move during the radiographic examination. Blurring prevents good visualization of the part and may warrant retaking of the radiograph. The following types of radiographic

views are used, and the methods used to position the patient for each are described.

Anteroposterior (AP) view. The x-rays are directed from the front toward the back of the body. The patient is positioned with the anterior aspect of the body facing the radiograph tube and the posterior aspect facing the radiographic film.

Posteroanterior (PA) view. The x-rays are directed from the back toward the front of the body. The patient is positioned with the posterior aspect of the body facing the radiograph tube and the anterior aspect facing the radiographic film (see Figure 14-1).

Lateral view. The x-ray beam passes from one side of the body to the opposite side.

Right lateral (RL) view. The right side of the body is positioned next to the radiographic film, and the x-rays are directed through the body from the left to the right side.

Left lateral (LL) view. The left side of the body is positioned next to the radiographic film, and the x-rays are directed through the body from the right to the left side.

Oblique view. The body is positioned at an angle or in a semilateral position.

Supine position. The patient is positioned on the back with the face upward.

Prone position. The patient is positioned on the abdomen with the head turned to one side.

SPECIFIC RADIOGRAPHIC EXAMINATIONS

The medical assistant should understand the purpose of commonly performed radiographic examinations and should be able to instruct a patient on the proper preparation for each (Figure 14-2). Frequently performed radiographic examinations and the special advance preparation necessary for each

Putting It All into Practice

My Name is Michelle Shockey, and I work for an orthopedic surgeon in a private practice. I assist the physician in minor office surgery, dressing changes, joint injections, and cast applications. When the physician performs surgery, I schedule the patients and do their preauthorizations. I have the opportunity to see a variety of problems, from sprains and strains to surgical conditions.

When our patients come to our orthopedic office, they are usually in a lot of pain. Pain plays a big part in how our patients feel on that specific day. We see patients with chronic problems that may never get better. Some patients come to our office in pain, but when their visits are over, they feel like they are on top of the world. Seeing a patient go from being unable to walk to being able to run a marathon is the best experience you can encounter. ∎

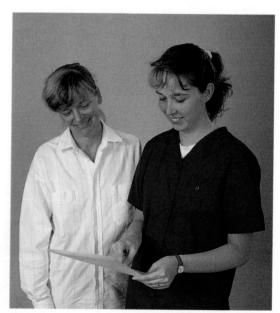

Figure 14-2. Michelle instructs a patient in proper preparation for a radiographic examination.

are described. The preparation may vary, depending on the medical office.

Mammography

Mammography is a radiographic examination of the breasts used to detect many forms of breast disease, such as benign breast masses, breast calcifications, fibrocystic breast disease, and particularly breast cancer. It also is used to monitor the effects of surgery and radiation therapy on breast tumors.

Mammography uses low doses of x-rays that pass through the breast and create an image on a film. On the radiograph, an abnormal area appears noticeably different from normal breast tissue. Mammography can be used to detect a breast tumor when the growth is less than 1 cm in diameter (about the size of a pea) and before it is clinically palpable. A malignant lump can be removed at an early stage; this usually results in conservative treatment with less disfigurement and a high survival rate. With early diagnosis and treatment, breast cancer survival rates for women can reach as high as 94%.

No specific preparation is necessary for mammography. The patient should not wear any lotions, powders, or deodorants because they may contain small amounts of metal that can be seen on the radiograph and may interfere with interpretation. For the mammogram, the patient must remove clothing from the waist up; the patient should be told to wear a two-piece outfit so that the procedure is easier and more comfortable.

A radiology technician generally performs the mammogram. The patient's breast is positioned on the mammography machine, and pressure is applied with a plastic compression paddle that flattens the breast (Figure 14-3). Compression of the breasts is necessary to obtain a clear radiograph and to lower the radiation dosage as much as possible. During the procedure, the patient must hold her breath and remain still momentarily because any type of motion, even breathing, can blur the image and make a repeat radiograph necessary.

Two radiographs are taken of each breast—one from above and one from the side. A radiologist then checks the mammogram (Figure 14-4) and occasionally orders additional images to obtain a more complete view of the breast tissue. After the procedure, the radiologist studies the mammogram for any signs of breast cancer or other breast problems and sends a written report of the findings to the patient's physician.

Bone Density Scan

A bone density scan is an enhanced form of x-ray technology that measures the bone mineral density of the human skeleton to detect bone loss. As individuals age, their bones may become less dense, causing them to become brittle and weak. This may lead to a bone fracture. Factors that cause bones to lose density include osteoporosis, thyroid and parathyroid conditions, and certain medications (e.g., corticosteroids). Postmenopausal women are at particular risk for osteoporosis; therefore, it is recommended that women above the age of 65 have a bone density scan every 2 years. *Osteoporosis* is a condition in which a gradual loss of calcium causes the bones to become thinner, more fragile, and more likely to break.

DEXA (dual energy x-ray absorptiometry) scanning is the most widely used bone density testing method. DEXA (pronounced "dexa") uses x-rays to determine the amount of bone in the human skeleton. During a DEXA scan, bone density measurements are taken at different parts of the body. The bone density measurements indicate if the patient has lost bone density. They also assist in detecting the

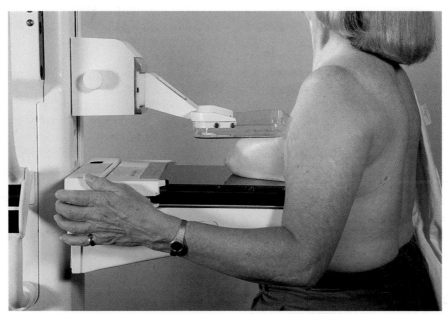

Figure 14-3. Patient positioning for mammography. (From Ballinger PW, Frank ED, eds: Merrill's atlas of radiographic positions and radiologic procedures, vol 2, ed 10, St Louis, 2003, Mosby.)

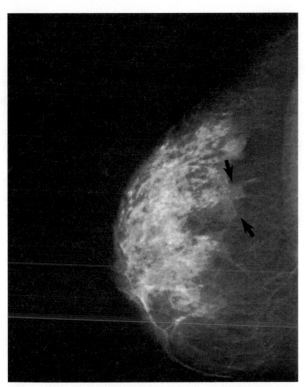

Figure 14-4. Mammogram. *Arrows* indicate suspicious area of increased density that needs further evaluation. (From Prue L: Atlas of mammographic positioning, Philadelphia, 1994, Saunders.)

presence of osteoporosis and can be used to predict the patient's risk of bone fracture. Patients on medication therapy for osteoporosis (e.g., Fosamax, Boniva) may also undergo DEXA to determine if the therapy is working.

The patient should be instructed to abstain from taking a calcium supplement or osteoporosis medication on the morning of the examination. These substances interfere with obtaining an accurate measurement of bone density. To perform the examination, the patient is positioned on an x-ray table and is instructed to remain as still as possible during the test. The radiologic technician then scans one or more areas of bone with the DEXA equipment. Areas that are typically scanned include the lower spine and hips.

Test results are in the form of two scores (a T score and a Z score), which are sent to the patient's physician. These scores assist the physician in diagnosing and treating the patient. The *T score* is derived by comparing the patient's measurements with those of healthy young normal adults with peak bone mass of the same gender and ethnic group as the patient. A score above −1 is considered normal. A score between −1 and −2.5 is classified as *osteopenia* or low bone mass. A score below −2.5 is defined as osteoporosis. The T score is used to estimate the patient's risk of developing a fracture. The *Z score* is derived by comparing the patient's measurements with an established database of normal individuals of the same age, gender, and ethnic group as the patient. An unusually high or low Z score may indicate the need for further testing.

PATIENT TEACHING   Mammography

Answer questions patients may have about mammography.

What is the purpose of mammography?
Mammography is a safe, low-dose radiographic examination used to screen for abnormal changes in the breasts. Mammography allows the physician to detect small lumps in the breast long before they can be felt. Although most breast lumps are not cancerous, breast cancer can be removed at an early stage when detected early, which usually results in treatment that is less deforming and has a much higher survival rate.

Who should have a mammogram?
The American Cancer Society recommends women 40 years old and older have an annual mammogram because the risk of breast cancer increases after this age. Women with a family history of, or other risk factors for, breast cancer should follow the advice of the physician regarding mammography; age guidelines do not apply because these women undergo examination on a more frequent basis.

What occurs during the mammography procedure?
During mammography, the breast is positioned on a special machine and is flattened with a compression paddle. Breast compression may be uncomfortable for some women. The discomfort can be reduced with avoidance of caffeine several days before the procedure and by scheduling the mammography the week after a menstrual period, when the breasts are less tender. Each breast is radiographed from above and from the side. A radiologist studies the resulting mammogram to detect any abnormalities. The results are reported to the physician.

Does mammography take the place of breast self-examination?
Mammography is not a substitute for breast self-examination. Women should continue to examine their breasts once a month and undergo a periodic breast examination by a physician. Most breast lumps are detected by women themselves.

- Encourage the patient to have a mammogram according to the schedule recommended by the American Cancer Society.
- Instruct the patient in the procedure for a breast self-examination.
- Provide the patient with educational materials on breast self-examination and mammography.

Gastrointestinal Series

Upper Gastrointestinal Radiography

An upper GI (UGI) is an examination of the upper digestive tract using fluoroscopy and radiography. The examination is helpful in the diagnosis of disorders of the esophagus, stomach, duodenum, and small intestine (e.g., gastroesophageal reflux disease [GERD]), hiatal hernia, peptic ulcer, benign and malignant tumors). The procedure may be ordered when the patient complains of difficulty in swallowing, vomiting, abdominal pain, gastric reflux (burping up food [GERD]), severe indigestion, and blood in the stool.

Proper patient preparation is important for this procedure. The patient's stomach must be empty at the beginning of the study, so food does not obscure the radiographic image. To prepare for the examination, the patient must eat a light evening meal and then not eat or drink anything, including water and medications, after midnight on the day before the examination. Food and fluid in the GI tract have a degree of density and could cause confusing shadows on the radiograph.

The stomach varies little in density from the structures around it, and to make it show up on a radiograph, a contrast medium must be used. The patient drinks a suspension of barium mixed with water and flavoring, which resembles a milkshake and has a chalky taste. Before drinking the barium, the patient may be asked to drink a carbonated beverage that consists of baking soda granules. This solution puts air into the stomach, causing it to expand. The combination of air and barium allows the radiologist to view the stomach in greater detail.

As the patient swallows the barium mixture, the radiologist observes its passage down the esophagus and into the stomach and duodenum with fluoroscopy. The barium coats the lining of the gastrointestinal tract, making it visible on the screen of the fluoroscope. Radiographs are taken periodically during the examination to allow a detailed study of the upper GI tract and to provide a permanent record. The patient's position is changed at various times so that the upper digestive tract can be visualized from different profiles. If the radiologist wants to observe the passage of barium through the small and large intestines, the patient must wait at the facility and return to the radiology examination room several times for additional radiographs. After the procedure, the radiologist prepares an upper GI report of the findings, which is sent to the patient's physician.

The medical assistant should explain to the patient that the barium suspension will appear in the stool for 1 to 3 days following the procedure and will cause the stool to have a whitish color. The barium mixture may cause constipation and the need for a laxative. To help prevent constipation, the patient should be instructed to increase fiber and fluid intake for several days following the procedure.

Lower Gastrointestinal Radiography

A lower GI involves filling the colon with a barium sulfate mixture with a catheter (tube) inserted into the rectum through the anus. Because of this, the procedure is sometimes called a barium enema. The examination uses fluoroscopy and radiography to observe and obtain permanent pictures of the colon and rectum (Figure 14-5). A lower GI

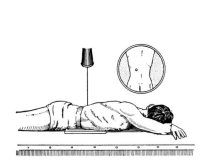
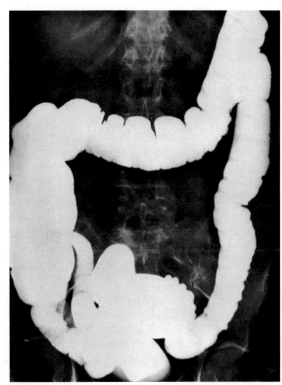

Figure 14-5. Lower GI. Colon is distended with barium. Positioning of patient and radiograph. (From Meschan I: Synopsis of radiologic anatomy with computed tomography, Philadelphia, 1980, Saunders.)

assists in diagnosis of disorders of the colon, such as polyps, cancerous tumors, diverticulosis, and the extent of inflammatory bowel disease (e.g., ulcerative colitis, Crohn's disease). The colon must be thoroughly cleansed in advance to remove gas and fecal material. Gas has a certain degree of density and shows up as confusing shadows on the radiograph. If fecal material appears on the film, the image of the colon is obscured.

Instructions for cleansing the colon may vary from one medical office to another, but in general, the patient is instructed to consume only clear liquids the day before the examination, such as water, plain coffee and tea, clear broth, and strained fruit juice. A laxative should be taken on the day before the scheduled examination; an **enema** also may be necessary. An **enema** is an injection of fluid into the rectum to aid in the elimination of feces from the colon. The patient should not drink anything (except water) after midnight on the day before the examination. On the morning of the examination, the patient may be required to perform a warm water cleansing enema until the returns are clear.

The patient should report at the scheduled time and is instructed to relax on one side while the rectal catheter is inserted. As the barium enters the colon, the radiologist watches it on the fluoroscopic screen and periodically takes radiographs. The patient has a sensation of fullness and the urge to defecate as the barium enters the colon. The catheter usually has a balloon on the tip of it to prevent the barium from coming back out. The patient is moved into various positions to allow the barium to fill the colon completely and to obtain better visualization of the colon. The patient is allowed to evacuate the barium, and another radiograph is taken to finish the radiographic examination. After the procedure, the radiologist prepares a lower GI report of the findings, which is sent to the patient's physician.

A *double-contrast barium enema radiographic study* is similar to a lower GI study; however (in addition to the barium), it also employs the use of air that is inserted into the colon through the same catheter as the barium. The air distends the wall of the colon and allows the radiologist to view the colon in greater detail, making it easier to detect polyps and small cancerous tumors.

Intravenous Pyelography

An intravenous pyelogram (IVP) is a radiograph of the kidneys, ureters, and bladder (Figure 14-6). An IVP is used to assist in the diagnosis of kidney stones, blockage or narrowing of the urinary tract, and growths within or near the urinary system.

The patient should consume only clear liquids starting at 4:00 PM the day before the examination. The evening before the examination, the patient must take a laxative such as magnesium citrate and/or Dulcolax tablets to remove gas and fecal material from the intestines. Removal of gas and fecal material permits proper visualization of the urinary tract. Starting at midnight the day before the examination, the patient should not eat, drink, smoke, or chew gum. Un-

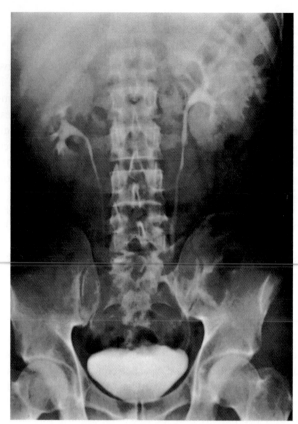

Figure 14-6. Intravenous pyelogram obtained 15 minutes after intravenous injection of a suitable contrast agent. (From Meschan I: Synopsis of radiologic anatomy with computed tomography, Philadelphia, 1980, Saunders.)

less the patient is allergic to iodine, a contrast medium consisting of iodine is used and is administered intravenously to the patient. As the iodine enters the bloodstream, the patient may feel warm and flushed and have a metallic or salty taste in the mouth. This reaction is normal and lasts for only a few minutes. If the patient is allergic to iodine, a different type of contrast medium must be used. After the procedure, the radiologist prepares an IVP report of the findings, which is sent to the patient's physician.

Other Types of Radiographs

Other types of radiographs that the medical assistant may encounter include the following:

Angiocardiogram: Radiograph of the heart in which valves and vessels are examined with radiography and fluoroscopy after introduction of a radiopaque contrast medium.

Bronchogram: Radiograph of the lungs after introduction of a radiopaque contrast medium.

Cerebral angiogram: Radiograph of the major arteries of the brain after injection of a radiopaque contrast medium.

Chest radiograph: Radiograph of the chest that does not use a contrast medium.

Cholangiogram: Radiograph of the bile ducts after administration of a radiopaque contrast medium.

Coronary angiogram: Radiograph of the coronary arteries after injection of a radiopaque contrast medium.

Cystogram: Radiograph of the urinary bladder after injection of a radiopaque contrast medium.

Hysterosalpingogram: Radiograph of the uterus and fallopian tubes after injection of a radiopaque contrast medium.

Myelogram: Radiograph of the spinal column after injection of a radiopaque contrast medium.

Retrograde pyelogram: Radiograph of the kidneys and urinary tract after injection of radiopaque contrast medium directly into the ureter through a ureteral catheter. The dye flows to the kidneys through the ureters.

Introduction to Diagnostic Imaging

Diagnostic imaging procedures are performed frequently because they allow for the visualization of internal body structures in great detail. The most common diagnostic imaging procedures are **ultrasonography** (US), computed tomography (CT), magnetic resonance imaging (MRI), and nuclear medicine. Diagnostic imaging procedures are usually performed in a hospital or a large clinic. The medical assistant, however, may need to relay information to a patient scheduled for such a procedure, including what to expect during the procedure and any patient preparation that may be required. The medical assistant should have a basic knowledge of diagnostic imaging procedures and the preparation necessary for each.

ULTRASONOGRAPHY

Ultrasonography, also called "ultrasound," is the oldest of the diagnostic imaging procedures. Ultrasound uses high-frequency sound waves for the study of soft tissue structures. Recent advances have been made in technology in ultrasound. These include three-dimensional (3-D) ultrasound, in which sound waves are formatted into 3-D images (Figure 14-7). Four-dimensional (4-D) ultrasound is another new technology that consists of 3-D ultrasound, but in motion.

Ultrasound is frequently used in the diagnosis of conditions of the abdominal and pelvic organs, particularly the liver, gallbladder, spleen, pancreas, kidneys, uterus, ovaries, and abdominal aorta. Some examples of conditions that can be detected using ultrasound include breast cysts, gallstones, and kidney stones.

An ultrasound examination of the heart is called an **echocardiogram** and is used to determine the size, shape, and position of the heart and the movement of the heart valves and chambers. Ultrasonography is also used for guiding a needle or other device during a minimally invasive procedure such as amniocentesis, a needle biopsy, cortisone injection into a joint, and needle aspiration of fluid in a joint.

Ultrasonography offers many advantages as a diagnostic imaging procedure. It shows movement, allows continuous viewing of a structure, uses sound waves rather than radia-

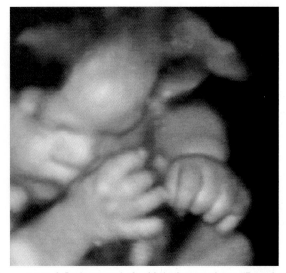

Figure 14-7. 3-D ultrasound of a third-trimester fetus. (From Leonard PC: Building a medical vocabulary: with Spanish translations, ed 7, St Louis, 2009, Saunders.)

tion, and is less expensive than other imaging procedures. Ultrasound does have some minor limitations. Because sound waves are unable to penetrate bone and air or gas-filled cavities such as the lungs, stomach, and intestines, ultrasound cannot be used in the evaluation of these structures. In addition, ultrasound may be difficult to use with obese patients because adipose tissue can interfere with sound wave transmission.

Before performing an ultrasound examination, a warm ultrasound gel must first be spread on the area to be examined. The purpose of the gel is to increase conductivity of the sound waves between the skin and the transducer. During the ultrasound examination, the examiner places a probe containing a transducer firmly on the patient's skin and moves it over the body areas to be examined. The transducer generates sound waves that are directed into the patient's tissues. The sound waves are reflected back to the transducer, similar to an echo. These sound waves are then transmitted to the ultrasound machine through a cable, where a computer converts them into an image. The size, shape, and consistency of the image are displayed on a video display screen; this image is known as a **sonogram** (Figure 14-8). The patient is often permitted to view the sonogram on the screen of the monitor as the procedure is performed. Selected images can be permanently recorded on paper, film, videotape, or a computerized storage medium. A radiologist reviews and interprets the images and prepares an ultrasound report that is sent to the patient's physician.

Although ultrasound is commonly used for a wide variety of noninvasive imaging procedures, individuals are most familiar with its use in obstetrics. Obstetric ultrasound is most frequently used to determine the gestational age of a fetus and to confirm the due date; to detect congenital abnormalities, ectopic pregnancy, and multiple pregnancy; and to determine the fetus' position and size late in pregnancy. If the fetus is old enough and is positioned correctly,

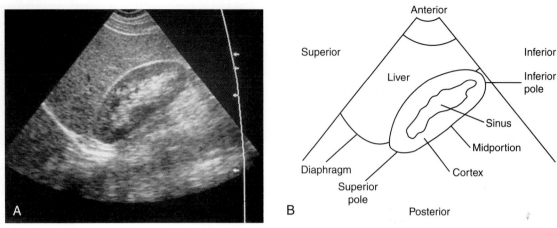

Figure 14-8. Sonogram of the right kidney. (From Tempkin BB: Ultrasound scanning: principles and protocols, ed 3, St Louis, 2009, Saunders.)

it also may be possible to determine its gender. Because the ultrasound machine is a compact unit, most obstetricians perform this procedure in their medical offices. Ultrasound is also used by gynecologists to evaluate and treat infertility problems.

Doppler ultrasound is a special application of ultrasound. It measures the direction and speed of blood as it flows through blood vessels, such as major arteries and veins in the abdomen, arms, legs, and neck. Doppler ultrasound images can assist the physician in diagnosing blood flow blockages, narrowing of blood vessels due to atherosclerosis, and congenital malformations.

Patient Preparation

The medical assistant should tell the patient what to expect during an ultrasound examination and instruct the patient in the preparation required for the procedure, as follows:
1. Ultrasound is a safe and painless procedure that takes approximately 15 to 45 minutes to complete, depending on the body part examined.

What Would You Do? What Would You *Not* Do?

Case Study 2

Sara-Jayne Monterey has been having heart palpitations. The physician ordered an electrocardiogram, and the results did not show any abnormalities. The physician then ordered a Holter monitor. Results showed the patient was having premature ventricular contractions, especially in the evening. The physician suspects that Sara-Jayne has a prolapsed mitral valve and has scheduled an echocardiogram at the local hospital. Sara-Jayne wants to know whether this procedure involves injecting a dye into her veins. She also wants to know whether the procedure will hurt. Two days before the appointment for the echocardiogram, Sara-Jayne calls the medical office to say that she just found out that she is pregnant and wants to know whether the procedure will have to be canceled. ■

---

2. The patient may need to prepare for the procedure, depending on the part of the body examined. An ultrasound of the gallbladder, liver, spleen, and pancreas necessitates that the patient fast for 8 to 12 hours. For an obstetric ultrasound, the patient needs to have a full bladder. The patient should be instructed to consume approximately 32 ounces of fluid about 1 hour before the procedure.
3. The patient must remain still when requested during the procedure because movement can interfere with accurate results. In addition, the patient may be asked to change positions so that the organs can be seen at different angles.

COMPUTED TOMOGRAPHY

Computed tomography (also known as a *CT* scan) is an advanced radiographic examination that uses only a minimal amount of radiation. It produces a series of cross-sectional images of a body part, permitting the imaging of structures that cannot be visualized with conventional radiographic procedures. A CT scan allows the radiologist to view the bones and organs of the head and body in fine detail and has been used most successfully in diagnostic studies of the brain, abdomen, and pelvis. CT scans are used primarily to detect and evaluate tumors and other abnormalities and to monitor the effects of surgery, radiation therapy, or chemotherapy on tumors.

The scan is conducted by a skilled diagnostic imaging technician. The patient is positioned on a special motorized table (Figure 14-9). From an adjoining room, the technician mechanically moves the table into a doughnut-shaped device known as the *CT scanner* until the part of the body to be examined is inside the tubular opening of the scanner.

During the scan, two examinations are often performed. The first examination is a plain scan, and the second is a repeat scan after a contrast medium has been injected

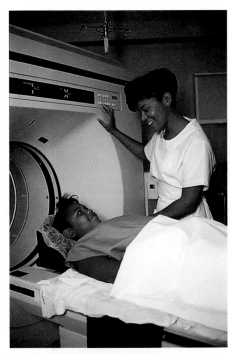

Figure 14-9. Positioning patient for computed tomography (CT) scan. (From Kowalczyk N, Donnett K: Integrated patient care for the imaging professional, St Louis, 1996, Mosby.)

through a vein in the arm. The contrast medium makes possible a sharper image of internal structures of the body. The x-ray tube within the CT scanner rotates around the patient, taking multiple radiographic images in a rapid sequence at different angles. The series of radiographs is processed with a computer to produce cross-sectional images of a body part similar to the slices of bread in a loaf. These images are permanently recorded on film or stored digitally on electronic media for evaluation by a radiologist (Figure 14-10). The radiologist reviews and interprets the images and prepares a CT report, which is sent to the patient's physician.

Patient Preparation

The medical assistant should tell the patient what to expect during the CT scan and should instruct the patient on the preparation required for the procedure, as follows:

1. Before the procedure, the patient must remove all radiopaque objects, such as dentures, eyeglasses, and jewelry, because they interfere with a clear image of the body part examined.
2. If a contrast medium is to be used, the patient may need to fast for several hours before the procedure. It is important to ask the patient whether he or she is allergic to radiographic contrast media to avoid an adverse reaction.
3. The patient should lie motionless and breathe normally during the procedure. When a radiograph is being taken, the patient is usually asked to hold his or her breath so that the radiograph is not blurred. The patient hears

mechanical clicking and whirring sounds from the scanner as pictures are taken.
4. Depending on the body part being examined, the procedure takes from 10 minutes to an hour to complete.

MAGNETIC RESONANCE IMAGING

MRI is used for imaging tissues of high fat and water content that cannot be seen with other radiologic techniques. MRI assists in the diagnosis of intracranial and spinal lesions and cardiovascular and soft tissue abnormalities, such as herniated discs and joint diseases. MRI allows the examiner to see through bone and view fluid-filled soft tissue in great detail.

MRI is a safe and painless procedure in which a strong magnetic field and ordinary radiowaves produce computer-processed images of internal body structures. Because MRI does not involve radiation, the U.S. Food and Drug Ad-

Memories *from* Externship

Michelle Shockey: My first externship was terrifying, but at the same time I was overwhelmed with excitement. I remember worrying how I was going to remember all my clinical and administrative skills. I was worried that I would hurt someone or forget to do something important.

One day a patient came into our office upset and crying. The examination rooms were full, so I took her into our staff lounge. I sat her down, fixed her a cup of coffee, and asked her if I could help. She told me that her son had drowned 2 years ago on that day, her mother had cancer, and her husband had passed away 8 months previously. I listened to everything she had to say, and I comforted her until the physician was ready to see her. She walked over to me, hugged me, and said my smile and people skills were the best treatment for her depression that she had ever had. Her telling me that made me feel good about my career choice, and it made me realize how fulfilling it was. It did not take me long to realize that all the hands-on skills that I had learned in the classroom were not forgotten. I also realized that a smile and listening to people are just as important as my skills. ∎

What Would You Do? What Would You *Not* Do?

Case Study 3

Michael Wendl is an 18-year-old high school varsity football player. For the past 3 months, he has had pain and swelling in his left shoulder. The physician schedules an MRI to assist in determining the cause of the problem. Michael has had several radiographs over the past 2 years and is worried about the radiation exposure to his body. He wants to know how much radiation will be involved with the procedure. Michael has problems with claustrophobia and wants to know whether he can play a game on his iPhone during the procedure to distract him. He also wants to know whether he is allowed to eat anything before the procedure. ∎

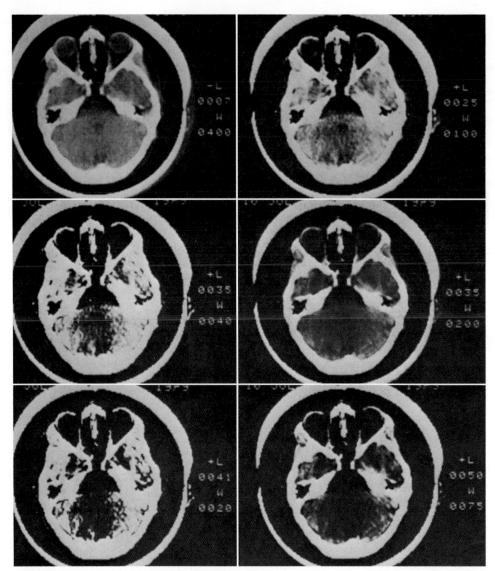

Figure 14-10. The computed tomography (CT) scanner takes multiple cross-sectional radiographic images. The images shown here are cross-sectional pictures of the head used to evaluate the orbits and sinuses. (From Snopek A: Fundamentals of special radiographic procedures, ed 4, Philadelphia, 1999, Saunders.)

ministration has classified the MRI machine as a low-risk device.

The patient lies on a table inside the bore of the cylindrical MRI machine while a diagnostic imaging technician in an adjoining room monitors the procedure (Figure 14-11). Because of the closed space, some patients may have difficulty with claustrophobia. The physician may order a sedative for these patients. Open MRI machines are less confining than traditional MRI machines; however, they are a newer technology and may not be available at some facilities.

The high-resolution, three-dimensional images that are obtained with MRI are permanently recorded on film or stored digitally on electronic media for evaluation by a radiologist. The radiologist reviews and interprets the images and prepares an MRI report, which is sent to the patient's physician.

Patient Preparation

The medical assistant should tell the patient what to expect during the MRI and instruct the patient in the preparation required for the procedure, as follows:

1. MRI is a safe and painless procedure with a usual completion time between 20 minutes and 1½ hours.
2. No special preparation is necessary for the MRI examination. The patient may eat or drink before the examination and take any prescribed medication. The patient should wear loose, comfortable clothing, such as a jogging suit, for the procedure.
3. Because the procedure involves a strong magnet, the patient should remove any metal or magnetic-sensitive objects, such as hairpins, eyeglasses, hearing aids, watches, rings, and credit cards. Avoid wearing cosmetics, as certain types of cosmetic preparations contain small amounts

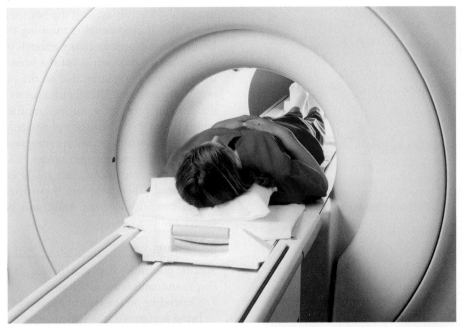

Figure 14-11. Magnetic resonance imaging (MRI). The patient lies on a table inside the bore of the cylindrical MRI machine while MRI technicians in an adjoining room monitor the procedure. (From Ballinger PW, Frank ED, eds: Merrill's atlas of radiographic positions and radiologic procedures, vol 3, ed 10, St Louis, 2003, Mosby.)

of metal. Individuals with a pacemaker or inner ear implant may not be able to undergo an MRI.

4. A contrast medium may be used for the procedure. It improves the resolution of the image by increasing the brightness in various parts of the body.

5. The patient must remain completely still for 15- to 20-minute intervals during the procedure. The patient hears a metallic clacking sound like a muffled drumbeat during the procedure. Earplugs or headphones are available for use if the patient desires.

NUCLEAR MEDICINE

Nuclear medicine is an advanced diagnostic imaging procedure in which a tiny bit of radioactive material is introduced into the patient. The radiation is introduced into the body by a diagnostic imaging technician using one of the following methods: intravenously, by ingestion, or by inhalation. The technologist positions the patient on a scanning table that works in association with a specialized piece of equipment known as a *gamma camera*. The gamma camera is positioned above or below the scanning table and is able to detect the radiation being given off by the body part that has been targeted by the radiation. This is accomplished through the use of scintillation crystals. These crystals convert the radiation being given off by the body into light. This light is converted into electrical impulses, which are interpreted by a computer program contained within the gamma camera. The resulting information is displayed as still images or functional animations of body parts and organs. Because it can show the actual function of organs,

nuclear medicine provides more detailed information for certain conditions than is provided by other diagnostic imaging examinations (e.g., CT scan, MRI).

The radioactive material used in nuclear medicine is known as a *radiopharmaceutical* (or radionuclide). Examples of commonly used radiopharmaceuticals include technetium-99m, iodine-123 and 131, and thallium-201. Most radiopharmaceuticals are chemically bound to a complex known as a *tracer*. A tracer is designed to be attracted to specific areas of the body or, in some cases, to types of diseased tissue.

The most common nuclear medicine procedures include bone scans and nuclear cardiac stress tests, which are described in more detail in the next section. Other types of nuclear medicine procedures that may be performed include gallbladder procedures, thyroid studies, brain scans, lung scans, and liver procedures.

Bone Scans

Bone scans are performed to detect small fractures (e.g., stress fractures) or lesions that may not be visible on other diagnostic imaging examinations. When a bone scan is performed, the patient is injected with a radiopharmaceutical. The patient must then wait at the facility for a predetermined period of time, based on the area being examined. The purpose of the waiting period is to allow the radiopharmaceutical to be absorbed sufficiently so that an accurate diagnosis can be made. The gamma camera detects the radiation given off by the small fracture, and it shows up as a "hot" spot on the nuclear images (Figure 14-12). The radiologist reviews the nuclear images and prepares a bone scan report, which is sent to the patient's physician.

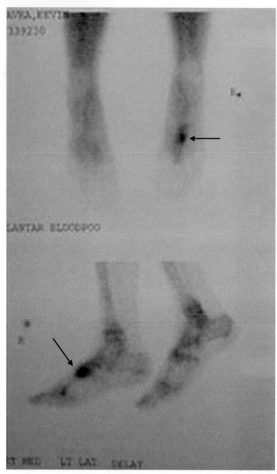

Figure 14-12. Bone scan of the foot. *Arrows* show the hot spot that indicates a stress fracture. (From Donatelli RA: Sports-specific rehabilitation, St Louis, 2007, Churchill Livingstone.)

Nuclear Cardiac Stress Test

A nuclear cardiac stress test is a diagnostic procedure used to evaluate the cardiovascular health of individuals with known heart disease or individuals at high risk for developing heart disease, particularly coronary artery disease (CAD). Although a nuclear stress test is more time consuming and expensive to perform than a simple stress test (described in Chapter 12), it provides more accuracy in diagnosing CAD.

The radiopharmaceutical used for a nuclear stress test is usually technetium-99mTc sestamibi (trade name is Cardiolite), which is administered intravenously and targets the heart. Nuclear images included in the stress test are taken by the gamma camera during two phases: a *resting phase* and a *stress phase* (which is a functional study). The resting phase is performed with the heart at a normal rate, whereas the stress phase is performed immediately after the patient exercises at his or her maximal (target) heart rate. The two sets of nuclear images—the resting images and the images taken under cardiac stress—are then compared with each other. These images assist the radiologist in determining which parts of the heart are healthy and functioning normally. The

images also identify areas of the heart that exhibit decreased blood flow during exercise, meaning that a portion of the heart muscle is not receiving enough oxygen. A decreased oxygen supply to a portion of the heart is known as cardiac ischemia and is typically due to the presence of coronary artery disease. The radiologist reviews and interprets the images and prepares a nuclear cardiac stress test report, which is sent to the patient's physician.

A PET (positron emission tomography) scan is a special type of nuclear imaging procedure. PET uses a special camera and computer to construct a 3-D image of the area being scanned. This procedure is particularly useful in diagnosing conditions of the brain and heart, such as brain cancer and heart disease.

Guidelines

Specific guidelines that may be required for nuclear medicine examinations are as follows:

1. Depending on the type of nuclear medicine examination being performed, the patient may be required to be in a fasting state or to abstain from consuming certain foods or substances such as caffeine for a period of time. The medical assistant should check with the facility performing the examination, so that proper dietary instructions can be relayed to the patient.

2. Nuclear medicine examinations are time consuming because most examinations require multiple scans. The interval between scans is determined by the part being examined and the type of equipment and radiopharmaceutical being used. There may be a delay between administration of the radiopharmaceutical and when the patient is actually placed on the scanning table. Follow-up images that may be done later the same day or, in some cases, the following morning also may be needed. Because of this, the medical assistant must inform the patient of the amount of time required for the examination, so that arrangements can be made with work and home schedules if needed.

3. Because most nuclear medicine examinations require that the patient lie still on a table for a prolonged time, the patient should be advised to wear comfortable clothing to the examination. If a nuclear medicine examination requires exercise as a component of the test, the patient should be instructed to wear appropriate exercise clothing, including athletic shoes.

DIGITAL RADIOLOGY

Modern advances in digital imaging technology have made inroads into the field of radiology. The result is the transformation of film-based radiology into a system of computer-displayed and stored digital images. To assist in understanding digital radiology, this transformation can be compared with the replacement of film cameras with digital cameras. Images can be taken and viewed immediately, and then sent electronically to a network of computers. These images can

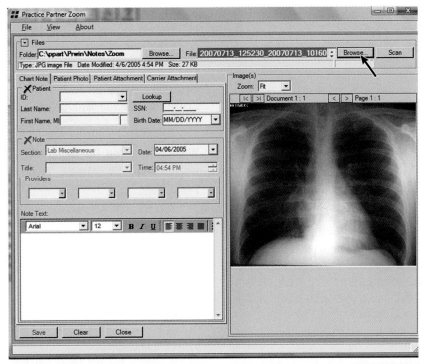

Figure 14-13. Digital image of a chest x-ray. (Screenshot used by permission of MCKESSON Corporation. All rights reserved. © MCKESSON Corporation, 2011.) (From Buck CJ: Electronic health record booster kit for the medical office, St Louis, 2009, Saunders.)

also be saved on a CD or DVD and given to the patient to take to his or her physician for review.

Digital radiology allows for increased efficiency and cost savings and better patient care. Higher-quality images and the ability to transfer these digital images electronically are two important benefits that affect the patient directly. As a result of this digital revolution, the medical assistant may be required to use the medical office computer to access, display (Figure 14-13), and permanently save images taken by the facilities providing digital imaging services.

℮volve *Check out the Evolve site to access additional interactive activities.*

MEDICAL PRACTICE *and the* LAW

Radiology and diagnostic imaging involve high-technology equipment and procedures that can be frightening and uncomfortable to the patient. Be aware of the patient's reactions, and provide assistance and comfort whenever possible. Be specific in providing the patient with instructions to ensure the best imaging results.

Procedures that involve injectable contrast media or that are invasive usually require written informed consent. Check office policy for procedures that require signed consent forms.

With procedures that use radiation, federal laws regulate usage and exposure testing and record-keeping. The acronym ALARA (As Low As Reasonably Able) reminds workers to minimize exposure to themselves and patients. Ask female patients whether they may be pregnant before beginning any radiologic procedure. ∎

What Would You Do? What Would You *Not* Do?   RESPONSES

Case Study 1
Page 573

What Did Michelle Do?

❏ Told Mrs. Ramirez that a role-playing game with Jose might help. Suggested that she play the "doctor" and pretend she is taking an x-ray of Jose.

❏ Told Mrs. Ramirez that the barium will have a flavoring in it but that it does taste chalky. Suggested that she explain to Jose why he needs to drink the barium—to help the doctor find what is wrong with him so that he will not get sick anymore.

❏ Told Mrs. Ramirez that Jose's truck is made of metal and would interfere with a good radiograph. Suggested that she bring the truck and tell Jose he could have it after the procedure.

❏ Explained that the barium might cause constipation and would cause Jose's next bowel movement to be white in color. Told her that she should encourage Jose to drink a lot of water after the procedure to help prevent constipation.

What Did Michelle Not *Do?*

❏ Did not tell Mrs. Ramirez that the barium solution would taste good and that she should not have any trouble getting Jose to drink it.

What Would You Do?/What Would You *Not* Do? Review Michelle's response and place a checkmark next to the information you included in your response. List additional information you included in your response.

_____
_____
_____
_____

Case Study 2
Page 580

What Did Michelle Do?

❏ Told Sara-Jayne that the procedure uses sound waves to visualize the heart. Explained that the procedure does not use a dye injected into the veins. Gave her an educational brochure on ultrasound imaging.

❏ Reassured Sara-Jayne that no pain is involved with an echocardiogram.

❏ Told Sara-Jayne that an ultrasound is normally safe during pregnancy because radiation is not used. The physician would be informed that she is pregnant, however, and if there is a change in his order, Sara-Jayne would be notified.

What Did Michelle Not *Do?*

❏ Did not allow Sara-Jayne to go ahead with the procedure without checking with the physician.

What Would You Do?/What Would You *Not* Do? Review Michelle's response and place a checkmark next to the information you included in your response. List additional information you included in your response.

_____
_____
_____
_____

Case Study 3
Page 581

What Did Michelle Do?

❏ Explained to Michael that an MRI does not use radiation, so he would not be exposed to any radiation during the procedure.

❏ Told Michael that he would not be able to play a game on his iPhone during the procedure. Explained that the MRI works with a strong magnet that might damage the iPhone and also interfere with a good image of the shoulder. Told Michael that he would need to lie still during the procedure.

❏ Told Michael the physician would be informed of his problem with claustrophobia. Explained that the physician may want to give him something to help him relax during the procedure.

❏ Told Michael that it was fine to eat before the procedure.

What Did Michelle Not *Do?*

❏ Did not overlook or minimize Michael's concern about claustrophobia.

What Would You Do?/What Would You *Not* Do? Review Michelle's response and place a checkmark next to the information you included in your response. List additional information you included in your response.

_____
_____
_____
_____

CERTIFICATION REVIEW

❏ **X-rays are used to visualize internal organs and structures** and serve as a diagnostic aid in determining the presence of disease. They also are used therapeutically in the treatment of malignant neoplasms. *Radiograph* is the term for the permanent record of the picture produced on radiographic film. Radiology is the branch of medicine that deals with the use of radiant energy in the diagnosis and treatment of disease.

❏ **A structure that permits the passage of x-rays is radiolucent.** A structure that obstructs the passage of x-rays is radiopaque. A contrast medium is used to make a particular structure visible on the radiograph. A fluoroscope is an instrument used to view internal organs and structures of the body directly on a display screen.

❏ **The position of the patient** is determined by the purpose of the examination and the area examined. Different types of radiographic views include anteroposterior (AP), posteroanterior (PA), lateral, oblique, supine, and prone.

❏ **Mammography** is a radiographic examination of the breasts used to detect breast disease. Mammography can be used to detect a breast tumor when the growth is less than 1 cm in diameter.

❏ **An upper GI** is an examination of the upper digestive tract with fluoroscopy and radiography. It is used in the diagnosis of disorders of the esophagus, stomach, duodenum, and small intestine.

❏ **A lower GI** involves filling the colon with a barium sulfate mixture with a catheter inserted into the rectum. This examination is used in the diagnosis of disorders of the colon, such as polyps, cancerous tumors, and diverticulosis, and to determine the extent of inflammatory bowel disease.

❏ **An intravenous pyelogram (IVP)** is a radiograph of the kidneys, ureters, and bladder. It is used to assist in the diagnosis of kidney stones, blockage or narrowing of the urinary tract, and growths within or near the urinary system.

❏ **Ultrasonography** uses high-frequency sound waves to study soft tissue structures. It is frequently used in the diagnosis of conditions of the abdominal and pelvic organs, particularly the liver, gallbladder, spleen, pancreas, kidneys, uterus, ovaries, and abdominal aorta. An ultrasound examination of the heart is called an *echocardiogram*. Ultrasound shows movement and allows continuous viewing of a structure. Obstetric ultrasound is used to determine the gestational age of a fetus and to confirm the date of delivery.

❏ **Computed tomography** (CT scan) is used to view the bones and organs of the head and body in fine detail. CT scans are used in the detection and evaluation of tumors and other abnormalities and in monitoring the effects of surgery, radiation therapy, or chemotherapy on tumors.

❏ **MRI** is used to assist in the diagnosis of intracranial and spinal lesions and of cardiovascular and soft tissue abnormalities, such as herniated discs and joint diseases. MRI allows the examiner to see through bone and view fluid-filled soft tissue in great detail.

❏ **Nuclear medicine** is an advanced diagnostic imaging procedure in which a tiny bit of radioactive material is introduced into the patient. A gamma camera is able to detect the radiation being given off by the body part that has been targeted by the radiation. Nuclear medicine has the ability to show the actual functions of organs. The most common nuclear medicine procedures include bone scans and cardiac studies. Other types of nuclear medicine procedures that may be performed include thyroid studies, brain scans, lung scans, and liver and gallbladder procedures.

TERMINOLOGY REVIEW

Medical Term	Word Parts	Definition
Contrast medium		A substance used to make a particular structure visible on a radiograph.
Echocardiogram	*ech/o-:* sound *cardi/o-:* heart *-gram:* record	An ultrasound examination of the heart.
Enema		An injection of fluid into the rectum to aid in the elimination of feces from the colon.
Fluoroscope	*fluor/o-:* fluorescence *-scope:* instrument used for visual examination	An instrument used to view internal organs and structures directly.
Fluoroscopy	*fluor/o-:* fluorescence *-scopy:* visual examination	Examination of a patient with a fluoroscope.

Continued

TERMINOLOGY REVIEW—cont'd

Medical Term	Word Parts	Definition
Radiograph	*radi/o-:* radiation *-graph:* instrument used to record, x-ray film	A permanent record of a picture of an internal body organ or structure produced on radiographic film.
Radiography	*radi/o-:* radiation *-graphy:* process of recording, x-ray filming	The taking of permanent records (radiographs) of internal body organs and structures by passing x-rays through the body to act on a specially sensitized film.
Radiologist	*radi/o-:* radiation *-ologist:* one who studies and practices (specialist)	A physician who specializes in the diagnosis and treatment of disease using radiation and other imaging techniques.
Radiology	*radi/o-:* radiation *-ology:* study of	The branch of medicine that deals with the use of radiation and other imaging techniques (such as ultrasound, CT scans, MRIs, and nuclear medicine) in the diagnosis and treatment of disease.
Radiolucent	*radi/o-:* radiation *-lucent:* transparent	Describing a structure that permits the passage of x-rays.
Radiopaque	*radi/o-:* radiation *-opaque:* opaque	Describing a structure that obstructs the passage of x-rays.
Sonogram	*son/o-:* sound *-gram:* record	The record obtained with ultrasonography.
Ultrasonography	*ultra-:* beyond, excess *sono-:* sound *-graphy:* process of recording	The use of high-frequency sound waves to produce an image of an organ or tissue.

ON THE WEB

For Information on Radiography and Diagnostic Imaging:

BrighamRAD: www.brighamrad.harvard.edu

Society for Computer Applications in Radiology: www.scarnet.org

Whole Brain Atlas: www.med.harvard.edu/AANLIB/home.html

Radiology Information: www.radiologyinfo.org

For Information on Breast Cancer:

American Cancer Society: www.cancer.org

Breast Cancer Treatment: AboutBreastCancerinfo.com

Breast Cancer: Cancercenter.com

Breast Cancer org: Breastcancer.org

Breast Cancer Site: www.thebreastcancersite.com

National Breast Cancer Foundation: www.nationalbreastcancer.org

Breast Cancer.Net: www.breastcancer.net

Breast Cancer Basics: breastcancer.about.com

15

Introduction to the Clinical Laboratory

LEARNING OBJECTIVES

Clinical Laboratory

1. Explain the general purpose of a laboratory test.
2. Identify and define the eight categories of a laboratory test on the basis of function. List examples of tests included under each category.
3. List and explain specific uses of laboratory test results.
4. Describe the relationship between the medical office and an outside laboratory.
5. List the information included in a laboratory directory.
6. Identify the purpose of a laboratory request form. List and explain the function of each type of information included on the form.
7. Identify the use of each of the following profiles, and list the tests included in each:
   - Comprehensive metabolic profile
   - Electrolyte profile
   - Hepatic function profile
   - Hepatitis profile
   - Lipid profile
   - Prenatal profile
   - Renal function profile
   - Rheumatoid profile
   - Thyroid function profile
8. Identify the purpose of the laboratory report form, and list the information included on it.
9. Describe the advantages of using a computer to send and receive laboratory documents.
10. Explain how an EMR program can be used to prepare a flow sheet for tests performed on a routine basis.

Collecting, Transporting, and Handling Specimens

1. Explain the purpose of advance patient preparation for the collection of a laboratory specimen.
2. List examples of specimens.
3. Identify and explain the guidelines that should be followed during specimen collection.
4. Explain why specimens must be handled and stored properly.
5. Identify the proper handling and storage techniques for each of the following specimens: blood, urine, microbiologic specimen, and stool specimen.

PROCEDURES

Use a laboratory directory.
Complete a laboratory request form.

Read a laboratory report.
Instruct a patient on the preparation necessary for a laboratory test that requires fasting.

Maintain laboratory test results using flow sheets.

Collect a specimen.

Handle and store a specimen.

Laboratory Testing in the Medical Office

1. Describe the following CLIA test categories: waived, moderately complex, and highly complex.
2. List and describe the information included in a product insert that accompanies a CLIA-waived testing kit.
3. List the advantages of an automated blood analyzer.
4. Explain the purpose of quality control in the laboratory, and list quality control methods that should be employed when a CLIA-waived laboratory test is performed.
5. List the laboratory safety guidelines that should be followed in the medical office to prevent accidents.

Perform a CLIA-waived laboratory test by following the manufacturer's instructions.
Perform quality control procedures when utilizing a CLIA-waived laboratory test.
Practice laboratory safety.

Introduction to the Clinical Laboratory
Laboratory Tests
Purpose of Laboratory Testing
Types of Clinical Laboratories
  Physician's Office Laboratory
  Physical Structure of the POL
  Outside Laboratories
  Laboratory Directory
  Collection and Testing Categories
Laboratory Requests
  Purpose
  Parts of Laboratory Request Form
Laboratory Reports
Laboratory Documents and the EMR
Patient Preparation and Instructions
  Fasting
  Medication Restrictions

Collecting, Handling, and Transporting Specimens
  Guidelines for Specimen Collection
Clinical Laboratory Improvement Amendments
  Purpose of CLIA 1988
  Categories of Laboratory Testing
  Requirements for Moderate-Complexity and
    High-Complexity Testing
CLIA-Waived Laboratory Testing
  CLIA-Waived Testing Kits
  CLIA-Waived Automated Analyzers
Quality Control
Categories of Test Results
  Qualitative Test Results
  Quantitative Test Results
Recording Test Results
Laboratory Safety

analyte
calibration
control
clinical diagnosis
fasting
homeostasis (hoe-mee-oh-STAY-sis)
in vivo (in-VEE-voe)
laboratory test
nonwaived test
plasma (PLAZ-ma)
product insert

profile
quality control
reagent
reference range
routine test
serum (SERE-um)
specimen (SPES-i-men)
test system
qualitative test
quantitative test
waived test

Introduction to the Clinical Laboratory

Clinical laboratory test results are often used along with a thorough health history and physical examination to obtain essential data needed by the physician for the accurate diagnosis and management of a patient's condition. Clinical **laboratory tests** provide objective and quantitative information regarding the status of body conditions and functions. When the body is healthy, its systems function normally, and a state of equilibrium of the internal environment is said to exist; this is termed **homeostasis.** When the body is in a state of homeostasis, the physical and chemical characteristics of body substances (e.g., fluids, secretions, excretions) are within an acceptable range known as the **reference range.**

When a pathologic condition exists, biologic changes occur within the body, altering the normal physiology or functioning of the body and resulting in an imbalance. These changes cause the patient to experience symptoms of that particular pathologic condition. Iron-deficiency anemia usually causes the patient to experience weakness, fatigue, pallor, irritability, and, in some cases, shortness of breath on exertion. In addition, these changes in the body's biologic processes may cause an alteration in the characteristics of body substances, such as an alteration in the chemical content of the blood or urine, an alteration in the antibody level, or an alteration in cell counts or cellular morphology.

Physical and chemical alterations of body substances become evident through abnormal values or results on laboratory tests—in other words, values outside the accepted reference range or limit for that particular test. Just as certain pathologic conditions cause specific symptoms to occur, certain pathologic conditions cause values outside of the reference range to occur for specific laboratory tests. Iron-deficiency anemia causes an alteration in normal red blood cell morphology and a decreased hemoglobin level.

An important realization is that a value outside of the reference range for a particular test may be seen with more than one pathologic condition. A decrease in the hemoglobin level is found with hyperthyroidism, cirrhosis of the liver, and autoimmune diseases. In this regard, the physician cannot rely solely on laboratory test results to make a diagnosis, but rather must rely also on the combination of data obtained from the health history, the physical examination, and diagnostic and laboratory test results.

LABORATORY TESTS

A **laboratory test** is defined as the clinical analysis and study of materials, fluids, or tissues obtained from patients to assist in the diagnosis and treatment of disease. Laboratory tests can be classified by function into one of the following categories: hematology, clinical chemistry, immunology and blood banking, urinalysis, microbiology, parasitology, cytology, and histology. Table 15-1 lists the definitions of each of these categories and provides examples of commonly performed tests in each. Use of these classifications makes it easier to refer to laboratory tests.

The number of laboratory tests ordered for a patient varies depending on the physician's clinical findings. A clinical diagnosis of streptococcal sore throat usually requires only a

Table 15-1 Categories of Laboratory Tests*			
Category	**Definition and Commonly Performed Tests**	**Category**	**Definition and Commonly Performed Tests**

Hematology	Hematology is a science dealing with the study of blood and blood-forming tissues. Laboratory analysis in hematology deals with examination of blood for detection of abnormalities and includes areas such as blood cell counts, cellular morphology, clotting ability of blood, and identification of cell types:
	    White Blood Cell Count (WBC)
	    Red Blood Cell Count (RBC)
	    Differential White Blood Cell Count (Diff)
	    Hemoglobin (Hgb)
	    Hematocrit (Hct)
	    Platelet Count
	    Reticulocyte Count
	    Prothrombin Time (PT)
	    Sedimentation Rate
		Immunology and blood banking	Laboratory analysis in immunology and blood banking deals with studying antigen-antibody reactions to assess the presence of a substance or to determine the presence of disease.
			Immunology
			    Antinuclear Antibody (ANA)
			    Antistreptolysin O (ASO)
			    C-Reactive Protein (CRP)
			    Hepatitis Tests
			    HIV Tests
			    Mononucleosis Test
			    Pregnancy Test
			    Rheumatoid Factor (RF)
			    Syphilis Tests (VDRL, RPR)
			Blood Banking
			    ABO Blood Typing
			    Rh Typing
			    Rh Antibody Test

*Categories of laboratory tests are listed, including definitions of each and commonly performed tests or pathologic conditions in each category. Tests commonly known by their abbreviations are listed this way.

Continued

Table 15-1 Categories of Laboratory Tests—cont'd

Category	Definition and Commonly Performed Tests	Category	Definition and Commonly Performed Tests

Clinical chemistry	Laboratory analysis in clinical chemistry determines the amount of chemical substances present in body fluids, excreta, and tissues (e.g., blood, urine, cerebrospinal fluid). The largest area in clinical chemistry is blood chemistry:
	
	Alanine Aminotransferase (ALT)
	Albumin
	Alkaline Phosphatase (ALP)
	Amylase
	Aspartate Aminotransferase (AST)
	Bilirubin
	Blood Alcohol
	Blood Lead
	Blood Urea Nitrogen (BUN)
	Calcium
	Carbon Dioxide
	Chloride
	Cholesterol
	Cortisol
	Creatine Kinase (CK)
	Creatinine
	Gamma-Glutamyltranspeptidase
	Globulin
	Glucose
	Inorganic Phosphorus
	Lactate Dehydrogenase (LD)
	Potassium
	Protein (Total)
	Sodium
	Thyroxine (T_4)
	Triiodothyronine (T_3) Uptake
	Triglycerides
	Uric Acid
		Urinalysis	Urinalysis involves physical, chemical, and microscopic analyses of urine.
			A. Tests included in physical analysis of urine:
			    Color
			    Appearance
			    Specific Gravity
			B. Tests included in chemical analysis of urine:
			    Glucose
			    Bilirubin
			    Blood
			    Ketones
			    Leukocytes
			    Nitrite
			    pH
			    Protein
			    Urobilinogen
			C. Tests included in microscopic analysis of urine:
			    Red Blood Cells
			    White Blood Cells
			    Epithelial Cells
			    Casts
			    Crystals

Microbiology	Microbiology is the scientific study of microorganisms and their activities. Laboratory analysis in microbiology deals with identification of pathogens present in specimens taken from the body (e.g., urine, blood, throat, sputum, wound, urethra, vagina, cerebrospinal fluid). Examples of infectious diseases diagnosed through identification of pathogens present in the specimen include the following: Candidiasis Chlamydia Diphtheria Gonorrhea Meningitis Pertussis Pneumonia Streptococcal Sore Throat Tetanus Tonsillitis Tuberculosis Urinary Tract Infection	Cytology	Laboratory analysis in cytology deals with detection of the presence of abnormal cells: Chromosome Studies Pap Test

Table 15-1	Categories of Laboratory Tests—cont'd		
Category	**Definition and Commonly Performed Tests**	**Category**	**Definition and Commonly Performed Tests**
Parasitology	Laboratory analysis in parasitology deals with detection of the presence of disease-producing human parasites or eggs present in specimens taken from the body (e.g., stool, vagina, blood). Examples of human diseases caused by parasites include the following: Amebiasis Ascariasis Hookworms Malaria Pinworms Scabies Tapeworms Toxoplasmosis Trichinosis Trichomoniasis	Histology	Histology is the microscopic study of the form and structure of various tissues that make up living organisms. Laboratory analysis in histology deals with the detection of diseased tissues: Biopsy Studies Tissue Analyses

strep test for confirmation. Many diseases cause more than one alteration in the physical and chemical characteristics of body substances, however, and a series of laboratory tests is often necessary to establish the pattern of abnormalities characteristic of a particular disease.

The medical assistant should realize that not all pathologic conditions necessitate the use of laboratory test results for arrival at a diagnosis; the information obtained from the patient's clinical signs and symptoms can be sufficient for a diagnosis of some conditions. In these instances, the physician is so certain of the clinical diagnosis that therapy can be instituted without laboratory confirmation. Most physicians diagnose acute purulent otitis media with the information obtained from patient symptoms (earache, fever, feeling of fullness in the ear) and from an otoscopic examination of the tympanic membrane (the tympanic membrane is red and bulging). Information obtained through the clinical signs and symptoms is sufficiently specific to otitis media to allow the physician to make a diagnosis and to prescribe treatment.

The medical assistant must acquire knowledge and skill in basic clinical laboratory methods and techniques. It is important that the medical assistant have knowledge of the laboratory tests that are performed most often, including the purpose of these tests, the reference range for each test, any advance patient preparation or special instructions, and any substances that might interfere with accurate test results, such as food or medication.

The medical assistant frequently works with this information when instructing a patient in advance preparation for a laboratory test, collecting, handling, and storing specimens; performing laboratory tests; and receiving and filing laboratory reports. It is essential that the medical assistant understand the value of laboratory tests and alert the physician to any abnormal results as soon as the test is performed or the laboratory report is received.

This chapter serves as an introduction to the clinical laboratory by providing an overview of methods and general guidelines to follow and by focusing on the relationship between the medical office and an outside laboratory. Specific information for collection, handling, storing, and testing of biologic specimens is presented in subsequent chapters.

PURPOSE OF LABORATORY TESTING

The most frequent use of laboratory test results is to assist in the diagnosis of a patient's condition. Laboratory test results also have many other significant medical uses. A summary of the purpose and function of laboratory testing follows:

1. Laboratory tests are most frequently ordered by the physician *to assist in the diagnosis of pathologic conditions.* Along with the health history and the physical examination, laboratory test results provide the physician with essential data needed to arrive at a diagnosis and prescribe treatment. After obtaining the health history and performing the physical examination, the physician may order laboratory tests for these reasons:

   - *To confirm a clinical diagnosis.* A **clinical diagnosis** is defined as a tentative diagnosis of a patient's condition obtained through the evaluation of the health history and the physical examination, without the benefit of laboratory or diagnostic tests.
   - The patient's signs and symptoms may provide a strong clinical diagnosis of a particular condition, and the physician may order laboratory tests simply to confirm that diagnosis. For example, the patient may have the typical signs and symptoms of diabetes mellitus, which would provide the physician with a fairly certain clinical diagnosis. In this instance, an oral glucose tolerance test (OGTT) may be ordered to confirm the diagnosis and to institute therapy.

- *To assist in the differential diagnosis of a patient's condition.* Two or more diseases may have similar signs and symptoms; the physician orders laboratory tests to assist in the differential diagnosis of the patient's condition. A diagnosis of streptococcal sore throat must be made with a laboratory test to differentiate it from other pathologic conditions with similar signs and symptoms, such as pharyngitis.

- *To obtain information regarding a patient's condition* when not enough concrete evidence exists to support a clinical diagnosis. The patient sometimes may have vague signs and symptoms, and laboratory tests are ordered to obtain information on what may be causing the patient's problem. For example, the patient may have nonspecific abdominal pain, and the physical examination may not yield enough information to support a clinical diagnosis. In this case, the physician may order a series of laboratory and diagnostic tests to assist in pinpointing the cause of the patient's problems.

2. *To evaluate the patient's progress and to regulate treatment.* When a diagnosis has been made, laboratory testing may be performed to evaluate the patient's progress and to regulate treatment. On the basis of the laboratory results, the therapy may need to be adjusted or further treatment prescribed. A patient undergoing iron therapy for iron-deficiency anemia should have a complete blood count (CBC) performed every month to assess the response to treatment and to ensure that the condition is improving. Another example is a patient who has had a cardiac valve replaced and is taking warfarin (Coumadin), an anticoagulant used to inhibit blood clotting. The patient must have a prothrombin time test at regular intervals to assess the clotting ability of the blood. On the basis of the test results, the medication may need to be adjusted to ensure the dosage is at a safe level. A patient with diabetes who measures his or her blood glucose level each day to regulate insulin dosage provides another example of laboratory tests used to regulate treatment.

3. *To establish a baseline level.* On the basis of such factors as age, gender, race, and geographic location, individuals have different normal levels within the established reference range for a particular test. In this respect, laboratory tests also can serve to establish each patient's baseline level with which future results can be compared. A patient who is going to receive warfarin (Coumadin) therapy should have a blood specimen drawn for a prothrombin time test before administration of this anticoagulant. The results serve as a baseline recording for that particular patient against which future prothrombin time test results can be compared.

4. *To prevent or reduce the severity of disease.* Laboratory tests also can help to prevent or reduce the severity of disease through early detection of abnormal findings. Certain conditions, such as high cholesterol, anemia, and diabetes, are relatively common disorders and sometimes may exist without symptoms in a patient, especially early in

the development of the disease. Laboratory tests known as **routine tests** are performed on a routine basis on apparently healthy patients (usually as part of a general physical examination) to assist in the early detection of disease. These tests are relatively easy to perform and present a minimal hazard to the patient. The most commonly used routine tests are urinalysis, CBC, and routine blood chemistries.

5. *To comply with state laws.* Another reason for a laboratory test is its requirement by state law. The statutes of most states require a gonorrhea and syphilis test to be performed on pregnant women. The purpose of these tests is to protect the mother and fetus from harm by screening for the presence of these sexually transmitted diseases.

TYPES OF CLINICAL LABORATORIES

The medical office may use an outside laboratory for testing, or the office may contain its own laboratory, known as a *physician's office laboratory* (POL), in which the medical assistant performs various tests. Most medical offices use a combination of the two to fulfill the physician's need for test results.

Physician's Office Laboratory

Generally, laboratory tests that are CLIA-waived and commonly required, such as glucose determination and urinalysis, are performed in the POL (Figure 15-1). CLIA (Clinical Laboratories Improvement Amendments) consists of regulations developed in 1988 by the federal government to improve the quality of laboratory testing in the United States. A **waived test** is a laboratory test that has been determined by CLIA to be a simple procedure that is easy to perform and has a low risk of erroneous test results. CLIA regulations are described in greater detail later in this chapter.

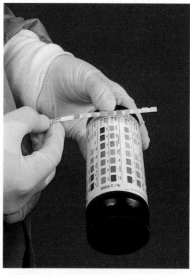

Figure 15-1. Urinalysis is frequently performed in a physician's office laboratory (POL).

Most physicians consider it too expensive in terms of equipment, supplies, and medical laboratory personnel to perform laboratory tests that are any more complex than waived tests in the medical office. These tests are usually performed at an outside laboratory. Outside laboratories use highly sophisticated automated equipment to perform the tests, providing the medical offices with fast and reliable test results.

Physical Structure of the POL

The physical structure of the POL should meet certain requirements to provide a safe and effective working environment for performing laboratory tests and storing laboratory equipment and supplies. The POL should be a separate room or work area in the medical office. Laboratory work counters should be large enough to provide ample space for testing specimens. Cabinets should be available for storing equipment and supplies. The medical assistant should check the supply inventory periodically and reorder supplies as needed. A refrigerator should be available in the POL for storing specimens that require refrigeration, such as blood tubes and urine awaiting pickup by a courier from an outside laboratory. In addition, certain testing components, such as controls and testing reagents, may require refrigeration. The temperature of the refrigerator must be maintained at between 36° F (2° C) and 46° F (8° C) to retard alterations in the physical and chemical compositions of specimens and to prevent deterioration of testing components that require refrigeration. The temperature of the refrigerator should be checked at least once each day and recorded on a refrigerator temperature log sheet. As specified by the Occupational Safety and Health Administration (OSHA) Standard, food must not be stored in the laboratory refrigerator, and a warning label must be attached to the refrigerator to alert employees to the presence of potentially infectious materials.

Equipment and supplies necessary to comply with the OSHA Standard should be readily accessible in the POL. These supplies include handwashing facilities, alcohol-based hand rubs, gloves, safety goggles and masks, safety-engineered syringes and needles, and biohazard sharps containers and biohazard trash bags. An eyewash station (Figure 15-2) is also recommended in the event of an exposure incident to the mucous membranes of the eyes, nose, or mouth.

The temperature of the room should be maintained within a range that is conducive to performing laboratory tests and storing testing materials that require room temperature storage. Temperatures outside of this range can cause deterioration of testing materials, such as controls and testing reagents. Some automated analyzers are able to operate only within a specific temperature range. When a specimen is tested, a chemical reaction occurs between the specimen and the testing reagents to produce the test results. With some analyzers, the chemical reaction can occur only within a certain temperature range. If the temperature is outside of the required range, the analyzer cannot perform the test, resulting in an error message that appears on the

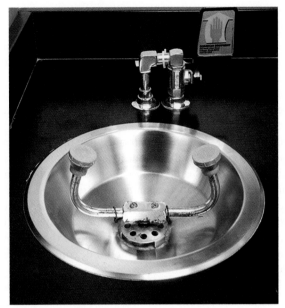

Figure 15-2. Eyewash station.

screen of the analyzer. The temperature range required for the storage of testing materials and for performing tests is stated in the instructions accompanying them. It is usually a room temperature that falls between 59° F (15° C) and 86° F (30° C).

Adequate lighting is essential to assist in the proper collection, handling, and testing of specimens. Good lighting is also needed for the proper interpretation of test results that use a visual color comparison method to determine test results, such as the dipstick method of urinalysis.

The medical assistant is responsible for making sure the POL is clean and free of clutter. Biohazard sharps containers and trash bags should be replaced as needed. A disinfectant should be readily available for disinfecting the laboratory work counters each day. The medical assistant should know how to care for each piece of laboratory equipment; this information is indicated in the operating manual that accompanies the equipment.

Outside Laboratories

Outside laboratories include hospital and privately owned independent laboratories, which employ individuals specifically trained in clinical laboratory techniques and methods such as medical laboratory technologists and technicians. Because the medical assistant usually works closely with an outside laboratory, a basic knowledge of the relationship between the medical office and the outside laboratory (as described in this section) is important. If the specimen is collected at the medical office, the laboratory usually provides the medical office with the supplies and forms necessary to collect the specimen and prepare it for transport to the laboratory. The medical assistant is responsible for checking these supplies periodically and for reordering them from the laboratory as needed.

Laboratory Directory

The outside laboratory provides the medical office with a laboratory directory (Figure 15-3), which serves as a valuable reference source for the proper collection and handling of specimens for transport to the outside laboratory. The laboratory may also maintain a website that includes a test menu of the specimen collection and handling requirements for each test performed by that laboratory. This allows the medical assistant to access this information easily and quickly using one or more of the following: a search box, an alphabetical index, or drop-down lists. If, after referring to the laboratory directory (or laboratory website), the medical assistant has a question regarding any aspect of the collection and handling of the specimen that is not clear, the laboratory should be contacted before proceeding.

Laboratory directories vary in organization, depending on the laboratory. The following information is generally included in the directory for each test performed by the laboratory:

- Name and CPT code of the test
- Reference range
- Amount and type of specimen required
- Supplies necessary for collection of the specimen (e.g., blood tubes)
- Techniques to be used for collection of the specimen
- Special instructions
- Patient preparation
- Proper handling and storage of the specimen
- Instructions for transporting the specimen
- Causes for rejection of the specimen by the laboratory
- Uses and limitations of the test
- Methodology used to perform the test

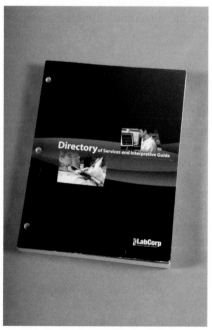

Figure 15-3. Laboratory directory.

Table 15-2 is a (modified) table of representative tests included in a laboratory directory to provide an overall understanding of the information included in a laboratory directory. The information presented in this modified directory includes all of the categories listed above with the exception of the following: special instructions, instructions for transporting the specimen, uses and limitations of the test, and methodology used to perform the test. (*Note:* Refer to Figure 15-8 for an example of a laboratory test exactly as it is presented in a laboratory directory.)

Collection and Testing Categories

Collection and testing of a specimen can be categorized as follows:

1. The specimen is collected and tested at the medical office.
2. The specimen is collected at the medical office and transferred to an outside laboratory for testing.
3. The patient is given a laboratory request to have the specimen collected and tested at an outside laboratory.

The medical assistant's responsibilities depend on which of these methods is used in the medical office. For example, a specimen collected at the medical office and transferred to an outside laboratory for testing involves a series of individual steps different from the steps followed when it is collected and tested at the medical office. The following clinical laboratory methods are presented in the remainder of this chapter to provide the student with the information needed to function competently in all three modes just described as follows:

1. Completing laboratory request forms and reviewing laboratory reports
2. Informing the patient of any necessary advance preparation or special instructions
3. Collecting, handling, and transporting specimens
4. Performing CLIA-waived tests in the medical office
5. Practicing quality control and laboratory safety

LABORATORY REQUESTS
Purpose

A laboratory request is a printed form that contains a list of the most frequently ordered laboratory tests (Figure 15-4). A laboratory request is required when the specimen is collected at the medical office and transferred to an outside laboratory for testing, or when the specimen is to be collected and tested at an outside laboratory, in which case the request is given to the patient at the medical office to take to the laboratory. The request provides the outside laboratory with essential information necessary for accurate testing, reporting of results, and billing. Organizational formats for the request forms vary, depending on the laboratory. In general, most outside laboratories find it more convenient and economical to provide the medical office with one form for designating all tests, with the possible exception of the Pap test, in which case a separate form, known as a *cytology request,* is provided.

Table 15-2 Representative Tests From a (Modified) Laboratory Directory

This table presents a modified table of representative tests included in a laboratory directory to provide you with an overall understanding of the components of a laboratory directory. The components presented in this modified directory include the name and CPT code of the test, reference range, amount and type of specimen required, supplies necessary for the collection of the specimen, techniques to use for collection of the specimen, patient preparation, proper handling and storage of the specimen, and causes for rejection of the specimen. This modified table does *not* include special instructions, instructions for transporting the specimen, uses and limitations of the test, and methodology used to perform the test. (*Note:* Refer to Figure 15-8 for an example of a laboratory test exactly as it is presented in a laboratory directory.)

Test and CPT Code	Specimen Requirements	Reference Range
ALT (alanine aminotransferase) CPT Code: 84460	2 ml serum in SST or transfer tube Centrifuge and separate serum within 45 minutes after collection. Refrigerate or store at RT.	45 U/L or less
AST (aspartate aminotransferase) CPT Code: 84450	2 ml serum in SST or transfer tube Centrifuge and separate serum from cells within 45 minutes after collection. Refrigerate or store at RT.	40 U/L or less
Bilirubin, total CPT Code: 82247	2 ml serum in SST or transfer tube Centrifuge and separate serum from cells within 45 minutes after collection. Refrigerate. Protect from light.	0.1-1.2 mg/dL
Blood group (ABO) and Rh Type CPT Codes: 86900, 86901	5 ml lavender-top tube A separate lavender-top tube is required for this test. Refrigerate or store at RT.	
BUN (blood urea nitrogen) CPT Code: 84520	2 ml serum in SST or transfer tube Centrifuge and separate serum within 45 minutes after collection. Refrigerate serum.	7-25 mg/dL
Calcium, serum CPT Code: 82310	2 ml serum in SST or transfer tube Centrifuge and separate serum from cells within 45 minutes after collection. Refrigerate or store at RT.	0-6 months: 8.9-11 mg/dL 7 months-adult: 8.5-10.6 mg/dL
CBC with differential CPT Code: 85025	5 ml lavender-top tube Gently invert tube 8-10 times immediately after drawing. Refrigerate or store at RT.	Values given with report
CK (creatine kinase) CPT Code: 82550	3 ml serum in SST or transfer tube Avoid exercise before venipuncture. Centrifuge and separate serum from cells within 45 minutes after collection. Refrigerate or store at RT.	Male: 17-148 U/L Female: 10-70 U/L
CRP (C-reactive protein) CPT Code: 86140	1 ml serum in SST or transfer tube Avoid hemolysis. Centrifuge and separate serum from cells within 45 minutes after collection. Refrigerate or store at RT.	0.0-4.9 mg/L
Glucose, plasma CPT Code: 82947	5 ml gray-top tube Patient should be fasting for 12 to 14 hours. Gently invert tube 8-10 times immediately after drawing. Refrigerate or store at RT.	65-99 mg/dL
LD (lactic acid dehydrogenase) CPT Code: 83615	3 ml serum in SST or transfer tube Hemolysis invalidates results. Centrifuge and separate serum from cells within 45 minutes after collection. Refrigerate or store at RT.	100-250 IU/L
PT/INR (prothrombin time) CPT Code: 85610	5-ml light blue-top tube Gently invert tube 3-4 times immediately after drawing. Clotting and hemolysis invalidate results. Store at RT.	PT/INR: 0.8-1.2 Patients on anticoagulant therapy: PT/INR: 2.0-3.0
RPR (rapid plasma reagin) CPT Code: 86592	1 ml serum in SST or transfer tube Centrifuge and separate serum from cells within 45 minutes after collection. Refrigerate.	Nonreactive

SST, Serum separator tube.

Continued

Table 15-2 Representative Tests From a (Modified) Laboratory Directory—cont'd

Test and CPT Code	Specimen Requirements	Reference Range
Sedimentation rate CPT Code: 85652	5 ml lavender-top tube Gently invert tube 8-10 times immediately after drawing. Refrigerate.	Male: 0-15 mm/hr Over 50 years: 0-20 mm/hr Female: 0-20 mm/hr Over 50 years: 0-30 mm/hr
Triiodothyronine (T₃) CPT Code: 84480	1 ml serum in SST or transfer tube Centrifuge and separate serum from cells within 45 minutes after collection. Refrigerate.	83-200 mg/dL
Thyroxine (T₄) CPT Code: 84436	2 ml serum in SST or transfer tube Centrifuge and separate serum from cells within 45 minutes after collection. Refrigerate.	4.5-12.0 μg/dL
Triglycerides CPT Code: 84478	2 ml serum in SST or transfer tube Patient should be fasting 12-14 hr. Centrifuge and separate serum from cells within 45 minutes after collection. Refrigerate or store at RT.	Less than 150 mg/dL
Urinalysis, routine CPT Code: 81003	Random sample in urine transport tube First morning specimen preferred (10 ml) Refrigerate.	Values given with report

Parts of Laboratory Request Form

The request form can be completed manually by the medical assistant by writing in all information required, or it may be completed on a computer screen by entering the information using a keyboard. Specific information that is required on the laboratory request form follows.

1. *Physician's name and address.* The physician's name and address should be clearly indicated on the laboratory request form to facilitate the reporting of test results to the physician. Laboratory request forms are usually prenumbered with the physician's account number, which assists in identification, reporting, and billing of laboratory tests.

2. *Patient's name and address.* The patient's name and address must be documented on the form as requested by the laboratory; for example, the laboratory may want the patient's name designated with the last name first, middle initial, and then first name. The patient's address is needed for billing purposes and must include the city, state, and zip code.

3. *Patient's age and gender.* The reference ranges for some tests vary depending on the patient's age and gender. The reference range for hemoglobin concentration varies according to gender (12 to 16 g/dL for a woman; 14 to 18 g/dL for a man).

4. *Date and time of collection of the specimen.* The date of the specimen collection indicates to the laboratory the number of days that have passed since the collection, providing the laboratory with information regarding the freshness of the specimen. A time lapse that is too long between collection and testing of a specimen may affect the accuracy of some test results. The time of collection is significant with respect to certain laboratory tests. The reference range for serum cortisol varies depending on whether the specimen is collected in the morning or in the afternoon.

5. *Laboratory tests desired.* The tests desired by the physician are usually indicated by marking a box adjacent to those tests (and their corresponding CPT code), as illustrated in Figure 15-3. A space designated as "additional tests" or "other tests" is provided on the laboratory request form for specifying the CPT code of a test that is desired but not listed on the request form. As previously indicated, the laboratory request form includes only the tests most frequently ordered. The laboratory directory contains a complete listing of all tests performed by the laboratory.

6. *Profiles.* Laboratory tests termed *profiles* may be ordered by the physician. A **profile** (also known as a *panel*) consists of an array of laboratory tests that have been determined to be the most sensitive and specific means of identifying a disease state or evaluating a particular organ or organ system. The profiles performed by an outside laboratory and the tests included in each are listed in the laboratory directory. A profile may be specific in nature, that is, all tests included relate to a specific organ of the body or a particular disease state. A specific profile is usually ordered when the physician does not have a definite clinical diagnosis but has a good idea of the patient's condition or what organ or organs are involved in the patient's condition. The physician orders a profile of the condition or organ in question. An example of a profile used to identify a disease state is the rheumatoid profile, which is used to assist in the diagnosis of rheumatoid arthritis. An example of a profile used to evaluate an organ is the hepatic function profile, which is used to assess liver function and to assist in the diagnosis of a pathologic condition that affects the liver.

LABORATORY REQUISITION
Biomedical Laboratories, Inc.
100 Main Street
Athens, Georgia 45760

☐ Fax Send additional copy of report to:

☐ Call Client Number/Physician's Name   Phone/Fax number

☐ Mail Physician's Address   City, State, Zip

Patient's Name (Last)	(First)	(MI)	Sex	Date of Birth MO DAY YEAR	Collection Time AM PM	Fasting YES NO	Collection Date MO DAY YEAR

NPI/UPIN	Physician's ID #	Patient's SS #	Patient's ID #	Urine hrs/vol hrs____ vol____

PATIENT

Physician's Name (Last, First)   Physician's Signature

Medicare # (Include prefix/suffix)   ☐ Primary ☐ Secondary

Medicaid #   State   Physician's Provider #

Diagnosis/Signs/Symptoms in ICD-9 Format (Highest Specificity)   REQUIRED

Patient's Address   Phone

City   State   ZIP

RESP. PARTY

Name of Responsible Party (if different from patient)

Address of Responsible Party (if different from patient)   APT #

City   State   ZIP

Patient's Relationship to Responsible Party: ■ 1–Self ☐ 2–Spouse ■ 3–Child ■ 4–Other

Performance Lab ☐   Carrier   Group #   Employee #   Mem

INSURANCE

Insurance Company Name   Plan   Carrier Code

Subscriber/Member #   Location   Group #

Insurance Address   Physician's Provider #

City   State   ZIP

Employer's Name or Number   Insured SS # (If not patient)   Worker's Comp ☐ Yes ☐ No

I hereby authorize the release of medical information related to the service subscribed herein and authorize payment directed to LabCorp.

X _____ Patient's Signature   Date

MEDICARE ADVANCE BENEFICIARY NOTICE

I have read the ABN on the reverse. If Medicare denies payment, I agree to pay for the identified test(s).

X _____ Patient's Signature   Date

NOTE: WHEN ORDERING TESTS FOR WHICH MEDICARE OR MEDICAID REIMBURSEMENT WILL BE SOUGHT, PHYSICIANS SHOULD ONLY ORDER TESTS THAT ARE MEDICALLY NECESSARY FOR THE DIAGNOSIS OR TREATMENT OF THE PATIENT. COMPONENTS OF THE ORGAN OR DISEASE PANELS/COMBINATIONS PRINTED BELOW ARE SHOWN ON THE REVERSE SIDE AND MAY ALSO BE ORDERED INDIVIDUALLY BELOW. COMPONENTS MAY BE BILLED SEPARATELY PER CARRIER POLICY.

PROFILES (See reverse for components)

80049	Basic Metabolic Profile	SST
80054	Comp Metabolic Profile	SST
80051	Electrolyte Profile	SST
80058	Hepatic Profile	SST
80059	Hepatitis Profile	SST
80061	Lipid Profile	SST
80091	Thyroid Profile	SST
80055	Prenatal Profile	RED LAV
80072	Rheumatoid Profile	SST

HEMATOLOGY

85025	CBC w Diff	LAV
85027	CBC w/o Diff	LAV
85014	Hematocrit	LAV
85018	Hemoglobin	LAV
85595	Platelet Count	LAV
85041	RBC Count	LAV
85048	WBC Count	LAV
85007	WBC Differential	LAV
89190	Nasal Smear, Eosin	Nasal Smear
85060	Pathologist Consult– Peripheral Smear	LAV

ALPHABETICAL/COMBINATION TESTS

86900 86901	ABO and Rh	LAV
82040	Albumin	SST
84075	Alkaline Phosphatase	SST
84460	ALT (SGPT)	SST
82150	Amylase, Serum	SST
86038	Antinuclear Antibodies	SST
84450	AST (SGOT)	SST
82607 82746	B₁₂ and Folate	SST
82250	Bilirubin, Total	SST

ALPHABETICAL TESTS CON'T

84520	BUN	SST
82310	Calcium	SST
80156	Carbamazepine (Tegretol®)	SER
82378	CEA	SST
82465	Cholesterol, Total	SST
82565	Creatinine	SST
80162	Digoxin	SER
82670	Estradiol	SST
82728	Ferritin, Serum	SST
82985	Fructosamine	SST
83001	FSH	SST
83001 83002	FSH and LH	SST
82977	GGT	SST
82947	Glucose, Plasma	GRY
82947	Glucose, Serum	SST
82950	Glucose, 2-hr. PP	SST
83036	Glycohemoglobin, Total	LAV
84703	hCG, Beta Subunit, Qual	SST
84702	hCG, Beta Subunit, Quant	SST
83718	HDL Cholesterol	SST
86677	Helicobacter pylori, IgG	SST
86706	Hep B Surface Antibody	SST
87340	Hep B Surface Antigen	SST
86803	Hep C Antibody	SST
83036	Hemoglobin A₁C	LAV
86701	HIV Antibodies	SST
83540	Iron, Total	SST
83540 83550	Iron and IBC	SST
83615	LDH	SST

ALPHABETICAL TESTS CON'T

83002	LH	SST
83690	Lipase	SER
80178	Lithium (Eskalith®)	SER
83735	Magnesium, Serum	SST
80184	Phenobarbital (Luminal®)	SER
80185	Phenytoin (Dilantin®)	SER
84132	Potassium	SST
84146	Prolactin, Serum	SST
84153	Prostate-Specific Antigen	SST
84066	Prostatic Acid Phos	SST
84155	Protein, Total	SST
85610	Prothrombin Time (PT)	BLU
85610 85730	PT and PTT Activated	BLU
85730	PTT Activated	BLU
86431	Rheumatoid Arthritis Factor	SST
86592	RPR	SST
86762	Rubella Antibodies, IgG	SST
85651	Sed Rate	LAV
84295	Sodium	SST
84403	Testosterone	SST
80198	Theophylline	SER
84436	Thyroxine (T₄)	SST
84478	Triglycerides	SST
84480	Triiodothyronine (T₃)	SST
84443	TSH, High Sensitivity	SST
84550	Uric Acid	SST
81003	Urinalysis Microscopic on Positives	URN
81001	Urinalysis with Microscopic	URN
80164	Valproic Acid (Depakene®)	SER

MICROBIOLOGY   See Reverse Side

■ ENDOCERVICAL ■ THROAT ■ URINE
■ STOOL ■ URETHRAL INDICATE SOURCE

87070	Aerobic Bacterial Culture	Bact Trnspt
87490 87590	Chlamydia/GC DNA Probe w/ Confirmation on Positives	Probe Trnspt
87490 87590	Chlamydia/GC DNA Probe Without Confirmation	Probe Trnspt
87490	Chlamydia DNA Probe	Probe Trnspt
87081	Genital, Beta-Hemolytic Strep Cult, Group B	Bact Trnspt
87070	Genital Culture, Routine	Bact Trnspt
87070	Lower Respiratory Culture	Steril Trnspt
87590	N. gonorrhoeae DNA Probe	Probe Trnspt
87015 87211	Ova and Parasites	O & P Kit
87081 X2 87045	Stool Culture	Fecal Trnspt
	Throat, Beta-Hemolytic Strep Cult, Group A	Bact Trnspt
87060	Upper Respiratory Culture, Routine	Bact Trnspt
87086	Urine Culture, Routine	Urn Cul Trnspt

Clinical Information/Comments

OTHER TESTS/INDIVIDUAL COMPONENTS

TEST #   TEST NAMES

LAB USE ONLY	STAT ☐ 998074	VENIPUNCTURE ☐ 998085	TRAVEL ☐ 998096	NON LABCORP ☐ 998239	VERBAL ORDER ☐ 998250	CHART ORDER ☐ 998261	HANDWRITTEN ☐ 998272	24 HR TUV ☐ 998283	PST/PSC #

CONTAINERS RECEIVED	SST SPUN	USST UNSPUN	SER SERUM TRNSPT	FRZ FRZ TRNS	RED RED	LAV LAVENDER	SLD SLIDE	BLU LT. BLUE	GRY GREY	GRN GREEN	RYB RYL BLU	YEL ACD	PLS PLASMA	URN URINE	24U 24 HR URINE	TA-U TART. ACID	FL FLUID	OT OTHER	BACT TRNSP	O & P KIT	PROBE TRNSP	URN CULT TRNSP	STERIL TRNSP	FECAL TRNSP	VIRAL TRNSP

300-0384

Figure 15-4. Laboratory request form.

A profile also may be general in nature. A general metabolic profile contains numerous routine laboratory tests and is used primarily in a routine health screen of a patient. General metabolic profiles are used to detect any changes in the body's biologic processes that may be present, although the patient may not have had any symptoms to indicate that these changes have occurred. General metabolic profiles also are used when the patient's symptoms are so vague that the physician does not have enough concrete evidence to support a clinical diagnosis of a specific organ or disease state. An example of a general profile is the comprehensive metabolic profile; refer to Table 15-3 for a list of the tests included in this profile.

The medical assistant should have knowledge of the names of common profiles and the tests generally contained in each, which are listed in Table 15-3. The tests contained in each profile may vary slightly from one laboratory to another.

7. *Source of the specimen.* Certain tests require that the source of the specimen (e.g., throat, wound, ear, eye, urine, vagina) be recorded on the laboratory request form. This is done for identification of the origin of the specimen for the laboratory, because this information is not available by looking at the specimen. In many instances, the source dictates the test method used by the laboratory to evaluate the specimen for the presence of a possible pathogen. The test method used to detect the presence of *Streptococcus* in a specimen obtained from the throat would be different from that used to detect *Candida albicans* in a vaginal specimen.

8. *Physician's clinical diagnosis (in International Classification of Diseases [ICD-9] format).* The clinical diagnosis assists the laboratory in correlating clinical laboratory data with the needs of the physician. In some instances, further testing is performed by the laboratory if one test method proves inconclusive with respect to providing the physician with the information necessary to confirm or reject the clinical diagnosis. Another function of the clinical diagnosis is to assure laboratory personnel that the test results are within the framework of the diagnosis. When the results of a test disagree with the physician's clinical diagnosis, the laboratory repeats the test on the same or another specimen. The clinical diagnosis also alerts laboratory personnel to the possibility of the presence of a potentially dangerous pathogen, such as the hepatitis virus. In addition, this information is necessary for third-party billing by the laboratory. If the laboratory bills an insurance company for these tests, the ICD-9 code for the clinical diagnosis needs to be on the insurance form. The processing of insurance forms is facilitated by having the information at hand and not having to contact the medical office to obtain it.

9. *Medications.* Certain medications may interfere with the accuracy and validity of test results. The laboratory should be notified on the request form of any medications taken by the patient.

10. *STAT.* Sometimes the physician wants the laboratory test results reported as soon as possible. In this case, "STAT" should be clearly indicated in bold letters (or the appropriate STAT box checked) on the laboratory request form. Requests that are marked STAT are performed as soon as possible after receipt by the laboratory, and the results are telephoned or faxed to the physician as soon as they are available.

After the specimen has been collected, the completed request form must be placed with the specimen for transport to the outside laboratory. The medical assistant should realize the significance of this simple but important step. Numerous possible tests can be performed on one particular specimen, and without the request form, the laboratory does not have the information it needs to carry out the physician's orders, causing delays in completing the tests and reporting results.

What Would You Do? What Would You *Not* Do?

Case Study 1

Three days ago, Hildy McNicle was given a laboratory requisition at the medical office to have blood drawn and tested at an outside medical laboratory. Hildy calls the medical office and says she is a little confused. She called the laboratory for her test results, and they would not give them to her. They told her to call the medical office. She does not understand this because her blood was collected and tested at the laboratory, and it would seem logical to her that they would give her the test results, especially because she is paying the laboratory to perform the tests. The test results have come back with abnormal values, and the physician is at a medical convention and will not return until tomorrow. ■

Putting It All into Practice

My Name is Korey McGrew, and I am employed by a group of physicians in a family practice medical office. Some of my duties include showing patients to examining rooms, taking the patient's vital signs, administering medications, transcription, filing, and many other duties that medical assistants perform. I have found that being a medical assistant has been challenging and rewarding, and I wish you the best of luck in reaching your goals.

When I first started working as a practicing medical assistant, I had a challenging venipuncture experience. The patient was a kind and personable 64-year-old man with hardening of the arteries. I tried to obtain the blood specimen from his arm but was not successful. The patient was calm and was not bothered at all by the unsuccessful stick. He said that it was hard to draw blood on him and to go ahead and try again. I decided to try taking blood from a vein on the back of his hand with a butterfly setup. To my relief, I obtained the blood specimen. I think that I was more nervous about this experience than the patient was. It is important to remain calm on the outside around patients even if you are nervous on the inside. ■

Table 15-3 Laboratory Profiles

Profile	Tests Included	Use
Comprehensive metabolic profile	Albumin ALP ALT AST Bilirubin (Total) BUN Calcium Carbon Dioxide Chloride Creatinine Glucose Inorganic Phosphorus Potassium Protein (Total) Sodium Triglycerides	General health screen that provides information on kidneys, liver, acid-base balance, blood glucose level, and blood proteins. Used to evaluate organ function and to check for conditions such as diabetes, liver disease, and kidney disease Routinely ordered as part of blood workup for physical examination or medical examination (particularly when patient's symptoms are vague) Abnormal test results are usually followed up with more specific tests before a diagnosis is made.
Electrolyte profile	Carbon Dioxide Chloride Potassium Sodium	Screen for electrolyte or acid-base imbalance and monitor effect of treatment on disease or condition that causes electrolyte imbalance. This profile also is used to evaluate patient taking medication that can cause electrolyte imbalance.
Hepatic profile	Albumin ALP ALT AST Bilirubin (Direct) Bilirubin (Total) Protein (Total)	Detection of pathologic conditions affecting the liver This test is often ordered when symptoms indicating a liver condition occur, such as jaundice, dark urine, light-colored bowel movements, or pain or swelling in the abdomen. This profile may be ordered when an individual has been exposed to hepatitis, has a family history of liver disease, has excessive alcohol consumption, or is taking medication that can result in liver damage.
Hepatitis profile	Hepatitis A Antibody, IgM Hepatitis B Core Antibody, total Hepatitis B Surface Antigen Hepatitis C Antibody	Detection of viral hepatitis
Lipid profile	Total Cholesterol LDL Cholesterol HDL Cholesterol Triglycerides VLDL Cholesterol (Calculation) Total Cholesterol/HDL Ratio (Calculation)	Determine risk of coronary artery disease.
Prenatal profile	ABO Grouping and Rh Typing CBC W/Diff and W/Plt Hepatitis B Surface Antigen Red Cell Antibody Screen Rubella Antibody Screen Syphilis Serology (RPR)	Establish baseline recordings and screenings of prenatal patients for disease or potential problems.
Renal function profile	Albumin BUN Calcium Carbon Dioxide Chloride Creatinine Glucose Phosphorus Potassium Sodium	Detection of kidney problems This profile shows how well the kidneys are functioning to remove excess fluid and waste. When a problem is detected, diagnostic imaging tests may be used for further evaluation and diagnosis
Rheumatoid profile	ANA CRP Rheumatoid Factor Sedimentation Rate Streptolysin O Uric Acid	Assist in diagnosis of rheumatoid arthritis and to help distinguish it from other forms of arthritis and conditions with similar symptoms This profile also is used to evaluate severity of rheumatoid arthritis, to monitor the condition and its complications, and to assess response to treatment.
Thyroid function profile	FTI Thyroxine (T_4) Triiodothyronine (T_3) Uptake	Detection of conditions affecting the thyroid gland

ALP, Alkaline phosphatase; ALT, alanine aminotransferase; ANA, antinuclear antibody; AST, aspartate aminotransferase; BUN, blood urea nitrogen; CBC, complete blood count; CRP, C-reactive protein; FTI, free thyroxine index; HDL, high-density lipoprotein; LDL, low-density lipoprotein; VLDL, very-low-density lipoprotein.

LABORATORY REPORTS

Laboratory report forms are used to relay the results of laboratory tests to the physician (Figure 15-5). The report is usually generated by a computer. It may consist of a preprinted form with the test results printed in the appropriate spaces on the form by a computer (as illustrated in Figure 15-5), or the entire report may be generated by the computer (Figure 15-6). The report includes the following information:

1. Name, address, and telephone number of the laboratory
2. Physician's name and address
3. Patient's name, age, and gender
4. Patient accession number
5. Date the specimen was received by the laboratory
6. Date the results were reported by the laboratory

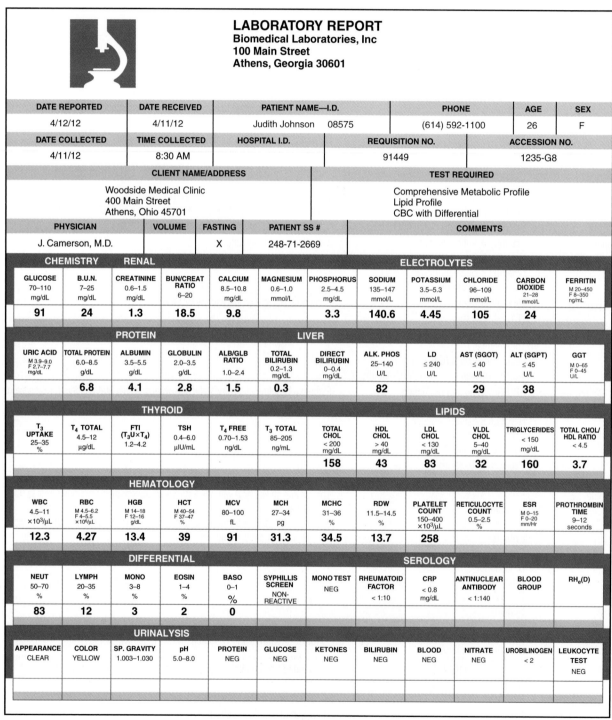

Figure 15-5. Laboratory report form.

Family Practice Health Care Center
3477 Arrowhead Ave
Phoenix, Arizona 78351
(942) 871-3746

ID#	SEX	PATIENT DEMOGRAPHICS	RESULTS PROVIDED BY
3368	F	Leah Percival	Medical Center Laboratory
		2973 Flint Dr.	
DOB		Phoenix, AZ 78366	ORDERING PROVIDER
4/28/78			Thomas Murphy, MD

AGE	ACCESSION #	LAB RECEIVED ON	LAB REPORTED ON
34	3380837630	12/07/2012 11:00:53	12/05/2012 14:08:00

LAB ID	SPECIMEN ID	COLLECTION DATE/TIME	FASTING
4739	30180906	12/04/2012 2:53:00	NO

NAME	VALUE	REFERENCE RANGE	UNITS	FLAG
CBC WITH DIFFERENTIAL/PLATELET				
-WBC	4.6	4.0-10.5	x10e3/uL	
-RBC	3.57	4.10-5.60	x10E3/uL	L
-Hemoglobin	11.2	12.5-17.0	g/dL	L
-Hematocrit	32.9	36.0-50.0	%	L
-MCV	92	80-98	fL	
-MCH	31.4	27.0-34.0	pg	
-MCHC	34.0	32.0-36.0	g/dL	
-RDW	15.6	11.7-15.0	%	H
-Platelets	308	140-415	x10E3/uL	
-Neutrophils	73	40-74	%	
-Lymphs	14	14-46	%	
-Monocytes	11	4-13	%	
-Eos	1	0-7	%	
-Basos	1	0-3	%	
-Neutrophils (Absolute)	3.4	1.8-7.8	x10E3/uL	
-Lymphs (Absolute)	0.6	0.7-4.5	x10E3/uL	L

Figure 15-6. Computer-generated laboratory report.

7. Names of the tests performed
8. Results of the tests
9. Reference range for each test performed

A patient accession number or laboratory number is assigned to each specimen received by the laboratory. Its purpose is to provide positive identification of each specimen within the laboratory and to allow easy access to the patient's laboratory records should a test result need to be located again. If the physician desires to have the laboratory test repeated, the accession number listed on the original report form must be included on the laboratory request form.

The **reference range** is also commonly referred to as a *reference interval* and a *reference value*. A reference range is defined as a certain established and acceptable parameter within which the laboratory test results of a healthy individual are expected to fall. The reference range is used to interpret laboratory test results for a particular patient. A range, rather than a single value, is necessary for laboratory test results because of individual differences among a general population caused by factors such as age, gender, race, and geographic location. In addition, no test can be so accurate that a single value is possible. The reference range for each test varies slightly from one laboratory to another, depending on the test method, equipment, and reagents used to perform the test. In this regard, it is essential that the medical assistant compare the test results with reference ranges supplied by the laboratory performing the test, rather than with a reference source such as a medical laboratory textbook.

Laboratory reports are delivered to the medical office using one or more of the following methods: faxed, mailed, hand-delivered by a laboratory courier, or sent electronically from the laboratory computer to the medical office computer. Abnormal results that pose a threat to the patient's health and laboratory reports marked STAT are telephoned or faxed to the medical office as soon as the tests are completed, and a complete written report follows immediately thereafter. The laboratory usually supplies the medical office with telephone reporting pads to transcribe results from the telephone report to reduce errors.

The medical assistant may be responsible for reviewing laboratory reports as they are received. The medical assistant should compare the patient's test results with the reference ranges supplied by the laboratory and notify the physician of any abnormal test results. Most laboratory computer systems automatically flag abnormal results on the laboratory report. The physician carefully reviews each laboratory report received by the office, and the data obtained are correlated with information obtained from the health history and physical examination. The physician indicates that he or she is finished with the report usually by placing his or her signature on it. The medical assistant is then responsible for filing the laboratory report in the patient's chart, according to the medical office policy.

LABORATORY DOCUMENTS AND THE EMR

Many medical offices communicate with outside laboratories electronically using a computer system that interfaces with the computer system in the outside laboratory. This provides distinct advantages for the medical office using an electronic medical record (EMR). Laboratory requisition forms can be completed on a request form displayed on the computer screen using fill-in boxes, drop-down lists, and check-boxes. Depending on the medical office policy, the form can then be transmitted electronically to the medical laboratory or printed out and placed with the specimen for transport to the laboratory.

Once the patient's tests have been completed, the laboratory test results are sent electronically to the medical office. The laboratory report is placed in the physician's "electronic review box" for his or her review and electronic signature. Abnormal values are often highlighted on the report as shown in Figure 15-6. If a critical result appears on the laboratory report, an urgent message is e-mailed to the physician. After the physician reviews the laboratory report and places his or her electronic signature on the report, the report is electronically filed in the patient's EMR.

Other advantages of the laboratory component of an EMR include the ability to quickly view laboratory results in chronological order. In addition, results of a laboratory test performed on a routine basis (e.g., glucose testing, cholesterol testing) can be accessed by the computer and plotted on a flow sheet (Figure 15-7). This permits an abnormal trend to be identified early, so that appropriate action can be taken.

If an EMR medical office is not networked through computers with an outside laboratory, the laboratory reports received by the office must be scanned into the computer and electronically filed in the patient's EMR. A scanned report has some limitations. The computer can display the report, but the data on the report cannot be accessed or manipulated. Because of this, laboratory data cannot be used for many of the functions previously described. For example, the data on a scanned report cannot be accessed and incorporated into a flow sheet for trend analysis.

PATIENT PREPARATION AND INSTRUCTIONS

Factors such as food consumption, medication, activity, and time of day affect the laboratory results of certain tests. For some laboratory tests, advance patient preparation is necessary to obtain a quality specimen suitable for testing, which leads to accurate results and assists the physician in accurate diagnosis and treatment. The quality of laboratory test results can be only as good as the quality of the specimen obtained from the patient. A specimen obtained from a patient who has not prepared properly may invalidate the test results and necessitate calling the patient back to collect the specimen again.

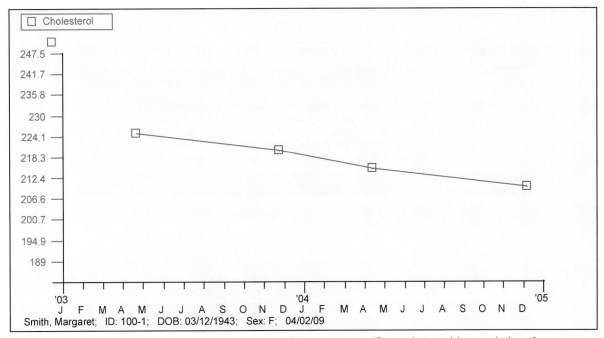

Figure 15-7. Cholesterol flow sheet generated by a computer. (Screenshot used by permission of MCKESSON Corporation. All rights reserved. © MCKESSON Corporation, 2011.) (From Buck CJ: Electronic health record booster kit for the medical office, St Louis, 2009, Saunders.)

The medical assistant is usually responsible for instructing the patient about the nature of the laboratory test and any advance preparation that might be necessary. A complete and thorough explanation of the information should be relayed clearly to the patient. The patient should be informed of the name of the test, how to prepare for the test, how the test is performed, and how and when to expect the test results. The medical assistant should make sure to explain the reason for the advance preparation, so the patient will be more likely to comply with the preparation necessary. It should be emphasized to the patient that the preparation is essential to obtain accurate test results and to avoid having to collect the specimen again.

After the instructions have been explained, the medical assistant needs to verify that the patient completely understands them and should offer to answer any questions. It also is advisable to provide the patient with a written information sheet (Figure 15-8) to serve as a reference, should the patient forget some of the information after leaving the medical office. Some specimen collections may require that the patient remain at the collection site for a specified time; an example of this is the OGTT, which requires several hours for the collection of multiple, timed specimens. The patient should be told in advance of the time requirement, so that any necessary arrangements can be made with an employer or babysitter.

Sometimes the patient collects the specimen at home. The medical assistant is responsible for explaining detailed instructions to the patient on proper techniques for collection of the specimen. For example, if a first-voided morning urine specimen is necessary for the laboratory test, the

medical assistant needs to provide the patient with the appropriate specimen container and to instruct the patient on proper collection, handling, and storage of the specimen until it reaches the medical office.

The specific type of preparation necessary for a particular test depends on the test ordered and the method used to run it. If the medical office uses an outside laboratory, the patient preparation necessary for each test can be found in the laboratory directory. If the test is performed in the medical office, the medical assistant should consult the manufacturer's instructions that accompany the test to obtain specific infor-

What Would You Do? What Would You *Not* Do?

Case Study 2

Hans Volkman is leaving the medical office after being seen by the physician. The physician gave him a laboratory requisition for a complete blood count and a lipid profile. Hans notices that the clinical diagnosis on the form indicates iron-deficiency anemia and wants to know why the physician did not prescribe any medication for him if he thought he had anemia. Hans says that he told the physician his father had a heart attack at age 53 years and asked whether he would order a cholesterol test. He says the physician must have forgotten because the test was not marked on the laboratory form. Hans has been instructed to fast for the laboratory tests. He says that he stops every morning at the Coffee Cup restaurant and has coffee with cream and sugar, orange juice, and two doughnuts. He would like to know whether he could just have the coffee before the tests. Hans says he has a hard time functioning in the morning without coffee. ■

ORAL GLUCOSE TOLERANCE TEST

PATIENT INFORMATION SHEET

General Information

Your physician has requested that you have an oral glucose tolerance test (OGTT). This test is performed to see how well your body processes glucose (sugar). Glucose is the primary source of energy for your body. The OGTT is primarily used to assist in diagnosis of diabetes. Your test is scheduled in the early morning because you will need to perform an overnight fast. The test generally lasts for a period of 3 hours.

Patient Preparation

It is very important that you prepare properly to ensure accurate test results. Patient preparation for this test includes the following:

1. For 3 days prior to the test you should consume a high-carbohydrate diet consisting of at least 150 grams of carbohydrate per day. Foods that are high in carbohydrate include bread, pasta, cereal, potatoes, rice, and crackers.
2. Do NOT drink or eat anything except water for 12 to 14 hours before the test.
3. Your physician will discuss what medications (if any) to discontinue before the test.

Testing Procedure

When you arrive at the testing facility, your blood will be drawn. You will then be given a glucose (sugar) solution to drink. Some people have a brief period of nausea after consuming the glucose solution. Your blood will be collected at intervals over a period of several hours.

During the testing procedure, you may experience some normal side effects such as weakness, a feeling of faintness, or perspiration. They are caused by a decrease in your body's glucose level as insulin is secreted in response to the glucose solution. These side effects are temporary and will only last for a short period of time. To ensure accurate test results, you need to adhere to the following during the testing procedure:

1. Sit quietly and do not leave the testing facility.
2. Do not eat or drink anything except water.
3. Do not smoke or chew gum during the procedure.

Following the Procedure

After the procedure you can eat and drink as usual and resume your normal activities. An appointment will be scheduled for you to discuss the test results with your physician.

Figure 15-8. Oral glucose tolerance test patient instruction sheet.

mation regarding patient preparation. Advance patient preparation usually consists of fasting, diet modification (e.g., low-fat diet), or medication restrictions.

Fasting

Some blood specimens require the patient to fast before collection. The composition of blood is altered by the consumption of food because digested food is absorbed into the circulatory system, changing the results of certain laboratory tests. Food intake causes blood glucose and triglyceride laboratory tests to yield falsely high results. Any individual test (e.g., fasting blood glucose [FBG], OGTT) or profile including these tests (e.g., comprehensive metabolic profile,

lipid profile) requires the patient to fast before the specimen is collected.

Fasting involves abstaining from food and fluids (except water) for a specified amount of time before the collection of the specimen (usually 12 to 14 hours). Fasting specimens are usually collected in the morning to allow food from the previous evening meal to be completely digested and absorbed. In addition, collection of the specimen in the morning causes the least amount of inconvenience to the patient in terms of abstaining from food and fluid.

The medical assistant must give detailed instructions to the patient, ensuring that the patient understands that fasting includes abstaining from food and fluid. The patient should be told, however, that it is permissible—in fact advisable—to drink water because dehydration caused by water abstinence can alter certain test results.

The medical assistant should indicate a specific time to the patient for initiation of the fast. If the specimen is to be collected in the morning, the patient should be instructed to begin fasting at 6:00 PM on the previous evening. The patient also must be told the time to report for collection of the specimen.

Medication Restrictions

Many medications affect the physical and chemical characteristics of body substances; medications taken by the patient may lead to inaccurate test results. Antibiotic therapy administered before collection of a throat specimen for strep testing may cause a falsely negative test result. The physician may ask the patient to avoid taking medication for a period of time before the collection of the specimen if discontinuing the medication would not cause any health threat or serious discomfort to the patient. Because medication is more likely to interfere with test results on urine than on blood, the patient is recommended to discontinue medication 48 to 72 hours before the collection of a urine specimen, and 4 to 24 hours before the collection of a blood specimen.

If the patient cannot be taken off medication, this information should be recorded on the laboratory request form for specimens transported to an outside laboratory for testing. This alerts the laboratory personnel to the presence of the medication. If the medication taken by the patient interferes with the method normally used to perform the test, the laboratory may be able to use an alternative method to obtain valid results. If the test is being performed in the medical office, the medical assistant should consult the manufacturer's instructions that accompany the test for the names of medications that interfere with test results.

The physician determines the need for a patient to discontinue medication before specimen collection. The medical assistant is responsible for ensuring that the patient understands any instructions regarding restrictions on medication and for recording medications the patient is taking on the laboratory request form.

COLLECTING, HANDLING, AND TRANSPORTING SPECIMENS

Clinical laboratory tests are performed on specimens obtained from the body. A **specimen** is a small sample or part taken from the body to represent the nature of the whole. Most laboratory tests are performed on specimens that are easily obtained from the body, such as blood, urine, feces, sputum, cervical and vaginal scrapings of cells, or samples of secretions or discharge from various parts of the body (e.g., nose, throat, wound, ear, eye, vagina, urethra), for microbiologic analysis. Other examples of specimens analyzed in the laboratory but more difficult to obtain from the body include gastric juices, cerebrospinal fluid, pleural fluid, peritoneal fluid, synovial fluid, and tissue specimens for biopsy. The source of the specimen may not be indicative of the pathologic condition in question, for example, triiodothyronine and thyroxine tests are performed on blood serum but are used to detect a condition that affects the thyroid gland.

The medical assistant is responsible for the collection of most specimens obtained from patients in the medical office; of these, blood and urine constitute the largest percentage of specimens collected. Certain specimens, such as a sample of vaginal or urethral discharge, cerebrospinal fluid, or a tissue specimen, must be collected by the physician; in these cases, the medical assistant assists with the collection.

The most important goal of specimen collection and handling is to provide the laboratory with a sample that is as biologically representative as possible of the body substance collected. If the specimen is collected or handled improperly, the **in vivo** characteristics of the specimen may be adversely affected, which may cause inaccurate and unreliable test results; this may interfere with the accurate diagnosis and treatment of the patient's condition.

Guidelines for Specimen Collection

Specific guidelines that should be used regarding specimen collection and handling follow. Procedure 15-1 describes collecting a specimen for transport to an outside laboratory.

1. *Review and follow the Occupational Safety and Health Administration (OSHA) Bloodborne Pathogens Standards* during specimen collection (see Chapter 2).
2. *Review the requirements for collection and handling of the specimen,* which include the collection supplies necessary, the type of specimen to be collected (e.g., **serum, plasma,** whole blood, clotted blood, urine), the amount

---

What Would You Do? What Would You *Not* Do?

Case Study 3

Kathleen O'Leary is scheduled for a follow-up appointment today at the office. She was seen last week with fatigue, shortness of breath, weight loss, increased urination, and blurred vision. Kathleen was given a laboratory requisition to have blood drawn at an outside medical laboratory. The physician ordered a complete blood count with differential and a comprehensive metabolic profile. When the charts are prepared for the day, Kathleen's laboratory results are not in her chart. Kathleen is contacted by phone; she says she knows she should have gone to the laboratory to have her blood drawn, but she is afraid of needles and panics at the sight of blood. She says that the last time she had her blood drawn she started feeling hot and light-headed and had to lie down on a table and was embarrassed. Kathleen says she also is worried the laboratory results might show something is wrong with her. She is thinking of not coming for her appointment today and hopes that she starts feeling better on her own. ■

necessary for laboratory analysis, the techniques to follow to collect the specimen, and proper handling and storage of the specimen. The medical assistant must refer to the appropriate reference source to determine the collection and handling requirements for each test ordered by the physician. If the specimen is transported to an outside laboratory, this information is indicated in the laboratory directory. Figure 15-9 shows an example of the collection and handling requirements for a triglycerides test exactly as it is presented in a laboratory directory. The collection and handling requirements necessary for specimens tested in the medical office are listed in the manufacturer's instructions that accompany the test system. A **test system** is defined as a setup that includes all of the test components required to perform a laboratory test such as testing devices, controls, and testing reagents.

3. *Assemble the equipment and supplies.* Use only the appropriate specimen containers as specified by the laboratory directory or manufacturer's instructions accompanying a test system. Substituting containers may not yield the proper type of specimen required or may affect the test results, as shown by the following examples. If serum is required and a tube containing an anticoagulant is used (instead of a tube without an anticoagulant), the blood separates into plasma and cells, rather than serum and cells, and the wrong type of blood specimen is obtained, which necessitates an-

Triglycerides	
CPT code:	84478
Type of specimen:	Serum
Amount:	2 ml
Collection supplies:	SST or transfer tube
Collection techniques:	Let stand for 30 minutes. Separate serum from cells within 45 minutes of collection.
Patient preparation:	Patient should fast for 12 to 14 hours prior to collection.
Handling and storage:	Refrigerate or store at room temperature. Stable at room temperature for up to 7 days.
Causes for rejection:	Nonfasting specimen, improper labeling of tube
Reference range:	Desirable: Less than 150 mg/dL
	Borderline high: 150-199 mg/dL
	High: 200-499 mg/dL
	Very high: 500 mg/dL or greater

Use:

Measurement of triglyceride levels assists with the diagnosis and treatment of diabetes mellitus, nephrosis, liver obstruction, and pancreatitis. In association with HDL cholesterol and total cholesterol, a triglyceride determination assists in the assessment of the risk for developing coronary artery disease. Elevated levels may occur with liver disease, nephritic syndrome, hypothyroidism, increased alcohol consumption, poorly controlled diabetes, and pancreatitis.

Limitations:

- Women on estrogens (high estrogen contraceptives can increase blood triglyceride levels).

- An increase in the triglyceride level may occur during pregnancy.

Methodology:

Enzymatic

Figure 15-9. Collection and handling requirements for a triglyceride test from a laboratory directory.

other specimen from the patient. Collection of a microbiologic specimen that may contain anaerobic pathogens with supplies meant for aerobic pathogens results in death of the anaerobic pathogen.

The specimen container should be sterile to prevent contamination of the specimen. Many specimens, especially microbiologic ones, are adversely affected by contaminants, such as extraneous microorganisms, which may affect the accuracy of the test results.

The medical assistant should check each container before use to ensure it is not broken, chipped, cracked, or otherwise damaged. Damaged containers are unsuitable for specimen collection and should be discarded. Some containers such as blood tubes have an expiration date (Figure 15-10). The medical assistant should make sure to check the expiration date on these containers to avoid using an outdated container.

4. *Label each specimen container.* The medical assistant should label each tube and specimen container. An unlabeled specimen is a cause for rejection of the specimen by an outside laboratory. Two *unique identifiers* should be used to label the specimen. A unique identifier is information that clearly identifies a specific patient, such as the patient's name and date of birth. A specimen can be labeled by attaching a computerized bar code label to the specimen (Figure 15-11, *A*). Laboratory instruments that do the testing are able to read the bar codes and automatically record results on a laboratory report for a particular patient using the demographic information supplied by the bar code. A specimen can also be labeled by hand-writing the information on the label, which should include the patient's name and date of birth, the date and time of collection, the medical assistant's initials, and any other information required by the laboratory, such as the source of the specimen (Figure 15-11, *B*). The information should be printed legibly, and the medical assistant should be certain that the information is accurate to avoid a mixup of specimens. The medical assistant must

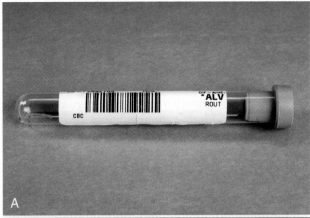

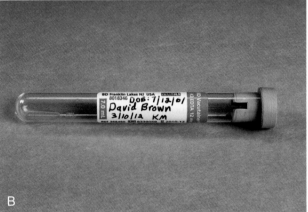

Figure 15-11. **A,** Computerized bar code label. **B,** Hand-labeled blood tube.

also complete a laboratory request form to accompany the specimen, as described earlier in this chapter. (*Note:* The medical assistant should follow the medical office policy as to when the tubes should be labeled. Some offices prefer that the tubes be labeled *before* the specimen is drawn; other offices want the tubes to be labeled *after* the specimen is drawn.)

5. *Identify the patient.* Proper patient identification is essential to avoid collecting a specimen on the wrong patient by mistake. After greeting the patient, the medical assistant should ask the patient to state his or her full name and date of birth. This information should be compared with the demographic data indicated in the patient's chart. The patient should *not* be asked whether he or she is a certain patient. For example, the patient should not be asked, "Are you Brad Thompson?" The patient may not hear the medical assistant correctly or may not be paying attention and may answer in the affirmative even if he is not that patient. A specimen that is not identified correctly could lead to an inaccurate patient diagnosis and the wrong treatment.

6. *Determine whether the patient has prepared properly.* If the patient was required to prepare before the specimen was collected, determine whether this was done prop-

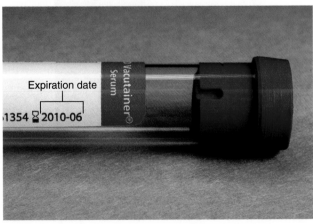

Figure 15-10. Blood tube showing expiration date.

erly. Improper preparation may lead to inaccurate test results. If a test that requires fasting, such as a FBG, is performed on a nonfasting specimen, the results are altered; in this case, they are falsely high. If the patient has not prepared properly, inform the physician; the physician may want the patient to prepare properly and return, or the physician may tell the medical assistant to go ahead with the collection but to alert the laboratory to the situation by marking the information on the laboratory request. In the example just given, "nonfasting specimen" would be written on the request form.

7. *Explain the procedure.* An explanation of the collection procedure helps relax and reassure the patient and gains the patient's confidence and cooperation, especially the first time the patient has a specimen collected.

8. *Collection of the specimen* involves a set of specific techniques for each type of specimen obtained. The information in this section is presented in general terms. Specific procedures for the collection of biologic specimens are included in this text in Chapters 16 through 20 (Urinalysis, Phlebotomy, Hematology, Blood Chemistry and Immunology, and Medical Microbiology).

Specimen collection involves a combination of medical and surgical aseptic techniques. Certain parts of the collection materials, such as needles, swabs, and the insides of specimen containers, must remain sterile. If a culture medium is used to collect a microbiologic specimen, the medical assistant must ensure that the lid of the container is removed only when the specimen is placed on the culture medium. Unnecessary removal of the lid results in contamination of the culture medium with extraneous microorganisms, which interferes with accurate test results. During the collection and handling of the specimen, the medical assistant must be careful to use medical and surgical asepsis to prevent contamination of the specimen, the patient, or the self (Figure 15-12).

The medical assistant must collect the specimen using proper technique. The proper type of specimen

must be collected as designated in the laboratory directory or by the instructions that accompany the test system. The collection procedure should be followed exactly to ensure a high-quality and reliable specimen. For example, collection of a random urine specimen when a clean-catch midstream specimen is required may affect the accuracy of the test results.

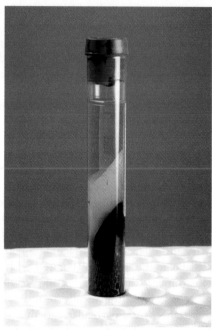

Figure 15-13. Serum specimen in a serum separator tube (SST) that has been centrifuged.

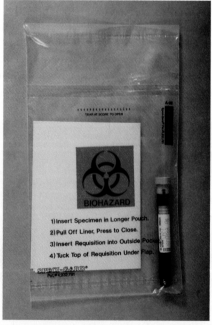

Figure 15-14. Biohazard specimen bag containing a specimen and laboratory request form.

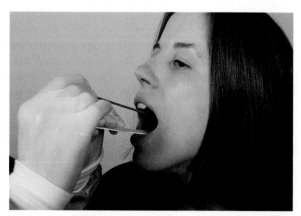

Figure 15-12. Medical and surgical asepsis must be used when collecting a specimen.

The medical assistant must be sure to collect the amount of specimen necessary for the test, which varies depending on the type of test being performed and the number of laboratory tests ordered on the specimen. If the medical assistant fails to collect the specified amount of a specimen that is being transported to an outside laboratory, the laboratory may not be able to perform the test, and the laboratory request is returned marked "quantity not sufficient" (QNS). This situation warrants calling the patient back for collection of another specimen.

9. *Process the specimen.* The specimen may need to be processed after collection. For example, when collecting a serum specimen using a serum separator tube (SST), the medical assistant must allow the tube to stand for 45 minutes and then centrifuge the specimen to separate the serum from the cells (with a gel barrier), as shown in Figure 15-13.

10. *Properly handle and store the specimen* to preserve its in vivo physical and chemical characteristics. Some specimens, such as microbiologic specimens, are more sensitive to environmental influences and must be handled with special care. Whenever possible, laboratory tests are best performed on fresh specimens (for most specimens, within 1 hour after collection) because they yield the most reliable test results. When this is not possible, the specimen must be stored; storage may be required until it can be tested at the medical office or picked up by a laboratory courier from an outside laboratory. If the specimen is being picked up by a laboratory courier, the OSHA standard requires that it be placed in a biohazard specimen bag (Figure 15-14) to protect the courier from the possibility of an exposure incident. General guidelines for handling and storing biologic specimens most frequently collected in the medical office are presented in Table 15-4.

Table 15-4 Handling and Storage of Biologic Specimens*

Specimen	Handling	Storage
Blood	**All Blood Specimens** Prevent hemolysis. Collect specimen in tube at room temperature.	**For Most Blood Specimens** Refrigerate at a temperature between 36° F (2° C) and 46° F (8° C) to retard alterations in physical and chemical composition of the specimen. (*Note:* Many blood specimens are stable at room temperature for up to 24 hours.) Plasma and serum may be frozen; however, whole blood should not be frozen because this would cause hemolysis.
	Serum Separate serum from cells within 45 min after collection.	
	Plasma Mix anticoagulant gently but thoroughly with blood specimen immediately after collection.	
Urine	Avoid contamination of inside of specimen container. Do not leave specimen standing out for longer than 1 hr after collection.	If urine specimen cannot be tested within 1 hr after collection, refrigerate it at a temperature between 36° F (2° C) and 46° F (8° C), or add an appropriate preservative.
Microbiologic specimens	Avoid contamination of swab used to collect specimen. Avoid contamination of inside of microbiologic specimen container. Protect yourself from contamination from microbiologic specimen. Protect anaerobic specimens from exposure to air.	Transport specimen as soon as possible. If not possible, place specimen in transport medium or inoculate it on appropriate culture medium, and (for most specimens) place it in refrigerator at a temperature between 36° F (2° C) and 46° F (8° C) to prevent drying and death of specimen or overgrowth of specimen with extraneous microorganisms.
Stool	Collect specimen in clean container. For detection of ova and parasites, keep stool warm.	For most accurate test results, deliver specimen to laboratory immediately. If transportation of specimen is delayed, mix stool with appropriate preservative or place it in transport medium.

*For all specimens: Do not expose to extreme temperature changes.

PROCEDURE 15-1

Outcome Collect a specimen for transport to an outside laboratory. A summary of the series of individual steps required for collecting a specimen in the medical office and transporting it to an outside laboratory is presented in this procedure.

1. Procedural Step. Inform the patient of any advance preparation or special instructions, which may include the following:
a. Diet modification
b. Fasting
c. Medication restriction
d. Collection of a specimen at home

Explain the instructions thoroughly, and provide the patient with written instructions to take home as a reference. Notify the patient of the time to report to the medical office for specimen collection.

Principle. The patient must prepare properly to provide a quality specimen that would lead to accurate test results and would avoid a return to have another specimen collected.

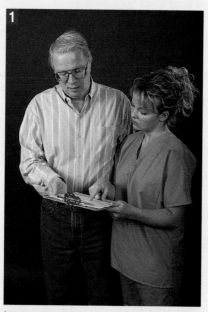

Instruct the patient on advance preparation.

2. Procedural Step. Review the requirements in the laboratory directory for the collection and handling of the specimens ordered by the physician, which include the following:
a. Collection materials required
b. Type of specimen to be collected
c. Amount of the specimen necessary for laboratory analysis
d. Procedure to follow to collect the specimen
e. Proper handling and storage of the specimen

Telephone the laboratory with any questions you have regarding any aspect of collection or handling of the specimen.

Principle. A review of the requirements beforehand prevents errors in collection and handling of the specimen.

3. Procedural Step. Complete the laboratory request form, which must include the following information:
a. Physician's name and address
b. Patient's name (and address if required)
c. Patient's age and gender
d. Date and time of the collection
e. Laboratory tests ordered by the physician
f. Type of specimen
g. Source of specimen
h. Physician's clinical diagnosis
i. Any medications the patient is taking
j. Third-party billing information

If the test results are needed by the physician as soon as possible, indicate "STAT" on the request in bold letters.

Principle. The completed form provides the laboratory with the information necessary to perform the tests accurately.

4. Procedural Step. Sanitize your hands.

5. Procedural Step. Assemble the equipment and supplies. Use the appropriate specimen container required by the outside laboratory. Ensure the container is sterile, and check that it is not broken, chipped, or cracked.

Principle. The appropriate specimen container must be used to ensure the collection of the proper type of specimen required by the laboratory. Damaged specimen containers are unsuitable for collection and should be discarded.

6. Procedural Step. Depending on the medical office policy, perform one of the following:
a. Attach a computer-generated bar code label to each tube or container and label it with your initials *or*
b. Clearly label the tubes and containers with the patient's name and date of birth, the date and time of collection, your initials, and any other information required by the laboratory, such as the source of the specimen.

(*Note:* The medical assistant should follow the medical office policy as to when the tubes should be labeled. Some offices prefer that the tubes be labeled *before* the specimen is drawn; other offices want the tubes to be labeled *after* the specimen is drawn.)

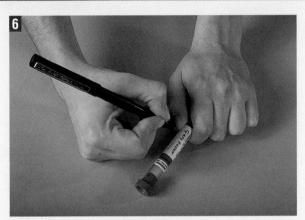

Label the tubes.

Principle. Two unique identifiers should be used when labeling the specimen (e.g., patient's name and date of birth). Properly labeled tubes and containers prevent mixups of specimens.

7. **Procedural Step.** Greet the patient and introduce yourself. Identify the patient by full name and date of birth, and explain the procedure. Verify that you have the correct patient. If patient preparation was required for the test, determine whether the patient prepared properly.

Principle. Identification of the patient prevents collection of a specimen from the wrong person by mistake. Specimen collection is often an anxiety-producing experience for the patient, and reassurance should be offered to help reduce apprehension.

8. **Procedural Step.** Collect the specimen according to the following guidelines:
   a. Follow the OSHA standard.
   b. Collect the specimen with the proper technique.
   c. Collect the proper type and amount of the specimen required for the test.

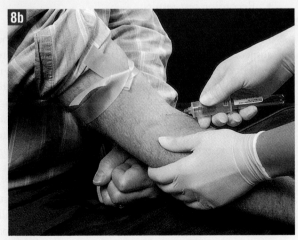

Collect the specimen.

d. If needed, place the lid tightly on the specimen container (e.g., urine specimen container).
e. Process the specimen further if required by the outside laboratory (e.g., centrifuging the specimen)

Principle. Proper collection of a specimen maintains its in vivo qualities and provides the laboratory with a biologically representative sample of the body substance collected.

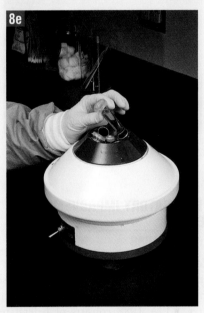

Centrifuge the specimen.

9. **Procedural Step.** Prepare the specimen for transport to an outside laboratory for testing by performing the following:
   a. Place the specimen in a biohazard specimen bag.
   b. Place the laboratory request in the outside pocket of the specimen bag.
   c. Properly handle and store the specimen while awaiting pickup by a laboratory courier.
   d. Record information in the patient's chart, including the date and time of collection, the type and source of the specimen, the laboratory tests ordered by the physician, and information indicating its transport to the outside laboratory, including the date the specimen was sent.

Principle. The biohazard bag protects the laboratory courier from the possibility of an exposure incident. The outside laboratory must have the completed request form to know which laboratory tests have been ordered by the physician. The specimen must be handled and stored properly to maintain the in vivo characteristics of the specimen.

Continued

PROCEDURE 15-1   Collecting a Specimen for Transport to an Outside Laboratory—cont'd

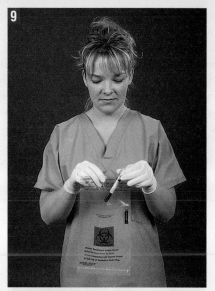

Prepare the specimen for transport.

CHARTING EXAMPLE	
Date	
3/10/12	8:00 a.m. Venous blood specimen collected from Ⓡ arm. Tests ordered: total cholesterol, HDL, and triglycerides. Pt was in a fasting state. Courier pick-up by Medical Center Laboratory on 3/10/12.
	———————— K. McGrew, CMA (AAMA)

CLINICAL LABORATORY IMPROVEMENT AMENDMENTS

Purpose of CLIA 1988

In 1988, Congress passed the Clinical Laboratory Improvement Amendments (CLIA 1988), which established standards for improving the quality of laboratory testing in the United States. CLIA 1988 consists of federal regulations governing all facilities that perform laboratory tests for health assessment or for the diagnosis, prevention, or treatment of disease. CLIA 1988 includes facilities not previously covered under federal legislation, such as medical offices, health departments, and nursing homes. Regulations for implementing CLIA were developed by the Department of Health and Human Services (HHS). The Centers for Medicare and Medicaid Services (CMS) is a division of HHS and is responsible for implementing and monitoring compliance with the CLIA regulations. In addition to CLIA regulations, a clinical laboratory must be in compliance with all other federal, state, and local laboratory legislation.

Categories of Laboratory Testing

CLIA regulations establish the following three categories of laboratory testing on the basis of the complexity of the testing methods.

1. *Waived tests*

    A **waived test** is a laboratory test that has been determined by HHS to meet the CLIA criteria for being a simple procedure that is easy to perform and has a low risk of erroneous test results. Waived tests include tests that have been approved by the Food and Drug Administration (FDA) for use by patients at home (e.g., blood

glucose testing). Physicians office laboratories (POLs) that perform only waived tests must apply for a certificate of waiver (CW) from CMS, which exempts them from many of the CLIA oversight requirements. The CW must be renewed every 2 years.

POLs holding a CW are still expected to adhere to good laboratory practices. The manufacturer's most *current* instructions that accompany the test system must be followed exactly; these include the following:
- Proper storage of the test system
- Adhering to expiration dates
- Proper collection and handling of the specimen
- Performing quality control procedures
- Properly testing the specimen
- Interpreting test results
- Recording test results

2. *Moderate-complexity tests*

    A moderate-complexity test is a **nonwaived test** that is subject to the CLIA 1988 regulations. Moderate-complexity tests account for 75% of the estimated 7 to 10 billion laboratory tests performed in the United States each year. Most of these tests are performed in outside laboratories which include hospital and independent laboratories. Some medical offices perform moderate-complexity tests known as *provider-performed microscopy* (PPM) procedures, which involve the examination of a specimen under the microscope. An example of a PPM procedure is the microscopic analysis of urine sediment. Other moderate-complexity tests that are occasionally performed in the medical office include urine and throat cultures and hematology and blood chemistry tests performed on nonwaived automated blood analyzers. Examples of these "benchtop" analyzers include the QBC hematology analyzer (Becton-Dickinson, Franklin Lakes, NJ), the Cell Dyn hematology analyzer (Abbott Laboratories, Abbott Park, Ill), the Ac*T hematology analyzer (Beckman Coulter, Brea, Calif), and the ATAT blood chemistry analyzer (GMI Inc., Ramsey, Minn).

3. ***High-complexity tests.***
   A high-complexity test is a nonwaived test that is subject to the CLIA 1988 regulations. High-complexity tests include all procedures related to cytogenetics, histopathology, histocompatibility, and cytology (includes Pap testing). These tests are not performed in medical offices; most are performed in laboratories already subject to federal regulations.

Requirements for Moderate-Complexity and High-Complexity Testing

Laboratories that perform nonwaived tests (moderate- and high-complexity tests) must meet CLIA regulations and are subject to unannounced inspections every 2 years by CMS. Major components of the CLIA 1988 regulations include the following:

1. *Patient test management.* A system must be established to maintain optimal integrity and identification of patient specimens throughout the testing process. This system must also ensure accurate reporting of results.

2. *Quality control.* To ensure accurate and reliable test results, each laboratory performing nonwaived tests must establish and follow written quality control procedures that monitor and evaluate the quality of each testing process. These include
   - *Developing a laboratory procedures manual.* The manual must include a clearly written procedure for each nonwaived test that is performed by the facility, following the manufacturer's instructions. The manual must be readily available and followed by laboratory personnel.
   - *Performing calibration procedures at least every 6 months* (or more frequently if indicated in the test system's operating manual) and documenting results in a quality control log. The calibration verification must be checked at a minimum of three levels that are within the reportable range of the test.
   - *Following the manufacturer's instructions for performing controls,* but at a minimum, performing two levels of controls daily and documenting results in a quality-control log. In addition, control procedures must be performed in the following situations: when there is a complete change of reagents, when major preventive maintenance is performed on an analyzer, or when any critical change occurs that may influence test performance.
   - *Performing and documenting actions taken when problems or errors are identified*
   - *Documenting all quality control activities*

3. *Quality assessment.* Each laboratory must establish and follow written policies and procedures to monitor and evaluate the overall quality of the total testing process to ensure the accuracy and reliability of patient test results.

4. *Proficiency testing.* Proficiency testing (PT) is a form of external quality control used to verify the accuracy and reliability of laboratory testing. Laboratory specimens are prepared by a CMS-approved proficiency testing agency. Three times a year, the POL must test a shipment of these unknown specimens using the same procedure as for testing a patient's specimen. The results are forwarded to the PT agency for evaluation. The PT agency grades the results using the CLIA grading criteria and sends the laboratory score to the POL, indicating how accurately it performed the testing.

5. *Personnel requirements.* CLIA regulations specify qualifications and responsibilities for personnel for laboratory directors, technical consultants, clinical consultants, and testing personnel. These regulations list specific education and training qualifications for the various positions and define responsibilities for persons who fill these positions. Personnel requirements are most stringent for high-complexity testing.

CLIA-WAIVED LABORATORY TESTING

Testing a laboratory specimen involves performing a series of steps to determine the presence or measurement of a specific substance in the specimen. Most POLs only perform tests that are CLIA-waived, and the medical assistant is usually responsible for performing these tests. Because of this, the remainder of this chapter focuses on guidelines that should be followed when CLIA-waived tests are performed.

Approximately 1600 CLIA-waived tests are commercially available that test for 76 different analytes. An **analyte** is a substance that is being identified or measured in a laboratory test, such as glucose, hemoglobin, and group A strep. The number of waived tests is expected to increase as new technology becomes available. To help the medical office keep current with new CLIA-waived tests, the HHS maintains the following website: www.cms.hhs.gov/clia. The FDA also maintains a website that provides information on all commercially available CLIA-waived test systems, categorized by analyte and the name of the test system. This website can be accessed at www.fda.gov/MedicalDevices/DeviceRegulationandGuidance/IVDRegulatoryAssistance/ucm124103.htm.

CLIA-waived tests that are performed most frequently in the medical office include the following:

- Blood glucose determination (using an FDA-approved blood glucose monitor)
- Dipstick urinalysis
- Fecal occult blood testing
- Urine pregnancy tests with visual color comparisons
- Group A rapid streptococcus testing
- Hemoglobin testing (using a CLIA-waived analyzer)
- Cholesterol testing (using a CLIA-waived analyzer)
- Triglyceride testing (using a CLIA-waived analyzer)
- Prothrombin time testing (using a CLIA-waived analyzer)
- Spun microhematocrit

CLIA-Waived Testing Kits

A laboratory testing kit consists of a box packaged with the devices and supplies needed to perform a laboratory test and generate test results. Each kit contains enough testing materials to perform a specific number of tests as indicated on the box label. Most of these tests are screening tests, and a positive result may indicate the need for further testing. Examples of CLIA-waived testing kits (Figure 15-15) include the Hemoccult fecal occult blood test (SmithKline Diagnostics, Inc., Palo Alto, Calif), the QuickVue HCG urine pregnancy test, and the QuickVue In-Line Strep A test (Quidel Corp., San Diego, Calif).

Each testing kit comes with a **product insert** (also known as a *package insert*). Information included in the product insert is outlined in Table 15-5. The medical assistant should read the entire product insert before performing the test and should follow the instructions *exactly* to ensure accurate and reliable test results. Of particular importance are the quality control procedures that must be carefully followed when working with a testing kit. This area is discussed in greater detail later in this section. The testing kit

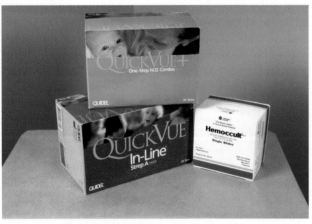

Figure 15-15. CLIA-waived testing kits.

may include a quick reference card, which is a condensed version of the steps in the testing procedure and can be used as a guide when performing the test. Because the quick reference card is only a synopsis of the testing procedure, it should never be substituted for the product insert when learning about the test and how to perform it.

Testing kits have specific stability and storage requirements that must be carefully followed. Before a testing kit is used, its expiration date must be checked. If the testing kit is outdated, the testing components may no longer be stable; expired components must not be used, to prevent inaccurate test results. Light, heat, and moisture can alter the effectiveness of a testing kit and cause premature expiration of the kit. The medical assistant should make sure to store testing kits according to the information in the product insert; this information is also indicated on the package label. Most testing kits are stored at room temperature.

Testing kits often use a *unitized testing device* to perform the test. A unitized testing device consists of a self-contained device, such as a cassette, to which a specimen is added directly and in which all of the steps of the testing procedure occur (Figure 15-16). A unitized device is used to perform one laboratory test (e.g., urine pregnancy testing) and is discarded after testing.

Many of the testing devices included in testing kits rely on a color change for interpretation of results. A color chart or color diagram is provided with the kit for making a visual comparison and interpreting results. When test results are recorded, the brand name of the testing kit should be specified. Some offices also require that the lot number of the testing kit be included with the recording.

CLIA-Waived Automated Analyzers

CLIA-waived automated analyzers have been developed for performing laboratory tests in the medical office; they are continually growing in number and are being modified as new technology becomes available. These analyzers consist of compact or handheld devices that permit the processing of a specimen in a short time with accurate test results. **Reagent** strips or test cassettes are often used with CLIA-waived analyzers. Test results are obtained through a direct (digital display or printed) readout (Figure 15-17).

The ease of operating automated systems should not lead to a false sense of security because these systems have limitations that must be recognized—the most critical one being the failure of the equipment. One of the most important aspects of use of an automated system is the ability to recognize signs that indicate the system is malfunctioning, because malfunctioning may lead to inaccurate test results.

The manufacturer of each automated system provides an operating manual (and sometimes an instructional video) with the instrument that includes information needed to collect and handle the specimen, perform quality control procedures, and test the specimen. In addition, the manufacturer typically has personnel available for on-site training and service. It is important that the medical assistant become completely familiar with all aspects of the automated

Table 15-5 Information Included in the Product Insert of a Testing Kit

Section	Information Included
Intended Use	A description of the purpose of the test and the reason for performing the test
Summary and Explanation	Provides a brief overview of the condition being detected by the test, including the symptoms, prevalence, and complications of the condition
Principles of the Procedure	A detailed explanation of how the test works to detect the substance in the patient's specimen
Precautions and Warnings	Outlines precautions that must be taken when running the test to ensure accurate and reliable test results. Also includes guidelines for safe handling, use, and disposal of chemical reagents included in the testing kit
Reagents and Materials Provided	A list of the collection devices, controls, reagents, and other supplies included in the testing kit. Describes each component in detail, including the number of tests in the kit and the types and amounts of reagents and supplies
Materials Not Provided	A list of the materials needed to perform the test, but not included in the testing kit
Storage and Stability	A description of the proper storage requirements of the testing kit such as temperature range. Also identifies how long each testing component is stable for both unopened and opened components
Specimen Collection and Handling	Type of specimen required and procedures that must be followed when collecting, handling, and storing the specimen to ensure a high-quality and reliable specimen. Also includes safety precautions to take when handling the specimen
Test Procedure	Presents a step-by-step procedure that must be followed to test the specimen. Diagrams and illustrations of the procedural steps are often included in this section.
Interpretation and Reading Results	Guidelines for reading and interpreting the test results. If a color change is involved in reading the results, a color comparison chart or color diagram is included with the testing kit. Also explains the action to take if the test results are invalid
Quality Control	An explanation of the quality control procedures that must be performed to ensure accurate and reliable test results. Includes instructions for performing control procedures. Also includes information on how often and when controls should be run and the expected results. Describes what should be done if the controls do not produce expected results
Limitations of the Procedure	A test system works only within certain prescribed conditions and situations. Identifies conditions or situations that might prevent the test from performing correctly and influence the test results, such as medications or the presence of certain medical conditions. Also identifies any supplemental testing needed to confirm a waived test
Expected Values	Identifies the test result(s) that should be expected by the user
Performance Characteristics	Presents the results of research studies that have been conducted to evaluate test performance

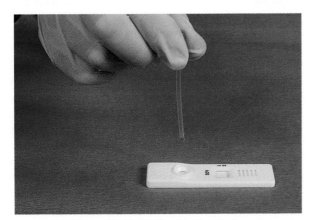

Figure 15-16. Unitized testing device

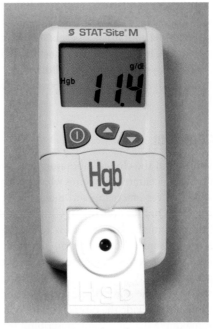

Figure 15-17. Digital readout of results on an automated analyzer.

systems used to perform laboratory tests in his or her medical office. Quality control procedures are of particular importance to ensure that the analyzer is functioning properly, and that the test results are reliable and accurate. Additional information on quality control procedures is presented later in this section.

When an automated analyzer is purchased, the testing components (e.g., controls, testing reagents) are usually

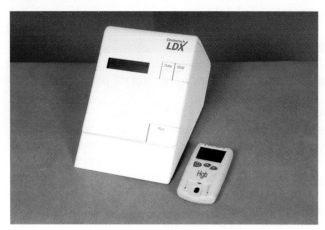

Figure 15-18. Clinical Laboratories Improvement Amendments (CLIA)-waived automated analyzers. Blood cholesterol analyzer *(left)* and hemoglobin analyzer *(right)*.

purchased separately. The medical assistant is responsible for checking the supplies periodically and reordering them as needed. Each testing component comes with a product insert, which indicates the proper storage and stability requirements. Most testing components are stored at room temperature. If a testing component needs to be stored in the refrigerator, it must be allowed to come to room temperature before it is used. Unopened controls are stable until the expiration date marked on the container. Once opened, some controls are stable only for a certain period of time (e.g., 30 days). For these controls, the medical assistant must write the date the control was opened *and* the date it should be discarded (expiration date) on the label of the control.

Some examples of brand names of CLIA-waived automated analyzers (Figure 15-18) include Cholestech LDX (Cholestech Corp., Hayward, Calif), STAT-Site Hemoglobin Meter (Stanbio Laboratory, Boerne, Tex), CoaguChek System and Accu-Chek (Roche Diagnostics, Branchburg, NJ), A1C Now (Bayer Corporation, Morrisville, NJ), and Clinitek urine analyzer (Siemens Corporation, New York City, NY).

QUALITY CONTROL

The ultimate goal in the clinical laboratory is to ensure that the laboratory test accurately measures what it is supposed to measure; this involves practicing and maintaining a quality control program. **Quality control (QC)** may be defined as the application of methods and means to ensure that test results are reliable and valid, and errors that may interfere with obtaining accurate test results are detected and eliminated. Practicing quality control methods ensures that test results represent the true status of the patient's condition and body functions and provide the physician with reliable information for making a diagnosis and prescribing treatment.

Quality control is an ongoing process that encompasses every aspect of patient preparation and specimen collection, handling, transport, and testing. The quality control meth-

ods that should be used to obtain precision and accuracy when using a CLIA-waived test system are presented here:

1. Storage and Handling of Test Systems
   a. Store the test system according to the manufacturer's instructions. Improper storage can cause deterioration of the testing components. Most test systems need to be stored at room temperature in a cool, dry area away from sources of heat and sunlight. Some testing components (e.g., controls, testing reagents) may need to be stored in the refrigerator.
   b. Allow time for refrigerated testing components to reach room temperature before using them. It usually takes 15 to 30 minutes for a testing component to reach room temperature.
   c. Controls often need to be shaken gently to mix them.
   d. Do not transfer testing components from one testing kit to another.
   e. Make sure environmental conditions are appropriate for running the test as specified in the manufacturer's instructions.

2. Stability of Testing Components
   a. Check the expiration date of each component in the test system before using it. Do not use a test component if it is past its expiration date.
   b. Unopened controls are stable until the expiration date marked on the container. Once opened, some controls are stable only for a certain period of time (e.g., 30 days). For these controls, the date the control is opened *and* the date it should be discarded (expiration date) must be written on the label of the control after it is opened. An opened control is stable until it reaches the expiration date stamped on the container or the expiration date indicated by the medical assistant on the container, whichever comes first.
   c. Discard outdated testing components as soon as they reach their expiration dates.

3. Calibration: **Calibration** is a mechanism used to check the precision and accuracy of a test system, such as an automated analyzer, to determine if the system is providing accurate results. A calibration check detects errors caused by laboratory equipment that is not working properly. Calibration is typically performed using a calibration device, often called a *standard.* The calibration device may come in the form of a calibration strip or cassette. The device is inserted into the analyzer (Figure 15-19, *A*), and the calibration results are displayed on the LCD screen of the analyzer or printed out by the analyzer. The calibration results are then compared with the expected results provided in the product insert or on the calibration device (Figure 15-19, *B*). Calibration guidelines include the following:
   a. Perform the calibration procedure by following the manufacturer's instructions. Instructions include information on the type of calibration device to use, how to perform the calibration procedure, and what action should be taken if the procedure does not perform as expected.

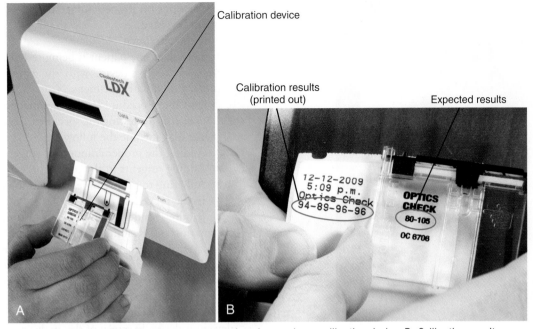

Calibration device

Calibration results
(printed out)

Expected results

Figure 15-19. **A,** Calibrating an automated analyzer using a calibration device. **B,** Calibration results are compared with expected results on the calibration device.

b. Document calibration results in a quality control log. This is a CLIA recommendation (not a requirement) for CLIA-waived test systems.

c. If the calibration procedure does not perform as expected, patient testing should not be conducted until the problem is identified and resolved.

d. The frequency of performing a calibration check is indicated in the manufacturer's instructions. At a minimum, a calibration check should be performed when a new lot number of testing reagents is put into use.

4. Controls: A **control** is a solution that is used to monitor a test system to ensure the reliability and accuracy of test results. Controls come with a product insert, which lists the expected ranges for control results. There are two categories of controls, which include *external controls* and *internal controls*.

Internal control: An internal control is built-in to some test systems (Figure 15-20). It evaluates whether certain aspects of the testing procedure are working properly. An internal control is performed at the same time that the testing procedure is performed. It checks for one or more of the following: whether a sufficient amount of the specimen was added, whether a sufficient amount of testing reagent was added, or whether the testing reagent migrated through the test device properly. If the internal control does not perform as expected, the test result is invalid and the specimen must be retested.

External controls: External controls are used to determine if the testing reagents are performing properly and to detect any errors in technique of the individual performing the test. External controls consist of commercially available solutions with known values. They

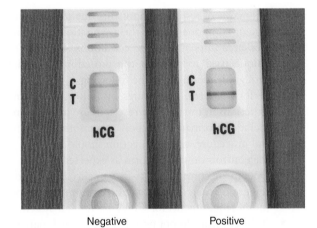

Negative | Positive

Figure 15-20. Internal control. The blue line next to the letter "C" indicates that the internal control has reacted as expected.

may be included with the test system or may need to be purchased separately. Generally, two levels of controls must be performed on a test system. A *low-level control* (also known as a *Level 1 control*) produces results that fall below the reference range for the test; a *high-level control* (also known as a *Level 2 control*) produces results that fall above the reference range for the test (Figure 15-21). The control procedure is performed in a manner similar to the procedure for performing the test on a specimen collected from a patient. Instead of adding the patient specimen to the testing device, however, the control is added to it. Control results are compared with expected results provided in the product insert. Failure of a control to produce expected results may be due to the following:

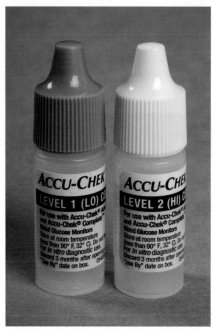

Figure 15-21. External controls. Low or level 1 control *(left)* and high or level 2 control *(right)*.

deterioration of testing components due to improper storage or components past their expiration date, improper environmental testing conditions, or errors in technique used to perform the procedure. External control guidelines include the following:

- Perform control procedures by following the instructions in the product insert. These instructions include information on how to perform the control procedure, and what action should be taken if the controls do not perform as expected.
- Document control results in a quality control log (Figure 15-22). This is a CLIA recommendation (not a requirement) for CLIA-waived test systems.
- If the controls do not perform as expected, patient testing should not be conducted until the problem is identified and resolved. Factors that can cause abnormal control results include outdated controls or testing reagents, improper storage of testing components, and an error in the technique used to perform the procedure.
- The frequency of performing external controls is indicated in the product insert. At a minimum, they should be performed on each new lot number of testing reagents and thereafter on a regular basis, such as monthly.

5. Collecting and Handling Specimens
   a. Use the appropriate collection devices to collect the specimen. Do not substitute other devices.
   b. Follow the manufacturer's instructions exactly for collecting and handling the specimen.
   c. If a specimen (e.g., urine) cannot be tested immediately, information is provided in the manufacturer's

instructions on proper storage of the specimen until it can be tested.

6. Testing the Specimen
   a. If more than one patient is being tested at a time, label each testing device with the patient's name to prevent mixup of specimens.
   b. Follow the procedure in the manufacturer's instructions *exactly* for testing the specimen. Specific requirements may include the following:
      - Adding the proper amounts of reagents
      - Adding reagents in the proper order
      - Adhering to proper time intervals for various steps in the procedure
      - Reading results within the proper time frame

7. Interpreting and Reading Test Results: Testing kits often rely on a color change for the interpretation of test results. The color change is compared with a color chart or a color diagram (Figure 15-23) included with the testing kit. Test results derived from an automated analyzer do not need to be interpreted and are printed out or displayed on the LCD screen of the analyzer. The following guidelines should be followed when test results from a testing kit are interpreted:
   a. Interpret the results according to instructions outlined in the product insert that accompanies the testing kit.
   b. Test results are usually interpreted as positive, negative, or invalid. Invalid results may be due to an improperly collected specimen or an error in technique in performing the testing procedure.
   c. If a test is invalid, retest a new sample with new testing materials. If the second test is invalid, contact the manufacturer.

CATEGORIES OF TEST RESULTS

Laboratory test results are categorized as qualitative or quantitative results.

Qualitative Test Results

Qualitative test results indicate whether or not a substance is present in the specimen being tested; they also provide an approximate indication of the amount of substance present. Interpretation of qualitative results usually involves the use of a color comparison chart or a color diagram. Results are recorded in terms of 1+, 2+, or 3+; trace, small, moderate, or large; negative or positive; or reactive or nonreactive. Testing kits usually provide qualitative test results.

Quantitative Test Results

Quantitative test results indicate the exact amount of a chemical substance that is present in the body; results are reported in measurable units (e.g., mg/dL). No interpretation is required to read quantitative results. Automated analyzers provide quantitative test results, with the results being printed out or displayed on the LCD screen of the analyzer.

QUALITY CONTROL LOG

BLOOD GLUCOSE TEST

Name of meter: *Accu-Check Advantage*	Controls

TEST STRIPS:

Lot number: _522677_

Exp date: _4/30/2013_

Code number _635_

LOW LEVEL CONTROL:

Lot number _63330_

Exp date _11/29/2013_

Expected range: _18 - 64_

HIGH LEVEL CONTROL:

Lot number _63330_

Exp date _11/29/2012_

Expected range: _270 - 324_

Date	Low level control	Accept	Reject	High level control	Accept	Reject	Technician
9/20/12	61	X		315	X		K. Mcgrew, CMA (AAMA)
9/21/12	53	X		310	X		K. Mcgrew, CMA (AAMA)
9/22/12	50	X		302	X		K. Mcgrew, CMA (AAMA)
9/23/12	48	X		300	X		K. Mcgrew, CMA (AAMA)
9/24/12	51	X		305	X		K. Mcgrew, CMA (AAMA)

Figure 15-22. Quality control log sheet for blood glucose testing.

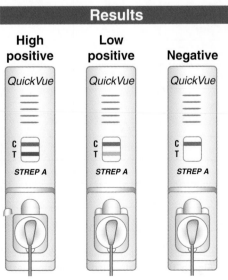

Figure 15-23. Color diagram used to interpret test results.

RECORDING TEST RESULTS

The medical assistant is responsible for recording laboratory test results. Careful recording is essential to avoid errors, which could affect the patient's diagnosis. It is usually unnecessary to chart results from laboratory reports returned from outside laboratories because the report itself is filed in the patient's record. In case of a STAT request or critical findings, the test results may be telephoned to the medical office, requiring the medical assistant to record results on a report form.

Results of laboratory tests performed by the medical assistant in the POL should be charted in the medical record and must include the date and time, name of the test, and test results. Quantitative test results should be recorded using the units of measurement of the test system (e.g., mg/dL). Qualitative test results should be recorded using words or abbreviations (e.g., positive, negative) and not symbols (e.g., +, −), because symbols can be accidentally changed or misinterpreted. The office may also maintain a log of the tests performed in the POL, which includes the patient's name, date and time, name of the test, the test results, and the name and credentials of the individual performing the test (Figure 15-24).

LABORATORY SAFETY

Laboratory safety is an important aspect of clinical laboratory testing in the medical office. Many of the laboratory tests performed in the medical office involve the use of haz-

QUALITY CONTROL LOG				
BLOOD GLUCOSE TEST				
ACCU-CHECK TEST STRIPS				
Lot number: _522677_				
Exp date: _4/30/2013_				
Code number _635_				
Date	Patient name	Patinet ID	Glucose results (in mg/dL0	Technician
9/20/12	Thomas Jeffers	1341	98	K. Mcgrew, CMA (AAMA)
9/20/12	Diana Woods	3744	74	K. Mcgrew, CMA (AAMA)
9/21/12	Lauren Campbell	6497	115	K. Mcgrew, CMA (AAMA)
9/21/12	Jason Coates	5310	78	K. Mcgrew, CMA (AAMA)
9/21/12	Chloe Pearson	2333	85	K. Mcgrew, CMA (AAMA)
9/22/12	Kathleen Dobson	1466	65	K. Mcgrew, CMA (AAMA)
9/22/12	Larry Wilson	5399	102	K. Mcgrew, CMA (AAMA)
9/23/12	Samantha Byran	2512	92	K. Mcgrew, CMA (AAMA)
9/24/12	Abbey Paulson	1788	88	K. Mcgrew, CMA (AAMA)
9/24/12	Michael Williams	3903	105	K. Mcgrew, CMA (AAMA)

Figure 15-24. Patient log of laboratory tests.

ardous chemical reagents, the handling of specimens that may contain pathogens, and the use of laboratory equipment. Practicing good technique in testing laboratory specimens and recognizing potential hazards help to reduce accidents in the laboratory. Some areas specifically related to laboratory safety in the medical office are described here.

Careful handling and storing of glassware to prevent breakage should be performed as follows:

1. Carefully arrange glassware in storage cabinets to prevent breakage.
2. Carefully remove glassware from storage cabinets.
3. If glassware does break, dispose of it in a puncture-resistant container to protect trash handlers from the shards.

The medical assistant should handle all chemical reagents carefully by adhering to the following instructions:

1. Ensure that all reagent containers are clearly and properly labeled.
2. If a label is loose, reattach it immediately.
3. Recap reagent containers immediately after use to prevent spills.

Laboratory specimens should be handled carefully as follows:

1. Follow the OSHA Bloodborne Pathogens Standard in collecting and handling laboratory specimens.
2. Wash hands immediately if some of the material contained in the specimen is accidentally touched.
3. Avoid hand-to-mouth contact, such as eating, drinking, or applying makeup, while working with specimens.
4. Immediately clean up any specimen spilled on the worktable, and cleanse the table with a disinfectant.
5. Properly dispose of all contaminated needles, syringes, specimen containers, and infectious waste used in specimen collection and testing.
6. Cover any break in the skin, such as a cut or scratch, with a bandage.
7. Ensure that all specimen containers are tightly capped to prevent leakage.
8. Do not store food in refrigerators where testing supplies or specimens are stored.
9. Handle all laboratory equipment and supplies properly and with care, as indicated by the manufacturer. For example, wait until the centrifuge comes to a complete stop before opening it.

evolve *Check out the Evolve site to access additional interactive activities.*

MEDICAL PRACTICE and the LAW

Laboratory procedures must be performed with precision to obtain accurate test results. Pay particular attention to each step in the procedure. Inaccurate laboratory results may cause the physician to incorrectly diagnose a patient's condition, which could lead to the wrong treatment. This situation can result in a lawsuit.

Certain federal regulations, including those from the Clinical Laboratories Improvement Amendments (CLIA) and the Occupational Safety and Health Administration (OSHA), govern laboratory testing. These regulations help ensure standardization of laboratory tests and safe handling of reagents, blood, and body fluids to prevent contamination of specimens and infection of health care workers. Know and follow all regulations. Failure to do so could result in legal liability. ■

What Would You Do? What Would You *Not* Do? RESPONSES

Case Study 1
Page 600

What Did Korey Do?
- ❏ Told Hildy that the laboratory cannot release test results. Explained that they are experts in performing tests but do not have the medical knowledge to know their meanings.
- ❏ Told Hildy that the physician needed to give her the test results. Explained that the physician was out of town today but that an appointment could be made for her for tomorrow to discuss the results with the physician.

What Did Korey Not Do?
- ❏ Did not give Hildy the test results.
- ❏ Did not alarm Hildy that something might be wrong.

What Would You Do?/What Would You *Not* Do? Review Korey's response and place a checkmark next to the information you included in your response. List additional information you included in your response.

_____

_____

_____

_____

Case Study 2
Page 605

What Did Korey Do?
- ❏ Told Hans that the term *clinical diagnosis* means what the physician "thinks" is wrong before the laboratory tests are performed.

Continued

❏ Explained that when the test results are returned, the physician would be able to make a diagnosis, and then he would determine what treatment is needed.

❏ Told Hans that a lipid profile includes several tests, and one of those tests is a cholesterol test. Explained that the tests in a lipid profile all help to determine whether someone is at risk for heart disease.

❏ Told Hans that he could not have any coffee until after his blood was drawn because it would affect the test results. Told him that his test could be scheduled first thing in the morning if that would help.

What Did Korey Not _Do?_

❏ Did not tell Hans he could have a cup of coffee before the laboratory tests.

❏ Did not tell Hans that he should not be eating doughnuts if he was concerned about his heart.

What Would You Do?/What Would You _Not_ Do? Review Korey's response and place a checkmark next to the information you included in your response. List additional information you included in your response.

_____
_____
_____
_____

Case Study 3
Page 607

What Did Korey Do?

❏ Stressed to Kathleen that if the laboratory test results are abnormal, it is better to know, so the physician can help make her better.

❏ Told Kathleen that many patients feel the same way about having blood drawn, so she is not alone. Relayed to her that her fear is normal, and she has no reason to be embarrassed.

❏ Told Kathleen that she should tell the laboratory about her last experience so they can make it easier for her. Explained that they would probably put her in a reclining position to draw her blood so that she would not get light-headed.

❏ Gave Kathleen some suggestions on how to relax during the venipuncture. Told her to turn her head when the blood was drawn.

❏ Asked Kathleen whether she had any additional symptoms.

❏ Checked with the physician to see whether he wanted to keep her appointment for today or have her appointment rescheduled after the laboratory work is completed.

What Did Korey Not _Do?_

❏ Did not ignore or minimize Kathleen's concerns and fears.

❏ Did not tell Kathleen that her test results would probably be fine.

What Would You Do?/What Would You _Not_ Do? Review Korey's response and place a checkmark next to the information you included in your response. List additional information you included in your response.

_____
_____
_____
_____

CERTIFICATION REVIEW

❏ **The purpose of laboratory testing** is to assist in the diagnosis of pathologic conditions, to evaluate a patient's progress, to regulate treatment, to establish a patient's baseline, to prevent or reduce the severity of disease, and to comply with state law if necessary. A routine test is a laboratory test performed on a routine basis on an apparently healthy patient to assist in the early detection of disease.

❏ **POL** consists of an in-house medical office laboratory. Laboratory tests that are CLIA-waived and commonly required are often performed in the POL. Outside laboratories include hospital and privately owned commercial laboratories.

❏ **A laboratory request** is a printed form that contains a list of the most frequently ordered laboratory tests. The laboratory request includes the physician's name and address; the patient's name, age, and gender; the date

and time of collection of the specimen; the laboratory tests desired; the source of the specimen; the clinical diagnosis; and medications taken by the patient. A profile consists of numerous laboratory tests that provide related information used to determine the health status of a patient.

❏ **The purpose of the laboratory report** is to relay the results of laboratory tests to the physician. Information included on a laboratory report is as follows: the name, address, and telephone number of the laboratory; the physician's name and address; the patient's name, age, and gender; the patient accession number; the date the specimen was received by the laboratory; the date the results were reported by the laboratory; the names of the tests performed; the results of the tests; and the reference range for each test performed. The reference range is a certain established and acceptable parameter or reference range within which the laboratory test results of a healthy individual are expected to fall.

❑ **Some laboratory tests** require advance patient preparation to obtain a quality specimen suitable for testing. A specimen obtained from a patient who has not prepared properly may invalidate the test results and necessitate calling the patient back to collect a specimen again. The specific type of preparation necessary for a particular test depends on the test ordered and the method used to perform it. A common patient preparation requirement for laboratory testing is fasting. Fasting means that the patient must abstain from food or fluids (except water) for a specified amount of time (usually 12 to 14 hours) before the collection of a specimen.

❑ **A specimen** is a small sample taken from the body to represent the nature of the whole. Examples of specimens include blood, urine, feces, sputum, cervical and vaginal scrapings of cells, and a sample of a secretion or discharge taken from various parts of the body such as the nose, throat, wounds, ear, eye, vagina, or urethra.

❑ **The purpose of CLIA** is to improve the quality of laboratory testing in the United States. CLIA consists of federal regulations governing all facilities that perform laboratory tests for health assessment or for the diagnosis, prevention, or treatment of disease.

❑ **CLIA regulations** establish three categories of laboratory testing—waived tests, moderate-complexity tests, and high-complexity tests. Laboratories that perform nonwaived tests must meet the CLIA 1988 regulations. Laboratories that perform only waived tests must apply for a certificate of waiver from CMS, which exempts them from many of the CLIA requirements.

❑ **Quality control** is the application of methods to ensure that test results are reliable and valid, and that errors are detected and eliminated. Quality control is an ongoing process that encompasses every aspect of patient preparation and specimen collection, handling, transport, and testing.

❑ **Laboratory safety** is an important aspect of clinical laboratory testing in the medical office. Practicing good techniques in testing laboratory specimens and recognizing potential hazard helps reduce accidents in the laboratory.

TERMINOLOGY REVIEW

Analyte A substance that is being identified or measured in a laboratory test.

Calibration A mechanism to check the precision and accuracy of a test system, such as an automated analyzer, to determine if the system is providing accurate results. Calibration is typically performed using a calibration device, often called a *standard.*

Clinical diagnosis A tentative diagnosis of a patient's condition obtained through evaluation of the health history and the physical examination, without the benefit of laboratory or diagnostic tests.

Control A solution that is used to monitor a test system to ensure the reliability and accuracy of test results.

Fasting Abstaining from food or fluids (except water) for a specified amount of time before the collection of a specimen.

Homeostasis The state in which body systems are functioning normally, and the internal environment of the body is in equilibrium; the body is in a healthy state.

In vivo Occurring in the living body or organism.

Laboratory test The clinical analysis and study of materials, fluids, or tissues obtained from patients to assist in diagnosis and treatment of disease.

Nonwaived test A complex laboratory test that does not meet the CLIA criteria for waiver and is subject to the CLIA regulations.

Plasma The liquid part of the blood, consisting of a clear, yellowish fluid that comprises approximately 55% of the total blood volume.

Product insert A printed document supplied by the manufacturer with a laboratory test product that contains information on the proper storage and use of the product.

Profile An array of laboratory tests for identifying a disease state or evaluating a particular organ or organ system.

Qualitative test A test that indicates whether or not a substance is present in the specimen being tested and also provides an approximate indication of the amount of the substance present.

Quality control The application of methods to ensure that test results are reliable and valid and that errors are detected and eliminated.

Quantitative test A test that indicates the exact amount of a chemical substance that is present in the body, with the results being reported in measurable units.

Reagent A substance that produces a reaction with a patient specimen that allows detection or measurement of the substance by the test system.

Reference range A certain established and acceptable parameter or reference range within which the laboratory test results of a healthy individual are expected to fall. (Also known as reference value and reference interval.)

Continued

TERMINOLOGY REVIEW—cont'd

Routine test A laboratory test performed routinely on apparently healthy patients to assist in the early detection of disease.

Serum The clear, straw-colored part of the blood (plasma) that remains after the solid elements and the clotting factor fibrinogen have been separated out of it.

Specimen A small sample of something taken to show the nature of the whole.

Test system A setup that includes all of the test components required to perform a laboratory test such as testing devices, controls, and testing reagents.

Waived test A laboratory test that meets the CLIA criteria for being a simple procedure that is easy to perform and has a low risk of erroneous test results. Waived tests include tests that have been FDA-approved for use by patients at home.

ON THE WEB

For Information on Aging:

National Institute on Aging: www.nia.nih.gov

Administration on Aging: www.aoa.gov

American Association of Retired Persons: www.aarp.org

Social Security Administration: www.ssa.gov

Centers for Medicare and Medicaid Services: www.cms.hhs.gov

Growth House: www.growthhouse.org

The AGS Foundation for Health in Aging: www.healthinaging.org

The Institute for Geriatric Social Work: www.bu.edu/igsw

Geriatrics at Your Fingertips: www.geriatricsatyourfingertips.org

Family Caregiver Alliance: www.caregiver.org

Medicare: www.medicare.gov

Aging Statistics: www.agingstats.gov

Alzheimer's Foundation of America: www.alzfdn.org

16

Urinalysis

LEARNING OBJECTIVES

Urinary System
1. Describe the structures that form the urinary system, and state the function of each.
2. List conditions that may cause polyuria and oliguria.
3. Define the terms used to describe symptoms of the urinary system.

Collection of Urine
1. Explain why a first-voided morning specimen is often preferred for urinalysis.

2. Explain the purpose of collecting a clean-catch midstream specimen.

3. Explain the purpose of a 24-hour urine collection.
4. List changes that may occur if urine is allowed to remain standing for longer than 1 hour.

Analysis of Urine
1. List factors that may cause urine to have an unusual color or become cloudy.
2. Identify the various tests that are included in the physical and chemical examination of urine.
3. List the structures that may be found in a microscopic examination of urine.

4. Explain the purpose of a rapid urine culture test.

Urine Pregnancy Testing
1. Explain the basis for urine pregnancy tests.
2. List the guidelines that must be followed in a urine pregnancy test to ensure accurate test results.

PROCEDURES

Instruct a patient in the procedure for collecting a clean-catch midstream urine specimen.
Instruct a patient on the procedure for collecting a 24-hour urine specimen.

Assess the color and appearance of a urine specimen.
Perform a chemical assessment of a urine specimen.

Prepare a urine specimen for microscopic analysis by the physician.
Perform a rapid urine culture test.

Perform a urine pregnancy test.

CHAPTER OUTLINE

Structure and Function of the Urinary System
Composition of Urine
    Terms Related to the Urinary System
Collection of Urine
    Guidelines for Urine Collection
    Urine Specimen Collection Methods
    Twenty-Four–Hour Urine Specimen
Analysis of Urine
    Physical Examination of Urine
    Chemical Examination of Urine

Reagent Strips
Microscopic Examination of Urine
Rapid Urine Cultures
Urine Pregnancy Testing
    Human Chorionic Gonadotropin
    Immunoassay Tests
    Guidelines for Urine Pregnancy Testing
Serum Pregnancy Test

anuria (ah-NOOR-ee-ah)
bilirubinuria (bill-ih-roo-bin-YUR-ee-ah)
bladder catheterization
diuresis (di-ah-REE-sis)
dysuria (dis-YUR-ee-ah)
frequency
glycosuria (glie-koe-SOO-ree-ah)
hematuria (hem-ah-TOOR-ee-ah)
ketonuria (kee-toe-NOO-ree-ah)
ketosis (kee-TOE-sis)
micturition (mik-tur-ISH-un)
nephron (NEF-ron)
nocturia (nok-TOOR-ee-ah)
nocturnal enuresis (nok-TOOR-nal en-YUR-ee-sas)

oliguria (oh-lig-YUR-ee-ah)
pH (PEE-AYCH)
polyuria (pol-ee-YUR-ee-ah)
proteinuria (proe-teen-YUR-ee-ah)
pyuria (pi-YUR-ee-ah)
renal threshold (REE-nul-THRESH-hold)
retention
specific gravity
supernatant (soo-per-NAY-tent)
suprapubic aspiration
urgency
urinalysis (yur-in-AL-ih-sis)
urinary incontinence
void (VOYD)

Structure and Function of the Urinary System

The function of the urinary system is to regulate the fluid and electrolyte balance of the body and to remove waste products. The urinary system consists of the kidneys, the ureters, the urinary bladder, and the urethra (Figure 16-1). The *kidneys* are bean-shaped organs approximately 4.5 inches (11.5 cm) long and 2 to 3 inches (5 to 8 cm) wide; they are located in the lumbar region of the body. Urine drains from the kidneys into the urinary bladder through two tubes known as *ureters.* Each ureter is approximately 10 to 12 inches long and ½ inch in diameter. The urine produced by the kidneys is propelled into the urinary bladder by the force of gravity and the peristaltic waves of the ureters. The *urinary bladder* is a hollow, muscular sac that can hold approximately 500 ml of urine. Its function is to store and expel urine. The *urethra* is a tube that extends from the urinary bladder to the outside of the body. The *urinary meatus* is the external opening of the urethra. In males, the urethra functions in transporting urine and reproductive secretions. In females, the urethra functions in urination only.

Each kidney contains approximately 1 million smaller units known as **nephrons** (Figure 16-2). The nephron is the functional unit of the kidney. It filters waste substances from the blood and dilutes them with water to produce urine. Another function of the nephron is reabsorption. Some substances filtered by the nephron, such as water, glucose, and electrolytes, are needed by the body and are reabsorbed or returned to the body for future use.

COMPOSITION OF URINE

A physiologic change in the body caused by disease can create a disturbance in one or more of the functions of the kidney. Detection of such a disturbance can be made with the examination of urine and other body fluids such as blood.

Urine is composed of 95% water and 5% organic and inorganic waste products. Organic waste products consist of urea, uric acid, ammonia, and creatinine. Urea is present in the greatest amounts and is derived from the breakdown of proteins. Inorganic waste products include chloride, sodium, potassium, calcium, magnesium, phosphate, and sulfate.

A normal adult excretes approximately 750 to 2000 ml of urine per day. This amount varies according to the amount of fluid consumed and the amount of fluid lost through other means, such as perspiration, feces, and water vapor from the lungs. An excessive increase in urine output is known as **polyuria,** with the urine volume exceeding 2000 ml in 24 hours. Polyuria may be caused by the excessive intake of fluids or the intake of fluids that contain caffeine (e.g., coffee, tea, cola), which is a mild diuretic. Certain drugs, such as diuretics, and the pathologic conditions of diabetes mellitus, diabetes insipidus, and renal disease also may result in polyuria. Decreased or scanty urine output is known as **oliguria.** In the case of oliguria, the urine volume is less than 400 ml in 24 hours. Oliguria may occur with decreased fluid intake, dehydration, profuse perspiration, vomiting, diarrhea, or kidney disease. The normal act of voiding urine is known as **micturition.**

Terms Related to the Urinary System

The medical assistant should have a thorough knowledge of the following terms used to describe symptoms associated with the urinary system:

Anuria Failure of the kidneys to produce urine.
Diuresis Secretion and passage of large amounts of urine.
Dysuria Difficult or painful urination.
Frequency The condition of having to urinate often.
Hematuria Blood present in the urine.
Nocturia Excessive (voluntary) urination during the night.
Nocturnal enuresis Inability of an individual to control urination at night during sleep (bedwetting).

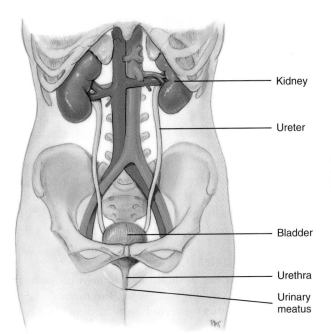

Figure 16-1. Structures that make up the urinary system. (Modified from Applegate EJ: The anatomy and physiology learning system, ed 3, St Louis, 2006, Saunders.)

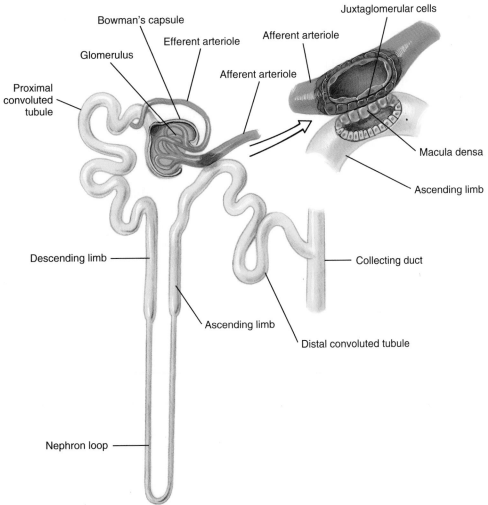

Figure 16-2. Nephron. (From Applegate EJ: The anatomy and physiology learning system, ed 3, St Louis, 2006, Saunders.)

Oliguria Decreased output of urine.

Polyuria Increased output of urine.

Pyuria Pus present in the urine.

Retention The inability to empty the bladder. The urine is being produced normally but is not being voided.

Urgency The immediate need to urinate.

Urinary incontinence The inability to retain urine.

COLLECTION OF URINE

The advantage of urine testing is that urine is readily available and obtaining it does not require an invasive procedure or the use of special equipment. For accurate test results, however, the medical assistant must adhere to proper urine collection procedures to obtain the proper specimen as ordered by the physician.

Guidelines for Urine Collection

The guidelines listed should be followed in collection of a urine specimen:

1. The medical assistant must obtain an adequate volume of urine as necessary for the type of test (usually 30 to 50 ml of urine).
2. Each specimen must be labeled properly with the patient's name and date of birth, the date and time of collection, and the type of specimen (i.e., urine) to avoid any mixups in specimens.
3. Any medication the patient is taking should be recorded on the laboratory requisition and in the patient's chart, because some medications may interfere with the accuracy of the test results.
4. If possible, the collection of a urine specimen should be avoided in women during menstruation and for several days thereafter because the specimen may become contaminated with blood. This results in a false-positive test result for blood in the urine.
5. The medical assistant should take into consideration that voiding may be difficult for patients under stress and anxiety. In these instances, understanding and patience should be conveyed to the patient.
6. A urine specimen may be difficult to obtain from a child, even with the assistance of a parent. In this case, the physician should be informed because another collection method may be used, such as a urine collection bag, suprapubic aspiration, or catheterization of the patient.

Urine Specimen Collection Methods

The type of test to be performed often dictates the method used to collect the urine specimen. A first-voided morning specimen is recommended for pregnancy testing, and a clean-catch midstream specimen is necessary for identification of the presence of a urinary tract infection (UTI).

Most offices use disposable plastic urine specimen containers. These containers are available in different sizes and come with lids to prevent spillage and to reduce bacterial and other types of contamination.

What Would You Do? What Would You Not Do?

Case Study 1

Yusuke Urameshi is at the office with fever and chills, frequency, and painful and difficult urination. The physician suspects that Mr. Urameshi has prostatitis and orders a clean-catch urine specimen for a complete urinalysis, including a microscopic examination of the sediment. Mr. Urameshi tries to collect the specimen but is able to collect only 5 ml of urine. He says that he is worried about what is wrong with him and he thinks his nervousness is making it hard to get a specimen. Mr. Urameshi says that it is probably just as well because he did not understand how to cleanse himself, and he is not sure that he did it right. ■

Random Specimen

Urine testing in the medical office is often performed on freshly voided, random specimens. The medical assistant instructs the patient to **void** into a clean, dry, wide-mouthed container, and the urine is tested immediately at the medical office.

First-Voided Morning Specimen

In many cases, a first-voided morning specimen may be desired for testing because it contains the greatest concentration of dissolved substances, and a small amount of an abnormal substance that is present would be more easily detected. The patient should be instructed to collect the first specimen of the morning after rising and to preserve the specimen by refrigerating it until it is brought to the medical office. It is important to provide the patient with a specimen container to prevent the patient's use of a container from home that might harbor contaminants and affect the test results.

Clean-Catch Midstream Specimen

The urinary bladder and most of the urethra are normally free of microorganisms, whereas the distal urethra and the urinary meatus normally harbor microorganisms. If the urine is being cultured and examined for bacteria, a clean-catch midstream specimen is necessary to prevent contamination of the specimen with these normally present microorganisms. Only microorganisms that may be causing the patient's condition are desired in the urine specimen. A clean-catch midstream collection may be ordered for the detection of a UTI and the evaluation of the effectiveness of drug therapy in a patient undergoing treatment for such an infection.

The purpose of the clean-catch midstream collection is the removal of microorganisms from the urinary meatus and the distal urethra. This is accomplished by instructing the patient to thoroughly cleanse the area surrounding the meatus and to void a small amount of urine into the toilet, which flushes out microorganisms in the distal urethra. The urine specimen is collected in a sterile container using medically aseptic techniques. A properly collected specimen reduces the possibility of having to do a bladder catheterization or a suprapubic aspiration of the bladder. **Bladder catheterization** involves the passing of a sterile tube (the catheter) through the urethra and into the bladder to remove urine. **Suprapubic aspiration** involves the passing of a sterile needle through the abdominal wall into the bladder to remove urine. Both of these procedures must be performed using sterile technique.

Guidelines

Guidelines that should be followed when collecting a clean-catch midstream specimen are listed:

1. A clean-catch midstream specimen is collected by the patient at the medical office. The medical assistant must provide complete instructions for collection of this specimen. Failure to instruct the patient adequately may necessitate a return to the medical office for the collection of another specimen because of bacterial contamination. Patient instructions for obtaining a clean-catch midstream specimen are presented in Procedure 16-1.

2. The medical assistant must label the container with the patient's name and date of birth, the date, the time of collection, and the type of specimen (clean-catch midstream specimen).

3. For reliable test results, the specimen should be tested immediately and should not be allowed to stand. If this is not possible, the specimen should be refrigerated, or a preservative should be added.

4. If the specimen is to be tested at an outside laboratory, completion of a laboratory requisition to accompany it is necessary. A urinalysis laboratory request form is shown in Figure 16-3.

5. The procedure is completed by sanitizing the hands and recording the procedure in the patient's chart. The information to be charted for specimens tested at the medical office includes the date and time, the type of specimen collected, and the laboratory test results. If the specimen is being transported to an outside laboratory for testing, record the date and time, the type of specimen collected, and the date the specimen was transported to the laboratory.

Twenty-Four–Hour Urine Specimen

A 24-hour urine specimen is used for quantitative measurement of specific urinary components. With collection of urine over a 24-hour period, greater accuracy of measurement exists than with a random specimen. This is because body metabolism, exercise, and hydration can affect the excretion rate of substances in the urine. In addition, at certain times during a 24-hour period, increased excretion of substances (e.g., electrolytes, hormones, proteins, urobilinogen) is seen, and at other times decreased excretion is seen. Examples of substances measured in a 24-hour specimen include calcium, cortisol, lead, potassium, protein, and urea nitrogen. A 24-hour specimen is often used in the diagnosis of the cause of kidney stone formation and in the

NAME:	ADDRESS:	UR- 183900	
		ICDA	
	DATE:	REQUESTING PHYSICIAN	
		PHYSICIAN HAS SEEN—INITIAL	

		ROUTINE URINALYSIS - 001				MICROSCOPIC - 022			QUANTITATIVE	
		APPEARANCE COLOR				WBC'S	/HPF	024	SULKOWITCH	
	023	SPECIFIC GRAVITY				RBC'S	/HPF	026	BILE	
	004	PH				CASTS (Hyaline)	/LPF		PHENYLPYRUVIC ACID	
		PROTEIN				CASTS (Granular)	/LPF	027	PHENESTIX	
		GLUCOSE				CASTS (Cellular)	/LPF	028	UROBILINOGEN	
	007	KETONES (ACETONE)				CASTS (Waxy)	/LPF	029	PORPHOBILINOGEN	
	3	OCCULT BLOOD				EPITHELIAL CELLS	/LPF	030	PORPHYRIN	
		BILE				BACTERIA		031	BENCE-JONES	
		UROBILINOGEN				MUCUS		025	TOTAL PROTEIN 24HR. SPECIMEN	
		LEUKOCYTE				CRYSTALS			TOTAL VOLUME REQUIRED:	
	COMMENTS					AMORPHOUS				
	URINALYSIS					OTHER:			SIGNATURE:	
	DMH-0067 (Rev. 3/83)			33		**F P N**			DATE:	

DMH-MedR-1065-A

Figure 16-3. Urinalysis laboratory request form.

control and prevention of new stone formation. It may also be used to perform a creatinine clearance test, which provides the physician with information on kidney function.

A large wide-mouthed container (3000 ml) is used to store the urine collected over the 24-hour period. To prevent changes in the quality of the urine specimen, the specimen must be kept refrigerated or placed in an ice chest. Some containers also contain a chemical preservative (in the form of crystals, tablets, or a liquid) to assist in maintaining the quality of the specimen. Examples of urine preservatives include hydrochloric acid, boric acid, acetic acid, and toluene. A hazardous chemical warning label should be attached to a specimen container with a preservative, and the patient should be instructed not to discard or touch the preservative in the container.

The patient is also provided with a container in which to collect each urine specimen. A female patient may be given a urine "hat," which is placed over the commode under the toilet seat; a male patient is often provided with a collection cup. After collection, the urine is poured into the large specimen container. This method makes collection easier and safer for the patient. If the patient voids urine directly into a specimen container that holds a preservative, the preservative could splash onto the patient's skin, resulting in a chemical burn.

The medical assistant should provide the patient with verbal and written instructions for collection of the urine specimen (Procedure 16-2). The patient should be advised to drink a normal amount of fluid during the collection period and to avoid alcohol intake for 24 hours before and during the collection period. The patient should be instructed to choose a 24-hour period when he or she will be at home, so that the urine will not have to be transported. The test should not be performed when the patient is menstruating. Certain medications, such as thiazides, phosphorus-binding antacids, allopurinol, and vitamin C, could alter the test results. The physician may want the patient to discontinue these medications for 1 week before the test.

PROCEDURE 16-1   Clean-Catch Midstream Specimen Collection Instructions

Outcome Instruct a patient in the procedure for collecting a clean-catch midstream urine specimen.

Equipment/Supplies

- Sterile specimen container and label
- Personal antiseptic towelettes
- Tissues

---

1. Procedural Step. Sanitize your hands. Greet the patient and introduce yourself. Identify the patient and explain the procedure.

2. Procedural Step. Assemble equipment. Label the specimen container with the patient's name and date of birth, the date, the type of specimen (clean-catch midstream), and your initials.

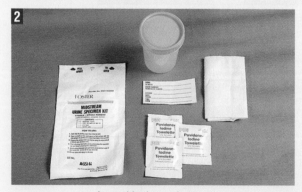

Assemble the equipment.

3. Procedural Step. Instruct a female patient on collection of the specimen as follows:

  a. Wash the hands, open the package of towelettes, and place them on their wrapper.

  b. Remove the lid from the specimen container and place it on a paper towel with the opening of the lid facing upward. Do not touch the inside of the lid or the inside of the specimen container.

  c. Pull undergarments down and sit on the toilet. Expose the urinary meatus by spreading apart the labia with one hand.

  d. Cleanse each side of the urinary meatus with an antiseptic towelette using a front-to-back motion (from pubis to anus). Use a separate antiseptic towelette for each side of the meatus. After use, discard each towelette in the toilet.

  Principle. Cleansing removes microorganisms from the urinary meatus. A front-to-back motion must be used for cleansing to avoid drawing microorganisms from the anal region into the area that is being cleansed.

  e. Cleanse directly across the meatus (front to back) with a third antiseptic towelette.

  f. Continue to hold the labia apart, and void a small amount of urine into the toilet.

  Principle. Voiding a small amount flushes microorganisms out of the distal urethra.

  g. Without stopping the urine flow, collect the next amount of urine by voiding into the sterile container. Do not touch the inside of the container. Fill the specimen container about half full with urine.

PROCEDURE 16-1   Clean-Catch Midstream Specimen Collection Instructions—cont'd

Principle. Touching the inside of the container contaminates it with microorganisms that normally reside on the skin.

   h. Void the last amount of urine into the toilet. This means that the first and last portions of the urine flow are not included in the specimen. Replace the lid of the specimen container.

   i. Wipe the area dry with a tissue, and discard it in the toilet. Flush the toilet and wash the hands.

4. Procedural Step. *Instruct a male patient as follows:*

   a. Wash the hands, open the towelettes, remove the lid from the specimen container, and remove undergarments.

   b. Stand in front of the toilet. Retract the foreskin of the penis (if uncircumcised).

   c. Cleanse the area around the meatus (glans penis) and the urethral opening (meatal orifice) by wiping each side of the meatus with a separate antiseptic towelette.

   d. Cleanse directly across the meatus with a third antiseptic towelette. After use, discard each towelette in the toilet.

   e. Void a small amount of urine into the toilet.

   f. Collect the next amount of urine by voiding into the sterile container without touching the inside of the container with the hands or penis. Fill the container about half full with urine.

   g. Void the last amount of urine into the toilet and replace the lid on the container.

   h. Wipe the area dry with a tissue, and discard it in the toilet. Flush the toilet and wash the hands.

5. Procedural Step. Provide the patient with instructions about what to do with the specimen after it has been collected (e.g., placing it in a designated area, directly handing it to the medical assistant).

6. Procedural Step. Record the procedure in the patient's chart. Include the date and time and the type of specimen collected (clean-catch midstream collection).

7. Procedural Step. Test the specimen at the office or prepare the specimen for transport to an outside laboratory for testing. If the specimen is to be transported to an outside laboratory, do the following:

   a. Place the specimen container in a biohazard specimen bag.

   b. Place the laboratory request in the outside pocket of the specimen bag.

   c. Properly preserve the specimen while awaiting pickup by a laboratory courier by placing it in a refrigerator.

   d. Chart the date the specimen was transported to the laboratory and the tests requested.

CHARTING EXAMPLE	
Date	
3/24/12	10:15 a.m. Clean-catch midstream collected
	by pt. Sent to Medical Center Laboratory for
	C & S on 3/24/12.——L. Proffitt, CMA (AAMA)

PROCEDURE 16-2   Collection of a 24-Hour Urine Specimen

Outcome   Collect a 24-hour urine specimen.

Equipment/Supplies

- Large urine collection container and label
- Collecting container
- Written instructions
- Laboratory requisition

1. Procedural Step. Sanitize your hands. Greet the patient and introduce yourself. Identify the patient, and explain the procedure.

2. Procedural Step. Assemble the equipment. Label the large specimen container with the patient's name and date of birth, the date, the type of specimen (24-hour urine specimen), and your initials.

Instruct the patient on collection of the specimen as follows.

3. Procedural Step. When you get up in the morning, empty your bladder into the toilet just as you normally do. In other words, this urine is not to be saved. Make a note of what time it is, and write the date and start time in the appropriate space on the label of the container.

Continued

PROCEDURE 16-2   Collection of a 24-Hour Urine Specimen—cont'd

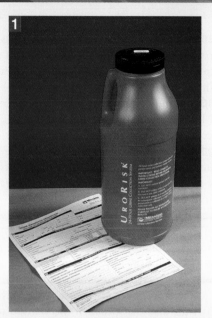

Assemble the equipment.

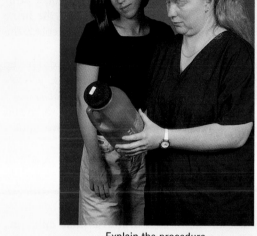

Explain the procedure.

Principle. This urine was produced before the collection period began and should not be included in the collection.

4. Procedural Step. The next time you need to urinate, void in the collecting container and then pour the urine into the large wide-mouthed specimen container.

5. Procedural Step. Tightly screw the lid onto the 24-hour specimen container, and put the container in your refrigerator or into an ice chest.

6. Procedural Step. Repeat procedural steps 4 and 5 each time you urinate.

7. Procedural Step. Emphasize the importance of the following to the patient:

a. The urine must be stored only in the designated container.

b. Collect all of the urine during the 24-hour period, including urine that you void if you get up during the night. The information this test provides would be inaccurate if any urine from the 24-hour period does not go into the container.

c. Urinate into the collection container before having a bowel movement to avoid losing urine you might pass during the bowel movement.

d. The collection must be started again from the beginning if any of the following occurs:

• You forget to collect the urine when you void.

• You spill some urine from the collection container.

• Your urine becomes contaminated with stool from a bowel movement.

• The child wets the bed (if the specimen is being obtained from a child).

• You go beyond the 24-hour collection period and collect too much urine.

8. Procedural Step. On the following morning, get up and void at the same time (exactly 24 hours after beginning the test). Void into the collection container for the last time and pour the urine into the large specimen container.

9. Procedural Step. Put the lid on the specimen container tightly, and write the date and time the test ended on the label in the appropriate space. Return the 24-hour specimen container to the office the same morning you complete the urine collection.

10. Procedural Step. Provide the patient with the 24-hour specimen container, a collection container, and written instructions. If the specimen container contains a chemical preservative, provide the patient with an MSDS (Material Safety Data Sheet) so that the patient has information regarding the chemical, its hazards, and measures to take to prevent injury and illness when handling the chemical. Chart this information in the patient's medical record.

11. Procedural Step. When the patient returns the 24-hour urine specimen container, ask the patient whether he or she encountered any difficulty in following the instructions for the 24-hour collection. If any problems occurred that resulted in undercollection or overcollection of urine, the entire collection process must be repeated.

PROCEDURE 16-2   Collection of a 24-Hour Urine Specimen—cont'd

12. Procedural Step. Prepare the specimen for transport to the laboratory. Complete a laboratory request form.

13. Procedural Step. Chart the results. Include the date and time, the type of specimen, and information on sending the specimen to the laboratory.

CHARTING EXAMPLE	
Date	
3/26/12	3:30 p.m. Container and verbal/written
	instructions provided on 24-hour specimen
	collection. ———————— L. Proffitt, CMA (AAMA)
3/28/12	10:00 a.m. 24-hour urine specimen sent to
	Medical Center Laboratory for kidney stone
	risk analysis. ———————— L. Proffitt, CMA (AAMA)

ANALYSIS OF URINE

Urinalysis is the analysis of urine and is the laboratory test most commonly performed in the medical office because a urine specimen is readily obtainable and can be easily tested. Urinalysis consists of *physical, chemical,* and *microscopic examinations.* Deviation from normal in any of the three areas assists the physician in the diagnosis and treatment of pathologic conditions, not only of the urinary system, but also of other body systems. Urinalysis may be performed as a screening measure as part of a general physical examination or to assist in the diagnosis of a pathologic condition. It also may assist in the evaluation of effectiveness of therapy after treatment has been initiated for a pathologic condition.

Urinalysis should be performed on a fresh or preserved specimen. If a specimen cannot be examined within 1 hour of voiding, it should be preserved at once in the refrigerator in a closed container and later returned to room temperature and mixed before testing. Chemical additives also are used to preserve urine specimens but generally are used only with specimens that require prolonged storage, such as specimens that must be shipped a long distance, because the chemical preservative sometimes interferes with the chemicals used to perform the urine test.

If the urine is allowed to stand at room temperature for longer than 1 hour, some of the following changes may occur:

1. Bacteria in the environment that get into the urine specimen work on the urea present in the urine, converting it to ammonia. Because ammonia is alkaline, an acid urine becomes alkaline, increasing the pH. In addition, an alkaline pH may result in a false-positive result on the protein test.
2. Bacteria multiply rapidly in the urine, resulting in a cloudy specimen and an increase in the nitrite.
3. If glucose is present in the specimen, it decreases in amount because microorganisms use the glucose as a source of food.

4. If any red or white blood cells are present, they may break down.
5. Casts decompose after several hours.

Physical Examination of Urine

The physical examination of urine includes determination of the color, appearance, and specific gravity. The color and appearance of the urine specimen may be evaluated during preparation for another testing procedure, such as chemical testing of the urine, or before centrifugation of the specimen in preparation for microscopic analysis. For an accurate evaluation of the color and appearance, the urine specimen must be collected in a clear plastic container.

Color

The normal color of urine ranges from almost colorless to dark yellow. Dilute urine tends to be lighter yellow in color, whereas concentrated urine is a darker yellow. The first-voided morning specimen is usually the most concentrated because consumption of fluids is decreased during the night. Urine becomes more dilute as the day progresses and more fluids are consumed.

The color of the urine is the result of the presence of a yellow pigment known as *urochrome,* produced by the breakdown of hemoglobin. It is common for the color of urine to vary among different shades of yellow within the course of a day. Classifications that can be used to describe the color of urine include light yellow, yellow, dark yellow, light amber, amber, and dark amber (Figure 16-4).

The color of the urine specimen assists in determining additional tests that may be necessary. Abnormal colors may be caused by the presence of hemoglobin or blood (resulting in a red or reddish color), bile pigments (resulting in a yellow-brown or greenish color), and fat droplets or pus (resulting in a milky color). Some foods and medications also may cause the urine to change to an abnormal color. Phenazopyridine (Pyridium), a urinary tract analgesic, causes the urine to change to an orange to red color.

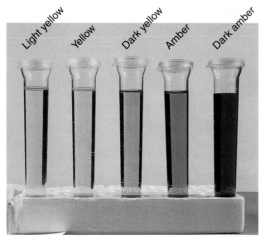

Figure 16-4. Color of urine.

Appearance

Evaluation of the appearance of urine is usually performed at the same time as the color evaluation. Fresh urine is usually clear, or transparent, but becomes cloudy on standing out too long. Cloudiness in a freshly voided specimen may be the result of the presence of bacteria, pus, blood, fat, yeast, sperm, mucous threads, or fecal contaminants. A microscopic examination of the urine sediment should be performed on all cloudy specimens to determine the cause of the cloudiness. Cloudiness resulting from bacteria may be caused by a UTI.

Classifications used to describe the appearance of urine include clear, slightly cloudy, cloudy, and very cloudy (Figure 16-5). The medical assistant should develop skill in recognizing the varying degrees of urine clarity.

Odor

Freshly voided urine normally should have a slightly aromatic odor. Urine that has been standing for a long time develops an ammonia odor from the breakdown of urea by

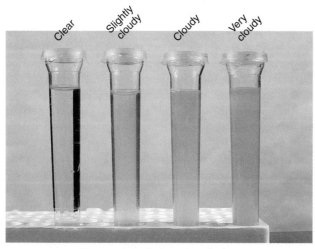

Figure 16-5. Appearance of urine.

bacteria in the specimen. The urine of a patient with diabetes mellitus may have a fruity odor from the presence of ketone. The urine of a patient with a UTI is usually foul-smelling, and the odor becomes worse on standing. Certain foods, such as asparagus, can cause the urine to have a musty smell. Although urine may have many characteristic odors, as a rule the odor of urine is not generally used in the diagnosis of a patient's condition.

Specific Gravity

The **specific gravity** of urine measures the weight of the urine compared with the weight of an equal volume of distilled water. Specific gravity indicates the amount of dissolved substance present in the urine, providing information on the ability of the kidneys to dilute or concentrate the urine. Specific gravity is decreased in conditions in which the kidneys cannot concentrate the urine, such as chronic renal insufficiency, diabetes insipidus, and malignant hypertension. The specific gravity is increased in patients with adrenal insufficiency, congestive heart failure, hepatic disease, diabetes mellitus with glycosuria, and conditions that cause dehydration, such as fever, vomiting, and diarrhea.

The normal specific gravity of urine ranges from 1.003 to 1.030, but is usually between 1.010 and 1.025 (the specific gravity of distilled water is 1.000). Specific gravity varies greatly with fluid intake and the state of hydration of an individual. Dilute urine contains fewer dissolved substances and has a lower specific gravity. Concentrated urine has a higher specific gravity because of the increased amount of dissolved substances. A urine specimen is generally more concentrated in the morning and becomes more dilute after fluid consumption.

In the medical office, specific gravity is most commonly measured using a reagent strip. This involves a color comparison determination with a reagent strip that contains a reagent area for specific gravity. The reagent strip is dipped into the urine specimen, and the results are compared with a color chart (see Procedure 16-3).

Chemical Examination of Urine

The chemical examination of urine is used to assist in the evaluation and diagnosis of kidney function, urinary tract infection, carbohydrate metabolism (diabetes mellitus), and liver function. Substances present in excessive (abnormal) amounts in the blood are usually removed by the urine. For example, glucose is normally present in the blood, but if it exceeds a certain level or threshold, the excess amount is excreted in the urine. Chemical testing of urine is an indirect means of detecting abnormal amounts of chemicals in the body, indicating a pathologic condition. The chemical examination of urine also can be used to detect the presence of substances that, in the absence of disease, do not normally appear in the urine, such as blood and nitrite.

Chemical tests that are routinely performed during a urinalysis include testing for pH, glucose, protein, and ketone. Other chemical tests that may be performed include testing for blood, bilirubin, urobilinogen, nitrite, and leukocytes.

- *Qualitative test results.* The chemical analysis of urine involves the use of qualitative and quantitative tests. Qualitative test results indicate whether a substance is present in the urine and also provide an approximate indication of the amount of the substance present. Interpretation of qualitative results usually involves the use of a color comparison chart, with results recorded in terms of 1+, 2+, or 3+; trace, small, moderate, or large; or negative or positive. Qualitative tests are useful for screening purposes in the medical office because they are easy to perform and can be used to screen large numbers of individuals—a procedure that otherwise might be too expensive and time consuming.

- *Quantitative test results.* Quantitative test results indicate the exact amount of a chemical substance that is present in the body; the results are reported in measurable units (e.g., mg/dL). Obtaining a quantitative test result on a urine specimen usually involves the use of more complex equipment and testing procedures than are found in the medical office; they also are more time-consuming to run.

Urine Testing Kits

Commercially prepared urine testing kits are most frequently used in the medical office for the chemical testing of urine. These kits are usually preferred because they contain premeasured reagents, the procedure is easy to follow, and they provide an immediate answer. Most of the test results are qualitative, and a positive result may indicate the need for further testing. Most of the tests are manufactured in the form of reagent strips, and they rely on a color change for interpretation of results. A color chart is provided with the kit for making a visual comparison.

For accurate and reliable test results, the medical assistant should carefully read and follow the instructions that accompany each kit. Test strips that contain more than one reagent may require different time intervals for reading results.

Putting It All into Practice

My Name is Linda Proffitt, and I work for a urologist and his wife, who is a pediatrician. I work primarily in the urology practice and only occasionally in pediatrics. I am responsible for having the charts ready when the patients are seen and for doing their urinalysis. Another one of my responsibilities is to assist with special procedures, such as catheter insertions, male and female dilations, ultrasound examinations of the bladder, and prostate examinations.

When I first started working in the urology office, I had to learn to assist with transrectal ultrasounds of the prostate in case the US technician was sick. When she retired, I inherited the position, whether I wanted it or not. At first I dreaded doing the procedures and would be so nervous that I would get the shakes and forget the order in which things were supposed to be done. My physician was understanding and would help by talking me through it. I think the main reason I was so nervous was that sometimes patients have trouble and we have to administer oxygen and run IVs. One time, a patient had a reaction to the pain medication we gave before the procedure.

Time, practice, and confidence in myself have improved my nerves, even with the occasional emergency situation. ■

sults. Certain medications that the patient is taking also may interfere with the test results. These medications are listed in the manufacturer's instructions accompanying the test.

Before a test is used, its expiration date must be checked. If the test is outdated, it must not be used to prevent inaccurate test results. Test material must not be used if a color change has occurred, or if the *tested* strip gives off a color that does not match the shades on the color chart. Light, heat, and moisture can alter the effectiveness of the strips; care must be taken to store the test materials in a cool, dry area. Most test materials are packaged in light-resistant containers to protect them from light. The test materials must never be transferred from their original container to another because the other container may harbor traces of moisture, dirt, or chemicals that could affect the test results.

When results are recorded, the brand name of the test that was used should be specified. Commercially available diagnostic kits for chemical tests on urine are presented in Table 16-1.

pH

The **pH** is the unit that indicates the acidity or alkalinity of a solution. The pH scale ranges from 0.0 to 14.0. The lower the number, the greater the acidity; the higher the number, the greater the alkalinity. A pH reading of 7.0 is neutral; a reading below 7.0 indicates acidity; and a reading above 7.0 indicates alkalinity.

The kidneys help regulate the acid-base balance of the body. For an accurate pH reading of the urine, the measure-

Table 16-1 Diagnostic Kits Used for Chemical Testing of Urine

Brand Name	Function
Products of Bayer Corporation	
Acetest	Reagent tablet to detect ketone
Albustix	Reagent strip to detect protein
Bili-Labstix	Reagent strip to detect pH, protein, glucose, ketone, bilirubin, and blood
Clinistix	Reagent strip to detect glucose
Combistix	Reagent strip to detect pH, protein, and glucose
Diastix	Reagent strip to detect glucose
Hema-Combistix	Reagent strip to detect pH, protein, glucose, and blood
Hemastix	Reagent strip to detect occult blood in urine
Ictotest	Reagent tablet to detect bilirubin
Keto-Diastix	Reagent strip to detect glucose and ketone
Ketostix	Reagent strip to detect ketone
Labstix	Reagent strip to detect pH, protein, glucose, ketone, and blood
Multistix	Reagent strip to detect pH, protein, glucose, ketone, urobilinogen, bilirubin, and blood
Multistix SG	Reagent strip to detect pH, protein, glucose, ketone, urobilinogen, bilirubin, blood, and specific gravity
Multistix 2	Reagent strip to detect leukocytes and nitrite
Multistix 5	Reagent strip to detect glucose, blood, protein, nitrite, and leukocytes.
Multistix 7	Reagent strip to detect pH, protein, glucose, ketone, blood, leukocytes, and nitrite
Multistix 8 SG	Reagent strip to detect pH, protein, glucose, ketone, blood, leukocytes, nitrite, and specific gravity
Multistix 9	Reagent strip to detect pH, protein, glucose, ketone, urobilinogen, bilirubin, blood, leukocytes, and nitrite
Multistix 9 SG	Reagent strip to detect pH, protein, glucose, ketone, bilirubin, blood, leukocytes, nitrite, and specific gravity
Multistix 10 SG	Reagent strip to detect pH, protein, glucose, ketone, urobilinogen, bilirubin, blood, leukocytes, nitrite, and specific gravity
Multistix PRO 10 LS	Reagent strip to detect pH, protein-high, protein-low, glucose, ketone, blood, leukocytes, nitrite, creatinine, and specific gravity
N-Multistix	Reagent strip to detect pH, protein, glucose, ketone, urobilinogen, bilirubin, blood, and nitrite
N-Multistix SG	Reagent strip to detect pH, protein, glucose, ketone, urobilinogen, bilirubin, blood, nitrite, and specific gravity
Uristix	Reagent strip to detect protein and glucose
Uristix 4	Reagent strip to detect protein, glucose, leukocytes, and nitrite
Products of Roche Laboratories	
Chemstrip 6	Reagent strip to detect pH, protein, glucose, ketone, blood, and leukocytes
Chemstrip 7	Reagent strip to detect pH, protein, glucose, ketone, bilirubin, blood, and leukocytes
Chemstrip 8	Reagent strip to detect pH, protein, glucose, ketone, urobilinogen, bilirubin, blood, and nitrite
Chemstrip 9	Reagent strip to detect pH, protein, glucose, ketone, urobilinogen, bilirubin, blood, leukocytes, and nitrite.
Chemstrip 10 SG	Reagent strip to detect pH, protein, glucose, ketone, urobilinogen, bilirubin, blood, leukocytes, nitrite, and specific gravity
Chemstrip 10 MD	Reagent strip to detect pH, protein, glucose, ketone, urobilinogen, bilirubin, blood, leukocytes, nitrite, and specific gravity (can be used with Roche urine analyzers)
Chemstrip 4 OB	Reagent strip to detect glucose, protein, blood, and leukocytes
Chemstrip 5 OB	Reagent strip to detect glucose, protein, blood, leukocytes, and nitrite.
Chemstrip 2 GP	Reagent strip to detect protein and glucose
Chemstrip 2 LN	Reagent strip to detect leukocytes and nitrite
Chemstrip μGK	Reagent strip to detect glucose and ketone
Chemstrip K	Reagent strip to detect ketone
Chemstrip Micral	Reagent strip to detect protein

Highlight on Drug Testing in the Workplace

Statistics

Statistics suggest that the problem of drug abuse is growing in the workplace. On any one day, 8.9 to 16 million employees are estimated to be working under the influence of drugs. The effects of on-the-job drug use extend into every segment of the population and touch every business and industry. The Occupational Safety and Health Administration (OSHA) estimates that 65% of all work-related accidents can be traced to substance abuse. The Metropolitan Insurance Company states that drug abuse costs industry $85 billion annually because of absenteeism, lowered productivity, and higher health care costs.

Testing Programs

Because of these economic and safety factors, businesses across the United States are adopting a less-permissive attitude toward drug use and are beginning compulsory drug testing in the workplace. Approximately one third of U.S. employers have implemented drug-testing programs in the workplace. These employers include utility companies, transportation operations, sports associations, and governmental agencies. Currently, many companies test blue-collar and white-collar employees for drug use. Companies with drug-testing programs report a significant reduction in employee accidents, fewer sick days, and healthier employees.

A comprehensive drug-testing program includes the detection of drug use in the workplace, policies to discourage further abuse, and the referral of employees for treatment and rehabilitation. Drug testing may be performed for one or more of the following purposes: (1) pre-employment drug screening, (2) testing for probable cause after unexplained behavior or incident (e.g., an accident on the job), and (3) random sample testing of the workforce to detect use of controlled substances by employees on the job.

Testing Methods

Blood testing is the best means for determining precise information concerning the amount of drug used and when the drug was taken. Blood tests are costly, however, and are time-consuming to perform. Urine drug testing offers the next best alternative; it is noninvasive and technically easier and cheaper to perform. Current urine screening tests target the most common drugs of abuse: amphetamines, barbiturates, benzodiazepines, cocaine, marijuana, opiates, PCP, methaqualone, and methadone.

Chain of Custody

The usual procedure for urine drug testing involves screening the specimen and confirming positive results with more specific urine tests. The specimen may be collected at the workplace, at the medical office, or at an outside laboratory. To help ensure reliable and valid drug-testing results, a security system or "chain of custody" must be followed in the collection and handling of the specimen. This typically includes ensuring the identification of the individual undergoing drug testing, taking precautions to avoid falsifying or tampering with specimens, properly labeling the urine specimen, sealing the sample in the specimen container after collection, and immediately sending it to the laboratory for analysis or refrigerating it at once for any delay in transport. Urine drug-testing kits are available for testing the specimen in the medical office. These kits provide immediate results and take only a few minutes to perform.

Disadvantages

The main disadvantage of urine drug testing is that a positive test result indicates only the presence of a drug in the urine; it does not provide any information regarding when the drug was taken. Drugs that are detected in the urine may or *may not* still be present in the blood, where they can affect an individual's behavior and impair performance. A positive urine test result does not reveal whether an individual is impaired by drugs. In addition, the initial urine screening tests are sometimes unreliable; unless positive results are confirmed with a more specific test, an individual may be unjustly accused of drug use. These factors and the violation of an individual's right to privacy are the main areas of dispute for individuals who oppose drug testing in the workplace.

Intervention

Companies with drug-testing programs have various options when results are positive, such as recommendations for drug treatment programs or disciplinary action. Many companies have established in-house employee assistance programs that include counseling and drug withdrawal therapy for employees who desire help. Most companies prefer to help current employees with rehabilitation instead of discharging them and hiring and training new employees. Studies show a 35% to 60% recovery rate for employees enrolled in drug treatment programs. ∎

---

ment should be performed on freshly voided urine. If the urine is allowed to remain standing, it becomes more alkaline as urea is converted to ammonia by bacterial action.

Although the pH of urine can normally range from 4.6 to 8.0, the pH of a freshly voided specimen of a patient on a normal diet is usually acidic and has a pH reading of about 6.0. An abnormally high pH reading on a fresh specimen (i.e., an alkaline urine) may indicate a bacterial infection of the urinary tract.

Glucose

Normally, no glucose should be detectable in the urine. Glucose in the blood is filtered through the nephrons and is reabsorbed into the body. If the glucose concentration in the blood becomes too high, the kidney is unable to reabsorb all of it back into the blood, the renal threshold is exceeded, and glucose is spilled into the urine—a condition known as **glycosuria.** (The **renal threshold** is the concentration at which a substance in the blood that is not normally excreted by the kidney begins to appear in the urine.) The renal threshold for glucose is generally 160 to 180 mg/dL (100 ml of blood), but this number may vary among individuals. Diabetes mellitus is the most common cause of glycosuria. Some individuals have a low renal threshold, and glucose may appear in their urine after the consumption of a large quantity of foods containing sugar. This condition is known as *alimentary glycosuria.*

Protein

The presence of protein in the urine is known as **proteinuria.** Protein in the urine usually indicates a pathologic condition if found in several samples over time. A temporary increase in urine protein may be caused by stress or strenuous exercise. Some of the conditions that may cause proteinuria include glomerular filtration problems, renal disease, and bacterial infection of the urinary tract. If proteinuria occurs, the physician usually requests an examination of the sediment to determine, through visual observation, what is causing protein to be in the urine.

Ketone

Three types of ketone bodies exist: beta-hydroxybutyric acid, acetoacetic acid, and acetone. *Ketones* are the normal products of fat metabolism and can be used by muscle tissue as a source of energy. When more than normal amounts of fat are metabolized by the body, the muscles cannot handle all of the ketones that result. Large amounts of ketone accumulate in the tissues and body fluids; this condition is known as **ketosis.** The body rids itself of these excess ketones by excreting them in the urine. **Ketonuria** is the term that refers to the presence of ketone bodies in the urine. Conditions that may lead to ketonuria include uncontrolled diabetes mellitus, starvation, and a diet composed almost entirely of fat.

Bilirubin

The average life span of a red blood cell is 120 days. When a red blood cell breaks down, one of the substances released from the breakdown of hemoglobin is a vivid yellow pigment known as *bilirubin.* Normally, bilirubin is transported to the liver and excreted into the bile, and it eventually leaves the body through the intestines in the feces. Certain liver conditions, such as gallstones, hepatitis, and cirrhosis, may result in the presence of bilirubin in the urine, or **bilirubinuria.** The urine becomes yellow-brown or greenish, and a yellow foam appears when the urine is shaken.

Urobilinogen

Normally, bilirubin is excreted by the liver into the intestinal tract. Bacteria present in the intestines convert it to urobilinogen. Approximately 50% of the urobilinogen is reabsorbed into the body for reexcretion by the liver. Small amounts may appear in the urine, but most of the urobilinogen is excreted in the feces. An increase in the production of bilirubin increases the amount of urobilinogen excreted in the urine. Conditions such as excessive hemolysis of red blood cells, infectious hepatitis, cirrhosis, congestive heart failure, and infectious mononucleosis may increase the level of urobilinogen in the urine.

Blood

Blood is considered an abnormal constituent of urine, unless it is present as a contaminant during menstruation. The condition in which blood is found in the urine is termed *hematuria.* Hematuria may be the result of injury or disorders such as cystitis, tumors of the bladder, urethritis, kidney stones, and certain kidney disorders.

Nitrite

Nitrite in the urine indicates the presence of a pathogen in the (normally sterile) urinary tract, which results in a UTI. The pathogen possesses the ability to convert nitrate, which normally occurs in the urine, to nitrite, which is normally absent. The nitrite test must be performed with urine that has been in the bladder for at least 4 to 6 hours to ensure that bacteria have converted nitrate to nitrite. Therefore, use of a first-voided morning specimen is recommended. The test should *not* be performed on specimens that have been left standing out because a false-positive result may occur from bacterial contamination from the environment. The nitrite test is a screening test and is usually followed by a quantitative culture and identification of the invading pathogen.

Leukocytes

The presence of leukocytes in the urine is known as *leukocyturia* and accompanies inflammation of the kidneys and the lower urinary tract. Examples of specific conditions include acute and chronic pyelonephritis, cystitis, and urethritis. Reagent strips are available that contain a reagent area that permits the chemical detection of intact and lysed leukocytes in the urine. The advantage of detecting lysed leukocytes is that these cells cannot be observed during a microscopic examination of urine sediment and would otherwise remain undetected. The recommended urine specimen, particularly for women, is a clean-catch midstream collection to prevent contamination of the specimen with leukocytes from vaginal secretions leading to false-positive test results.

Reagent Strips

In the medical office, reagent strips are the most commonly used diagnostic urine testing kit. Reagent strips consist of disposable plastic strips on which separate reagent areas are affixed for testing specific chemical constituents that may be present in the urine during pathologic conditions. The results provide the physician with information to assist in diagnosis of the following:

- Conditions affecting kidney function (e.g., kidney stones)
- Urinary tract infection
- Conditions affecting carbohydrate metabolism (e.g., diabetes mellitus)
- Conditions affecting liver function (e.g., hepatitis)

Test results also provide the physician with information related to the status of the patient's acid-base balance and urine concentration. Reagent strips are considered qualitative tests, and a positive result necessitates further testing. Table 16-2 presents an outline of reagent strip parameters and the diagnoses in which they assist.

The number and type of reagent areas included on the reagent strip depend on the particular brand of reagent strips. Multistix 10 SG (Bayer Corporation, Tarrytown, NY) contains 10 reagent areas for testing pH, protein, glucose, ketone, bilirubin, blood, urobilinogen, nitrite, specific gravity, and leukocytes. Other brands and the tests included for each are listed in Table 16-1.

The reagent strip urine testing procedure presented in this chapter (Procedure 16-3) is specifically for Multistix 10 SG; however, this procedure can be followed for the chemical testing of urine with most reagent strips. In all instances, the medical assistant should read the manufacturer's instructions before performing the test.

Guidelines for Reagent Strip Urine Testing

Testing urine with reagent strips is a relatively easy procedure to perform. Specific guidelines must be followed, however, to obtain accurate test results.

1. *Type of specimen.* The best results are obtained with a freshly voided and thoroughly mixed urine specimen. If the medical assistant is unable to test the specimen within 1 hour of voiding, the specimen should be refrigerated immediately and then allowed to return to room temperature before testing.
2. *Type of collection.* Most reagent strips are designed to be used with a random specimen collection; however, clean-catch midstream and first-voided morning specimens are suggested for specific tests. The nitrite test results are optimized with a first-voided morning specimen, whereas a clean-catch midstream collection is recommended for the leukocyte test.
3. *Specimen container.* The specimen container used must be thoroughly clean and free from any detergent or disinfectant residue because cleansing agents contain oxidants that react with the chemicals on the reagent strip, leading to inaccurate test results. The container should be large enough to allow for complete immersion of all reagent strip areas.
4. *Time intervals.* Read the test results at the exact time intervals specified on the color chart. Do not read any test results after 2 minutes.
5. *Interpretation of results.* Of particular importance is the comparison of the reagent strip with the color chart. The reagent strip must be compared with the color chart in good lighting to obtain a good visual match of the color reactions with the color chart provided with the test kit.
6. *Storage of reagent strips.* The reagents on the strips are sensitive to light, heat, and moisture, and the bottle containing the strips must be stored in a cool, dry area away from direct sunlight, with the cap tightly closed to main-

tain reactivity of the reagent. The bottle may contain a desiccant that should not be removed because its purpose is to promote dryness by absorbing moisture. The bottle of reagent strips must be stored at a temperature between 59° F (15° C) and 86° F (30° C). The strips should not be stored in the refrigerator or freezer. A tan-to-brown discoloration or darkening on the reagent areas indicates deterioration of the chemical reagent strips, in which case the strips should not be used because the test results would be inaccurate.

Quality Control Testing

Quality control testing should be used in a chemical examination of urine with a reagent strip. Quality control testing ensures the reliability of test results by (1) determining whether the reagent strips are reacting properly, and (2) confirming that the test is being properly performed and accurately interpreted.

To check the reliability of Multistix reagent strips, the Chek-Stix control (Bayer Corporation) should be used. Each Chek-Stix control consists of a firm plastic strip to which are affixed synthetic ingredients (Figure 16-6). The control strip is reconstituted by immersing it in distilled water for 30 minutes, which allows the ingredients on the strip to dissolve in the water. After reconstitution, the resulting solution is tested in the same manner as a urine specimen. The values to be expected are outlined in the product insert that accompanies the control strips. The results of the control test should be recorded in a quality control log. If the expected values are not obtained, the cause of the problem must be determined and corrected. Factors that can cause a problem include outdated reagent strips, improper storage of the strips, and an error in testing

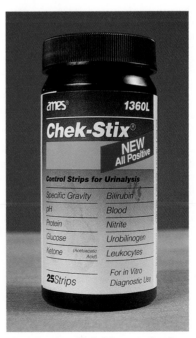

Figure 16-6. Chek-Stix control strips.

Table 16-2 Urine Test Strip Parameters and the Diagnoses They Assist*

System/Source	Leukocytes	Nitrite	Urine pH		Protein
Genitourinary	Renal infection or inflammation • Acute/chronic pyelonephritis • Glomerulonephritis • Urolithiasis • Tumors • Lower urinary tract infection (cystitis, urethritis, prostatitis)	Bacteriuria • Urinary tract infection (cystitis, urethritis, prostatitis, pyelonephritis)	Up (greater than 6) in: • Renal failure • Bacterial infection (e.g., *Proteus* bacteriuria) • Renal tubular acidosis		Renal, glomerular, or tubular disease • Glomerulonephritis • Glomerulosclerosis (e.g., in diabetes) • Nephrotic syndrome • Pyelonephritis • Renal tuberculosis
Hepatobiliary					
Gastrointestinal			Up in: • Pyloric obstruction	Down in: • Diarrhea • Malabsorption	
Cardiovascular					Congestive heart failure
Hormonal, metabolic, and other systems			Up in: • Alkalosis (metabolic, respiratory)	Down in: • Acidosis (metabolic, respiratory, diabetic) • Pulmonary emphysema • Dehydration	Gout Hypokalemia Preeclampsia Severe febrile infection
Environmental (diet, drugs, stress)	Phenacetin-induced nephritis		Up in: • Diet high in vegetables, citrus fruits • Alkalizing drug use (sodium bicarbonate, acetazolamide)	Down in: • Diet high in meats or other protein, cranberries • Acidifying drug use (e.g., ammonium chloride, methenamine mandelate therapy)	Nephrotoxic drugs

*Reagent strip detection of abnormal urine constituent or concentration characteristic of disease (e.g., glycosuria in diabetes mellitus) may provide useful screen or monitor, but requires confirmation with other laboratory and clinical evidence.
Courtesy Boehringer-Mannheim Diagnostics, Indianapolis, Ind.
Modified from Conn HF, Conn RB (eds): Current diagnosis 5, Philadelphia, 1977, Saunders; Davidson I, Henry JB (eds): Todd-Stanford clinical diagnosis by laboratory methods, ed 15, Philadelphia, 1974, Saunders; Raphael SS, et al: Lynch's medical laboratory technology, ed 3, Philadelphia, 1976, Saunders; Wallach J: Interpretation of diagnostic tests, ed 2, Boston, 1974, Little, Brown; Widmann FK: Goodale's clinical interpretation of laboratory tests, ed 7, Philadelphia, 1973, Davis.

Glucose	Ketone	Urobilinogen	Bilirubin	Blood, Erythrocytes (Hematuria)	Hemoglobin
Renal glycosuria (e.g., during pregnancy) Renal tubular disease (e.g., in Fanconi's syndrome) Decreased renal glucose threshold (e.g., in old age)				Renal infection, inflammation, or injury • Renal tuberculosis • Renal infarction • Calculi (urethral, renal) • Polycystic kidneys • Tumors (bladder, renal pelvis, prostate) • Salpingitis • Cystitis	Renal intravascular Hemolysis Acute glomerulonephritis
		Liver cell damage Chronic liver stasis Cirrhosis Dubin-Johnson syndrome *Note:* May be 0 or down in biliary obstruction	Biliary dysfunction • Gallstones Obstructive jaundice Hepatitis (viral toxic) Dubin-Johnson syndrome	Cirrhosis	
	Vomiting Diarrhea	*Note:* May be negative with inhibition of intestinal flora by antimicrobial agents		Colon tumor Diverticulitis	
Myocardial infarction				Bacterial endocarditis	
Diabetes mellitus Hemochromatosis Hyperthyroidism Cushing's syndrome Pheochromocytomas	Diabetic ketosis Glycogen storage disease Preeclampsia Acute fever	Sickle cell anemia Hemolytic disease • Pernicious anemia Leptospirosis	Hemolytic disease Leptospirosis	Blood dyscrasias • Hemophilia • Thrombocytopenia • Sickle cell anemia Disseminated lupus erythematosus Malignant hypertension	Hemolytic disease Plasmodium (malaria) Clostridium (tetanus)
Sudden shock or pain Steroid therapy	Weight-reducing diet Ketogenic diet (e.g., in anticonvulsant therapy) Starvation			Hemorrhagenic drugs (e.g., anticoagulant, salicylate) Nephrotoxic agents Internal injury or foreign body Vitamin C or K deficiency	Overexertion Exposure to cold Incompatible blood transfusion Drug-induced hemolysis

technique. The quality control test should be performed when each bottle of strips is opened for the first time, or when a question of reliability arises regarding the testing strips.

Urine Analyzer

Urine analyzers are used to perform an automatic chemical examination of urine with reagent strips. They offer the advantage of the ability to perform the chemical analysis quickly and to interpret results automatically. These analyz-

ers are used most often in medical offices that perform moderate-volume to large-volume urine testing.

The Clinitek Analyzer (Bayer Corporation) is an example of a urine analyzer that automatically reads Multistix SG and other (Bayer) urinalysis reagent strips (Figure 16-7, *A*). The results are printed out, and abnormal results are flagged to call attention to them (Figure 16-7, *B*). Different models are available; some can be used to perform a color and appearance analysis and a microscopic examination of the urine.

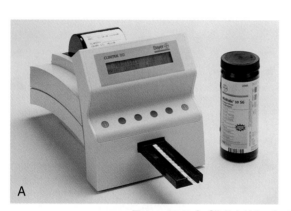

```
ID: __Erika Seager_____
          11-16-12    5:37 PM
CLARITY: __Clear_____
COLOR: YELLOW

MULTISTIX 10 SG

GLU     NEGATIVE
BIL     NEGATIVE
KET     NEGATIVE
SG      1.025
BLO*    TRACE-LYSED
pH      5.5
PRO     NEGATIVE
URO     0.2 E.U./dl
NIT     NEGATIVE
LEU     NEGATIVE
```

A   B

Figure 16-7. A, Clinitek Urine Analyzer. **B,** Clinitek printout.

---

see DVD   **PROCEDURE 16-3   Chemical Testing of Urine With the Multistix 10 SG Reagent Strip**

Outcome Perform a chemical assessment of a urine specimen.

Equipment/Supplies

- Disposable gloves
- Multistix 10 SG reagent strips
- Urine container

- Timer
- Laboratory report form

1. **Procedural Step.** Perform the quality control testing procedure if using a new bottle of testing strips.
   Principle. Performing the quality control procedure ensures the reliability of test results.
2. **Procedural Step.** Obtain a freshly voided urine specimen from the patient with a clean container. The specimen should be uncentrifuged and at room temperature.
   Principle. The best results are obtained with a freshly voided specimen. The container should be clean because contaminants could affect the results. Uncentrifuged specimens ensure a homogeneous sample.

3. **Procedural Step.** Sanitize your hands.
4. **Procedural Step.** Assemble the equipment. Check the expiration date of the reagent strips.
   Principle. Outdated reagent strips may lead to inaccurate test results.
5. **Procedural Step.** Apply gloves. Remove a reagent strip from its plastic container, and recap the container immediately. Do not touch the test areas with your fingers or lay the strip on the table. It is permissible, however, to lay the reagent strip on a clean, dry paper towel.

PROCEDURE 16-3 Chemical Testing of Urine With the Multistix 10 SG Reagent Strip—cont'd

Principle. Recapping the container is necessary to prevent exposing the strips to environmental moisture, light, and heat, which cause altered reagent reactivity. Contamination of test areas by the hands or table surface may affect the accuracy of test results.

6. Procedural Step. Thoroughly mix the urine specimen and remove the lid from the container. Using the dominant hand, completely immerse the reagent strip in the urine specimen, and remove it immediately. While removing, run the edge of the strip against the rim of the urine container to remove excess urine.

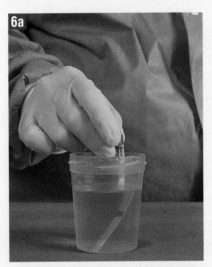

Completely immerse the reagent strip in the urine.

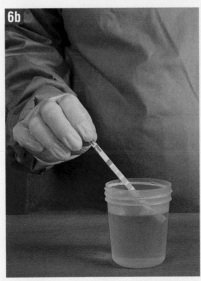

Run the edge of the strip against the urine container.

Principle. The strip should be completely immersed to ensure that all test areas are moistened for accurate test results. Prolonged immersion of the reagent strip and failure to remove excess urine may cause the reagents to dissolve and leach onto adjacent test areas, affecting the accuracy of the test results.

7. Procedural Step. With the nondominant hand, start the timer, pick up the reagent strip container, and rotate it to the color chart. Hold the reagent strip in a horizontal position and place it as close as possible to the corresponding color blocks on the color chart. Do not lay the strip directly on the color chart because this will result in soiling of the chart by the urine. Read the results carefully and at the exact reading times, starting with the shortest time specified on the color chart and as indicated here:

Glucose, 30 seconds   Bilirubin, 30 seconds
Ketone, 40 seconds   Specific gravity, 45 seconds
Blood, 60 seconds   pH, 60 seconds
Protein, 60 seconds   Urobilinogen, 60 seconds
Nitrite, 60 seconds   Leukocytes, 2 minutes

Principle. Holding the strip in a horizontal position avoids soiling your gloves with urine and prevents reagents from running over into adjacent testing areas, causing inaccurate test results. The strip must be read at the proper time interval to avoid dissolving out reagents, leading to inaccurate test results.

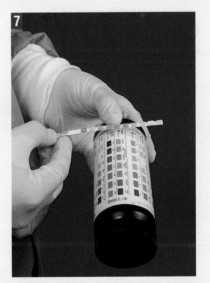

Hold the strip horizontally and read the results.

8. Procedural Step. Dispose of the strip in a regular waste container.

9. Procedural Step. Remove gloves, and sanitize your hands.

Continued

PROCEDURE 16-3

**PROCEDURE 16-3   Chemical Testing of Urine
With the Multistix 10 SG Reagent Strip—cont'd**

10. Procedural Step. Chart the results. Results should be charted by following the interpretation guide provided above each color block on the color chart. Most offices use a preprinted reporting form to make it easier to record results. The recording should include the date and time, the brand name of the test used (Multistix 10 SG), and the results.

10

Multistix® 10 SG

2161

COLOR CHART

Reagent Strips for Urinalysis
For In Vitro Diagnostic Use

READ PRODUCT INSERT BEFORE USE.
IMPORTANT: Do not expose to direct sunlight.
Do not use after 4/01.

Bayer

TESTS AND READING TIME

TEST	NEGATIVE						
LEUKOCYTES 2 minutes	NEGATIVE		TRACE	SMALL +	MODERATE ++	LARGE +++	
NITRITE 60 seconds	NEGATIVE		POSITIVE	POSITIVE	(Any degree of uniform pink color is positive)		
UROBILINOGEN 60 seconds	NORMAL 0.2	NORMAL 1	mg/dL 2	4	8	(1 mg ≈ approx. 1EU)	
PROTEIN 60 seconds	NEGATIVE	TRACE	mg/dL 30 +	100 ++	300 +++	2000 or more ++++	
pH 60 seconds	5.0	6.0	6.5	7.0	7.5	8.0	8.5
BLOOD 60 seconds	NEGATIVE	NON-HEMOLYZED TRACE	NON-HEMOLYZED MODERATE	HEMOLYZED TRACE	SMALL +	MODERATE ++	LARGE +++
SPECIFIC GRAVITY 45 seconds	1.000	1.005	1.010	1.015	1.020	1.025	1.030
KETONE 40 seconds	NEGATIVE	mg/dL	TRACE 5	SMALL 15	MODERATE 40	LARGE 80	LARGE 160
BILIRUBIN 30 seconds	NEGATIVE		SMALL +	MODERATE ++	LARGE +++		
GLUCOSE 30 seconds	NEGATIVE	g/dL (%) mg/dL	1/10 (tr.) 100	1/4 250	1/2 500	1 1000	2 or more 2000 or more

Do not use this chart for interpreting test results.
©1999 Bayer Corporation, Diagnostics Division, Tarrytown, NY 10591   Rev. 4/99   0401123

CHARTING EXAMPLE

Multistix *10 SG Reagent Strips for Urinalysis*

PATIENT   Annette Ross

DATE   3/22/12   TIME   9:45 a.m.

LEUKOCYTES	NEGATIVE ☑		TRACE ☐	SMALL + ☐	MODERATE ++ ☐	LARGE +++ ☐	
NITRITE	NEGATIVE ☑		POSITIVE ☐	POSITIVE ☐	(Any degree of uniform pink color is found)		
UROBILINOGEN	NORMAL 0.2 ☑	NORMAL 1 ☐	mg/dL 2 ☐	4 ☐	8 ☐	(1mg = approx. 1 BU)	
PROTEIN	NEGATIVE ☐	TRACE ☑	mg/dL 30 * ☐	100 ++ ☐	300 +++ ☐	2000 OR MORE ☐	
pH	5.0 ☑	6.0 ☐	6.5 ☐	7.0 ☐	7.5 ☐	8.0 ☐	8.5 ☐
BLOOD	NEGATIVE ☑	NON-HEMOLYZED TRACE ☐	NON-HEMOLYZED MODERATE ☐	HEMOLYZED TRACE ☐	SMALL + ☐	MODERATE ++ ☐	LARGE +++ ☐
SPECIFIC GRAVITY	1.000 ☐	1.006 ☐	1.010 ☐	1.015 ☑	1.020 ☐	1.025 ☐	1.030 ☐
KETONE	NEGATIVE ☑	mg/dL	TRACE 5 ☐	SMALL 15 ☐	MODERATE 40 ☐	LARGE 80 ☐	LARGE 160 ☐
BILIRUBIN	NEGATIVE ☑		SMALL + ☐	MODERATE ++ ☐	LARGE +++ ☐		
GLUCOSE	NEGATIVE ☑	g/L (%) mg/dL	1/10 tr. 100 ☐	1/6 250 ☐	1/2 500 ☐	1 1000 ☐	2 or more 2000 or more ☐

(Modified and printed by permission of Siemens Medical Solutions Diagnostics, Tarrytown, NY.)

PROCEDURE 16-3

Microscopic Examination of Urine

Urine sediment is the solid material contained in the urine. A microscopic examination of the urine sediment performed by the physician helps clarify results of the physical and chemical examinations. A first-voided morning specimen is generally preferred because it is more concentrated and contains more dissolved substances; small amounts of abnormal substances are more likely to be detected. Use of a fresh specimen is important because changes occur in a specimen left standing out, as was previously discussed. These changes affect the reliability of the test results. The medical assistant is responsible for preparing the urine specimen for microscopic examination by the physician, as presented in Procedure 16-4. Structures that may be found in a microscopic examination of urine are described next. Tables 16-3 to 16-6 provide an outline of these structures and of the possible causes of their presence.

Red Blood Cells

Red blood cells appear as round, colorless, biconcave discs that are highly refractile. The presence of 0 to 5 per high-power field (HPF) is considered normal. More than this

amount may indicate bleeding somewhere along the urinary tract. Table 16-3 lists the possible causes of an abnormal number of red blood cells in the urine. Concentrated urine causes the red blood cells to become shrunken or *crenated,* whereas dilute urine causes them to swell and become rounded, which may cause them to hemolyze. If the red blood cells have hemolyzed, they cannot be seen under the microscope. The presence of blood in the urine still can be identified, however, with a reagent strip, such as Multistix, which is designed to detect free hemoglobin.

Memories *from* **Externship**

Linda Proffitt: My main problem as a student on externship was that I was a little shy. I learned that when your patient is relaxed, he or she is more likely to give you additional and important information about what is wrong. If your patient tenses up during a procedure, this can cause pain for the patient and make the procedure more difficult. When I started to make myself talk more to the patients and staff, things went more smoothly. ∎

PATIENT TEACHING   Urinary Tract Infections

Answer questions patients may have about UTIs.

What is a UTI?

UTI is a general term for the presence of bacteria in any portion of the urinary tract. UTIs, particularly those involving the bladder (cystitis) and urethra (urethritis), are common and treatable. A UTI is usually treated with an antibiotic. Use of all of the antibiotic for the full number of days prescribed by the physician is important, even if the symptoms disappear. If the medication is stopped too soon, the infection may recur and may be more difficult to treat than the original infection.

What are the symptoms of a UTI?

The symptoms of a simple UTI (cystitis) commonly include the frequent need to urinate, urgency (meaning the immediate need to urinate), a burning sensation during urination, and sometimes blood in the urine. Symptoms of a more complicated UTI involving the kidneys (pyelonephritis) include the above symptoms as well as lower abdominal discomfort, low back pain, fever, cloudy or foul-smelling urine, and blood in the urine.

Why do women have UTIs more frequently than men?

Women are more prone than men to the type of UTI called *cystitis* because the urethra of a woman is much shorter than that of a man, which makes travel up the urethra and into the bladder easier for bacteria. The most common source of infection is bacteria *(Escherichia coli).* This organism is normally found in the large intestine but can travel from the anal area to the urinary bladder, often as the result of poor hygienic practices. Cystitis occurs if *E. coli* organisms

are able to overcome the body's natural defenses when the bacteria reach the urinary bladder and set up an infection.

What can women do to prevent a UTI?

Women prone to development of UTIs should practice the following prevention measures:

- Practice good hygienic measures by always cleaning the genital area from front to back after a bowel movement.
- Avoid possible irritants, such as bubble baths, perfumed soaps, feminine hygiene sprays, and the use of strong powders and bleaches for washing underclothes.
- Avoid clothing that traps moisture and encourages the growth of microorganisms, such as tight, constricting clothing; nylon panties; and panty hose.
- Avoid activities that can contribute to irritation of the urinary meatus, such as prolonged bicycling, motorcycling, horseback riding, and travel that involves prolonged sitting.
- Urinate as soon as possible when you feel the urge. Holding urine in the bladder gives the bacteria more time to grow, which can cause more infection. The more often you urinate, the more quickly the bacteria are removed from the bladder.
- Seek prompt treatment if you experience any of the symptoms of a UTI.
- Encourage the patient with a UTI to drink plenty of water to help flush the bacteria out of the urinary tract.
- Emphasize to the patient the importance of taking all of the antibiotic for the duration of time prescribed by the physician.
- Emphasize the importance of practicing preventive measures to prevent the occurrence of UTIs.
- Provide the patient with educational materials on UTIs.

Table 16-3 Cells in Urine Sediment

Type	Presence in Normal Urine	Possible Causes of Abnormal Numbers of Cells in Urine	Microscopic Appearance
Red blood cells	0-5 cells per high-power field (depending on preparation of urine sediment)	Inflammatory diseases Acute glomerulonephritis Pyelonephritis Hypertension Renal infarction Trauma Stones Tumor Bleeding diseases Use of anticoagulants	 Red blood cells
White blood cells	0-8 cells per high-power field (depending on preparation of urine sediment)	Pyelonephritis Cystitis Urethritis Prostatitis Transplant rejection (manifested by lymphocytes in urine) Tissue injury accompanied by severe inflammation (manifested by monocytes in urine) Inflammation, immune mechanisms, and other host defense mechanisms (manifested by histiocytes in urine)	 White blood cells
Squamous epithelial cells	Often present, depending on collection technique	Vaginal contamination	 Squamous epithelial cells
Transitional epithelial cells	Moderate number of cells present	Disease of the bladder or renal pelvis Catheterization	 Transitional epithelial cells
Renal tubular epithelial cells	Present in small numbers, higher numbers in infants	Acute tubular necrosis Glomerulonephritis Acute infection Renal toxicity Viral infection	 Renal tubular epithelial cells

Text courtesy Boehringer Mannheim Diagnostics, Indianapolis, Ind.
Photomicrographs courtesy Bayer Corporation, Elkhart, Ind.

Table 16-3 Cells in Urine Sediment—cont'd

Type	Presence in Normal Urine	Possible Causes of Abnormal Numbers of Cells in Urine	Microscopic Appearance
Cytomegalic inclusion bodies	Not normally present in urine	Cytomegalic inclusion disease	
Tumor cells	Not normally present in urine	Tumors of: Renal pelvis Renal parenchyma Ureters Bladder	

White Blood Cells

White blood cells are round and granular and have a nucleus. They are approximately 1.5 times as large as a red blood cell. The presence of 0 to 8 per HPF is considered normal. More than this amount may indicate inflammation of the genitourinary tract. Table 16-3 lists the possible causes of an abnormal number of white blood cells in the urine.

Epithelial Cells

Most structures that make up the urinary system are composed of several layers of epithelial cells. The outer layer is constantly sloughed off and replaced by the cells underneath it. *Squamous epithelial cells* are large, clear, flat cells with an irregular shape. They contain a small nucleus and come from the urethra, bladder, and vagina. Squamous epithelial cells are normally present in small amounts in the urine. *Renal epithelial cells* are round and contain a large nucleus. They come from the deeper layers of the urinary tract, and their presence in the urine is considered abnormal. Table 16-3 lists the types of epithelial cells and possible causes of the presence of abnormal amounts in the urine.

Casts

Casts are cylindrical structures formed in the lumen of the tubules that make up the nephron. Materials in the tubules harden, are flushed out, and appear in the urine in the form of casts. Various types of casts may be present in the urine. Their presence generally indicates a diseased condition.

Casts are named according to what they contain. *Hyaline casts* are pale, colorless cylinders with rounded edges that vary in size. *Granular casts* are hyaline casts that contain granules and are described as "coarsely granular" or "finely granular," depending on the size of the granules. *Fatty casts* are hyaline casts that contain fat droplets. *Waxy casts* are light yellow and have serrated edges; their name is derived from the fact that they appear to be made of wax. *Cellular casts* contain organized structures and are named according to what they contain. Examples include red blood cell casts, which are hyaline casts containing red blood cells; white blood cell casts, which are hyaline casts containing white blood cells; epithelial casts, which are hyaline casts containing epithelial cells; and bacterial casts, which are hyaline casts containing bacteria. Table 16-4 lists the types of casts and possible causes of their presence in urine.

Crystals

A variety of crystals may be found in the urine. The type and number vary with the pH of the urine. Abnormal crystals include leucine, tyrosine, cystine, and cholesterol. Crystals that commonly appear in acid urine include amorphous urates, uric acid, and calcium oxalate. Crystals that commonly appear in alkaline urine include amorphous phosphate, triple phosphate, calcium phosphate, and ammonium urate crystals. Table 16-5 lists the types of urine crystals and their significance when found in urine.

Miscellaneous Structures

Mucous threads are normally present in small amounts in the urine. They appear as long, wavy, threadlike structures with pointed ends.

Bacteria should not normally exist in the urinary tract. The presence of more than a few bacteria may indicate either contamination of the specimen during collection or a UTI. Bacteria are small structures that may be rod-shaped or round.

Yeast cells are smooth, refractile bodies with an oval shape. A distinguishing feature of yeast cells is small buds that project from the cells involved with reproduction. Yeast cells in the urine of female patients are usually a vaginal contaminant caused by the yeast *Candida albicans* and produce the vaginal infection known as *candidiasis*. They also may be present in the urine of patients with diabetes mellitus.

Parasites may be present in the urine sediment as a contaminant from fecal or vaginal material. *Trichomonas vaginalis* is a parasite that causes trichomoniasis vaginitis.

Spermatozoa may be present in the urine of a man or woman after intercourse. The spermatozoa have round heads and long, slender, hairlike tails.

Table 16-6 lists the miscellaneous structures that may be present in the urine and the significance when found.

Table 16-4 Casts in Urine Sediment

Type	Description	Possible Causes	Microscopic Appearance
Hyaline casts	Colorless, transparent Low refractive index	Normal urine Strenuous exercise Acute glomerulonephritis Acute pyelonephritis Malignant hypertension Chronic renal disease	 Hyaline cast
Red blood cell casts	Red blood cells in hyaline matrix Yellow-orange color High refractive index	Acute glomerulonephritis Lupus nephritis Severe nephritis Collagen diseases Renal infarction Malignant hypertension	 Red blood cell cast
White blood cell casts	Neutrophils in hyaline matrix High refractive index	Acute pyelonephritis Acute glomerulonephritis Chronic renal disease	 White blood cell cast
Epithelial cell casts	Renal tubular epithelial cells in hyaline matrix High refractive index	Glomerulonephritis Vascular disease Toxin Virus	 Epithelial cell cast
Granular casts	Opaque granules in matrix	Heavy proteinuria (nephrotic syndrome) Orthostatic proteinuria Congestive heart failure with proteinuria Acute or chronic renal disease	 Granular cast

Text courtesy Boehringer Mannheim Diagnostics, Indianapolis, Ind.
*Photomicrographs from Stepp CA, Woods M: Laboratory procedures for medical office personnel, Philadelphia, 1998, Saunders.
†Photomicrographs courtesy Bayer Corporation, Diagnostics Division, Elkhart, Ind.
‡Photomicrographs from Henry JB: Clinical diagnosis and management by laboratory methods, ed 21, Philadelphia, 2006, Saunders.

Table 16-4 Casts in Urine Sediment—cont'd

Type	Description	Possible Causes	Microscopic Appearance
Waxy casts	Sharp, refractile outlines Irregular "broken-off" ends Absence of differentiated structures	Severe chronic renal disease Malignant hypertension Kidney disease resulting from diabetes mellitus Acute renal disease	* Waxy cast
Fatty casts	Fat globules in transparent matrix	Nephrotic syndrome Diabetes mellitus Mercury poisoning Ethylene glycol poisoning	‡ Fatty cast
Broad casts	Larger diameter than other casts	Acute tubular necrosis Severe chronic renal disease Urinary tract obstruction	† Broad cast
Mixed casts	Combination of any of the above	Any of the above, depending on cellular constituents	† Mixed cast

Table 16-5 **Urine Crystals**

Type of Urine	Type of Crystals	Description of Crystals	Significance When Found in Urine	Microscopic Appearance
Normal acid urine	Amorphous urate	Colorless or yellow-brown granules (pink macroscopically)	Nonpathologic	Amorphous urate crystals
	Uric acid	May be colorless, yellow-brown, or red-brown; may be square, diamond-shaped, wedge-shaped, or grouped in rosettes	Usually nonpathologic; in large numbers, may indicate gout	Uric acid crystals
	Calcium oxalate	Octahedral or dumbbell-shaped; possess double refractive index	Usually nonpathologic; may be associated with stone formation	Calcium oxalate crystals
Normal alkaline urine	Amorphous phosphates	Small, colorless granules	Nonpathologic	Amorphous phosphate crystals
	Triple phosphates	Colorless prisms with three to six sides ("coffin lids") or feathery, shaped like fern leaves	Usually nonpathologic; may be associated with urine stasis or chronic urinary tract infection	Triple phosphate crystals

Text courtesy Boehringer Mannheim Diagnostics, Indianapolis, Ind.
*Photomicrographs courtesy Bayer Corporation, Diagnostics Division, Elkhart, Ind.
†Photomicrographs from Stepp CA, Wood M: Laboratory procedures for medical office personnel, Philadelphia, 1998, Saunders.
‡Photomicrographs from Henry JB: Clinical diagnosis and management by laboratory methods, ed 21, Philadelphia, 2006, Saunders.

Table 16-5 Urine Crystals—cont'd

Type of Urine	Type of Crystals	Description of Crystals	Significance When Found in Urine	Microscopic Appearance
	Ammonium biurate	Yellow-brown "thorny apple" appearance or yellow-brown spheres	Nonpathologic	* Ammonium biurate crystals
	Calcium phosphate	Colorless prisms or rosettes	Usually nonpathologic; may be associated with urine stasis or chronic urinary tract infection	‡ Calcium phosphate crystals
	Calcium carbonate	Usually appear colorless and amorphous; may be shaped like dumbbells, rhombi, or needles	Usually nonpathologic; may be associated with inorganic calculi formation	§ Calcium carbonate crystals
Abnormal urine	Tyrosine	Thin, dark needles, arranged in sheaves or clumps; usually colorless, but may be pale yellow-brown	Liver disease or inherited metabolic disorder	* Tyrosine crystals
	Leucine	Yellow-brown spheres with radial striations	Liver disease or inherited metabolic disorder	* Leucine crystals

§Photomicrograph from Brunzel NA: Fundamentals of urine and body fluid analysis, ed 2, St Louis, 2004, Saunders.   *Continued*

Table 16-5 Urine Crystals—cont'd

Type of Urine	Type of Crystals	Description of Crystals	Significance When Found in Urine	Microscopic Appearance
	Cystine	Clear, hexagonal plates	Cystinuria	* Cystine crystals
	Hippuric acid	Star-shaped clusters of needles, rhombic plates, or elongated prisms; may be colorless or yellow-brown	Usually nonpathologic	¶ Hippuric acid crystals
	Bilirubin	Delicate needles or rhombic plates; red-brown in color; birefringent	Bilirubinuria	* Bilirubin crystals
	Cholesterol	Colorless, transparent plates with regular or irregular corner notches	Chyluria, urinary tract infections, nephritic syndrome	† Cholesterol crystals
	Creatine	Pseudohexagonal plates with positive birefringence	Destruction of muscle tissue owing due to muscular dystrophies, atrophies, and myositis	
	Aspirin	Distinctive prismatic or starlike forms; usually colorless, show positive birefringence	Ingestion of aspirin or other salicylates	

¶Photomicrograph from Lehmann CA: Saunders manual of clinical laboratory science, Philadelphia, 1998, Saunders.

Table 16-5 Urine Crystals—cont'd

Type of Urine	Type of Crystals	Description of Crystals	Significance When Found in Urine	Microscopic Appearance
	Sulfonamide	Yellow-brown dumbbells, asymmetric sheaves, rosettes, or hexagonal plates	Ingestion of sulfonamide drugs	Sulfonamide crystals
	Ampicillin	Long, thin, clear crystals	Parenteral administration of ampicillin	Ampicillin crystals
	X-ray media	Long, thin rectangles or flat, four-sided, notched plates	X-ray procedure with contrast media	X-ray media crystals

Table 16-6 Microorganisms and Artifacts in the Urine

Microorganisms/Artifacts	Significance When Found in the Urine	Microscopic Appearance
Bacteria	More than 100,000 bacteria per ml indicates urinary tract infection. 10,000–100,000 bacteria per ml indicates that tests should be repeated. Less than 10,000 bacteria per ml may signify urine in which any bacteria are due to urethral organisms or contamination. Bacteria accompanied by white blood cells or white blood cell or mixed casts may indicate acute pyelonephritis.	Bacteria (small rod structures)
Yeast	May indicate contamination by yeasts from skin or hair May indicate diabetes mellitus or urinary tract infection *Candida albicans* may occur in patients with diabetes mellitus or in the contaminated urine of female patients with candidal vaginitis.	*Candida albicans* (yeast)

Text courtesy Boehringer Mannheim Diagnostics, Indianapolis, Ind.
*Photomicrographs courtesy Bayer Corporation, Diagnostics Division, Elkhart, Ind.

Continued

Table 16-6 Microorganisms and Artifacts in the Urine—cont'd

Microorganisms/Artifacts	Significance When Found in the Urine	Microscopic Appearance
Parasites and parasitic ova	Usually indicate fecal or vaginal contamination and should be reported *Trichomonas* may be found in patients with urethritis and in contaminated urine of women with *Trichomonas* vaginitis. Pinworm is a common contaminant and should be reported.	 *Trichomonas* (parasite)
Spermatozoa	Nonpathologic	 Spermatozoa

Urinary artifacts
  Hair (a)
  Pollen grains
  Bubbles
  Oil droplets
  Fibers (b)
  Powder (c)
  Dust
  Mucous threads (d)
  Glass particles
	Nonpathologic
	May result from improper urine collection, improper slide preparation, or outside contamination
		(a)
		
		Hair
		(b)
		
		Fiber
		(c)
		
		Powder
		(d)
		
		Mucous threads

†Photomicrograph from Lehman CA: Saunders manual of clinical laboratory science, Philadelphia, 1998, Saunders.
‡Photomicrograph from Stepp CA, Woods M: Laboratory procedures for medical office personnel, Philadelphia, 1998, Saunders.

PROCEDURE 16-4   Prepare a Urine Specimen for Microscopic Examination: Kova Method

Outcome Prepare a urine specimen for microscopic analysis by the physician.

Equipment/Supplies

- Disposable gloves
- Urine specimen (first-voided morning specimen)
- Kova urine centrifuge tube
- Kova cap
- Kova pipet

- Kova slide
- Kova stain
- Test tube rack
- Urine centrifuge
- Mechanical stage microscope

Preparing the Specimen

1. Procedural Step. Sanitize the hands, and assemble the equipment.

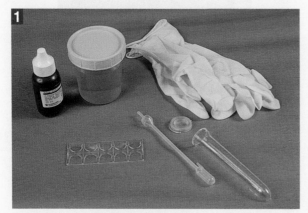

Assemble the equipment.

2. Procedural Step. Apply gloves. Mix the urine specimen with the Kova pipet.
Principle. The specimen must be well mixed to ensure accurate test results.

3. Procedural Step. Pour the urine specimen into the urine centrifuge tube. Fill it to the 12-ml graduation mark, and cap the tube.

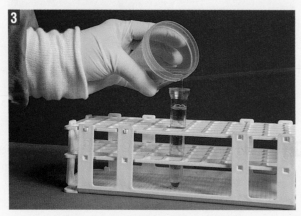

Pour the specimen into the urine tube.

4. Procedural Step. Centrifuge the tube for 5 minutes at approximately 1500 revolutions per minute (rpm).
Principle. Centrifuging the specimen causes the solid elements in the urine to settle to the bottom of the tube.

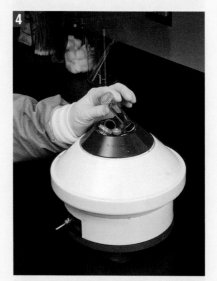

Centrifuge the specimen.

5. Procedural Step. Remove the urine tube from the centrifuge; do not disturb or dislodge the sediment.

6. Procedural Step. Remove the cap. Insert the Kova pipet into the urine tube, and push it to the bottom of the tube until it seats firmly. Ensure that the clip on the bulb is hooked over the outside edge of the tube.

7. Procedural Step. Decant the specimen by inverting the tube and pouring off the **supernatant** fluid. Approximately 1 ml of sediment is retained in the bottom of the tube.

8. Procedural Step. Remove the pipet from the tube. Add 1 drop of Kova stain to the tube. Place the pipet back in the tube, and mix the sediment and stain together vigorously with the pipet. Ensure that the sediment and the stain are well mixed. Place the urine tube in a test tube rack.

Continued

PROCEDURE 16-4   Prepare a Urine Specimen for Microscopic Examination: Kova Method—cont'd

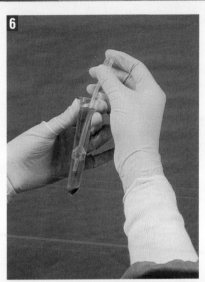

Insert the pipet until it seats firmly.

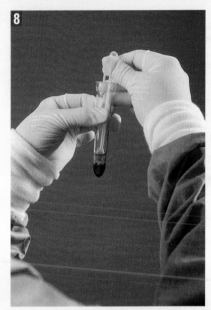

Mix the sediment and stain.

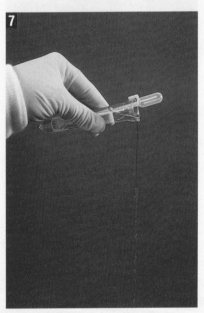

Pour the supernatant fluid.

d. Gently squeeze the bulb to allow the specimen to fill the well. Do not overfill or underfill the well.

e. Place the pipet in the urine tube.

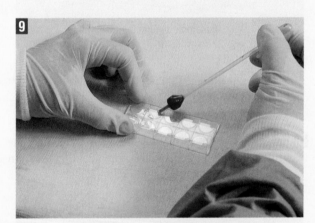

Fill the well with the specimen.

Principle. Kova stain improves the detail of the sediment for better visualization of structures under the microscope.

9. Procedural Step. Transfer a sample of the sediment to the Kova slide as follows:

a. Place the Kova slide on a flat surface with the open "envelope" areas facing upward.

b. Squeeze the bulb of the pipet to draw a sample of the sediment into the tip of the pipet.

c. Place the tip of the pipet so that it just touches the notched corner edge of the slide.

10. Procedural Step. Allow the specimen to sit for 1 minute to permit the sediment to settle in the well.

Principle. Allowing the sediment to settle prevents structures from moving when the slide is viewed under the microscope.

11. Procedural Step. Place the slide on the stage of the microscope. Focus the specimen for the physician under the microscope by following the procedure presented in Procedure 20-1: *Using the Microscope.*

PROCEDURE 16-4   Prepare a Urine Specimen for Microscopic Examination: Kova Method—cont'd

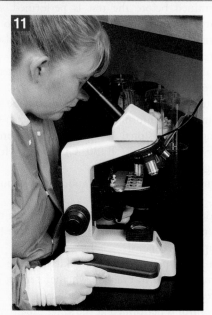

Examine the specimen.

12. Procedural Step. When the physician is finished examining the urine sediment, remove the slide from the stage.

13. Procedural Step. Dispose of the plastic slide and pipet in a regular waste container. Rinse the remaining urine down the sink. Cap the empty plastic urine tube, and dispose of it in a regular waste container.

14. Procedural Step. Remove gloves, and sanitize your hands.

LAB REPORT

Date	Time	Name
3/18/12	10:00 a.m.	Tanya Howe

MICROSCOPIC	
WBCs	20/HPF
RBCs	3/HPF
CASTS (Hyaline)	0/LPF
CASTS (Granular)	0/LPF
CASTS (Cellular)	0/LPF
CASTS (Waxy)	0/LPF
EPITHELIAL CELLS	0/LPF
BACTERIA	Freq
MUCUS	Occ
CRYSTALS	0

_____ T. Bach, MD

RAPID URINE CULTURES

A urine culture is used to assist in diagnosis of a UTI and the assessment of the effectiveness of antibiotic therapy for a patient with a UTI. Rapid urine culture tests are sometimes used in the medical office to culture a urine specimen; brand names include Uricult and Urichek. They provide more immediate results compared with sending the specimen to an outside laboratory for culture. Rapid urine cultures consist of a slide attached to a screw cap. Each side of the slide is coated with an agar medium suitable for the growth of urinary bacteria. If the surface of the agar medium is dehydrated, or if evidence of mold or bacterial growth is present, the culture test should not be used but should be discarded in an appropriate receptacle. The slide is suspended in a clean plastic vial, which protects it from contamination during inoculation, storage, or handling.

The type of urine specimen that provides the most accurate results is a clean-catch midstream specimen collected after the urine has been in the bladder at least 4 to 6 hours. The procedure for performing a rapid urine culture test is presented in Procedure 16-5.

URINE PREGNANCY TESTING

The diagnosis of pregnancy can be accomplished several ways. By the eighth week after fertilization, pregnancy can be confirmed with the medical history and physical examination. The physician may desire an earlier diagnosis, however, with a pregnancy test to initiate early prenatal care. A pregnancy test also may be necessary before certain medications are ordered or procedures are performed that may cause injury to a fetus.

In the medical office, immunologic tests are often used for pregnancy testing. These tests are performed on a concentrated urine specimen and rely on the presence of a hormone known as *human chorionic gonadotropin* (HCG) for a positive reaction.

Human Chorionic Gonadotropin

HCG is produced by the developing fertilized egg, and small amounts of it are secreted into the urine and blood. Immediately after conception and implantation of the fertilized egg, the plasma level of HCG increases rapidly and can be used to detect pregnancy with a serum pregnancy test as early as 6 days before the first missed menstrual period. The highest plasma levels of HCG occur at about 8 weeks after conception. After this time, the production of HCG declines and remains at a lower level for the duration of the pregnancy. Within 72 hours of delivery, HCG disappears entirely from the plasma. As a result, pregnancy tests are more sensitive during the first trimester and may show a negative reaction when the level of HCG begins to decline during the second and third trimesters.

Immunoassay Tests

Immunoassay tests are used in the medical office for the detection of pregnancy. These tests are convenient to perform and provide immediate test results. Positive and negative reactions are evidenced by a specific visible reaction that is observed and interpreted by the individual performing the test.

Immunoassay tests are commercially available in testing kits that contain the required reagents and supplies to perform the test. Each kit can be used to perform a specific number of tests, ranging from 25 to 50. The instructions in the product insert accompanying the testing kit should be followed exactly to prevent inaccurate test results. When performed correctly, most urine pregnancy tests are 99% accurate with low occurrences of false-positive test results.

Immunoassay tests provide for the rapid, qualitative detection of HCG in a urine specimen; brand names include QuickVue One-Step (Quidel, San Diego, Calif), OSOM (Genzyme Diagnostics, Cambridge, MA), and Clearview (Inverness Medical, Princeton, NJ). Early prediction pregnancy tests may be able to detect pregnancy as early as 2 to 3 days before a first missed menstrual period. Urine pregnancy tests performed this early, however, may show a false-negative result and should be repeated later to confirm the results. Accurate results are much more probable if the urine is tested 1 week after a missed period.

Immunoassay tests take approximately 5 minutes to perform, and the test results are easily observed as a color change. Specific instructions for interpreting the test results are included in the product insert. The procedure for performing an immunoassay test with QuickVue (Quidel) is outlined in Procedure 16-6.

Guidelines for Urine Pregnancy Testing

Specific guidelines must be followed in a urine pregnancy test to ensure accurate test results:

1. Use clean, preferably disposable, urine containers to collect the specimen. Traces of detergent in the specimen container may cause inaccurate test results.
2. The preferred specimen for a urine pregnancy test is a first-voided morning specimen because it contains the highest concentration of HCG; however, a random urine specimen can also be used. If the urine specimen cannot be tested immediately after voiding, it should be preserved in the refrigerator. A patient who collects the specimen at home should be given instructions on preserving the specimen.
3. The specific gravity of the urine specimen should be determined before the test is performed. A specific gravity of less than 1.007 is considered too dilute for pregnancy testing because it may lead to a false-negative test result.
4. The urine specimen should be at room temperature before the procedure is performed.
5. The urine pregnancy testing kit should be stored according to the information in the product insert. Most testing kits are stored at a room temperature between 59° F (15° C) and 86° F (30° C) and away from direct sunlight.
6. Testing kits past their expiration dates should not be used.
7. If more than one patient is being tested at a time, label each testing device with the patient's name to prevent mixup of specimens.
8. Most urine pregnancy testing kits include a built-in internal control to evaluate whether certain aspects of the testing procedure are working properly. The internal control is performed at the same time that the testing procedure is performed. The urine pregnancy internal control determines whether a sufficient amount of the specimen was added to the testing cassette, and if the correct procedural technique was followed. If the internal control does not perform as expected, the test result is invalid and the specimen must be retested. It is recommended that the internal control be documented in a quality control log for the first pregnancy test run each day.

What Would You Do? What Would You Not Do?

Case Study 3

Rita Lavelle is 8½ months pregnant and is at the clinic for a prenatal appointment. Lately, she has been having difficulty obtaining a urine specimen at the medical office because of her enlarged abdomen. At her last appointment, the office provided her with a urine specimen container so that she could obtain her specimen more easily at home. Rita brings in a first-voided urine specimen in a glass jar. She says her dog chewed up the specimen container from the office, so she used an empty peanut butter jar. The urine testing results from her specimen show that her glucose level is normal, but her protein level is 4+. Until this time, her urine test results all have been normal. Rita is concerned about her baby. She says that she was cleaning her bathroom cabinet yesterday and came across a pregnancy test; just for the fun of it, she decided to run the test. The results were negative, and now she is worried that something is wrong. Rita says that she has not been sleeping as well at night, and that she has noticed more Braxton-Hicks contractions, but the baby has been kicking and moving as usual. ∎

QUALITY CONTROL LOG

URINE PREGNANCY TEST

	Date	Name of test	Control lot #	Control expiration date	External positive control	External negative control	Technician
1	3/25 2012	Quick Vue One Step HCG	140400	3/16/13	+	−	L. Proffit CMA (AAMA)
2	4/22 2012	Quick Vue One Step HCG	140400	3/16/13	+	−	L. Proffit CMA (AAMA)
3	5/27 2012	Quick Vue One Step HCG	140400	3/16/13	+	−	L. Proffit CMA (AAMA)
4							
5							
6							
7							
8							
9							
10							

Figure 16-8. Quality control log for urine pregnancy testing.

9. It is recommended that a positive and a negative external control be performed with each new lot of shipment of urine pregnancy testing kits, and then monthly thereafter. External controls are used to determine if the testing reagents are performing properly and to detect any errors in technique of the individual performing the test. External controls consist of commercially available solutions and may be included with the test system or may need to be purchased separately. The control procedure is performed in a similar manner to the procedure for performing the test on a specimen collected from a patient. Instead of adding the patient specimen to the testing device, however, the control is added to it. The positive control should produce a positive result, and the negative control should produce a negative result. The results should be documented in a quality control log (Figure 16-8). Failure of an external control to produce expected results may be due to the following: deterioration of testing components due to improper storage, improper environmental testing conditions, or errors in technique used to perform the procedure.

10. Conditions other than a normal pregnancy that can result in a positive result include ectopic pregnancy and molar pregnancy.

SERUM PREGNANCY TEST

The radioimmunoassay (RIA) for HCG is a quantitative test used to detect HCG in the serum of the blood. This test can detect pregnancy earlier and with greater accuracy than a urine pregnancy test. A serum pregnancy test can usually detect pregnancy at approximately the eighth day after fertilization, which is 6 days before the first missed menstrual period. This test uses a radioisotope technique and is capable of detecting minute amounts of HCG in the blood. This test is generally used to diagnose abnormalities, such as ectopic pregnancy; to follow the course of early pregnancy when abnormalities of embryonic development are suspected; and to provide an early diagnosis of pregnancy in individuals at high risk, such as patients with diabetes.

PROCEDURE 16-5 Performing a Rapid Urine Culture Test

Outcome Perform a rapid urine culture test.

Equipment/Supplies

- Disposable gloves
- Rapid urine culture kit
- Urine specimen (clean-catch midstream specimen)
- Incubator
- Biohazard waste container

Preparing the Specimen

1. Procedural Step. Sanitize your hands, and assemble the equipment. Check the expiration date on the rapid culture test. It should not be used if the expiration date has passed. Label the vial with the patient's name and date of birth and the date and time of inoculation.
Principle. An expired urine culture test may produce inaccurate test results.

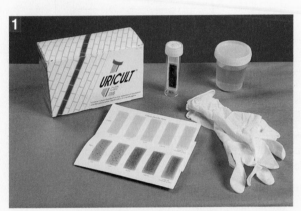

Assemble the equipment.

2. Procedural Step. Apply gloves. Remove the slide from its protective vial by unscrewing the cap of the vial; do not touch the culture media.

3. Procedural Step. Dip the agar-coated slide into the urine specimen; it must be completely immersed. If the urine volume is not sufficient to immerse the agar slide fully, the urine may be poured over the agar surfaces.

4. Procedural Step. Allow excess urine to drain from the slide.

5. Procedural Step. Immediately replace the inoculated slide in its protective vial. Screw the cap on loosely.

6. Procedural Step. Place the vial upright in an incubator for 18 to 24 hours at 93° F to 100° F (35° C to 38° C).
Principle. Incubation for longer than 24 hours may cause erroneous test results.

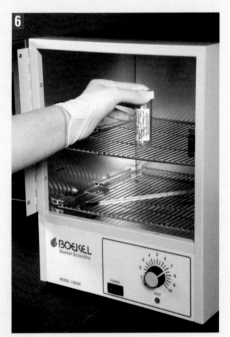

Incubate the specimen.

Reading Test Results

7. Procedural Step. Apply gloves. Remove the vial from the incubator after the incubation period. Remove the slide from its protective vial, and compare the bacterial colony count density on the agar surface with the colony density reference chart provided by the manufacturer. The bacterial colony density on the agar surface should be matched with the printed example it most closely resembles on the colony density chart. (No actual bacterial colony counting is necessary.)

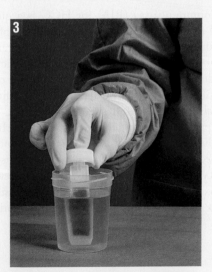

Dip the slide into the urine specimen.

PROCEDURE 16-5   Performing a Rapid Urine Culture Test—cont'd

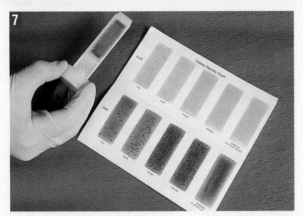

Compare the slide with the reference chart.

8. Procedural Step. Interpret results. The results of rapid urine tests are interpreted as follows:

Normal: Less than 10,000 bacteria/ml of urine. *Significance:* A normal result indicates the absence of infection.

Borderline: 10,000 to 100,000 bacteria/ml of urine. *Significance:* A borderline result may be caused by chronic and relapsing infections, and it is recommended that the test be repeated.

Positive:

a. More than 100,000 bacteria/ml of urine.

b. Confluent growth, or complete coverage of the agar surface with bacterial colonies, which may occur occasionally when a colony count is more than 100,000 bacteria/ml.

Significance: A positive result indicates that a bacterial infection is present.

9. Procedural Step. Return the slide to the vial, and screw on the cap. (*Note:* To aid in the safe disposal of inoculated slides, it is recommended that the slide be immersed in a disinfectant solution, such as 3% phenol solution or Cidex, before the slide is placed in the vial.)

10. Procedural Step. Dispose of the rapid culture test in a biohazard waste container. Remove the gloves, and sanitize the hands.

11. Procedural Step. Chart the results. Include the date and time, the name of the test (e.g., Uricult), and the results.

CHARTING EXAMPLE	
Date	
3/21/12	10:00 a.m. Uricult: Normal. ———————— ———————————— L. Proffitt, CMA (AAMA)

PROCEDURE 16-6

---

see DVD

PROCEDURE 16-6   Performing a Urine Pregnancy Test

Outcome Perform a urine pregnancy test.

Equipment/Supplies

- Disposable gloves
- Urine pregnancy testing kit (QuickVue by Quidel)
- Urine specimen (first-voided morning specimen)

1. Procedural Step. Sanitize the hands, and assemble the equipment. Check the expiration date on the urine pregnancy testing kit. It should not be used if the expiration date has passed. When a new testing kit is opened (and thereafter on a monthly basis), external positive and negative controls should be performed according to the instructions in the product insert accompanying the controls. Document the control results in a quality control log. If the controls do not perform as expected, patient testing should not be conducted until the problem is identified and resolved.

Principle. An expired pregnancy test may produce inaccurate test results. Running positive and negative

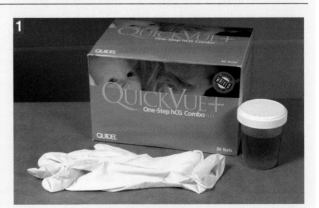

Assemble the equipment.

external controls ensures that the test results are valid and reliable. Factors that can cause abnormal control results include outdated controls or testing reagents, improper storage of testing components, and an error in the technique used to perform the procedure.

2. **Procedural Step.** Apply gloves. Rotate the urine specimen cup to mix the urine. Inspect the foil pouch containing the cassette. If it is torn or punctured, discard the test and obtain another one from the testing kit. Remove the test cassette from its foil pouch, and place it on a clean, dry, level surface.

   Principle. The foil pouch should not be opened until it is time to perform the test.

3. **Procedural Step.** Add 3 drops of urine to the round sample well on the test cassette with a disposable pipet supplied with the kit. The test cassette should not be handled or moved again until the test is ready for interpretation. Dispose of the pipet in a regular waste container.

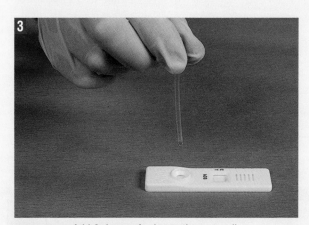

Add 3 drops of urine to the test well.

4. **Procedural Step.** Wait 3 minutes, and read the results by observing the test result window.

5. **Procedural Step.** Interpret the test results as follows:

   Negative: The appearance of the blue procedural control line next to the letter "C" only and no pink to purple test line next to the letter "T" in the test result window. In addition, the background of the test window should be clear and not interfere with the ability to read the test results. (*Note:* If the test result is negative and pregnancy is suspected, another specimen should be collected and tested 48 to 72 hours later.)

   Positive: The appearance of any pink to purple line next to the letter "T" along with a blue procedural control line next to the letter "C" in the test result window. In addition, the background of the test window should be clear and should not interfere with the ability to read test results.

   Invalid result: If no blue procedural control line appears within 3 minutes, or if the background of the test window interferes with reading the results, the test result is invalid, and the specimen must be retested with a new cassette.

   Principle. The blue procedural control line is a positive internal quality control indicator designating that a sufficient urine sample was added to the cassette well and that the test is working properly. A background in the test window that is clear and does not interfere with reading the test results is a negative internal quality control indicator and also indicates that the test is working properly.

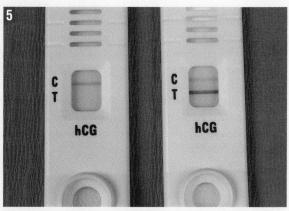

Negative　　　　　Positive

Interpret the results.

6. **Procedural Step.** Dispose of the test cassette in a regular waste container. Remove gloves, and sanitize your hands.

7. **Procedural Step.** Chart the results. Include the date and time of the patient's last menstrual period (LMP), the name of the test, and the results recorded as either positive or negative.

CHARTING EXAMPLE

Date	
3/25/12	10:30 a.m. LMP: 2/20/12.
	QuickVue preg test: Positive.
	L. Proffitt, CMA (AAMA)

evolve *Check out the Evolve site to access additional interactive activities.*

MEDICAL PRACTICE *and the* LAW

In collection and analysis of patient urine, meticulous attention should be paid to patient instructions, such as cleansing and collecting first morning, midstream, or 24-hour specimens. Patients are often embarrassed to have someone else see their urine, so handle urine specimens in a professional, matter-of-fact manner, with universal precautions to protect yourself. As with all diagnostic procedures, care must be taken to perform the test correctly and treat results confidentially.

Civil versus Criminal Law

Civil law involves a conflict with another person, and if found guilty by a preponderance of evidence (greater than 50%), the loser may lose money or property. Malpractice is a type of civil law. Civil law is divided into *torts,* or wrongs, and *contracts,* or promises. Malpractice is a tort, and nonpayment for services is a contract.

Criminal law involves a conflict with society as a whole (local, state, or federal law). If found guilty beyond a reasonable doubt, the loser may lose money, property, freedom (jail), or life (execution). Violation by the physician of licensure laws and failure to report child abuse are criminal suits. ■

What Would You Do? What Would You Not Do? RESPONSES

Case Study 1
Page 630

What Did Linda Do?
❏ Took some time to try to calm and relax Mr. Urameshi. Reassured him that the physician would do everything he could to make him better.
❏ Offered Mr. Urameshi something to drink and told him it might help him obtain a specimen.
❏ Went over the directions again with Mr. Urameshi.
❏ Asked Mr. Urameshi if he would try again to obtain a specimen.

What Did Linda Not Do?
❏ Did not tell Mr. Urameshi that he was not trying hard enough.

What Would You Do?/What Would You *Not* Do? Review Linda's response and place a checkmark next to the information you included in your response. List additional information you included in your response.

_____
_____
_____
_____

Case Study 2
Page 637

What Did Linda Do?
❏ Asked Nora whether she takes all of the antibiotic she is prescribed when she has a UTI.
❏ Explained to Nora in terms she can understand why women seem to be more prone to development of UTIs.
❏ Explained to Nora what she could do to help prevent UTIs. Gave her a patient education brochure on UTIs to take home.

❏ Told Nora that the physician is not legally or ethically permitted to call in a prescription for her without seeing her. Also explained that it is in the best interests of her health care to be seen by the physician.

What Did Linda Not Do?
❏ Did not tell Nora that she could not test her urine at home.

What Would You Do?/What Would You *Not* Do? Review Linda's response and place a checkmark next to the information you included in your response. List additional information you included in your response.

_____
_____
_____

Case Study 3
Page 660

What Did Linda Do?
❏ Told Rita that some peanut butter residue might have been left in the jar she used and might have affected the test results. Asked her to try to collect another specimen at the office so that the urine could be tested again.
❏ Told Rita that if something happens to the specimen container again, she should come to the office and get another one.
❏ Told Rita that several things could have caused her pregnancy test result to be negative. Explained to her that the test could have been outdated or not stored properly. Also explained that as a pregnancy gets further along, less of the hormone that causes the test to be positive is secreted, so negative test results at the end of a pregnancy are not unusual.

❑ Reassured Rita that many women have trouble sleeping during the last month of pregnancy, and that it is normal to have more Braxton-Hicks contractions as she gets closer to delivery.

❑ Told Rita that Linda would inform the physician of her symptoms so that he could discuss them in greater detail with her.

What Did Linda Not *Do?*

❑ Did not criticize Rita for collecting her specimen in a peanut butter jar.

❑ Did not ignore or minimize Rita's concerns.

What Would You Do?/What Would You *Not* Do? Review Linda's response and place a checkmark next to the information you included in your response. List additional information you included in your response.

_____

_____

_____

_____

CERTIFICATION REVIEW

❑ **The function of the urinary system** is to regulate the fluid and electrolyte balance of the body and to remove waste products. The urinary system comprises the kidneys, the ureters, the urinary bladder, and the urethra.

❑ **The nephron** is considered the functional unit of the kidney. Each kidney is composed of approximately 1 million nephrons. The nephron filters waste substances from the blood and dilutes them with water to produce urine. Another function of the nephron is reabsorption.

❑ **Urine is composed of** 95% water and 5% organic and inorganic waste products. The normal adult excretes approximately 750 to 2000 ml of urine per day.

❑ **An excessive increase in urine output** is known as *polyuria* and may be caused by excessive intake of fluids, certain drugs, diabetes mellitus, and renal disease. Decreased output of urine is known as oliguria and may be caused by decreased fluid intake, dehydration, profuse perspiration, vomiting, diarrhea, or kidney disease.

❑ **The type of test to be performed** often dictates the method used to collect the urine specimen. A first-voided morning specimen contains the greatest concentration of dissolved substances and is recommended for microscopic examination of urine. A clean-catch midstream specimen is recommended for the detection of a UTI. A 24-hour specimen is used to measure quantitatively specific substances in the urine.

❑ **A complete urinalysis** consists of physical, chemical, and microscopic examinations of urine. Deviation from normal in any of the three areas assists the physician in the diagnosis and treatment of pathologic conditions. A urine specimen should not be left standing out for longer than 1 hour because changes take place that affect the test results.

❑ **Physical examination of urine** involves determination of the color, appearance, and specific gravity of the urine. Dilute urine tends to be lighter yellow in color, whereas concentrated urine is a darker yellow. Fresh urine is usually clear and transparent.

❑ **The specific gravity of urine** ranges from 1.003 to 1.030 but is usually between 1.010 and 1.025. Dilute urine contains fewer dissolved substances and has a lower specific gravity; concentrated urine has a higher specific gravity from the increased amount of dissolved substances.

❑ **Chemical testing of urine** is a means of detecting abnormal amounts of chemicals in the body, which may indicate a pathologic condition. Chemical tests include pH, glucose, protein, ketone, blood, bilirubin, urobilinogen, nitrite, and leukocytes.

❑ **Microscopic examination** of the urine sediment helps clarify results of the physical and chemical examination. Structures that may be found in microscopic examination of urine include red and white blood cells, epithelial cells, casts, crystals, and miscellaneous structures, such as mucous threads, bacteria, yeast cells, parasites, and spermatozoa.

❑ **A urine culture** is used to assist in diagnosis of a UTI and to assess the effectiveness of antibiotic therapy for a patient with a UTI.

❑ **Human chorionic gonadotropin (HCG)** is produced by the developing fertilized egg, and small amounts of it are secreted into the urine and blood. Urine pregnancy tests are used to detect the presence of HCG and can be used to detect pregnancy as early as 2 to 3 days after the first missed menstrual period.

↻ TERMINOLOGY REVIEW

Medical Term	Word Parts	Definition
Anuria	*an-:* without, absence of *ur/o-:* urine *-ia:* condition of disease or abnormal state	Failure of the kidneys to produce urine.
Bilirubinuria	*bilirubino/o:* bilirubin *ur/o-:* urine *-ia:* condition of disease or abnormal state	The presence of bilirubin in the urine.
Bladder catheterization		The passing of a sterile catheter through the urethra and into the bladder to remove urine.
Diuresis		Secretion and passage of large amounts of urine.
Dysuria	*dys-:* difficult, labored, painful *ur/o-:* urine *-ia:* condition of disease or abnormal state	Difficult or painful urination.
Frequency		The condition of having to urinate often.
Glycosuria	*glyc/o-:* sugar *ur/o-:* urine *-ia:* condition of disease or abnormal state	The presence of glucose in the urine.
Hematuria	*hemat/o-:* blood *ur/o-:* urine *-ia:* condition of disease or abnormal state	Blood present in the urine.
Ketonuria	*keton/o-:* ketone *ur/o-:* urine *-ia:* condition of disease or abnormal state	The presence of ketone bodies in the urine.
Ketosis	*keton/o-:* ketone *-osis:* abnormal condition	An accumulation of large amounts of ketone bodies in the tissues and body fluids.
Micturition		The act of voiding urine.
Nephron		The functional unit of the kidney.
Nocturia	*noct/i-:* night *ur/o-:* urine *-ia:* condition of disease or abnormal state	Excessive (voluntary) urination during the night.
Nocturnal enuresis		Inability of an individual to control urination at night during sleep (bedwetting).
Oliguria	*olig/o-:* scanty, few *ur/o-:* urine *-ia:* condition of disease or abnormal state	Decreased or scanty output of urine.
pH		The unit that describes the acidity or alkalinity of a solution.
Polyuria	*poly-:* many *ur/o-:* urine *-ia:* condition of disease or abnormal state	Increased output of urine.
Proteinuria	*protein-:* protein *ur/o-:* urine *-ia:* condition of disease or abnormal state	The presence of protein in the urine.

Continued

TERMINOLOGY REVIEW—cont'd

Medical Term	Word Parts	Definition
Pyuria	*py/o-:* pus *ur/o-:* urine *-ia:* condition of disease or abnormal state	The presence of pus in the urine.
Renal threshold		The concentration at which a substance in the blood that is not normally excreted by the kidneys begins to appear in the urine.
Retention		The inability to empty the bladder. The urine is being produced normally but is not being voided.
Specific gravity		The weight of a substance compared with the weight of an equal volume of a substance known as the standard. In urinalysis, the *specific gravity* refers to the measurement of the amount of dissolved substances present in the urine compared with the same amount of distilled water.
Supernatant	*super:* over, above	The clear liquid that remains at the top after a precipitate settles.
Suprapubic aspiration	*supra-:* above *pub/o-:* pubis *-ic:* pertaining to	The passing of a sterile needle through the abdominal wall into the bladder to remove urine.
Urgency		The immediate need to urinate.
Urinalysis	*urin/o-:* urine	The physical, chemical, and microscopic analyses of urine.
Urinary incontinence		The inability to retain urine.
Void		To empty the bladder.

ON THE WEB

For Information on Kidney Disease:

National Kidney Foundation: www.kidney.org

National Institute of Diabetes and Digestive and Kidney Diseases: www.niddk.nih.gov

For Information on Drug Abuse:

National Institute on Drug Abuse: www.nida.nih.gov

American Council for Drug Education: www.acde.org

Research Institute on Addictions: www.ria.buffalo.edu

Alcohol and Drug Free Workplace: www.dol.gov/workingpartners

Alcohol and Drug Abuse: www.alcoholanddrugabuse.com

DARE: www.dare.com

Dependency Free: www.dependencyfree.com

17

Phlebotomy

LEARNING OBJECTIVES

Venipuncture

1. List and describe the general guidelines that should be followed when performing a venipuncture.
2. Explain how each of the following blood specimens is obtained:
   - Clotted blood
   - Serum
   - Whole blood
   - Plasma
3. List the layers the blood separates into when an anticoagulant is added to the specimen.
4. List the layers the blood separates into when an anticoagulant is not added to the specimen.
5. List the OSHA safety precautions that must be followed during venipuncture and when separating serum or plasma from whole blood.
6. State the additive content of each of the following vacuum tubes, and list the types of blood specimens that can be obtained from each: red, lavender, gray, light blue, green, royal blue.
7. Identify and explain the order of draw for the vacuum tube and butterfly methods of venipuncture.
8. List and describe the guidelines for use of evacuated tubes.
9. Identify possible problems during a venipuncture.
10. List four ways to prevent a blood specimen from becoming hemolyzed.
11. Explain how the serum separator tube functions in the collection of a serum specimen.

Skin Puncture

1. Explain when a skin puncture would be preferred over a venipuncture.
2. Describe each of the following skin puncture devices: disposable semiautomatic lancet and reusable semiautomatic lancet.
3. List and describe the guidelines for performing a finger puncture.

PROCEDURES

Perform a venipuncture using the vacuum tube method.
Perform a venipuncture using the butterfly method.
Perform a venipuncture using the syringe method.
Separate serum from a blood specimen.

Obtain a capillary blood specimen using a disposable semiautomatic lancet.
Obtain a capillary blood specimen using a reusable semiautomatic lancet.

CHAPTER OUTLINE

Introduction to Phlebotomy
Venipuncture
General Guidelines for Venipuncture
  Patient Preparation for Venipuncture
  Review Collection and Handling Requirements
  Identification of the Patient
  Assemble the Equipment and Supplies

Reassuring the Patient
Patient Position for Venipuncture
Application of the Tourniquet
Site Selection for Venipuncture
Alternative Venipuncture Sites
Types of Blood Specimens
OSHA Safety Precautions

KEY TERMS

antecubital space (an-tih-KYOO-bih-tul SPAYS)
anticoagulant (an-tih-koe-AG-yoo-lent)
buffy coat
evacuated tube
hematoma (hee-mah-TOE-mah)
hemoconcentration (hee-moe-kon-sen-TRAY-shun)
hemolysis (hee-MOL-ih-sis)
osteochondritis (OS-tee-oh-kon-DRY-tis)

osteomyelitis (OS-tee-oh-mie-LIE-tis)
phlebotomist (fleh-BOT-oe-mist)
phlebotomy (fleh-BOT-oe-mee)
plasma
serum
venipuncture (VEN-ih-punk-chur)
venous reflux (VEEN-us-REE-fluks)
venous stasis (VEEN-us-STAE-sis)

Introduction to Phlebotomy

The purpose of phlebotomy is to collect a blood specimen for laboratory analysis. The word *phlebotomy* is derived from the Greek words for "vein" *(phlebos)* and "incision" *(otomy)* and literally means making an incision into a vein. As used in the clinical laboratory sciences, **phlebotomy** is defined generally as the collection of blood. An individual who collects a blood sample is a **phlebotomist.**

Some blood specimens are tested in the medical office, and others are picked up and taken to an outside laboratory for testing. The latter specimens need to placed in a biohazard specimen bag along with a laboratory request (Figure 17-1), so that laboratory personnel know what type of test the physician desires. The medical assistant may be responsible for completing the laboratory request form either on the computer or manually. The request form includes the physician's name and address; the patient's name, address, age, and gender; the date and time of collection of the specimen; the International Classification of Diseases (ICD)-9 code of the clinical diagnosis; and a mark next to the type of test or tests to be performed.

Phlebotomy encompasses three major areas of blood collection:
- Arterial puncture
- Venipuncture
- Skin puncture

An arterial puncture is typically performed in a hospital to assess the oxygen level, carbon dioxide level, and acid-base balance of arterial blood; medical assistants do not perform arterial punctures. In the medical office, medical assistants perform venipunctures and skin punctures. This chapter focuses on these two ways to obtain blood.

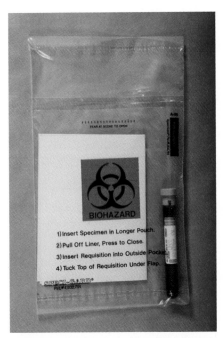

Figure 17-1. Specimen in a biohazard specimen bag along with the laboratory request form.

VENIPUNCTURE

Venipuncture means the puncturing of a vein for the removal of a venous blood sample. In the medical office, a venipuncture is performed when a large blood specimen is needed for testing. Venipuncture can be performed by the following three methods:

- Vacuum tube method
- Butterfly method
- Syringe method

The vacuum tube method is the fastest and most convenient of the three methods and is used most often. This method relies on the use of an **evacuated tube,** which is a closed glass or plastic tube that contains a vacuum. The butterfly and syringe methods are used for difficult draws, such as when a vein is small or sclerosed (hardened). This chapter presents the theory and procedure for each method.

GENERAL GUIDELINES FOR VENIPUNCTURE

General guidelines that are common to all three methods of venipuncture include any advance preparation, reviewing specimen collection and handling requirements, identification of the patient, reassuring the patient, assembling equipment and supplies, positioning the patient, applying the tourniquet, selecting a site for the venipuncture, obtaining the type of blood specimen required, and following the Occupational Safety and Health Administration (OSHA) Bloodborne Pathogens Standard.

Patient Preparation for Venipuncture

The patient should be given instructions an appropriate number of days before the specimen collection on any advance preparation that is required. Although most tests require no preparation, some tests require fasting or the avoidance of certain medications. *Fasting* involves abstaining from food or fluids (except water) for a specified amount of time before the collection of a specimen. If the medical assistant is unsure whether a laboratory test requires advance patient preparation, an appropriate reference source should be consulted. If the specimen is being tested at an outside laboratory, references consist of a laboratory directory and the laboratory's technical support staff. If the specimen is being tested at the medical office, references include the manufacturer's operating manual and/or product inserts included with blood analyzers and testing kits.

When a laboratory test requires advance preparation, before performing the venipuncture, verify that the patient has prepared properly. If the patient has not properly prepared, do not collect the specimen unless directed otherwise by the physician. If the venipuncture is to be rescheduled, carefully review the preparation requirements with the patient.

Review Collection and Handling Requirements

The medical assistant must review the requirements for collecting and handling the blood specimen. These include the collection supplies necessary, the type of specimen to be collected (e.g., **serum, plasma,** whole blood, clotted blood), the amount necessary for laboratory analysis, the techniques to follow to collect the specimen, and the proper handling and storage of the specimen. The medical assistant must refer to the appropriate reference source to determine the collection and handling requirements for each test ordered by the physician. If the specimen is transported to an outside laboratory, this information is indicated in the laboratory directory. Figure 17-2 shows an example of the collection and handling requirements for a complete blood count (CBC) as it is presented in a laboratory directory. The collection and handling requirements necessary for specimens tested in the medical office are listed in the manufacturer's instructions that accompany the test system.

Identification of the Patient

It cannot be emphasized enough how important it is to identify the patient using two forms of identification (e.g., name and date of birth) before performing a venipuncture. Proper patient identification is essential to avoid collecting a specimen on the wrong patient by mistake. After greeting the patient, the medical assistant should ask the patient to state his or her full name and date of birth. This information should be compared with the demographic data indicated in the patient's chart. The patient should *not* be asked whether he or she is a certain patient. For example, the patient should not be asked: "Are you Brad Thompson?" The patient may not hear the medical assistant correctly or may not be paying

---

CBC (with differential and platelet count)

CPT Code: 85025

Tests included: WBC, RBC, hemoglobin, hematocrit, platelet count, differential, and red blood cell indices (MCV, MCH, MCHC, and RDW). If abnormal cells are observed on a manual differential or if the automated differential results meet specific flagging criteria, a full manual differential will be performed.

Type of specimen: Whole blood

Amount: 7 ml

Collection supplies: 7-ml lavender (EDTA) stoppered tube

Collection techniques: Red-stoppered and SST tubes should be collected before the lavender-stoppered tube. Completely fill tube to the exhaustion of the vacuum to ensure a proper blood to anticoagulant ratio. Gently invert tube 8-10 times immediately after drawing to mix the anticoagulant with the blood.

Patient preparation: None

Handling and storage: Store at room temperature for up to 24 hours following collection. Store in refrigerator for up to 48 hours following collection.

Causes for rejection: Hemolyzed or clotted specimen, under-filled tube, improper labeling of tube. Specimen collected in any tube other than an EDTA (lavender-stoppered) tube or a specimen that is more than 48 hours old.

Reference range: Values given with report

Use:
The CBC is used as a screening test to assess the overall health of an individual and to detect a wide range of hematologic conditions such as anemia, leukemia, and inflammatory processes. The CBC is also used to assist in managing medication and chemotherapeutic decisions.

Limitations:
- A manual differential can identify cells that may be misidentified by an automated analyzer
- Red blood cell indices are not a substitute for the direct examination of a blood smear

Methodology: Automated cell counter and microscopy

Figure 17-2. Collection and handling requirements for a complete blood count (CBC) from a laboratory directory.

---

attention and may answer in the affirmative even if he is not that patient. If the patient is not properly identified, this, in turn, could lead to incorrect labeling of the specimen. A specimen that is not identified correctly could lead to an inaccurate patient diagnosis and the wrong treatment.

Assemble the Equipment and Supplies

Use only the appropriate blood tubes as specified by the laboratory directory or manufacturer's instructions accompanying a test system. Substituting blood tubes may not yield the proper type of specimen required or may affect the test results, as shown by the following examples. If serum is required and a tube containing an anticoagulant is used (instead of a tube without an anticoagulant), the blood separates into plasma and cells, rather than serum and cells, and the wrong type of blood specimen is obtained, which necessitates obtaining another specimen from the patient.

The medical assistant should check each blood tube before use to ensure that it is not broken, chipped, cracked, or otherwise damaged. Damaged blood tubes are unsuitable for specimen collection and should be discarded. Blood tubes have an expiration date (Figure 17-3). The medical assistant should make sure to check the expiration date on the tube to avoid using an outdated blood tube.

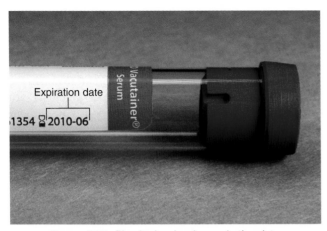

Figure 17-3. Blood tube showing expiration date.

The medical assistant must be sure to label each blood tube. An unlabeled specimen is a cause for rejection of the specimen by an outside laboratory. Two *unique identifiers* should be used to label the specimen. A unique identifier is information that clearly identifies a specific patient, such as the patient's name and date of birth. A specimen can be labeled by attaching a computerized bar code label to the specimen (Figure 17-4, *A*). The bar code label includes (at least) two unique patient identifiers. A specimen can also be labeled by hand writing the information on the label, which should include the patient's name and date of birth (two unique identifiers), the date and time of collection, the medical assistant's initials, and any other information required by the laboratory (Figure 17-4, *B*). The information should be printed legibly, and the medical assistant should be certain that the information is accurate to avoid a mixup of specimens. The medical assistant must also complete a laboratory request form to accompany the blood specimen. (*Note:* The medical assistant should follow the medical office policy as to when the tubes should be labeled. Some offices prefer the tubes be labeled *before* the specimen is drawn; other offices want the tubes to be labeled right *after* the specimen is obtained.)

Reassuring the Patient

Venipuncture is often a frightening experience for the patient. For many patients, the anticipation of the procedure is worse than the actual drawing of the blood. The medical assistant should take time to explain the procedure to the patient in an unhurried and confident manner. This helps to alleviate the patient's fears, which relaxes the patient's veins. Relaxed veins make venipuncture easier to perform and result in less pain for the patient.

Instruct the patient to remain still during the procedure. Explain to the patient that a small amount of pain is associated with a venipuncture, but it is brief. Never tell the patient that the venipuncture will not hurt. Just before inserting the needle, tell the patient that he or she will "feel a small stick." This prevents startling the patient, which could cause the patient to move. Movement causes pain for the patient, and it may damage the venipuncture site.

Patient Position for Venipuncture

The patient position for venipuncture is especially important to the successful collection of a blood specimen. Proper positioning allows easy access to the vein and is more comfortable for the patient. The patient position depends on the vein to be used. The most common site for venipuncture is the **antecubital space,** and the information presented next refers to this site.

The patient should be seated comfortably in a chair. The arm should be extended downward to form a straight line from the shoulder to the wrist with the palm facing up; the arm should not bend at the elbow. The arm should be well supported on the armrest by a rolled towel or by having the patient place the fist of the other hand under the elbow (Figure 17-5).

A venipuncture should never be performed with the patient sitting on a stool or standing. The patient may faint and injure himself or herself. If the patient appears nervous or has fainted in the past from a venipuncture, it is best to place the patient in a semireclining position (semi-Fowler's position) on the examining table. A pillow or a cushion

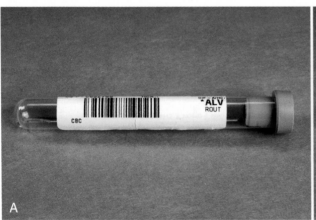

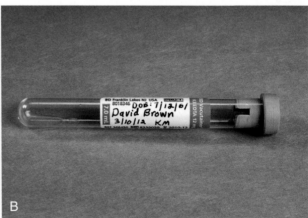

Figure 17-4. **A,** Computerized bar code label. **B,** Hand-labeled blood tube.

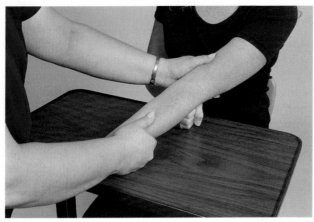

Figure 17-5. Patient position for obtaining a blood specimen from the antecubital veins.

should be placed under the patient's arm to support the arm in a straight line from the shoulder to the wrist.

Although unusual, it is possible for blood to flow from the evacuated tube back into the patient's vein during the procedure. This condition is known as **venous reflux**. Venous reflux could cause the patient to have an adverse reaction to a tube additive, particularly if the additive in the tube is ethylenediaminetetraacetic acid (EDTA). Venous reflux can occur only if the contents of the evacuated tube are in contact with the tube stopper while the specimen is being drawn. Venous reflux is prevented by keeping the patient's arm in a downward position so that the evacuated tube remains below the venipuncture site and fills from the bottom up.

Application of the Tourniquet

An important step in the venipuncture procedure is the application of the tourniquet. The tourniquet makes the patient's veins stand out so that they are easier to palpate. The tourniquet acts as a "dam," which causes the venous blood to slow down and pool in the veins in front of the tourniquet. This pooling of blood makes the veins more prominent so that they are more visible and can be palpated.

When applying a tourniquet, it is important to obtain the correct tourniquet tension. The tourniquet should be applied with enough tension to slow the venous flow without affecting the arterial flow. A tourniquet that is too tight obstructs both venous blood flow and arterial flow, which may result in a specimen that produces inaccurate test results. A tourniquet that is too loose fails to cause the veins to stand out enough to be palpated. A correctly applied tourniquet should fit snugly and not pinch the patient's skin.

Guidelines for Applying the Tourniquet

The following guidelines help to ensure successful application of the tourniquet:

1. Do not apply the tourniquet over sores or burned skin.
2. Place the tourniquet 3 to 4 inches above the bend in the elbow. This allows adequate room for cleansing the site and performing the venipuncture without the tourniquet getting in the way.
3. Apply the tourniquet so that it is snug, but not so tight that it pinches the patient's skin or is otherwise painful to the patient.
4. When applying the tourniquet, ask the patient to clench his or her fist. This pushes blood from the lower arm into the veins and makes them easier to palpate. You can ask the patient to clench and unclench the fist a few times; however, vigorous pumping should be avoided because it could lead to hemoconcentration, which could produce inaccurate test results.
5. Never leave the tourniquet on for longer than 1 minute because this would be uncomfortable for the patient. In addition, prolonged application of the tourniquet causes the venous blood to stagnate, or pool in one place too

---

Putting It All into Practice

My Name is Dori Glover, and I work in a very busy, fast-paced family practice office for two physicians. I love my job. The physicians are great, with very different styles; the pace is fast; and the time flies by. I am constantly challenged, learning new things, meeting and helping people, and being a part of a team that works well together.

While performing a venipuncture for a routine blood chemistry profile (a procedure I have performed many times), I accidentally stuck myself. I could see the blood inside my glove, and I could see the patient's blood clinging to the point of the needle—my heart sank. I placed the needle and holder in the sharps container and tried to keep my cool and not alarm the patient. I mentally assessed the patient. He was an older man from a rural community, but I know you cannot always judge a book by its cover.

I excused myself and immediately proceeded to wash my hands thoroughly with soap and water and rinse, rinse, rinse! I then notified the physician. The physician questioned the patient regarding

operations he had had in the previous year. He had undergone bypass surgery and had received 2 units of blood. Although blood is effectively screened, I thought about that one-in-a-zillion chance that it could have been contaminated. Thankfully, I had received the hepatitis B immunization series, but there was still concern regarding hepatitis C and, of course, HIV.

The patient was gracious and complied with our request to be tested for hepatitis and HIV. The physician and I discussed the situation, and we determined the risk to be low, but he nonetheless offered me the option of getting the HIV postexposure prophylactic treatment. This treatment is very toxic and is not something you want to receive needlessly. I declined and proceeded to wait in agony for the patient's test results. The word **_relief_** hardly describes how I felt when the patient's laboratory results came back negative!

This incident confirmed the importance of getting the hepatitis B immunization and paying attention to good technique when performing procedures involving blood. ∎

long—a condition known as **venous stasis.** When venous stasis occurs, the plasma portion of the blood filters into the tissues, causing hemoconcentration. **Hemoconcentration** is an increase in the concentration of nonfilterable blood components in the blood vessels, such as red blood cells, enzymes, iron, and calcium, as a result of a decrease in the fluid content of the blood. This can result in inaccurate results for a variety of laboratory tests.

6. Ideally, you should remove the tourniquet as soon as a good blood flow is established; however, this may not be practical when you are first learning the venipuncture procedure. Removing the tourniquet may cause the needle to move such that no more blood can be obtained, and the blood has to be redrawn. When you are learning the venipuncture procedure, it is better to wait until just before the needle is removed to remove the tourniquet.

7. *Always* remove the tourniquet before removing the needle from the patient's arm. If the needle is removed first, the pressure of the tourniquet causes blood to be forced out of the puncture site and into the surrounding tissue, resulting in a hematoma. A **hematoma** is defined as a swelling or mass of coagulated blood caused by a break in a blood vessel.

8. After use, wipe a tourniquet thoroughly with a disinfectant such as alcohol. Disposable tourniquets are available that are thrown away after one use.

Types of Tourniquets

The most common tourniquets are the *rubber* tourniquet and the *Velcro-closure* tourniquet. The type of tourniquet used is a matter of individual preference.

Rubber Tourniquet

The rubber tourniquet consists of a flat, soft band of rubber approximately 1 inch (2.5 cm) wide and 15 to 18 inches (38 to 45 cm) long. Rubber tourniquets are commercially available in latex or non-latex rubber. They offer the advantage of being easily removable with one hand. The technique for applying a rubber tourniquet is described next and is illustrated in Figure 17-6.

Procedure: Rubber Tourniquet

1. Hold each end of the tourniquet with one hand. Position the tourniquet 3 to 4 inches (7.5 to 10 cm) above the bend in the elbow, making sure that the tourniquet lies flat against the patient's skin. Pull the ends away from each other to create tension (see Figure 17-6, *A*).

2. Bring the ends of the tourniquet toward each other and cross one over the other at the point of your grasp, with enough tension so that the tourniquet is snug but is not pinching the patient's skin (see Figure 17-6, *B*).

3. Tuck a portion of the top length into the bottom length, forming a loop between the tourniquet and the patient's arm. This allows for a one-handed release of the tourniquet when pulled on one end. Make sure the flaps are directed upward so that they do not dangle into the working area (see Figure 17-6, *C*).

Velcro-Closure Tourniquet

The Velcro-closure tourniquet consists of a band of rubber or elastic material with Velcro attached at the ends. This type of tourniquet is easier to apply and is more comfortable for the patient than the rubber tourniquet. The disadvantage of the Velcro-closure tourniquet is that it is more

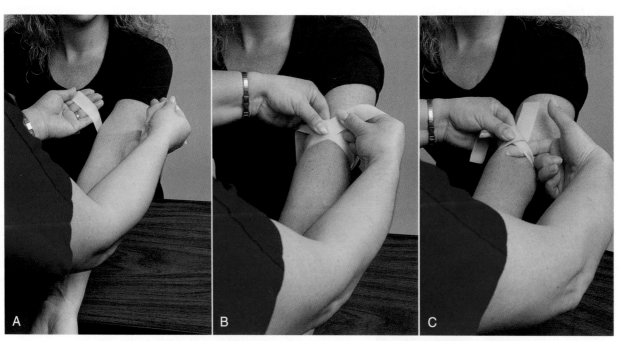

Figure 17-6. Application of a rubber tourniquet. **A,** Create tension by pulling the ends of the tourniquet away from each other. **B,** With tension, cross one flap over the other at the point of your grasp. **C,** Form a loop by tucking a portion of the top length into the bottom length.

difficult to remove with one hand than the rubber tourniquet. In addition, this type of tourniquet may not fit around the arms of extremely obese patients. The technique for applying a Velcro-closure tourniquet is described next and is illustrated in Figure 17-7.

Procedure: Velcro-Closure Tourniquet

1. Hold each end of the tourniquet with one hand. Position the tourniquet 3 to 4 inches (7.5 to 10 cm) above the bend in the elbow.
2. Wrap the tourniquet around the arm, and secure it with the Velcro fastener. The tourniquet should be applied with enough tension so that it is snug but is not pinching the patient's skin.

Site Selection for Venipuncture

For most patients, the best site to use is the veins in the antecubital space (Figure 17-8). If the patient has large, visible antecubital veins, drawing blood is easy. If the patient has small veins or veins that cannot be palpated, obtaining a blood specimen can be quite a challenge, even for the most experienced medical assistant.

The antecubital space is the surface of the arm in front of the elbow. The antecubital veins generally have a wide lumen and are close to the surface of the skin, which makes them easily accessible. In addition, these veins typically have thick walls, making them less likely to collapse. Using the antecubital space spares the patient unnecessary pain because the skin is less sensitive there than at other sites, such as the back of the hand. The medical assistant should not be misled by the presence in some patients of many small, very blue "spidery" veins that lie close to the surface of the skin. These veins are not suitable for performing a venipuncture. The antecubital veins lie beneath these veins.

The best vein to use in the antecubital space is the *median cubital.* The median cubital is a prominent vein in the

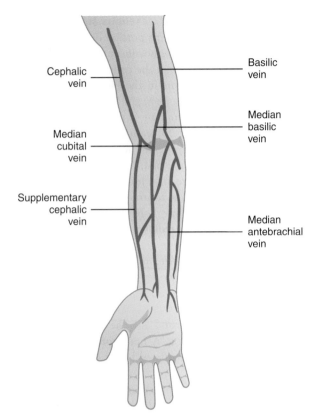

Figure 17-8. Antecubital veins.

middle of the antecubital space and does not roll (see Figure 17-8). At times, however, the median cubital vein cannot be used, for example, when it lies deep in the tissues and cannot be palpated or is scarred from repeated venipunctures.

The *cephalic* and *basilic* veins are located on opposite sides of the antecubital space and provide an alternative site when the median cubital vein is unavailable. The cephalic vein is located on the thumb side of the antecubital space, and the basilic vein is located on the little finger side of the antecubital space. The disadvantage of these "side" veins is that they tend to roll or move away from the needle, escaping puncture. To prevent rolling, firm pressure should be applied below and to the side of the vein to stabilize it as the needle is inserted.

The brachial artery also is located in the antecubital space, but it lies deeper in the tissues. This is the artery that is used to measure blood pressure. Before performing a venipuncture, palpate for the presence of this artery. In contrast to a vein, an artery pulsates, is more elastic, and has a thicker wall than a vein. If the brachial artery is inadvertently punctured, the patient feels more than the usual amount of pain, and the blood is bright red and comes out in pulsing movements. If this situation occurs, the tourniquet should be removed and then the needle. Pressure with a gauze pad should be applied for 4 to 5 minutes.

Guidelines for Site Selection

Specific guidelines should be followed to facilitate the selection of a good vein:

1. Ensure that the lighting is adequate. Good lighting facilitates inspection of the veins.

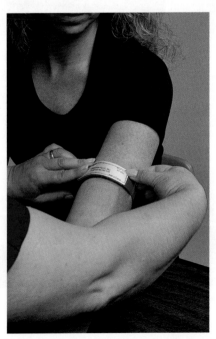

Figure 17-7. Application of a Velcro-closure tourniquet.

2. Ensure that the veins "stand out" as much as possible. Before locating a venipuncture site, always apply the tourniquet, and have the patient make a fist. This combination makes the veins more prominent.

3. Examine the antecubital veins of both arms. The best site to perform a venipuncture varies with each individual. The patient may have larger veins in one arm than in the other. It is advisable to ask the patient whether he or she has had a venipuncture before. Most adults have had previous venipunctures and know which of their veins are best to use and which should be avoided. Listen to and evaluate information offered by the patient.

4. Use inspection and particularly palpation to select a vein. A vein does not have to be seen to be a good selection. If you cannot see a vein, palpation alone can be used to locate it. A vein feels like an elastic tube that "gives" under the pressure of the fingertips.

5. Always palpate for the median cubital vein (middle vein) first. It usually is bigger, is anchored better, bruises less, and poses the smallest risk of injuring underlying structures (e.g., nerves and arteries) than the other veins. Because of this, if the patient's median cubital vein cannot be seen but still can be palpated, it should be used as the first choice when selecting a vein. If the median cubital vein is good in both arms, select the one that appears the fullest. The cephalic vein located on the thumb side is the next best vein choice because it does not roll and bruise as easily as the basilic vein. The basilic vein, located on the little finger side of the antecubital space, is the least desirable venipuncture site in the antecubital space. Branches of the median nerve may lie close to this vein in some individuals. In addition, the basilic vein lies in close proximity to the brachial artery. Both of these conditions pose a risk of injury to underlying structures when blood is drawn from the basilic vein.

6. Thoroughly assess the patient's veins. To assess a vein as a possible site for venipuncture, place one or two fingertips (index and middle fingers) over it and press lightly, then release pressure. Do not use your thumb to palpate the vein because it is not as sensitive as the index finger. To be suitable for a venipuncture, the vein should feel round, firm, elastic, and engorged. When you depress and release an engorged vein, it should spring back in a rounded, filled state.

7. Determine the size, depth, and direction of the vein. When a suitable vein has been located, it should be palpated thoroughly and carefully to determine the direction of the vein and to estimate the size and depth of the vein. Palpate and trace the path of the vein several times by rolling your index finger back and forth over the vein to determine its size. Inspect and palpate the vein for problems. Some veins that appear suitable at first sight feel small, hard, bumpy, or flat when palpated.

8. Map the location of the site. After locating an acceptable vein, mentally "map" the location of the puncture site on the patient's arm with "skin marks." This technique is particularly helpful if the vein cannot be seen, but only palpated. The puncture site may be located on or next to a skin mark, such as a freckle, a small wrinkle, or a pigmented area.

9. Do not leave the tourniquet on for longer than 1 minute. When first learning the venipuncture procedure, you may need to perform numerous assessments of the patient's arms to locate the best vein. After each assessment, remove the tourniquet for approximately 2 minutes to allow normal circulation of the blood to occur. This prevents patient discomfort and hemoconcentration, which can lead to inaccurate results for a variety of laboratory tests.

10. If a good vein cannot be found, the following techniques can be employed to make the veins more prominent:
   • Remove the tourniquet, and have the patient dangle the arm over the side of the chair for 1 to 2 minutes.
   • Tap the vein site sharply a few times with your index finger and second finger.
   • Gently massage the arm from the wrist to the elbow.
   • Apply a warm, moist washcloth to the area for 5 minutes.

Alternative Venipuncture Sites

If it is impossible to locate a suitable vein in the antecubital space, alternative sites are available, including the inner forearm, the wrist area above the thumb, and the back of the hand (Figure 17-9). These alternative veins are smaller and have thinner walls than the antecubital veins and should be used for venipuncture only when all possibilities for obtaining the blood specimen at the antecubital site have been considered. If the medical assistant is able to palpate a small vein in the antecubital space, it may be possible to obtain blood there using the butterfly method of venipuncture.

The hand veins, in particular, should be used only as a last resort. The veins of the hand have a tendency to roll because they are not supported by much tissue and are close to the surface of the skin. This makes them more difficult to stick. In addition, an abundant supply of nerves is present in the hands, which makes this procedure more uncomfortable for the patient. Hand veins tend to have thin walls, which makes them more susceptible to collapsing, bruising, and phlebitis. In some patients, however, especially the obese and the elderly, the hand veins may be the only accessible site.

Types of Blood Specimens

The type of blood specimen required depends on the type of test to be performed. Serum is required for most blood chemistry studies, whereas whole blood is required for a complete blood count. The various types of blood specimens that the medical assistant would be required to obtain through the venipuncture procedure are as follows:

1. *Clotted blood.* Clotted blood is obtained from a tube that does not contain an anticoagulant. A tube without an anticoagulant causes the blood cells to clot.

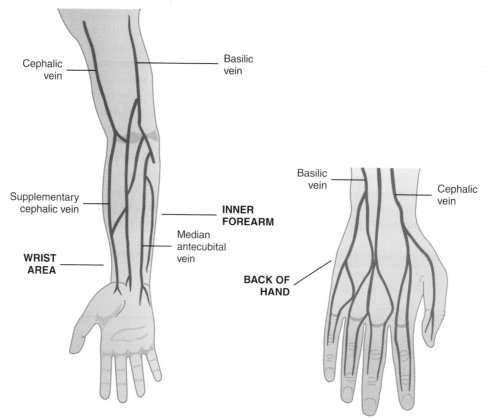

Figure 17-9. Alternative venipuncture sites: the inner forearm, the wrist area above the thumb, and the back of the hand.

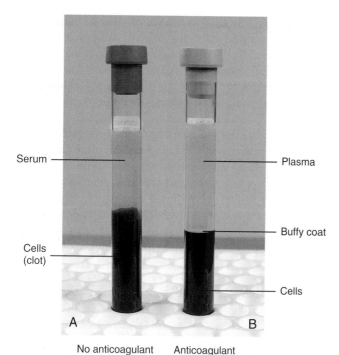

Figure 17-10. Layers into which the blood separates when there is no anticoagulant (**A**) and when an anticoagulant is present (**B**).

2. *Serum.* Serum is obtained from clotted blood by allowing the specimen to stand and then centrifuging it. Centrifuging a blood specimen that does not contain an anticoagulant causes the blood to separate into the following layers (Figure 17-10, *A*):
   - Top layer—serum
   - Bottom layer—clotted blood cells
3. *Whole blood.* Whole blood is obtained by using a tube that contains an **anticoagulant.** An anticoagulant is a substance that inhibits blood clotting. It is important to mix the anticoagulant with the blood by gently inverting the tube back and forth 8 to 10 times after collection.
4. *Plasma.* Plasma is obtained from whole blood that has been centrifuged. Centrifuging a blood specimen that contains an anticoagulant causes the blood to separate into the following layers (Figure 17-10, *B*):
   - Top layer—plasma
   - Middle layer—**buffy coat** (contains white blood cells and platelets)
   - Bottom layer—red blood cells

OSHA Safety Precautions

The OSHA Bloodborne Pathogens Standard presented in Chapter 2 must be carefully followed during the venipuncture procedure to avoid exposure to bloodborne pathogens. The following OSHA requirements apply specifically to the venipuncture procedure and to separation of serum or plasma from whole blood (see later):

1. Wear gloves when it is reasonably anticipated that you will have hand contact with blood.
2. Avoid hand-to-mouth contact, such as eating, drinking, or applying makeup, while working with blood specimens.
3. Wear a face shield or mask in combination with an eye protection device whenever splashes, spray, splatter, or droplets of blood may be generated.
4. Perform all procedures involving blood in a manner so as to minimize splashing, spraying, splattering, and generating droplets of blood.
5. Bandage cuts and other lesions on the hands before gloving.
6. Sanitize hands as soon as possible after removing gloves.
7. If your hands or other skin surfaces come in contact with blood, wash the area as soon as possible with soap and water.
8. If your mucous membranes (e.g., eyes, nose, mouth) come in contact with blood, flush them with water as soon as possible.
9. Do not bend, break, or shear contaminated venipuncture needles.
10. Do not recap a contaminated venipuncture needle.
11. Locate the sharps container as close as possible to the area of use. Immediately after use, place the contaminated venipuncture needle (and plastic holder) in the biohazard sharps container.
12. Place blood specimens in containers that prevent leakage during collection, handling, processing, storage, transport, and shipping.
13. Handle all laboratory equipment and supplies properly and with care as indicated by the manufacturer. For example, wait until the centrifuge comes to a complete stop before opening it.
14. Do not store food in refrigerators where testing supplies or specimens are stored.
15. If you are exposed to blood, report the incident immediately to your physician-employer.

What Would You Do? What Would You *Not* Do?

Case Study 1

Angela Castillo is 21 years old and comes to the office at 9:00 AM to have her blood drawn for a CBC and a thyroid profile. She has brought a friend along with her. Angela seems nervous, and her voice is shaking. She says this is the first venipuncture she has ever had. Angela asks whether her friend could stay with her to give her moral support while her blood is being drawn. Angela says that the blood has to be taken out of her left arm. She says she is right-handed and has a softball game this evening. When the veins of Angela's left arm are examined, a suitable vein cannot be located; however, she has a good median cubital vein in her right arm. Angela then wants to know whether the blood could be drawn from her left hand like they do on hospital television shows. ■

VACUUM TUBE METHOD OF VENIPUNCTURE

The vacuum tube method is frequently used to collect venous blood specimens. This method is considered ideal for collecting blood from normal healthy antecubital veins that are adequate in size to withstand the pressure of the vacuum in the evacuated tube. Procedure 17-1 outlines the venipuncture vacuum tube method. The vacuum tube system consists of a collection needle, a plastic holder, and an evacuated tube (Figure 17-11). One commercially available vacuum tube system is the Vacutainer System (Becton Dickinson, Franklin Lakes, NJ).

Needle

The needle used with the vacuum tube method consists of a double-pointed stainless steel needle with a threaded hub near its center (Figure 17-12). The needle is coated with silicon, enabling it to penetrate the skin smoothly. The threaded hub of the needle screws into the plastic holder. Vacuum tube needles are packaged in sealed twist-apart plastic containers. The needle gauge and length are printed on the paper seal on the container (see Figure 17-12). A needle should not be used if the seal has been broken.

The double-pointed needle consists of an anterior needle and a posterior needle. The *anterior needle* is longer and has a beveled point designed to facilitate entry into the skin and the vein. The *posterior needle* is shorter, and its purpose is to pierce the rubber stopper of the evacuated tube. The posterior needle has a rubber sleeve that functions as a valve. Pushing the tube stopper of an evacuated tube onto the posterior needle compresses this rubber sleeve and exposes the opening of the needle, allowing blood to enter the tube. When a tube is removed, the sleeve slides back over the needle opening and stops the flow of blood.

Vacuum tube needles are available in sizes 20 G to 22 G, with 21 G needles used most often for a routine venipunc-

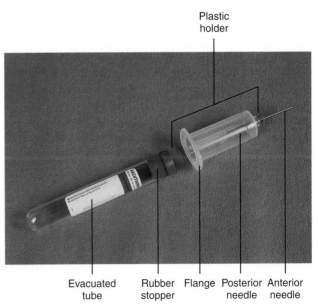

Figure 17-11. Vacuum tube system.

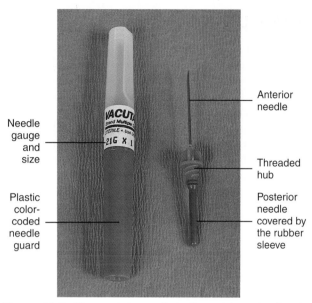

Needle gauge and size

Plastic color-coded needle guard

Anterior needle

Threaded hub

Posterior needle covered by the rubber sleeve

Figure 17-12. Vacuum tube needle in its container showing the gauge and size of the needle. The gauge of this needle is 21 G, and the size is 1 inch.

ture. A 22 G needle is recommended for children and adults with smaller veins, and a 20 G needle is sometimes used when a large-volume tube is used to collect a blood specimen. Manufacturers often color-code the needle guard and hub of venipuncture needles by gauge for easier identification, for example, Becton Dickinson uses the following color-coding system: yellow for 20 G needles, green for 21 G needles (see Figure 17-12), and black for 22 G needles. Vacuum tube needles come in two lengths: 1 inch and 1½ inches. The length used is based on individual preference; most medical assistants prefer the 1-inch needle for routine venipunctures. A 1-inch needle is less intimidating to the patient and tends to offer greater control because it allows the medical assistant to rest the fourth and fifth fingers on the patient's arm for stability. A 1½-inch needle allows more room for stabilizing the vein.

Safety-Engineered Venipuncture Devices

OSHA stipulates requirements to reduce needlestick and other sharps injuries among health care workers. As discussed in Chapter 2, employers are required to evaluate and implement commercially available safer medical devices that reduce occupational exposure to the lowest extent feasible.

Safer medical devices include safety-engineered venipuncture devices. These devices incorporate a built-in safety feature to reduce the risk of a needlestick injury. Figure 17-13 illustrates a safety-engineered venipuncture device and the method for using it.

Plastic Holder

The plastic holder consists of a plastic cylinder with two openings. The small opening is used to secure the double-pointed needle, and the large opening is used to hold the evacuated tube. The large opening has a plastic extension

known as the *flange*. The flange assists in the insertion and removal of evacuated tubes and prevents the plastic holder from rolling when it is placed on a flat surface.

The plastic holder has an indentation about ½ inch from the hub of the needle. This marks the point at which the posterior needle starts to enter the rubber stopper of the tube. If a tube stopper is inserted past this point before the vein is entered, the tube fills with air, which prevents blood from entering the tube.

Evacuated Tubes

Evacuated tubes consist of a glass or plastic tube with either a rubber stopper or a *Hemogard closure* stopper. The tube contains a premeasured vacuum that creates suction to pull the blood specimen into the tube. Evacuated tubes use a color-coded stopper system for ease in identifying the additive (or no additive) content of the tube. The additive content of evacuated tubes is described in the box *Additive Content of Evacuated Tubes* and is illustrated in Figures 17-14 and 17-15. A tube additive must not alter the blood components or affect the laboratory test to be performed.

The color of the tube stopper used depends on the type of test to be performed. The medical assistant must determine the correct stopper color to use for each collection. The color-coded stoppered tubes must not be substituted for one another because inaccurate test results could occur. If a CBC has been ordered by the physician, a lavender-stoppered tube must be used and a different color–stoppered tube cannot be substituted for it.

Evacuated tubes are available in varying capacities that range between 2 milliliters and 10 milliliters (see Figure 17-14). The capacity of the tube used depends on the amount of the specimen required for the test. If the medical assistant is working with an outside laboratory, information on the amount of specimen required for a laboratory test and the stopper color of the tube required is indicated in the laboratory directory. If the test is being performed in the medical office, this information is indicated in the instructions accompanying the blood analyzer or testing kit.

Information regarding additive content, expiration date, and tube capacity is on the label of each package of evacuated tubes (Figure 17-16). In addition, evacuated tubes have a label affixed to them indicating the additive content, expiration date, and tube capacity, as well as a fill indicator to indicate when the vacuum has been exhausted and the tube is full.

A Hemogard closure stopper consists of a special rubber stopper and a plastic closure that overhangs the outside of the tube. Together, these components act as a single unit to reduce the likelihood of coming in contact with the contents of the tube. After collecting a blood specimen, the medical assistant may need to gain access to the blood in the tube for testing it or for further processing, such as in separating serum from whole blood. A conventional rubber stopper–evacuated tube "pops" as the top is removed, which may result in splattering of blood. The design of the Hemogard stopper works to prevent splattering of blood when the

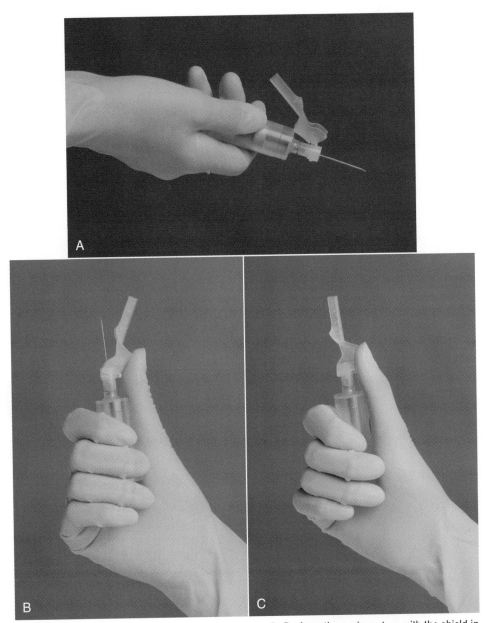

Figure 17-13. Safety-engineered venipuncture device. **A,** Perform the venipuncture with the shield in a downward position. **B,** After performing the venipuncture, push the shield forward. **C,** Continue pushing until the needle tip is fully covered by the shield. Discard the needle and holder in a biohazard sharps container.

top is removed. The color coding of Hemogard closure stoppers is similar to that of rubber-stoppered tubes (see Figure 17-15).

Additive Content of Evacuated Tubes

Evacuated tubes use a color-coded system for ease in identifying the additive content of each type of tube. The most frequently used evacuated tubes in the medical office are classified here according to the color of the stopper and the additive content:

1. **Red.** Red-stoppered tubes do not contain an anticoagulant and are used to obtain clotted blood or serum.

Serum is required for serologic tests and most blood chemistries.

2. **Red/gray-speckled tube (often called a "tiger top" tube).** The tube has a gold stopper if Hemogard tubes are used. These tubes are used to obtain serum. These tubes do not contain an anticoagulant; however, they do contain an additive known as a clot activator. A *clot activator* consists of a substance that makes the red blood cells in the tube clot more quickly to yield serum. Red/gray and gold–stoppered tubes also contain a gel that separates the cells from the serum when the tube is centrifuged. A tube with a clot activator must be inverted

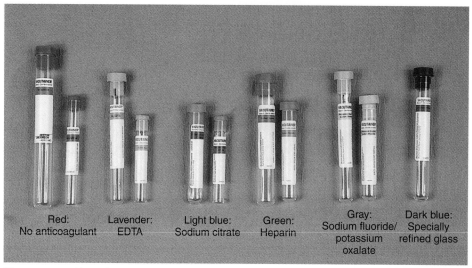

Figure 17-14. Vacutainer evacuated tubes. The stoppers of the evacuated tubes are color-coded for ease in identifying the additive content. The lavender-, light blue–, green-, gray-, and royal blue–stoppered tubes contain an anticoagulant and are used to obtain whole blood or plasma. The red-stoppered tube contains no additive and is used to obtain clotted blood or serum.

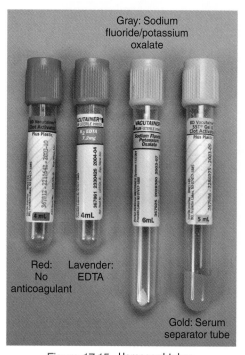

Figure 17-15. Hemogard tubes.

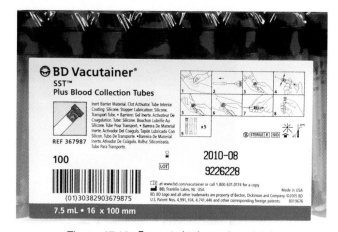

Figure 17-16. Evacuated tube package label.

5 times after it is drawn to mix the clot activator with the blood specimen.

3. **Lavender.** Lavender-stoppered tubes contain the anticoagulant *ethylenediaminetetraacetic acid* (EDTA) and are used to obtain whole blood or plasma. The most common use is to collect a blood specimen for a complete blood count (CBC).

4. **Light blue.** Light blue–stoppered tubes contain the anticoagulant sodium citrate and are used to obtain whole blood or plasma; the most common use is for coagulation tests, such as prothrombin time.

5. **Green.** Green-stoppered tubes contain the anticoagulant heparin and are commonly used to collect blood specimens to perform blood gas determinations and pH assays.

6. **Gray.** Gray-stoppered tubes contain sodium fluoride (a preservative) and potassium oxalate (an anticoagulant) and are used to obtain whole blood or plasma; the most common use is to collect blood specimens to perform a glucose tolerance test (GTT).

7. **Royal blue.** Royal blue–stoppered tubes contain either EDTA or no additive at all. These tubes are made of a specially refined glass and rubber stopper and are used for the detection of trace elements, such as lead, zinc, arsenic, and copper, which are contracted through occupational or environmental exposure.

Order of Draw for Multiple Tubes

When the vacuum tube system is used, and when multiple tubes of blood are to be drawn, the following order of draw (Table 17-1) is recommended by the *Clinical Laboratory Standards Institute (CLSI):*

1. **Blood culture tube:** Yellow-stoppered glass tube that contains the anticoagulant sodium polyanethol sulfonate (SPS), which is used for blood cultures and other tests that require sterile specimens.
   - *Rationale:* To prevent contamination of the specimen by other tubes, which may lead to inaccurate test results.
2. **Coagulation tube:** Light blue–stoppered tube for coagulation tests.
   - *Rationale:* To prevent additives from other tubes from getting into the tube.
   - *Note:* The tubing of the butterfly setup contains 0.3 to 0.5 ml of air. If a light blue–stoppered tube is the first or only tube to be drawn, a 5-ml red-stoppered tube must be drawn first and discarded. This is because some of the tube's vacuum is exhausted by the air in the tubing (rather than blood), resulting in underfilling of the tube. If the light blue–stoppered tube is filled first, the underfilled tube results in an incorrect

anticoagulant-to-blood ratio. An incorrect ratio when performing a coagulation test leads to inaccurate coagulation test results. It is also important to completely fill coagulation tubes to the exhaustion of the vacuum; failure to do so leads to erroneous coagulation test results.

What Would You Do? What Would You *Not* Do?

Case Study 2

Buzz Braydon had a heart attack 4 weeks ago and is taking the anticoagulant warfarin (Coumadin). He is at the office for a checkup and to have his prothrombin time tested. Blood is collected from a small vein in Buzz's left arm using the butterfly method. After the specimen is collected, Buzz wants to know why a red-stoppered tube was used to draw blood from him and then thrown away. Buzz says that he is going on vacation in North Carolina for 2 weeks. He says that they explained to him at the hospital why he should have his blood tested every week, but he's not sure where to go to get his blood tested while he's on vacation. Buzz wants to know if, as long as he takes his medication exactly as he should, it would be all right to skip his weekly prothrombin test during that time. ■

Table 17-1 Order of Draw for Collection of Multiple Evacuated Tubes

Order of draw by color of stopper	Additive or anticoagulant	Number of inversions after collection
Yellow	Sterile blood culture tube that contains SPS (sodium polyanethol sulfonate)	8 to 10 inversions
Light blue	Sodium citrate	3 to 4 inversions
Red	Glass: no additive Plastic: clot activator	No inversions 5 inversions
Red/gray	Serum separator gel and clot activator	5 inversions
Gold		
Green	Heparin	
Light green/gray	Plasma separator gel and lithium heparin	8 to 10 inversions
Light green		
Lavender	EDTA	8 to 10 inversions
Royal blue	EDTA No additive	8 to 10 inversions No inversions
Gray	Sodium fluoride/potassium oxalate	8 to 10 inversions

EDTA, Ethylenediaminetetraacetic acid; SPS, sodium polyanethol sulfonate.

3. **Serum tubes:** Tubes with or without a clot activator, and tubes with or without a gel barrier (e.g., red-stoppered tube; red/gray- or gold-stoppered tubes)
   - *Rationale:* To prevent contamination of serum tubes by tubes with an anticoagulant.
4. **Anticoagulant tubes** in this order of stopper color: green, lavender, royal blue (that contains EDTA), and gray
   - *Rationale:* To prevent cross-contamination between different types of anticoagulants, which may lead to inaccurate test results.

Evacuated Tube Guidelines

Certain guidelines should be followed when using evacuated tubes, as follows:

1. Select the proper evacuated tubes according to the tests to be performed and the amount of specimen required.
2. Check to ensure that the tube is not cracked. A cracked tube no longer has a vacuum.
3. Check the expiration date on each tube. Outdated tubes may no longer contain a vacuum, and, as a result, they would not be able to draw blood into the tube.
4. Make sure each tube is properly labeled. Proper labeling avoids mixing up specimens. Advances in specimen identification include the use of computer bar codes to identify specimens. Laboratory instruments that do the testing are able to read the bar codes and automatically record results onto the laboratory report form for a particular patient using the identification number supplied by the bar code. Along with the bar code, additional printed information is included on a bar code label (Figure 17-17). It is important to attach the correct bar code label to the blood tube. Inspect the label for printed information indicating the color-stopper tube (e.g., LV for lavender) or type of tube (e.g., SST for serum separator tube) to which the label must be attached. For example, the bar code label illustrated in Figure 17-17 must be placed on a lavender (LV) tube that is being collected to perform a CBC.
5. Before using tubes that contain powdered additives (e.g., gray-stoppered tube), gently tap the tube just be-low the stopper so that all of the additive is dislodged from the stopper. If an additive remains trapped in the stopper, erroneous test results may occur.
6. Take precautions to avoid premature loss of the tube's vacuum. Premature loss of vacuum can occur from the following:
   - Dropping the tube
   - Pushing the posterior needle through the tube stopper before puncturing the vein
   - Partially pulling the needle out of the vein after penetrating the patient's vein
7. Use a continuous, steady motion to make the puncture. Performing the puncture with a slow, timid motion or a rapid, jabbing motion is painful for the patient. In addition, a rapid motion could cause the needle to go completely through the vein, resulting in failure to obtain blood and possibly a hematoma.
8. When multiple tubes are to be drawn, follow the proper *order of draw.* This prevents contamination of nonadditive tubes by additive tubes and cross-contamination between different types of additive tubes, which could lead to inaccurate test results.
9. Fill evacuated tubes until the vacuum is exhausted, as evidenced by cessation of blood flow into the tube. The tube is almost, but not quite, full when the vacuum is exhausted. If the evacuated tube is removed before the vacuum is exhausted, a rush of air enters the tube, damaging the red blood cells. A tube that contains an anticoagulant must be filled completely to ensure the proper ratio of anticoagulant to the blood specimen.
10. Remove the last tube from the plastic holder before removing the needle from the patient's vein. This prevents blood from dripping out of the tip of the needle after it is withdrawn from the patient's skin.
11. Mix tubes that contain a clot activator or an anticoagulant immediately after drawing by gently inverting them. Gentle inversion provides adequate mixing without causing **hemolysis,** or breakdown of blood cells. One inversion consists of one complete turn of the

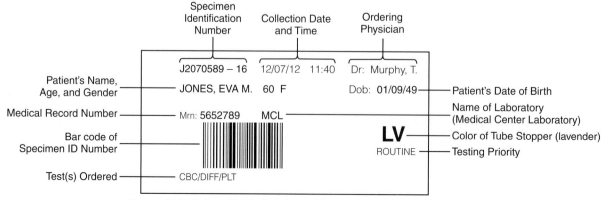

Figure 17-17. Information included on a laboratory specimen bar code label.

wrist (180 degrees) and then back again. Tubes with a clot activator should be inverted 5 times, and tubes with an anticoagulant (with the exception of sodium citrate tubes) should be inverted 8 to 10 times. Tubes containing sodium citrate (light-blue stopper) should be gently inverted 3 to 4 times. (see Table 17-1). Inad-

equate mixing or not mixing tubes with an anticoagulant immediately after drawing them may result in clotting of the blood, leading to inaccurate test results.

12. After the venipuncture, the top of the stopper may contain residual blood. Take precautions by following the OSHA Standard when handling these tubes.

PROCEDURE 17-1   Venipuncture—Vacuum Tube Method

Outcome Perform a venipuncture using the vacuum tube method.

Equipment/Supplies

- Disposable gloves
- Tourniquet
- Antiseptic wipe
- Double-pointed needle
- Plastic holder
- Evacuated tubes with labels

- Sterile 2 × 2 gauze pad
- Adhesive bandage
- Biohazard sharps container
- Biohazard specimen bag
- Laboratory request form

1. **Procedural Step.** Review the requirements for collecting and handling the blood specimen as ordered by the physician. Sanitize your hands.

2. **Procedural Step.** Greet the patient and introduce yourself. Identify the patient by asking the patient to state his or her full name and date of birth. Compare this information with the demographic data in the patient's chart. If the patient was required to prepare for the test (e.g., fasting, medication restriction), determine whether he or she has prepared properly. If the patient has not followed the patient preparation requirements, notify the physician for instructions on handling this situation.

   Principle. It is important to confirm that you have the correct patient to avoid collecting a specimen on the wrong patient. The patient must prepare properly to obtain a quality specimen that would lead to accurate test results.

3. **Procedural Step.** Assemble the equipment. Select the proper evacuated tubes for the tests to be performed. Check the expiration date on the tubes. Label each tube using one of the following methods: (a) attaching a computer bar code label to each tube to be drawn and labeling it with your initials, or (b) manually labeling each tube with the patient's name and date of birth, the date, and your initials. If the specimen is to be tested at an outside laboratory, complete a laboratory request form. (*Note:* Follow the medical office policy as to when the tubes should be labeled. Some offices prefer that tubes be labeled *before* the specimen is drawn; other offices want the tubes to be labeled right *after* the specimen is drawn.)

   Principle. Outdated tubes may no longer contain a vacuum, and, as a result, they may not be able to draw blood into the tube. Proper labeling of blood specimens avoids a mixup of specimens.

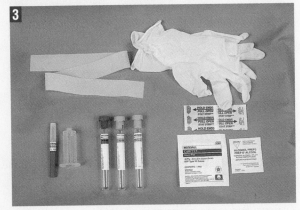

Assemble the equipment.

4. **Procedural Step.** Prepare the vacuum tube system. Remove the cap from the posterior needle using a twisting and pulling motion. Insert the posterior needle into the small opening on the plastic holder. Screw the plastic holder onto the Luer adapter, and tighten it securely.

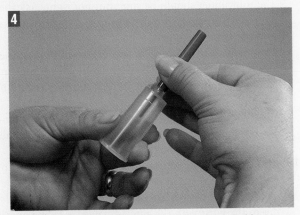

Insert the posterior needle into the plastic holder.

Continued

PROCEDURE 17-1   Venipuncture—Vacuum Tube Method—cont'd

Principle. An unsecured needle can fall out of its plastic holder.

5. Procedural Step. Open the sterile gauze packet, and lay it flat to allow the gauze pad to rest on the inside of its wrapper. Position the evacuated tubes in the correct order of draw. If the evacuated tube contains a powdered additive, tap the tube just below the stopper to release any additive adhering to the stopper.

Principle. If an additive remains trapped in the stopper, erroneous test results may occur.

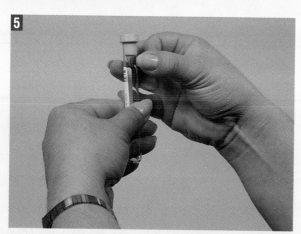

Tap tubes with powdered additives.

6. Procedural Step. Place the first tube loosely in the plastic holder.

7. Procedural Step. Explain the procedure to the patient, and reassure the patient. Perform a preliminary assessment of both arms to determine the best vein to use. It also is helpful to ask the patient which arm has been used in the past to obtain blood.

Principle. Venipuncture is often a frightening experience for the patient, and reassurance should be offered to reduce apprehension.

8. Procedural Step. Apply the tourniquet. Position the tourniquet 3 to 4 inches above the bend in the elbow. The tourniquet should be snug but not tight. Ask the patient to clench the fist of the arm to which the tourniquet has been applied.

Principle. The combined effect of the pressure of the tourniquet and the clenched fist should cause the antecubital veins to stand out so that accurate selection of a puncture site can be made.

9. Procedural Step. With a tourniquet in place, thoroughly assess the veins of first one arm and then the other to determine the best vein to use.

10. Procedural Step. Position the patient's arm. The arm with the vein selected for the venipuncture should be extended and placed in a straight line from the shoulder to the wrist with the antecubital veins facing ante-

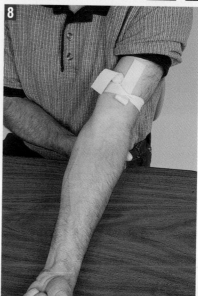

Apply the tourniquet.

riorly. The arm should be supported on the armrest by a rolled towel or by having the patient place the fist of the other hand under the elbow.

Principle. This position allows easy access to the antecubital veins.

11. Procedural Step. Thoroughly palpate the selected vein. Gently palpate the vein with the fingertips to determine the direction of the vein and to estimate its size and depth. Never leave the tourniquet on an arm for longer than 1 minute at a time. (*Note:* If you need to perform several assessments to locate the best vein,

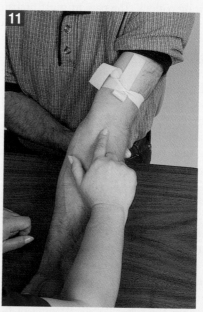

Palpate the vein.

PROCEDURE 17-1   Venipuncture—Vacuum Tube Method—cont'd

the tourniquet must be removed and reapplied after a 2-minute waiting period.)

Principle. Leaving the tourniquet on for longer than 1 minute is uncomfortable for the patient and may alter the test results.

12. **Procedural Step.** Remove the tourniquet and cleanse the site with an antiseptic wipe. Cleansing should be done in a circular motion, starting from the inside and moving away from the puncture site. Allow the site to air-dry; after cleansing, do not touch the area, wipe the area with gauze, or fan the area with your hand. Place the remaining supplies within comfortable reach of your nondominant hand.

Principle. Using a circular motion helps carry foreign particles away from the puncture site. The site must be allowed to air-dry to allow the alcohol enough time to destroy microorganisms on the patient's skin. Residual alcohol entering the blood specimen can cause hemolysis, leading to inaccurate test results. In addition, residual alcohol causes the patient to experience a stinging sensation when the puncture is made. Touching or fanning the area causes contamination of the puncture site, and the cleansing process must be repeated. Items used during the procedure should be positioned so that you do not have to reach over the patient and possibly move the needle, resulting in pain, injury, or both.

13. **Procedural Step.** Reapply the tourniquet. Apply gloves. If you are using a needle with a safety shield, rotate the shield backward toward the holder (refer to Figure 17-13, *A*). Remove the cap from the needle using a twisting and pulling motion. Hold the vacuum tube system by placing the thumb of the dominant hand on top of the plastic holder and the pads of the first three fingers underneath the holder and evacuated tube. The needle should be positioned with the bevel facing up. Position the evacuated tube so that the label is facing down.

Principle. Gloves provide a barrier against bloodborne pathogens. Positioning the needle with the bevel up allows easier entry into the skin and the vein, resulting in less pain for the patient. With the label facing down, you would be able to observe the blood as it fills the tube, which allows you to know when the tube is full.

14. **Procedural Step.** Anchor the vein. Grasp the patient's arm with the nondominant hand. Your thumb should be placed 1 to 2 inches below and to the side of the puncture site. Using your thumb, draw the skin taut over the vein in the direction of the patient's hand.

Principle. The thumb helps hold the skin taut for easier entry and helps stabilize the vein to be punctured. Placing the thumb to the side keeps it out of

the way of the vacuum tube setup, so that you can maintain a 15-degree angle when entering the vein.

15. **Procedural Step.** Position the needle at a 15-degree angle to the arm. Rest the backs of the fingers on the patient's forearm. Ensure that the needle points in the same direction as the vein to be entered. The needle should be positioned so that it enters the vein approximately ⅛ inch below the place where the vein is to be entered.

Principle. An angle of less than 15 degrees may cause the needle to enter above the vein, preventing puncture. An angle of more than 15 degrees may cause the needle to go through the vein by puncturing the posterior wall. This could result in a hematoma.

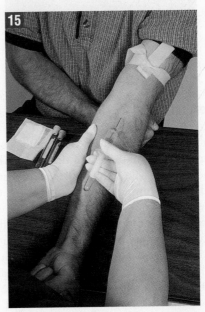

Position the needle.

16. **Procedural Step.** Tell the patient that he or she will "feel a small stick," and with one continuous steady motion, enter the skin and then the vein. You will feel a sensation of resistance followed by a "release" as the vein is entered. When the "release" is felt, you have entered the vein and should not advance the needle any farther.

Principle. Using one continuous steady motion helps to prevent tissue damage.

17. **Procedural Step.** Stabilize the vacuum tube setup by firmly grasping the holder between the thumb and the underlying fingers to prevent the needle from moving. Do *not* change hands during the procedure.

Principle. Stabilizing the holder helps prevent the needle from moving when a tube is inserted or removed. Changing hands may cause the needle to move, which is painful for the patient.

Continued

PROCEDURE 17-1   Venipuncture—Vacuum Tube Method—cont'd

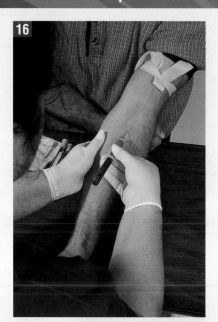

Make the puncture.

can cause the needle to come out of the vein prematurely, resulting in blood being forced out of the puncture site. A tube containing an anticoagulant must be inverted immediately to prevent the blood from clotting. Careful mixing of the blood with a clot activator or an anticoagulant prevents hemolysis.

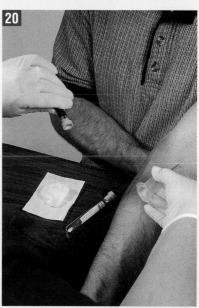

Invert tubes with additives back and forth 8 to 10 times.

18. Procedural Step. With the nondominant hand, place the first two fingers on the underside of the flange on the plastic holder, and with the thumb, slowly push the tube forward to the end of the holder. This allows the posterior needle to puncture the rubber stopper. Blood begins flowing into the tube if the (anterior) needle is in a vein.

Principle. Not using the flange may cause the needle to advance forward and go completely through the vein, resulting in failure to obtain blood; internal bleeding also may occur, resulting in a hematoma.

19. Procedural Step. Allow the evacuated tube to fill to the exhaustion of the vacuum, as indicated by cessation of the blood flow into the tube. The suction of the evacuated tube automatically draws the blood into the tube.

Principle. If the evacuated tube is removed before the vacuum is exhausted, a rush of air enters the tube, damaging the red blood cells. Also, a tube containing an additive, such as an anticoagulant, must be filled completely to ensure accurate test results.

20. Procedural Step. Remove the tube from the holder by grasping the tube with the fingers, placing the thumb or index finger against the flange, and pulling the tube off the posterior needle. Do not change the position of the needle in the vein. If the tube contains a clot activator, gently invert the tube back and forth 5 times before laying it down. If the tube contains an anticoagulant, gently invert the tube 8 to 10 times.

Principle. The rubber sheath covers the point of the needle, stopping the flow of blood until the next tube is inserted. Not using the flange to remove the tube

21. Procedural Step. Using the flange, carefully insert the next tube into the holder. Continue in this manner until the last tube has been filled.

22. Procedural Step. Remove the tension from the tourniquet by pulling upward on one of the flaps of the tourniquet. Ask the patient to unclench the fist.

Principle. The tourniquet tension must be removed before the needle. Otherwise, the pressure on the vein from the tourniquet could cause internal and external bleeding around the puncture site.

23. Procedural Step. Remove the last tube from the holder. Immediately invert the tube back and forth 5 times if it contains a clot activator and 8 to 10 times if it contains an anticoagulant.

Principle. Removing the last tube prevents blood from dripping out of the tip of the needle after it is removed from the patient's arm.

24. Procedural Step. Place a sterile gauze pad slightly above the puncture site, and carefully withdraw the needle at the same angle as for penetration. Immediately move the gauze over the puncture site, and apply firm pressure. (Do not apply any pressure to the puncture site until the needle is completely removed.) If you are using a needle with a safety shield, push the shield forward with your thumb until you hear an audible click, which indicates the shield has locked into place. Do not push the shield forward by pressing it against a hard surface. (See Figure 17-13, *B, C*.)

Principle. Placing the gauze pad above the puncture helps prevent tissue movement as the needle is withdrawn and reduces patient discomfort. Careful withdrawal prevents further tissue damage.

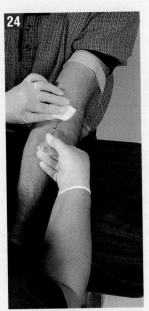

Remove the tourniquet and withdraw the needle.

25. Procedural Step. Immediately discard the plastic holder and attached needle in a biohazard sharps container. Do not remove the needle from the holder; the holder must be discarded and not reused.

Principle. Immediate disposal of the needle and holder unit is required by the OSHA Standard to prevent a needlestick injury; even if a safety shield has been activated to encase the anterior needle, a needlestick injury can still occur from the posterior needle, which is only covered with a rubber sleeve. Plastic holders are often contaminated with blood and must not be reused.

26. Procedural Step. Continue to apply pressure with the gauze pad. Cooperative patients can be asked to assist by applying pressure with the gauze pad for 1 to 2 minutes. The arm can be elevated to facilitate clot formation. Do not allow the patient to bend the arm at the elbow because this increases blood loss from the puncture site.

Principle. Applying pressure reduces the leakage of blood from the puncture site externally or internally.

Internal leakage of blood into the tissues could result in a hematoma.

27. Procedural Step. Stay with the patient until the bleeding has stopped. Remove the gauze, and inspect the puncture site to ensure that the opening is sealed with a clot. Apply an adhesive bandage to the puncture site. As an alternative, the gauze pad can be folded into quarters and taped on the puncture site to be used as a pressure bandage. Instruct the patient not to pick up anything heavy for about an hour. (*Note:* If swelling or discoloration occurs, apply an ice pack to the site after bandaging it.)

Principle. Lifting a heavy object causes pressure on the puncture site, which could result in bleeding.

28. Procedural Step. Place the tubes in an upright position in a test tube rack. Remove the gloves, and sanitize your hands.

29. Procedural Step. Chart the procedure. Include the date and time, which arm and vein were used, unusual patient reaction, and your initials.

30. Procedural Step. If needed, process the specimen (e.g., centrifuging the specimen to separate serum from the cells). Test the specimen or prepare the specimen for transport to an outside laboratory for testing according to the medical office policy. If the specimen is to be transported to an outside laboratory, do the following:

a. Place the specimen tube in a biohazard specimen bag.

b. Place the laboratory request in the outside pocket of the specimen bag.

c. Properly handle and store the specimen while awaiting pickup by a laboratory courier.

d. Chart the date the specimen was transported to the laboratory in the patient's record.

Principle. The biohazard bag protects the laboratory courier from the possibility of an exposure incident. The outside laboratory must have the completed request form to know which laboratory tests have been ordered by the physician. The specimen must be handled and stored properly to maintain the in vivo characteristics of the specimen.

CHARTING EXAMPLE

Date	
4/5/12	9:00 a.m. Venous blood specimen collected from (L) arm. Picked up by Medical Center Laboratory on 4/5/12. _____
	_____ D. Glover, CMA (AAMA)

BUTTERFLY METHOD OF VENIPUNCTURE

The butterfly method of venipuncture is also called the *winged infusion method.* This is because a winged infusion set is used to perform the procedure. The term *butterfly* is derived from the plastic "wings" located between the needle and the tubing of the winged infusion set (Figure 17-18).

The butterfly method is used to collect blood from patients who are difficult to stick by conventional methods because it provides better control when making the puncture, and less pressure is exerted on the vein wall from the evacuated tube. The butterfly method is recommended for adults with small antecubital veins and children, who typically have small antecubital veins. The butterfly method also is used when the antecubital veins are unavailable and veins in the forearm, wrist area, or back of the hand are used, as may occur with elderly and obese patients. These alternative veins are usually smaller and sometimes have a thin wall (e.g., hand veins), making them more likely to collapse when using the vacuum tube method of venipuncture. With the vacuum tube method, the "sucking action" exerted on the vein when the pressure in the vacuum is released causes the vein to collapse, blocking the flow of blood into the tube. The butterfly method results in less pressure on the vein wall because the pressure exerted by the evacuated tube must travel through a length of tubing before reaching the vein. Because the pressure against the vein wall is minimized, the vein is less likely to collapse with the butterfly method. Procedure 17-2 describes the venipuncture procedure using the butterfly method.

The gauge of the winged infusion needle used to collect a blood specimen ranges from 21 G to 23 G, and the length of the needle ranges from ½ to ¾ inch. The needle is short and sharp, making it easier to stick difficult veins. For extremely small veins, a 23 G needle should be used to prevent rupture of the vein by a larger needle. In this case, it is preferable to use smaller-volume tubes (e.g., 2-ml evacuated tubes) because large evacuated tubes may put too much vacuum pressure on the vein, causing it to collapse. Manufacturers often color-code the wings of the infusion setup by gauge for easier identification; for example, Becton Dickinson uses the following color coding system: green for 21 G needles and light blue for 23 G needles (see Figure 17-18).

The winged infusion needle is attached to a 7- or 12-inch length of tubing and a *Luer adapter,* which is attached to a (posterior) needle with a rubber sleeve. A plastic holder is screwed onto the Luer adapter, which allows it to be used with evacuated tubes (see Figure 17-18, *A*). Winged infusion sets also are available with a hub adapter that allows them to be used with a syringe (see Figure 17-18, *B*). Safety needles are available with a shield that covers the contaminated needle after it is withdrawn from the patient's vein (Figure 17-19).

Guidelines for the Butterfly Method

Certain guidelines should be followed when performing the butterfly method of venipuncture, as follows:

1. Position the patient according to the site selected for the venipuncture as follows:
   - **Antecubital, wrist and forearm veins.** Position the arm in a straight line from the shoulder to the wrist as described in the vacuum tube method of venipuncture.
   - **Hand veins.** Position the patient's hand on the armrest, and ask the patient to make a loose fist or to grasp a rolled towel. This combination causes the hand veins to stand out so that accurate selection of a puncture site can be made. Locate a suitable vein between the knuckles and the wrist bones. Hand veins are usually visible and easy to locate.
2. Position the tourniquet according to the venipuncture site as follows: If the veins of the forearm or wrist are used, apply the tourniquet to the forearm, approximately 3 inches above the puncture site. For hand veins, posi-

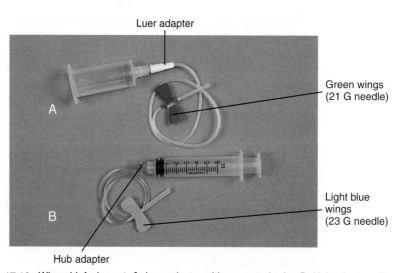

Figure 17-18. Winged infusion set. **A,** Luer adapter with evacuated tube. **B,** Hub adapter with syringe.

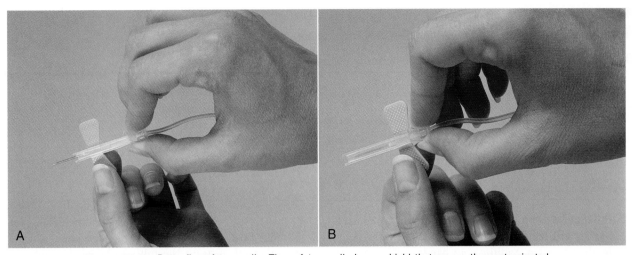

Figure 17-19. Butterfly safety needle. The safety needle has a shield that covers the contaminated needle after it is withdrawn from the patient's vein. **A,** The medical assistant has covered one half of the needle with the shield. **B,** The needle is completely covered with the shield.

tion the tourniquet on the arm just above the wrist bone (Figure 17-20).

3. Grasp the needle by compressing the plastic wings together. Insert the needle with the bevel facing up at a 15-degree angle to the skin. When the vein has been entered, decrease the angle to 5 degrees.

4. After decreasing the needle angle to 5 degrees, slowly thread the needle inside the vein an additional ¼ inch. This anchors or seats the needle in the center of the vein and allows the medical assistant to use both hands to change tubes.

5. To prevent venous reflux, keep the evacuated tube and holder in a downward position as in the vacuum tube venipuncture procedure. This technique ensures that the blood fills from the bottom up and not near the rubber stopper.

6. When multiple tubes are to be drawn, follow the proper order of draw. The order of draw for the butterfly method is identical to that for the vacuum tube method (previously presented). Following this order of draw prevents contamination of nonadditive tubes and cross-contamination of additive tubes.

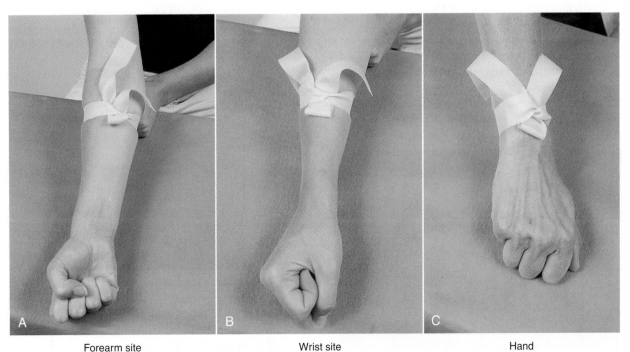

Forearm site   Wrist site   Hand

Figure 17-20. Application of the tourniquet for alternative venipuncture sites.

PROCEDURE 17-2   Venipuncture—Butterfly Method

Outcome Perform a venipuncture using the butterfly method.

Equipment/Supplies

- Disposable gloves
- Tourniquet
- Antiseptic wipe
- Winged infusion set with a Luer adapter
- Plastic holder
- Evacuated tubes with labels

- Sterile 2 × 2 gauze pad
- Adhesive bandage
- Biohazard sharps container
- Biohazard specimen bag
- Laboratory request form

1. **Procedural Step.** Review the requirements for collecting and handling the blood specimen as ordered by the physician. Sanitize your hands.

2. **Procedural Step.** Greet the patient and introduce yourself. Identify the patient by asking the patient to state his or her full name and date of birth. Compare this information with the demographic data in the patient's chart. If the patient was required to prepare for the test (e.g., fasting, medication restriction), determine whether he or she has prepared properly. If the patient has not followed the patient preparation requirements, notify the physician for instructions on handling this situation.

    Principle. It is important to confirm that you have the correct patient to avoid collecting a specimen on the wrong patient. The patient must prepare properly to obtain a quality specimen that would lead to accurate test results.

3. **Procedural Step.** Assemble the equipment. Select the proper evacuated tubes for the tests to be performed. Check the expiration date on the tubes. Label each tube using one of the following methods: (a) attaching a computer bar code label to each tube and labeling it with your initials, or (b) manually labeling each tube with the patient's name and date of birth, the date, and your initials. If the specimen is to be tested at an outside laboratory, complete a laboratory request form. (*Note:* Follow the medical office policy as to

when the tubes should be labeled. Some offices prefer that tubes be labeled *before* the specimen is drawn; other offices want the tubes to be labeled right *after* the specimen is drawn.)

    Principle. Outdated tubes may no longer contain a vacuum, and, as a result, they may not be able to draw blood into the tube. Proper labeling of blood specimens avoids the mixup of specimens.

4. **Procedural Step.** Prepare the winged infusion set. Remove the winged infusion set from its package. Extend the tubing to its full length, and stretch it slightly to prevent it from recoiling. Insert the posterior needle into the small opening on the plastic holder. Screw the plastic holder onto the Luer adapter, and tighten it securely.

    Principle. Extending the tubing straightens it to permit a free flow of blood in the tubing. An unsecured needle can fall out of its plastic holder.

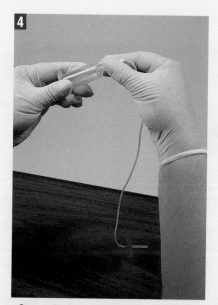

Screw the Luer adapter into the holder.

5. **Procedural Step.** Open the sterile gauze packet, and lay it flat to allow the gauze pad to rest on the inside of its wrapper. Position the evacuated tubes in the correct order of draw. If the evacuated tube contains a

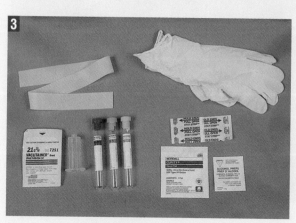

Assemble the equipment.

powdered additive, tap the tube just below the stopper to release any additive adhering to the stopper.

Principle. If an additive remains trapped in the stopper, erroneous test results may occur.

6. **Procedural Step.** Place the first tube loosely in the plastic holder with the label facing down.

Principle. With the label facing down, you can observe the blood as it fills the tube, which allows you to know when the tube is full.

7. **Procedural Step.** Explain the procedure to the patient, and reassure the patient. Perform a preliminary assessment of both arms to determine the best vein to use. It also is helpful to ask the patient which arm has been used in the past to obtain blood.

Principle. Venipuncture is often a frightening experience for the patient, and reassurance should be offered to reduce apprehension.

8. **Procedural Step.** Apply the tourniquet. Position the tourniquet 3 to 4 inches above the bend in the elbow. The tourniquet should be snug but not tight. Ask the patient to clench the fist of the arm to which the tourniquet has been applied.

Principle. The combined effect of the pressure of the tourniquet and the clenched fist should cause the antecubital veins to stand out so that accurate selection of a puncture site can be made.

9. **Procedural Step.** With a tourniquet in place, thoroughly assess the veins of first one arm and then the other to determine the best vein to use.

10. **Procedural Step.** Position the patient's arm. The arm with the vein selected for the venipuncture should be extended and placed in a straight line from the shoulder to the wrist with the antecubital veins facing anteriorly. The arm should be supported on the armrest by a rolled towel or by having the patient place the fist of the other hand under the elbow.

Principle. This position allows easy access to the antecubital veins.

11. **Procedural Step.** Thoroughly palpate the selected vein. Gently palpate the vein with the fingertips to determine the direction of the vein and to estimate its size and depth. Never leave the tourniquet on an arm for longer than 1 minute at a time. (*Note:* If you need to perform several assessments to locate the best vein, the tourniquet must be removed and reapplied after a 2-minute waiting period.)

Principle. Leaving the tourniquet on for longer than 1 minute is uncomfortable for the patient and may alter the test results.

12. **Procedural Step.** Remove the tourniquet and cleanse the site with an antiseptic. Cleansing should be done in a circular motion, starting from the inside and moving away from the puncture site. Allow the site to air-dry,

and after cleansing, do not touch the area, wipe the area with gauze, or fan the area with your hand. Place your remaining supplies within comfortable reach.

Principle. Using a circular motion helps carry foreign particles away from the puncture site. The site must be allowed to air-dry to allow the alcohol enough time to destroy microorganisms on the patient's skin. Residual alcohol entering the blood specimen can cause hemolysis, leading to inaccurate test results. In addition, residual alcohol causes the patient to experience a stinging sensation when the puncture is made. Touching or fanning the area causes contamination of the puncture site, and the cleansing process must be repeated. Items used during the procedure should be positioned so that you do not have to reach over the patient and possibly move the needle, resulting in patient pain, injury, or both.

13. **Procedural Step.** Reapply the tourniquet. Apply gloves. With the dominant hand, grasp the winged infusion set by pressing the butterfly tips together. Remove the protective sheath from the needle of the infusion set. The needle should be positioned with the bevel facing up.

Principle. Gloves provide a barrier against bloodborne pathogens. Positioning the needle with the bevel up allows easier entry into the skin and the vein, resulting in less pain for the patient.

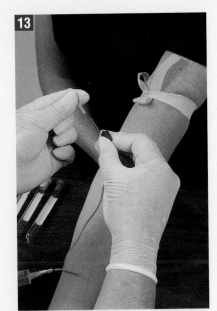

Remove the protective shield from the needle.

14. **Procedural Step.** Anchor the vein. Grasp the patient's arm with the nondominant hand. The thumb should be placed 1 to 2 inches below and to the side of the

Continued

puncture site. Using the thumb, draw the skin taut over the vein in the direction of the patient's hand.

Principle. The thumb helps hold the skin taut for easier entry and helps stabilize the vein to be punctured. Placing the thumb to the side keeps it out of the way of the winged infusion setup so that you can maintain a 15-degree angle when entering the vein.

15. **Procedural Step.** Position the needle at a 15-degree angle to the arm. Rest the backs of the fingertips on the patient's skin. Make sure the needle points in the same direction as the vein to be entered. The needle should be positioned so that it enters the vein approximately ⅛ inch below the place where the vein is to be entered.

Principle. An angle of less than 15 degrees may cause the needle to enter above the vein, preventing puncture. An angle of more than 15 degrees may cause the needle to go through the vein by puncturing the posterior wall. This could result in a hematoma.

16. **Procedural Step.** Tell the patient that he or she will "feel a small stick," and with one continuous steady motion, enter the skin and then the vein. You will feel a sensation of resistance followed by a "release" as the vein is entered. After penetrating the vein, decrease the angle of the needle to 5 degrees. If the needle is in the vein, a flash of blood appears at the top of the tubing.

Principle. Using one continuous motion reduces tissue damage.

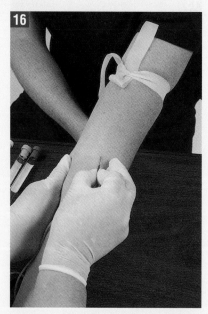

Make the puncture.

17. **Procedural Step.** Seat the needle by threading it forward an additional ¼ inch inside the center of the vein so that it does not twist out of the vein, even if

you let go of it. Open the butterfly wings and securely rest the wings flat against the skin. Ensure that the needle does not move.

Principle. Seating the needle anchors the needle in the center of the vein and allows the use of both hands for changing tubes. Moving the needle is painful for the patient.

18. **Procedural Step.** Keep the tube and holder in a downward position so that the tube fills from the bottom up and not near the rubber stopper. Slowly push the tube forward to the end of the holder. This allows the needle to puncture the rubber stopper. Blood begins to flow into the tube. Allow the evacuated tube to fill to the exhaustion of the vacuum, as indicated by cessation of the blood flow into the tube. The suction of the evacuated tube automatically draws the blood into the tube.

Principle. The tube must fill from the bottom up to prevent venous reflux. If the evacuated tube is removed before the vacuum is exhausted, a rush of air enters the tube, damaging the red blood cells. Also, a tube containing an anticoagulant must be filled completely to ensure accurate test results.

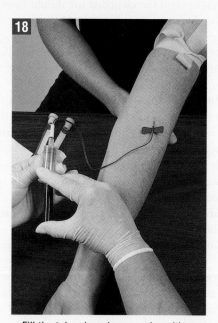

Fill the tubes in a downward position.

19. **Procedural Step.** Remove the tube from the plastic holder. If the tube contains a clot activator, gently invert the tube back and forth 5 times before laying it down. If the tube contains an anticoagulant, gently invert the tube 8 to 10 times.

Principle. The rubber sheath covers the point of the needle, stopping the flow of blood until the next tube is inserted. A tube containing an anticoagulant must

PROCEDURE 17-2

PROCEDURE 17-2   Venipuncture—Butterfly Method—cont'd

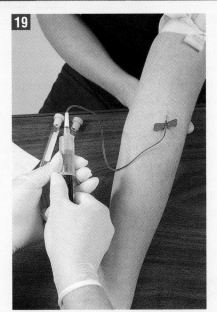

Remove the tube from the holder.

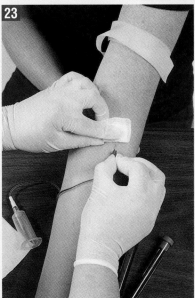

Release the tourniquet and remove the needle.

be inverted before laying it down to prevent the blood from clotting. Careful mixing of the blood with a clot activator or an anticoagulant prevents hemolysis.

20. **Procedural Step.** Using the flange, carefully insert the next tube into the holder. Continue in this manner until the last tube has been filled.

21. **Procedural Step.** Remove the tension from the tourniquet by pulling upward on one of the flaps of the tourniquet. Ask the patient to unclench the fist.

    Principle. The tourniquet tension must be removed before the needle. Otherwise, pressure on the vein from the tourniquet could cause internal and external bleeding around the puncture.

22. **Procedural Step.** Remove the last tube from the holder. Immediately invert the tube back and forth 5 times if it contains a clot activator and 8 to 10 times if it contains an anticoagulant.

    Principle. Removing the last tube from the holder prevents blood from dripping out of the tip of the needle after it is removed from the patient's arm.

23. **Procedural Step.** Place a sterile gauze pad slightly above the puncture site. Grasp the setup just below the wings, and slowly withdraw the needle at the same angle as for penetration. Immediately move the gauze over the puncture site, and apply firm pressure. (*Note:* Do not apply pressure to the puncture site until the needle is completely removed.) Cooperative patients can be asked to assist by applying pressure with the gauze pad. If you are using a butterfly needle with a safety shield, grasp the base of the shield with the thumb and index fingers of one hand and, with the other hand, grasp either wing. Slide the wing back

into the rear slot of the safety shield until you hear an audible click, which indicates the shield has locked into place (see Figure 17-18, *A, B*).

Principle. Placing the gauze pad above the puncture site helps prevent tissue movement as the needle is withdrawn and reduces patient discomfort. Careful withdrawal prevents further tissue damage.

24. **Procedural Step.** Immediately discard the winged infusion set and attached plastic holder. Holding onto the plastic holder, first drop the needle into a biohazard sharps container followed by the tubing and holder. Do not remove the plastic holder from the setup; the plastic holder must be discarded and not reused.

    Principle. Proper disposal is required by the OSHA Standard to prevent a needlestick injury; even if a safety shield has been activated to encase the butterfly needle, a needlestick injury can still result from the posterior needle, which is covered with only a rubber sleeve. Plastic holders are often contaminated with blood and must not be reused.

25. **Procedural Step.** Continue to apply pressure with the gauze pad. The arm can be elevated to facilitate clot formation. Do not allow the patient to bend the arm at the elbow because this increases blood loss from the puncture site.

    Principle. Applying pressure reduces the leakage of blood from the puncture site externally or internally. Internal leakage into the tissues could result in a hematoma.

26. **Procedural Step.** Stay with the patient until the bleeding has stopped. Remove pressure, and inspect

Continued

PROCEDURE 17-2   Venipuncture—Butterfly Method—cont'd

the puncture site to ensure that the opening is sealed with a clot. Apply an adhesive bandage to the puncture site. As an alternative, the gauze pad can be folded into quarters and taped onto the puncture site to be used as a pressure bandage. Instruct the patient not to pick up anything heavy for about an hour. (*Note:* If swelling or discoloration occurs, apply an ice pack to the site after bandaging it.)

Principle. Lifting a heavy object causes pressure on the puncture site, which could result in bleeding.

27. **Procedural Step.** Place the tubes in an upright position in a test tube rack. Remove the gloves, and sanitize your hands.

28. **Procedural Step.** Chart the procedure. Include the date and time, which arm and vein were used, unusual patient reactions, and your initials.

29. **Procedural Step.** If needed, process the specimen (e.g., centrifuging the specimen to separate serum from the cells). Test the specimen or prepare the specimen for transport to an outside laboratory for testing according to the medical office policy. If the specimen is to be transported to an outside laboratory, do the following:
    a. Place the specimen tube in a biohazard specimen bag.

b. Place the laboratory request in the outside pocket of the specimen bag.
c. Properly handle and store the specimen while awaiting pickup by a laboratory courier.
d. Chart the date the specimen was transported to the laboratory in the patient's record.

Principle. The biohazard bag protects the laboratory courier from the possibility of an exposure incident. The outside laboratory must have the completed request form to know which laboratory tests have been ordered by the physician. The specimen must be handled and stored properly to maintain the in vivo characteristics of the specimen.

CHARTING EXAMPLE

Date	
4/10/12	10:30 a.m. Venous blood specimen collected from Ⓛ arm. Picked up by Medical Center Laboratory on 4/10/12 _____
	_____ D. Glover, CMA (AAMA)

Memories *from* Externship

Dori Glover: One of the most terrifying things for me as a student was learning venipuncture. Even though I would practice during classroom laboratory hours and felt comfortable with it, it still scared me to know I would have to draw on a real person one day. When the day arrived to draw on my laboratory partner, I became sick to my stomach. In the end, we both got through it just fine and walked away without hurting each other. I spent days trying to prepare myself for that first experience, but after it was over, I felt more confident and relaxed that I could do this. At my externship site, I was able to perform several venipunctures a day, which raised my confidence level. Today venipuncture is my favorite responsibility of all. I would draw blood all day if I could. I know I could even draw with my eyes closed, but never would, of course! ∎

What Would You Do? What Would You *Not* Do?

Case Study 3

Maud Gabriel is at the office complaining of persistent headaches and abdominal pain over the past 3 months. The physician gives Mrs. Gabriel a laboratory requisition to have her blood drawn and tested at an outside laboratory. Mrs. Gabriel says that her daughter who lives with her works as a phlebotomist at the local hospital. Mrs. Gabriel wants to know whether her daughter can draw her blood at home and then drop it off at the laboratory. She says that the last time she had her blood drawn, they had to stick her 2 times and then she got a big bruise on her arm afterward. She says the laboratory technician kept digging around in her arm to find the vein and that it was quite painful. ∎

SYRINGE METHOD OF VENIPUNCTURE

The syringe method is the least used method of venipuncture. This is because the amount of blood that can be collected is limited by the capacity of the syringe being used. In addition, after the blood specimen is obtained, it must be transferred from the syringe to an evacuated tube. This

requires an additional step in the venipuncture procedure, which is time-consuming.

The syringe method is used primarily to obtain blood from small veins that are likely to collapse from the use of the vacuum tube method. Because the rate of blood flow into the syringe is not dictated by the premeasured vacuum of an evacuated tube, the syringe method offers better control than other methods of venipuncture. When the vein has been punctured, the specimen is obtained by pulling back on the plunger of the syringe. Pulling the plunger back slowly minimizes pressure against the vein wall, so that the vein is less likely to collapse.

The setup for the syringe method includes a disposable needle and syringe. The gauge of the needle ranges from 21 G to 23 G, and the length of the needle ranges from 1 to 1½ inches. For extremely small veins, a 23 G needle should be used to prevent rupture of the vein by a larger needle. The capacity of the syringe depends on the amount of specimen required and ranges from 5 ml to 20 ml. If more than 20 ml is required, a second venipuncture must be performed; this is another disadvantage of this method.

After the blood specimen is collected, it must be transferred to an evacuated tube. The OSHA Bloodborne Pathogens Standard requires the use of a needleless device to transfer the blood specimen from the syringe to an evacuated tube. Transferring the specimen with the needle used to collect the specimen is prohibited by OSHA because it increases the risk of a needlestick injury. The needle must be removed from the syringe, and a needleless device must be attached to the syringe. The evacuated tube can then be safely filled. Procedure 17-3 describes the venipuncture procedure using a syringe, including the proper method for transferring the blood specimen to an evacuated tube.

When multiple tubes are to be filled, follow the proper order of fill. The order of fill recommended by the Clinical and Laboratory Standards Institute (CLSI) for the syringe method is identical to the order of draw for the vacuum tube and butterfly methods (previously presented). Following this order of fill prevents contamination of nonadditive tubes and cross-contamination of additive tubes. Tubes with additives should be gently inverted back and forth 8 to 10 times immediately after they are filled.

PROCEDURE 17-3   Venipuncture—Syringe Method

Outcome Perform a venipuncture using the syringe method.

Equipment/Supplies

- Disposable gloves
- Tourniquet
- Antiseptic wipe
- Syringe and needle with a safety shield
- Evacuated tubes with labels
- Needleless blood transfer device

- Test tube rack
- Sterile 2 × 2 gauze pad
- Adhesive bandage
- Biohazard sharps container
- Biohazard specimen bag
- Laboratory request form

1. Procedural Step. Follow procedural steps 1 through 3 of the butterfly method of venipuncture (see Procedure 17-2).

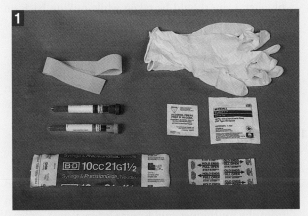

Assemble the equipment.

2. Procedural Step. Prepare the needle and syringe, making sure to keep the needle and the inside of the syringe sterile. Break the seal on the syringe by moving the plunger back and forth several times. Loosen the cap on the needle, and check that the hub is screwed tightly into the syringe.

3. Procedural Step. Place the evacuated tubes to be filled in a test tube rack on a work surface. If an evacuated tube contains a powdered additive, tap the tube just below the stopper to release any additive adhering to the stopper. Ensure that the tubes are placed in the correct order to be filled. Open the sterile gauze packet, and place the gauze pad on the inside of its wrapper.
Principle. If an additive remains trapped in the stopper, erroneous test results may occur.

4. Procedural Step. Follow procedural steps 7 through 12 of the butterfly method of venipuncture.

5. Procedural Step. Reapply the tourniquet. Apply gloves. Remove the cap from the needle. Hold the syringe by placing the thumb of the dominant hand on top of the syringe while supporting the underside of the syringe with the pads of the first three fingers. The needle should be positioned with the bevel facing up.
Principle. Gloves provide a barrier against bloodborne pathogens. Positioning the needle with the bevel up allows easier entry into the skin and the vein, resulting in less pain for the patient.

Continued

6. **Procedural Step.** Anchor the vein. Grasp the patient's arm with the nondominant hand. The thumb should be placed 1 to 2 inches below and to the side of the puncture site. Using the thumb, draw the skin taut over the vein in the direction of the patient's hand.
   Principle. The thumb helps hold the skin taut for easier entry and helps stabilize the vein to be punctured.

7. **Procedural Step.** Rest the backs of the fingertips on the patient's forearm. Position the needle at a 15-degree angle to the arm. Make sure the needle points in the same direction as the vein to be entered. Position the needle so that it enters the vein approximately ⅛ inch below the place where the vein is to be entered.
   Principle. An angle of less than 15 degrees may cause the needle to enter above the vein, preventing puncture. An angle of more than 15 degrees may cause the needle to go through the vein by puncturing the posterior wall. This could result in a hematoma.

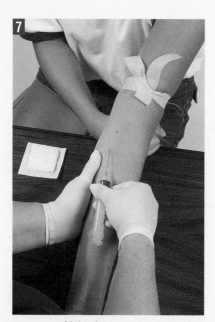

Make the puncture.

8. **Procedural Step.** Tell the patient that he or she will "feel a small stick," and with one continuous steady motion, enter the skin and then the vein. You will feel a sensation of resistance followed by a "release" as the vein is entered. When the "release" is felt, you have entered the vein and should not advance the needle any farther.
   Principle. Using one continuous motion helps to prevent tissue damage.

9. **Procedural Step.** Stabilize the syringe by firmly grasping it between the thumb and the underlying fingers to prevent the needle from moving. Do *not* change hands during the procedure. Blood may enter the top of the syringe spontaneously. If not, pull back gently on the plunger until blood begins to enter the syringe.
   Principle. Stabilizing the syringe prevents the needle from moving when blood is pulled into the syringe with the plunger. Changing hands may cause the needle to move, which is painful for the patient.

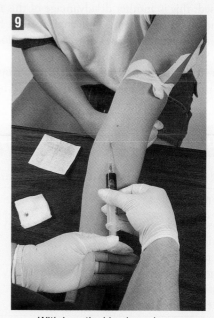

Withdraw the blood specimen.

10. **Procedural Step.** Remove the desired amount of blood by pulling back slowly and gently on the plunger. Care should be taken while pulling back on the plunger to prevent the accidental withdrawal of the needle from the patient's arm.
    Principle. Pulling back on the plunger causes a suction effect, which draws the blood into the syringe. The blood should be withdrawn slowly from the vein to prevent hemolysis and to prevent the vein from collapsing.

11. **Procedural Step.** Remove the tension from the tourniquet by pulling upward on one of the flaps of the tourniquet. Ask the patient to unclench the fist.
    Principle. The tourniquet tension must be removed before the needle. Otherwise, the pressure on the vein from the tourniquet could cause internal and external bleeding around the puncture site.

12. **Procedural Step.** Place a sterile gauze pad slightly above the site, and slowly withdraw the needle at the same angle as for penetration. Immediately move the gauze pad over the puncture site, and apply firm pressure. (*Note:* Do not apply pressure to the puncture site until the needle is completely removed.)

PROCEDURE 17-3 Venipuncture—Syringe Method—cont'd

Principle. Placing the gauze pad over the puncture site helps prevent tissue movement as the needle is withdrawn and reduces patient discomfort. Careful withdrawal prevents further tissue damage.

13. Procedural Step. Activate the safety shield on the needle, and place the needle and syringe on the tray. Inspect the shield to make sure it has locked into place. *Principle.* The safety shield must be activated to prevent an accidental needlestick when the needle is removed from the syringe.

14. Procedural Step. Continue to apply pressure with the gauze pad. Cooperative patients can be asked to assist by applying pressure with the gauze pad for 1 to 2 minutes. The arm can be elevated to facilitate clot formation. Do not allow the patient to bend the arm at the elbow because this increases blood loss from the puncture site. *Principle.* Applying pressure reduces the leakage of blood from the puncture site externally or internally. Internal leakage into the tissues could result in a hematoma.

15. Procedural Step. Transfer the blood to the labeled evacuated tubes as soon as possible, as follows:
a. Double-check that the tubes are in the correct order of fill in the test tube rack.
b. Remove the needle encased in the safety shield from the syringe, using a mechanical unwinder (e.g., a mechanical unwinder on a sharps container), and discard it in a biohazard sharps container.
c. Hold the syringe vertically, and immediately insert the tip of the syringe into the hub of the needleless

blood transfer device. Turn the syringe clockwise to secure it.
d. Insert the first evacuated tube into the blood transfer device/syringe assembly, and allow the vacuum to fill the tube. Do not apply pressure to the plunger of the syringe.
e. If the blood is added to a tube containing a clot activator, it must be mixed immediately by gently inverting the tube back and forth 5 times.
f. If the blood is added to a tube containing an anticoagulant, it must be mixed immediately by gently inverting the tube back and forth 8 to 10 times.
g. Continue until all evacuated tubes have been filled.
Principle. OSHA requires the use of a needleless transfer device to transfer blood from a syringe to an evacuated tube to reduce the risk of a needlestick injury. A delay in transferring the blood to the evacuated tubes causes clotting of the blood in the syringe. The suction action of the vacuum tube automatically draws the blood into the tube. Tubes that contain an anticoagulant must be inverted immediately to prevent the blood from clotting. Careful mixing of the blood with the anticoagulant prevents hemolysis.

16. Procedural Step. Properly dispose of the entire assembly (syringe and blood transfer device) in a biohazard sharps container. *Principle.* Proper disposal is required by the OSHA Standard.

17. Procedural Step. Follow procedural steps 26 through 29 of the butterfly method of venipuncture.

PROBLEMS ENCOUNTERED WITH VENIPUNCTURE

Sometimes the medical assistant encounters problems when attempting to draw blood from a patient. The appropriate response depends on the type of problem.

Failure to Obtain Blood

Periodically, even individuals highly skilled at performing venipuncture have difficulty obtaining blood. Although large and prominent veins make it easier to collect the blood specimen, conditions often exist that make the procedure more difficult.

It is often difficult to draw blood from obese patients who have small, superficial veins and whose veins suitable for venipuncture are buried in adipose tissue. Elderly patients with arteriosclerosis may have veins that are thick and hard, making them difficult to puncture. Other patients have veins that are small or have a thin wall, making the veins likely to collapse. After two unsuccessful attempts at venipuncture, the medical assistant should seek assistance in obtaining the blood specimen.

Factors that result in failure to obtain blood after the needle has been inserted include not inserting the needle far enough, preventing it from entering the vein (Figure 17-21); insertion of the needle too far, causing it to go through the vein; and the bevel opening becoming lodged against the wall of the vein. In these instances, most authorities recommend removal of the needle, rather than trying to probe the vein. Probing is often uncomfortable for the patient and can affect the integrity of the blood specimen, leading to inaccurate test results. Occasionally, an evacuated tube loses its vacuum because of a manufacturing defect or through improper handling of the tube. If suspected, this problem can be corrected by removing the defective tube and inserting another vacuum tube.

Inappropriate Puncture Sites

If a patient complains of pain or soreness in a potential venipuncture site, this area should be avoided. In addition, any skin areas that are scarred, bruised, burned, or adjacent to areas of infection should not be used. A venipuncture should not be performed on an arm with edema or an arm

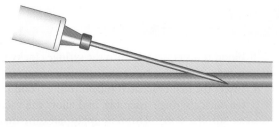

A. Correct insertion of the needle into the vein.

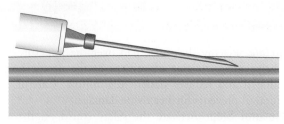

B. Improper angle of insertion (<15°), causing the needle to enter above the vein.

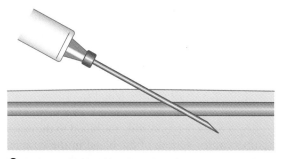

C. Improper angle of insertion (>15°), causing the needle to go through the vein.

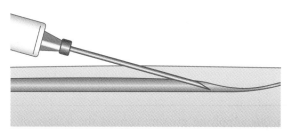

D. Collapsed vein (most likely to occur in persons with small veins).

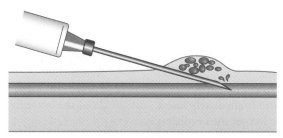

E. The beveled opening is partially within and partially outside of the vein, causing a hematoma.

Figure 17-21. Problems encountered with venipuncture.

on the same side as a mastectomy. Swelling makes is more difficult to locate a vein and results in a longer time for healing of the puncture site to occur. Other sites to avoid include an arm that has a cast applied to it and an arm on the same side as a radical mastectomy.

Scarred and Sclerosed Veins

An individual who has had many venipunctures over a period of years often develops scar tissue in the wall of the vein. Elderly patients may have veins that have become thickened from arteriosclerosis. In both cases, the veins feel stiff and hard when palpated. A scarred or sclerosed vein is difficult to stick, and the blood return may be poor owing to a narrowed lumen; it is recommended that another vein be used for the venipuncture. If this is impossible, the needle should be inserted with careful pressure to avoid going completely through the vein.

Rolling Veins

The median cubital vein, located in the center of the antecubital space, is considered the best vein for a venipuncture. Sometimes it is impossible to use this vein, however, such as when it lies deep in the tissues and cannot be palpated or is scarred from repeated venipunctures. The veins on either side of the median cubital (cephalic or basilic) can be used, but they have a tendency to "roll," or move away from the needle, escaping puncture. To prevent rolling, firm pressure should be applied below and to the side of the vein to stabilize it as the needle is inserted.

Collapsing Veins

Veins are most likely to collapse in individuals who have small veins or veins with thin walls. This is particularly true when the vacuum tube method is used. The "sucking action" exerted on the vein when the pressure in the vacuum is released causes the vein to collapse, blocking the flow of blood into the tube (see Figure 17-21). The typical result observed is that a small amount of blood enters the tube and then stops. Because better control and less pressure on the vein is possible, the butterfly or syringe method of venipuncture is recommended to obtain the specimen in patients with small veins.

Premature Needle Withdrawal

Patient movement or improper venipuncture technique can cause the needle to come out of the vein prematurely. Because of the pressure exerted by the tourniquet, blood may be forced out of the puncture site, and immediate action is required to prevent a hematoma. The tourniquet should be removed at once, a gauze pad placed on the puncture site, and pressure applied until the bleeding has stopped.

Hematoma

A hematoma is caused by blood leaking from the puncture site of the vein and into the surrounding tissues, resulting in a bruise. A hematoma is caused by a needle that is inserted too far and goes through the vein, a bevel opening that is partially in the vein and partially out of the vein (see Figure 17-21), and insufficient pressure applied to the puncture site after removing the needle. The first sign of a hematoma is a sudden swelling around the puncture site. If this occurs when the needle is in the patient's vein, first the tourniquet and then the needle should be removed immediately, and pressure should be applied to the puncture site until the bleeding stops.

Hemolysis

The blood specimen should be handled carefully at all times. Blood cells are fragile, and rough handling may cause hemolysis, or breakdown of the blood cells. Hemolyzed blood specimens produce inaccurate test results. To prevent hemolysis, these guidelines should be followed:

1. Store the vacuum tubes at room temperature because chilled tubes can result in hemolysis.
2. Allow the alcohol to air-dry completely before performing the venipuncture. Alcohol entering a blood specimen can cause hemolysis.
3. Use an appropriate-gauge needle to collect the specimen. Using a small-gauge needle (e.g., 25 G) can cause the blood cells to rupture as they pass through the lumen of the needle.
4. Practice good technique in collecting the specimen; excessive trauma to the blood vessel can result in hemolysis.
5. Always handle the blood tube carefully; do not shake it or handle it roughly.

Fainting

Occasionally, a patient experiences dizziness or fainting during or after a venipuncture. Should this occur, the most immediate concern is to protect the patient from injury, for example, by preventing the patient from falling. The patient should be placed in a position that promotes blood flow to the brain, and the physician should be notified for further treatment; see the box *Highlight on Vasovagal Syncope (Fainting)*.

Highlight on Vasovagal Syncope (Fainting)

Most people experience no change in their sense of well-being when they have blood taken. A very small percentage of individuals experience a type of fainting, however, known as *vasovagal syncope.*

Cause and Symptoms

Vasovagal syncope is caused by unpleasant physical or emotional stimuli, such as pain, fright, and the sight of blood. A sudden pooling of blood occurs, which results in a sudden decrease in blood pressure. This momentarily deprives the brain of blood, causing a temporary loss of consciousness, usually lasting only 1 to 2 minutes. Vasovagal syncope usually occurs when an individual is in an upright position, as in standing or sitting. Before fainting, the patient usually experiences some warning signals, such as sudden light-headedness, nausea, weakness, yawning, paleness, blurred vision, a feeling of warmth, and sweating followed by drooping eyelids; a weak, rapid pulse; and finally unconsciousness.

Treatment

A person who is about to faint should be placed in a position that facilitates blood flow to the brain and told to breathe deeply. The preferred position is lying down (supine) with the legs elevated and the collar and clothing loosened. This position may not always be possible, such as when a patient is seated and the venipuncture needle has already been inserted. In this case, the tourniquet and then the needle should be removed, and the patient's head should be lowered between the legs. An individual who has fainted should be protected from injury by falling and should be placed in a position that facilitates blood flow to the brain, as just described.

Prevention

Fainting during or after venipuncture is more likely in the following individuals: patients having a venipuncture for the first time, young patients, thin patients, patients with a low diastolic or high systolic blood pressure, patients with a history of fainting, nervous and apprehensive patients, and patients who are very quiet or very talkative. Fainting often can be prevented by identifying and closely observing individuals who are more likely to faint (as described). Talking to the patient often helps relax the patient and divert attention from the venipuncture procedure. If a patient has a history of fainting, he or she should be in a semi-Fowler's position for the venipuncture procedure because people rarely faint in this position. Other factors that contribute to fainting and that should be avoided include fatigue, lack of sleep, hunger, and environmental factors, such as a noisy, crowded, or overheated room. ■

OBTAINING A SERUM SPECIMEN
Serum

Serum is plasma from which the clotting factor fibrinogen has been removed. A brief discussion of serum is presented here, and a thorough discussion of plasma is presented later in this chapter.

Serum is normally clear in appearance and light yellow to yellow in color. Serum contains many dissolved substances, such as glucose, cholesterol, sodium, potassium, chloride, antibodies, hormones, and enzymes. As a result, many laboratory tests require a serum specimen to determine whether these substances are within normal limits and to detect substances that should not normally be in the serum, and that, if present, indicate a pathologic condition.

Tube Selection

A tube without an anticoagulant (e.g., red-stoppered or SST) must be used to collect the blood specimen, to allow the specimen to separate into serum and clotted blood cells. Because the amount of serum recovered is only a portion of the specimen, a blood specimen must be drawn that is 2.5 times the amount required for the test. If 2 ml of serum is required, a 5-ml tube of blood must be collected; if 3 ml of serum is required, an 8-ml tube is collected, and if 4 ml of serum is required, a 10-ml tube is collected.

Preparation of the Specimen

After the blood specimen has been collected, the red-stoppered tube or SST must be allowed to stand upright at room temperature for 30 to 45 minutes before being centrifuged. This allows clot formation of the blood cells, which yields more serum from the specimen. If the specimen is centrifuged too soon after collection of the blood specimen, the clotting factors do not have an opportunity to settle down into the cell layer to form a whole blood clot. The result of this is the formation of a *fibrin clot* in the serum layer. A fibrin clot is a spongy substance that occupies space, interfering with adequate serum collection (Figure 17-22). The blood specimen should not be allowed to stand for longer than 1 hour, however, because leaching of substances from the cell layer into the serum may occur. This leaching of substances changes the integrity of the serum, leading to inaccurate test results.

Removal of Serum

After the blood cells have clotted by allowing the specimen to stand, the specimen is centrifuged for 10 minutes. If a red-stoppered tube has been used to collect the specimen, the serum is removed from the clot using a pipet and is placed in a separate transfer tube. It is important that proper technique be employed in removing the serum, to avoid disturbing the cell layer of the clot and drawing red blood cells into the serum layer. If cells do enter the serum, the entire specimen must be recentrifuged.

When the serum has been removed from the blood specimen, the medical assistant should hold the specimen

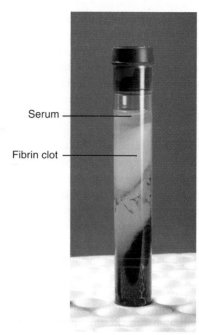

Figure 17-22. A fibrin clot may interfere with adequate collection of serum.

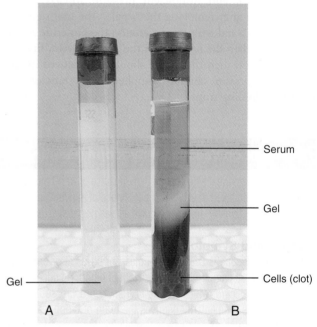

Figure 17-23. Serum separator tubes. **A,** An unused tube that contains the thixotropic gel in the bottom of the tube. **B,** A tube that has been used to collect a blood specimen. During centrifugation, the gel temporarily becomes fluid and moves to the dividing point between the serum and blood cells in a fibrin clot.

in the transfer tube up to good light. The serum specimen should be inspected for the presence of intact red blood cells or hemolyzed blood; in both cases, the specimen has a reddish appearance. A specimen that has a reddish appearance must be recentrifuged. If the specimen contains intact red blood cells, they settle to the bottom of the tube, and the serum can be removed. If the blood is hemolyzed, recentrifugation would not make the red color disappear because the red blood cells have ruptured and released hemoglobin into the serum. Hemolyzed serum is unsuitable for laboratory tests because the results would be inaccurate; another blood specimen must be collected. Procedure 17-4 presents the method for separating serum from whole blood using a conventional red-stoppered evacuated tube.

Serum Separator Tubes

A serum separator tube (SST), which is also known as a gel barrier tube, is an evacuated tube specially designed to facilitate the collection of a serum specimen. The SST tube is identified by a red/gray stopper (or gold stopper if using Hemogard tubes) and is used for collection and separation of blood. The serum separator tube contains a thixotropic gel, which is in a solid state at the bottom of the unused tube (Figure 17-23, A).

The blood specimen is collected and processed following the appropriate venipuncture method. The specimen must be allowed to stand in an upright position for 30 to 45 minutes for proper clot formation of the blood cells and centrifuged as previously described. During centrifugation, the gel temporarily becomes fluid and moves to the dividing point between the serum and clotted cells, where it re-forms into a solid gel, serving as a physical and chemical barrier between the serum and the clot (Figure 17-23, B). It is important to centrifuge the specimen for the proper length of time (i.e., 10 minutes). Centrifuging the specimen for less than 10 minutes can result in an incomplete gel barrier between the serum and the clot.

The serum can be transported or stored in the separator tube; the medical assistant must inspect the tube carefully to ensure that the gel barrier is firmly attached to the glass wall. If a complete barrier has not formed, the serum specimen must be removed and placed in a properly labeled transfer tube to prevent leaching of substances from the cell layer into the serum, affecting the accuracy of the test results.

PROCEDURE 17-4 Separating Serum from a Blood Specimen

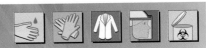

Outcome Separate serum from a blood specimen.

Equipment/Supplies

- Red evacuated tube setup
- Test tube rack
- Disposable pipet
- Transfer tube and label

- Disposable gloves
- Face shield or mask and an eye protection device
- Centrifuge
- Biohazard sharps container

1. Procedural Step. Collect the blood specimen by following the venipuncture procedure. Use a tube containing no anticoagulants (red-stoppered) to collect the specimen. The tube selected should have a capacity of 2½ times the amount of serum required. Label the red-stoppered tube and the transfer tube with the patient's name and date of birth, the date, and your initials. In addition, the transfer tube should bear the

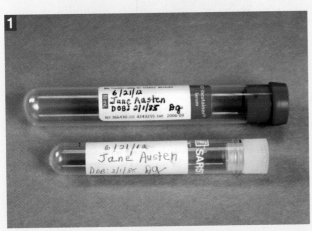

Label the tubes.

word "serum." Allow the tube to fill until the vacuum is exhausted.

Principle. To obtain serum, a tube containing no additives must be used. The tube must be allowed to fill completely to obtain the proper amount of serum. Several types of specimen, such as serum, plasma, and urine, are straw-colored; the transfer tube containing serum must be labeled as such to avoid confusion and mixup among these specimens.

2. Procedural Step. Place the blood specimen tube in an upright position in a test tube rack for 30 to 45 minutes at room temperature. To prevent evaporation of the serum sample, do not remove the tube's stopper.

Principle. Specimens must be placed in an upright position and allowed to stand to permit clot formation of the blood cells and avoid the formation of a fibrin clot in the serum, which yields more serum from the specimen. Evaporation of the sample leads to falsely elevated test results.

3. Procedural Step. Place the specimen in the centrifuge, stopper end up. Balance the specimen with the same type and weight of tube or another specimen tube. Make sure the tube is stoppered to prevent

Continued

PROCEDURE 17-4   **Separating Serum from a Blood Specimen—cont'd**

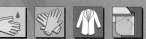

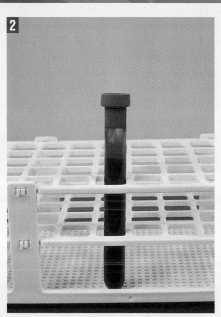

Allow the specimen to stand for 30 to 45 minutes.

Centrifuge the specimen.

evaporation of the sample during centrifugation. Centrifuge the specimen for 10 minutes. Allow the centrifuge to come to a complete stop after the timer goes off. Do not open the lid or try to stop the centrifuge with your hand.

Principle. Centrifuging packs the cells and causes them to settle at the bottom of the tube, yielding more serum. If the centrifuge is not balanced, it may vibrate and move across the table top. An unbalanced centrifuge also can cause specimen tubes to break.

Centrifuging the specimen for longer than 10 minutes can result in hemolysis of blood cells.

4. **Procedural Step.** Put on a face shield or a mask and an eye protection device such as goggles or glasses with solid side shields. Apply gloves. Carefully remove the tube from the centrifuge without disturbing the contents.

   Principle. The OSHA Standard requires the use of personal protective equipment whenever spraying or splashing of blood might be generated. Disturbing the contents may cause the cells to enter the serum, and the specimen will need to be recentrifuged.

5. **Procedural Step.** Using a twisting and pulling motion, carefully remove the stopper from the tube, pointing the stopper away from you. Squeeze the bulb of the pipet to push the air out, then insert it into the serum. Place the tip of the pipet against the side of the tube approximately ¼ inch above the cell layer. Release the bulb to suction serum into the pipet. Do not allow the tip of the pipet to touch the cell layer.

   Principle. Pointing the stopper away prevents accidental spraying or splashing of the specimen onto the medical assistant. The air should be removed from the bulb before inserting the pipet into the serum to prevent disturbance of the cell layer. If the cell layer is disturbed, red blood cells would enter the serum, and the specimen would need to be recentrifuged.

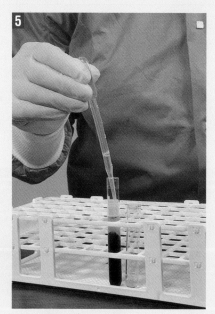

Pipet the serum.

6. **Procedural Step.** Transfer the serum in the pipet to the transfer tube. Continue pipetting until as much serum as possible is removed without disturbing the

PROCEDURE 17-4   Separating Serum from a Blood Specimen—cont'd

cell layer. Tightly cap the transfer tube to prevent sample evaporation.

7. Procedural Step. Hold the serum specimen up to the light, and examine it for the presence of hemolysis. Ensure that the proper amount of serum has been obtained.

Principle. Hemolyzed serum is unsuitable for laboratory testing.

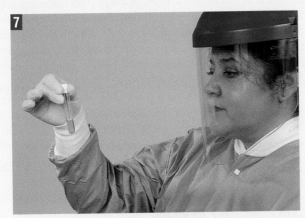

Examine the serum.

8. Procedural Step. Properly dispose of equipment. Following the OSHA Standard, the evacuated tube (containing the blood specimen) and the disposable pipet must be discarded in a biohazard sharps container.

9. Procedural Step. Remove the gloves, and sanitize your hands.

10. Procedural Step. Test the specimen, or prepare the specimen for transport to an outside laboratory for testing according to the medical office policy. If the specimen is to be transported to an outside laboratory, do the following:
   a. Place the specimen tube in a biohazard specimen bag.
   b. Place the laboratory request in the outside pocket of the biohazard bag.
   c. Properly store the specimen while awaiting pickup by a laboratory courier.
   d. Chart the date the specimen was transported to the laboratory in the patient's record.

OBTAINING A PLASMA SPECIMEN

Plasma

Plasma is the liquid portion of the blood and has the same appearance (clear) and color (light yellow to yellow) as serum. It serves as a transportation medium in which various substances are dissolved and blood cells are suspended for circulation through the body. Approximately 92% of plasma consists of water; the remaining 8% is dissolved solid substances (solutes) that are carried by the blood to and from the tissues.

The solutes present in greatest amounts are the *plasma proteins,* which include serum albumin, globulins, fibrinogen, and prothrombin. Serum albumin is synthesized in the liver and regulates the volume of plasma in the blood vessels. Globulins play an important role in the immunity mechanism of the body, and fibrinogen and prothrombin are essential for proper blood clotting.

Various *electrolytes* are carried by the plasma and are needed for normal cell functioning and maintenance of the normal fluid and acid-base balance of the body. Some of these electrolytes are sodium, chloride, potassium, calcium, phosphate, bicarbonate, and magnesium. *Nutrients* derived from the breakdown of food substances are carried by the plasma to nourish the tissues of the body and include glucose, amino acids, and lipids. *Waste products* formed as the by-products of metabolism are carried by the plasma to be excreted and include urea, uric acid, lactic acid, and creati-

nine. *Respiratory gases* are dissolved in and carried by the plasma and include carbon dioxide and a small amount of oxygen. Substances in the plasma that help regulate and control body functions include hormones, antibodies, enzymes, and vitamins.

Tube Selection

Sometimes a plasma specimen is required for a laboratory test. The procedure for separating plasma from whole blood is essentially the same as that for separating serum from whole blood, with minor variances, which are described here.

A tube containing an anticoagulant must be used to obtain plasma. The medical assistant should check the laboratory directory or the medical office laboratory procedures manual to determine the type of anticoagulant to be used, which is specified by the color of the tube stopper. The tube used to collect the specimen *and* the transfer tube should be properly labeled with a bar code label or manually labeled with the patient's name and date of birth, the date, and the medical assistant's initials. In addition, the transfer tube should bear the word "plasma."

Preparation and Removal of the Specimen

As with serum, a blood specimen must be collected that is 2.5 times the amount required for the test. Before collecting the specimen, evacuated tubes containing a powdered additive (e.g., gray-stoppered tube) should be tapped just below the stopper to release any of the anticoagulant that may have adhered to the stopper. It is important to allow the specimen to fill to the exhaustion of the vacuum to ensure the proper ratio of anticoagulant to blood, which ensures accurate test results.

Immediately after the specimen is drawn, the tube should be gently inverted back and forth 8 to 10 times to mix the anticoagulant with the blood specimen. The specimen is placed in a centrifuge with the stopper on for 10 minutes. (The specimen does not need to stand before it is centrifuged.) Centrifuging the specimen packs the blood cells and causes the blood to separate into three layers: a top layer of plasma, a middle layer (the buffy coat), and a bottom layer of red blood cells. The plasma is separated from the blood specimen using the same procedure as that outlined for the separation of serum from whole blood.

Plasma Separator Tube

A plasma separator tube (PST) containing the anticoagulant lithium heparin and a gel barrier may be required by the outside laboratory for the collection of plasma. When using conventional rubber stopper tubes, the color of the stopper is light green/gray, and when using a Hemogard closure tube, the color of the stopper is light green. The PST tube used to collect the specimen should be properly labeled with a bar code label or manually labeled with the patient's name and date of birth, the date, and the medical assistant's initials.

Immediately after the specimen is drawn, the PST tube should be gently inverted back and forth 8 to 10 times to mix the anticoagulant with the blood specimen. The specimen is placed in a centrifuge with the stopper on for 10 minutes. (The specimen does not need to stand before it is centrifuged.) During centrifugation, the gel temporarily becomes fluid and moves to the dividing point between the plasma and cells, where it re-forms into a solid gel, serving as a physical and chemical barrier between the plasma and the cells. The plasma must be removed and placed in a properly labeled transfer tube within 2 hours of collection.

SKIN PUNCTURE

A skin puncture is used to obtain a capillary blood specimen and is also called a *capillary puncture*. Laboratory testing of a capillary blood specimen is usually performed at the medical office. Examples of such tests are hemoglobin, hematocrit, blood glucose, mononucleosis, and prothrombin time.

A skin puncture is performed when a test requires only a small blood specimen. Skin puncture is the method preferred for obtaining blood from infants and young children. Collecting blood in this age group by venipuncture is often difficult and may damage veins and surrounding tissues. In addition, infants and young children have such a small blood volume that removing large quantities of blood may cause anemia. A skin puncture also might be performed as a last resort on an adult when a blood specimen is needed and there are no acceptable veins. Before collecting a capillary blood specimen, the medical assistant must (1) select a puncture site, (2) select the skin puncture device, and (3) obtain the proper microcollection device to collect the specimen.

PUNCTURE SITES

The puncture site varies depending on the age of the patient. The fingertip of the third or fourth finger is the preferred site for a skin puncture on an adult. In the past, the earlobe also was recommended as a skin puncture site for an adult. This is no longer true. Blood obtained by puncturing the earlobe has been found to contain a higher concentration of hemoglobin than fingertip blood. In addition, the earlobe produces a slower flow of blood, making it more difficult to obtain a blood specimen.

In an infant (birth to 1 year old), the skin puncture should be performed on the plantar surface of the heel. A finger puncture should *never* be performed on infants. The amount of tissue between skin surface and bone is so small that an injury to the bone is likely. After a child is walking, the skin puncture can be performed on the fingertip.

SKIN PUNCTURE DEVICES

According to OSHA, a skin puncture should be performed in the medical office using either a disposable or a reusable semiautomatic retractable lancet device. The device used to perform the skin puncture is a matter of personal preference, and the technique for performing the puncture depends on the device that is used. A description of skin puncture devices is presented next, and procedures for using them are presented at the end of this section.

Regardless of the skin puncture device, the puncture must not penetrate deeper than 3.1 mm on adults and 2.0 mm on infants (plantar surface of the heel) and children. If the puncture is deeper than this, the bone may be penetrated, which could result in the painful and serious conditions of osteochondritis or osteomyelitis. **Osteochondritis** is inflammation of bone and cartilage, and **osteomyelitis** is inflammation of the bone or bone marrow caused by bacterial infection. To avoid these complications, skin puncture devices are used with a spring-loaded blade (available in different lengths) to control the depth of puncture. The blade length used to perform a skin puncture is based on the sizes of the patient's fingers and the amount of blood specimen required. Adults with thin fingers and children require a shorter blade to avoid penetrating the bone. A longer blade must be used to obtain enough blood to fill a microcollection device, whereas a shorter blade can be used if only a drop of blood is needed.

OSHA does not recommend the use of lancets that are not retractable. A lancet that is not retractable increases the possibility that the medical assistant will stick himself or herself accidentally, resulting in an exposure incident. A disadvantage of a lancet that is spring-loaded and does not retract automatically is that some patients may become apprehensive and flinch when they see the point of the lancet. Children might pull their hands out of the medical assistant's grasp.

Disposable Semiautomatic Lancet

A disposable semiautomatic retractable lancet consists of a spring-loaded plastic holder with a metal blade inside the holder. Disposable lancets are available in different lengths of blades to control the depth of the puncture. The plastic holder may be color-coded by the manufacturer for ease in identifying the blade length of the lancet device, such as Surgilance Safety Lancets (Surgilance, Inc., Norcross, Ga) (Figure 17-24, *A*). The plastic holder conceals the blade so the patient cannot see it during the puncture, as with the CoaguChek Lancet (Roche Diagnostics, Branchburg, NJ) (Figure 17-24, *B*). Another example is the Quikheel Infant

Lancet (Becton Dickinson), which is used for heel punctures on infants.

To perform the skin puncture, the lancet device is placed on the patient's skin, and the device is activated. Depending on the brand, this is accomplished by one of the following methods:
- Depressing an activation button located on the top of the lancet until an audible click is heard (e.g., CoaguChek Lancet)
- Pushing the lancet firmly onto the puncture site until an audible click is heard (e.g., Surgilance Safety Lancet)

When the device is activated, the spring forces the blade into the skin and retracts the blade into the holder. The concealed blade and automatic puncture tend to result in less patient apprehension. After the puncture, the entire lancet device is discarded in a biohazard sharps container. Procedure 17-5 describes the skin puncture procedure using a disposable semiautomatic lancet.

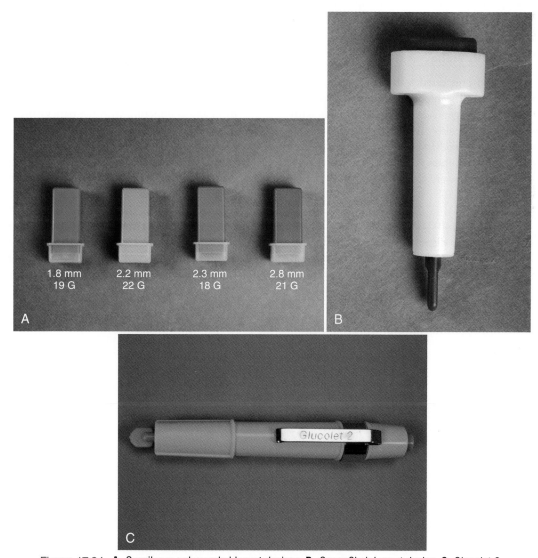

Figure 17-24. **A,** Surgilance color-coded lancet devices. **B,** CoaguChek Lancet device. **C,** Glucolet 2.

Reusable Semiautomatic Lancet

A wide variety of reusable semiautomatic lancets are commercially available; however, not all are appropriate for use in the medical office. Some of these devices are suitable for use only by an individual patient to perform home blood glucose monitoring. When used by more than one patient in the medical office, they have been associated with the transmission of hepatitis B. The safest reusable device is one in which the part that becomes contaminated is retractable and can be disposed of easily. This type of device reduces the risk of a sharps injury and infection from a contaminated sharp. An example of a reusable lancet that is safe to use in the medical office is the Glucolet II (Bayer Corporation, Morristown, NJ).

The Glucolet II consists of a plastic spring-loaded lancet holder and a retractable lancet/endcap (Figure 17-24, *C*). The lancet holder is reusable, whereas the lancet/endcap is retractable and disposable and is meant for only one use. To perform the puncture, the lancet/endcap is placed on the patient's skin, and a release button is depressed. The spring forces the blade into the skin and retracts the blade into the endcap. After the procedure, the lancet/endcap is discarded in a biohazard sharps container (Procedure 17-6).

MICROCOLLECTION DEVICES

After the skin has been punctured, a capillary blood specimen must be collected. The blood specimen can be collected directly onto a reagent strip, such as occurs with blood glucose monitors. It also can be collected in a small container known as a *microcollection device*. The device depends on the laboratory equipment running the test. Common microcollection devices are capillary tubes and microcollection tubes.

Capillary Tubes

A capillary tube consists of a disposable glass or plastic tube (see Figure 17-25). Depending on the size of the tube, it can hold 5 to 75 µl of blood. In the medical office, a capillary tube is used to collect a blood specimen for a hematocrit determination. This procedure is presented in Chapter 18.

Microcollection Tubes

A microcollection tube consists of a small plastic tube with a removable blood collector tip. The tip is designed to collect capillary blood from a skin puncture, which results in a relatively large blood specimen. After the specimen has been collected, the collector tip is removed, discarded, and replaced by a plastic plug. Microcollection tubes are available with or without anticoagulants. The plugs are color-coded and correspond to the color-coded evacuated tube system used in venipuncture. One such device is the Microtainer (Becton Dickinson) (Figure 17-25).

GUIDELINES FOR PERFORMING A FINGER PUNCTURE

1. If a laboratory test requires advance preparation, before you perform the finger puncture, verify that the patient has prepared properly. If this is not the case, do not collect the specimen unless directed otherwise by the physician. If the finger puncture is to be rescheduled, carefully review the preparation requirements with the patient.

2. The patient should be seated comfortably in a chair. The arm should be firmly supported and extended with the palmar surface of the hand facing up. Never perform a skin puncture with the patient sitting on a stool or standing. The patient may faint and injure himself or herself.

3. Instruct the patient to remain still during the procedure. Explain to the patient that the procedure should be relatively quick and only slightly uncomfortable. Just before making the puncture, tell the patient that he or she will "feel a small stick." This prevents startling the patient, which could cause the patient to move.

4. Use the lateral part of the tip of the third or fourth finger (middle or ring finger) of the nondominant hand for

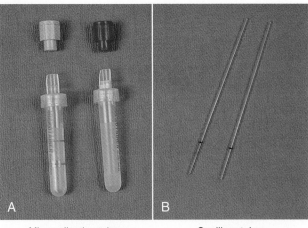

Microcollection tubes   Capillary tubes

Figure 17-25. Microcollection devices.

the puncture site. The capillary beds in these fingers are large, and the skin is easy to penetrate. The puncture site should be free of lesions, scars, bruises, and edema. The index finger is not recommended as a puncture site. The index finger is more calloused, which makes it harder to penetrate than the other fingers. Also, the patient uses that finger more and would notice the pain longer. The little finger also should not be used as a puncture site. The amount of tissue between the skin surface and the bone is so small that using this finger as a puncture site could result in injury to the bone.

5. After selecting the puncture site, warm the site to increase the blood flow to the capillary bed. Warming the site can be accomplished by gently massaging the finger 5 or 6 times from base to tip, or by placing the hand in warm water for a few minutes (105° F [40° C]). Warming the site promotes bleeding after an effective puncture.

6. Cleanse the site with an antiseptic wipe, and allow it to dry thoroughly. The site must be dry to allow a round drop of blood to form on the finger. Otherwise, the drop would leach out onto the skin of the patient's finger and be difficult to collect. In addition, alcohol entering the capillary specimen contaminates it, leading to inaccurate test results. Alcohol also causes the patient to experience a stinging sensation when the puncture is made.

7. Firmly grasp the finger in front of the most distal knuckle joint. Apply enough pressure to cause the fingertip to become hard and red so that adequate penetration and depth of puncture will occur.

8. Make the puncture in the fleshy portion of the fingertip, slightly to the side of center. To prevent injury to the bone, do not puncture the side or very tip of the finger. The blade of the lancet should be positioned so that the puncture is perpendicular to the lines of the fingerprint rather than parallel to the fingerprint (Figure 17-26). This facilitates the formation of a well-formed drop of blood that is easy to collect. A puncture that is not perpendicular causes the blood flow to follow the lines of the fingerprint and run down the finger, making it difficult to collect.

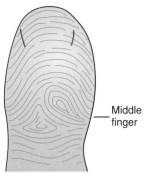

Figure 17-26. Recommended sites for a finger puncture.

9. Firmly press the lancet device against the puncture site, and activate the spring-loaded puncturing device. If a good puncture has been made, the blood flows freely. When learning this procedure, many individuals do not apply enough pressure to obtain a puncture that is deep enough. If this occurs, a poor blood flow results, and the patient has to be punctured again. A deep puncture hurts no more than a superficial one and provides a much better blood flow.

10. Wipe away the first drop of blood with a gauze pad. The first drop of blood is diluted with alcohol and tissue fluid and is not a suitable specimen for testing. Using the first drop of blood may lead to inaccurate test results.

11. Allow a large drop of blood to form by applying continual gentle pressure near the puncture site. Collect the blood specimen using a reagent strip or the appropriate microcollection device. If the required amount of blood is not obtained, you can gently massage the tissue surrounding the puncture site to promote blood flow. Do not squeeze or massage excessively because doing so causes dilution of the blood specimen with tissue fluids, which can affect the accuracy of the test results.

12. Check the puncture site to make sure the bleeding has stopped. Apply an adhesive bandage, if needed. A bandage is not recommended for children younger than 2 years old. The bandage may irritate the skin of a young child, and the child might put the bandage in his or her mouth, aspirate it, and choke.

PROCEDURE 17-5 Skin Puncture—Disposable Semiautomatic Lancet Device

Outcome Obtain a capillary blood specimen.

Equipment/Supplies

- Disposable gloves
- Antiseptic wipe
- CoaguChek lancet

- Sterile 2 × 2 gauze pad
- Adhesive bandage
- Biohazard sharps container

Continued

**PROCEDURE 17-5   Skin Puncture—Disposable Semiautomatic
Lancet Device—cont'd**

1. **Procedural Step.** Sanitize your hands.
2. **Procedural Step.** Greet the patient and introduce yourself. Identify the patient by asking the patient to state his or her full name and date of birth. Compare this information with the demographic data in the patient's chart. If the patient was required to prepare for the test (e.g., fasting, medication restriction), determine whether he or she has prepared properly. If the patient has not followed the patient preparation requirements, notify the physician for instructions on handling this situation.
3. **Procedural Step.** Assemble the equipment. Open the sterile gauze packet and lay it flat to allow the gauze pad to rest on the inside of its wrapper.

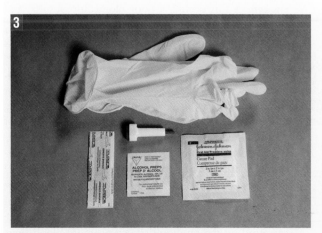

Assemble the equipment.

4. **Procedural Step.** Explain the procedure to the patient, and reassure the patient.
   Principle. Reassurance should be offered to reduce apprehension.
5. **Procedural Step.** Seat the patient comfortably in a chair. The patient's arm should be firmly supported and extended with the palmar surface of the hand facing up.
6. **Procedural Step.** Select an appropriate puncture site. Use the lateral part of the tip of the third or fourth finger of the nondominant hand to make the puncture. If the patient's finger is cold, you can warm it by gently massaging the finger 5 or 6 times from base to tip, or by placing the hand in warm water for a few minutes.
   Principle. Warming the site increases the blood flow to the area and promotes bleeding from the puncture site.
7. **Procedural Step.** Cleanse the site with an antiseptic wipe. Allow the site to air-dry, and after cleansing it, do not touch the area, wipe the area with gauze, or fan the area with your hand.

Principle. The site must be allowed to air-dry to allow enough time for the alcohol to destroy microorganisms on the patient's skin. If the site is dry, a round drop of blood forms on the finger, making it easy to collect the specimen. If the site is not dry, the blood leaches out and runs down the finger, making it difficult to collect. Residual alcohol entering the blood specimen can cause hemolysis, leading to inaccurate test results. In addition, residual alcohol causes the patient to experience a stinging sensation when the puncture is made. Touching or fanning the area causes contamination, and the cleansing process has to be repeated.

8. **Procedural Step.** Apply gloves. Using a twisting motion, remove the plastic post from the lancet.
   Principle. Gloves provide a barrier precaution against bloodborne pathogens.
9. **Procedural Step.** Without touching the puncture site, firmly grasp the patient's finger in front of the most distal knuckle joint. Apply enough pressure to cause the fingertip to become hard and red. Position the blade of the lancet perpendicular to the lines of the fingerprint on the fleshy portion of the fingertip, slightly to the side of center.
   Principle. The site must be grasped with enough pressure so that adequate penetration and depth of puncture can occur. Punctures that are not perpendicular cause the blood to run down the finger, making it difficult to collect. Puncturing the side or tip of the finger may cause the lancet to penetrate the bone.

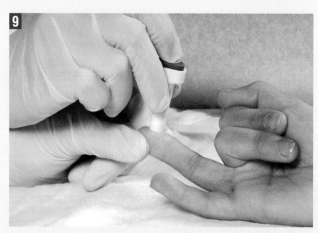

Make the puncture.

10. **Procedural Step.** Firmly depress the activation button, without moving the lancet or finger, until an audible click is heard. Pressing the activation button causes the lancet to puncture the skin and then retract into its plastic casing. A well-made puncture results in

a free-flowing wound that needs only slight pressure to make it bleed.

Principle. Moving the lancet or finger before the process is complete can result in an inadequate puncture and poor blood flow.

11. **Procedural Step.** Immediately dispose of the lancet device in a biohazard sharps container.

Principle. Proper disposal of contaminated sharps is required by the OSHA Standard to prevent exposure to bloodborne pathogens.

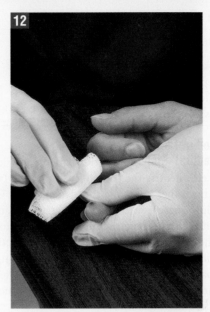

Wipe away the first drop of blood.

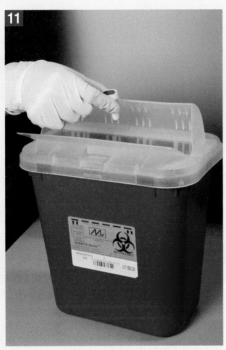

Discard the lancet.

12. **Procedural Step.** Wait a few seconds to allow blood flow to begin. Wipe away the first drop of blood with a gauze pad.

Principle. The first drop of blood is diluted with alcohol and tissue fluid and is not a suitable specimen.

13. **Procedural Step.** Use the second drop of blood for the test. Allow a large well-rounded drop of blood to form by holding the hand in a downward position and applying gentle continuous pressure without squeezing the finger. You can massage the tissue surrounding the puncture firmly but gently to encourage blood flow.

Principle. Squeezing or massaging the site excessively causes dilution of the blood sample with tissue fluid, leading to inaccurate test results.

14. **Procedural Step.** Collect the blood specimen on a test strip or in the appropriate microcollection device.

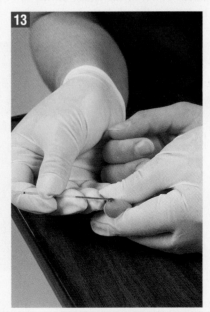

Collect the specimen.

15. **Procedural Step.** Have the patient hold a gauze pad over the puncture and apply pressure until the bleeding stops. As a safety precaution, remain with the patient until the bleeding stops. If needed, apply an adhesive bandage.

16. **Procedural Step.** Test the blood specimen by following the manufacturer's instructions that accompany the blood analyzer or testing kit.

17. **Procedural Step.** Remove the gloves, and sanitize your hands.

PROCEDURE 17-6   Skin Puncture—Reusable Semiautomatic Lancet Device

Outcome Obtain a capillary blood specimen.

Equipment/Supplies

- Disposable gloves
- Antiseptic wipe
- Glucolet II lancet device
- Disposable retractable lancet/endcap

- Sterile 2 × 2 gauze pad
- Adhesive bandage
- Biohazard sharps container

1. **Procedural Step.** Sanitize your hands.
2. **Procedural Step.** Greet the patient and introduce yourself. Identify the patient by asking the patient to state his or her full name and date of birth. Compare this information with the demographic data in the patient's chart. If the patient was required to prepare for the test (e.g., fasting, medication restriction), determine whether he or she has prepared properly. If the patient has not followed the patient preparation requirements, notify the physician for instructions on handling this situation.
3. **Procedural Step.** Assemble the equipment. Push the transparent barrel of the lancet device toward the release button until it clicks into place.

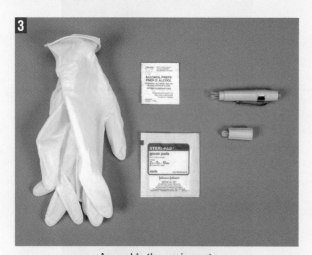

Assemble the equipment.

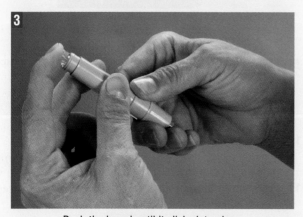

Push the barrel until it clicks into place.

4. **Procedural Step.** Insert the retractable lancet/endcap onto the lancet device. Open the sterile gauze packet and lay it flat to allow the gauze pad to rest on the inside of its wrapper.

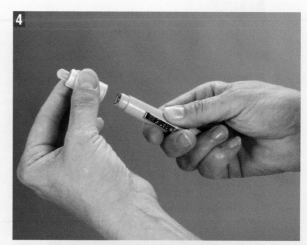

Insert the retractable lancet onto the device.

5. **Procedural Step.** Explain the procedure to the patient, and reassure the patient.
   Principle. Reassurance should be offered to reduce apprehension.
6. **Procedural Step.** Seat the patient comfortably in a chair. The patient's arm should be firmly supported and extended with the palmar surface of the hand facing up.
7. **Procedural Step.** Select an appropriate puncture site. Use the lateral part of the tip of the third or fourth finger of the nondominant hand to make the puncture. If the patient's finger is cold, you can warm it by gently massaging the finger 5 or 6 times from base to tip, or by placing the hand in warm water for a few minutes.
   Principle. Warming the site increases the blood flow to the area and promotes bleeding from the puncture site.
8. **Procedural Step.** Cleanse the site with an antiseptic wipe. Allow the site to air-dry, and after cleansing it, do not touch the area or fan the area with your hand.

PROCEDURE 17-6   Skin Puncture—Reusable Semiautomatic Lancet Device—cont'd

Principle. The site must be allowed to air-dry to allow enough time for the alcohol to destroy microorganisms on the patient's skin. If the site is dry, a round drop of blood forms on the finger, making it easy to collect the specimen. If the site is not dry, the blood leaches out and runs down the finger, making it difficult to collect. Residual alcohol entering the blood specimen can cause hemolysis, leading to inaccurate test results. In addition, residual alcohol causes the patient to experience a stinging sensation when the puncture is made. Touching or fanning the area causes contamination, and the cleansing process has to be repeated.

9. Procedural Step. Apply gloves. Using a twisting motion, remove the plastic post from the lancet/endcap.

Principle. Gloves provide a barrier against bloodborne pathogens.

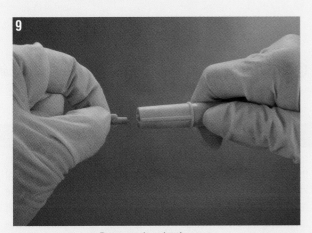

Remove the plastic post.

10. Procedural Step. Without touching the puncture site, firmly grasp the patient's finger in front of the most distal knuckle joint. Apply enough pressure to cause the fingertip to become hard and red. Position the blade of the lancet perpendicular to the lines of the fingerprint on the fleshy portion of the fingertip slightly to the side of center.

Principle. The site must be grasped with enough pressure so that adequate penetration and depth of puncture can occur. Punctures that are not perpendicular cause the blood to run down the finger, making it difficult to collect. Puncturing the side or tip of the finger may cause the lancet to penetrate the bone.

11. Procedural Step. Firmly press the activation button without moving the Glucolet or finger. Pressing the activation button causes the lancet to puncture the skin and then retract into the endcap. A well-made

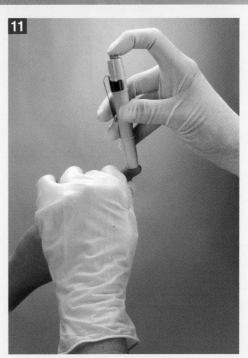

Make the puncture.

puncture results in a free-flowing wound that needs only slight pressure to make it bleed.

Principle. Moving the lancet or finger before the process is complete can result in an inadequate puncture and poor blood flow.

12. Procedural Step. Wait a few seconds to allow blood flow to begin. Wipe away the first drop of blood with a gauze pad.

Principle. The first drop of blood is diluted with alcohol and tissue fluid and is not a suitable specimen.

13. Procedural Step. Use the second drop of blood for the test. Allow a large well-rounded drop of blood to form by holding the hand in a downward position and applying gentle continuous pressure without squeezing the finger. The tissue surrounding the puncture site can be massaged firmly but gently to encourage blood flow.

Principle. Squeezing or massaging the site excessively causes dilution of the blood sample with tissue fluid, leading to inaccurate test results.

14. Procedural Step. Collect the blood specimen on a test strip or in the appropriate microcollection device as required by the test being performed.

15. Procedural Step. Have the patient hold a gauze pad over the puncture site, and apply pressure until the bleeding stops. As a safety precaution, remain with the patient until the bleeding stops. If needed, apply an adhesive bandage.

Continued

PROCEDURE 17-6

PROCEDURE 17-6   Skin Puncture—Reusable Semiautomatic Lancet Device—cont'd

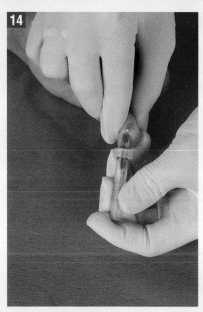

Collect the specimen.

16. **Procedural Step.** Remove the endcap from the lancet device, and discard it in a biohazard sharps container.
17. **Procedural Step.** Test the blood specimen by following the manufacturer's instructions that accompany the blood analyzer or testing kit.
18. **Procedural Step.** Remove the gloves, and sanitize your hands.
19. **Procedural Step.** Sanitize and disinfect the Glucolet II according to the manufacturer's instructions. Store the Glucolet II in its resting position.

℮volve *Check out the Evolve site to access additional interactive activities.*

MEDICAL PRACTICE *and the* LAW

Phlebotomy is an invasive procedure that can harm the patient if performed incorrectly. Sharps and medical waste contaminated with blood must be disposed of according to federal regulations. Laboratory tests involving blood must be performed correctly for accurate results. Incorrect results can lead to inaccurate diagnosis and treatment. Currently, performing HIV testing requires the patient's written consent. If the patient has questions regarding HIV, refer him or her to the physician for discussion. Never give out laboratory results without checking with the physician. Medical assistants are usually given permission by the physician to relay negative laboratory test results; however, abnormal laboratory results should be relayed by the physician. The medical assistant does not have the medical knowledge to answer the questions the patient may have when the results are abnormal. HIV results (negative or positive) should be given only by the physician. Never speculate to the patient or coworkers about the results of any test. All test results must remain confidential.

Use appropriate personal protective equipment to prevent the transmission of bloodborne pathogens to protect yourself, your coworkers, and your patients. ■

What Would You Do? What Would You *Not* Do?   RESPONSES

Case Study 1
Page 679

What Did Dori Do?
❑ Told Angela that it was fine to have her friend there while she gets her blood drawn.
❑ Told Angela that she could not have the blood drawn out of her left arm because a good vein could not be located in that arm.
❑ Told Angela that using the hand veins is always the last choice when drawing blood. Explained that there are a lot of nerve endings in the hand, which makes it hurt more.

❑ Explained to Angela that there will just be a small stick and that it will heal quickly, and there should be no reason it would affect her softball game this evening.
❑ Tried to relax and reassure Angela before the venipuncture. Carefully explained the procedure to her because it was her first one.
❑ Because Angela was nervous, took precautions to prevent her from fainting by placing her in a semi-Fowler's position on the examining table.
❑ Had Angela's friend stand near the head of the table to help calm her down.

What Would You Do? What Would You *Not* Do? RESPONSES—cont'd

What Did Dori Not Do?

❏ Did not try to draw Angela's blood from her left arm or hand.

❏ Did not ignore the fact that Angela was nervous about the venipuncture.

What Would You Do?/What Would You *Not* Do? Review Dori's response and place a checkmark next to the information you included in your response. List additional information you included in your response.

_____

_____

_____

_____

Case Study 2
Page 683

What Did Dori Do?

❏ Told Buzz that when a butterfly setup is used, the air in the tubing alters the test results. Explained that the red tube is used to get rid of the air, and because it is not needed for testing, it is thrown away.

❏ Stressed to Buzz how important it is to have his blood tested every week to ensure there is not too much or too little of the Coumadin in his body. Explained to him again what might occur if his Coumadin were at the wrong level.

❏ Told Buzz that the office would help him locate a medical laboratory where he will be vacationing, so he can have his test done.

❏ Made sure that Buzz had a laboratory requisition so that he could have his test done while he was on vacation.

What Did Dori Not Do?

❏ Did not tell Buzz that it would be all right to skip his prothrombin test during his vacation.

What Would You Do?/What Would You *Not* Do? Review Dori's response and place a checkmark next to the information you included in your response. List additional information you included in your response.

_____

_____

_____

_____

Case Study 3
Page 696

What Did Dori Do?

❏ Told Mrs. Gabriel that the laboratory can accept only specimens drawn at the laboratory or at the medical office.

❏ Told Mrs. Gabriel that if it would make her feel more comfortable, the laboratory could drop off the blood-drawing supplies at the office, and her blood could be drawn tomorrow at the office.

❏ Informed the physician about Mrs. Gabriel's experience at the laboratory.

What Did Dori Not Do?

❏ Did not tell Mrs. Gabriel that probing a vein could cause the test results to be inaccurate.

What Would You Do?/What Would You *Not* Do? Review Dori's response and place a checkmark next to the information you included in your response. List additional information you included in your response.

_____

_____

_____

_____

CERTIFICATION REVIEW

❏ **Phlebotomy is the collection of blood,** and the individual collecting the blood sample is known as a *phlebotomist. Venipuncture* means the puncturing of a vein for removal of a venous blood sample. Venipuncture can be performed by the following methods: vacuum tube, butterfly, and syringe.

❏ **The antecubital space** is generally used as the site for drawing blood. The antecubital veins typically have a wide lumen and are close to the surface of the skin, which makes them easily accessible. The best vein to use in the antecubital space is the median cubital. This vein is usually bigger, is anchored better, bruises less, and poses the smallest risk of injury to underlying structures compared with other veins. The cephalic and basilic veins are located on either side of the antecubital space and are considered an alternative when the me-

dian cubital vein is unavailable. The cephalic vein is located on the thumb side of the antecubital space, and the basilica vein is located on the little finger side of the antecubital space.

❏ **The various types of blood specimens** that the medical assistant would be required to obtain through the venipuncture procedure include clotted blood, serum, whole blood, and plasma. The blood specimen should be handled carefully at all times. Blood cells are fragile, and rough handling may cause hemolysis. Hemolyzed blood specimens produce inaccurate test results.

❏ **The vacuum tube method** is frequently used to collect venous blood specimens. Vacuum tube needles are available in sizes 20 G to 22 G and come in two lengths: 1 inch and 1½ inch. Evacuated tubes consist of a glass tube with a rubber stopper and a vacuum to pull the

Continued

CERTIFICATION REVIEW—cont'd

blood specimen into the tube. Evacuated tubes use a color-coded system to identify their additive content.

❏ **The butterfly method** of venipuncture is also called the *winged infusion method.* It is used to collect blood from patients who are difficult to stick by conventional methods, such as adult patients with small antecubital veins and children.

❏ **The syringe method** is the least used method of venipuncture. This is because after the blood specimen is obtained, it must be transferred from the syringe to an evacuated tube, which presents the risk of an accidental needlestick. The syringe method is used primarily to obtain blood from small veins.

❏ **Plasma** is the straw-colored liquid portion of the blood. It serves as a transportation medium in which various substances are dissolved and in which blood cells are suspended for circulation through the body. Approximately 92% of plasma consists of water; the remaining 8% is dissolved solid substances that are carried by the blood to and from the tissues.

❏ **A skin puncture** is used to obtain a capillary blood specimen. A skin puncture is performed when a test requires only a small blood specimen. Also, skin puncture is the method preferred for obtaining blood from infants and young children. The fingertip is the preferred site for a skin puncture on an adult.

❏ **When the skin has been punctured,** a capillary blood specimen must be collected. The blood specimen can be collected directly onto a reagent strip, or it can be collected in a microcollection device. Examples of microcollection devices are capillary tubes and microcollection tubes.

TERMINOLOGY REVIEW

Medical Term	Word Parts	Definition
Antecubital space	*ante-:* before	The surface of the arm in front of the elbow.
Anticoagulant	*anti-:* against	A substance that inhibits blood clotting.
Buffy coat		A thin, light-colored layer of white blood cells and platelets that lies between a top layer of plasma and a bottom layer of red blood cells when an anticoagulant has been added to a blood specimen.
Evacuated tube		A closed glass or plastic tube that contains a premeasured vacuum.
Hematoma	*hemat/o-:* blood *-oma:* tumor or swelling	A swelling or mass of coagulated blood caused by a break in a blood vessel.
Hemoconcentration	*hem/o-:* blood	An increase in the concentration of the nonfilterable blood components in the blood vessels, such as red blood cells, enzymes, iron, and calcium, as a result of a decrease in the fluid content of the blood.
Hemolysis	*hem/o-:* blood *-lysis:* breakdown	The breakdown of blood cells.
Osteochondritis	*oste/o-:* bone *myel/o-:* bone marrow *-itis:* inflammation	Inflammation of bone and cartilage.
Osteomyelitis	*oste/o-:* bone *myel/o-:* bone marrow *-itis:* inflammation	Inflammation of the bone or bone marrow as a result of bacterial infection.
Phlebotomist	*phleb/o-:* vein *tomist:* specialist	A health care professional trained in the collection of blood specimens.
Phlebotomy	*phleb/o-:* vein *-otomy:* incision	Incision of a vein for the removal of blood; the collection of blood.
Plasma		The liquid part of the blood consisting of a clear, straw-colored fluid that comprises approximately 55% of the blood volume.
Serum		Plasma from which the clotting factor fibrinogen has been removed.

TERMINOLOGY REVIEW—cont'd

Medical Term	Word Parts	Definition
Venipuncture	*ven/o-:* vein	Puncturing of a vein.
Venous reflux	*ven/o-:* vein *-ous:* pertaining to	The backflow of blood (from an evacuated tube) into the patient's vein.
Venous stasis	*ven/o-:* vein *stasis:* control, stop	The temporary cessation or slowing of the venous blood flow.

ON THE WEB

For Information on Phlebotomy:

Clinical Laboratory Standards Institute: www.clsi.org

Lab Explorer: www.labexplorer.com

American Society for Clinical Laboratory Science (ASCLS): www.ascls.org

American Society for Clinical Pathology (ASCP): www.ascp.org

American Society of Phlebotomy Technicians (ASPT): www.aspt.org

Becton Dickinson: www.bd.com

National Phlebotomy Association (NPA): www.nationalphlebotomy.org

The Safety Lady: www.safetylady.com

My Blood Draw: www.myblooddraw.com

Phlebotomy Pages: www.phlebotomypages.com

18

Hematology

LEARNING OBJECTIVES

Hematology Tests

1. List the tests included in a complete blood count.
2. Describe the shape of an erythrocyte and explain how it acquires this shape.
3. Describe the composition of hemoglobin and explain its function.
4. Describe the normal appearance of leukocytes and explain how they fight infection in the body.
5. State the reference range for each of the following hematologic tests:
   - Hemoglobin
   - Hematocrit
   - Red and white blood cell counts
   - Differential cell count
   - Platelet count
   - PT/INR
6. State the purpose of the hematocrit, and list the layers into which the blood separates after it has been centrifuged.
7. Explain how the RBC indices can help diagnose the various types of anemia.
8. Explain the purpose of the differential cell count.
9. Describe the appearance of the five types of white blood cells.
10. State the purpose of the PT/INR test.
11. List the advantages of PT/INR home testing.

PROCEDURES

Perform a hemoglobin determination using a CLIA-waived automated analyzer and the manufacturer's operating manual.

Perform a hematocrit determination.

Prepare a blood smear.

Collect a specimen for a PT/INR test.

Perform a PT/INR test on a CLIA-waived analyzer.

CHAPTER OUTLINE

Introduction to Hematology

Hematology is the study of blood, including the morphologic appearance and function of blood cells and diseases of the blood and blood-forming tissues. Laboratory analysis in hematology is concerned with the examination of blood for the purpose of detecting pathologic conditions. It includes performing blood cell counts, evaluating the clotting ability of the blood, and identifying cell types. These tests are valuable tools that allow the physician to determine whether each blood component falls within its reference range.

Examples of hematologic tests include hemoglobin, hematocrit, white blood cell count, red blood cell count, differential white blood cell count, prothrombin time, erythrocyte sedimentation rate, and platelet count. Table 18-1 summarizes common hematologic tests, purposes of the tests, reference ranges, and conditions that cause values outside of the reference range.

Certain hematologic laboratory tests may be performed in the medical office. Advances in CLIA-waived automated blood analyzers designed for use in the medical office have made this possible. Automated blood analyzers perform laboratory tests with accurate test results in a short time. Each automated analyzer is accompanied by a detailed operating manual that explains its operation, test parameters, care, and maintenance.

The most frequently performed hematologic laboratory test is the *complete blood count* (CBC). A CBC is routinely performed on new patients and on patients with a pathologic condition. The test results provide valuable information to assist the physician in making a diagnosis, evaluating the patient's progress, and regulating treatment. The tests included in a CBC are as follows:

- White blood cell (WBC) count
- Red blood cell (RBC) count
- Platelet count
- Hemoglobin (Hgb)
- Hematocrit (Hct)
- Differential white blood cell count (Diff)
- Red blood cell indices

An example of a laboratory report indicating the results of a CBC is presented in Figure 18-1.

COMPONENTS AND FUNCTIONS OF BLOOD

Blood consists of two parts—liquid and solid. Plasma, the liquid portion of the blood, consists of a clear yellowish fluid that makes up approximately 55% of the blood volume. The plasma transports nutrients to the tissues of the body to nourish and sustain them, and it picks up wastes from the tissues. These wastes are eliminated through the kidneys. The plasma also transports antibodies, enzymes, and hormones to help regulate normal body functioning.

The solid portion of the blood consists of three types of cells: erythrocytes, leukocytes, and thrombocytes. The solid portion of the blood accounts for 45% of the total blood volume. The average adult body contains 10 to 12 pints (5 to 6 L) of blood.

Erythrocytes

In an adult, erythrocytes, or red blood cells, are formed in the red bone marrow of the ribs, sternum, skull, and pelvic bone and in the ends of the long bones of the limbs. The immature form of an erythrocyte contains a nucleus. As the cell develops and matures, however, it loses its nucleus and acquires the shape of a biconcave disc, thicker at the rim than at the center. This shape provides the erythrocyte with a greater surface area for the exchange of substances. An erythrocyte is approximately 7 to 8 mm in diameter. The average number of erythrocytes ranges from 4 to 5.5 million per cubic millimeter of blood in a woman, and from 4.5 to 6.2 million per cubic millimeter of blood in a man.

A major portion of the erythrocyte consists of **hemoglobin,** a complex compound that transports oxygen and is responsible for the red color of the erythrocyte. The amount of hemoglobin in the blood averages 12 to 16 g/dL for a woman and 14 to 18 g/dL for a man. A hemoglobin molecule consists of a globin, or protein, and an iron-containing pigment called *heme.* One hemoglobin molecule loosely combines with four oxygen molecules in the lungs to form a substance called **oxyhemoglobin.** Oxyhemoglobin is transported and

Table 18-1 Common Hematologic Tests

Name of Test (Abbreviation)	Purpose	Reference Range	Increased With	Decreased With
White blood cell count (WBC)	Assists in diagnosis and prognosis of disease	4500-11,000/mm^3 (or 10^9 cells/L)	**Leukocytosis** Acute infections (appendicitis, chickenpox, diphtheria, infectious mononucleosis, meningitis, pneumonia, rheumatic fever, smallpox, tonsillitis) Hemorrhaging Trauma Malignant disease Leukemia Polycythemia vera	**Leukopenia** Viral infections Hypersplenism Bone marrow depression Infectious hepatitis Cirrhosis Chemotherapy Radiation therapy
Red blood cell count (RBC)	Assists in diagnosis of anemia and polycythemia	*Male:* 4.5-6.2 million/mm^3 (or 10^{12} cells/L) *Female:* 4-5.5 million/mm^3 (10^{12} cells/L) MCV: 80-100 fL MCH: 27-31 pg MCHC: 32%-36% RDW: 11.5%-14.5%	Polycythemia vera Secondary polycythemia Severe diarrhea Dehydration Acute poisoning Pulmonary fibrosis Severe burns	Iron-deficiency anemia Hodgkin's disease Multiple myeloma Leukemia Hemolytic anemia Pernicious anemia Lupus erythematosus Addison's disease
Hemoglobin (Hgb or Hb)	To screen for anemia, determine its severity, monitor response to treatment	*Male:* 14-18 g/dL (SI units: 2.17-2.79 mmol/L) *Female:* 12-16 g/dL (SI units: 1.86-2.48 mmol/L)	Severe burns Chronic obstructive pulmonary disease Congestive heart failure	Anemia Hyperthyroidism Cirrhosis Severe hemorrhage Hemolytic reactions Hodgkin's disease Leukemia
Hematocrit (Hct)	Assists in diagnosis and evaluation of anemia	*Male:* 40%-54% *Female:* 37%-47%	Polycythemia vera Severe dehydration Shock Severe burns	Anemia Leukemia Hyperthyroidism Cirrhosis Acute blood loss Hemolytic reactions
Differential white blood cell count (diff)	Assists in diagnosis and prognosis of disease	Neutrophils 50%-70% Eosinophils 1%-4% Basophils 0-1% Lymphocytes 20%-35% Monocytes 3%-8%	**Neutrophilia** Acute bacterial infections Parasitic infections Liver disease **Eosinophilia** Allergic conditions Parasitic infections Addison's disease Lung and bone cancers **Basophilia** Leukemia Chronic inflammation Polycythemia vera Hemolytic anemia Hodgkin's disease	**Neutropenia** Acute viral infections Blood diseases Hormone diseases Chemotherapy **Eosinopenia** Infectious mononucleosis Hypersplenism Congestive heart failure Aplastic and pernicious anemia **Basopenia** Acute allergic reactions Hyperthyroidism Steroid therapy

Table 18-1 Common Hematologic Tests—cont'd

Name of Test (Abbreviation)	Purpose	Reference Range	Increased With	Decreased With
			Lymphocytosis Acute and chronic infections Hematopoietic disorders Addison's disease Carcinoma Hyperthyroidism	**Lymphopenia** HIV infection Cardiac failure Cushing's disease Hodgkin's disease Leukemia
			Monocytosis Viral infections Bacterial and parasitic infections Collagen diseases Cirrhosis Polycythemia vera Polycythemia	**Monocytopenia** Prednisone treatment Hairy cell leukemia
Prothrombin time/INR (PT/INR)	To screen for coagulation disorders and regulate treatment of patients taking oral anticoagulant therapy with warfarin sodium (Coumadin)	0.8-1.2	**Thrombocytosis** Prothrombin deficiency Vitamin K deficiency Hemorrhagic disease of the newborn Liver disease Anticoagulant therapy Biliary obstruction Acute leukemia Polycythemia vera	**Thrombocytopenia** Acute thrombophlebitis Diuretics Multiple myeloma Pulmonary embolism Vitamin K therapy
Erythrocyte sedimentation rate (ESR)	Nonspecific test for connective tissue diseases, malignancy, and infectious diseases; also used to evaluate progress of inflammatory diseases (elevated test results warrant further testing)	Westergren's method: *Male:* younger than age 50, 0-20 mm/hr; age 50 or older, 0-20 mm/hr *Female:* younger than age 50, 0-20 mm/hr; age 50 or older, 0-30 mm/hr	Collagen diseases Infections Inflammatory diseases Carcinoma Cell or tissue destruction Rheumatoid arthritis	Polycythemia vera Sickle cell anemia Congestive heart failure
Platelet count (Plt)	Assists in evaluation of bleeding disorders that occur with liver disease, thrombocytopenia, uremia, and anticoagulant therapy	150,000-400,000/mm³ (SI units: 150-400 × 10⁹/L)	**Thrombocytosis** Cancer Leukemia Polycythemia vera Splenectomy Acute blood loss Rheumatoid arthritis Trauma (fractures)	**Thrombocytopenia** Pernicious anemia Aplastic anemia Hemolytic anemia Pneumonia Allergic conditions Infection Bone marrow–depressant drugs

distributed to the tissues, where the oxygen is easily released from the hemoglobin. The blood picks up carbon dioxide, a waste product, and transports it back to the lungs to be expelled. When oxygen combines with hemoglobin, a bright red color results that is characteristic of arterial blood. Venous blood is darker red owing to its lower oxygen content.

The average life span of a red blood cell is 120 days. Toward the end of this time, it becomes more and more fragile and eventually ruptures and breaks down; this process is known as **hemolysis.** Hemoglobin, liberated from the red blood cell, also breaks down. The iron is stored and later is reused to form new hemoglobin, and the protein is metabolized by the body. **Bilirubin** is formed by metabolism of the heme units and is transported to the liver, where it is eventually excreted as a waste product in the bile.

Leukocytes

Leukocytes, or white blood cells, are clear, colorless cells that contain a nucleus. The number of leukocytes in the healthy adult ranges from 4500 to 11,000 per cubic millimeter of blood. **Leukocytosis** is the condition of having an abnormal increase in the number of leukocytes (greater

Family Practice Health Care Center
3477 Arrowhead Ave
Phoenix, Arizona 78351
(942) 871-3746

LAB REPORT

ID#	SEX	PATIENT DEMOGRAPHICS	RESULTS PROVIDED BY
3569	M	Laurence F. Dodds	Medical Center Laboratory
		1073 Longview Dr.	
DOB		Brighton, Arizona 78351	ORDERING PROVIDER
06/17/1989			Thomas Murphy, MD

AGE	ACCESSION #	LAB RECEIVED ON	LAB REPORTED ON
20	33972405	12/07/2012 11:00:53	12/05/2012 14:08:00

LAB ID	SPECIMEN ID	COLLECTION DATE/TIME	FASTING
5701	82540339	12/04/2012 2:53:00	NO

NAME	VALUE	REFERENCE RANGE	UNITS	FLAG
CBC WITH DIFFERENTIAL/PLATELET				
-WBC	4.6	4.0-10.5	x10E3/uL	
-RBC	3.57	4.10-5.60	x10E3/uL	L
-Hemoglobin	11.2	12.5-17.0	g/dL	L
-Hematocrit	32.9	36.0-50.0	%	L
-MCV	92	80-98	fL	
-MCH	31.4	27.0-34.0	pg	
-MCHC	34.0	32.0-36.0	g/dL	
-RDW	15.6	11.7-15.0	%	H
-Platelets	308	140-415	x10E3/uL	
-Neutrophils	73	40-74	%	
-Lymphocytes	14	14-46	%	
-Monocytes	11	4-13	%	
-Eosinophils	1	0-7	%	
-Basophils	1	0-3	%	

Figure 18-1. Computer-generated laboratory report for a complete blood count (CBC).

than 11,000 per cubic millimeter), and **leukopenia** is the condition of having an abnormal decrease in the number of leukocytes (less than 4500 per cubic millimeter).

The function of leukocytes is to defend the body against infection. Pathogens can gain entrance to the body in a variety of ways (review the infection process cycle in Chapter 2). Leukocytes attempt to destroy invading pathogens and remove them from the body. In contrast to erythrocytes, leukocytes do their work in the tissues; they are transported to the site of infection by the circulatory system.

During inflammation, the blood vessels in the infected area dilate, resulting in an increased blood supply. More oxygen, nutrients, and white blood cells can be delivered to the infected area to aid in the healing process. The cells in the capillary walls spread apart, enlarging the pores between the cells. White blood cells squeeze through the pores by **ameboid movement** and move out into the tissues to fight the infection. This movement of the leukocytes through the pores of the capillaries and out into the tissues is known as **diapedesis.**

Leukocytes (especially the granular forms) are phagocytic, and when they arrive at the site of infection, they begin the process of **phagocytosis,** the engulfing and destruction of pathogens and damaged cells. In some conditions, pus forms in the infected area (suppuration); pus contains dead leukocytes, dead bacteria, and dead tissue cells.

Thrombocytes

Platelets, also known as *thrombocytes,* are small, clear, and disc-shaped. They lack a nucleus and are formed in the red bone marrow from giant cells known as *megakaryocytes.* Platelets function by participating in the blood-clotting mechanism. The number of platelets in a healthy adult ranges from 150,000 to 400,000 per cubic millimeter of blood.

HEMOGLOBIN DETERMINATION

Hemoglobin (Hgb) is a major component of red blood cells. Hemoglobin transports oxygen to the tissue cells of the body and is responsible for the color of the red blood cell.

The hemoglobin determination is used to measure indirectly the oxygen-carrying capacity of the blood. The reference range for an adult female is 12 to 16 g/dL, and the reference range for an adult male is 14 to 18 g/dL. A hemoglobin determination is performed as an individual test or as part of the CBC. A hemoglobin determination is often performed as a routine test on individuals, such as children younger than 2 years of age and pregnant women, who are at risk for developing anemia.

A decreased hemoglobin level occurs with **anemia** (especially iron-deficiency anemia), hyperthyroidism, cirrhosis of the liver, severe hemorrhaging, hemolytic reactions, and certain systemic diseases, such as leukemia and Hodgkin's disease. Increased levels of hemoglobin are present with **polycythemia,** chronic obstructive pulmonary disease, and congestive heart failure.

The hemoglobin determination can be performed on capillary or venous blood. Hemoglobin can be measured in the medical office using a hemoglobin analyzer. A hemoglobin analyzer permits processing of the specimen in a short time with accurate and reliable test results, allowing the physician to evaluate the condition while the patient is still at the medical office. Examples of CLIA-waived hemoglobin analyzers often used in the medical office include the Hemoglobin Hb 201+ Analyzer (HemoCue, Inc., Lake Forest, Calif.) and the Stat-Site Hgb Meter (Stanbio Laboratory, Boerne, Tex.) (Figure 18-2).

One of the primary advantages of using a hemoglobin analyzer is that it requires only a finger puncture to perform the test rather than a venous blood specimen collected through a venipuncture. The manufacturer of each hemoglobin analyzer provides an operating manual (and sometimes an instructional video) with the instrument that includes information needed to perform quality control procedures, precautions to take when running the test, and information on storage and stability of the testing devices (e.g., testing cards or cuvettes) and control reagents, collection of the specimen, and the procedure for testing the specimen. It is important that the medical assistant become completely familiar with all aspects of the hemoglobin analyzer. Quality control procedures are of particular importance to ensure that the analyzer is functioning properly, and that test results are reliable and accurate. (Refer to

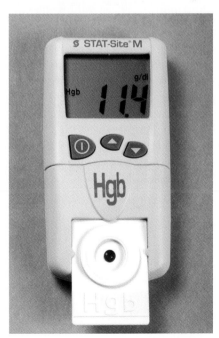
Figure 18-2. CLIA-waived hemoglobin analyzer.

Chapter 15, Quality Control, to review quality control guidelines for laboratory testing.)

The medical assistant must follow the hemoglobin procedure *exactly* as presented in the operating manual. The basic procedure for performing a hemoglobin test involves placing a testing device in the analyzer. A skin puncture is performed on a finger, and a drop of the patient's blood is placed on the testing device. After a countdown period in which the analyzer determines the hemoglobin test results, the hemoglobin results are displayed on the LCD screen of the analyzer. The medical assistant should record the results in the patient's chart, including the date and time, the name of the test (hemoglobin), and the results measured in g/dL.

HEMATOCRIT

The hematocrit (Hct) is a simple, reliable, and informative test that is frequently performed in the medical office. The word *hematocrit* means "to separate blood." The solid or cellular elements are separated from the plasma by centrifuging an anticoagulated blood specimen. The heavier red blood cells become packed and settle to the bottom of a tube. The top layer contains the clear, straw-colored plasma. Between the plasma and the packed red blood cells is a small, thin, yellowish-gray layer known as the *buffy coat,* which contains the platelets and white blood cells (Figure 18-3).

The purpose of the hematocrit is to measure the percentage volume of packed red blood cells in whole blood. The normal hematocrit range for a woman is 37% to 47%; for a man, 40% to 54%. A low hematocrit reading may indicate anemia, and a high reading may indicate polycythemia. The hematocrit, in conjunction with other hematologic

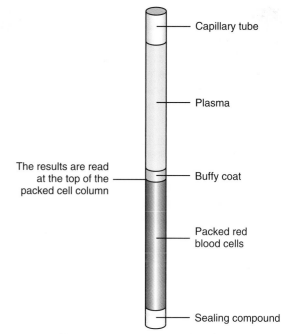

Figure 18-3. Hematocrit test results. The blood cells are separated from the plasma by centrifuging an anticoagulated blood specimen, and the results are read at the top of the packed cell column.

tests, is an aid to the physician in the diagnosis of a patient's condition. The hematocrit also is used as a screening measure for the early detection of anemia and is often included in a general physical examination.

The *microhematocrit method* is used most often in the medical office to perform a hematocrit determination. Through capillary action, blood is drawn directly from a free-flowing skin puncture into a disposable capillary tube lined with an **anticoagulant**. An anticoagulated blood specimen collected by venipuncture also can be used; through capillary action, the blood specimen is drawn into the capillary tube from the evacuated collection tube. After the specimen is collected, one end of the capillary tube is sealed with a commercially prepared sealing compound (e.g., Cha-Seal [Chase Scientific, Langley, Wash.], Seal-Ease [Becton Dickinson, Franklin Lakes, NJ]). The capillary tube is then placed in a microhematocrit centrifuge. The centrifuge spins the blood at an extremely high speed; only 3 to 5 minutes are required to pack the red blood cells. The results are read at the top of the packed cell column. Procedure 18-1 describes how to perform a hematocrit determination.

What Would You Do? What Would You *Not* Do?

Case Study 1

Theodore Pascal is at the office for a general physical examination. The physician orders a routine urinalysis and a hemoglobin determination be done on Theodore at the office. Theodore wants to know whether the physician thinks there is something wrong with him. He also wants to know the purpose of the blood test and how it is done. When Theodore realizes that a hemoglobin determination involves a finger-stick, he says that he does not like having his finger stuck and wants to know whether the blood can be taken out of his earlobe instead. ■

PATIENT TEACHING Iron-Deficiency Anemia

Answer questions patients have about iron-deficiency anemia.

What is anemia?

Anemia is a shortage of red blood cells or hemoglobin. Hemoglobin, the part of the blood that gives red blood cells their color, carries oxygen to all the cells in the body. There are many types of anemia, of which iron-deficiency anemia is the most common. Other types of anemia include pernicious anemia, sickle cell anemia, hemolytic anemia, and aplastic anemia.

What causes iron-deficiency anemia?

In general, iron-deficiency anemia is caused by conditions that deplete the iron stored in the body; it can result from an increased need for iron by the body or an increased loss of iron from the body. Iron-deficiency anemia may occur in children younger than 2 years old if their diet does not include enough iron to meet the demands of rapid growth. This is especially true in children whose main source of nutrition during these years is breast milk or bottle milk, because milk contains very little iron. Adolescent girls are prone to iron-deficiency anemia because of growth spurts during puberty and blood loss through menstruation. In adults, the most common cause of anemia is chronic blood loss, such as from a bleeding ulcer or bleeding hemorrhoids and heavy menstrual bleeding. Pregnant women also are at increased risk because of the demands of the growing fetus.

What can be done for individuals at risk for iron-deficiency anemia?

Individuals prone to developing iron-deficiency anemia are encouraged to increase foods in their diet that contain iron, such as beef, liver, spinach, eggs, and iron-fortified breads and cereals. As a preventive measure, the physician usually prescribes vitamin supplements for individuals who are at increased risk for developing iron-deficiency anemia, such as pregnant women, infants, and young children. Infant formulas and cereals that have been supplemented with iron are also available.

What are the symptoms of anemia?

All types of anemia have the same general symptoms. Often these symptoms do not develop right away; when they do develop, feeling tired and run down may be the only sign of anemia. Other symptoms that may occur, particularly as the anemia becomes worse, are paleness of the skin, fingernail beds, and mucous membranes; shortness of breath, especially during physical activity; dizziness; headache; irritability; and inability to concentrate. These symptoms result from the diminished ability of the blood to carry oxygen to the cells of the body. Blood tests are necessary to diagnose anemia and to determine the specific type of anemia present.

How is iron-deficiency anemia treated?

The most important part of treating anemia is to determine its cause, such as not enough iron consumed in the diet or chronic blood loss, and to correct that condition. The physician usually prescribes an iron supplement to replace the iron that has been depleted from the body. It is generally prescribed in oral form, but it is given through an injection in special situations. An oral iron supplement causes the stool to turn a black, tarlike color. This is normal and should not be a cause for concern. Also, an effort should be made to consume foods high in iron content.

- For patients who have had a vitamin supplement prescribed to *prevent* iron-deficiency anemia, such as children younger than 2 years old and pregnant women: Emphasize to the patient the importance of taking the vitamin supplement every day to prevent the development of iron-deficiency anemia.
- For patients who have had an iron supplement prescribed to treat iron-deficiency anemia: Emphasize to the patient the importance of taking the iron supplement for the period of time prescribed by the physician, because replacement of iron takes time.
- Instruct patients to keep iron supplements out of the reach of children to prevent iron poisoning.
- Provide patients with written educational materials about anemia.

PROCEDURE 18-1 Hematocrit

Outcome Perform a hematocrit determination.

Equipment/Supplies

- Microhematocrit centrifuge
- Disposable gloves
- Lancet
- Antiseptic wipe
- Gauze pads

- Capillary tubes
- Sealing compound
- Adhesive bandage
- Biohazard sharps container

1. **Procedural Step.** Sanitize your hands. Greet the patient and introduce yourself. Identify the patient by full name and date of birth, and explain the procedure.

2. **Procedural Step.** Assemble equipment. Open the gauze packet. Cleanse the puncture site with an antiseptic wipe, and allow it to air-dry. Apply gloves and

Continued

PROCEDURE 18-1   Hematocrit—cont'd

perform a finger puncture, then dispose of the lancet in a biohazard sharps container.

Principle. Personal protective equipment and proper disposal of the lancet are required by the OSHA standard to prevent exposure to bloodborne pathogens.

3. Procedural Step. Wipe away the first drop of blood with a gauze pad. Fill the first capillary tube by holding one end of it horizontally, but slightly downward, next to the free-flowing puncture. Keep the tip of the capillary tube in the blood, but do not allow it to press against the patient's skin. Calibrated tubes are filled to the calibration line; uncalibrated tubes are filled approximately three quarters (within 10 to 20 mm of the end of the tube). The blood is drawn into the tube through capillary action. Fill a second tube using the method just described. Place a gauze pad over the puncture site and apply pressure.

Principle. Not keeping the tip of the capillary tube in the blood can cause air bubbles in the stem of the tube, which leads to inaccurate test results. Allowing the capillary tube to press against the skin closes the opening of the capillary tubes and does not allow blood to enter. The type of tube (calibrated or uncalibrated) is based on the method used to read the test results. The hematocrit should be performed in duplicate to ensure accurate and reliable test results.

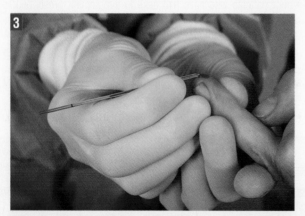

Fill the capillary tube.

4. Procedural Step. Push the dry end of the tube (end opposite the filling end that does not contain blood) down into the sealing compound. This seals the end of the capillary tube. The sealing compound can be used to hold the capillary tubes until they are ready to be placed in the microhematocrit centrifuge. To do this, the sealing compound should be placed on a flat surface with the tubes in a vertical position. Before removing a capillary tube from the sealing compound, rotate the tube between the thumb and index finger to prevent the sealing compound from pulling out when the tube is lifted out of the sealing compound.

Principle. Blood in the capillary tube at the end being sealed prevents a successful closure, which may cause leakage of the blood specimen, leading to inaccurate test results. Capillary tubes must be sealed properly to prevent leakage of the blood specimen during centrifugation.

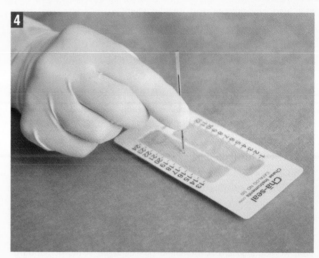

Seal one end of the tube.

5. Procedural Step. Check the patient's puncture site for bleeding and apply an adhesive bandage, if needed.

6. Procedural Step. Place the capillary tubes in the microhematocrit centrifuge with the sealed end facing out. Balance one tube, with the other capillary tube placed on the opposite side of the centrifuge.

Principle. Placing the sealed end toward the outside prevents the blood specimen from spinning out of the capillary tube when the centrifuge is in operation.

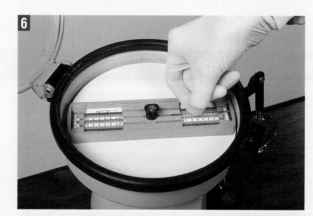

Place the tube in the centrifuge.

7. Procedural Step. Place the cover on the centrifuge, and lock it securely. Centrifuge the blood specimen for 3 to 5 minutes at a speed of 10,000 rpm.

PROCEDURE 18-1 Hematocrit—cont'd

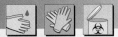

Principle. Centrifuging the blood specimen causes the red blood cells to become packed and to settle on the bottom of the tube.

8. Procedural Step. Allow the centrifuge to come to a complete stop. Read the results, as follows:

Calibrated tube. If a capillary tube with a calibration line was used, read the results using the special graphic reading device that is part of the centrifuge. Adjust the capillary tube so that the bottom of the red blood cell column (just above the sealing compound) is placed on the 0 line. With a magnifying glass, read the results at the top of the packed red blood cell column, and you will see a percentage on the reading device.

Uncalibrated tube. If an uncalibrated tube was used, you must use a microhematocrit reader card to determine the results; place the top of the plasma column on the 100% mark and the bottom of the cell column on the 0 line. Read the results on the scale, which corresponds to the top of the packed cell column.

In both cases, the buffy coat should not be included in the reading. The answer represents the percentage of blood volume occupied by the red blood cells. (The hematocrit determination on this reading device is 38.)

Principle. Stopping the centrifuge with your hands can injure you and can damage the machine.

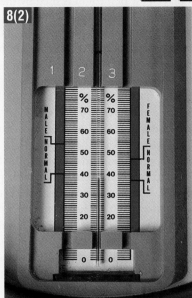

8(2)

Read the results.

9. Procedural Step. Read the second tube in the manner just described; the results of the tubes should agree within 4 percentage points. If not, the hematocrit procedure must be repeated. If they are within 4 percentage points, the two values are averaged to derive the test results.

10. Procedural Step. Properly dispose of the capillary tubes in a biohazard sharps container. Remove gloves and sanitize your hands. Chart the results. Include the date and time and the hematocrit results.

11. Procedural Step. Return the equipment to its proper storage place. Store the sealing compound at room temperature. Exposing it to a temperature above 80° F adversely affects its consistency.

Reference Range for Hematocrit:
Female: 37% to 47%
Male: 40% to 54%

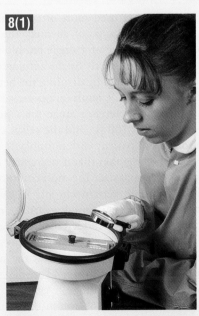

8(1)

Align the bottom of the red cell column with the 0 line.

CHARTING EXAMPLE

Date	
5/5/12	11:15 a.m. Hct: 38%._____
	_____ L. Sharpe, CMA (AAMA)

PROCEDURE 18-1

WHITE BLOOD CELL COUNT

The white blood cell (WBC) count is used by the physician to assist in the diagnosis and prognosis of disease. The white blood cell count is an approximate measurement of the number of white blood cells in the circulating blood. The reference range for a white blood cell count is 4500 to 11,000 white blood cells per cubic millimeter of blood, which is expressed as 4.5 to 11 ($\times 10^3/mm^3$) on laboratory reports. An increase in the white blood cell count, or leukocytosis, is most commonly seen in acute infection such as appendicitis, chickenpox, diphtheria, infectious mononucleosis, meningitis, and rheumatic fever. Normal elevation of the white blood cell count can occur with pregnancy, strenuous exercise, stress, and treatment with corticosteroids. Conditions that result in leukopenia, or a decrease in the white blood cell count, include viral infections, chemotherapy, and radiation therapy.

If performed in the medical office, a (CLIA-nonwaived) automated blood cell counter must be used to obtain the WBC count, which is a moderately complex test. Blood cell counters also are able to perform a red blood cell count, platelet count, hemoglobin, hematocrit, and differential white blood cell count, as well as calculation of red blood cell indices. Examples of nonwaived blood cell counters include the QBC Autoread (Beckton Dickinson), the Cell-Dyn (Abbott, Santa Clara, Calif.), and the Coulter (Coulter Company, Brea, Calif.) (Figure 18-4).

RED BLOOD CELL COUNT

The red blood cell (RBC) count is a measurement of the number of red blood cells in whole blood. The range for the red blood cell count in a healthy woman is 4 to 5.5 million red blood cells per cubic millimeter of blood, expressed on laboratory reports as 4 to 5.5 ($\times 10^6/mm^3$). The range for a healthy man is 4.5 to 6.2 million red blood cells per cubic millimeter of blood, expressed on a laboratory report as 4.5 to 6.2 ($\times 10^6/mm^3$). In the medical office, the red blood cell count is performed using a blood cell counter.

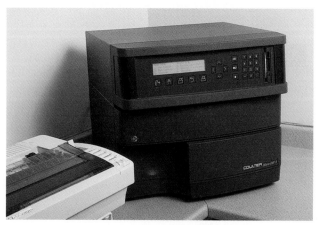

Figure 18-4. Coulter blood cell counter.

Conditions that cause a decrease in the red blood cell count include anemia, Hodgkin's disease, and leukemia; conditions that cause an increase in red blood cells include polycythemia, dehydration, and pulmonary fibrosis.

RED BLOOD CELL INDICES

The red blood cell (RBC) indices are measurements that are reported as part of the CBC (complete blood count) test. RBC indices provide the physician with information about the size and hemoglobin content of a patient's red blood cells. The RBC indices include the MCV, MCH, MCHC, and the RDW, which are described in greater detail below. The RBC indices are obtained from calculations performed on certain test results included in a CBC, specifically, the RBC count, hemoglobin, and hematocrit. The calculation is automatically performed by the blood cell analyzer that performs the CBC.

A decrease in the number of red blood cells or in the amount of hemoglobin is known as anemia. More than 400 types of anemia have been identified, but many of them are rare conditions. Each of the various forms of anemia (e.g., iron-deficiency anemia, pernicious anemia) may alter one or more of the RBC indices in a particular way. This information is used by the physician to assist in the diagnosis of the type of anemia a patient has and in determination of its cause. The RBC indices are discussed in the following sections.

MCV: Mean Corpuscular Volume

The MCV is the index used most often to assist in the diagnosis of a particular type of anemia. The MCV is a measure of the average size of a single red blood cell. The MCV can be measured directly by the automated cell analyzer, or it can be calculated by dividing the hematocrit by the RBC count. The MCV results are expressed in femtoliters (fL). The MCV reference range for a normal-sized red blood cell is 80 to 100 fL, and the cell is described as being **normocytic.** A patient with normocytic anemia has a RBC count or hemoglobin that is decreased, but the red blood cells are of normal size. The most common causes of normocytic anemia are certain chronic diseases such as kidney disease, cancer, rheumatoid arthritis, and thyroiditis. It can also be caused by sudden blood loss and aplastic anemia.

An MCV result below 80 means that the patient's red blood cells are smaller than normal and are described as being **microcytic.** The most common cause of microcytic anemia (low MCV) is a lack of iron in the diet, known as iron-deficiency anemia. Microcytic anemia may also be due to *thalassemia,* which is a hereditary type of anemia. An MCV result greater than 100 fL means that the cells are larger than normal, or **macrocytic.** The most common causes of macrocytic anemia (high MCV) are folic acid deficiency and a lack of vitamin B_{12} in the body, known as *pernicious anemia.*

MCH: Mean Corpuscular Hemoglobin

The MCH measures the average weight of hemoglobin within a red blood cell. The MCH is calculated by dividing the hemoglobin value by the RBC count; the results are expressed in pictograms (pg). The reference range for an MCH is 27 to 31 pg. Because microcytic red blood cells (low MCV) typically have less hemoglobin (low MCH), and macrocytic red blood cells (high MCV) typically have more hemoglobin (high MCH), the causes for values outside of the reference range are the same as those for MCV values outside of the reference range. For example, iron-deficiency anemia is associated with both a decreased MCV and a decreased MCH.

MCHC: Mean Cell Hemoglobin Concentration

The MCHC measures the average concentration of hemoglobin within a single red blood cell. The MCHC is calculated by dividing the hemoglobin value by the hematocrit value; the results are expressed as a percentage. The MCHC reference range for a red blood cell with a normal concentration of hemoglobin is 32% to 36%, and the cell is described as being **normochromic.** An example of a type of anemia that exhibits normochromia is pernicious anemia, which is caused by a lack of vitamin B_{12} in the body. An MCHC result below 32% means that the patient's red blood cells contain less than the normal concentration of hemoglobin or are **hypochromic,** a condition that occurs with iron-deficiency anemia and thalassemia. Because there is a physical limit to the amount of hemoglobin that can fit into a RBC, an MCHC level above 36% does not occur (and therefore, RBCs cannot be *hyperchromic*).

RDW: Red Cell Distribution Width

Normally, all the red blood cells in a patient's specimen should be the same size, with very little variation. The RDW measures any variation in the size of the red blood cells in a patient's specimen. The RDW is calculated by using the MCV and RBC count values. The RDW reference range is 11.5% to 14.5%. Certain anemias, such as iron-deficiency anemia, can change the size of some of the red blood cells, resulting in an increase in the RDW. *Anisocytosis* is the term used to describe a variation in the size of red blood cells.

WHITE BLOOD CELL DIFFERENTIAL COUNT

There are five types of white blood cells, or leukocytes, each having a certain size, shape, appearance, and function (Figure 18-5). The purpose of the differential cell count is to

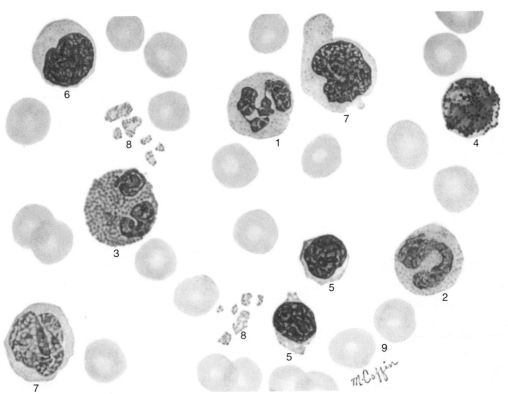

Figure 18-5. Types of human blood cells. *1* to *7,* White blood cells (leukocytes) stained as they are in the laboratory to show the many types. They play the active role in immune response or in defense against disease. *1,* Neutrophil; *2,* neutrophilic band; *3,* eosinophil; *4,* basophil; *5,* lymphocyte; *6,* (large) lymphocyte; *7,* monocyte; *8,* platelets (thrombocytes), which are responsible for clotting; and *9,* red blood cells (erythrocytes), which carry oxygen. (From Custer RP: An atlas of the blood and bone marrow, ed 2, Philadelphia, 1974, Saunders.)

identify and count the five types of white blood cells in a representative blood sample. An increase or decrease in one or more types may occur in pathologic conditions; this assists the physician in making a diagnosis.

The differential cell count can be performed automatically or manually. The automatic method is faster and more convenient; however, the manual method allows for closer inspection of abnormal white blood cells. If a differential cell count is performed on an automated analyzer at an outside laboratory and abnormalities are flagged by the analyzer, the laboratory will then perform a differential cell count by using the manual method.

Automatic Method

The automatic method involves the use of a blood cell counter, such as the Coulter cell counter (see Figure 18-4). The specimen requirement is an ethylenediaminetetraacetic acid (EDTA)-anticoagulated blood specimen, which is obtained through venipuncture using a lavender-stoppered tube. The blood cell counter automatically performs the differential cell count, and the results are printed on a laboratory report.

Manual Method

If a physician orders a manual differential cell count on a blood specimen, the medical assistant must prepare two blood smears at the medical office for transport to the outside laboratory. The preparation of a blood smear is outlined in Procedure 18-2. Fresh whole blood is preferred for blood smears; however, a satisfactory smear can be made from an EDTA-anticoagulated blood specimen, provided that the smear is made within 24 hours after collection. Other anticoagulants should not be used because they could alter the morphology and staining reaction of the white blood cells. After preparing the blood smear, the medical assistant places the slides in a protective slide container for transport to an outside laboratory.

The blood smear is evaluated at the laboratory by medical laboratory personnel. Because white blood cells are clear and colorless, they must be stained with an appropriate dye (usually Wright's stain) before a differential count is performed.

What Would You Do? What Would You *Not* Do?

Case Study 2

Baylee Frasure brings in her 6-month-old son, Travis, for a well-child visit. Mrs. Frasure has been breastfeeding Travis since he was born, and he is not yet on solid food. She says that Travis has been doing just fine, but he did not like his liquid vitamins, so she stopped giving them to him. Mrs. Frasure says that she is eating a well-balanced diet and takes a multivitamin every day, so she did not think this would be a problem. Travis' hemoglobin is checked during the visit, and it is 8 g/dL. The physician prescribes ferrous sulfate drops for Travis. After the physician leaves the room, Mrs. Frasure becomes quite upset. She says she does not understand why Travis' hemoglobin is so low. She says that she thought that breast milk provided the best nutrition possible for infants. ■

The nucleus, the cytoplasm, and any granules in the cytoplasm take on the characteristic color of their cell type; this aids in proper identification. A minimum of 100 white blood cells is identified on the blood smear using a microscope, and each is assigned to its appropriate category (neutrophil, eosinophil, basophil, lymphocyte, or monocyte). The number of each type of leukocyte is recorded as a percentage and reflects the overall distribution of white blood cells in the patient's bloodstream. During the manual evaluation of the blood smear, the laboratory technologist will also examine the slide for abnormalities in the morphology of the red blood cells, including their size, shape, and structure.

Types of White Blood Cells

Leukocytes are classified into two major categories—granular and nongranular. *Granular leukocytes* contain distinct granules in the cytoplasm and include neutrophils, eosinophils, and basophils. Nongranular leukocytes contain few or no granules in the cytoplasm and include lymphocytes and monocytes. The five types of white blood cells are described here, along with their reactions to Wright's stain.

The *neutrophils* are the most numerous of the white blood cells. A neutrophil has a purple, multilobed nucleus that may contain three to five lobes or segments; neutrophils also are known as "segs." The cytoplasm of a neutrophil stains a faint pink and contains many fine granules that stain a violet pink. Neutrophils exhibit a high degree of ameboid movement and are actively phagocytic. Immature forms of neutrophils known as *bands* can be identified by their curved, nonsegmented nuclei. Normally, 0% to 5% of the neutrophils present are in the immature band form. When the percentage of band forms increases, this condition is often referred to as a "shift to the left." An increase in the number of neutrophils, including band forms, is generally seen during an acute infection.

An *eosinophil* contains a segmented nucleus, generally of no more than two lobes. Large granules are found in the cytoplasm; they stain a bright reddish orange. An increase in eosinophils is often seen in allergic conditions and parasitic infestations.

Basophils are the least numerous of the white blood cells. A basophil contains an S-shaped nucleus. The cytoplasm contains large, coarse, dark bluish-black granules that almost completely obscure the details of the nucleus.

Lymphocytes are the smallest white blood cells. A lymphocyte has a round or slightly indented nucleus that almost fills the cell and stains a deep purplish blue. There is a small rim of sky-blue cytoplasm surrounding the nucleus that contains few or no granules. Lymphocytes are involved with the immune system and the production of antibodies. An increase in lymphocytes generally occurs with certain viral diseases, including infectious mononucleosis, mumps, chickenpox, rubella, and viral hepatitis.

Monocytes are the largest white blood cells. A monocyte has a large nucleus that is usually kidney-shaped or horseshoe-shaped, but it can be round or oval. Monocytes contain abundant cytoplasm that stains grayish blue.

Memories *from* Externship

Latisha Sharpe: During my externship experience, I had a female patient who drank too much the night before and had been vomiting for 3 hours before coming to the physician's office. Although this incident was self-inflicted, I still found myself feeling deeply sorry for the patient. She was so weak she could not hold her head up, so I stayed with her and held her head up while she was vomiting. I stayed with her throughout this time, and my sympathy for her really made a difference. No matter what the situation is, I always let the patient know that I care. ∎

Reference Range

The healthy adult reference range for each type of white blood cell making up the total number of leukocytes is listed here:

Neutrophils: 50% to 70%
Eosinophils: 1% to 4%
Basophils: 0% to 1%
Lymphocytes: 20% to 35%
Monocytes: 3% to 8%

What Would You Do? What Would You *Not* Do?

Case Study 3

Marjorie Merrick comes to the office for a follow-up visit to discuss her laboratory results with the physician. Marjorie is in perimenopause and has been having problems with heavy menstrual periods, hot flashes, insomnia, fatigue, and shortness of breath. Marjorie's laboratory tests indicate that she has iron-deficiency anemia. The physician orders an injection of iron dextran, Z-track technique, and instructs Marjorie to take an iron supplement every day and to return in 3 months for a recheck. Marjorie says she has heard that an iron injection can stain the skin and wants to know whether that is true. She says she has a friend who has anemia, and he has to go in every week for a vitamin B_{12} shot. Marjorie wants to know whether she will have to do that, too. Marjorie signed up to donate blood this week at her church's Red Cross blood drive. She wants to know whether it is all right for her to donate. ∎

PROCEDURE 18-2 Preparation of a Blood Smear for a Differential Cell Count

Outcome Prepare a blood smear for a differential white blood cell count.

Equipment/Supplies

- Disposable gloves
- Supplies to perform a finger puncture or venipuncture
- Lavender-stoppered evacuated tube
- Slides with a frosted edge
- Slide container
- Biohazard specimen bag
- Laboratory request form
- Biohazard sharps container

1. Procedural Step. Sanitize your hands. Greet the patient and introduce yourself. Identify the patient by full name and date of birth, and explain the procedure.

2. Procedural Step. Assemble the equipment. Using a pencil, label two slides on the frosted edge with the patient's name and date of birth, and the date.

Principle. Laboratories request the preparation of two blood smears as a means of quality control.

3. Procedural Step. Open the gauze packet. Cleanse the puncture site with an antiseptic wipe. Apply gloves, obtain a blood sample from the patient, and place a drop of fresh whole blood on each slide as follows:

From a venipuncture. You can obtain the blood specimen from the fresh whole blood left in the needle immediately after performing a venipuncture for a CBC (using a lavender-stoppered tube) as follows: After withdrawing the needle from the patient's arm, deposit the drops of blood remaining in the needle onto the middle of each slide, approximately ¼ inch from the slide's frosted edge. The lavender tube can be used to

help push the blood out of the needle. The drop of blood should be approximately 1 to 2 mm in diameter, which is about the size of the head of a matchstick. Immediately discard the venipuncture needle and attached holder in a biohazard sharps container.

From a skin puncture. Perform a finger puncture, and wipe away the first drop of blood. Place a drop of blood from the patient's finger in the middle of each slide, approximately ¼ inch from the slide's frosted edge, by touching the slide to the drop of blood. Do not allow the patient's finger to touch the slide.

Principle. If the patient's finger touches the slide, it will spread out the blood specimen, producing an uneven smear. In addition, moisture or oil from the patient's finger could interfere with the smear.

4. Procedural Step. Make the blood smear as follows:

a. Hold a second "spreader" slide between the thumb and index finger of the dominant hand. Position a nondominant finger (or fingers) at the end of the slide (end opposite the frosted edge). Position the

Continued

PROCEDURE 18-2

PROCEDURE 18-2   Preparation of a Blood Smear
for a Differential Cell Count—cont'd

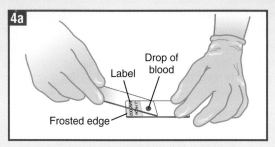

Hold the spreader slide in front of the drop of blood.

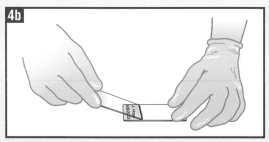

Move the spreader into the drop of blood.

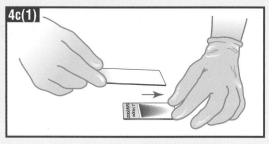

Spread the blood across the slide.

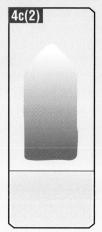

Properly prepared blood smear. (From Rodak BF: Hematology: clinical principles and applications, Philadelphia, 1995, Saunders.)

spreader slide in front of the drop of blood and at a 30-degree angle to the first slide.

b. Move the spreader slide until it touches the drop of blood. The blood distributes itself along the edge of the spreader by capillary action.

c. Using a smooth, continuous motion, with a light, but firm pressure, spread the blood thinly and evenly across the surface of the first slide, ending the motion by lifting the spreader slide off the specimen in a smooth, low arc. The smear should be approximately 1½ inches long. The blood smear is thickest at the beginning and gradually thins to a very fine "feathered" edge.

d. Repeat the above procedure to prepare the second blood smear. If the blood smear has been prepared correctly, it exhibits the following characteristics: (a) It is smooth and even with no ridges, holes, lines, streaks, or clumps; (b) it is not too thick or too thin; (c) a feathered edge is seen at the thin end of the smear; and (d) a margin is evident on all sides of the smear. Repeat this step with the other slide.

Principle. An angle of more than 30 degrees causes the smear to be too thick; the cells overlap, do not stain well, and are smaller than normal, making them difficult to count. If the angle were smaller than 30 degrees, the smear would be too thin, and the cells would be spread out, increasing the time needed to count them.

5. Procedural Step. Dispose of the spreader slide in a biohazard sharps container.

6. Procedural Step. Lay the blood smears on a flat surface, and allow them to air-dry. Never blow on the slides to dry them.

Principle. The blood smears must be dried immediately to prevent shrinkage of the blood cells, which makes them difficult to identify. Blowing on the slide might cause exhaled water droplets to make holes in the smears.

7. Procedural Step. Once the slides are completely dry, place them in a protective slide container. Prepare the blood tube and slides for transport to the laboratory. Place the lavender-stoppered tube and slide container in a biohazard specimen bag and seal the bag.

8. Procedural Step. Remove your gloves, and sanitize your hands. Complete a laboratory request form. Place a copy of the laboratory request in the outside pocket of the specimen bag.

9. Procedural Step. Chart the procedure. Include the date and time, the type of collection and the date the specimen was transported to the laboratory. File a copy of the laboratory request in the patient's chart. Place the specimen bag in the appropriate location for pickup by a courier.

PROCEDURE 18-2   Preparation of a Blood Smear for a Differential Cell Count—cont'd

4c(3)

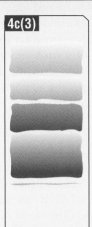 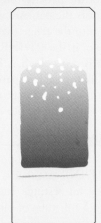 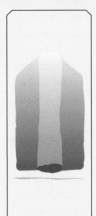 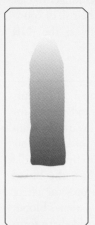 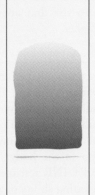 

Slide contains gaps or ridges Cause:	Slide contains holes Cause:	Slide contains streaks Cause:	Slide is too thin Cause:	Slide is too thick Cause:	The length of the smear is too short Cause:
• Too much pressure applied to spreader slide • Uneven pressure used to push spreader slide	• Dirt or finger-prints on the slide • Fat globules or lipids in the specimen • Blood is contaminated with powder from glove	• Uneven pressure used to push spreader slide • Drop of blood started to dry out	• Blood drop is too small • Angle of less than 30 degrees is used	• Blood drop is too large • Angle of less than 30 degrees is used	• Blood drop is too small • Angle of more than 30 degrees is used • Spreader slide is pushed too quickly and not far enough along the slide

Improperly prepared blood smears. (Modified from Rodak BF: Hematology: clinical principles and applications, Philadelphia, 1995, Saunders.)

CHARTING EXAMPLE

Date	
5/05/12	11:15 a.m. Venous blood specimen collected from Ⓡ arm. Specimen to Medical Center Laboratory for CBC c̄ diff on 5/05/12.———— ————————— L. Sharpe, CMA (AAMA)

PROCEDURE 18-2

PT/INR

The PT/INR test is a combination of a PT (prothrombin time) test and a mathematical calculation performed on the PT test to arrive at a standardized value known as an INR (International Normalized Ratio). The PT test result measures how long it takes an individual's blood to form a clot. PT test results are measured in seconds. The reference range for aPT for an adult is 10 to 20 seconds; this means that the blood of a healthy adult should clot within 10 to 20 seconds.

A variety of testing reagents can be used to measure PT. Each of these reagents works in a slightly different way to assess the clotting ability of the blood. Because of this, a PT result obtained when one reagent is used at a particular laboratory cannot be compared with a PT result that has been tested using a different reagent at another laboratory. To account for these differences, the coagulation analyzer running a PT test performs a mathematical calculation on the PT results to convert the results to a standardized ratio. This ratio, known as an INR, is obtained by comparing the patient's PT results with those of a normal (control) sample. The INR allows a patient's PT test results to be compared regardless of the testing reagent or laboratory used to run the test.

The PT/INR result is expressed as a number, and because the value is a ratio, the result does not have a unit of measurement attached to it. A healthy individual with a normal clotting ability should have a PT/INR result that falls between 0.8 and 1.2. The higher the number, the longer it takes for the blood to clot. For example, an individual with a PT/INR of 3.0 would have blood that takes longer to clot than an individual with a PT/INR of 1.0. The risk of spontaneous bleeding begins to rise dramatically as the INR reaches a level of 4.0 or higher.

Purpose

The PT/INR test is most commonly performed on patients undergoing long-term warfarin therapy. Brand names for warfarin include Coumadin and Jantoven. Warfarin is an anticoagulant, which inhibits the formation of blood clots in the body. An anticoagulant works by interfering with the blood clotting mechanism in the body; thus, the blood takes longer to clot. The PT/INR test measures the effect that warfarin has on the clotting ability of a patient's blood.

Warfarin is prescribed for patients who are likely to form clots. The most common conditions for which warfarin is prescribed include heart attack, stroke, and thrombophlebitis (also known as *deep vein thrombosis,* or DVT). Patients who experience recurrent atrial fibrillation are often placed on warfarin therapy. Atrial fibrillation is an irregular heartbeat, which can cause blood to pool in the heart; the pooled blood may cause a blood clot to form, which can travel to the brain, resulting in a stroke. Patients who have had a heart valve replaced with a mechanical valve are also placed on long-term warfarin therapy because of the increased risk that a clot may form on the mechanical valve, causing heart blockage. A PT/INR test also may be ordered on patients who are exhibiting signs and symptoms of a coagulation disorder, such as unexplained nosebleeds, excessive bleeding from the gums, easy bruising, heavy menstrual periods, and unexplained blood in the stool or urine.

The physician determines the ideal PT/INR range for a patient on long-term warfarin therapy, which depends on the condition being treated. The usual desired PT/INR range for a patient on warfarin therapy following a stroke or heart attack, or for a patient with recurring atrial fibrillation, is between 2.0 and 3.0. The PT/INR for a patient with a mechanical valve replacement has a higher range, which falls between 2.5 and 3.5. The goal of warfarin therapy is to increase the clotting time to a level that prevents the formation of blood clots without causing excessive bleeding or bruising.

To ensure that a patient remains in his or her ideal PT/INR range and thereby minimize complications of warfarin therapy, the patient must undergo periodic PT/INR testing. The frequency of testing depends on several factors, which include the stability of the patient's previous test results and the occurrence of conditions that may cause the test results to fall outside of the patient's desired range. When a patient is first placed on warfarin therapy, a PT/INR test is performed once or twice a week to assess the patient's response to the warfarin. Based on the PT/INR results, the dosage is adjusted so that the patient's results become stable and consistently fall within his or her ideal

PT/INR range. Once the test results become stabilized, a patient on long-term warfarin therapy should have a PT/INR test performed every 2 to 4 weeks. If the PT/INR result is outside of the patient's predetermined ideal range, the physician adjusts the patient's warfarin dosage to bring the patient back into the range that is optimal for that patient. For example, if the PT/INR of a stroke patient on warfarin therapy is 3.6, which is higher than the desired range (2.0 to 3.0) for such a patient, the physician will lower the patient's warfarin dosage until the patient returns to a value that is within his or her desired range.

Collection of the Specimen

The medical assistant may be responsible for collecting the specimen for a PT/INR test that is to be transported to an outside laboratory for testing. The PT/INR test requires only a small (4 to 5 ml) tube of blood. The blood must be collected in a tube containing sodium citrate, which is a light blue–stoppered tube (Figure 18-6). The sodium citrate prevents the specimen from clotting without affecting the test results.

As described in Chapter 17, when the butterfly method is used to collect the specimen, a red-stoppered discard tube must first be drawn, followed by collection in the light blue tube. If a light blue–stoppered tube is the first or only tube to be drawn, a 5-ml red-stoppered tube must be drawn first and discarded. This is because some of the tube's vacuum is exhausted by the air in the butterfly tubing setup (rather than blood), resulting in underfilling of the tube. A butterfly setup with 7-inch tubing contains 0.3 ml of air, and a setup with 12 inches of tubing contains 0.5 ml of air. If the light blue–stoppered tube is filled first, the underfilled tube results in an incorrect anticoagulant-to-blood ratio. An incorrect ratio when performing a PT/INR test leads to inaccurate test results.

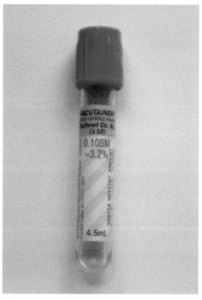

Figure 18-6. Light blue–stoppered tube used to collect a specimen for a PT/INR test.

When collecting a specimen for a PT/INR, it is very important to fill the tube to the exhaustion of the vacuum. Failure to do so results in an underfilled tube and, as described above, leads to inaccurate test results. Most light blue–stoppered tubes have a fill indicator, so the medical assistant can determine if the tube has been completely filled. Once the tube has been drawn, it should be imme-diately and gently inverted 3 to 4 times to mix the antico-agulant with the blood. The tube should then be placed in a biohazard specimen bag, along with a laboratory request for pickup by a laboratory courier. Complete instructions for collection and handling of a specimen for a PT/INR test as presented in a laboratory directory are outlined in Figure 18-7.

PT/INR

CPT Code: 85610

Type of specimen: Whole blood or plasma

Amount: 5 ml

Collection supplies: Light blue–stoppered tube (sodium citrate)

Collection techniques: Blood must be collected in a light blue–stoppered tube containing 3.2% buffered sodium citrate. When collecting the specimen using a winged infusion set, a red 5-ml discard tube should be drawn first. The citrate tube must be filled completely to ensure a proper blood to anticoagulant ratio. Gently invert tube 3-4 times immediately after drawing to mix the anticoagulant with the blood. Any tube containing a clot activator or an anticoagulant should be collected after the light blue–stoppered tube. SST tubes should also be collected after the light blue–stoppered tube.

Patient preparation: None

Handling and storage: Specimen is stable at room temperature for up to 24 hours. If testing cannot be performed within 24 hours, specimen should be centrifuged for 15 minutes and the plasma removed using a plastic pipet and placed in a transfer tube, being careful not to disturb the buffy coat. Place the plasma in a labeled transfer tube and place in a freezer.

Causes for rejection: Hemolyzed or clotted specimen, underfilled tube (less than 90% full), improper labeling of tube. Specimen collected in any tube other than a sodium citrate (light blue–stoppered) tube.

Reference range:	Patients not on warfarin therapy:	0.8-1.2
	Patients on moderate-intensity warfarin therapy:	2.0-3.0
	Patients on high-intensity warfarin therapy for a mechanical heart valve	2.5-3.5

Use:
- Therapeutic monitoring of patients on warfarin therapy
- Detection of coagulation disorders

Limitations:
- Barbiturates, oral contraceptives and hormone-replacement therapy, and vitamin K can decrease the PT/INR.
- Consumption of large amounts of food containing vitamin K can decrease the PT/INR.
- Hematocrits in the range of 24%-54% have been demonstrated not to affect results.

Methodology: Photo-optical clot detection analyzer

Figure 18-7. Specimen collection and handling requirements for a PT/INR test from a laboratory directory.

Performing a PT/INR Test

CLIA-waived handheld coagulation analyzers are commercially available for performing a PT/INR test in the medical office. Brand names include HemoSense INRatio 2 (Inverness Medical Innovations, Inc., Waltham, Mass) and CoaguChek System (Roche Diagnostics, Branchburg, NJ) (Figure 18-8). One of the primary advantages of these coagulation analyzers is that they require only a finger puncture to perform the test, rather than a venous blood specimen collected through a venipuncture. The manufacturer of each coagulation analyzer provides an operating manual (and sometimes an instructional video) with the instrument that includes information needed to perform quality control procedures, precautions to take when running the test, and information on storage and stability of the testing strips, collection of the specimen, and the procedure for testing the specimen. It is important that the medical assistant become completely familiar with all aspects of the coagulation analyzer used to perform a PT/INR test. Quality control procedures are of particular importance to ensure that the analyzer is functioning properly and that the test results are reliable and accurate. (Refer to Chapter 15, Quality Control, to review quality control guidelines for laboratory testing.)

The medical assistant must follow the PT/INR procedure *exactly* as presented in the operating manual. The basic procedure for performing a PT/INR test involves placing a testing strip in the analyzer. A skin puncture is performed on a finger, and a drop of the patient's blood is placed on the strip. After a countdown period in which the analyzer determines the PT test results and calculates the INR, the PT/INR results are displayed on the LCD screen of the analyzer. The medical assistant should record the results in the patient's chart, including the date and time, the name of the test (PT/INR), and the ratio value.

PT/INR Home Testing

The health insurance company of a patient on long-term warfarin therapy may provide the patient with a coagulation analyzer to test his or her blood at home (Figure 18-9). Home testing provides the patient with the convenience of not having to make periodic visits to a laboratory or medical office to have a PT/INR test performed. In addition, the patient is able to test his or her blood without a laboratory order from the physician. This provides a distinct advantage because patients are able to check their PT/INR immediately when conditions occur that might indicate a problem, such as nosebleeds, bleeding gums, or unexplained bruising. In these situations, treatment can be instituted immediately to prevent the problem from getting worse. Other factors that can affect the PT/INR results and cause them to be outside of the patient's ideal range include the following: a change in diet; use of prescription or over-the-counter medications that interact with warfarin; vitamins and herbal preparations; a change in the level of exercise; illness; smoking; and alcohol consumption. It is important that the patient keep his or her physician informed of any factors that may alter the body's response to warfarin.

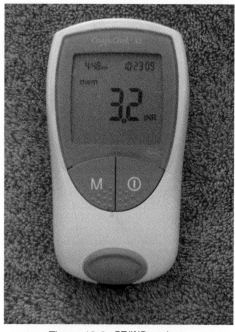

Figure 18-8. PT/INR analyzer.

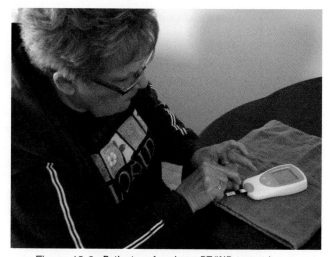

Figure 18-9. Patient performing a PT/INR test at home.

evolve *Check out the Evolve site to access additional interactive activities.*

MEDICAL PRACTICE *and the* LAW

Any blood specimen can contain bloodborne pathogens, such as hepatitis B and HIV. If spraying or splashing of blood is a possibility, use personal protective equipment, including gloves, mask, and goggles.

Laboratory test results are confidential. Giving out results without the patient's permission can result in an invasion of privacy lawsuit. Usually only the physician gives these results, so he or she can explain their meaning to the patient. ■

What Would You Do? What Would You *Not* Do? RESPONSES

Case Study 1
Page 724

What Did Latisha Do?
- ❏ Told Theodore that the physician was running some routine screening tests on him to make sure he is in good health. Explained that all patients have these tests run as part of a physical examination.
- ❏ Told Theodore that it was not possible to get the specimen from the earlobe. Explained that the earlobe is not recommended as a good site from which to obtain blood.
- ❏ Reassured Theodore that the finger-stick would be made on the least sensitive part of his finger. Told him that it would hurt for just a second, and then it would be all over and it would heal quickly.
- ❏ Told Theodore that the purpose of the blood test is early detection of anemia. Explained that if anemia is present, it can be caught early and treated before symptoms develop.

What Did Latisha Not *Do?*
- ❏ Did not collect the specimen from Theodore's earlobe.
- ❏ Did not tell Theodore that he is healthy and does not have anything wrong with him.

What Would You Do?/What Would You *Not* Do? Review Latisha's response and place a checkmark next to the information you included in your response. List additional information you included in your response.

_____

_____

_____

_____

Case Study 2
Page 730

What Did Latisha Do?
- ❏ Commended Mrs. Frasure on eating nutritiously.
- ❏ Told Mrs. Frasure that breast milk does not contain very much iron. Explained that because of this, it is important to give Travis his liquid vitamins, which have iron in them.
- ❏ Reassured Mrs. Frasure that breastfeeding does provide very good nutrition for Travis.
- ❏ Explained to Mrs. Frasure that the iron supplement may cause Travis' stool to be a dark, tarlike color, and she should not be alarmed because this is normal.

What Did Latisha Not *Do?*
- ❏ Did not criticize Mrs. Frasure for not giving Travis his vitamins or make her feel it was her fault that his hemoglobin was low.

What Would You Do?/What Would You *Not* Do? Review Latisha's response and place a checkmark next to the information you included in your response. List additional information you included in your response.

_____

_____

_____

_____

Case Study 3
Page 731

What Did Latisha Do?
- ❏ Told Marjorie that the iron injection can stain the skin but that it would be given in a special way to prevent that from happening.
- ❏ Told Marjorie that vitamin B_{12} injections are given for pernicious anemia and that her type of anemia is iron-deficiency anemia.
- ❏ Gave Marjorie a patient education brochure on iron-deficiency anemia to take home with her.
- ❏ Told Marjorie that the Red Cross requires that a blood donor's hemoglobin level be within the normal range. Explained that she could not donate this time, but that when her hemoglobin is back to normal, she will be able to donate.
- ❏ Explained to Marjorie that the iron supplement may cause her stool to be a dark, tarlike color, and she should not be alarmed because this is normal.

What Did Latisha Not *Do?*
- ❏ Did not tell Marjorie that her friend has pernicious anemia because there is no way of knowing this.

What Would You Do?/What Would You *Not* Do? Review Latisha's response and place a checkmark next to the information you included in your response. List additional information you included in your response.

_____

_____

_____

_____

CERTIFICATION REVIEW

- ❑ **Hematology involves the study of blood,** including its morphologic appearance and function, and diseases of the blood and blood-forming tissues. The most frequently performed hematologic laboratory test is the complete blood count (CBC). The tests included in a CBC are hemoglobin, hematocrit, white blood cell count, red blood cell count, differential white blood cell count, and red blood cell indices.

- ❑ **Blood consists of plasma and cells.** The function of plasma is to transport nutrients to the tissues of the body and to pick up wastes from the tissues.

- ❑ **The three types of cells in the blood** are erythrocytes, leukocytes, and thrombocytes. Erythrocytes are formed in the red bone marrow. The average number of erythrocytes in a woman is 4 to 5.5 million per cubic millimeter of blood; in a man it is 4.5 to 6.2 million per cubic millimeter of blood.

- ❑ **Hemoglobin transports oxygen** and is responsible for the red color of the erythrocyte. The amount of hemoglobin in the blood averages 12 to 16 g/dL for a woman and 14 to 18 g/dL for a man. The average life span of a red blood cell is 120 days.

- ❑ **Leukocytes are clear, colorless cells** that contain a nucleus. The number of leukocytes in a healthy adult ranges from 4500 to 11,000 per cubic millimeter of blood. Leukocytosis is an abnormal increase in the number of leukocytes, and leukopenia is an abnormal decrease in the number of leukocytes. The function of leukocytes is to defend the body against infection.

- ❑ **Thrombocytes, or platelets,** participate in the blood-clotting mechanism. The normal number of platelets in an adult is 150,000 to 400,000 per cubic millimeter.

- ❑ **The hemoglobin determination** measures indirectly the blood's oxygen-carrying capacity. A hemoglobin determination is often performed as a routine test on individuals at risk for developing anemia, such as children younger than 2 years old and pregnant women.

- ❑ **The purpose of the hematocrit** is to measure the percentage volume of packed red blood cells in whole blood. The normal hematocrit range for a woman is 37% to 47%; for a man it is 40% to 54%. A low hematocrit reading may indicate anemia, whereas a high reading may indicate polycythemia.

- ❑ **The white blood cell count** assists in the diagnosis and prognosis of disease. Leukocytosis is most commonly seen in acute infection. Conditions that result in leukopenia include viral infections, chemotherapy, and radiation therapy.

- ❑ **The red blood cell count** is a measurement of the number of red blood cells in whole blood. Conditions that cause a decrease in red blood cells include anemia, Hodgkin's disease, and leukemia. Conditions that cause an increase include polycythemia, dehydration, and pulmonary fibrosis.

- ❑ **The RBC indices** are measurements that are reported as part of the CBC; they provide the physician with information about the size and hemoglobin content of a patient's red blood cells. RBC indices include the MCV, MCH, MCHC, and the RDW. They are obtained from calculations performed on certain test results included in a CBC, specifically, the RBC count, hemoglobin, and hematocrit. Each of the various forms of anemia alters the RBC indices in a particular way. This information is used by the physician to assist in the diagnosis of the type of anemia a patient has and in determination of its cause.

- ❑ **The purpose of the differential cell count** is to identify and count the five types of white blood cells in a representative blood sample, which assists the physician in making a diagnosis. An increase or decrease in one or more types can occur in pathologic conditions.

- ❑ **The five types of white blood cells** are neutrophils, eosinophils, basophils, lymphocytes, and monocytes. Neutrophils are the most numerous of the white blood cells. An increase in the number of neutrophils is generally seen during an acute infection. Basophils are the least numerous of the white blood cells. Lymphocytes are the smallest white blood cells and are involved with the immune system and the production of antibodies. An increase in lymphocytes generally occurs with certain viral diseases. Monocytes are the largest white blood cells.

- ❑ **The PT/INR test** is a combination of a PT (prothrombin time) test and a mathematical calculation performed on the PT test to arrive at a standardized value known as an INR (International Normalized Ratio). The PT/INR test is most commonly performed on patients undergoing long-term warfarin therapy. A PT/INR test also may be ordered on patients who are exhibiting signs and symptoms of a coagulation disorder.

⟲ TERMINOLOGY REVIEW

Medical Term	Word Parts	Definition
Ameboid movement		Movement used by leukocytes that permits them to propel themselves from the capillaries into the tissues.
Anemia	*an-:* without or absence of *-emia:* blood condition	A condition in which there is a decrease in the erythrocytes or amount of hemoglobin in the blood.
Anisocytosis	*anis/o-:* unequal, dissimilar *cyt/o:* cell *-osis:* abnormal condition	A variation in the size of red blood cells.
Anticoagulant	*anti-:* against *-coagulant:* clotting	A substance that inhibits blood clotting.
Bilirubin	*bili-:* bile	An orange-colored bile pigment produced by the breakdown of heme from the hemoglobin molecule.
Diapedesis	*dia-:* through	The ameboid movement of blood cells (especially leukocytes) through the wall of a capillary and out into the tissues.
Hematology	*hemat/o-:* blood *-ology:* study of	The study of blood and blood-forming tissues.
Hemoglobin	*hem/o-:* blood *-globin:* protein	The protein- and iron-containing pigment of erythrocytes that transports oxygen in the body.
Hemolysis	*hem/o-:* blood *-lysis:* breakdown	The breakdown of erythrocytes with the release of hemoglobin into the plasma.
Hypochromic	*hypo-:* below, deficient *chrom/o:* color *-ic:* pertaining to	A red blood cell with a decreased concentration of hemoglobin.
Leukocytosis	*leuk/o-:* white *cyt/o:* cell *-osis:* abnormal condition (means increased when used with blood cell word parts)	An abnormal increase in the number of white blood cells (greater than 11,000 per cubic millimeter of blood).
Leukopenia	*leuk/o-:* white *-penia:* abnormal reduction in number	An abnormal decrease in the number of white blood cells (less than 4500 per cubic millimeter of blood).
Microcytic	*micro-:* small *cyt/o:* cell *-ic:* pertaining to	An abnormally small red blood cell.
Macrocytic	*macr/o-:* abnormally large *cyt/o:* cell *-ic:* pertaining to	An abnormally large red blood cell.
Normochromic	*norm/o-:* normal *chrom/o:* color *-ic:* pertaining to	A red blood cell with a normal concentration of hemoglobin.
Normocytic	*norm/o:* normal *cyt/o:* cell *-ic:* pertaining to	A normal-sized red blood cell.
Oxyhemoglobin	*oxy/i-:* oxygen *hem/o:* blood *-globin:* protein	Hemoglobin that has combined with oxygen.
Phagocytosis	*phag/o-:* eat, swallow *cyt/o:* cell *-osis:* abnormal condition	The engulfing and destruction of foreign particles, such as bacteria, by special cells called *phagocytes*.
Polycythemia	*poly-:* many *cyt/o:* cell *hem/o:* blood *-ia:* condition of diseased or abnormal state	A disorder in which there is an increase in the red blood cell mass.

ON THE WEB

For Information on Anemia:

National Anemia Action Council: www.anemia.org

Anemia Education: www.anemia.com

For Information on Leukemia:

The Leukemia and Lymphoma Society: www.leukemia.org

Leukemia Research Foundation: www.leukemia-research.org

Leukemia: www.oncologychannel.com

For Information on Clotting Disorders:

Clotting Disorders: www.coagulation-factors.com

National Alliance for Thrombosis and Thrombophilia: www.stoptheclot.org

Clot Care Online Resource: www.clotcare.com

19

Blood Chemistry and Immunology

LEARNING OBJECTIVES

Blood Chemistry

1. Explain the purpose of a blood chemistry test.
2. Explain the functions of glucose and insulin in the body.
3. State the patient preparation for a fasting blood glucose test.
4. Identify the normal range for a fasting blood glucose test.
5. State the purpose of each of the following tests: fasting blood glucose test, 2-hour postprandial glucose test, and oral glucose tolerance test.
6. Describe the procedure for a 2-hour postprandial blood glucose test.
7. Identify the patient preparation required for an oral glucose tolerance test.
8. State the restrictions that must be followed by the patient during an oral glucose tolerance test.
9. List three advantages of self-monitoring of blood glucose by diabetic patients.
10. Explain the purpose of the hemoglobin A_{1c} test.
11. State the hemoglobin A_{1c} level for an individual without diabetes.
12. State the recommended blood glucose level and hemoglobin A_{1c} percentage for an individual with diabetes.
13. Explain the storage requirements for blood glucose test strips.
14. Describe the functions of LDL cholesterol and HDL cholesterol in the body.
15. State the desirable ranges for each of the following tests: total cholesterol, LDL cholesterol, and HDL cholesterol.
16. State the patient preparation for a triglyceride test.

Immunology

1. Explain the purpose of each of the following immunologic tests: hepatitis tests, HIV tests, syphilis tests, mononucleosis test, rheumatoid factor, antistreptolysin test, C-reactive protein, cold agglutinins, ABO and Rh blood typing, and Rh antibody titer.
2. List the symptoms of infectious mononucleosis.
3. Identify the locations of the blood antigens and antibodies.
4. Explain how the blood antigen-antibody reaction is used for blood typing in vitro.
5. List the antigens and antibodies in the following blood types: A, B, AB, and O.
6. Explain the difference between Rh-positive and Rh-negative blood.

PROCEDURES

Perform a fasting blood glucose test using a glucose monitor.
Demonstrate the proper care and maintenance of a glucose monitor.
Instruct a patient on how to measure blood glucose using a glucose monitor.
Perform blood chemistry testing, using an automated blood chemistry analyzer and operating manual.

Perform a rapid mononucleosis test.

KEY TERMS

agglutination (ah-gloo-ti-NAY-shun)
analyte
antibody (AN-ti-bod-ee)
antigen (AN-ti-jen)
antiserum (AN-ti-sere-um)
blood antibody
blood antigen
donor
gene (jeen)
glycogen (GLIE-koe-jen))

glycosylation
HDL cholesterol
hemoglobin A_{1c}
hyperglycemia (hie-per-glie-SEE-me-ah)
hypoglycemia (hie-poe-glie-SEE-me-ah)
in vitro (in-VEE-troe)
in vivo (in-VEE-voe)
LDL cholesterol
lipoprotein (lie-poe-PROE-teen)
recipient (ree-SIP-ee-ent)

Introduction to Blood Chemistry and Immunology

CLIA-waived blood chemistry and immunologic laboratory tests are often performed in the medical office. Advances in CLIA-waived automated blood analyzers and testing kits designed specifically for use in the medical office have made this possible. Automated blood analyzers perform laboratory tests in a short time with accurate test results.

This chapter is divided into two units. The first presents blood chemistry laboratory tests, and the second presents immunologic tests. The material in this chapter about blood testing is intended to serve only as a basic guide for the medical assistant and should be supplemented by much

well-supervised practice in a classroom laboratory, the medical office, or both.

BLOOD CHEMISTRY

Blood chemistry testing involves the quantitative measurement of chemical substances in the blood. These chemicals are dissolved in the liquid portion (plasma) of the blood. Numerous types of blood chemistry tests are available; the type of test (or tests) the physician orders depends on the clinical diagnosis. Table 19-1 lists common blood chemistry tests with specimen requirements, normal values, and conditions that cause abnormal test results. The blood chemistry tests that are most frequently performed are described in greater detail in this chapter.

Table 19-1 Common Blood Chemistry Tests

Name of Test (Abbreviation)	Purpose	Reference Range	Increased With	Decreased With
Alanine aminotransferase (ALT)	To detect liver disease	45 U/L or less	Hepatocellular disease Active cirrhosis Metastatic liver tumor Obstructive jaundice Pancreatitis	
Alkaline phosphatase (ALP)	Assists in diagnosis of liver and bone diseases	25-140 U/L	Liver disease Bone disease Hyperparathyroidism Infectious mononucleosis	Hypophosphatasia Malnutrition Hypothyroidism Chronic nephritis
Aspartate aminotransferase (AST)	To detect tissue damage	40 U/L or less	Myocardial infarction Liver disease Acute pancreatitis Acute hemolytic anemia	Beriberi Uncontrolled diabetes with acidosis
Blood urea nitrogen (BUN)	Screens for renal disease, especially glomerular functioning	7-25 mg/dL	Kidney disease Urinary obstruction Dehydration Gastrointestinal bleeding	Liver failure Malnutrition Impaired absorption
Calcium (Ca)	To assess parathyroid functioning and calcium metabolism and evaluate malignancies	8.5-10.8 mg/dL	**Hypercalcemia** Hyperparathyroidism Bone metastases Multiple myeloma Hodgkin's disease Addison's disease Hyperthyroidism	**Hypocalcemia** Hypoparathyroidism Acute pancreatitis Renal failure
Chloride (Cl)	Assists in diagnosing disorders of acid-base and water balance	96-109 mmol/L	Dehydration Cushing's syndrome Hyperventilation Preeclampsia Anemia	Severe vomiting Severe diarrhea Ulcerative colitis Pyloric obstruction Severe burns Heat exhaustion
Cholesterol (Chol)	To screen for atherosclerosis related to coronary artery disease; secondary aid in study of thyroid and liver functioning	**Total Cholesterol** *Desirable:* Less than 200 mg/dL *Borderline high:* 200-239 mg/dL *High:* 240 mg/dL or greater **LDL Cholesterol** *Optimal:* Less than 100 mg/dL *Near optimal:* 100-129 mg/dL *Borderline high:* 130-159 mg/dL *High:* 160-189 mg/dL *Very high:* 190 mg/dL or greater **HDL Cholesterol** *Optimal:* 60 mg/dL or greater *Desirable:* Men: 40-50 mg/dL Women: 50-60 mg/dL *Increased risk for coronary artery disease:* Men: Less than 40 mg/dL Women: Less than 50 mg/dL	Atherosclerosis Cardiovascular disease Obstructive jaundice Hypothyroidism Nephrosis	Malabsorption Liver disease Hyperthyroidism Anemia
Creatinine (Creat)	Screening test of renal functioning	0.6-1.5 mg/dL	Impaired renal function Chronic nephritis Obstruction of urinary tract Muscle disease	Muscular dystrophy

Continued

Table 19-1 Common Blood Chemistry Tests—cont'd

Name of Test (Abbreviation)	Purpose	Reference Range	Increased With	Decreased With
Globulin (Glob)	To identify abnormalities in rate of protein synthesis and removal	2-3.5 g/dL	Brucellosis Chronic infections Rheumatoid arthritis Dehydration Hepatic carcinoma Hodgkin's disease	Agammaglobulinemia Severe burns
Glucose	To detect disorders of glucose metabolism		**Hyperglycemia**	**Hypoglycemia**
Fasting blood glucose (FBG)		*Normal:* 70-99 mg/dL *Pre-diabetes:* 100-125 mg/dL *Diabetes:* 126 mg/dL or above	Diabetes	Excess insulin
2-Hour postprandial blood sugar (2-hr PPBS)		**2-hr PPBS:** Less than 140 mg/dL (SI units: Less than 7.8 mmol/L)	Hepatic disease	Addison's disease
Oral glucose tolerance test (OGTT)		**(2 hr)** *Normal:* 139 mg/dL and below *Pre-diabetes:* 140-199 mg/dL *Diabetes:* 200 mg/dL or above	Diabetes Brain damage Cushing's syndrome	Hypoglycemia Bacterial sepsis Pancreatic carcinoma Hepatic necrosis Hypothyroidism
Lactate dehydrogenase, 30° C (LD)	Assists in confirming myocardial or pulmonary infarction; also used in differential diagnosis of muscular dystrophy and pernicious anemia	240 U/L or less	Acute myocardial infarction Acute leukemia Muscular dystrophy Pernicious anemia Hemolytic anemia Hepatic disease Extensive cancer	
Phosphorus (P)	Assists in proper evaluation and interpretation of calcium levels; used to detect disorders of endocrine system, bone diseases, and kidney dysfunction	2.5-4.5 mg/dL	**Hyperphosphatemia** Renal insufficiency Severe nephritis Hypoparathyroidism Hypocalcemia Addison's disease	**Hypophosphatemia** Hyperparathyroidism Rickets and osteomalacia Diabetic coma Hyperinsulinism
Potassium (K)	To diagnose disorders of acid-base and water balance in the body	3.5-5.3 mmol/L	**Hyperkalemia** Renal failure Cell damage Acidosis Addison's disease Internal bleeding	**Hypokalemia** Diarrhea Pyloric obstruction Starvation Malabsorption Severe vomiting Severe burns Diuretic administration Chronic stress Liver disease with ascites
Sodium (Na)	To detect changes in water and salt balance in the body	135-147 mmol/L	**Hypernatremia** Dehydration Conn's syndrome Primary aldosteronism Coma Cushing's disease Diabetes insipidus	**Hyponatremia** Severe burns Severe diarrhea Addison's disease Severe nephritis Pyloric obstruction

Table 19-1 Common Blood Chemistry Tests—cont'd

Name of Test (Abbreviation)	Purpose	Reference Range	Increased With	Decreased With
Total bilirubin (TB)	To evaluate liver functioning and hemolytic anemia	0.2-1.3 mg/dL	Liver disease Obstruction of common bile or hepatic duct Hemolytic anemia	
Total protein (TP)	Screens for diseases that alter protein balance and assesses state of body hydration	6-8.5 g/dL	Dehydration (vomiting, diarrhea) Chronic infections Acute liver disease Multiple myeloma Lupus erythematosus	Severe hemorrhaging Hodgkin's disease Severe liver disease Malabsorption
Total thyroxine (Total T$_4$)	To assess thyroid functioning and evaluate thyroid replacement therapy	4.5-12 μg/dL	**Hyperthyroidism** Graves' disease Thyrotoxicosis Thyroiditis	**Hypothyroidism** Cretinism Goiter Myxedema Hypoproteinemia
Triglycerides (Trig)	To evaluate patients with suspected atherosclerosis	*Desirable:* Less than 150 mg/dL *Borderline high:* 150-199 mg/dL *High:* 200-499 mg/dL *Very high:* 500 mg/dL or greater	Liver disease Kidney disease Obesity Hypothyroidism Poorly controlled diabetes Pancreatitis	Malnutrition Congenital lipoproteinemia Hyperthyroidism
Uric acid (UA)	To evaluate renal failure, gout, and leukemia	*Male:* 3.9-9 mg/dL *Female:* 2.2-7.7 mg/dL	Renal failure Gout Leukemia Severe eclampsia Lymphomas	Patients undergoing treatment with uricosuric drugs

COLLECTION OF A BLOOD CHEMISTRY SPECIMEN

Most blood chemistry tests performed at an outside laboratory require a serum specimen for analysis (Figure 19-1). If the specimen is collected at the medical office, the medical assistant will need to perform a venipuncture using a serum separator tube (SST) or a red-stoppered tube. An example of a blood chemistry profile frequently ordered on patients in the medical office is a *comprehensive metabolic profile* (CMP). A CMP contains numerous blood chemistry tests and is used primarily in routine health screening of a patient. It is frequently used to detect any changes in the body's biologic processes that may be present, although the patient may not have had any symptoms to indicate that these changes have occurred. A comprehensive metabolic profile is also used when the patient's symptoms are so vague that the physician does not have enough concrete evidence to support a clinical diagnosis of a specific organ or disease state. Specimen collection and handling requirements for a comprehensive metabolic profile as presented in a laboratory directory are outlined in Figure 19-2.

AUTOMATED BLOOD CHEMISTRY ANALYZERS

Automated blood chemistry analyzers are used to perform blood chemistry testing. A blood chemistry analyzer consists of a reflectance photometer that quantitatively mea-

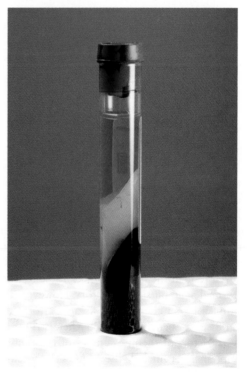

Figure 19-1. Most blood chemistry tests are performed on a serum specimen collected in a serum separator tube (SST).

Comprehensive Metabolic Profile

CPT Code:	80053

Tests included: albumin, albumin/globulin ratio (calculated), alkaline phosphatase, ALT, AST, BUN/creatinine ratio (calculated), calcium, carbon dioxide, chloride, creatinine, globulin, glucose, potassium, sodium, total bilirubin, total protein.

Type of specimen:	Serum
Amount:	4 ml
Collection supplies:	SST (send entire tube)
Collection techniques:	Let SST stand for 30 minutes. Centrifuge SST within 45 minutes of collection to separate serum from cells with gel barrier.
Patient preparation:	Patient should fast for 12 to 14 hours prior to collection.
Handling and storage:	Refrigerate or store at room temperature. Stable at room temperature for 24 hours and stable in the refrigerator for 72 hours.
Causes for rejection:	Nonfasting specimen, hemolysis, improper labeling of tube
Reference range:	Values given with report.

Use:
The CMP is used as a screening test to assess the overall health of an individual. It is used to detect any changes in the body's biologic processes that may be present, although the patient may not have had any symptoms to indicate these changes have occurred. Also see uses of individual tests.

Limitations:	See individual tests for limitations.
Methodology:	See individual tests for methodologies.

Figure 19-2. Specimen collection and handling requirements for a comprehensive metabolic profile as presented in a laboratory directory.

sures the amount of chemical substances, or analytes, in the blood. An *analyte* is defined as a substance that is being identified or measured in a laboratory test. Specifically, a reflectance photometer measures light intensity to determine the exact amount of an analyte in a specimen.

Most physicians consider it too expensive in terms of equipment, supplies, and medical laboratory personnel to perform blood chemistry tests that are any more complex than waived tests in the medical office. These tests are usually performed at an outside laboratory. However, if moderately complex blood chemistry tests are performed in the medical office, a "benchtop" blood chemistry analyzer is typically used to run them; examples of these nonwaived "benchtop" analyzers include the ATAC Lab System (Clinical Data, Inc., Newton, Mass) (Figure 19-3) and the Reflotron Analyzer (Roche Diagnostics, Branchburg, NJ). Examples of CLIA-waived blood chemistry analyzers that are more commonly used to run blood chemistry tests in the medical office include the Accu-Check Advantage blood glucose meter (Roche Diagnostics), A_{1c} Now (Bayer Corporation, Morrisville, NJ), and the Cholestech LDX Cholesterol System (Cholestech Corporation, Hayward, Calif).

The manufacturer of each blood chemistry analyzer provides an operating manual (and sometimes an instructional video) with the instrument that includes information needed to collect and handle the specimen, perform quality control procedures, and test the specimen. The manufacturer also has personnel available for on-site training and service. Because most medical offices use CLIA-waived blood chemistry analyzers (rather than nonwaived analyzers), the remainder of this chapter focuses on CLIA-waived blood chemistry analyzers used in the medical office.

It is important that the medical assistant become completely familiar with all aspects of the CLIA-waived analyzer

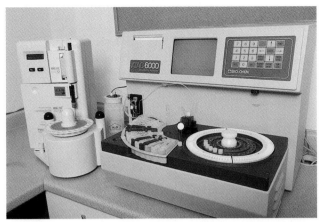

Figure 19-3. Blood chemistry analyzer (ATAC Lab System by Clinical Data, Inc.).

used to perform blood chemistry testing in his or her medical office. Medical offices running CLIA-waived tests are required to follow the manufacturer's instructions *exactly* for each testing procedure. Instructions include information on the quality control procedures that must be performed when running the test. Quality control procedures are of particular importance to ensure that the analyzer is functioning properly, and that the test results are reliable and accurate. Additional information on quality control procedures is presented below (also refer to the Quality Control section in Chapter 15, pages 618 to 620).

Quality Control

The ultimate goal when performing blood chemistry testing is to ensure that the test accurately measures what it is supposed to measure; this involves practicing and maintaining

a quality control program. Quality control consists of methods and means to ensure that test results are reliable and valid. Two important quality control measures must be performed routinely when a blood chemistry analyzer is used: calibration of the instrument and running controls.

Calibration

Calibration is a mechanism used to check the precision and accuracy of a blood chemistry analyzer, to determine if the system is providing accurate results. A calibration check detects errors caused by laboratory equipment that is not working properly. Calibration is typically performed using a calibration device, often called a *standard.* The calibration device may come in the form of a calibration strip or cassette. The device is inserted into the analyzer (Figure 19-4, *A*) and the calibration results are displayed on the LCD screen of the analyzer. The calibration results are then compared with the expected results provided in the product insert or on the calibration device (Figure 19-4, *B*). If the calibration procedure does not perform as expected, patient testing should not be conducted until the problem has been identified and resolved. The frequency of performing a calibration check is indicated in the manufacturer's instructions. At a minimum, a calibration check should be performed when a new lot number of testing reagents is put into use.

Controls

A blood chemistry control consists of a solution that is used to monitor a blood chemistry analyzer to ensure the reliability and accuracy of the test results. Controls consist of commercially available solutions with known values. Controls usually come with a product insert, which lists the expected

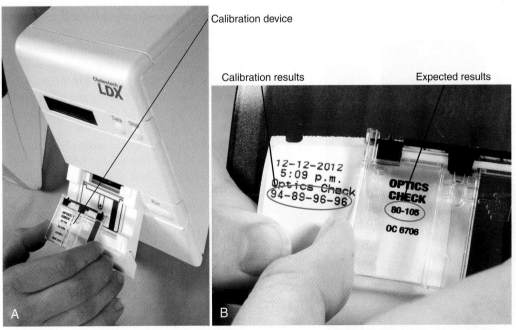

Figure 19-4. **A,** Calibrating a blood chemistry analyzer using a calibration device. **B,** The calibration results are compared with the expected results on the calibration device.

ranges for control results (Figure 19-5); however, expected ranges may sometimes be printed on the containers of the testing reagents. Controls are used to determine if the testing reagents are performing properly and to detect any errors in technique by the individual performing the test.

Generally, two levels of controls must be performed on a blood chemistry analyzer. A *low-level control* (also known as a *Level 1 control*) produces results that fall below the reference range for the test; a *high-level control* (also known as a *Level 2 control*) produces results that fall above the reference range for the test. The control procedure is performed in a similar manner to the procedure for performing the test on a specimen collected from a patient. Instead of the patient specimen being added to the testing device, however, the control is added to it (Figure 19-6). The control results are compared with ex-

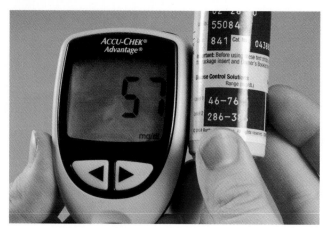

Figure 19-7. The control results are compared with the expected results.

pected results provided in the product insert (see Figure 19-5) or on the container of the testing reagents (Figure 19-7).

Failure of a control to produce expected results may be due to the following: deterioration of testing components due to expired testing components or improper storage, improper environmental testing conditions, or errors in the technique used to perform the procedure. If the controls do not perform as expected, patient testing should not be conducted until the problem has been identified and resolved. The frequency of performing controls is indicated in the manufacturer's instructions. At a minimum, they should be performed on each new lot number of testing reagents, and thereafter on a regular basis, such as monthly.

BLOOD GLUCOSE

Glucose is the end product of carbohydrate metabolism; it is the chief source of energy for the body. Energy is needed to perform normal functions and to maintain body temperature. The body maintains a constant blood glucose level to ensure a continuous source of energy for the body. Ingested glucose that is not needed for energy can be stored for later use in the form of **glycogen** in muscle and liver tissue. When no more tissue storage is possible, excess glycogen is converted to triglycerides (a form of fat) and is stored as adipose tissue.

Insulin is a hormone secreted by the beta cells of the pancreas that is required for normal use of glucose in the body. Insulin enables glucose to enter the body's cells and be converted to energy. Insulin also is needed for the proper storage of glycogen in liver and muscle cells.

Blood Glucose Testing

Measuring the amount of glucose in a blood specimen is one of the most commonly performed blood chemistry tests. It is used to detect abnormalities in carbohydrate metabolism such as those that occur in pre-diabetes, diabetes, gestational diabetes, **hypoglycemia,** and liver and adrenocortical dysfunction. Blood glucose is measured by several different testing methods, which include the fasting blood

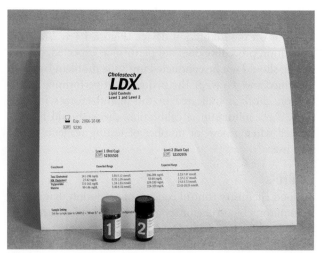

Figure 19-5. Controls come with a product insert, which lists the expected ranges for control results.

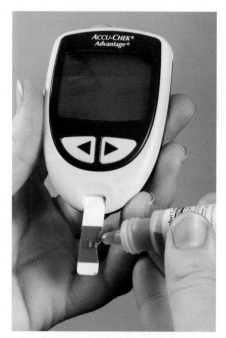

Figure 19-6. The control solution is added to a testing strip.

glucose, the 2-hour postprandial blood sugar test, and the oral glucose tolerance test. Each of these methods serves a specific role in diagnosing and evaluating abnormalities in carbohydrate metabolism, and each is described in greater detail here.

Fasting Blood Glucose Test

Blood glucose is usually measured when the patient is in a fasting state. This type of test, termed a *fasting blood glucose* (FBG), involves collecting a fasting blood sample and measuring the amount of glucose in it. The patient should not have anything to eat or drink except water for 12 hours preceding the test. Certain medications, such as oral contraceptives, salicylates, diuretics, and steroids, may affect the test results; the physician may place the patient on medication restrictions for a specific period before the test—usually 3 days. The patient should be scheduled for the test in the morning to minimize the inconvenience of abstaining from food and fluid.

A FBG is often performed on patients diagnosed with diabetes to evaluate their progress and regulate treatment, and on other patients as a routine screening test to detect pre-diabetes and diabetes. *Pre-diabetes* is the term used to describe the condition in which glucose levels are higher than normal, but not high enough to be classified as diabetes. An individual with pre-diabetes has an increased risk of developing type 2 diabetes. The American Diabetes Association (ADA) recommends the following guidelines for interpretation of FBG test results:

70-99 mg/dL:	Normal
100-125 mg/dL:	Pre-diabetes (also termed *impaired fasting glucose*)
126 mg/dL or above:	Diabetes (confirm by repeating the FBG test on another day)

Two-Hour Postprandial Blood Glucose Test

The 2-hour postprandial blood glucose (2-hour PPBG) test is used to screen for diabetes and to monitor the effects of insulin dosage in patients with diabetes. The patient is required to fast, beginning at midnight preceding the test and continuing until breakfast. For breakfast, the patient must consume a prescribed meal that contains 100 g of carbohydrate, which consists of orange juice, cereal with sugar, toast, and milk. An alternative to this is the consumption of a 100-g test-load glucose solution. A blood specimen is collected from the patient exactly 2 hours after consumption of the meal or glucose solution.

In a nondiabetic patient, the glucose level returns to the fasting level within 1½ to 2 hours of glucose consumption, whereas the glucose level in a diabetic patient does not return to the fasting level. A postprandial glucose level of 140 g/dL or higher suggests diabetes and warrants further testing, such as the oral glucose tolerance test.

Oral Glucose Tolerance Test

The oral glucose tolerance test (OGTT) provides more detailed information about the ability of the body to metabolize glucose by assessing the insulin response to a glucose load. The OGTT is used to assist in the diagnosis of pre-diabetes, diabetes, gestational diabetes, hypoglycemia, and liver and adrenocortical dysfunction. It provides a more thorough analysis of glucose use than is provided by the FBG or the 2-hour PPBG test.

Testing Requirements

The patient is usually required to consume a high-carbohydrate diet, consisting of 150 g of carbohydrate per day, for 3 days before the oral glucose tolerance test. The patient must be in a fasting state when the test begins. On the morning of the test, a blood specimen is drawn from the patient for an FBG. If the FBG indicates **hyperglycemia,** the physician should be notified because this situation is a contraindication for the administration of a large test load of glucose.

After the FBG has been performed, the patient is instructed to drink a solution containing 75 grams of glucose. At regular intervals thereafter a blood specimen is taken to determine the patient's ability to handle the increased

---

Putting It All into Practice

My Name is Michelle Villers, and I work for a physician in an internal medicine medical office. My primary job responsibility includes running the laboratory at the office. I mainly draw blood and perform blood chemistry tests. I also work up patients, run electrocardiograms, apply Holter monitors, and perform pulmonary function tests.

When performing a venipuncture, you need to make sure all the necessary equipment is on hand and ready. Sometimes you may have a tube that has no vacuum in it. In cases like these, it is always better to have a couple of spare tubes on hand. I recently had an experience in which one of my tubes had no vacuum. Luckily, I had a few extra tubes within arm's reach, so I did not have to interrupt the procedure to get a new one. I have learned that you can never be too prepared. ■

What Would You Do? What Would You *Not* Do?

Case Study 1

Crystal Louellen is at the medical office for an oral glucose tolerance test. She says that she tried not to eat anything, but she started shaking, so she stopped at McDonald's on the way over and got a sausage biscuit and orange juice. Crystal gets quite upset when she learns that she has to come back again to have her test run. She said that she hired a babysitter to watch her four preschool-age children. She demands to know why this test takes so long and why she can't have anything to eat before the test. Crystal wants to know if she can bring her children next time, so she doesn't have to hire a babysitter. Crystal says that she's a "nicotine" addict, and when she's not needed for testing, she could take the kids outside to play. She says that way the kids won't bother anyone and she can have a cigarette at the same time. ■

amount of glucose. Each blood specimen must be labeled carefully with the exact time of collection. The patient is permitted to eat and drink normally after completion of the test.

It is important that the patient adhere to certain restrictions during the test to ensure accurate results. Because food and fluid affect blood glucose levels, the patient must not eat or drink anything except water during the test. Smoking is not permitted during the test because tobacco is a stimulant that increases the blood glucose level. The patient should remain at the testing site so that he or she is present when needed for collection of blood specimens and to minimize activity. Activity affects the test results by using up glucose; the patient should remain relatively inactive during the test. Sitting and reading is an activity that would be recommended.

Side Effects

During the test, the patient may experience some normal side effects, including weakness, a feeling of faintness, and perspiration. These are considered normal reactions of the body to a decrease in the glucose level as insulin is secreted in response to the glucose load. The patient should be reassured that this is a temporary condition. Serious symptoms of severe hypoglycemia should be reported immediately to the physician; these may include headache; pale, cold, and clammy skin; irrational speech or behavior; profuse perspiration; and fainting.

Interpretation of Results

As glucose is absorbed into the bloodstream, the blood glucose level of a nondiabetic individual increases to a peak level of 160 to 180 mg/dL approximately 30 to 60 minutes after the glucose solution is consumed. The pancreas secretes insulin to compensate for this rise, and the blood glucose returns to the fasting level within 2 hours of ingestion of the glucose solution.

The individual with diabetes does not exhibit the normal use of glucose just described. This is because individuals with diabetes are unable to remove glucose from the bloodstream at the same rate as nondiabetic individuals. The blood glucose peaks at a much higher level. In addition, blood glucose levels are above normal throughout the test because of the lack of insulin.

Two hours after the glucose solution is consumed, the test results are interpreted as follows, according to guidelines set forth by the American Diabetes Association (ADA):

139 and below:	Normal
140-199 mg/dL:	Pre-diabetes (also known as *impaired glucose tolerance*)
200 mg/dL or above:	Diabetes (confirm by repeating the OGTT test on another day)

Hypoglycemia

Hypoglycemia is a condition in which the glucose in the blood is abnormally low (FBG below 70 mg/dL). During the OGTT, patients with this condition exhibit an abnor-

mally low blood glucose level, beginning at the 2-hour interval and continuing for 4 or 5 hours. Hypoglycemia results from removal of glucose from the blood at an excessive rate, or from decreased secretion of glucose into the blood, which can be caused by an overdose of insulin, Addison's disease, bacterial sepsis, carcinoma of the pancreas, hepatic necrosis, or hypothyroidism.

TESTS FOR MANAGEMENT OF DIABETES

It is important for individuals with diabetes to manage their condition effectively. This is best accomplished by keeping blood glucose levels as close to normal as possible. Diabetic patients who maintain good blood glucose control generally experience fewer symptoms and delay or prevent long-term complications of the disease; these results can lead to a longer life.

Two testing methods are used for the management of diabetes—self-monitoring of blood glucose and the hemoglobin A_{1c} test. Self-monitoring of blood glucose, which is performed by diabetic patients at home, measures day-to-day fluctuations in blood glucose levels. The hemoglobin A_{1c} test must be ordered by the physician and provides an average or overall picture of the patient's blood glucose levels over time. These testing methods assist the patient and the physician in determining whether the diabetes management plan is working, or whether it needs to be adjusted.

Self-Monitoring of Blood Glucose

Individuals with diabetes cannot usually tell by the way they feel whether or not their blood glucose levels are within normal range. The only way for them to know for certain is by self-monitoring of blood glucose (SMBG). SMBG not only provides diabetic patients with feedback for maintaining normal blood glucose levels, it also assists them in anticipating and treating day-to-day, or even hour-

Memories *from* **Externship**

Michelle Villers: During my externship experience, I was assigned to a four-physician pediatric practice. The office was constantly busy with screaming children. As if I were not nervous enough, I was asked to assist in the removal of sutures. When I walked into the room with the physician, beads of sweat began to form on my forehead. A child was lying on the examining table—a little boy no more than 7 years old. He was there to have sutures removed from a recent surgery. The sutures had been tied very well, and it was difficult for the physician to cut them. The little boy lay there with tears streaming down his cheeks. I reassured him and talked to him, and his tears began to subside. "A few more minutes and it will be all over," I told him. And within those next few minutes, the physician cut the last suture. The little boy eagerly hopped down off the examining table and gave me a big hug. I learned that day how a little reassurance can make everyone involved feel better. ■

PATIENT TEACHING　Diabetes

Answer questions patients have about diabetes.

What is diabetes?

Diabetes is a lifelong condition that occurs when the body is not able to use glucose for energy because of a problem with insulin. Diabetes develops when the body produces little or no insulin, or when the body cannot use the insulin it does produce (known as *insulin resistance*). According to the American Diabetes Association, almost 24 million Americans have diabetes; of these, nearly 6 million are not yet diagnosed and are unaware that they have diabetes. An additional 57 million people have pre-diabetes. Pre-diabetes is a condition in which the glucose levels of an individual are higher than normal, but not high enough to be classified as diabetes. An individual with pre-diabetes has an increased risk of developing type 2 diabetes.

The cause of diabetes is not completely understood, but it seems that the predisposition to develop diabetes is inherited. Diabetes increases the risk of developing serious complications, including heart disease, blindness (retinopathy), nerve damage (neuropathy), kidney damage (nephropathy), and poor circulation, which can result in amputation of a limb.

What is the function of insulin?

Insulin is a hormone produced and secreted by the beta cells of the pancreas. The pancreas is a gland located just behind the stomach and is about the size of a hand. Insulin is required for the normal use of glucose in the body. Through the process of digestion, carbohydrates are broken down into glucose. Shortly after a meal containing carbohydrates is consumed, glucose levels in the blood begin to increase. This sends a message to the pancreas to secrete insulin. Insulin "unlocks" the cells of the body and allows glucose to enter the cells. Inside the cells, glucose is converted into energy. Glucose is the main source of energy for the body and is needed to carry out normal body functions and to assist in maintaining body temperature.

What are the symptoms of diabetes?

Individuals with diabetes produce little or no insulin or cannot use the insulin they do produce. Without insulin, glucose cannot get into the cells of the body, and it builds up in the bloodstream, resulting in a high blood glucose level, known as *hyperglycemia*. Although blood glucose levels are increased, the body is unable to use the glucose for energy. This results in increased hunger, weight loss, and fatigue. The body attempts to get rid of the excess glucose by expelling it in the urine. To be excreted, the glucose must be diluted in large amounts of water. This results in increased urination and increased thirst to replace the water being lost. A summary of the symptoms of diabetes follows:

Increased urination
Excessive thirst
Weight loss
Constant hunger
Nausea and vomiting
Abdominal pain
Fatigue
Blurred vision

What is the difference between type 1 diabetes and type 2 diabetes?

Two main categories of diabetes have been identified: type 1 diabetes and type 2 diabetes. Type 2 diabetes is the most common form of diabetes. Approximately 90% of individuals with diabetes have type 2 diabetes.

Type 1 diabetes

Type 1 diabetes can occur at any age but is most apt to begin in childhood, adolescence, or early adulthood (before age 30). Type 1 diabetes is an autoimmune disease in which the body produces antibodies that attack and gradually destroy the insulin-producing beta cells of the pancreas. This results in an inability of the body to produce any insulin at all, or it may produce very little insulin. The symptoms are usually severe and occur rapidly—typically over weeks or months. Individuals with type 1 diabetes almost always require insulin therapy. The insulin is administered subcutaneously using an insulin syringe/needle or an insulin pen. An insulin pen is an insulin injection device that contains a needle and holds a vial of insulin. Insulin also can be administered through an insulin pump, which is a small, battery-operated device about the size of a cell phone that is clipped to a belt or carried in a pocket (see illustration). The pump is connected to plastic tubing that continuously delivers insulin into the subcutaneous tissue of the abdomen. An insulin pump also can be programmed to deliver varying doses of insulin as a patient's need for insulin changes during the day (e.g., before exercise or meals).

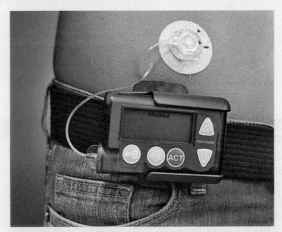

Insulin pump. (From Lewis S: Medical-surgical nursing, ed 7, St Louis, 2007, Mosby.)

Type 2 diabetes

Type 2 diabetes can affect people at any age, but the chance of developing it increases with age, and it is more likely to occur in individuals who are 40 years of age or older. The biggest risk factor for developing type 2 diabetes is excess body weight. As a result of the recent increase in childhood obesity combined with a sedentary

Continued

lifestyle, type 2 diabetes is starting to appear in younger age groups. Individuals with type 2 diabetes do not produce enough insulin or are not able to use the insulin they do produce (insulin resistance), resulting in high blood glucose levels. Type 2 diabetes almost always has a slow onset with mild symptoms that appear gradually over a long time (often years). Some individuals have no symptoms at all (except for high blood glucose levels). Because of this, they may be unaware that they have diabetes until a complication from prolonged hyperglycemia occurs, such as a vision problem or foot pain. Type 2 diabetes is first treated by dietary adjustments, weight reduction, and exercise. These changes sometimes can restore insulin sensitivity, even if the weight loss is modest. Approximately 20% of cases of type 2 diabetes can be managed by lifestyle changes alone. The next step, if necessary, is treatment with oral hypoglycemics, which are medications taken by mouth that stimulate the release of insulin from the pancreas, help the body use its own insulin better, or both. If this treatment is ineffective, insulin therapy becomes necessary to maintain normal or near-normal glucose levels.

What factors increase the risk of developing type 2 diabetes?

The cause of type 2 diabetes is unknown, although certain factors, known as *risk factors,* make a person more prone to developing type 2 diabetes. The more risk factors present, the more likely it is that an individual will develop type 2 diabetes. Some of these factors can be controlled, and others cannot.

Risk factors that can be controlled
1. **Weight.** The risk factor that contributes most to the development of type 2 diabetes is excess body weight. Approximately 80% of individuals with type 2 diabetes are overweight. Being overweight (body mass index of 25 or greater) makes it harder for the body to use insulin. A research study by the Diabetes Prevention Program showed that people who followed a low-fat, low-calorie diet; lost a moderate amount of weight; and engaged

in regular physical activity (five times a week for 30 minutes) sharply reduced their chances of developing type 2 diabetes.
2. **Smoking.** Smoking makes it harder for the body to control the blood glucose level.
3. **Lack of physical activity.** Regular exercise helps the body to use insulin normally, whereas a sedentary lifestyle contributes to insulin resistance.
4. **High blood pressure, abnormal lipid profile, or both.** The following factors contribute to insulin resistance: blood pressure greater than 130/80 mm Hg, HDL cholesterol of 35 mg/dL or less, and triglyceride level of 250 mg/dL or greater. Decreasing blood pressure also can reduce the risk of cardiovascular complications.

Risk factors that cannot be controlled
1. **Family history.** The risk of developing type 2 diabetes is increased if a close relative (parent, brother, sister) has diabetes.
2. **Gestational diabetes or giving birth to a large infant.** Women who have diabetes during pregnancy or gave birth to an infant weighing more than 9 lb are at greater risk for developing type 2 diabetes.
3. **Age.** Type 2 diabetes is more common in people 40 years and older, but it is increasing among young people who are overweight and inactive.
4. **Ethnic group.** The following ethnic groups are more likely to develop type 2 diabetes: African Americans, Latinos, Hispanics, Native Americans, Asian Americans, and Pacific Islanders.

Can diabetes be cured?

There is no cure for diabetes, but the outlook for individuals with this condition is improving. This is primarily due to better patient education, advances in blood glucose monitoring, and newer methods of insulin delivery that help simplify management of the disease. Today, most individuals with diabetes under good control have life expectancies comparable with those of individuals without diabetes. ■

Case Study 2

Dave Felden has recently been diagnosed with type 1 diabetes and is taking insulin. He has come to the office for an FBG. A fingerstick will be performed to collect the specimen, and a glucose meter will be used to test the specimen. Dave has been performing this test on himself at home now for 2 weeks and wants to know whether he can stick his own finger. Dave says that he's been having a few problems giving himself his insulin injections. He says that he has been getting some very large air bubbles in his syringe when he draws up the insulin. He says he's been having trouble getting them out and wants to know how important that is. Dave says he is on a limited income and wants to know whether he could use his needle and syringe for more than one injection. He also wants to know whether he should throw his used needle and syringes in the regular trash. ■

to-hour, fluctuations in glucose levels brought on by food, exercise, stress, and infection.

Diabetic patients who take insulin (insulin-dependent) must monitor their blood glucose levels each day. Based on the results of SMBG, decisions can be made regarding insulin and dietary adjustments that may be necessary to maintain normal glucose levels and to avoid the extremes of hypoglycemia and hyperglycemia (see Chapter 21). Satisfactory control of the blood glucose level on a day-to-day basis through SMBG reduces symptoms of the disease and helps delay or prevent long-term complications that can occur with diabetes.

Frequency of Testing

The frequency of blood glucose testing depends on numerous factors, including the severity of the diabetes, diet, activity level, and special conditions such as pregnancy. Ideally, the blood glucose level for an insulin-dependent diabetic patient should be measured 4 times a day: in the morning (after an 8-hour fast), before lunch, before dinner, and at bedtime. The FBG test result (obtained in the morning) is the best overall indicator of control, and the other determinations provide guidance for adjusting insulin dosage, diet, and exercise.

Test Results

Blood glucose levels are measured using a glucose meter, and the results are displayed in mg/dL. Table 19-2 lists recommended blood glucose levels for patients with diabetes based on when the testing is performed. Diabetic patients should be instructed to maintain a cumulative record of their daily SMBG test results for periodic review by the physician. This record assists the physician in making decisions regarding the patient's diabetes management plan.

Advantages

Research shows that SMBG is the most effective way for a diabetic patient to maintain a normal blood glucose level and delay or prevent long-term complications associated with diabetes. High blood glucose levels (greater than 180 mg/dL) for a long time can cause progressive damage to the body organs, resulting in blindness, kidney disease, nerve damage, and circulation problems. Because of the necessity of performing a skin puncture and the fact that the patient must assume responsibility in self-management decisions, the medical assistant may need to reinforce the advantages of self-monitoring of blood glucose, as follows:

1. **Convenience of testing.** The patient is able to test his or her blood at any time of the day without a laboratory order from the physician. This provides a distinct advantage because patients are able to check their blood glucose level when a side effect common to diabetes occurs, such as hypoglycemia. In these situations, treatment can be instituted immediately to prevent the problem from getting worse.
2. **Greater involvement in self-management decisions.** The patient is able to become more involved in self-management decisions regarding insulin dosage, meal planning, and physical activity. Initially some patients lack confidence in making insulin and dietary adjustments based on the blood glucose test results. The medical assistant should provide encouragement and stress the benefits to be derived in terms of improved regulation of the blood glucose level.

3. **Reliable decision making regarding insulin dosage.** More reliable decisions regarding insulin needs can be made during situations that affect the blood glucose level, such as illness, emotional stress, increased physical activity, or suspected hypoglycemia.
4. **Delay in or prevention of long-term complications.** The medical assistant should emphasize to patients how important it is to perform daily SMBG testing to increase their chances of staying healthy. As previously discussed, diabetic patients who maintain good blood glucose control generally experience fewer symptoms and a delay in or prevention of long-term complications of the disease.

Hemoglobin A_{1c} Test

The hemoglobin A_{1c} test (Hb A_{1c} test or A_{1c} test) provides valuable information for determining whether a diabetic patient's blood glucose level is under control. The A_{1c} test supplies the physician with an assessment of the average amount of glucose in the blood over a 3-month period.

When an individual consumes food containing glucose, the glucose is absorbed from the digestive tract and into the circulatory system. Glucose (sugar) has a "sticky" quality to it and thus has a tendency to stick to protein in the body. One of the proteins it attaches to is the protein included in hemoglobin. Hemoglobin is found in red blood cells and functions in transporting oxygen in the body. The process of glucose attaching to hemoglobin is known as *glycosylation.*

When glucose attaches or glycosylates to the protein in hemoglobin, it forms a compound known as **hemoglobin A_{1c}.** Glycosylation occurs in all individuals—hemoglobin A_{1c} is formed in diabetic patients and healthy individuals. The amount of glucose that attaches to hemoglobin is proportional to the amount of glucose in the blood; the more glucose in the blood, the more hemoglobin becomes glycated and the higher the A_{1c} level. Individuals with undiagnosed or poorly controlled diabetes have a higher than normal blood glucose level, and more hemoglobin A_{1c} forms in these individuals. The percentage of hemoglobin A_{1c} in the blood can be measured by the A_{1c} laboratory test. The attachment of the glucose to the hemoglobin is permanent for the life of the red blood cell (90 to 120 days); the A_{1c} test result is able to provide an overall picture of the patient's blood glucose level for the past 3 months. CLIA-waived analyzers are available for performing a hemoglobin A_{1c} test in the medical office; an example is the A1c Now (Bayer Corporation).

Interpretation of Results

The normal A_{1c} level for an individual without diabetes is 4% to 6%. Patients with diabetes usually have a higher A_{1c} level than this. The American Diabetes Association (ADA) strongly recommends that patients with diabetes maintain an A_{1c} level of less than 7%. Table 19-3 shows the correlation between hemoglobin A_{1c} percentages and average blood glucose levels. A change in a patient's diabetes man-

Table 19-2 Recommended Blood Glucose Levels for Patients With Diabetes	
Time of Day	Recommended Blood Glucose Level (mg/dL)
Before meals	80-120
1-2 hr after meals	100-180
At bedtime	100-140

Table 19-3	Comparison of Hemoglobin A$_{1c}$ Percentages With Average Blood Glucose Levels	
Hemoglobin A$_{1c}$ (%)	**Average Daily Blood Glucose Level (mg/dL)**
4	65
5	100
6	135
7	170
8	205
9	240
10	275
11	310
12	345

agement plan is almost always required if the A$_{1c}$ test result is greater than 8%.

Patients who keep their hemoglobin A$_{1c}$ levels close to 7% have a much better chance of delaying or preventing diabetic complications than do patients with A$_{1c}$ levels that are 8% or greater. Studies show that for every 1 percentage point drop in the A$_{1c}$ value, a 35% reduction in risk for diabetes-related complications occurs.

The physician orders an A$_{1c}$ test when a patient is first diagnosed with diabetes to determine how elevated the blood glucose level has been before the condition was diagnosed. The test is usually ordered several times after a diabetes management plan has been prescribed to verify that blood glucose control is being achieved. The A$_{1c}$ test is ordered periodically for patients already diagnosed with diabetes to evaluate the effectiveness of their diabetes management plan. For stable diabetic patients under good control, the test is typically ordered at least 2 times a year (every 6 months). The test is usually ordered on a more frequent basis for patients who have difficulty maintaining control of their blood glucose levels. The A$_{1c}$ test also is ordered when the physician makes an adjustment to a patient's diabetic management plan to assess the effectiveness of the change in treatment.

GLUCOSE METERS

In the medical office, a CLIA-waived glucose meter is often used to measure the blood glucose level quantitatively. The test most frequently performed using the glucose meter is the FBG, although some offices also perform the OGTT and the 2-hour postprandial test. By measuring the blood glucose concentration in the medical office, better patient care can be provided. On-site testing eliminates the time required for an outside laboratory to provide the results, allowing the physician to make decisions immediately regarding diagnosis, treatment, and follow-up care. Procedure 19-1 describes how to measure blood glucose using the Accu-Chek Advantage glucose meter.

Reagent Test Strips

A reagent test strip must be used with the glucose meter; it consists of a plastic strip with a reaction pad. The pad contains chemicals that react with the glucose in whole blood to determine the blood glucose level in mg/dL. Through an electronic signal, the glucose results are displayed as a digital readout. The manufacturer's instructions accompanying the glucose meter must be followed exactly to ensure accurate and reliable test results.

It is important to store the container of test strips properly to prevent their deterioration, which affects the test results. The chemical reagents on the strips are sensitive to heat, light, and moisture and must be stored in a cool, dry area at room temperature (less than 90° F [32° C]) with the cap tightly closed. Strips that are discolored or that have darkened should be discarded to prevent inaccurate test results. The container of test strips includes a desiccant. Its purpose is to promote dryness by absorbing moisture.

Calibration Procedure

A calibration procedure may be required for a glucose meter. Because the Accu-Chek Advantage glucose meter is presented in Procedure 19-1, the calibration method discussed here relates specifically to this meter.

The calibration procedure is a coding procedure that is performed to ensure accurate and reliable test results; most glucose meters require this calibration procedure. The coding procedure must be performed each time a new container of test strips is opened. It is performed to compensate for variables that occur in the manufacturing process, which cause one batch of test strips to be a little different from another batch. The coding procedure programs the electronics of the glucose meter to match the reactivity of the container of strips that are in current use.

The coding procedure for the Accu-Chek Advantage is performed using a plastic code key that accompanies each container of Accu-Chek Advantage test strips (Figure 19-8). Accu-Chek requires lot-specific calibration, meaning that the calibration procedure needs to be performed only once per container of test strips. This is possible because the Accu-Chek glucose meter has a built-in memory system that enables it to retain a point of reference after it has been calibrated. This reference point is retained until the glucose meter is reprogrammed for a new container of test strips. The coding procedure delineated next should be followed when a new container of Accu-Chek test strips is opened:

1. Ensure that the meter is turned off.
2. Turn the meter over so that the back of the meter is facing you.
3. Remove the old code key, if one is installed, and discard it in a waste container.
4. Insert a new code key by sliding it into the code key slot until it snaps into place (see Figure 19-8, *A*).
5. Turn the meter on. A three-digit code number appears on the display screen. This number must match the code

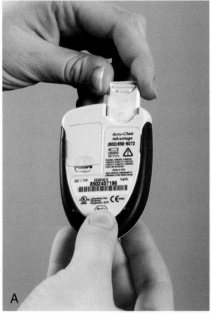
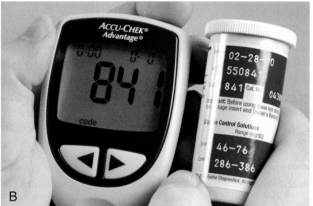

Figure 19-8. Accu-Chek Advantage code key calibration procedure. **A,** The code key is inserted into the monitor. **B,** The code number must match the code number of the vial of test strips.

number of the vial of test strips (see Figure 19-8, *B*). If it does not, repeat steps 1 through 3.

Control Procedure

A control test should be run to ensure that test results are reliable and valid, and that errors that might interfere with test results are detected and eliminated. A control check is performed on the Accu-Chek Advantage using commercially available glucose control solutions. Two levels of controls (high and low) (Figure 19-9) should be used.

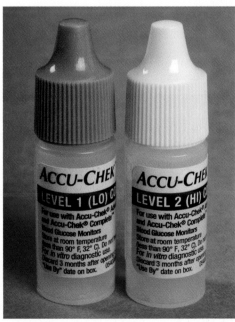

Figure 19-9. Glucose controls.

The control solution is effective for 3 months from the date it is opened. When the control solution is opened, the medical assistant must write the date on the container label. The control solution can then be used for 3 months from that date (which should also be written on the container) or until the manufacturer's expiration date (stamped on the container) is reached, whichever comes first. The control solution is sensitive to heat, light, and moisture and must be stored with the cap tightly closed in a cool, dry area at room temperature between 36° F (2° C) and 86° F (30° C).

A control test should be performed under the following circumstances:
1. When the meter is new
2. Daily, before the meter is used for the first time
3. When a new container of test strips is opened
4. If the cap is left off the vial of test strips for any length of time
5. If the meter is dropped
6. If the test result does not agree with the way the patient feels
7. If a test has been repeated, and the blood glucose result is still lower or higher than expected

If Level 1 or Level 2 control results are not within the acceptable range, the following should be performed:
1. Check the expiration date of the test strips and control solutions to make sure they are not outdated.
2. Determine whether the test strips and control solutions were stored at room temperature.
3. Make sure the container lids were tight on the test strips container and the control solution containers.
4. Check to make sure the code on the meter matches the code on the test strip vial.

5. Review the technique used to run the control to make sure it was followed correctly.

Any errors should be corrected, and the control should be run again. If the results are still not within acceptable range, the manufacturer of the glucose meter should be contacted.

Care and Maintenance

The glucose meter must be handled carefully. It is a delicate instrument, and a severe physical jar could result in a malfunction. The glucose meter should not be placed in an area of high humidity, such as a bathroom. In addition, the meter should not be exposed to severe variations in environmental temperature, such as would occur if it is left in a closed vehicle on a hot or cold day.

Proper cleaning of the glucose meter is essential for its accurate and reliable operation. On a regular basis, the exterior of the glucose meter, including the display screen, should be cleaned with a soft, clean cloth slightly dampened with a mild cleaning agent, and it should be dried thoroughly. Acceptable cleaning agents include alcohol and mild dishwashing liquid mixed with water. Do not allow water or cleaning solution to run into the glucose meter; this could damage the internal components.

Because glucose meters are battery operated, periodic replacement of the battery is required. The glucose meter alerts the user to low battery voltage by displaying a special notation on the screen. The type of battery required is specified in the operating manual, along with directions for installation.

PATIENT TEACHING Obtaining a Capillary Blood Specimen

The medical assistant may need to instruct the patient in the procedure for obtaining and testing a capillary blood specimen for blood glucose measurement. Properly educating the patient to perform the procedure is the most important factor in obtaining accurate test results.

1. **Obtaining the capillary blood specimen.** Inform the patient of the sites available for obtaining the blood specimen, including the fingers and the side of the hand that has no calluses. Most patients prefer to use an automatic lancet to perform the skin puncture. Using such a device makes the puncture less painful, and the preset puncture depth generally ensures a successful stick. For a finger puncture, instruct the patient to obtain the blood specimen from the lateral side of the fingertip because this area contains fewer nerve endings, and less pain results. If the patient's hands are cold, tell him or her to rub them together or place them in warm water, which improves blood flow to the area. Instruct the patient in the proper procedure for obtaining enough blood to ensure accurate test results.

2. **Performing the blood glucose test.** The patient performs the test with a test strip using a glucose meter. Instruct the pa-

tient in the proper procedure for performing the test, making sure he or she understands that accurate test results assist in achieving greater glucose control. Patients also should be given detailed instructions on proper care and maintenance of the glucose meter.

3. **Recording results.** Instruct the patient to record each test result in a log book between office visits to provide a permanent record. In addition, most glucose meters are equipped with a memory system that stores test results for later retrieval. Keeping track of these factors helps explain a shift in the blood glucose level and provides the basis for sound self-management decisions. The following information should be included with each recording:
   - Date and time
   - Number of hours since the patient last ate
   - Time of the last insulin injection or oral hypoglycemic medication
   - Any feeling of physical or emotional stress
   - Amount of exercise the patient has had

 PROCEDURE 19-1 Blood Glucose Measurement Using the Accu-Chek Advantage Glucose Meter

Outcome Perform a fasting blood glucose (FBG) test.

Equipment/Supplies

- Disposable gloves
- Accu-Chek Advantage glucose meter
- Accu-Chek Advantage test strips
- Code key
- Control solutions

- Lancet
- Antiseptic wipe
- Gauze pad
- Biohazard sharps container

---

1. Procedural Step. Sanitize your hands. Assemble the equipment. Check the expiration date on the container of test strips. Check to make sure the environ-

mental temperature falls between 57° F (14° C) and 104° F (40° C).

PROCEDURE 19-1 Blood Glucose Measurement Using the Accu-Chek Advantage Glucose Meter—cont'd

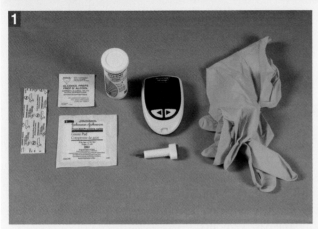

Assemble the equipment.

Principle. Outdated test strips can cause inaccurate test results. If the temperature is outside of the required range, the meter cannot perform the test, causing an error message to appear on the screen of the analyzer.

2. Procedural Step. If necessary, calibrate the glucose meter using the code key that accompanies the container of test strips.

a. Ensure that the meter is turned off.

b. Turn the meter over so that the back of the meter is facing you.

c. Insert the code key into the slot on the back of the meter.

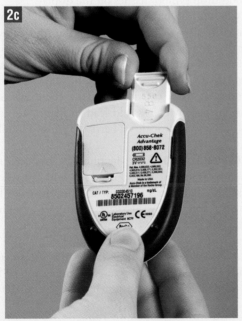

Insert the code key.

d. Push on the code key until it snaps into place.

e. Turn on the meter.

f. A three-digit code number appears on the display screen. The number must match the code number on the container of test strips.

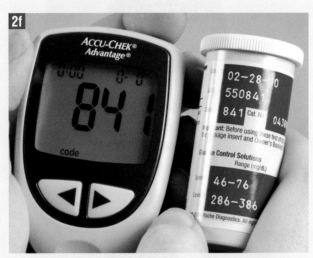

Check the code number.

Principle. Calibrating with the code key compensates for variables that occur in the manufacturing process of the test strips and must be performed before strips from a new container are used.

3. Procedural Step. Run a Level 1 (low) and Level 2 (high) control check on the glucose meter using Accu-Chek Advantage control solutions as follows:

a. Check the expiration date on the control solutions. (*Note:* The expiration date for the test strips was checked previously and therefore does not need to be checked again.)

b. Remove a test strip from the container and immediately recap the container.

c. Gently insert the end of the test strip with the silver-colored bars into the test strip guide with the yellow target area facing up. This automatically turns on the meter.

d. Check to make sure the code number matches the number displayed on the container of strips.

e. When the strip is inserted correctly, a blood drop symbol flashes on the display screen, indicating that it is ready to accept the control solution.

f. Roll the Level 1 low control solution between the palms of your hands to mix it.

g. Press and release the right arrow button once to select the Level 1 control.

h. Hold the control solution at an angle to the edge of the yellow target area of the test strip. Squeeze

Continued

PROCEDURE 19-1   Blood Glucose Measurement Using the Accu-Chek Advantage Glucose Meter—cont'd

the container, and touch and hold a drop of control solution to the edge (not the top) of the yellow target area. Promptly replace the cap for the control solution.

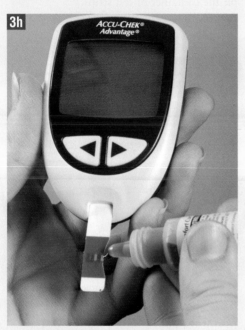

Apply the control solution.

i. After a short time, the control result is displayed on the screen of the glucose meter.

j. If the low control result is within the acceptable range, the result will alternate with the word "OK" on the display screen. The result will also fall within the expected range listed on the test strip container.

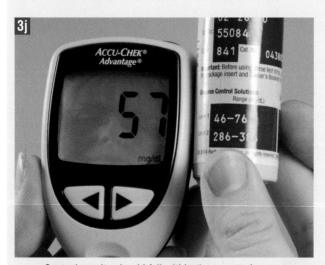

Control results should fall within the expected range.

k. Repeat the control procedure outlined above using a Level 2 high control.

l. Record the control results in the Quality Control log.

Principle. Running a low and a high control check ensures that the test results are reliable and valid. Gloves do not need to be worn because the control consists of a glucose solution.

4. **Procedural Step.** Sanitize your hands. Greet and introduce yourself. Identify the patient by full name and date of birth. Explain the procedure.

5. **Procedural Step.** Ask the patient whether he or she has had anything to eat or drink (besides water) for the past 12 hours.

Principle. Consumption of food or fluid increases the blood glucose level, leading to inaccurate interpretation of FBG test results.

6. **Procedural Step.** Remove a test strip from the container. Promptly replace the lid of the container to prevent the strips from being exposed to moisture.

Principle. The reagent pads are moisture sensitive and could be affected by environmental moisture, leading to inaccurate test results.

7. **Procedural Step.** Gently insert the end of the test strip with the silver-colored bars into the test strip guide with the yellow target area facing up. Check that the code number displayed matches the code number on the vial of test strips that you are using. When the test strip symbol flashes on the display, the meter is ready to accept a blood specimen.

Principle. When the strip is correctly inserted, a blood drop symbol flashes on the display.

8. **Procedural Step.** Open the gauze packet. Cleanse the puncture site with an antiseptic wipe, and allow it to air-dry. Apply gloves, and perform a finger puncture. Dispose of the lancet in a biohazard sharps container.

Principle. The antiseptic must be allowed to dry to prevent it from reacting with the chemicals on the reagent pad, which would lead to inaccurate test results. Gloves provide a barrier against bloodborne pathogens.

9. **Procedural Step.** After the puncture has been made, wipe away the first drop of blood with a gauze pad. Place the hand in a dependent position (palm facing down), and gently massage the finger around the puncture site until a large drop of blood forms.

Principle. The first drop of blood contains a large amount of serum, which dilutes the specimen and leads to inaccurate test results. A large drop of blood is needed to cover the target area of the test strip completely.

PROCEDURE 19-1 Blood Glucose Measurement Using the Accu-Chek Advantage Glucose Meter—cont'd

10. Procedural Step. Apply the drop of blood to the Comfort Curve test strip as follows:

a. Touch and hold a drop of blood to the edge (not the top) of the yellow target area.

b. Completely fill the yellow target area. You will hear a beeping sound when sufficient blood has been applied. If any yellow mesh is visible after you have applied the initial drop of blood, a second drop of blood may be applied to the target area within 15 seconds of the first drop. If more than 15 seconds has passed, the test result may be erroneous, and you should discard the test strip and repeat the test.

Principle. The entire yellow target area must be completely covered with blood to ensure accurate and reliable test results.

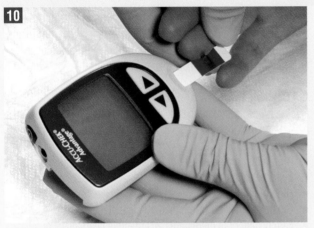

Apply a drop of blood.

11. Procedural Step. Have the patient hold a gauze pad over the puncture site and apply pressure until the bleeding stops.

12. Procedural Step. When the blood is correctly applied to the strip, an hourglass flashes on the screen while the meter analyzes the blood specimen. After a short time, the glucose value is displayed in milligrams per deciliter (mg/dL). If the glucose value is higher or lower than expected, or if the screen displays something other than the glucose value, see the Troubleshooting Guide section of the operator's manual to obtain instructions for correcting the problem. (The glucose result indicated on this glucose meter is 98 mg/dL.)

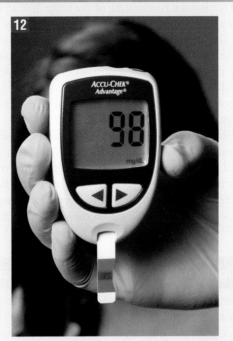

Read the glucose results.

13. Procedural Step. Remove the test strip from the meter, and discard it in a biohazard waste container. Turn the meter off.

14. Procedural Step. Check the puncture site and apply an adhesive bandage to the patient's finger if needed.

15. Procedural Step. Remove your gloves, and sanitize your hands. Chart the results. Include the date and time, the type of glucose test (e.g., FBG), the glucose test results, and when the patient last ate. If the patient has diabetes, also record the time of his or her last insulin injection or last consumption of oral hypoglycemic medication.

16. Procedural Step. Properly store the glucose meter according to the manufacturer's instructions.

CHARTING EXAMPLE

Date	
5/18/12	8:30 a.m. FBG: 98 mg/dL. Pt last ate on
	5/17 @ 7:00 p.m.
	————————————M. Villers, CMA (AAMA)

PROCEDURE 19-1

CHOLESTEROL

Cholesterol is a white, waxy, fatlike substance (lipid) that is essential for normal functioning of the body. It is an important component of all cell membranes in the body and is used in the production of essential hormones and bile. Most of the cholesterol circulating in the blood is manufactured by the liver; however, a portion of it comes from an individual's diet and is known as *dietary cholesterol*. Dietary cholesterol is found only in animal products, such as organ meats, egg yolk, and dairy products.

High blood cholesterol means an excessive amount of cholesterol is present in the blood. An individual's cholesterol level is determined by his or her genetic makeup and by the amounts of dietary cholesterol, saturated fat, and *trans* fat consumed. High blood cholesterol may cause fatty deposits, or plaque, to build up on the walls of the arteries,

a condition known as *atherosclerosis*. As the atherosclerosis progresses, the arteries become more occluded, which eventually could lead to a heart attack or stroke. Because of this, high blood cholesterol is considered a risk factor for coronary artery disease (see *Highlight on Heart Disease With a Focus on Coronary Artery Disease*), and efforts should be made to reduce the cholesterol level (see *Highlight on Lowering Cholesterol*).

HDL and LDL Cholesterol

Cholesterol is transported in the blood as a complex molecule known as a **lipoprotein.** Two types of lipoproteins contain cholesterol: low-density lipoprotein (LDL) and high-density lipoprotein (HDL).

LDL picks up cholesterol from ingested fats and the liver and delivers it to blood vessels and muscles, where it is deposited in the cells. **LDL cholesterol** is often referred to as

---

Highlight on Heart Disease With a Focus on Coronary Artery Disease

Heart disease is a general term used to refer to a variety of medical conditions that affect the heart. The primary forms of heart disease include coronary artery disease (CAD), high blood pressure, heart attacks, strokes, congestive heart failure, congenital heart disease, and rheumatic heart disease. These various forms of heart disease are interrelated and have elements in common, for example, atherosclerosis can lead to a stroke or heart attack.

Heart disease is the number one killer of adults in the United States today. Because of the national focus on heart disease and cholesterol reduction, since 1985 a decline in heart attacks by 25% has been reported, as well as a decline in strokes by nearly 40%; however, heart disease is likely to remain the number one cause of death until more Americans adopt a more heart-healthy lifestyle.

Coronary Artery Disease

The most common symptom of coronary artery disease is chest pain, which is known as angina pectoris. Angina pectoris is a symptom, or a set of symptoms, rather than a disease. Angina pectoris occurs when the muscle tissue of the heart does not receive enough oxygenated blood, resulting in discomfort or pain under the sternum.

Cause

For most patients, the cause of angina is atherosclerosis of the coronary arteries. *Atherosclerosis* of the coronary arteries is a condition in which fibrous plaques of fatty deposits and cholesterol build up on the inner walls of the coronary arteries. This causes narrowing and partial blockage of the lumen of these arteries, along with hardening of the arterial wall. CAD results in a reduction of oxygenated blood flow to the heart muscle. Despite the narrowing, enough oxygen may still reach the heart muscle for normal needs. More oxygen is needed, however, when situations occur that increase the workload of the heart, such as physical activity, emotional stress, a heavy meal, and exposure to cold weather. If the coronary arteries cannot deliver enough oxygen to the heart muscle during

these times of increased need, angina pectoris may result. Severe and prolonged anginal pain generally suggests a myocardial infarction (heart attack) caused by complete blockage of the coronary arteries and requires immediate medical attention.

CAD Risk Factors

Not everyone is equal when it comes to CAD. Some individuals have a much higher risk of developing it than others. The following are risk factors for CAD:

- High total blood cholesterol (greater than 200 mg/dL confirmed by repeated measurement)
- High blood pressure
- Cigarette smoking (more than 10 cigarettes per day)
- Family history of premature CAD (definite heart attack or sudden death in a parent or sibling before age 55 years)
- Diabetes
- History of blood vessel disease
- Obesity and overweight
- Low HDL cholesterol (less than 40 mg/dL confirmed by repeated measurement)
- Elevated triglyceride level (greater than 150 mg/dL)
- Being a man older than 45 years
- Being a woman older than 55 years or postmenopausal

Some of these risk factors can be modified; others, such as age, gender, and a family history of CAD, cannot be modified or controlled. The three major risk factors for CAD are high total blood cholesterol, high blood pressure, and cigarette smoking, all of which are modifiable.

Each person's overall risk of CAD must be assessed individually by the physician, based on the type and number of risk factors present. A 47-year-old man with a cholesterol level of 220 mg/dL who smokes a pack of cigarettes a day and is overweight is at greater risk than a 28-year-old man who is within a normal weight range, does not smoke, and exercises regularly but has a cholesterol level of 250 mg/dL. ∎

"bad" cholesterol because an excess amount of it in the blood can cause plaque to build up on the arterial walls, resulting in atherosclerosis. See Table 19-1 for an interpretation of LDL cholesterol values.

HDL removes excess cholesterol from the cells and carries it to the liver to be excreted. Because HDL removes excess cholesterol from the walls of the blood vessels, it is protective and beneficial to the body and is often called "good" cholesterol. A high **HDL cholesterol** level has been shown to reduce the risk of coronary artery disease, whereas a low level of HDL cholesterol (less than 40 mg/dL) is a risk factor for coronary artery disease.

Cholesterol Testing

All adults older than 20 years of age should have a cholesterol test at least once every 5 years. Initial testing includes a *total cholesterol* determination, which is a combined measurement of LDL cholesterol and HDL cholesterol in the blood. To obtain a fuller picture of a patient's cholesterol status, physicians typically also order an HDL cholesterol determination, which measures only the HDL cholesterol in the blood. Cholesterol tests are considered screening tests, and elevated results usually require confirmation through repeat testing before a diagnosis of high blood cholesterol is made.

Interpretation of Results

Cholesterol test results are interpreted as follows: Total cholesterol levels less than 200 mg/dL are desirable. Levels between 200 and 239 mg/dL are borderline high, and levels of 240 mg/dL and greater are high. Based on confirmed testing, individuals in the high category are clearly at increased risk for coronary artery disease, and individuals in the borderline high category are at increased risk if they have other risk factors, such as being overweight or smoking. According to the American Heart Association, an HDL cholesterol level less than 40 mg/dL for men and less than 50 mg/dL for women is considered a risk factor for coronary artery disease. An HDL cholesterol level between 40 and 50 mg/dL for men and between 50 and 60 mg/dL for women is desirable, whereas an HDL cholesterol level greater than 60 mg/dL is considered optimal and provides some protection against heart disease.

Although the primary use of cholesterol testing is to screen for the presence of high blood cholesterol related to coronary artery disease, this test also is used as a secondary aid in the study of thyroid and liver function. See Table 19-1 for a list of specific conditions that cause abnormal cholesterol test results.

Patient Preparation

Because total cholesterol and HDL cholesterol determinations are not affected significantly by food consumption, the patient usually is not required to fast before collection of the blood specimen. Some physicians prefer the patient to be in a fasting state, however.

If the total cholesterol level is 200 mg/dL or greater, the physician usually orders a *lipid profile,* which includes total

cholesterol, HDL cholesterol, LDL cholesterol, and triglycerides. (The LDL cholesterol level is usually determined as a calculation from the triglyceride and HDL cholesterol levels.) Because triglyceride levels are affected by the consumption of food, the patient must be instructed to fast for at least 12 hours before the blood specimen is collected. An elevated triglyceride level (150 mg/dL or higher) is considered a risk factor for coronary artery disease, particularly when the LDL cholesterol is high and the HDL cholesterol is low.

Although the primary use of cholesterol testing is to screen for the presence of high blood cholesterol related to coronary artery disease, this test also is used as a secondary aid in the study of thyroid and liver function. See Table 19-1 for a list of specific conditions that cause abnormal cholesterol test results.

CLIA-Waived Cholesterol Analyzers

CLIA-waived analyzers are available for performing cholesterol testing in the medical office; an example is the Cholestech LDX Cholesterol System (Cholestech Corporation) (Figure 19-10).

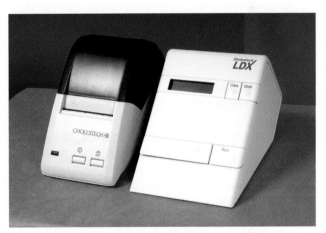

Figure 19-10. Cholestech LDX Cholesterol System.

What Would You Do? What Would You *Not* Do?

Case Study 3

Karen Scrimshaw is at the office. She is 20 years old and is mildly obese. Karen had her cholesterol tested at a health fair, and it was 325. The physician orders a CBC, lipid profile, and thyroid profile on Karen and instructs her to return in 1 week for a follow-up visit to discuss the test results. Karen is very concerned about her cholesterol. She says that she had a candy bar and some potato chips before going to the health fair and wants to know whether that could have caused her cholesterol to be so high. She also wants to know the accuracy of machines that are used at health fairs. Karen says that if she has to go on cholesterol medication, it would be hard to decide between Lipitor and Zocor. She says she has seen them advertised on television, and they both seem pretty good to her. ■

Highlight on Lowering Cholesterol

Research has shown, beyond doubt, that high total blood cholesterol is a major risk factor for coronary artery disease, and the higher the cholesterol, the greater the risk. The National Institutes of Health (NIH) has established guidelines on safe levels of blood cholesterol. The NIH recommends that adults not exceed 200 mg/dL of blood cholesterol.

The National Cholesterol Educational Program (NCEP) was established in 1985 by the federal government to reduce the prevalence of elevated blood cholesterol levels in the United States by educating the public about the health risks associated with high blood cholesterol and to make recommendations for helping individuals reduce their cholesterol levels. It has been shown that for every 1% that an individual lowers his or her total blood cholesterol, the risk of coronary artery disease is reduced by 2%. Taking the following measures can help individuals reduce their level of "bad" LDL cholesterol and increase their level of "good" HDL cholesterol.

Diet

Dietary therapy is the first line of treatment for high blood cholesterol. The NCEP recommends that all individuals (older than 2 years of age) reduce dietary cholesterol, *trans* fat, and saturated fats. Many foods high in fat tend to be high in cholesterol. Nutrition labels on packaged products provide information on the cholesterol and fat content of a food.

Dietary Cholesterol

The body manufactures all the cholesterol it needs for normal functioning, and dietary intake of cholesterol (in foods) serves only to increase the blood cholesterol. According to the NCEP, dietary cholesterol should be limited to 300 mg daily, which is slightly more than the amount of cholesterol in one egg (270 mg). Cholesterol is found only in animal foods and shellfish. Egg yolks, dairy products, and organ meats such as liver and kidneys are especially high in cholesterol.

Saturated Fat

The intake of saturated fat is the most important dietary factor leading to high blood cholesterol, even more so than consuming dietary cholesterol. In general, the more saturated a fat is, the harder and more solid it is at room temperature. The main source of saturated fat is animal products, including meat fat, poultry skin, and the fat in dairy products (butter, cream, ice cream, cheese, whole milk). Unsaturated fats have little or no effect on the blood cholesterol level; they include olive oil, canola oil, peanut oil, and sunflower,

safflower, and corn oils. The NCEP recommends that no more than 30% of the calories consumed each day come from fat, with no more than 10% of calories coming from saturated fat and the remaining 20% from unsaturated fat.

Soluble Fiber

Soluble fiber has been shown to lower the cholesterol level by keeping the cholesterol consumed from being absorbed by the body. Examples of foods high in soluble fiber are bran, oats, and beans.

Weight Reduction

It is estimated that one in four Americans is overweight. It is recommended that these individuals follow a sensible eating plan along with an exercise program to reach and maintain desirable weight. Losing weight reduces total cholesterol and triglyceride levels. Overweight and obese people are at very high risk for heart disease because their hearts have to work harder to pump blood through the body.

Exercise

An aerobic exercise program is especially beneficial for weight control because it improves cardiovascular fitness and lowers blood cholesterol level. People who exercise regularly generally have higher HDL cholesterol levels and lower triglyceride levels in their blood. The American Heart Association recommends that healthy individuals perform any moderate-to-vigorous intensity aerobic activity for at least 30 minutes on most days of the week at 50% to 85% of their maximum heart rate. These activities can include brisk walking, jogging, hiking, bicycling, swimming, and stair climbing.

Smoking Cessation

Smoking is one of the three main risk factors for coronary artery disease. By quitting smoking, an individual may be able to strengthen the heart and lower the cholesterol level. Also, nonsmokers tend to have higher HDL levels in their blood. A variety of smoking cessation programs are usually available in the community. Some people have succeeded by using nicotine patches, which help them adjust gradually to lower levels of nicotine.

Generally, the cholesterol level begins to decrease 2 to 3 weeks after a cholesterol-lowering diet and other cholesterol-lowering measures are begun. Over time, it is possible to reduce the total cholesterol level by 30 to 55 mg/dL or even more through these lifestyle changes. If the blood cholesterol level cannot be lowered to an acceptable level, the physician may prescribe cholesterol-lowering medications along with continuation of the aforementioned measures. ■

The manufacturer of each cholesterol analyzer provides an operating manual (and sometimes an instructional video) with the instrument that includes information needed to collect and handle the specimen, perform quality control procedures, and test the specimen. The manufacturer may also have personnel available for on-site training.

It is important that the medical assistant become completely familiar with all aspects of the CLIA-waived analyzer used to perform cholesterol testing in his or her medical office. Medical offices running CLIA-waived tests are required to follow the manufacturer's instructions *exactly* for each testing procedure. These instructions include the quality control procedures that must be performed when the test is run. Quality control procedures are of particular importance to ensure that the analyzer is functioning properly, and that the test results are reliable and accurate.

TRIGLYCERIDES

Triglycerides are the chemical form in which most fat exists in food, as well as in the body. Triglycerides are derived from two sources. The first is synthesis by the body. Ingested glucose that is not needed for energy can be stored in the form of **glycogen** in muscle and liver tissue for later use. When no more tissue storage is possible, most of the excess glycogen is synthesized by the body into triglycerides (a form of fat) and stored as adipose tissue. Excess protein not needed by the body is also converted to triglycerides and stored as adipose tissue. The second source of triglycerides is food. Excess triglycerides consumed by eating foods containing fat are also stored as adipose tissue.

Some of the triglycerides in the body are not stored as fat, but remain in the bloodstream, specifically in the plasma. Most triglycerides in the bloodstream are carried by a lipoprotein known as very low density lipoprotein (VLDL). In normal amounts, triglycerides are essential to good health. Triglycerides carried by the blood serve as a major source of energy for the body. An excess of blood triglycerides, however, places an individual at increased risk for coronary artery disease, particularly when the LDL cholesterol is high and the HDL cholesterol is low. Triglyceride levels in the blood are usually measured as part of a lipid profile and are interpreted as follows:

Normal:	Less than 150 mg/dL
Borderline high:	150 to 199 mg/dL
High:	200 to 499 mg/dL
Very high:	500 mg/dL or higher

Conditions that result in elevated blood triglyceride levels include obesity, type 2 diabetes, being physically inactive, excessive alcohol consumption, smoking, hypothyroidism, kidney disease, and liver disease.

BLOOD UREA NITROGEN

The blood urea nitrogen (BUN) is a kidney function test. Urea is the end product of protein metabolism and is normally present in the blood. Certain kidney diseases may interfere with the ability of the body to excrete the urea properly, causing an increased level of urea in the blood. See Table 19-1 for a list of specific conditions that cause abnormal BUN test results.

IMMUNOLOGY

Immunology (also known as serology) is the scientific study of antigen and antibody reactions. An **antigen** is a substance that is capable of stimulating the formation of antibodies in an individual. Antigens may consist of protein, glycoprotein, complex polysaccharides, or nucleic acid. Specific examples of antigens include bacteria and viruses, bacterial toxins, allergens, and blood antigens. An **antibody** is a substance that is capable of combining with an antigen, resulting in an antigen-antibody reaction.

Laboratory testing in immunology deals with studying antigen-antibody reactions to assess the presence of a substance (e.g., ABO blood typing) or to assist in the diagnosis of disease (e.g., mononucleosis testing). Immunologic tests are often used for the early diagnosis of disease and are used to follow the course of the disease.

IMMUNOLOGIC TESTS

Specific examples of immunologic tests are described next.

Hepatitis Tests

Hepatitis testing is performed to detect viral hepatitis. There are five types of viral hepatitis—A, B, C, D, and E—which are described in detail in Chapter 2. Hepatitis testing not only detects the presence of viral hepatitis, it also determines the type of hepatitis present.

HIV Tests

The enzyme immune assay (EIA) test and the enzyme-linked immunosorbent assay (ELISA) test are used as screening tests for the presence of HIV. Newer rapid screening HIV testing kits are also commercially available; brand names include Uni-Gold Recombigen HIV (Trinity Biotech Plc, Bray County Wicklow, Ireland), Clearview HIV (Inverness Medical Innovations, Inc., Waltham, Mass), and the OraQuick Rapid HIV test (OraSure Technologies, Bethlehem, Pa). Because of the possibility of a false-positive result, a second screening test is always performed if a blood specimen tests positive. If the second test also is positive, a more specific test, such as the Western blot test, is performed to confirm the test results. An individual who tests positive for HIV is seropositive.

A negative HIV test is not conclusive for the absence of HIV infection. If an individual has recently been infected with HIV, the antibodies may not have had time to develop. It generally takes 2 to 12 weeks (but possibly as long as 6 months) for the HIV antibodies to appear in the blood.

Syphilis Tests

Syphilis is a sexually transmitted disease (STD) caused by the microorganism *Treponema pallidum*. The most common tests used to detect the presence of syphilis are the Venereal Disease Research Laboratories (VDRL) test and the rapid plasma reagin (RPR) test. Test results are reported as nonreactive, weakly reactive, or reactive. Weakly reactive and reactive results are considered positive for the presence of syphilis antibodies. These tests are screening tests, and a positive result warrants more specific testing to arrive at a diagnosis of syphilis.

Mononucleosis Test

The mononucleosis test ("mono test") is used to detect the presence of infectious mononucleosis. The theory and procedure for this test are discussed in detail in this chapter.

Rheumatoid Factor

Rheumatoid arthritis is a chronic inflammatory disease that affects the joints of the body. The blood of patients with rheumatoid arthritis contains a type of antibody called *rheumatoid factor* (RF). This test detects the presence of rheumatoid factor antibodies and assists in the diagnosis of rheumatoid arthritis.

Antistreptolysin O Test

The antistreptolysin O (ASO) test is used to detect ASO antibodies in the serum. It is the most widely used immunologic test for the detection of conditions resulting from streptococcal infections and diseases that occur secondary to a streptococcal infection. This test is useful in assisting in the diagnosis of rheumatic fever, glomerulonephritis, bacterial endocarditis, and scarlet fever.

C-Reactive Protein

During inflammation and tissue destruction, an abnormal protein called *C-reactive protein* (CRP) appears in the blood. Patients with inflammatory conditions or disorders accompanied by tissue destruction have positive results to this test. Because of this, the CRP test is used to assist in diagnosing or charting the progress of rheumatoid arthritis, acute rheumatic fever, widespread malignancy, and bacterial infections.

Cold Agglutinins

The cold agglutinins test is used to detect the presence of antibodies called *cold agglutinins.* This test is performed by incubating the patient's serum with erythrocytes at cold temperatures. If cold agglutinins are present, this causes **agglutination** of the erythrocytes. Cold agglutinins are found in patients with infectious mononucleosis, mycoplasmal pneumonia, chronic parasitic infections, and lymphoma.

ABO and Rh Blood Typing

Blood typing is performed to determine an individual's ABO and Rh blood type. Knowledge of blood type helps to prevent transfusion and transplant reactions and to identify problems such as hemolytic disease of the newborn. The theory and procedure for ABO and Rh blood typing are presented in this chapter.

Rh Antibody Titer

The Rh antibody titer test detects the amount of circulating Rh antibodies in the blood. These antibodies can occur in a pregnant woman who is Rh-negative and is carrying an Rh-positive fetus. This test is most frequently used to detect the presence of an Rh incompatibility problem with a mother and her unborn child.

RAPID MONONUCLEOSIS TESTING

Infectious mononucleosis is an acute infectious disease caused by the Epstein-Barr virus (EBV). Infectious mononucleosis most frequently affects children and young adults. It is transmitted through saliva by direct oral contact, and because of this, it is often called the "kissing disease." Symptoms of infectious mononucleosis include mental and physical fatigue, fever, sore throat, severe weakness, headache, and swollen lymph nodes.

The (CLIA-waived) rapid mono test is often performed in the medical office and is used to assist in the diagnosis of infectious mononucleosis. Rapid mono tests are easy to perform and provide reliable results in a short time. Patients with infectious mononucleosis produce an antibody called *heterophile antibody,* usually by 6 to 10 days into the illness. Rapid mono tests detect this antibody. The presence of the heterophile antibody along with patient symptoms can provide the basis for the diagnosis of infectious mononucleosis.

Figure 19-11 illustrates the QuickVue+ Mononucleosis Test setup (Quidel Corporation, San Diego, Calif), and Figure 19-12 outlines the procedure for performing a rapid mono test using the QuickVue+ Mononucleosis Test. Figure 19-13 is an illustration of positive and negative test results for the QuickVue+ Mononucleosis Test.

BLOOD TYPING
Blood Antigens

Each individual has a blood type. Blood type depends on the presence of certain factors, or antigens, on the surface of the red blood cells. **Blood antigens** consist of protein and are inherited through **genes,** which program the body to produce a particular antigen. If a blood antigen is present, it appears on the surface of all the red blood cells in the body.

Many types of antigens can appear in the blood. These antigens can be grouped into categories known as *blood group systems.* The blood group systems that are most likely to cause problems in blood transfusions and in Rh disease of the newborn are the ABO and Rh blood group systems. These are the blood group systems most commonly tested for in the medical laboratory.

Within the ABO blood group system are four main blood types—A, B, AB, and O. The blood type depends on which antigens are present on the surface of the red blood cells.

- If the A antigen is present, the blood type is A.
- If the B antigen is present, the blood type is B.
- If A and B antigens are present, the blood type is AB.
- If neither the A nor the B antigen is present, the blood type is O.

Figure 19-14 illustrates this principle.

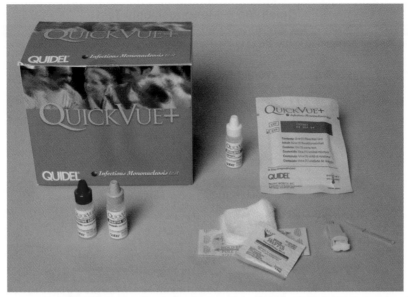

Figure 19-11. QuickVue+ mononucleosis test setup. (From Garrels M, Oatis CS: Laboratory testing for ambulatory settings, ed 2, St Louis, 2011, Saunders.)

Blood Antibodies

Blood antibodies are proteins that are naturally present in the plasma of the blood. An antibody is a substance that is capable of combining with an antigen. The body never produces an antibody to combine with its own blood antigen. If the blood type is A, the plasma does not contain the A antibody. The B antibody naturally occurs in that plasma, however. The B antibody cannot combine with the A antigen. If a blood antigen and its corresponding antibody combine (in this case, the A antigen combining with the A antibody), a serious antigen-antibody reaction occurs that could be life-threatening.

- If the blood type is A, the plasma contains the B antibody.
- If the blood type is B, the plasma contains the A antibody.
- If the blood type is AB, neither the A nor the B antibody appears in the plasma.
- If the blood type is O, the A and B antibodies appear in the plasma. Type O blood has neither the A nor the B antigen on the surface of its red blood cells. The A and B antibodies in the plasma would not have an A or B antigen to combine with them (Table 19-4).

Rh Blood Group System

In 1940, Landsteiner and Wiener discovered the Rh blood group system while working with rhesus monkeys. Most people in the United States have the Rh antigen present on the red blood cells and have type Rh-positive

Table 19-4	ABO Blood Group System	
Blood Type	Antigen Present on Red Blood Cell	Antibody Present in Plasma
A	A	B
B	B	A
AB	A, B	Neither A nor B
O	Neither A nor B	A, B

blood. The remaining 15% of the Caucasian population and 7% of the African American population do not have the Rh antigen present on the red blood cells and have type Rh-negative blood. In contrast to the A and B antibodies, the Rh antibodies do not normally occur in the plasma.

BLOOD ANTIGEN AND ANTIBODY REACTIONS

When a blood antigen and its corresponding antibody unite, the result is the clumping, or agglutination, of red blood cells. Agglutination of red blood cells can be serious and fatal if it occurs **in vivo** (in the living body). The clumped red blood cells cannot pass through the small tubules of the kidneys, and this may lead to kidney failure. Also, the clumping of the red blood cells eventually leads to hemolysis, or breakdown of the red blood cells.

QuickVue + Mononucleosis Test

FOR INFORMATIONAL USE ONLY ■ FOR INFORMATIONAL USE ONLY ■ FOR INFORMATIONAL USE ONLY
Not to be used for performing assay. Refer to most current package insert accompanying your test kit.

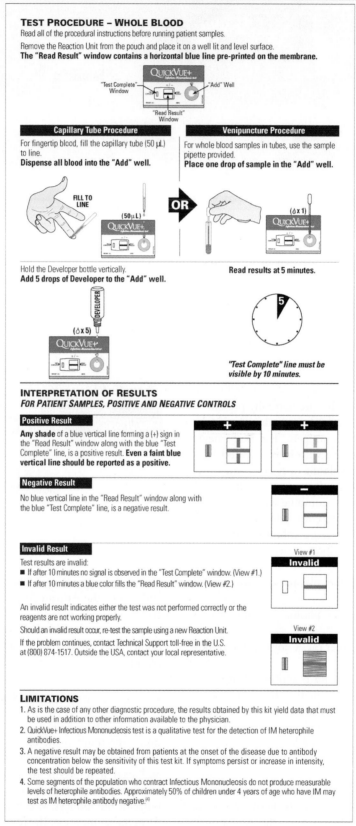

Figure 19-12. Procedure for performing the QuickVue+ Mononucleosis Test. (Courtesy of and modified from Quidel Corporation, San Diego, Calif.)

Highlight on Blood Donor Criteria

Every year, approximately 5 million Americans require blood transfusions, resulting in transfusion of 13.5 million units of blood. A safe, readily available blood supply is essential for lifesaving medical procedures, such as replacing blood loss from hemorrhages or surgical procedures, replacing plasma in burn and shock victims, and providing platelets to control bleeding. In an average population, 75% of the people are physically and medically eligible to donate blood; only 5% of those eligible donate.

Basic blood donor criteria have been established on a national basis to ensure donor safety and a quality blood donation. All blood collection facilities, such as the American Red Cross, must follow these regulations. In general, blood donors must be in good health and must be of a certain age and weight.

Health History

To protect the donor and the recipient, each donor is asked to give a brief health history. The prospective donor is asked to provide information related to diseases that may be transmitted through the blood (e.g., hepatitis, AIDS) and medications being taken that could affect the quality of the blood donation. Information also is obtained related to medical conditions that might jeopardize the health of the donor if he or she were to donate.

Based on this information, a prospective donor could be *temporarily deferred* from donating blood because of the following: blood transfusion, treatment for cancer, a human bite in which the skin was broken, certain immunizations, organ transplant, pregnancy, treatment for syphilis or gonorrhea, a skin infection, certain medical conditions such as a recent heart attack or active tuberculosis, taking of certain prescription medications (e.g., anticoagulants), and travel to a malaria-prone area. Temporarily deferred donors are told how long they must wait and are encouraged to donate blood when the waiting period is over. The waiting period varies based on the condition or situation; the waiting period is at least 12 months after treatment for syphilis or gonorrhea is received, whereas only a 7-day wait is required after the potential donor has been immunized for hepatitis B.

A prospective donor is *permanently deferred* from giving blood for any of the following reasons: leukemia, a clotting disorder, hepatitis, infection with the AIDS virus (HIV infection) and behavior associated with the spread of the AIDS virus, and a history of IV drug use. An individual also is permanently deferred if he or she spent 3 months or longer in the United Kingdom between 1980 and 1996 (a country where "mad cow disease" is found).

Age

An individual must be at least 17 years old to donate blood. With written parental consent, however, some states permit 16-year-olds to donate blood. No upper age limit has been established for blood donation, as long as the individual feels well and has no restrictions or limitations on his or her activities.

Date of Last Donation

At least 56 days (8 weeks) must elapse between donations.

Weight

The donor must weigh at least 110 lb. (In some states, the minimum weight is 105 lb.) For the average individual, the total volume of blood is approximately 8% of body weight. Underweight donors are not accepted because a full donation would result in a proportionately greater reduction in blood volume and might precipitate a reaction. No upper weight limit is in place as long as the individual's weight is not greater than the weight limit of the blood donor bed being used.

Temperature

Body temperature of donors may not exceed 99.5° F (37.5° C). The primary purpose of temperature measurement is to eliminate donors who are ill.

Pulse

The acceptable range for the pulse rate is 50 to 110 beats per minute. If the pulse rate seems to be elevated because of physical exertion, the donor may be asked to remain seated for 5 to 10 minutes, with a recheck taken after the rest period.

Blood Pressure

The acceptable limit for blood pressure is a reading no higher than 180 mm Hg for the systolic pressure and a reading no higher than 100 mm Hg for the diastolic pressure.

Hemoglobin

The hemoglobin must be 12.5 g/dL or greater for men and women.

Blood-Donating Process

It takes approximately 1 hour to donate blood. The process begins with the health history, followed by a mini-physical check of temperature, pulse, blood pressure, and hemoglobin level. Next, 1 unit (1 pint) of blood is collected using a sterile needle and a sterile plastic bag that contains an additive. A donor should feel no pain during the blood collection procedure, which takes approximately 8 to 10 minutes. It is not possible to contract AIDS or any other infectious disease by donating blood. After the unit of blood has been collected, the donor is encouraged to have refreshments to begin replenishing the fluids and nutrients temporarily lost during the donation.

Processing the Blood

Each blood donation is tested for AIDS, hepatitis, and syphilis. Any unit of blood that tests positive is rejected for transfusion. The unit of blood is typed and labeled with its ABO and Rh blood type. It is then available for distribution to hospitals for transfusing purposes. ■

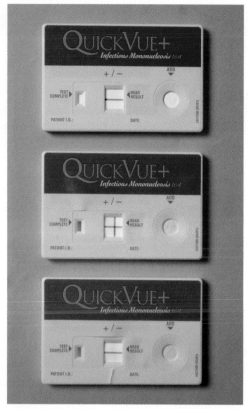

Figure 19-13. QuickVue+ mononucleosis test results. (From Garrels M, Oatis CS: Laboratory testing for ambulatory settings, ed 2, St Louis, 2011, Saunders.)

Blood antigen-antibody reactions can occur if the wrong blood type is administered to a patient during a blood transfusion. If an individual with type A blood is given a transfusion of type B blood, the B antibody of the **recipient** (person receiving the blood) would combine with the B antigen of the **donor** (person donating the blood), and an antigen-antibody reaction would occur, resulting in agglutination of red blood cells. We say that type A blood is incompatible with type B blood.

AGGLUTINATION AND BLOOD TYPING

Agglutination of red blood cells is the basis for the ABO and Rh blood typing procedure. The antigen-antibody reaction occurs **in vitro,** or "in glass" in the laboratory, so there is no threat to life.

To test for the ABO blood group system, a commercially prepared antiserum is used. An antiserum is a serum that contains antibodies. An **antiserum** containing the A antibody is added to an unknown blood specimen. If the A antigen is present, it combines with the A antibody, resulting in agglutination. An antiserum containing the B antibody is added to another sample of the unknown blood. If the B antigen is present, it combines with the B antibody, resulting in agglutination. If agglutination occurs in both instances, the sample is type AB. If no agglutination occurs, this indicates the absence of blood antigens, or type O blood. Agglutination that occurs in vitro is visible to the naked eye. The antigen-antibody reaction that occurs when the unknown blood sample is type A is diagrammed in Figure 19-15.

Unknown blood sample containing Type A blood: **The antiserum containing the A antibody:**

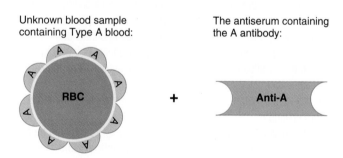

The bridge forming between the antigen and antibody represents the antigen-antibody reaction. This reaction leads to agglutination of red blood cells, which is visible to the naked eye.

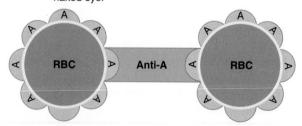

Figure 19-15. The antigen-antibody reaction that occurs in vitro when the unknown blood sample is type A.

Type A blood:
A antigen is present

Type B blood:
B antigen is present

Type AB blood:
A and B antigens are both present

Type O blood:
Neither A nor B antigens are present

Figure 19-14. Blood type depends on which antigens are present on the surface of the red blood cells (RBCs).

℮volve *Check out the Evolve site to access additional interactive activities.*

MEDICAL PRACTICE *and the* LAW

When running laboratory tests, you must ensure that all equipment is functioning properly. This is done by periodic calibration or running of controls on each piece of equipment. Know when and how often to calibrate or run controls, and document appropriately. Without these quality controls, results cannot be trusted to be accurate. Inaccurate results can lead to inaccurate diagnosis and treatment. Use personal protective equipment appropriate to each test to avoid transmission of disease and cross-contamination of specimens.

Who Can Sue?

Anyone can sue for anything. The important thing to know is "Can they win?" The person filing the lawsuit is called the *plaintiff,* and the one being sued is called the *defendant.* To win a malpractice lawsuit, four things are necessary:

1. The defendant must have had a duty to the plaintiff, that is, a physician-patient relationship must exist.

2. Care must have been provided that was not consistent with that of a "reasonably prudent" physician or medical assistant. In other words, a mistake was made, and the individual who made it should have known better. If you work in a specialty area, you are expected to know more about that specialty than if you worked in a general practice office. Be very familiar with your office's policy and procedures manual.

3. The plaintiff must prove proximate cause. This means the patient's problem is a direct cause of the physician's or medical assistant's actions.

4. The plaintiff must have been injured by the mistake. Damages may include pain and suffering, loss of income, and medical bills.

To avoid personal lawsuits, practice good care, document everything you do, and maintain good relationships with patients. Some patients who are hurt may sue, but most patients who are hurt and are angry *will* sue. ■

What Would You Do? What Would You *Not* Do? RESPONSES

Case Study 1
Page 749

What Did Michelle Do?

❑ Apologized to Crystal for the inconvenience. Explained to her that it takes 3 to 4 hours to run an oral glucose tolerance test because several specimens must be collected over time to see how her body handles sugar.

❑ Explained to Crystal that eating and smoking cause the test results to be inaccurate. Told her that she could eat and smoke as soon as the test was over.

❑ Told Crystal that she needs to sit quietly during the test, so it would not be possible for her to bring her children.

❑ Informed the physician of Crystal's situation to see whether he had any suggestions.

What Did Michelle Not Do?

❑ Did not become defensive or intimidated by Crystal's behavior.

❑ Did not tell Crystal that the staff would watch Crystal's children during the test.

❑ Did not tell Crystal that it was not a good idea for her to smoke around her children.

What Would You Do?/What Would You *Not* Do? Review Michelle's response and place a checkmark next to the information you included in your response. List additional information you included in your response.

_____

_____

_____

_____

Case Study 2
Page 752

What Did Michelle Do?

❑ Told Dave that it would be fine for him to perform his own finger-stick.

❑ Made sure that his finger was cleansed with an antiseptic wipe and that he wiped away the first drop of blood.

❑ Explained to Dave that the air bubbles take up space that the insulin should occupy, and that if he does not get rid of them, he will not get his full dose of insulin.

❑ Demonstrated how to remove air bubbles, and had Dave practice it at the office.

❑ Told Dave he must not reuse his needle and syringe. Explained that a used needle could cause him to get an infection. Asked Dave whether he had checked to see if his insurance would cover the cost of the needles and syringes.

❑ Told Dave that he should put his used needles and syringes in a thick plastic container such as an empty detergent container. After the container is full, he should close it tightly with a screw lid, then it can be thrown out with his regular trash. Explained that this will protect his family and the trash handlers from getting stuck while disposing of the trash.

What Did Michelle Not Do?

❑ Did not tell Dave he didn't need to worry about the air bubbles in the syringe.

Continued

What Would You Do? What Would You *Not* Do? RESPONSES—cont'd

What Would You Do?/What Would You *Not* Do? Review Michelle's response and place a checkmark next to the information you included in your response. List additional information you included in your response.

_____

_____

_____

_____

Case Study 3
Page 761

What Did Michelle Do?
❑ Tried to calm and reassure Karen.
❑ Explained to Karen that the cholesterol results are not affected by food, so eating before the health fair should not have affected her results.
❑ Told Karen that before a cholesterol analyzer is used, it is usually checked to ensure that it is working properly.
❑ Reassured Karen that the physician was checking her cholesterol again and was running some additional tests to determine whether she is having any problems.

❑ Told Karen that if she must take medication, the physician will determine what drug is best for her.

What Did Michelle Not Do?
❑ Did not tell Karen that her cholesterol is extremely high.
❑ Did not tell Karen that she should be more careful about what she eats because she is overweight.
❑ Did not tell Karen that there was no way to know whether the cholesterol analyzer used at the health fair was calibrated and had controls run on it.

What Would You Do?/What Would You *Not* Do? Review Michelle's response and place a checkmark next to the information you included in your response. List additional information you included in your response.

_____

_____

_____

_____

CERTIFICATION REVIEW

❑ **Blood chemistry testing** involves the quantitative measurement of chemical substances in the blood. These chemicals are dissolved in the liquid portion of the blood; most blood chemistry tests require a serum specimen for analysis. In the medical office, CLIA-waived automated blood chemistry analyzers are often used to perform blood chemistry testing.

❑ **Quality control** consists of methods and means to ensure that test results are reliable and valid.

❑ **Calibration** involves the use of a standard to check the precision of the blood chemistry analyzer. If an analyzer is not properly calibrated, it cannot produce accurate test results.

❑ **A control** consists of a sample of a known value. Normal controls fall within the normal range, whereas abnormal controls fall outside the normal range.

❑ **Glucose** is the end product of carbohydrate metabolism; its function is to serve as the chief source of energy for the body. Glucose that is not needed for energy can be stored in the form of glycogen in muscle and liver tissue for later use. Insulin is a hormone secreted by the pancreas and is required for normal use of glucose in the body.

❑ **Measuring the glucose** in a blood specimen is one of the most common blood chemistry tests. It is used to detect abnormalities in carbohydrate metabolism, such as occur in pre-diabetes, diabetes, gestational diabetes, hypoglycemia, and liver and adrenocortical dysfunction.

❑ **Blood glucose** is usually measured when the patient is in a fasting state. This type of test is termed a *fasting blood glucose* (FBG). The patient should not have anything to eat or drink except water for 12 hours preceding the test. The normal range for FBG is 70 to 99 mg/dL. FBG is often performed on patients with diabetes to evaluate their progress and regulate treatment, and as a routine screening procedure in patients to detect pre-diabetes and diabetes.

❑ **The 2-hour postprandial blood sugar** (2-hour PPBS) test is used to screen for diabetes and to monitor the effects of insulin dosage in diagnosed diabetic patients.

❑ **The oral glucose tolerance test** (OGTT) provides more detailed information about the ability of the body to metabolize glucose by assessing the insulin response to a glucose load. The OGTT is used in the diagnosis of pre-diabetes, diabetes, gestational diabetes, hypoglycemia, and liver and adrenocortical dysfunction.

❑ **The hemoglobin A_{1c} test** (abbreviated as Hb A_{1c} test or simply A_{1c} test) provides valuable information for determining that a diabetic patient's blood glucose level is under control. The A_{1c} test furnishes the physician with an assessment of the average amount of glucose in the blood over a 3-month period. The normal A_{1c} level for an individual without diabetes is 4% to 6%. The American Diabetes Association strongly recommends that individuals with diabetes maintain a hemoglobin A_{1c} level of less than 7%.

CERTIFICATION REVIEW—cont'd

❑ **Cholesterol** is a white, waxy, fatlike substance that is essential for normal functioning of the body. Most of the cholesterol circulating in the blood is manufactured by the liver; a portion of it is dietary. Dietary cholesterol is found only in animal products.

❑ **High blood cholesterol** may cause fatty deposits, or plaque, to build up on the walls of the arteries, a condition known as *atherosclerosis*. LDL cholesterol is often referred to as "bad" cholesterol because an excess amount of it in the blood can cause atherosclerosis. HDL cholesterol is often referred to as "good" cholesterol because it removes excess cholesterol from the walls of the blood vessels.

❑ **Cholesterol test results** are interpreted as follows: Total cholesterol levels less than 200 mg/dL are desirable. Levels between 200 and 239 mg/dL are borderline high, and levels of 240 mg/dL and greater are high. An HDL cholesterol level greater than 60 mg/dL is optimal, and a level less than 40 mg/dL is a risk factor for coronary artery disease.

❑ **Immunology** is the scientific study of the serum of the blood. Immunologic tests include hepatitis tests, HIV tests, syphilis tests, mono test, rheumatoid factor, antistreptolysin O test, C-reactive protein, cold agglutinins, ABO and Rh blood typing, and Rh antibody titer.

❑ **Infectious mononucleosis** is an acute infectious disease caused by the Epstein-Barr virus (EBV). Symptoms include mental and physical fatigue, fever, sore throat, severe weakness, headache, and swollen lymph nodes.

❑ **Blood antigens** consist of protein and are inherited through genes. Within the ABO blood group system are four main blood types—A, B, AB, and O. Blood antibodies are proteins that are naturally present in the plasma of the blood. An antibody is a substance that is capable of combining with an antigen. When a blood antigen and its corresponding antibody unite, the result is the clumping, or agglutination, of red blood cells. Agglutination of red blood cells can be serious and fatal if it occurs in the living body.

TERMINOLOGY REVIEW

Medical Term	Word Parts	Definition
Agglutination (as it pertains to blood)		Clumping of blood cells.
Analyte		A substance that is being identified or measured in a laboratory test.
Antibody	*anti-:* against	A substance that is capable of combining with an antigen, resulting in an antigen-antibody reaction.
Antigen	*anti-:* against *-gen:* substance or agent that produces or causes	A substance capable of stimulating the formation of antibodies.
Antiserum (*pl.* antisera)	*anti-:* against	A serum that contains antibodies.
Blood antibody	*anti-:* against	A protein present in the blood plasma that is capable of combining with its corresponding blood antigen to produce an antigen-antibody reaction.
Blood antigen	*anti-:* against *-gen:* substance or agent that produces or causes	A protein present on the surface of red blood cells that determines a person's blood type.
Donor		One who furnishes something, such as blood, tissue, or organs, to be used in another individual.
Gene		A unit of heredity.
Glycogen	*glyco-:* sugar *-gen:* substance or agent that produces or causes	The form in which carbohydrate is stored in the body.
Glycosylation	*glyco-:* sugar	The process of glucose attaching to hemoglobin.
HDL cholesterol		A lipoprotein, consisting of protein and cholesterol, that removes excess cholesterol from the cells.
Hemoglobin A_{1c}	*hemo-:* blood	Compound formed when glucose attaches or glycosylates to the protein in hemoglobin.

Continued

↻ TERMINOLOGY REVIEW—cont'd

Medical Term	Word Parts	Definition
Hyperglycemia	*hyper-:* above, excessive *glyc/o:* sugar *-emia:* blood condition	An abnormally high level of glucose in the blood.
Hypoglycemia	*hypo-:* below, deficient *glyc/o:* sugar *-emia:* blood condition	An abnormally low level of glucose in the blood.
In vitro		Occurring in glass. Refers to tests performed under artificial conditions, as in the laboratory.
In vivo		Occurring in the living body or organism.
LDL cholesterol		A lipoprotein, consisting of protein and cholesterol, that picks up cholesterol and delivers it to the cells.
Lipoprotein	*lipo-:* fat	A complex molecule consisting of protein and a lipid fraction such as cholesterol. Lipoproteins function in transporting lipids in the blood.
Recipient		One who receives something, such as a blood transfusion, from a donor.

🖰 ON THE WEB

For Information on Diabetes:

American Diabetes Association: www.diabetes.org

Joslin Diabetes Center: www.joslin.org

National Diabetes Education Initiative: www.ndei.org

The National Institute of Diabetes: www.niddk.nih.gov

20

Medical Microbiology

LEARNING OBJECTIVES

PROCEDURES

Microorganisms and Disease

1. List and explain the stages of an infectious disease.
2. List and describe the three classifications of bacteria based on shape.
3. Give examples of infectious diseases caused by the following types of cocci:
   - Staphylococci
   - Streptococci
   - Diplococci
4. State examples of infectious diseases caused by bacilli, spirilla, and viruses.

Microscope

1. Explain the function of each of the following parts of a compound microscope: base, arm, stage, light source, substage condenser, iris diaphragm, body tube, coarse adjustment, and fine adjustment.
2. Identify the function of each of the following microscope lenses: low-power, high-power, and oil-immersion.
3. List the guidelines for proper care of the microscope.

Use a microscope.
Properly handle and care for a microscope.

Microbiologic Specimen Collection

1. Explain the purpose of obtaining a specimen, and identify body areas from which a specimen can be taken for microbiologic examination.
2. List ways to prevent contamination of a specimen by extraneous microorganisms.
3. Explain the precautions a medical assistant should take to prevent infection from a pathogenic specimen.
4. Explain the purpose of and describe the procedure for culturing a microbiologic specimen.

Collect a throat specimen.

Microbiologic Tests

1. Explain the importance of the early diagnosis of streptococcal pharyngitis.
2. Explain the purpose of and describe the procedure for a sensitivity test.
3. Explain the purpose of a microbiologic smear.
4. Explain the purpose of Gram staining.
5. Identify infectious diseases caused by gram-positive bacteria and gram-negative bacteria.
6. Give examples of methods to prevent and control infectious diseases in the community.

Perform a streptococcus test using a rapid strep test.
Perform a streptococcus test using the bacitracin susceptibility test.
Prepare a wet mount.
Prepare a microbiologic smear.

KEY TERMS

bacilli (bah-SILL-ie)
cocci (KOK-sie)
colony (KOL-oe-nee)
contagious (kon-TAE-jus)
culture
culture medium
false-negative
false-positive
fastidious (fas-TID-ee-us)
immunization (im-yoo-ni-ZAY-shun)
incubate (IN-kyoo-bate)
incubation period
infectious disease

inoculate (in-NOK-yoo-late)
microbiology (mie-kroe-bie-OL-oe-jee)
mucous membrane (MYOO-kus MEM-brain)
normal flora
resistance
sequela (SEK-kwe-lah)
smear
specimen (SPESS-ih-men)
spirilla (spa-RILL-ah)
streaking
streptolysin (strep-toe-LIE-sin)
susceptible (suh-SEP-tih-bul)

Introduction to Microbiology

Microbiology is the scientific study of microorganisms and their activities. As described in Chapter 2, microorganisms are tiny living plants and animals that cannot be seen by the naked eye, but must be viewed under a microscope. Anton van Leeuwenhoek (1632-1723) designed a magnifying glass strong enough for viewing microorganisms. He was the first individual to observe and describe protozoa and bacteria (Figure 20-1). Leeuwenhoek's magnifying glass was the precursor of modern microscopes used today to study microorganisms. A microscope allows the observer to see individual microbial cells and to differentiate and identify microorganisms.

For the most part, microbiology deals with unicellular, or one-celled, microscopic organisms. All of the life processes necessary to sustain the microbe are performed by one cell. Among them are the ingestion of food substances and their use for energy, growth, reproduction, and excretion.

Microorganisms are *ubiquitous;* they are found almost everywhere—in the air, in food and water, in the soil, and in association with plants, animals, and human life. Although vast numbers of microorganisms exist, only a relatively small number are pathogenic and able to cause disease.

When a pathogen infects a host, it often produces a set of symptoms peculiar to that disease. Scarlet fever is characterized by a sore throat, swelling of the lymph nodes in the neck, a red and swollen tongue, and a bright red rash covering the body. These symptoms aid the physician in diagnosing the disease. The medical assistant must be alert to all symptoms that the patient describes and must relay this information to the physician through careful and concise charting of these symptoms in the patient's medical record.

If the physician is not able to diagnose the disease from the patient's clinical signs and symptoms, laboratory tests may be used to help the physician identify the pathogen. Identification of the pathogen leads to proper treatment of

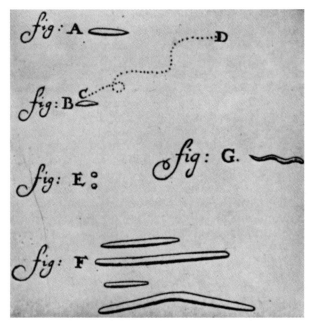

Figure 20-1. Bacteria drawn by van Leeuwenhoek in 1684. (From Fuerst R: Frobisher and Fuerst's microbiology in health and disease, ed 15, Philadelphia, 1983, Saunders.)

the disease. Categories of laboratory tests used to identify a pathogen include the following:

- Microbial culture
- Biochemical tests
- Microscopy
- DNA testing (also known as PCR testing)

Although most laboratory tests used to identify a pathogen are performed at an outside laboratory, the medical assistant is frequently responsible for collection of the specimen that will be transported to the outside laboratory.

This chapter provides an introduction to microbiology, including a description of proper microbiologic collection and handling techniques that must be followed to ensure a quality specimen. Identification of a pathogen using microbial culturing, biochemical testing, and microscopy is also discussed in this chapter. DNA testing to detect pathogens (e.g., chlamydia and gonorrhea) was previously described in Chapter 8. Before undertaking this study, the medical assistant should review Chapter 2, which discusses introductory concepts that are basic to this chapter.

NORMAL FLORA

Every individual has a **normal flora,** which consists of the harmless microorganisms that normally reside in many parts of the body but do not cause disease. The surface of the skin, the **mucous membrane** of the gastrointestinal tract, and parts of the respiratory and genitourinary tracts all have an abundant normal flora. Some microorganisms that make up the normal flora are beneficial to the body, such as those that inhabit the intestinal tract that feed on other potentially harmful microscopic organisms. Other examples are microorganisms found in the intestinal tract

that synthesize vitamin K, an essential vitamin needed by the body for proper blood clotting. In rare instances, if the opportunity arises (e.g., lowered body **resistance**), certain microorganisms of the normal flora can become pathogenic and cause disease.

INFECTION

Invasion of the body by pathogenic microorganisms is known as *infection.* Under conditions favorable to the pathogens, they grow and multiply, resulting in an **infectious disease** (also known as a communicable disease) that produces harmful effects on the host. Not all pathogens that enter a host are able to cause disease, however. When a pathogen enters the body, it attempts to invade the tissues so that it can grow and multiply. The body tries to stop the invasion with its second line of natural defense mechanisms,* which includes inflammation, phagocytosis by white blood cells, and the production of antibodies. These defense mechanisms work to destroy the pathogen and remove it from the body. If the body is successful, the pathogens are destroyed, and the individual experiences no adverse effects. If the pathogen is able to overcome the body's natural defense mechanisms, an infectious disease results.

Many infectious diseases are **contagious,** meaning that the pathogen that causes the disease can be spread from one person to another directly or indirectly. Frequently, *droplet infection* is the mode of transmission of a contagious disease.

Droplet infection refers to an infection that is indirectly transmitted by tiny contaminated droplets of moisture expelled from the upper respiratory tract of an infected individual. When an individual exhales (as during breathing, talking, coughing, or sneezing), a fine spray of moisture droplets is emitted by that individual from the upper respiratory tract. If the individual has a contagious disease that is transmitted by droplet infection, the pathogens are carried into the air by these tiny moisture droplets. Another individual may inhale these contaminated droplets and become infected with the disease. To help prevent the spread of droplet infections, contagious individuals should cover their mouths and noses while coughing or sneezing. See Figure 2-1 for examples of other means of pathogen transmission.

Stages of an Infectious Disease

When a pathogen becomes established in the host, a series of events generally ensues. The stages of an infectious disease are as follows:

1. The *infection* is the invasion and multiplication of pathogenic microorganisms in the body.
2. The *incubation period* is the interval of time between the invasion by a pathogenic microorganism and the appearance of the first symptoms of the disease. Depending on the type of disease, the **incubation period** may range

---

*The first line of natural defense mechanisms, which work to prevent the entrance of pathogens into the body (e.g., coughing, sneezing), is described in Chapter 2.

from a few days to several months. During this time, the pathogen is growing and multiplying.

3. The *prodromal period* is a short period in which the first symptoms that indicate an approaching disease occur. Headache and a feeling of illness are common prodromal symptoms.

4. The *acute period* is when the disease is at its peak and symptoms are fully developed. Fever is a common symptom of many infectious diseases.

5. The *decline period* is when symptoms of the disease begin to subside.

6. The *convalescent period* is the stage in which the patient regains strength and returns to a state of good health.

MICROORGANISMS AND DISEASE

The groups of microorganisms known to contain species capable of causing human disease include bacteria, viruses, protozoa, fungi (including yeasts), and animal parasites. Bacteria and viruses are most frequently responsible for causing human diseases and are discussed next.

Bacteria

Bacteria are microscopic single-celled organisms. Of the 1700 species known to dwell in humans, only approximately 100 produce human disease. The discovery of antibiotics has helped immensely in combating and controlling bacterial infections. Antibiotics are not effective against viral infections, however.

Bacteria can be classified according to their shape into three basic groups (Figure 20-2). Round bacteria are known as **cocci.** Cocci can be categorized further as diplococci, streptococci, or staphylococci, depending on their pattern of growth. Rod-shaped bacteria are **bacilli.** Spiral and curve-shaped bacteria are **spirilla,** and they include spirochetes and vibrios.

Cocci

Staphylococci are round bacteria that grow in grapelike clusters (Figure 20-3, *A*). The species *Staphylococcus epidermidis* is widely distributed and is normally present on the surface of the skin and the mucous membranes of the mouth, nose,

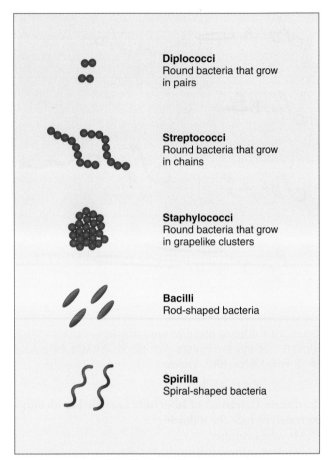

Diplococci
Round bacteria that grow in pairs

Streptococci
Round bacteria that grow in chains

Staphylococci
Round bacteria that grow in grapelike clusters

Bacilli
Rod-shaped bacteria

Spirilla
Spiral-shaped bacteria

Figure 20-2. Classification of bacteria based on shape.

throat, and intestines. *S. epidermidis* is usually nonpathogenic; however, a cut, abrasion, or other break in the skin can allow invasion of the tissues by the organism, resulting in a mild infection.

Staphylococcus aureus is commonly associated with pathologic conditions such as boils, carbuncles, pimples, impetigo, abscesses, *Staphylococcus* food poisoning, and wound infections. Infections caused by staphylococci usually cause much pus formation (suppuration) and are termed *pyogenic* infections.

Streptococci are round bacteria that grow in chains (Figure 20-3, *B*). Before the advent of antibiotics, streptococcal infections were a major cause of human death. Diseases caused by streptococci include streptococcal sore throat ("strep throat"), scarlet fever, rheumatic fever, pneumonia, puerperal sepsis, erysipelas, and skin conditions such as carbuncles and impetigo.

Diplococci are round bacteria that grow in pairs. Pneumonia, gonorrhea, and meningitis are infectious diseases caused by diplococci.

Bacilli

Bacilli are rod-shaped bacteria that are frequently found in the soil and air (Figure 20-3, *C*). Some bacilli are able to form spores, a characteristic that enables them to resist adverse conditions such as heat and disinfectants. Diseases

---

What Would You Do? What Would You *Not* Do?

Case Study 1

Paula Hutchinson brings her 8-year-old daughter Caitlin to the medical office. Caitlin has had a fever, sore throat, and difficulty eating for the past 2 days. The physician orders a rapid strep test. Caitlin refuses to open her mouth so that the specimen can be collected. She says that she doesn't want that "swab thing" in her mouth because she's afraid it will make her throw up. Paula wants to know why the strep test must be run. She says that Caitlin's throat is very red with white patches and wants to know why the physician doesn't just prescribe an antibiotic for her without running the test. ■

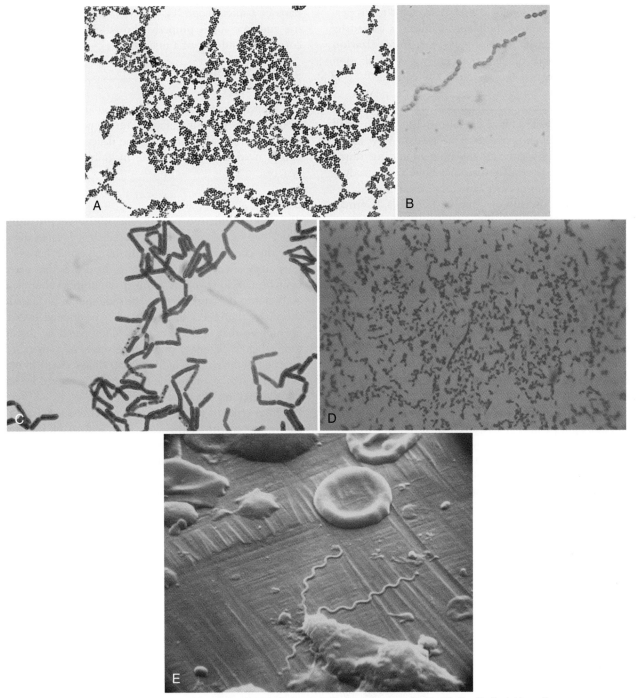

Figure 20-3. Types of bacteria. **A,** Staphylococci. **B,** Streptococci. **C,** Bacilli. **D,** *Escherichia coli.* **E,** Spirilla. (**A, B,** and **D** from Mahon CR, Manuselis G Jr: Textbook of diagnostic microbiology, ed 2, Philadelphia, 2000, Saunders; **C** courtesy Cathy Bissonette; **E** courtesy Dr. Andrew G. Smith.)

caused by bacilli include botulism, tetanus, gas gangrene, gastroenteritis produced by *Salmonella* food poisoning, typhoid fever, pertussis (whooping cough), bacillary dysentery, diphtheria, tuberculosis, leprosy, and plague.

Escherichia coli is a species of bacillus that is found among the normal flora of the large intestine in enormous numbers (Figure 20-3, *D*). It is normally a harmless bacterium; however, if it enters the urinary tract as a result of lowered resistance, poor hygiene practices, or both, it may cause a urinary tract infection.

Spirilla

Spirilla are spiral or curve-shaped bacteria. *Treponema pallidum,* a spirochete, is the causative agent of syphilis (Figure 20-3, *E*). This microorganism cannot be grown in commonly available culture media; the diagnosis of syphilis is generally made using serologic tests. A serologic test is performed on the serum of the blood. Cholera is caused by another type of spirillum, *Vibrio cholerae.* **Immunization** and proper methods of sanitation and water purification have all but eliminated cholera in the United States.

Viruses

Viruses are the smallest living organisms. They are so small that an electron microscope must be used to view them. Viruses infect plants, animals, and humans and use nutrients inside the host's cells for their metabolic and reproductive needs. Infectious diseases caused by viruses include influenza, chickenpox, rubeola (measles), rubella (German measles), mumps, poliomyelitis, smallpox, rabies, herpes simplex, herpes zoster, yellow fever, hepatitis, and most infectious diseases of the upper respiratory tract, including the common cold.

MICROSCOPE

Many kinds of microscopes are available, but the type used most often for office laboratory work is the *compound microscope.* The compound microscope consists of a two-lens system, and the magnification of one system is increased by the other. A source of bright light is required for proper illumination of the object to be viewed. This combination of lenses and light permits visualization of structures that cannot be seen with the unaided eye, such as microorganisms and cellular forms. The compound microscope consists of two main components—the support system and the optical system. The medical assistant should be able to identify the parts of a microscope (Figure 20-4) and should be able to use and care for it properly. Procedure 20-1 outlines the correct use and care of a microscope.

Support System

Frame

The working parts of the microscope are supported by a sturdy frame consisting of a *base* for support and an *arm* for carrying it without damaging the delicate parts. The arm also is needed to support the magnifying and adjusting systems.

Stage

The *stage* of a microscope is the flat, horizontal platform on which the microscope slide is placed. It is located directly over the condenser and beneath the objective lenses. The stage has a small round opening in the center that permits light from below to pass through the object being viewed and up into the lenses above. The slide should be placed on the stage; the object to be viewed is positioned over this opening so that it is satisfactorily illuminated by the light source below. Standard microscope stages have metal clips attached to the stage to hold the glass slide securely in place. With this type of stage, the slide must be moved by hand for examination of various areas on it.

Other types of microscopes have a *mechanical stage* that allows movement of the slide in a vertical or horizontal position by using adjustment knobs. The mechanical stage provides precise positioning of the slide, which is essential for performing certain procedures, such as differential white blood counts and inspection of Gram-stained smears.

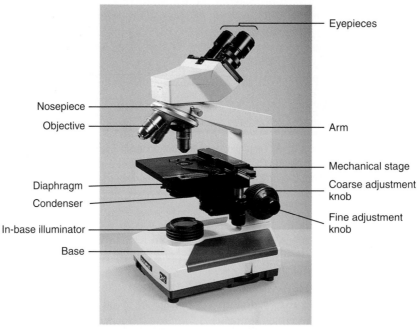

Figure 20-4. Parts of the microscope.

Light Source

The light source is at the base of the microscope and consists of a built-in illuminator, along with a switch for turning it on and off. The light is directed to the condenser above it and then through the object to be viewed.

Condenser

Compound microscopes have a lens system between the light source and object, known as the *substage condenser.* A popular condenser is the *Abbé condenser,* which consists of two lenses used to illuminate objects with transmitted light. The condenser collects and concentrates the light rays and directs them up, bringing them to a focus on the object so that it is well illuminated.

Diaphragm

The amount of light focused on the object also can be controlled by the *diaphragm,* located beneath or inside the condenser. The diaphragm consists of a series of horizontally arranged interlocking plates with a central opening, or *aperture.* The diaphragm has a lever that is used to increase or decrease the amount of light admitted by increasing or decreasing the aperture.

Appropriate intensity of light is essential for proper viewing of the specimens, especially at a higher magnification. A general rule is that as the desired magnification increases, the more intense the light must be. Increased light intensity is required for good visualization of a specimen with the oil-immersion objective. With the low-power objective, the light must be diminished to produce the appropriate contrast for specimen detail and to reduce glare. The degree of illumination also is influenced by the density of the object; stained structures (e.g., a Gram-stained smear of bacteria) usually require more light than do unstained specimens.

Adjustment Knobs

Two adjustment knobs are used to bring the specimen into focus: the coarse adjustment knob and the fine adjustment knob. The *coarse adjustment* is used first to obtain an approximate focus quickly. The *fine adjustment* is then used to obtain the precise focusing necessary to produce a sharp, clear image. On some microscope models, the adjustment knobs are mounted as two separate knobs; on others, they are placed together with the smaller fine adjustment knob extending from a larger coarse adjustment wheel.

Optical System

Compound microscopes have a two-lens magnification system. *Magnification* is defined as the ratio of the apparent size of an object viewed through the microscope to the actual size of the object.

Eyepiece

The first lens system is the eyepiece, or ocular lens, located at the top of the body tube and marked 10×, meaning that it magnifies 10 times. Microscopes that have one eyepiece only are called *monocular* microscopes, and microscopes with two eyepieces are called *binocular.* A binocular microscope is recommended for medical office laboratory work because it causes less eye fatigue than the monocular type. The binocular eyepieces can be adjusted to the individual by moving the eyepieces apart or together as needed.

Objective Lenses

The second lens system consists of three objective lenses located on the revolving *nosepiece,* each with a different degree of magnification. The metal shafts of the objective lenses differ in length and are identified by power of magnification. The short objective is known as the *low-power objective* and has a magnification of 10×. The *high-power objective* is known as the "high-dry objective" because it does not require the use of immersion oil; it has a magnification of 40×. The *oil-immersion objective* has the highest power of magnification, which is 100×.

The degree of magnification is engraved onto the metal shaft of each objective. In addition, some microscope manufacturers identify each objective lens by colored rings that encircle the metal shaft of the objective. Yellow is used for low power, blue for high power, and white for oil immersion. If the objective is not color-coded, it can be identified by the length of the metal shaft; the low-power objective is the shortest, and the oil-immersion objective is the longest.

The objective lens magnifies the specimen, and the ocular lens magnifies the image produced by the objective lens. The *total magnification* of each objective is determined by multiplying the ocular magnification by the objective magnification. The total magnification of the low-power objective is 100 times (100×) the actual size of the object being viewed (10 × 10). The total magnification of the high-power objective is 400× (10 × 40), and that of the oil-immersion magnification is 1000× (10 × 100).

Focus

Depending on the type of microscope, two ways may be used to focus on a specimen. Some microscopes are equipped with a *barrel focus.* With this type of microscope, the body tube (or barrel) moves, while the stage remains stationary during focusing. Other microscopes focus on the specimen using *stage focus.* With this type of microscope, the stage moves while the body tube remains stationary during focusing.

Low and High Power

The low-power objective is used for the initial focusing and light adjustment of the microscope. The low-power objective also is used for the initial observation and scanning requirements needed for most microscopic work. Urine sediment is first examined using the low-power objective to scan the specimen for the presence of casts.

The high-power objective is used for a more thorough study, such as observing cells in greater detail. The *working distance,* defined as the distance between the tip of the lens and the slide, is short when using this objective. Because of this, care must be taken in focusing the high-power objective to prevent it from striking and breaking the slide or damaging the lens.

Most compound microscopes are *parfocal*. This means that when the specimen is focused with the low-power objective, the nosepiece can be rotated to the high-power objective and focused simply with the fine adjustment knob.

Oil Immersion

The oil-immersion objective provides the highest magnification and is used to view very small structures or the detail of larger structures, such as microorganisms and blood cells. The oil-immersion objective has a very short working distance, and when it is in use, the lens nearly rests on the microscope slide itself. A special grade of oil, known as *immersion oil,* must be used with this lens. Oil has the advantage of not drying out when exposed to air for a long time. A drop of oil is placed on the slide and resides between the oil-immersion objective and the slide. The oil provides a path for the light to travel on between the slide and the lens and prevents the scattering of light rays, which permits clear viewing of very small structures. The oil also improves the resolution of the objective lens, that is, its ability to provide sharp detail, which is particularly necessary at high magnifications. Procedures that require oil immersion include differential white blood cell counts and examination of Gram-stained smears.

Care of the Microscope

The microscope is a delicate instrument and must be handled carefully. These guidelines should be followed to care for the microscope properly:

1. Always carry the microscope with two hands. Place one hand firmly on the arm and the other hand under the base for support. Place the microscope down gently to prevent jarring it, which could damage delicate parts.

2. Always handle the microscope in such a way that your fingers do not touch the lenses to avoid leaving fingerprints on them. When using a microscope, avoid wearing mascara because it is difficult to remove from the ocular lens.

3. When it is not in use, keep the microscope covered with its plastic dust cover and stored in a case or cupboard. Store it with the nosepiece rotated to the low-power objective and as close as possible to the stage.

4. Periodically clean the microscope by washing the enameled surfaces with mild soap and water and drying them thoroughly with a soft cloth. Never use alcohol on the enameled surfaces because it might remove the finish.

5. After each use, wipe the metal stage clean with gauze or tissue. If immersion oil comes in contact with the stage, remove it with a piece of gauze that is slightly moistened with xylene.

6. The ocular, objectives, and condenser consist of hand-ground optical lenses, which must be kept spotlessly clean by using clean, dry lens paper. Optical glass is softer than ordinary glass; to prevent scratching the lens, do not use tissues or gauze. If the lenses are especially dirty, use a commercial lens cleaner or xylene in the cleaning process. Apply a small amount of cleaner to the lens paper, followed by thorough drying and polishing with a clean piece of lens paper.

7. Keep the light source free of dust, lint, and dirt by periodic polishing with lens paper.

8. A malfunctioning microscope should be repaired only by a qualified service person. Attempting to fix the microscope yourself may result in further damage.

PROCEDURE 20-1   Using the Microscope

Outcome Use a microscope.

Equipment/Supplies

- Microscope
- Lens paper
- Specimen slide
- Tissue or gauze

- Immersion oil
- Xylene
- Soft cloth

---

1. Procedural Step. Clean the ocular and objective lenses with lens paper.

2. Procedural Step. Turn on the light source.

3. Procedural Step. Rotate the nosepiece to the low-power objective (10×), clicking it into place. Use the coarse adjustment knob to provide sufficient working space for placing the slide on the stage and to avoid damaging the objective lens as follows:

   a. **Barrel focus:** Raise the objective all the way up using the coarse adjustment knob.

   b. **Stage focus:** Lower the stage all the way down using the coarse adjustment knob.

4. Procedural Step. Place the slide on the stage specimen side up, and make sure it is secure.

5. Procedural Step. Position the low-power objective until it almost touches the slide using the coarse adjustment knob. Be sure to observe this step to prevent the objective from striking the slide.

6. Procedural Step. Look through the ocular. If a monocular microscope is being used, keep both eyes open

PROCEDURE 20-1 Using the Microscope—cont'd

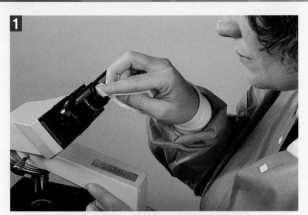

Clean the lens.

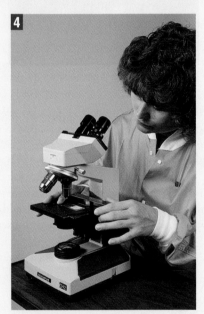

Place the slide on the stage.

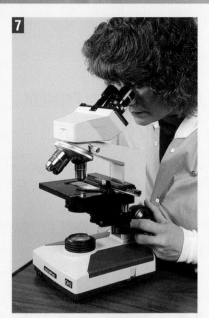

Focus the specimen.

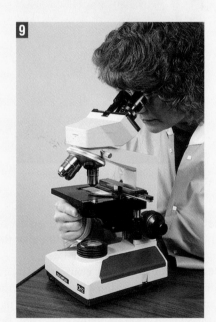

Adjust the light.

to prevent eyestrain. With a binocular microscope, adjust the two oculars to the width between your eyes until a single circular field of vision is obtained.

7. **Procedural Step.** Bring the specimen into coarse focus as follows:

   a. **Barrel focus:** Slowly raise the objective using the coarse adjustment knob.

   b. **Stage focus:** Slowly lower the stage using the coarse adjustment knob.

Observe the specimen through the ocular until it comes into focus.

8. Procedural Step. Use the fine adjustment knob to bring the specimen into a sharp, clear focus.

9. **Procedural Step.** Adjust the light as needed, using the iris diaphragm to provide maximal focus and contrast.

10. Procedural Step. Rotate the nosepiece to the high-power objective, making sure it clicks into place.

Proper focusing with the low-power objective ensures that the objective does not hit the slide during this operation. Use the fine adjustment knob to bring the specimen into a precise focus. Do not use the coarse adjustment to focus the high-power objective to prevent the objective from moving too far and striking the slide.

11. Procedural Step. Examine the specimen as required by the test or procedure being performed.

12. Procedural Step. Turn off the light after use, and remove the slide from the stage.

Continued

13. **Procedural Step.** Clean the stage with a tissue or gauze.
14. **Procedural Step.** Properly care for and store the microscope.

Using the Oil-Immersion Objective

1. **Procedural Step.** Rotate the nosepiece to the oil-immersion objective. Do not click it into place, but move it to one side.
2. **Procedural Step.** Place a drop of immersion oil on the slide directly over the center opening in the stage.

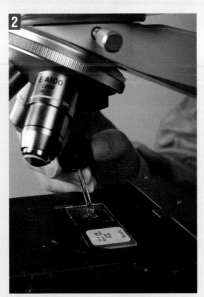

Place a drop of oil on the slide.

3. **Procedural Step.** Move the oil-immersion objective into place until a click is heard. Ensure that the objective does not touch the stage or slide.
4. **Procedural Step.** Using the coarse adjustment, slowly position the oil-immersion objective until the tip of the lens touches the oil but does not come in contact with the slide. A "pop" of light is observed. Be sure to observe carefully this step of the procedure.
5. **Procedural Step.** Look through the eyepiece, and focus slowly using the coarse adjustment until the object is visible.
6. **Procedural Step.** Use the fine adjustment to bring the object into sharp focus to view fine details.
7. **Procedural Step.** Adjust the light as needed, using the iris diaphragm to provide maximal focus and contrast. Increased light intensity is required for good visualization of the specimen with the oil-immersion objective.
8. **Procedural Step.** Examine the specimen as required by the test or procedure being performed.

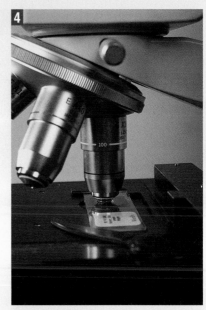

Move the lens until it just touches the oil.

9. **Procedural Step.** Turn off the light after use. Remove the slide from the stage, being careful not to get oil on the high-power objective or the stage.
10. **Procedural Step.** Using a piece of clean, dry lens paper, gently clean the oil-immersion objective. The lens must be cleaned immediately after use to prevent oil from drying on the lens surface. In addition, the oil may seep into the lens and perhaps loosen it.

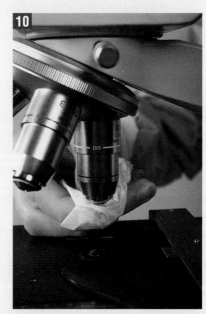

Clean the oil from the lens.

11. **Procedural Step.** Clean the oil from the slide by immersing it in xylene and wiping it off with a soft cloth.

MICROBIOLOGIC SPECIMEN COLLECTION

If the physician suspects that a particular disease is caused by a pathogen, he or she may want to obtain a specimen for microbiologic examination. This examination identifies the pathogen causing the disease and aids in diagnosis. If a urinary tract infection is suspected, a urine specimen is obtained for bacterial examination. In this instance, a clean-catch midstream collection is required to obtain a specimen that excludes the normal flora of the urethra and urinary meatus.

A **specimen** is a small sample or part taken from the body to represent the whole. The medical assistant is often responsible for collecting specimens from certain areas of the body, such as the throat, nose, and wounds. The medical assistant may be responsible for assisting the physician in the collection of specimens from other areas, such as the cervix, vagina, urethra, and rectum. In most instances, a sterile swab is used to collect the specimen. A *swab* is a small piece of cotton wrapped around the end of a slender wooden or plastic stick. It is passed across a body surface or opening to obtain a specimen for microbiologic analysis.

To prevent inaccurate test results, good techniques of medical and surgical asepsis must be practiced when a specimen is obtained. The medical assistant must be careful not to contaminate the specimen with *extraneous microorganisms*. These are undesirable microorganisms that can enter the specimen in various ways; they grow and multiply and possibly obscure and prevent identification of pathogens that might be present. To prevent extraneous microorganisms (i.e., normal flora) from contaminating the specimen, all supplies used to obtain the specimen (e.g., swabs, specimen containers) must be sterile. In addition, the specimen should not contain microorganisms from areas surrounding the collection site. When obtaining a throat specimen, the

Putting It All into Practice

My Name is Natalie Moorehead, and I work for a physician who specializes in family practice. Working as a medical assistant, one can encounter many challenges. One experience that I had involved a 4-year-old boy. The patient came into the office with a very sore throat and a high fever. He did not think that his office visit had gone too badly until he found out that the physician had ordered a rapid strep test to check for strep throat. That's when he decided he did not care for me, my tongue depressor, or my swab. He decided to protest by keeping his mouth tightly shut. Rather than forcing the procedure on the child, I took my time and kept my patience. I managed to convince the child that even though the procedure was uncomfortable and tasted bad, it was the only way we would know if he was really sick or not. I also explained that the test was the only way the doctor would know what kind of medicine to prescribe so he could get well and feel like playing again. It took a while, but we got our specimen, and the patient received the right antibiotic that he needed to get better. ■

swab should not be allowed to touch the inside of the mouth.

The OSHA Bloodborne Pathogens Standard presented in Chapter 2 should be carefully followed when performing microbiologic procedures. Specifically, the medical assistant must wear gloves when it is reasonably anticipated that hand contact might occur with blood or other potentially infectious materials. Eating, drinking, smoking, and applying makeup are strictly forbidden when one is working with microorganisms because pathogens can be transmitted to the medical assistant through hand-to-mouth contact. In addition, labels for specimen containers should not be licked, and any break in the skin, such as a cut or scratch, must be covered with a bandage. If the medical assistant accidentally touches some of the material in the specimen, the area of contact should be washed immediately and thoroughly with soap and water. If the specimen comes in contact with the worktable, the table should be cleaned immediately with soap and water, followed by a suitable disinfectant, such as phenol. The worktable also should be cleaned with a disinfectant at the end of each day.

After collection, the specimen must be placed in its proper container with the lid securely fastened. The container must be clearly labeled with the patient's name and date of birth, the date, the source of the specimen, the medical assistant's initials, and any other required information. Procedure 20-2 outlines the procedure for collecting a specimen for a throat culture.

Handling and Transporting Microbiologic Specimens

After the microbiologic specimen has been collected, care should be taken in handling and transporting it. Delay in processing the specimen may cause the death of pathogens or overgrowth of the specimen by microorganisms that are part of the normal flora usually collected along with the pathogen from the specimen site. If the specimen is to be analyzed in the medical office, it should be examined under the microscope or cultured immediately. Otherwise, it should be preserved (if possible) with the method used by the medical office.

Specimens transported to an outside medical laboratory by a courier service are usually placed in a transport medium. The transport medium prevents drying of the specimen and preserves it in its original state until it reaches its destination. Transport media are discussed in greater detail in the section on "Collection and Transport Systems."

Outside laboratories provide the medical office with specific instructions on the care and handling of specimens being transported to them. These specimens must be accompanied by a laboratory request that designates the physician's name and address; the patient's name, age, and gender; the date and time of collection; the type of microbiologic examination requested; the source of the specimen (e.g., throat, wound, urine); and the physician's clinical diagnosis. The form usually includes a space to indicate whether the patient is receiving antibiotic therapy. Antibiotics may suppress the growth of bacteria, a factor that could produce **false-negative** results.

Wound Specimens

Wound specimens are collected using many of the techniques described previously. In many cases, two swabs are used to collect the specimen. The specimen is obtained by inserting the swab into the area of the wound that contains the most drainage and gently rotating the swab from side to side to allow it to absorb completely any microorganisms present. The swab is placed in the specimen container, and the process is repeated using a second swab. To obtain accurate and reliable test results, it is important to collect a specimen from within the wound, rather than from the surface.

Collection and Transport Systems

Microbiologic collection and transport systems are available to facilitate the collection of a specimen to be transported to an outside laboratory for analysis; examples include Culturette (Becton Dickinson, Franklin Lakes, NJ) and Starswab II (Starplex Scientific, Beverly, Mass) (Figure 20-5). These systems consist of a sterile swab and a plastic tube that contains a transport medium. The transport medium prevents drying of the specimen and preserves it in its original state until it reaches its destination. The collection and transport system comes packaged in a peel-apart envelope and should be stored at room temperature. The procedure for the use of a microbiologic collection and transport system is outlined next.

1. Sanitize your hands, and apply gloves.
2. Check the expiration date on the peel-apart envelope.
3. Peel back the package, and remove the cap from the collection tube. Remove the cap/swab unit from the peel-apart package. The cap is permanently attached to the sterile swab.
4. Using aseptic technique, collect the specimen. Do not allow the swab to touch any area other than the collection site.
5. Insert the swab into the collection tube.
6. Push the cap/swab in as far as it will go to immerse the swab completely in the transport medium. Make sure the cap is tightly in place.

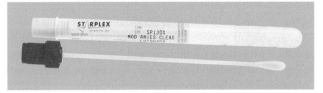

Figure 20-5. Starswab II Collection and Transport System.

Case Study 2

Hollie Dolley, age 18, is at the medical office complaining of fatigue, fever, headache, and a terrible sore throat. She just enrolled in a medical assisting program and has been really worried about doing well in her classes. Hollie says that she stays up until midnight every night studying, and she works 30 hours at a drugstore on the weekends. The physician orders a rapid mononucleosis test on Hollie, and it is positive. Hollie says she has never felt so awful in her whole life and wants to know whether she is going to die from this. She says it hurts really bad to swallow and she cannot eat. Hollie says that she has heard one gets mono from kissing, and she does not have a boyfriend, so she doesn't understand how she could possibly have mono. Hollie wants to know why the physician did not prescribe an antibiotic for her so that she could get well sooner and not have to miss any of her classes. ■

7. Remove gloves, and sanitize your hands.
8. Label the tube with the patient's name and date of birth, the date, the source of the specimen (e.g., throat, wound), and your initials. Place the tube in a biohazard specimen transport bag. Place the laboratory request in the outside pocket of the bag.
9. Complete a laboratory request form.
10. Place the collection tube in a biohazard specimen bag with the laboratory requisition form in the outside pocket.
11. Chart the procedure.
12. Transport the specimen to the laboratory within 24 hours.

Memories *from* Externship

Natalie Moorehead: Terrified and excited at the same time to be experiencing my first externship, I found myself in a busy pediatric office. After a few days of watching and learning, I prepared to work up an infant for a well-child examination. Before entering the room, I was told by a staff member that the HIV status of the infant's mother was questionable. Alarmed at first as to how I would feel in this situation, I immediately remembered all the precautions we had talked about in class. As I took the infant from the mother to weigh and measure him, I have to admit many thoughts ran through my mind, but again I was calmed because of all the information we had received in school regarding OSHA precautions. Faced with that situation today, after practicing wisely and safely for 5 years, I would not think twice about it because I know from my education and experience that these types of situations can be handled without alarm. ■

PROCEDURE 20-2   Collecting a Throat Specimen

Outcome Collect a throat specimen for a rapid strep test.

A throat specimen is obtained by using a sterile swab. It is commonly collected to aid in the diagnosis of infections such as streptococcal sore throat, pharyngitis, and tonsillitis. Less frequently, it is used to diagnose whooping cough and diphtheria. These latter diseases are not prevalent today because of the availability of immunizations against them. This procedure outlines the steps necessary to obtain a throat specimen to perform a rapid streptococcus test, which is discussed later in the chapter.

Equipment/Supplies

- Disposable gloves
- Tongue depressor
- Sterile swab
- Waste container

1. **Procedural Step.** Sanitize your hands, and assemble the equipment.
2. **Procedural Step.** Greet the patient and introduce yourself. Identify the patient by full name and date of birth and explain the procedure.
3. **Procedural Step.** Position the patient, and adjust the light to provide clear visualization of the throat.
   Principle. The throat must be clearly visible so that the medical assistant is able to determine the proper area for obtaining the specimen.
4. **Procedural Step.** Apply gloves. Remove the sterile swab from its peel-apart package, being careful not to contaminate it.
   Principle. Contamination of the swab may lead to inaccurate test results.

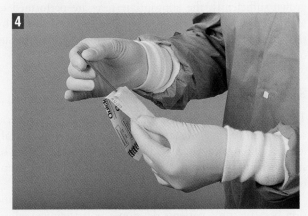

Remove the swab.

5. **Procedural Step.** Depress the tongue with the tongue depressor.
   Principle. The tongue depressor holds the tongue down and facilitates access to the throat.
6. **Procedural Step.** Place the swab at the back of the throat (posterior pharynx), and firmly rub it over any lesions or white or inflamed areas of the mucous membrane of the tonsillar area and posterior pharyngeal wall. Rotate the swab constantly as you collect the specimen, making sure there is good contact with the tonsillar area. Do not allow the swab to touch any areas other than the throat, such as the inside of the mouth.

Principle. The swab should be rubbed over suspicious-looking areas where pathogens are likely to be found. A rotating motion is used to deposit the maximal amount of material possible on the swab. Touching it to any areas other than the throat contaminates the specimen with extraneous microorganisms.

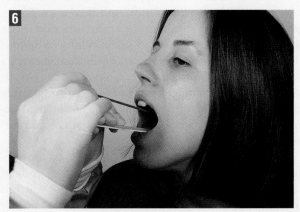

Collect the specimen.

7. **Procedural Step.** Keeping the patient's tongue depressed, withdraw the swab, and remove the tongue depressor from the patient's mouth.
8. **Procedural Step.** Properly dispose of the tongue depressor in a regular waste container to prevent transmission of microorganisms.
9. **Procedural Step.** Process the swab according to the directions accompanying the rapid strep test.
10. **Procedural Step.** Remove gloves, and sanitize your hands. Chart the test results.

CHARTING EXAMPLE	
Date	
7/12/12	10:30 a.m. Throat specimen collected.
	QuickVue Strep Test: Positive. ————
	———————— N. Moorehead, CMA (AAMA)

PROCEDURE 20-2

MICROBIAL CULTURES

After a microbiologic specimen is collected, it may be examined to determine the type of microorganisms present. Because most specimens generally contain only a few pathogens, it is often desirable to induce any pathogens that are present to grow and multiply.

Most microorganisms, especially bacteria, can be grown on a culture medium. A **culture medium** is a mixture of nutrients on which microorganisms are grown in the laboratory. The culture medium and the environment in which it is placed must meet the requirements to support and encourage the growth of the suspected pathogen. These growth requirements include the presence or the absence of oxygen (depending on the microorganism); proper nutrition, temperature, and pH; and moisture.

The culture medium may be solid or liquid. Blood agar is one of the most frequently used solid culture media. It is prepared by adding sheep's blood to a substance known as *agar,* which is transparent and colorless. Blood added to the agar provides nutrients that support the growth of a variety of bacteria. When heated, it melts and becomes a liquid. On cooling, agar solidifies, forming a firm surface on which microorganisms can be grown. A liquid culture medium is often referred to as a *broth* and is usually contained in a tube; an example is nutrient broth. Culture media must be stored in the refrigerator and warmed to room temperature before use. A cold culture medium must not be used because the cold temperature results in the death of microorganisms placed on it.

A *Petri plate* is frequently used to hold solid culture medium. The plate consists of a shallow circular dish made of glass or clear plastic with a cover, the diameter of which is greater than that of the base. Microorganisms can be cultured on the surface of the medium in the plate (Figure 20-6). Petri plates allow examination of a culture while preventing microorganisms from entering or escaping. A

culture is a mass of microorganisms growing in a laboratory culture medium.

Most medical offices use commercially prepared culture media in disposable plastic Petri plates. The plates come packaged in a plastic bag and must be stored in the refrigerator with the medium side facing upward. The plastic bag prevents the medium from drying out; storing the plates with the medium side facing upward prevents condensation on the medium surface. The plate has an expiration date that must be checked before using. Plates that are past the expiration date or are dried out or contaminated should not be used.

The solid culture medium in a Petri plate is **inoculated** by lightly rolling the swab containing the specimen over the surface of the medium; this process is known as **streaking.** The cover of the Petri plate should be removed only when the specimen is being spread on the culture medium. Unnecessary removal of the cover results in contamination of the medium with extraneous microorganisms. The culture is **incubated** for 24 to 48 hours in conditions that encourage the growth of the suspected pathogen.

Most specimens taken for analysis contain a mixture of organisms because of the presence of normal flora in most parts of the body. When this is the case, the resulting culture is known as a *mixed culture,* or one that contains two or more types of microorganisms. To analyze most microbiologic specimens, the suspected pathogen must be separated from the mixed culture and permitted to grow alone. This establishes a *pure culture,* or a culture that contains only one type of microorganism. After the culture has grown sufficiently, the appropriate tests are performed to identify the pathogen. It is impossible to grow viruses by this method; rather, they must be cultured on living tissue or identified using serologic tests.

STREPTOCOCCUS TESTING

The most common streptococcal condition is streptococcal sore throat, or *streptococcal pharyngitis,* which primarily affects children and young adults. The causative agent of streptococcal pharyngitis is a group A beta-hemolytic streptococcus known as *Streptococcus pyogenes.*

Streptococcal pharyngitis is a potentially serious condition because some patients develop a poststreptococcal sequela. A **sequela** is a morbid secondary condition that occurs as a result of a less serious primary infection. A few patients with streptococcal pharyngitis (primary infection) develop rheumatic fever; the rheumatic fever is considered a poststreptococcal sequela. Owing to the risk of a sequela, early diagnosis and treatment with antibiotics of streptococcal pharyngitis is important. In the medical office, commercially available tests are often used for identification of group A beta-hemolytic streptococci. The most frequently used testing methods are presented next.

Rapid Streptococcus Tests

Rapid streptococcus tests are biochemical tests that directly detect group A streptococcus from a throat swab in a very short time. Most tests require only 4 to 10 minutes to pro-

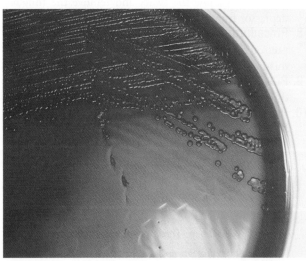

Figure 20-6. Streptococcal colonies growing on a blood agar culture medium contained in a Petri plate. (From Mahon CR, Manuselis G Jr: Textbook of diagnostic microbiology, ed 2, Philadelphia, 2000, Saunders.)

cess; diagnosis can often be made and antibiotics prescribed, if necessary, before the patient leaves the office.

The most frequently used rapid streptococcus test is the direct antigen identification test, which confirms the presence of group A streptococcus through an antigen-antibody reaction. The test works by combining particles sensitized to the streptococcus antibody with the throat specimen. If group A streptococcal antigen is in the specimen, it combines with the antibody-sensitized particles to produce a color change that can be observed with the unaided eye. Rapid streptococcus tests also include a control that determines whether the test results are accurate and reliable.

The advantage of the direct antigen identification test is that it provides the physician with immediate test results rather than requiring an overnight culture. Specific instructions are included with every commercially avail-

able antigen identification test; examples of these tests include QTest Strep (Becton Dickinson, Franklin Lakes, NJ), Clearview Strep A (Wampole Laboratories, Princeton, NJ), and QuickVue In Line Strep A (Quidel, San Diego, Calif) (Figure 20-7).

Hemolytic Reaction and Bacitracin Susceptibility Test

Streptococci are classified according to their hemolytic properties exhibited on a blood agar medium into three types: *alpha*, *beta*, and *gamma*. They are further divided according to their antigenic properties into 15 subgroups designated by the letters *A* through *O*. The hemolytic reaction and bacitracin susceptibility test is a biochemical culture test that relies on these hemolytic and antigenic properties of streptococci for the interpretation of test results.

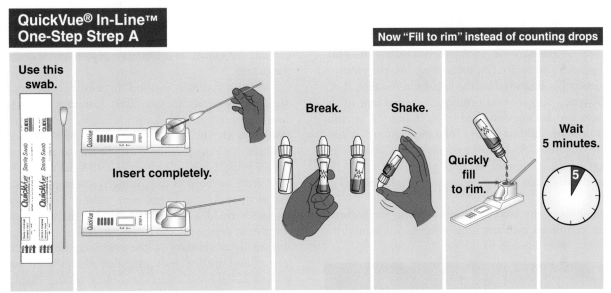

If liquid has not moved across the Result Window in 1 minute, completely remove the swab and reinsert.

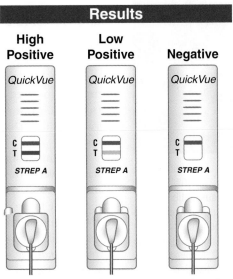

Figure 20-7. Procedure for performing the QuickVue In-Line One-Step Strep A test. (Courtesy Quidel Corporation, San Diego, Calif.)

The testing procedure involves placing a filter paper disc impregnated with 0.04 U of bacitracin on the surface of a sheep blood agar medium previously inoculated with the throat specimen. The medium is incubated for 18 to 24 hours to allow growth of the bacteria and to permit diffusion of the bacitracin into the culture medium surrounding the disc.

After the 18- to 24-hour incubation period, the plate is examined for its *hemolytic reaction.* As stated, the causative agent of streptococcal pharyngitis is a (group A) beta-hemolytic streptococcus. Beta-hemolytic streptococci produce and secrete **streptolysin,** an exotoxin that completely hemolyzes red blood cells; a clear, wide, colorless zone of hemolysis (with no intact red blood cells) around the bacterial colonies indicates their presence. A greenish halo around the colonies indicates the less pathogenic alpha-hemolytic streptococci. The generally nonpathogenic gamma-type streptococci do not cause a reaction on the blood agar medium.

If the hemolytic property exhibited is of the beta type, the area around the bacitracin disc is next inspected for *bacitracin susceptibility.* Group A streptococci are **susceptible** or sensitive to bacitracin; because of this, the group A streptococcus is destroyed by the bacitracin. Groups B, C, and G (which also are beta-hemolytic) are resistant to the bacitracin and are not destroyed by it. If group A streptococcus is present, a clear zone of inhibition appears around the disc (Figure 20-8, *A*). Because groups B, C, and G are resistant to the bacitracin, bacteria grow right up to the edge of the disc, that is, there is no zone of inhibition (Figure 20-8, *B*).

Hemolysis of the blood agar surrounding the bacterial colonies combined with any zone of inhibition around the bacitracin disc is considered presumptive positive for group A beta-hemolytic streptococci. The test is considered presumptive because a small percentage of bacterial strains included in groups B, C, and G are sensitive to bacitracin; a fraction (less than 5%) of the test results are false-positive. A **false-positive** is a test result indicating that a condition is present when it actually is not.

The bacitracin disc test is a convenient, reliable, and cost-effective method used in the medical office to determine the presence of streptococcal pharyngitis. Since the development of the rapid streptococcus tests, however, it is not used as frequently.

SENSITIVITY TESTING

The physician may request not only that the laboratory identify the infecting pathogen, but also that a sensitivity test be performed on it to determine the best antibiotic to treat the condition. The test is always performed on a pure rather than a mixed culture. A sensitivity test determines the susceptibility of pathogenic bacteria to various antibiotics; only the growth of the infectious pathogen is desired on the culture.

The most common method for sensitivity testing is the *disc-diffusion method* (Figure 20-9). Commercially prepared discs impregnated with known concentrations of various antibiotics are dropped on the surface of a solid culture medium in a Petri plate inoculated with the pathogen. The culture is incubated, allowing the antibiotics to diffuse into the culture medium. If the pathogen is susceptible or sensitive to an antibiotic, a clear zone without bacterial growth surrounds the disc. This indicates that the antibiotic was effective in destroying the pathogen. If the pathogen is unaffected by or resistant to the antibiotic, no clear zone is seen around the disc, indicating that the antibiotic was unable to kill the pathogen. Sensitivity testing enables the physician to decide which antibiotics would most likely be effective against the infectious disease in question.

MICROSCOPIC EXAMINATION OF MICROORGANISMS

Microorganisms can be examined under a microscope in the fixed state or in the living state. Examination in the fixed state involves the preparation of a smear through heat fixation, followed by a staining process such as Gram stain (see later). Most microorganisms are examined in the fixed state because it is easier to examine them when they are stained.

Some microorganisms require examination in the living state, however, owing to special circumstances, such as their inability to be readily stained or difficulty in culturing them. The living state also allows visualization of the movement of motile microorganisms. This is especially helpful in the identification of certain motile microorganisms, such as *Trichomonas vaginalis,* which is the causative agent of the vaginal infection trichomoniasis. To observe the motility of microorganisms, they first must be suspended in a liquid

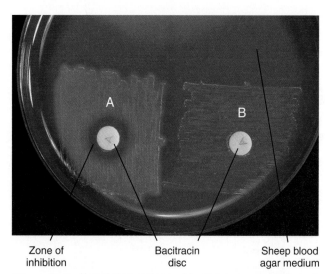

| Zone of inhibition | Bacitracin disc | Sheep blood agar medium |

Figure 20-8. Hemolytic reaction and bacitracin susceptibility test. **A,** Positive reaction for group A beta-hemolytic streptococcus, as evidenced by a clear zone of inhibition present around the bacitracin disc. **B,** Negative reaction as evidenced by bacteria growing right up to the edge of the disc. (Modified from Mahon CR, Manuselis G Jr: Textbook of diagnostic microbiology, ed 2, Philadelphia, 2000, Saunders.)

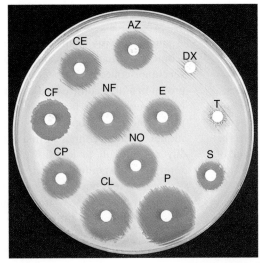

AZ: Azithromycin
CE: Cephalothin
CF: Ciprofloxacin
CL: Clarithromycin
CP: Ciprozil
DX: Doxycycline
E: Erythromycin
NF: Nitrofurantoin
NO: Norfloxacin
P: Penicillin
S: Sulfisoxazole
T: Tetracycline

Figure 20-9. Sensitivity testing. (From Mahon CR, Manuselis G Jr: Textbook of diagnostic microbiology, ed 2, Philadelphia, 2000, Saunders.)

PATIENT TEACHING Strep Throat

Answer questions patients have about strep throat.

What is strep throat?

Strep throat is a contagious and acute infection that is medically known as *streptococcal pharyngitis.* It is caused by the bacterium group A streptococcus. Strep throat is transmitted directly from one person to another through droplets of saliva or nasal secretions. It most frequently occurs in children 5 to 10 years old and during the months of October through April. Strep infections are different from most other infectious diseases because having one strep infection does not prevent the development of another at a future date.

What are the symptoms of strep throat?

The symptoms of strep throat are a sore throat with severe pain on swallowing, a bright red pharynx (called "beefy red pharynx"), fever, white patches on the tonsils, swollen glands in the neck, muscular aches and pains, and a feeling of tiredness.

How is strep throat diagnosed and treated?

Strep throat is diagnosed by taking a throat specimen and running a laboratory test on it to determine whether group A streptococcus is present. Strep throat usually is treated by antibiotics taken orally for 10 days. It is important to take all of the antibiotic prescribed by the physician to prevent complications that can occur from strep throat. A patient with strep throat should rest in bed and avoid contact with others to prevent spreading it.

What are the complications of strep throat?

Severe complications can result from strep throat if it is not adequately treated, including rheumatic fever and glomerulonephritis, which is a kidney disorder. These complications are rare because most patients seek early treatment for strep infections.

- Encourage the patient to complete the entire prescribed course of antibiotics.
- Instruct the patient to notify the physician if new symptoms develop.
- Provide the patient with educational materials about strep throat.

What Would You Do? What Would You *Not* Do?

Case Study 3

John Seimer calls the medical office. He says that he is not a patient at the office but would like some assistance. He says that for the past 3 days he has had a headache, fever, chills, and aching muscles. He says that a week ago he pulled a tick off his lower leg, and several days later he found a red rash around the tick bite. He says that he went on the Internet and looked up his symptoms, and he is sure that he has Lyme disease. The Internet site recommended taking doxycycline for 3 weeks to treat Lyme disease. John says that he does not like to go to the doctor and has not been to see a doctor for over 10 years. He wants to know whether the doctor could call in a prescription for doxycycline for him. He says that he has health insurance and the doctor could bill him for an appointment, just as long as he does not have to come in. ∎

medium so that they are free to move about. The most common method of examining microorganisms in the living state is the wet mount method, which is described next.

Wet Mount Method

In the wet mount method, the medical assistant places a drop of fluid containing the organism on a glass slide and covers it with a coverslip (Figure 20-10). The coverslip may be ringed with petroleum jelly to provide a seal between the slide and the coverslip. The purpose is to reduce the rate of evaporation through air currents that lead to drying and possible death of the specimen.

The slide is placed under the microscope for examination by the physician using the high-power objective. For satisfactory visualization, the intensity of the light must be diminished by partially closing the diaphragm of the microscope. The slide and coverslip should be properly disposed of in a biohazard sharps container.

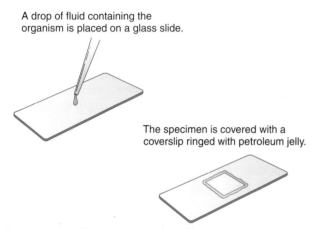

A drop of fluid containing the organism is placed on a glass slide.

The specimen is covered with a coverslip ringed with petroleum jelly.

Figure 20-10. Wet mount method of slide preparation for examining microorganisms in the living state.

Smears

A **smear** consists of material spread on a slide for microscopic examination. It can be prepared directly from the specimen collected on the swab, or the specimen can be grown first on a culture medium and a smear then prepared. Most smears must be stained before they can be viewed under the microscope, using one of many staining techniques. Bacteria contained in a smear are colorless and usually are difficult to identify under the microscope unless some type of staining is used.

Smears are often helpful when time is a factor because a smear can be prepared immediately from the specimen. This procedure gives the physician a preliminary clue to the causative agent while other, more time-consuming tests are being performed. Procedure 20-3 outlines the method to prepare a microbiologic smear.

Gram Stain

Gram stain is often used in combination with other tests to help in the diagnosis and treatment of infectious diseases. As already discussed, bacteria contained in a smear are colorless and usually are difficult to identify under the microscope unless some type of staining is used. Gram stain allows the observer to view directly the size, shape, and growth patterns of the bacteria.

In 1883, Christian Gram, a Danish physician, discovered a way to differentiate bacteria on the basis of their color reactions to various stains. Gram stain is based on the fact that when treated with crystal violet dye, cerain bacteria permanently retain this dye after undergoing a decolorization process. These bacteria exhibit a purple color when viewed under the microscope and are known as *gram-positive* bacteria (Figure 20-11, *A*). Other bacteria are unable to retain this dye after being decolorized and become colorless. They must be counterstained with a red dye to become visible under the

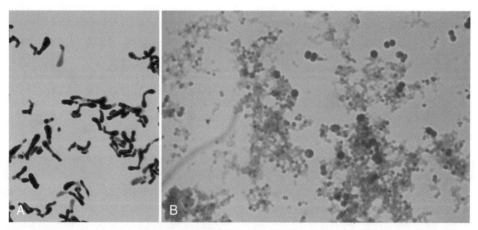

Figure 20-11. Gram-positive and gram-negative bacteria. **A,** Diphtheria is caused by a gram-positive bacillus. **B,** Gonorrhea is caused by a gram-negative diplococcus. (**A** courtesy Cathy Bissonette; **B** from Mahon CR, Manuselis G Jr: Textbook of diagnostic microbiology, ed 2, Philadelphia, 2000, Saunders.)

microscope. These bacteria exhibit a pink or red color and are known as *gram-negative* bacteria (Figure 20-11, *B*). These staining characteristics are due to differences in the chemical composition of the bacterial cell walls.

Gram stain allows for the division of most bacteria into two groups—gram-positive and gram-negative. Infectious diseases caused by gram-positive bacteria include streptococcal sore throat, scarlet fever, rheumatic fever, diphtheria, lobar pneumonia, tetanus, and botulism. Infectious diseases caused by gram-negative bacteria include whooping cough, gonorrhea, meningitis, bacillary dysentery, cholera, typhoid fever, and plague.

Bacteria that are Gram-stained also are observed for their characteristic shape and fall into one of the following categories: gram-positive rods, gram-negative rods, gram-positive cocci, or gram-negative cocci. The causative agent of gonorrhea is a gram-negative diplococcus.

PREVENTION AND CONTROL OF INFECTIOUS DISEASES

Individuals in the community can help prevent and control infectious diseases by practicing good techniques of medical asepsis, by obtaining proper nutrition and rest, and by using good hygienic measures. In addition, infected individuals should contact their physicians in an effort to ensure early diagnosis and treatment of the infectious disease. Immunizations are available to prevent a wide range of infectious diseases. The medical assistant has a responsibility to help educate community members about practices that reduce the transmission of pathogens and help control and prevent infectious diseases.

PROCEDURE 20-3 Preparing a Smear

Outcome Prepare a microbiology smear.

Equipment/Supplies

- Disposable gloves
- Bunsen burner
- Clean glass slide
- Microbiologic specimen
- Slide forceps
- Sterile swab
- Biohazard waste container

1. Procedural Step. Sanitize your hands.

2. Procedural Step. Assemble the equipment. Label the slide with the patient's name and date of birth, and the date.

3. Procedural Step. Apply gloves. Hold the edges of the slide between your thumb and index finger. Starting at the right side and using a rolling motion, gently and evenly spread the material from the specimen over the slide. The material should cover approximately one half to two thirds of the slide. Do not rub the material vigorously over the slide. Properly dispose of the contaminated swab in a biohazard waste container.

Principle. The specimen may contain pathogens that are capable of infecting the medical assistant; it is important to wear gloves. A rolling motion is used to deposit the maximal amount of material possible on the slide. Rubbing may disintegrate the cellular structures making up the microorganisms in the specimen.

4. Procedural Step. Allow the smear to air-dry in a flat position for at least 30 minutes. Heat should not be applied at this time.

Principle. Air-drying allows the bacterial cells to dry slowly. Applying heat at this stage would burst the bacterial cells, resulting in an inappropriate smear.

5. Procedural Step. Holding the slide with the slide forceps, heat-fix the smear by quickly passing the slide back and forth (approximately 3 times) through the flame of a Bunsen burner. The slide has been fixed properly if the back of the slide feels uncomfortable (but not too hot) when touched to the back of your hand. Excessive heat should be avoided. Allow the slide to cool completely. An alternative to heat-fixing the slide is to apply ethyl alcohol to the slide and allow it to air-dry.

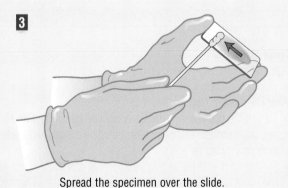

Spread the specimen over the slide.

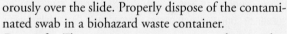

Continued

PROCEDURE 20-3

PROCEDURE 20-3   Preparing a Smear—cont'd

Principle. Heat-fixing the slide kills the microorganisms and attaches them firmly to the slide so that they do not wash off during the staining process. An excessive amount of heat could result in distortion of the bacterial cells.

6. **Procedural Step.** Prepare the slide for examination under the microscope. Inform the physician that the slide is ready for examination.

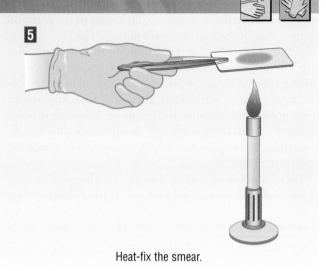

Heat-fix the smear.

evolve *Check out the Evolve site to access additional interactive activities.*

MEDICAL PRACTICE *and the* LAW

This chapter addresses the collection and identification of microorganisms that cause infections. You must maintain standard precautions whenever handling potentially infectious material to protect yourself, your coworkers, and your patients. Microbiology is an exact science—one stray microorganism can contaminate the entire specimen. Sanitize hands thoroughly, and apply new gloves between handling of specimens to avoid cross-contamination. If specimen contamination occurs, immediately discard the specimen and collect a new one. Be precise in your labeling—a mislabeled specimen can cause unnecessary concern, treatment, or both for the patient.

Maintain confidentiality of information. Certain infectious diseases must be reported to the Centers for Disease Control and Prevention (CDC) or the local board of health. Otherwise, do not give information to anyone other than the patient or legal guardian. ■

What Would You Do? What Would You *Not* Do? RESPONSES

Case Study 1
Page 776

What Did Natalie Do?
❑ Told Paula that it is important that the physician find out whether Caitlin has strep throat because strep can sometimes develop into a more serious infection. Explained that if Caitlin does have strep throat, the doctor would want to prescribe the best antibiotic to treat the infection.
❑ Talked with Caitlin about the reason for the test. Explained that it will help the doctor find the best way to treat her so that she starts feeling better as soon as possible.
❑ Reassured Caitlin that the procedure would be very quick and it would be over before she knew it.
❑ Told Caitlin that after the specimen was obtained, she could choose a prize from the treasure box.

What Did Natalie Not *Do?*
❑ Did not force the collection swab into Caitlin's mouth.

What Would You Do?/What Would You *Not* Do? Review Natalie's response and place a checkmark next to the information you included in your response. List additional information you included in your response.

_____

_____

_____

_____

Case Study 2
Page 784

What Did Natalie Do?
❑ Told Hollie that mononucleosis is usually transmitted by kissing, but it sometimes can be transmitted by coughs and sneezes from an infected person.
❑ Sympathized with Hollie and told her that it probably feels like she is going to die, but she should start to feel better as her body begins to fight off the disease.

PROCEDURE 20-3

What Would You Do? What Would You *Not* Do? RESPONSES—cont'd

- ❑ Explained to Hollie that mononucleosis is caused by a virus and that antibiotics do not work against viruses.
- ❑ Told Hollie to try drinking cold fluids or sucking on a Popsicle until she feels more like eating.

What Did Natalie Not *Do?*
- ❑ Did not ignore or minimize Hollie's concerns.

What Would You Do?/What Would You *Not* Do? Review Natalie's response and place a checkmark next to the information you included in your response. List additional information you included in your response.

_____

_____

_____

_____

Case Study 3
Page 789

What Did Natalie Do?
- ❑ Sympathized with John and told him that a lot of people do not like coming to see the doctor. Told him that the doctor could not

legally or ethically prescribe medication for him without seeing him.
- ❑ Told John that the office could not bill him for an appointment that he did not have.
- ❑ Asked John whether he wanted to make an appointment to see the doctor.

What Did Natalie Not *Do?*
- ❑ Did not tell John he should not be diagnosing himself with information he found on the Internet.

What Would You Do?/What Would You *Not* Do? Review Natalie's response and place a checkmark next to the information you included in your response. List additional information you included in your response.

_____

_____

_____

_____

CERTIFICATION REVIEW

- ❑ **Microbiology** is the scientific study of microorganisms and their activities. Each individual has a normal flora, which consists of the harmless, nonpathogenic microorganisms that normally reside in many parts of the body but do not cause disease.
- ❑ **The invasion of the body** by pathogenic microorganisms is known as *infection.* Many infectious diseases are contagious, meaning that the pathogen causing the disease can be spread from one person to another directly or indirectly. Frequently, droplet infection is the mode of transmission of pathogens.
- ❑ **The incubation period** is the interval of time between the invasion by a pathogenic microorganism and the appearance of the first symptoms of the disease. The prodromal period is when the first symptoms of a disease occur. The acute period is when the disease is at its peak and the symptoms are fully developed. The decline period is when the symptoms of the disease begin to subside. The convalescent period is the stage in which the patient regains strength and returns to health.
- ❑ **Bacteria** can be classified into three basic groups according to their shape. Staphylococci are round bacteria that grow in grapelike clusters. Streptococci are round bacteria that grow in chains. Diplococci are round bacteria that grow in pairs. Bacilli are rod-shaped bacteria that are frequently found in the soil and air. Spirilla are

spiral and curve-shaped bacteria. Viruses are the smallest living organisms, and an electron microscope must be used to view them.
- ❑ **A compound microscope** is used for office laboratory work. It contains three objective lenses. The low-power objective has a magnification of 10× and is used in the initial observation and scanning requirements needed for most microscopic work. The high-power objective has a magnification of 40× and is used for a more thorough study. The oil-immersion objective has the highest power of magnification, which is 100×.
- ❑ **A specimen** is a small sample taken from the body to represent the nature of the whole. Throat specimens are frequently collected in the medical office to aid in the diagnosis of streptococcal sore throat. Specimens also can be collected from wounds and from the eye, ear, cervix, vagina, urethra, and rectum.
- ❑ **A culture medium** is a mixture of nutrients on which microorganisms are grown in the laboratory. A culture is a mass of microorganisms growing in a laboratory culture medium. A mixed culture contains two or more different types of microorganisms. A pure culture contains only one type of microorganism.
- ❑ **The most common streptococcal condition** is streptococcal sore throat. A sequela is a morbid secondary condition that occurs as a result of a less serious primary infection. A small percentage of patients with strepto-

Continued

CERTIFICATION REVIEW—cont'd

coccal pharyngitis develop rheumatic fever; rheumatic fever is considered a poststreptococcal sequela.

❏ **A sensitivity test** determines the best antibiotic to treat a condition caused by a pathogenic bacterium. A sensitivity test must be performed on a pure culture.

❏ **Microorganisms** can be examined under a microscope in the fixed state or in the living state. Examination in the fixed state involves the preparation of a smear followed by a staining process such as Gram stain. A smear consists of material spread on a slide for microscopic examination. The wet mount method is used to examine microorganisms in the living state.

❏ **Gram stain** is used to differentiate bacteria on the basis of their color reactions to various stains. Bacteria exhibiting a purple color when they are viewed under the microscope are known as *gram-positive bacteria*. Bacteria exhibiting a pink or red color are known as *gram-negative bacteria*.

TERMINOLOGY REVIEW

Medical Term	Word Parts	Definition
Bacilli (*sing.* bacillus)		Bacteria that have a rod shape.
Cocci (*sing.* coccus)	*-cocci:* berry-shaped	Bacteria that have a round shape.
Colony		A mass of bacteria growing on a solid culture medium that have arisen from the multiplication of a single bacterium.
Contagious		Capable of being transmitted directly or indirectly from one person to another.
Culture		The propagation of a mass of microorganisms in a laboratory culture medium.
Culture medium		A mixture of nutrients on which microorganisms are grown in the laboratory.
False-negative		A test result denoting that a condition is absent when it is actually present.
False-positive		A test result denoting that a condition is present when it is actually absent.
Fastidious		Extremely delicate, difficult to culture, and involving specialized growth requirements.
Immunization	*-immuno:* immune	The process of becoming protected from a disease through vaccination.
Incubate		In microbiology, the act of placing a culture in a chamber (incubator) that provides optimal growth requirements for the multiplication of the organisms, such as the proper temperature, humidity, and darkness.
Incubation period		The interval of time between the invasion by a pathogenic microorganism and the appearance of first symptoms of the disease.
Infectious disease		A disease caused by a pathogen that produces harmful effects on its host (also known as a communicable disease).
Inoculate		To introduce microorganisms into a culture medium for growth and multiplication.
Microbiology	*micro-:* small *bi/o:* life *-ology:* study of	The scientific study of microorganisms and their activities.
Mucous membrane		A membrane lining body passages or cavities that open to the outside.
Normal flora		Harmless, nonpathogenic microorganisms that normally reside in many parts of the body but do not cause disease.
Resistance		The natural ability of an organism to remain unaffected by harmful substances in its environment.
Sequela		A morbid (secondary) condition occurring as a result of a less serious primary infection.

☺ TERMINOLOGY REVIEW—cont'd

Medical Term	Word Parts	Definition
Smear		Material spread on a slide for microscopic examination.
Specimen		A small sample or part taken from the body to show the nature of the whole.
Spirilla (*sing.* spirillum)		Bacteria that have a spiral or curved shape.
Streaking		In microbiology, the process of inoculating a culture to provide for the growth of colonies on the surface of a solid medium. Streaking is accomplished by skimming a wire inoculating loop that contains the specimen across the surface of the medium, using a back-and-forth motion.
Streptolysin		An exotoxin produced by beta-hemolytic streptococci, which completely hemolyzes red blood cells.
Susceptible		Easily affected, lacking resistance.

☺ ON THE WEB

For Information on Disease and Infection Control:

American Society for Microbiology: www.asm.org

Association for Professionals in Infection Control and Epidemiology: www.apic.org

Centers for Disease Control and Prevention: www.cdc.gov

World Health Organization (WHO): www.who.int/en

Infection Control Today: www.infectioncontroltoday.com

Infectious Diseases Society of America (IDSA): www.idsociety.org

National Multiple Sclerosis Society: www.nmss.org

Cystic Fibrosis Foundation (CFF): www.cff.org

Disease Information: www.disease.com

21

Emergency Medical Procedures

LEARNING OBJECTIVES	PROCEDURES

First Aid

1. State the purpose of first aid.
2. Explain the purpose of the emergency medical services (EMS) system.
3. List the OSHA standards for administering first aid.
4. List the guidelines that should be followed when providing emergency care.

Common Emergency Situations

1. List and describe conditions that cause respiratory distress.
2. List the symptoms of a heart attack and a stroke.
3. Explain the causes of each of the following types of shock: cardiogenic, neurogenic, anaphylactic, and psychogenic.
4. Identify and describe the three classifications of external bleeding.
5. Explain the difference between an open wound and a closed wound.
6. Describe the characteristics of each of the following fractures: impacted, greenstick, transverse, oblique, comminuted, and spiral.
7. Identify the characteristics of each of the following burns: superficial, partial-thickness, and full-thickness.
8. Explain the difference between a partial seizure and a generalized seizure.
9. List examples of each of the following types of poisoning: ingested, inhaled, absorbed, and injected.
10. Identify factors that place an individual at higher risk for developing heat-related and cold-related injuries.
11. Describe the differences between type 1 and type 2 diabetes mellitus.
12. Explain the causes of insulin shock and diabetic coma.
13. Identify the symptoms and describe emergency care for each of the following conditions: respiratory distress, heart attack, stroke, shock, bleeding, wounds, musculoskeletal injuries, burns, seizures, poisoning, heat and cold exposure, and diabetic emergencies.

Respond to common emergency situations.

CHAPTER OUTLINE

Introduction to Emergency Medical Procedures
Office Crash Cart
Emergency Medical Services System
First Aid Kit
OSHA Safety Precautions
Guidelines for Providing Emergency Care
  Respiratory Distress
  Emphysema
  Hyperventilation
  Heart Attack

Stroke
Shock
Bleeding
Wounds
Musculoskeletal Injuries
Burns
Seizures
Poisoning
Heat and Cold Exposure
Diabetic Emergencies

burn
crash cart
crepitus (KREP-it-us)
dislocation
emergency medical services (EMS) system
first aid
fracture (FRAK-shur)
hypothermia (hie-poe-THER-mee-ah)

poison
pressure point
seizure (SEE-zhur)
shock
splint
sprain
strain
wound

Introduction to Emergency Medical Procedures

Medical emergencies often arise inside and outside of the workplace that can result in sudden loss of life or permanent disability. If an emergency situation occurs in the medical office, the physician provides immediate medical care for the patient. Some medical offices maintain a crash cart for this purpose. In these situations, the medical assistant may be required to assist the physician in providing emergency medical care.

The medical assistant may need to administer first aid for medical emergencies that occur outside of the medical office environment. **First aid** is defined as the immediate care administered before complete medical care can be obtained to an individual who is injured or suddenly becomes ill. The medical assistant is most likely to administer first aid to a family member or friend. The purposes of first aid are to save a life, reduce pain and suffering, prevent further injury, reduce the incidence of permanent disability, and increase the opportunity for an early recovery.

This chapter focuses on common emergency situations that the medical assistant may encounter and the first aid required for each. It is not intended, however, as a substitute for thorough first aid instruction through the American Red Cross, National Safety Council, or American Heart Association.

OFFICE CRASH CART

A **crash cart** is a specially equipped cart for holding and transporting medications, equipment, and supplies needed to perform lifesaving procedures in an emergency. A growing number of physicians are incorporating crash carts into their medical offices. Patients who are injured or suddenly become ill might be brought to the medical office for emergency medical care. In addition, a patient might develop a sudden illness at the medical office that requires emergency medical care. Examples of these situations include life-threatening cardiac dysrhythmias, shock, cardiac arrest, poisoning, and traumatic injury.

The items on an office crash cart vary widely among medical offices depending on the extent of the emergency medical care that is likely to be administered. This is directly related to the time it takes for emergency medical personnel to arrive and the location of the nearest hospital. Table 21-1 is a general list of the medications, equipment, and supplies that may be included on an office crash cart. The medical assistant may be responsible for regularly checking the crash cart to replenish supplies and to check the expiration dates on medications.

EMERGENCY MEDICAL SERVICES SYSTEM

The **emergency medical services (EMS) system** is a network of community resources, equipment, and emergency medical technicians (EMTs) that provides emergency care to victims of injury or sudden illness. An *EMT* is a professional provider of prehospital emergency care, which includes care at the scene and during transportation to the hospital. An EMT-basic (EMT-B) has received formal training and is certified to provide basic life support measures. An *EMT-paramedic* (EMT-P) is qualified to provide advanced life support care, including advanced airway maintenance, starting intravenous drips, administration of medication, cardiac monitoring and interpretation, and cardiac defibrillation.

Activating EMS is often the most important step in an emergency. Rapid arrival of EMTs increases the patient's chances of surviving a life-threatening emergency. In most urban and in some rural areas in the United States, the medical assistant can activate the local EMS by dialing 911 on the telephone. Other areas have a local seven-digit number, in which case it is important to keep the number at hand.

When calling local EMS, the medical assistant speaks with an *emergency medical dispatcher* (EMD). An EMD has had formal training in handling emergency situations over the phone. The responsibility of the EMD is to answer the emergency call, listen to the caller, obtain critical information, determine what help is needed, and send the appropriate personnel and equipment. The EMD also is responsible for relaying instructions to the caller about providing emergency care until the EMTs arrive.

Table 21-1 Office Crash Cart

Name	Drug Category	Emergency Use
Medications Used in Cardiovascular Emergencies		
Epinephrine (Adrenalin)	Sympathomimetic*	Helps restore cardiac rhythm in cardiac arrest
Sodium bicarbonate	Alkalinizing agent	To correct metabolic acidosis after cardiac arrest
Lidocaine (Xylocaine)	Antiarrhythmic	For rapid control of acute ventricular arrhythmias after myocardial infarction
Bretylium tosylate	Antiarrhythmic	For treatment of ventricular fibrillation or ventricular tachycardia that fails to respond to lidocaine
Procainamide (Pronestyl)	Antiarrhythmic	Alternative drug when lidocaine fails to suppress ventricular arrhythmias
Atropine	Parasympatholytic†	For treating bradycardia associated with hypotension
Isoproterenol (Isuprel)	Sympathomimetic	To increase heart rate in bradycardia that fails to respond to atropine
Dopamine (Intropin)	Sympathomimetic	For treatment of hypotension associated with cardiogenic shock
Dobutamine (Dobutrex)	Sympathomimetic	To manage congestive heart failure when increase in heart rate is not desired
Nitroprusside (Nitropress)	Antihypertensive-vasodilator	For immediate reduction of blood pressure in hypertensive crisis and cardiogenic shock
Norepinephrine (Levophed)	Sympathomimetic	To increase blood pressure in cardiogenic shock and other hypotensive emergencies
Adenosine (Adenocard)	Antiarrhythmic	To manage complex paroxysmal supraventricular tachycardia
Verapamil (Calan, Isoptin)	Antiarrhythmic	For treatment of supraventricular tachycardia that fails to respond to adenosine
Furosemide (Lasix)	Diuretic	For treatment of congestive heart failure and acute pulmonary edema
Nitroglycerin (Nitrostat)	Coronary vasodilator	For treatment of chest pain associated with angina pectoris and acute myocardial infarction
Intravenous Solutions		
5% Dextrose (D5W)	Glucose	Solution of 5% glucose in water used to replace fluid and nutrients
Isotonic saline	Electrolyte	Solution of sodium chloride in purified water used to replace lost fluid, sodium, and chloride
Lactated Ringer's solution	Electrolyte	Sterile solution of sodium chloride, potassium chloride, and calcium chloride in purified waters, used to replace fluids and electrolytes
Medications Used in Breathing Emergencies		
Epinephrine (Adrenalin)	Sympathomimetic	For symptomatic relief in acute attacks of bronchial asthma or bronchospasm associated with chronic bronchitis and emphysema
Terbutaline (Brethine)	Sympathomimetic	For symptomatic relief of bronchial asthma and reversible bronchospasm associated with bronchitis and emphysema
Aminophylline	Bronchodilator	For symptomatic relief in acute attacks of bronchial asthma or reversible bronchospasm associated with chronic bronchitis and emphysema
Albuterol (Proventil, Ventolin)	Sympathomimetic	For symptomatic relief of bronchial asthma and reversible bronchospasm associated with chronic bronchitis and emphysema
Medications Used in Anaphylactic Reactions		
Epinephrine (Adrenalin)	Sympathomimetic	For treatment of hypersensitivity reactions caused by medications, allergens, or insect stings
Diphenhydramine (Benadryl)	Antihistamine	To counteract histamine in treatment of hypersensitivity reactions
Methylprednisolone (Solu-Medrol)	Glucocorticoid	
Medications Used for Poisoning		
Ipecac syrup	Emetic	To induce vomiting of ingested poisons
Activated charcoal	Antidote, adsorbent	Used as general purpose antidote to adsorb swallowed poisons; to decrease absorption of poison or drug by binding with any unabsorbed drug from digestive tract
Naloxone (Narcan)	Narcotic antagonist	For treatment of overdoses caused by narcotics or synthetic narcotic agents

*A drug that stimulates the sympathetic nervous system; also called an *adrenergic*.
†A drug that inhibits the action of the parasympathetic nervous system; also called an *anticholinergic*.

Name	Drug Category	Emergency Use
Table 21-1 Office Crash Cart—cont'd		
Medications Used in Neurologic Emergencies		
Diazepam (Valium)	Anticonvulsant, antianxiety	For treatment of convulsions in major motor seizures, status epilepticus, and acute anxiety states
Phenytoin (Dilantin)	Anticonvulsant	For controlling status epilepticus; for management of generalized tonic-clonic seizures, complex partial seizures, and critical focal seizures
Phenobarbital	Anticonvulsant, sedative-hypnotic	For management of generalized tonic-clonic seizures and partial seizures, and in the control of acute convulsive episodes (status epilepticus, febrile seizures)
Medications Used in Metabolic Emergencies		
Glucose (e.g., orange juice)	Glucose	To provide glucose for conscious patients with hypoglycemia
50% Dextrose	Glucose	To provide glucose for unconscious patients with hypoglycemia

Equipment and Supplies

Cardiac Equipment
Defibrillator
Defibrillator pads

Intravenous Equipment
Tourniquet
Surgical tape
IV catheters
IV cannulas
IV tubing and needles
Armboard
IV cut-down tray

Surgical Equipment
Scalpel
Curved and straight hemostats
Needle holder
Tissue forceps
Small scissors
Local anesthetic
Gauze squares

Airway Equipment
Suction equipment
Suction pumps
Suction tubing
Suction catheters
Oral and nasal airways
Oxygen equipment
Oxygen
Oxygen face mask
Nasal cannula
Oxygen tubing
Laryngoscope handle and blades
Endotracheal tubes
Lubricant

Miscellaneous Supplies
Sterile gloves
Clean gloves
Biohazard containers
Syringes (assorted sizes)
Needles (assorted sizes)
Filter needles
Tubex syringe
Alcohol swabs
Betadine (povidone-iodine) swabs
Sterile dressings
Roller gauze (various widths)
Adhesive tape
Adhesive strip bandages
Bandage scissors
Local anesthetic (lidocaine [Xylocaine])
Lidocaine ointment
Lidocaine spray
Lubricant
Tongue blades
Flashlight
Cold packs
Sphygmomanometer
Stethoscope

These guidelines should be followed when calling EMS:
- Speak clearly and calmly to the EMD. Identify the problem as accurately and concisely as possible so that proper equipment and personnel can be sent. The EMD needs to know the number of victims, the condition of the victim or victims, and the emergency care that has already been administered.
- The EMD will ask you for your phone number and address. In responding, relay to the dispatcher the exact location of the victim, including the correct street name and house number and (if applicable) the building name, floor, and room number. With the 911 enhanced emergency system, the address automatically appears on a monitor; however, there is a chance that the address will not show up on the monitor. In addition, the emergency may not be happening in the same location as the caller. If possible, have someone meet the ambulance personnel and direct them to the scene.
- Do not hang up until the EMD gives you permission to do so. The dispatcher may need additional information

or may give you instructions on treating the patient until EMTs arrive.

FIRST AID KIT

The medical assistant should acquire and maintain a first aid kit. A first aid kit contains basic supplies to provide emergency care to individuals who have been injured or become suddenly ill (Figure 21-1). It is recommended that a first aid kit be kept at home and in the car.

First aid kits are available at most drug stores. It also is possible to make your own. Along with the items shown in Figure 21-1, the first aid kit should include the phone numbers of the local emergency medical service, the poison control center, and the police and fire departments. It is important to check the first aid kit regularly and replace supplies as needed.

OSHA SAFETY PRECAUTIONS

To avoid exposure to bloodborne pathogens and other potentially infectious materials, the OSHA Bloodborne Pathogens Standard presented in Chapter 2 should be followed when performing first aid. The following guidelines help reduce or eliminate the risk of infection:

1. Make sure that your first aid kit contains personal protective equipment, such as gloves, a face shield and mask, and a pocket mask.

2. Wear gloves when it is reasonably anticipated that your hands will come into contact with the following: blood and other potentially infectious materials, mucous membranes, nonintact skin, and contaminated articles or surfaces.

3. Perform all first aid procedures involving blood or other potentially infectious materials in a manner that minimizes splashing, spraying, spattering, and generation of droplets of these substances.

4. Wear protective clothing and gloves to cover cuts or other lesions of the skin.

5. Sanitize your hands as soon as possible after removing gloves.

6. Avoid touching objects that may be contaminated with blood or other potentially infectious materials.

7. If your hands or other skin surfaces come in contact with blood or other potentially infectious materials, wash the area as soon as possible with soap and water.

8. If your mucous membranes (in eyes, nose, and mouth) come in contact with blood or other potentially infectious materials, flush them with water as soon as possible.

9. Avoid eating, drinking, and touching your mouth, eyes, and nose while providing emergency care or before you sanitize your hands.

10. If you are exposed to blood or other potentially infectious materials, report the incident as soon as possible to your physician so that postexposure procedures can be instituted.

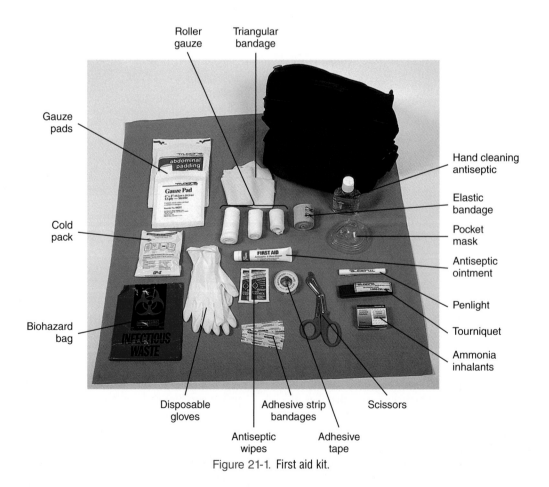

Figure 21-1. First aid kit.

GUIDELINES FOR PROVIDING EMERGENCY CARE

The remainder of this chapter presents specific emergency situations that may be encountered by the medical assistant and the emergency care required for each. These guidelines should be followed when providing emergency care:

1. Remain calm, and speak in a normal tone of voice. These measures help calm and reassure the patient.

2. Make sure that the scene is safe before approaching the patient. It is important that you protect yourself from harm in an emergency situation.

3. Before administering emergency care to a conscious patient, you must first have permission or consent. To obtain consent, you must inform the patient who you are, your level of training, and what you are going to do to help. *Never* administer care to a conscious patient who refuses it. When a life-threatening condition exists, and the patient is unconscious or otherwise unable to give consent, consent is assumed or implied. Under law, it is implied that if the patient could give consent to care, he or she would.

4. Follow the OSHA standards when providing emergency care to reduce or eliminate exposure to bloodborne pathogens or other potentially infectious materials.

5. Know how to activate your local EMS system. Activating the EMS is often the most important step you can take to help a patient who has experienced an injury or sudden illness.

6. Do not move the patient unnecessarily. Unnecessary movement can result in further injury or can be life-threatening to a patient with a serious condition.

7. Obtain information as to what happened from the patient, family members, coworkers, or bystanders.

8. Look for a medical alert tag on the patient's wrist or neck. A medical alert tag provides information on a medical condition the patient may have.

9. Continue caring for the patient until more highly trained personnel arrive. On the arrival of emergency medical personnel or a physician, relay the condition in which you found the patient and the emergency care that has been administered.

Respiratory Distress

Respiratory distress indicates that the patient is breathing but is having great difficulty in doing so. Respiratory distress sometimes may lead to respiratory arrest. It is important that the medical assistant be alert for the signs and symptoms of respiratory distress, which may include noisy breathing, such as gasping for air or rasping, gurgling, or whistling sounds; breathing that is unusually fast or slow; and breathing that is painful. The general care for respiratory distress is to place the patient in a comfortable position that facilitates breathing. Most patients prefer a sitting or semireclining position. Remain calm, and reassure the patient to help reduce anxiety. Calming the patient may help the patient breathe easier. If the patient's condition worsens or does not resolve within a few minutes, activate the local EMS. Examples of conditions that frequently cause respiratory distress are described next.

Asthma

Asthma is a condition characterized by wheezing, coughing, and dyspnea. During an asthmatic attack, the bronchioles constrict and become clogged with mucus, which accounts for many of the symptoms of asthma.

Asthma may occur at any age, but it is more common in children and young adults. If the condition is not treated, it can lead to serious complications, such as permanent lung damage. It is frequently, but not always, associated with a family history of allergies. Any of the common allergens, such as house dust, pollens, molds, or animal danders, may trigger an asthmatic attack. Asthmatic attacks also may be caused by nonspecific factors, such as air pollutants, tobacco smoke, chemical fumes, vigorous exercise, respiratory infections, exposure to cold, and emotional stress. Normally, an individual with asthma easily controls attacks with medications. These medications stop the muscle spasms and open the airway, making breathing easier.

Some patients may develop a severe prolonged asthmatic attack that is life-threatening, which is known as *status asthmaticus*. These patients can move only a small amount of air. Because so little air is being moved, the typical breathing sounds associated with asthma may not be audible. The patient may have a bluish discoloration of the skin and extremely labored breathing. Status asthmaticus is a true emergency and requires immediate transportation of the patient to an emergency care facility by the fastest way possible.

Emphysema

Emphysema is a progressive lung disorder in which the terminal bronchioles that lead into the alveoli become plugged with mucus. Because of this problem, the alveoli become damaged, resulting in less surface area to diffuse oxygen into the blood. Eventually, this condition results in loss of elasticity of the alveoli, causing inhaled air to become trapped in the lungs. This makes breathing difficult, particularly during exhalation.

Emphysema usually develops over many years and is found most frequently in heavy smokers. It also occurs in patients with chronic bronchitis and in elderly patients whose lungs have lost their natural elasticity. Chronic emphysema is one of the major causes of death in the United States. As the lungs progressively become less efficient, breathing becomes more and more difficult. Patients with advanced cases may go into respiratory or cardiac arrest.

Hyperventilation

Hyperventilation literally means "overbreathing." Hyperventilation is a manner of breathing in which the respirations become rapid and deep, causing an individual to exhale too much carbon dioxide. Low carbon dioxide levels in the body account for many of the symptoms of hyperventilation. Hyperventilation is often the result of fear or anxiety and is more likely to occur in individuals who are tense and nervous. It also is caused by serious organic conditions, such as diabetic coma, pneumonia, pulmonary edema, pulmonary embolism, head injury, high fever, and aspirin poisoning.

In addition to rapid and deep respirations, the signs and symptoms of hyperventilation include dizziness, faintness, and light-headedness; visual disturbances; chest pain; tachycardia; palpitations; fullness in the throat; and numbness and tingling of the fingers, toes, and the area around the mouth. Despite their rapid breathing efforts, patients complain that they cannot get enough air. They often think they are having a heart attack.

Treatment for hyperventilation caused by emotional factors is as follows: Calm and reassure the patient, and encourage him or her to slow the respirations, allowing the carbon dioxide level to return to normal. In the past, breathing into a paper bag was advocated as a remedy for hyperventilation. More recent studies no longer recommend this practice because it could be harmful if an underlying medical condition exists, or if the patient is not actually hyperventilating. If the medical assistant suspects that hyperventilation has been caused by an organic problem, EMS should be activated immediately.

Heart Attack

A heart attack, also known as a *myocardial infarction* (MI), is caused by partial or complete obstruction of one or both of the coronary arteries or their branches. In most cases, the severity of the attack depends on the size of the obstructed artery and the amount of myocardial tissue nourished by that artery. If a small branch of a coronary artery is obstructed, myocardial damage and symptoms may be mild, whereas the damage is usually extensive and the symptoms intense if a coronary artery is completely blocked.

The principal symptom of a heart attack is chest pain or discomfort. Patients describe the chest pain as squeezing or crushing pressure, severe indigestion or burning, heaviness, or aching. Chest discomfort can range in severity from feel-ing only mildly uncomfortable to being intense and accompanied by a feeling of suffocation and doom. The pain is usually felt behind the sternum and may radiate to the neck, throat, or jaw, or to both shoulders and both arms. The pain associated with a heart attack is prolonged and usually is not relieved by resting or taking nitroglycerin. Other signs and symptoms of a heart attack include shortness of breath, profuse perspiration, nausea, and fainting.

If the medical assistant suspects that the patient is having a heart attack, EMS should be activated immediately. Meanwhile, loosen tight clothing and have the patient rest in a comfortable position that facilitates breathing. If cardiac arrest occurs, the medical assistant should begin CPR immediately.

Stroke

A stroke, also called a *cerebrovascular accident* (CVA), results when an artery to the brain is blocked or ruptures, causing an interruption of blood flow to the brain. The signs and symptoms of a stroke include sudden weakness or numbness of the face, arm, or leg on one side of the body; difficulty in speaking; dimmed vision or loss of vision in one eye; double vision; dizziness; confusion; severe headache; and loss of consciousness.

If the medical assistant suspects that the patient is having a stroke, EMS should be activated immediately. Meanwhile, loosen tight clothing and have the patient rest in a comfortable position. If respiratory arrest, cardiac arrest, or both occur, begin rescue breathing cardiopulmonary resuscitation (CPR) as required.

Shock

For the body to function properly, adequate blood flow must be maintained to all of the vital organs. This is accomplished by the three important cardiovascular functions, as follows:
- Adequate pumping action of the heart
- Sufficient blood circulating in the blood vessels
- Blood vessels being able to respond to blood flow

When an individual experiences a severe injury or illness, one or more of these cardiovascular functions may be affected, which can lead to shock.

Shock is defined as the failure of the cardiovascular system to deliver enough blood to all of the body's vital organs. Shock accompanies different types of emergency situations, such as hemorrhaging, a myocardial infarction, and severe allergic reaction. The five major types of shock are categorized according to cause: hypovolemic, cardiogenic, neurogenic, anaphylactic, and psychogenic. Each type of shock is described in this section. If not treated, most types of shock become life-threatening. This is because shock is progressive—when it reaches a certain point, it becomes irreversible, and the patient's life cannot be saved.

The signs and symptoms of shock are caused by the failure of the vital organs to receive enough oxygen and nutrients. The organs most affected are the heart, brain, and lungs, which can be irreparably damaged in 4 to 6 minutes.

The general signs and symptoms of shock are weakness, restlessness, anxiety, disorientation, pallor, cold and clammy skin, rapid breathing, and rapid pulse.

If not treated, these symptoms can progress rapidly to a significant drop in blood pressure, cyanosis, loss of consciousness, and death. The signs and symptoms of shock may be subtle or pronounced. In addition, no single sign or symptom determines accurately the presence or severity of the shock. Because of this, it is crucial to consider the nature of the illness or injury in determining whether the patient is a possible victim of shock. If a patient has a traumatic injury to the abdomen, shock should be considered a possibility, even if the patient's signs and symptoms do not suggest shock.

Shock (with the exception of psychogenic shock) requires immediate medical care. The medical assistant should activate EMS without delay so that proper medical care can be obtained as soon as possible.

Hypovolemic Shock

Hypovolemic shock is caused by loss of blood or other body fluids. Conditions that result in this type of shock include external and internal hemorrhaging; plasma loss from severe burns; and severe dehydration from vomiting, diarrhea, or profuse perspiration. The first priority in hypovolemic shock is to control bleeding. A patient in hypovolemic shock must have the volume of fluid that was lost replaced and must be transported to an emergency care facility immediately.

Cardiogenic Shock

Cardiogenic shock is caused by the failure of the heart to pump blood adequately to all of the body's vital organs. This type of shock occurs when the heart has been injured or damaged. Cardiogenic shock is most frequently seen with myocardial infarction. Other causes include dysrhythmias, severe congestive heart failure, acute valvular damage, and pulmonary embolism. When a patient develops cardiogenic shock, it is difficult to reverse and has a high fatality rate (80% to 90%).

Neurogenic Shock

Neurogenic shock occurs when the nervous system is unable to control the diameter of the blood vessels. In normal situations, the nervous system instructs the blood vessels to constrict or dilate, which controls blood pressure. In neurogenic shock, that control is lost, and the blood vessels dilate, causing the blood to pool in peripheral areas of the body away from vital organs.

This type of shock is most often seen with brain and spinal injuries. The blood vessels become dilated, and not enough blood is present in the circulatory system to fill the dilated vessels, which causes the blood pressure to drop significantly.

Anaphylactic Shock

Anaphylactic shock is a life-threatening reaction of the body to a substance to which an individual is highly allergic. Allergens that are most apt to result in anaphylaxis are drugs (e.g., penicillin), insect venoms, foods, and allergen extracts used in hyposensitization injections.

An anaphylactic reaction causes the release of large amounts of histamine, resulting in dilation of the blood vessels throughout the entire body and a decrease in blood pressure. The symptoms of anaphylactic shock begin with sneezing, hives, itching, angioedema, erythema, and disorientation and progress to difficulty in breathing, dizziness, fainting, and loss of consciousness. Medical care should be obtained immediately because most fatalities occur within the first 2 hours.

The emergency care for anaphylactic shock is the administration of epinephrine. Because time is a factor, individuals known to have a severe allergy carry an anaphylactic emergency treatment kit that contains injectable epinephrine (Figure 21-2) and oral antihistamines. With the kit, treatment for a severe allergic reaction can be started immediately.

Psychogenic Shock

Psychogenic shock is the least serious type of shock. It is caused by unpleasant physical or emotional stimuli, such as pain, fright, and the sight of blood. With psychogenic shock, sudden dilation of the blood vessels causes blood to pool in the abdomen and extremities. This temporarily deprives the brain of blood, causing a temporary loss of consciousness (fainting), usually lasting 1 to 2 minutes. Fainting generally occurs when an individual is in an upright position. Before fainting, the patient usually experiences some warning signals such as sudden light-headedness, pallor, nausea, weakness, yawning, blurred vision, a feeling of warmth, and sweating.

An individual who is about to faint should be placed in a position that facilitates blood flow to the brain and told to breathe deeply. The preferred position is to move the patient into a supine position with the legs elevated approximately 12 inches and the collar and clothing loosened (Figure 21-3). This position is not always possible, such as when a patient is seated; in this case, the patient's head should be lowered between the legs (Figure 21-4). A patient who has fainted should be placed in the supine position with the legs elevated. It is recommended that a patient who has fainted should contact her or his physician for further evaluation.

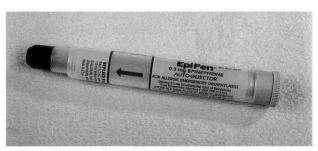

Figure 21-2. Anaphylactic emergency epinephrine injector.

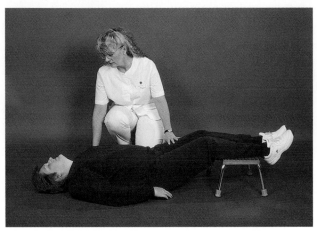

Figure 21-3. Prevention and treatment of fainting.

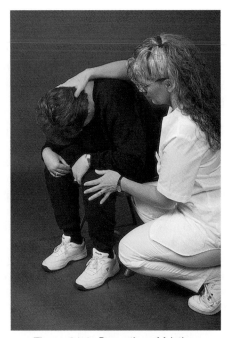

Figure 21-4. Prevention of fainting.

Bleeding

Bleeding, or hemorrhaging, is the escape of blood from a severed blood vessel. Bleeding can range from very minor to very serious, leading to shock and death. The amount of blood that can be lost before bleeding becomes life-threatening varies according to each individual. In general, loss of 25% to 40% of an individual's total blood volume can be fatal. This equates to approximately 2 to 4 pints of blood for the average adult.

External Bleeding

External bleeding is bleeding that can be seen coming from a wound. Common examples of external bleeding include bleeding from open fractures, lacerations, and the nose. Individuals with serious external bleeding exhibit the following symptoms: obvious bleeding, restlessness, cold and clammy skin, thirst, increased and thready pulse, rapid and shallow respirations, a drop in blood pressure (a late symptom), and decreasing levels of consciousness. Three types of external bleeding can be classified according to the type of blood vessel that has been injured: capillary, venous, and arterial.

Capillary Bleeding

Capillary bleeding, the most common type of external bleeding, consists of a slow oozing of bright red blood. This type of bleeding occurs with minor cuts, scratches, and abrasions.

Venous Bleeding

Venous bleeding occurs when a vein has been punctured or severed. This type of bleeding is characterized by a slow and steady flow of dark red blood.

Arterial Bleeding

Arterial bleeding, the most serious type of external bleeding, occurs when an artery is punctured or severed. It is the least common type of bleeding because arteries are situated deeper in the body and are protected by bone. Arterial bleeding is characterized by bright red blood that spurts. The arteries most frequently involved in accidents are the carotid, brachial, radial, and femoral arteries.

Emergency Care for External Bleeding

The most effective way to control bleeding is to apply direct pressure to the bleeding site. The pressure functions by slowing down or stopping the flow of blood. The amount of pressure required depends on the type of bleeding. A small amount of pressure is usually sufficient to control capillary bleeding, whereas significant pressure is often required to control arterial bleeding.

If bleeding cannot be controlled with direct pressure, a pressure point can be used. A **pressure point** is a site on the body where an artery lies close to the surface of the skin and can be compressed against an underlying bone. Figure 21-5 illustrates pressure points. Using a pressure point helps slow or stop the flow of blood from the wound. The pressure points used most often are found on the brachial and femoral arteries. The brachial artery is located on the inside of the upper arm midway between the elbow and the shoulder. Squeezing the brachial artery helps control severe bleeding in the arm. The femoral artery is located in the groin, and squeezing helps control severe bleeding in the leg.

The specific steps for controlling bleeding are as follows:
1. Apply direct pressure to the wound with a clean covering such as a large, thick gauze dressing (Figure 21-6, *A*). If gauze is unavailable, a clean material such as a sanitary napkin, washcloth, handkerchief, or sock can be used. If the wound is located on an extremity, elevate the limb while continuing to apply direct pressure.
2. Apply additional dressings if needed. If the dressing soaks through, apply another dressing over the first one, and continue to apply pressure (Figure 21-6, *B*). (Never remove a dressing after it has been applied because this could result in more bleeding.) If bleeding cannot be

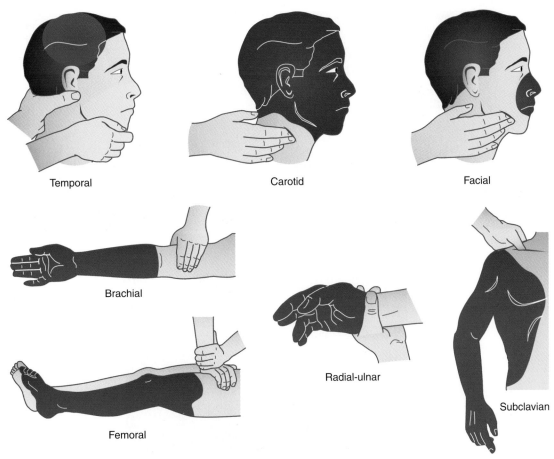

Temporal

Carotid

Facial

Brachial

Radial-ulnar

Femoral

Subclavian

Figure 21-5. Locations of pressure points. *Shaded areas* show the regions in which bleeding may be controlled by pressure at the points indicated. (From Miller BF, Keane CB: Encyclopedia and dictionary of medicine, nursing, and allied health, ed 7, Philadelphia, 2003, Saunders.)

controlled with direct pressure, apply pressure to the appropriate pressure point while continuing to apply direct local pressure.
3. Apply a pressure bandage. When bleeding has been controlled, apply a bandage snugly over the dressing to maintain pressure on the wound (Figure 21-6, *C*).
4. Transport the patient to an emergency care facility, or, if the case is serious enough, activate the local emergency medical services.

Nosebleeds

A nosebleed, or epistaxis, is a common form of external bleeding that usually is not serious but is more of a nuisance. Nosebleeds are usually caused by an upper respiratory infection but can result from a direct blow from a blunt object, hypertension, strenuous activity, and exposure to high altitudes.

Emergency Care for a Nosebleed
1. Position the patient in a sitting position with the head tilted forward. This prevents the blood from running down the back of the throat, which may result in nausea.
2. Apply direct pressure by pinching the nostrils together (Figure 21-7, *A*). Do not release the pressure too soon because the bleeding may resume. Adequate clot forma-

tion usually takes about 15 minutes. An ice pack can be applied to the bridge of the nose to help control the bleeding (Figure 21-7, *B*). If these measures do not control the bleeding, apply pressure on the upper lip, just below the nose.

Putting It All into Practice

My Name is Judy Markins, and I work at a large clinic in the family medicine department with 12 physicians. We also have 6 to 10 physicians who do their internships and residency programs with us.

One day as I was performing my usual morning duties of getting the office ready for that day's patients, the office door opened. There stood a mother with her very ill child. I immediately took them back to a room. When I took the boy's temperature, it was 104° F. I asked the mother if she had been giving him any type of fever reducer. She said she had, but that it was not helping. Under the direction of our physician, I immediately started trying to reduce the fever. The fever started to come down, and the look of relief on the mother's face was beyond words. That was one of the many days that reinforced how satisfied I am with my career choice. ■

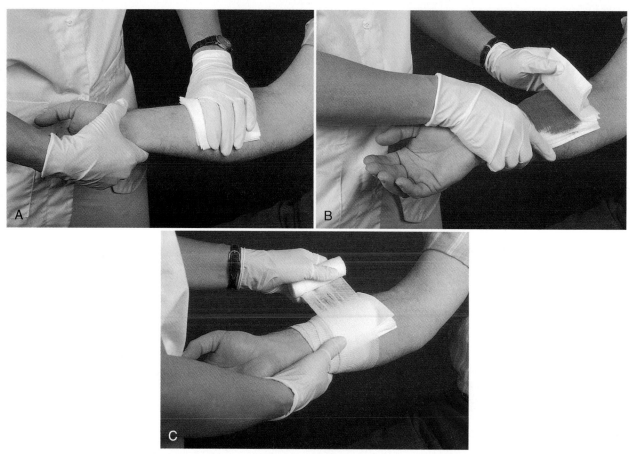

Figure 21-6. Control of bleeding. **A,** Apply direct pressure to the wound with a large, thick gauze dressing. **B,** If blood soaks through the dressing, apply another dressing over the first one, and continue to apply pressure. **C,** When bleeding has been controlled, apply a pressure bandage.

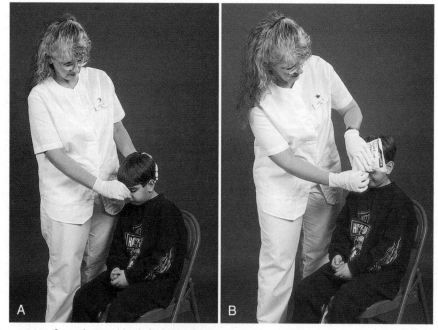

Figure 21-7. Care of a nosebleed. **A,** Apply direct pressure by pinching the nostrils together. **B,** An ice pack can be applied to the bridge of the nose to help control the bleeding.

3. After the bleeding has stopped, tell the patient not to blow the nose for several hours because this could loosen the clot, causing the bleeding to start again.
4. If bleeding cannot be controlled, transport the patient to an emergency care facility for further treatment.

Internal Bleeding

Internal bleeding is bleeding that flows into a body cavity or an organ, or between tissues. It may be minor, as in the case of a contusion, or it may be very serious, such as with a severe, blunt blow to the abdomen.

Severe internal bleeding is a life-threatening emergency. Because no obvious blood flow occurs, the nature of the injury and the signs and symptoms of bleeding must be used to recognize internal bleeding. Signs and symptoms include bruises, pain, tenderness, or swelling at the site of the injury; rapid weak pulse; cold, clammy skin; nausea and vomiting; excessive thirst; a drop in blood pressure; and a decreased level of consciousness.

If a patient is suspected to have internal bleeding, the local EMS should be activated immediately. Until emergency medical personnel arrive, the patient should be kept quiet and treated for shock.

Wounds

A **wound** is a break in the continuity of an external or internal surface, caused by physical means. Wounds may be open or closed.

Open Wounds

An open wound is a break in the skin surface or mucous membrane that exposes the underlying tissues. Because the skin is broken, hemorrhaging and wound contamination are primary concerns with open wounds. Open wounds include incisions, lacerations, punctures, and abrasions (Figure 21-8). An individual with an open wound should receive prompt medical attention by a physician if any of the following occur: spurting blood; bleeding that cannot be controlled; a break in the skin that is deeper than just the outer skin layers; embedded debris or an embedded object in the wound; involvement of nerves, muscles, or tendons; and occurrence on the mouth, tongue, face, genitals, or other area where scarring would be apparent.

Incisions and Lacerations

An incision is a clean, smooth cut caused by a sharp cutting instrument, such as a knife, a razor, or a piece of glass. Deep incisions are accompanied by profuse bleeding; in addition, damage to muscles, tendons, and nerves may occur. Because the edges of the wound are smooth and straight, incisions usually heal better than lacerations.

A laceration is a wound in which the tissues are torn apart, rather than cut, leaving ragged and irregular edges. Lacerations are caused by dull knives, large objects that have been driven into the skin, and heavy machinery. Deep lacerations result in profuse bleeding, and a scar often results from jagged tearing of the tissues.

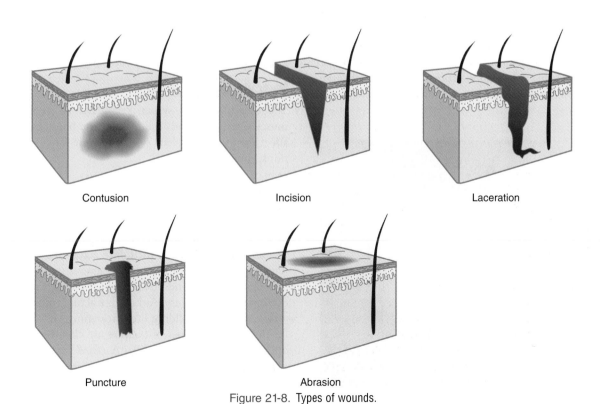

Contusion   Incision   Laceration

Puncture   Abrasion

Figure 21-8. Types of wounds.

Emergency Care for Incisions and Lacerations

Minor Incisions and Lacerations

1. Assess the length, depth, and location of the wound.
2. Control bleeding by covering the wound with a dressing and applying firm pressure.
3. Clean the wound with soap and water to remove dirt and other debris (Figure 21-9).
4. Cover the wound with a dry, sterile dressing. Instruct the patient to check the wound for redness, swelling, discharge, or an increase in pain, and to contact a physician if any of these problems occur.

Serious Incisions and Lacerations

1. Control bleeding by covering the wound with a large, thick gauze dressing and applying firm pressure. Do not clean or probe the wound because this may result in more bleeding.
2. Transport the individual to a physician, or, if the wound is serious enough, activate the local EMS.

Punctures

A puncture is a wound made by a sharp, pointed object piercing the skin layers and sometimes the underlying structures. Objects that cause a puncture wound include a nail, splinter, needle, wire, knife, bullet, and animal bite. A puncture wound has a very small external skin opening, and for this reason bleeding is usually minor. A tetanus booster may be administered because the tetanus bacteria grow best in a warm, anaerobic environment, as would be found in a puncture wound.

Emergency Care for Puncture Wounds

1. Allow the wound to bleed freely for a few minutes to help wash out bacteria.
2. Clean the wound with soap and water.
3. Apply a dry, sterile dressing to prevent contamination.
4. Transport the individual to a physician so that medical care can be provided to prevent infection and to ensure that the patient's tetanus toxoid immunization is up to date.

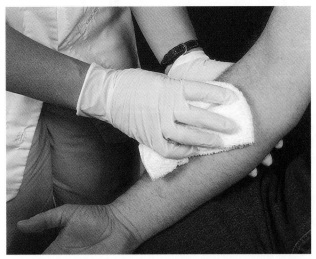

Figure 21-9. Minor incisions and lacerations should be cleaned with soap and water to remove dirt and other debris.

Abrasions

An abrasion, or scrape, is a wound in which the outer layers of the skin are scraped or rubbed off. Blood may ooze from ruptured capillaries; however, the bleeding usually is not severe. Abrasions are caused by falls, resulting in floor burns and skinned knees and elbows. Dirt and other debris are frequently rubbed into the wound; it is important to clean scrapes thoroughly to prevent infection.

Emergency Care for Abrasions

1. Rinse the wound with cold running water.
2. Wash the wound gently with soap and water to remove dirt and other debris. A physician should remove embedded debris.
3. Cover large abrasions with a dry, sterile dressing. Small minor abrasions do not require a dressing.
4. Instruct the patient to check the wound for signs of inflammation, including redness, swelling, discharge, or increased pain, and to contact a physician if they occur.

Closed Wounds

A closed wound involves an injury to the underlying tissues of the body without a break in the skin surface or mucous membrane; an example is a contusion or a bruise. A contusion results when the tissues under the skin are injured (see Figure 21-8); it is often caused by a sudden blow or force from a blunt object. Blood vessels rupture, allowing blood to seep into the tissues, which results in a bluish discoloration of the skin and swelling. Most contusions heal without special treatment, but cold compresses may reduce bleeding, reduce swelling and discoloration, and relieve pain. After several days, the color of the contusion turns greenish or yellow, owing to oxidation of blood pigments. Contusions commonly occur with injuries such as fractures, sprains, strains, and black eyes. These injuries, along with the corresponding emergency care, are discussed next.

Musculoskeletal Injuries

The musculoskeletal system comprises all of the bones, muscles, tendons, and ligaments of the body. Injuries that affect the musculoskeletal system include fractures, dislocations, sprains, and strains.

Fracture

A **fracture** is any break in a bone. The break may range in severity from a simple chip or a crack to a complete break or shattering of the bone. Fractures can occur anywhere on the surface of the bone, including across the surface of a joint such as the wrist or ankle. Fractures result from a direct blow, a fall, bone disease, or a twisting force as may occur in a sports injury. Although fractures often cause severe pain, they are seldom life-threatening.

The two basic types of fracture are closed fractures and open fractures (Figure 21-10). A *closed fracture,* the most common type, occurs when there is a break in a bone but no break in the skin over the fracture site. An *open fracture* involves a break in the bone along with penetration of the overlying skin surface. Open fractures are more serious ow-

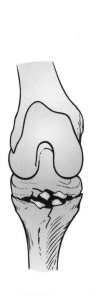
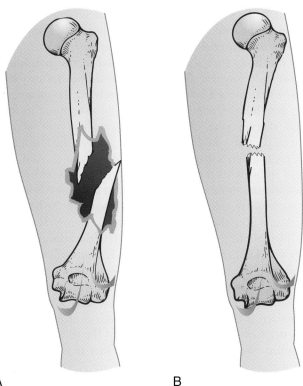

A   B

Figure 21-10. Fractures. **A,** Open fracture. **B,** Closed fracture. (From Connolly JF: DePalma's the management of fractures and dislocations: an atlas, Philadelphia, 1981, Saunders.)

ing to the risk of blood loss and contamination leading to infection.

The signs and symptoms of a fracture include pain and tenderness, deformity, swelling and discoloration, loss of function of the body part, and numbness or tingling. The patient usually guards the injured part and may relay to you that he or she heard the bone break or snap or felt a grating sensation. This grating sensation, known as **crepitus,** is caused by the bone fragments rubbing against each other.

Fractures also can be classified according to the nature of the break: impacted, greenstick, transverse, oblique, comminuted, and spiral. Figure 21-11 illustrates and describes these types of fracture.

Dislocation

A **dislocation** is an injury in which one end of a bone making up a joint is separated or displaced from its normal position. A dislocation is caused by a violent pulling or pushing force that tears the ligaments. Dislocations usually result from falls, sports injuries, and motor vehicle accidents. Signs and symptoms of a dislocation include significant deformity of the joint, pain and swelling, and loss of function.

Sprain

A **sprain** is the tearing of ligaments at a joint. Sprains may result from a fall, a sports injury, or a motor vehicle accident. The joints most often sprained are the ankle, knee,

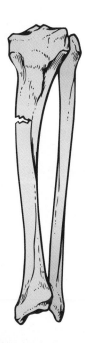
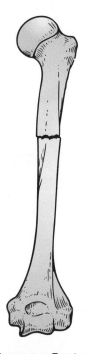
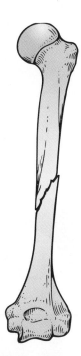
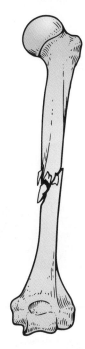
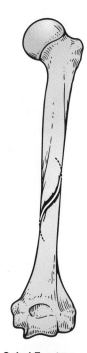

Impacted Fracture
The broken ends of the bones are forcefully jammed together.

Greenstick Fracture
The bone remains intact on one side, but broken on the other, in much the same way that a "green stick" bends; common in children, whose bones are more flexible than those of adults.

Transverse Fracture
The break occurs perpendicular to the long axis of the bone.

Oblique Fracture
The break occurs diagonally across the bone; generally the result of a twisting force.

Comminuted Fracture
The bone is splintered or shattered into three or more fragments; usually caused by an extremely traumatic direct force.

Spiral Fracture
The bone is broken into a spiral or S-shape; caused by a twisting force.

Figure 21-11. Types of fractures.

wrist, and fingers. Signs and symptoms of a sprain include pain, swelling, and discoloration. Sprains can vary in seriousness from mild to severe, depending on the amount of damage to the ligaments.

Strain

A **strain** is the stretching and tearing of muscles or tendons. Strains are most likely to occur when an individual lifts a heavy object or overworks a muscle, as during exercise. The muscles most commonly strained are those of the neck, back, thigh, and calf. Signs and symptoms of a strain are pain and swelling. Strains do not usually cause the intense symptoms associated with fractures, dislocations, and sprains.

Emergency Care for a Fracture

It is often difficult to determine whether a patient has a fracture, a dislocation, or a sprain because the symptoms of these injuries are similar. Because of this, any serious musculoskeletal injury to an extremity should be treated as though it were a fracture.

The primary goal of emergency care for a fracture is to immobilize the body part. Immobilization reduces pain and prevents further damage. A **splint** is any item that immobilizes a body part. In an emergency situation, items such as a length of wood, cardboard, or rolled newspapers or magazines can be used for splinting. The splint should be padded with a soft material such as a rolled-up towel.

The body part should be splinted in the position in which you found it. Severely angulated fractures may have to be straightened before splinting, however. If you attempt to straighten an angulated fracture, be careful not to force the affected part. A dislocated bone end can become "locked" and would have to be realigned at the hospital. If you straighten an angulated bone and encounter pain, stop and splint it in the position in which you found it. The splint also should immobilize the area above and below the injury. When splinting an injury to the wrist, the hand and forearm also should be immobilized (Figure 21-12, *A*). When splinting an injury to the shaft of the bone, the joints above and below the injury should be immobilized. When splinting the forearm, the elbow joint and the wrist joint should be immobilized.

The splint should be held in place with a roller gauze bandage or other suitable material, such as neckties, scarves, or strips of cloth (Figure 21-12, *B*). The splint should be applied snugly, but not so tightly that it interferes with proper circulation. After applying the splint, check the pulse below the splint to ensure the splint has not been applied too

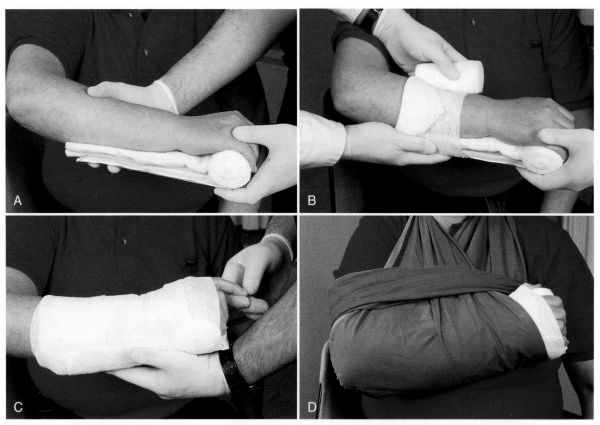

Figure 21-12. Emergency care of a fracture. **A,** The splint should immobilize the area above and below the injury. **B,** The splint is held in place with a roller gauze bandage. **C,** After the splint is applied, the pulse below the splint should be checked to ensure that the splint has not been applied too tightly. **D,** A sling can be used to elevate the extremity to reduce swelling. (From Henry M, Stapleton E: EMT prehospital care, ed 2, Philadelphia, 1997, Saunders.)

tightly. If you cannot detect a pulse, immediately loosen the splint until you can feel the pulse (Figure 21-12, *C*).

Whenever possible, elevate an injured extremity after it has been immobilized to reduce swelling (Figure 21-12, *D*). An ice pack also can be applied to the injured part. Cold limits the accumulation of fluid in the body tissues by constricting blood vessels and reducing leakage of fluid into the tissues. In addition, cold temporarily relieves pain through its anesthetic or numbing effect, which reduces stimulation of nerve receptors.

After you have properly immobilized the injury, transport the patient to an emergency care facility, or if the injury is serious enough, activate the local EMS. In any situation in which an injury to the spine is suspected, activate EMS.

Burns

A **burn** is an injury to the tissues caused by exposure to thermal, chemical, electrical, or radioactive agents. The severity of a burn depends on the depth of the burn, the percentage of the body involved, the type of agent causing the burn, the duration and intensity of the agent, and the part of the body affected. Burns are classified according to the depth of tissue injury, as illustrated in Figure 21-13.

Superficial (First-Degree) Burn

A superficial burn is the most common type of burn. It involves only the top layer of skin, the epidermis. With this type of burn, the skin appears red, is warm and dry to the touch, and is usually painful. Sunburn is a common example of a superficial burn. A superficial burn heals in 2 to 5 days of its own accord and does not cause scarring.

Partial-Thickness (Second-Degree) Burn

A partial-thickness burn involves the epidermis and extends into the dermis but does not pass through the dermis to the underlying tissues. The burned area usually appears red, mottled, and blistered. In most cases, the blisters should not be broken because they provide a protective barrier against infection. Partial-thickness burns are usually very painful, and the area often swells. This type of burn usually heals within 3 to 4 weeks and may result in some scarring.

Full-Thickness (Third-Degree) Burn

A full-thickness burn completely destroys the epidermis and the dermis and extends into the underlying tissues, such as fat, muscle, bone, and nerves. The affected area appears charred black, brown, and cherry red, with the damaged tissues underneath often pearly white. The patient

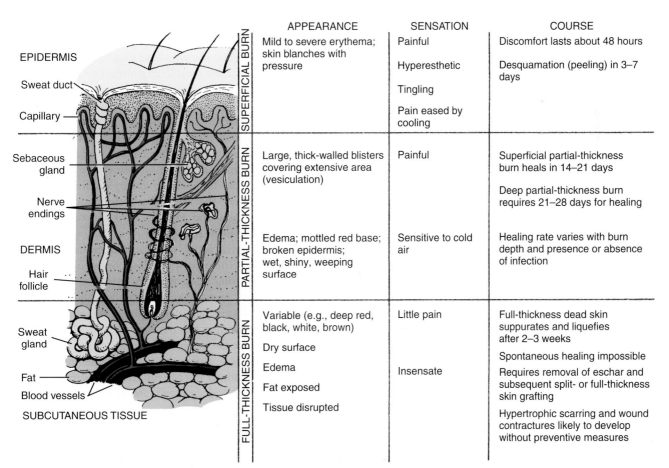

Figure 21-13. Types of burns. (From Polaski AL, Tatro SE: Luckmann's core principles and practice of medical-surgical nursing, Philadelphia, 1996, Saunders.)

may experience intense pain; however, if damage to the nerve endings is substantial, the patient may feel no pain at all. During the healing process, dense scars typically result. Infection is a major concern, and the patient must be carefully monitored.

Thermal Burns

Thermal burns usually occur in the home, often as a result of fire, scalding water, or coming into contact with a hot object such as a stove or curling iron.

Emergency Care for Major Thermal Burns

1. Stop the burning process to prevent further injury. If the individual is on fire, wrap him or her in a blanket, rug, or heavy coat and push him or her to the ground to help smother the flames. If a covering is unavailable, shout at the individual to drop to the ground and roll around to smother the flames.
2. Cool the burn, using large amounts of cool water from a faucet or garden hose. Do not use ice or ice water because this may result in further tissue damage; it also causes heat loss from the body. If the burn covers a large surface area (greater than 20%), do not use water. The loss of a large amount of skin surface places the patient at risk for hypothermia (generalized body cooling). With large surface area burns, you may cool the most painful areas, but not an area greater than 20% of the body (i.e., two arms, one leg).
3. Activate the local EMS.
4. Cover the patient with a clean, nonfuzzy material such as a tablecloth or sheet. The cover maintains warmth, reduces pain, and reduces the risk of contamination. Do not apply any type of ointment, antiseptic, or other substance to the burned area.

Emergency Care for Minor Thermal Burns

1. Immerse the affected area in cold water for 2 to 5 minutes. Be careful not to break any blisters because they provide a protective barrier against infection.
2. Cover the burn with a dry sterile dressing.

Chemical Burns

Chemical burns occur in the workplace and at home. The severity of the burn depends on the type and strength of the chemical and the duration of exposure to the chemical. The main difference between a chemical burn and a thermal burn is that the chemical continues to burn the patient's tissues as long as it is on the skin. Because of this factor, it is important to remove the chemical from the skin as quickly as possible and then to activate the local EMS.

Liquid chemical burns should be treated by flooding the area with large amounts of cool running water until emergency personnel arrive. If a solid substance such as lime has been spilled on the patient, it should be brushed off before flooding the area with water. This is because a dry chemical may be activated by contact with water.

Seizures

A **seizure** is a sudden episode of involuntary muscular contractions and relaxation, often accompanied by changes in sensation, behavior, and level of consciousness. A seizure results when the normal electrical activity of the brain is disturbed, causing the brain cells to become irritated and overactive. Specific conditions that trigger a seizure include epilepsy, encephalitis, a recent or old head injury, high fever in infants and young children, drug and alcohol abuse or withdrawal, eclampsia associated with toxemia of pregnancy, diabetic conditions, and heatstroke.

Seizures are classified as partial or generalized according to the location of the abnormal electrical activity in the brain. *Partial seizures* are the most common type, occurring in approximately 80% of individuals who have seizures. With a partial seizure, the abnormal electrical activity is localized into specific areas of the brain; only the brain functions in those areas are affected.

Partial seizures are further classified as simple or complex, depending on whether the patient's level of consciousness is affected. The symptoms of a *simple partial seizure* include twitching or jerking in just one part of the body. This type of seizure lasts less than 1 minute, and the patient remains awake and alert during the seizure. With a *complex partial seizure,* the patient's level of consciousness is affected, and the patient has little or no memory of the seizure afterward. Symptoms of this type of seizure include abnormal behavior such as confusion, a glassy stare, aimless wandering, lip smacking or chewing, and fidgeting with clothing, which lasts from a few seconds to a minute or two. A simple and a complex partial seizure can progress to a generalized seizure.

With a *generalized seizure,* the abnormal electrical activity spreads through the entire brain. The best-known type of generalized seizure is a *tonic-clonic seizure* (formerly known as a "grand mal seizure"). With this type of seizure, the patient exhibits tonic-clonic activity followed by a postictal state. During the tonic phase, the patient suddenly loses consciousness and exhibits rigid muscular contractions, which result in odd posturing of the body. Respirations are inhibited, which may cause cyanosis around the mouth and lips. The patient may lose control of the bladder or bowels, resulting in involuntary urination and defecation. The tonic phase lasts 30 seconds, followed by the clonic phase. During the clonic phase, the patient's body jerks about violently. The patient's jaw muscles contract, which may cause the patient to bite the tongue or lips. The final phase of the seizure is the postictal state, lasting 10 to 30 minutes, in which the patient exhibits a depressed level of consciousness, is disoriented, and often has a headache. The patient generally has little or no memory of the seizure and feels confused and exhausted for several hours after the seizure.

In some instances of seizures, particularly in patients with epilepsy, an aura precedes the seizure. An *aura* is a sensation perceived by the patient that something is about to happen; examples include a strange taste, smell, or sound; a twitch; or a feeling of dizziness or anxiety. An aura provides the patient with a warning signal that a seizure is about to begin.

Although seizures are frightening to observe, they usually are not as bad as they look. Most patients fully recover within a few minutes after the seizure begins. An exception to this is *status epilepticus,* in which seizures are prolonged or come in rapid succession without full recovery of consciousness between them. Status epilepticus is a potentially life-threatening situation that requires immediate medical care.

Emergency Care for Seizures

The most important criterion in caring for a patient in a seizure is to protect the patient from harm. Remove hazards from the immediate area to protect the patient from injury sustained by striking a surrounding object. Do not restrain the patient. Loosen restrictive clothing that may interfere with breathing, such as collars, neckties, scarves, and jewelry. The seizure will occur no matter what you do; restraining the patient could seriously injure the patient's muscles, bones, or joints. Do not insert anything into the patient's mouth during the seizure because this could damage the teeth or mouth or interfere with breathing. In addition, it could trigger the gag reflex, causing the patient to vomit and possibly aspirate the vomitus into the lungs. If the patient vomits, roll him or her onto one side so that the vomitus can drain from the mouth.

If you are uncertain as to the cause of the seizure, or if you suspect that the patient is having status epilepticus, activate your local EMS immediately. Otherwise, transport the patient to an emergency medical care facility for further evaluation and treatment after the seizure is over.

Poisoning

A **poison** is any substance that causes illness, injury, or death if it enters the body. Most poisoning episodes occur in the home, are accidental, and occur in children younger than 5 years of age. Poisoning usually involves common substances, such as cleaning agents, medications, and pesticides. For most poisonous substances, the reaction is more serious in children and the elderly than in adults. A poison can enter the body in four ways: ingestion, inhalation, absorption, or injection.

Poison control centers are valuable resources that are easily accessible to medical personnel and the community. More than 500 regional poison control centers have been established across the United States; most are located in the emergency departments of large hospitals. These centers are staffed by personnel who have access to information about almost all poisonous substances. Most centers are staffed 24 hours a day, and calls are toll-free. In addition, a National Poison Control Hotline number (1-800-222-1222) can be called 24 hours a day.

Memories *from* Externship

Judy Markins: As it turned out, one of my most terrible moments during my externship was a great learning experience. I was drawing blood (which was not my favorite procedure) and missed the vein—not once, but twice. You could see the sweat under my gloves. My stomach was in my throat, and I did not want to try again. Thank goodness my patient was understanding, and I had an excellent externship supervisor. She insisted that I try again, encouraging me that I could do it and suggesting some techniques that she had learned from her many years of experience. I got the blood specimen, along with some new-found confidence.

In most situations, someone can help you if you have questions. Use your resources when you need to. Be honest, know your procedure, and have confidence in yourself. ■

What Would You Do? What Would You *Not* Do?

Case Study 1
Beth Eaton calls the office. She says that she thinks her 3-year-old daughter, Olivia, has eaten some chewable vitamins. Beth was taking a shower, and when she came out, Olivia was holding an empty vitamin bottle and saying "Good candy." Beth says she does not know how Olivia got the child-proof top off. She thinks the bottle was about a third of the way full. Beth says that Olivia is complaining that her tummy hurts. Beth says she has syrup of ipecac and wants to know whether she should give some to Olivia. ■

Ingested Poisons

Poisons that are ingested enter the body by being swallowed. Ingestion is the most common route of entry for poisons. Examples of poisons that are often ingested include cleaning products, pesticides, contaminated food, petroleum products (e.g., gasoline, kerosene), and poisonous plants. Abuse of drugs, alcohol, or both also can result in poisoning from an accidental or intentional overdose. Signs and symptoms of poisoning by ingestion are based on the specific substance that has been consumed but often include strange odors, burns or stains around the mouth, nausea, vomiting, abdominal pain, diarrhea, difficulty in breathing, profuse perspiration, excessive salivation, dilated or constricted pupils, unconsciousness, and convulsions.

Emergency Care for Poisoning by Ingestion

1. Acquire as much information as possible about the type of poison, the amount ingested, and when it was ingested.
2. Call your poison control center or local EMS. *Never* induce vomiting unless directed to do so by a medical authority. Vomiting is often contraindicated—when an individual is unconscious, has swallowed a petroleum

product, or has swallowed a corrosive poison such as a strong acid or base. Corrosive poisons may cause more injury to the esophagus, throat, and mouth if they are vomited back up. If it is available, you may be directed by the poison control center to administer activated charcoal. Activated charcoal is used to absorb the poison that remains in the stomach and prevents absorption by the intestine.

3. If the individual vomits, collect some of the vomitus for transport with the patient to the hospital for analysis by a toxicologist, if necessary. In addition, bring along containers of any substances ingested, such as empty medication bottles and household cleaner containers, because the label of the container often lists the ingredients in the product.

Inhaled Poisons

A poison that is inhaled is breathed into the body in the form of gas, vapor, or spray. The most commonly inhaled poison is carbon monoxide, such as from car exhausts, malfunctioning furnaces, and fires. Other inhaled poisons include carbon dioxide from wells and sewers and fumes from household products such as glues, paints, insect sprays, and cleaners (e.g., ammonia, chlorine). Signs and symptoms of inhaled poisoning often include severe headache; nausea and vomiting; coughing or wheezing; shortness of breath; chest pain or tightness; facial burns; burning of the mouth, nose, eyes, throat, or chest; cyanosis; confusion; dizziness; and unconsciousness.

Emergency Care for Inhaled Poisons

1. Determine whether it is safe to approach the patient. Toxic gases and fumes also can be dangerous to individuals helping the patient.
2. Remove the individual from the source of the poison and into fresh air as quickly as possible.
3. Call your poison control center or local EMS.
4. If oxygen is available, you may be directed to administer it under the supervision of a physician. Oxygen is the primary antidote for carbon monoxide poisoning.

Absorbed Poisons

A poison that is absorbed enters the body through the skin. Examples of absorbed poisons include fertilizers and pesticides used for lawn and garden care. Signs and symptoms of absorbed poisoning include irritation, burning and itching, burning of the skin or eyes, headache, and abnormal pulse or respiration or both.

Emergency Care for Absorbed Poisons

1. Remove the patient from the source of the poison. Avoid contact with the toxic substance.
2. Call your poison control center or local EMS. In most cases, you will be instructed to flood the area that has been exposed to the poison with water. Dry chemicals should be brushed from the skin before flooding with water.

What Would You Do? What Would You *Not* Do?

Case Study 2

Anita Alland calls the office and says that her son, Garon, was stung by a yellow jacket about an hour ago while mowing the grass. She says that his entire arm and back are red and swollen, and that he has a lot of redness and swelling around his eyes. Garon is itching all over and seems fuzzy-headed. Anita says she has never seen anyone do this after being stung. She says she had Garon take a cold shower to see if it would help. After the shower, he started feeling faint and dizzy, and now he is having trouble breathing. Anita wants to know whether she can bring him to the office so that he can be seen by the physician. ■

Injected Poisons

An injected poison enters the body through bites, through stings, or by a needle. Examples of injected poisons include the venom of insects, spiders, snakes, and marine creatures such as jellyfish and the bite of rabid animals. The poison also may be a drug that is self-administered with a hypodermic needle, such as heroin. General signs and symptoms of injected poisoning include an altered state of awareness; evidence of stings, bites, or puncture marks on the skin; mottled skin; localized pain or itching; burning, swelling, or blistering at the site; difficulty in breathing; abnormal pulse rate; nausea and vomiting; and anaphylactic shock.

Insect Stings

It is estimated that 1 of every 125 Americans is allergic to insect stings. Approximately 40 people in the United States die every year from a severe allergic reaction to insect stings. The incidence of deaths is low because most people know they need to obtain medical attention immediately if an allergic reaction begins.

Almost all of the insects whose venom can cause allergic reactions belong to a group called *Hymenoptera*, which includes honeybees and bumblebees, wasps, yellow jackets, and hornets. When a honeybee stings, its stinger remains embedded in the victim's skin, causing the bee to die as it tries to tear itself away. Wasps, yellow jackets, and hornets are more aggressive than bees and can sting repeatedly. Hornets are the most aggressive of the group and may sting even when not provoked. Yellow jackets are close behind in aggressiveness, and wasps usually sting only if someone interferes with them near their nest.

If an insect sting does not cause an allergic reaction within 30 minutes, chances are excellent that no problem will occur. A normal reaction to an insect sting includes localized pain, redness, swelling, and itching lasting 1 to 2 days. Any generalized reaction not arising directly from the area of the sting is almost certain to be an allergic reaction, which begins with symptoms such as sneezing, hives, itching, angioedema, erythema, and disorientation and progresses to difficulty in breathing, dizziness, faintness, and loss of consciousness.

Medical care should be sought immediately because these are the symptoms of an anaphylactic reaction, and most fatalities occur within 2 hours of the sting. Because time is a factor, individuals known to have a severe allergy to insect stings carry an anaphylactic emergency treatment kit containing injectable epinephrine and oral antihistamines (see Figure 21-2). With this kit, treatment for a severe allergic reaction can be started immediately.

Emergency Care for Insect Stings

1. Remove the stinger and attached venom sac. Scrape the stinger off the patient's skin with your fingernail or a plastic card such as a credit card (Figure 21-14). Do not use tweezers or forceps because squeezing the venom sac may cause more venom to be injected into the patient's tissues.
2. Wash the site with soap and water.
3. Apply a cold pack to the affected area to reduce pain and swelling.
4. Observe the patient for signs of an anaphylactic reaction.

Spider Bites

Although spiders are numerous throughout the United States, most do not cause injuries or serious complications. Only two spiders have bites that cause serious or life-threatening reactions: the black widow spider and the brown recluse spider. Both of these spiders prefer dark, out-of-the-way places such as in woodpiles, in brush piles, under rocks, and in dark garages and attics. Because of this, bites usually occur on the hands and arms of individuals reaching into places where the spiders are hiding. Often the individual does not know that he or she has been bitten until he or she begins to feel ill or notices swelling and a bite mark on the skin.

The black widow spider is approximately 1 inch long and is black with a distinctive bright-red hourglass shape on its

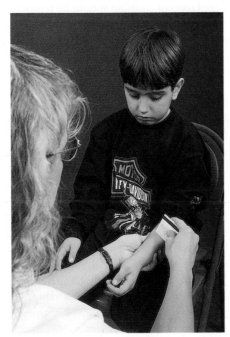

Figure 21-14. Removing a honeybee stinger and venom sac using the edge of a credit card.

abdomen. The venom injected when this spider bites an individual is toxic to the central nervous system. Signs and symptoms of a black widow bite include swelling and a dull pain at the injection site; nausea and vomiting; a rigid, boardlike abdomen; fever; rash; and difficulty in breathing or swallowing. Although the symptoms are severe, they are not usually fatal. An antivenin is available; however, because of its undesirable and frequent side effects, it generally is administered only to individuals with severe bites and to those who may have a heightened reaction, such as elderly individuals and children younger than 5 years old.

The brown recluse spider is light brown with a dark-brown violin-shaped mark on its back. The bite of a brown recluse causes severe local effects, including tenderness, redness, and swelling at the injection site. Systemic effects, such as difficulty in breathing or swallowing, seldom occur.

Emergency Care for Spider Bites

1. Wash the wound.
2. Apply a cold pack to the affected area to reduce pain and swelling.
3. Obtain medical help immediately if you suspect the individual has been bitten by a black widow spider or a brown recluse spider, or if a severe reaction begins to occur.

Snakebites

Snakebites kill very few people in the United States. Every year, approximately 45,000 persons are bitten by a snake; however, only 7000 of these bites involve a poisonous snake, and fewer than 15 of the individuals die. Species of poisonous snakes in the United States include rattlesnakes, copperheads, cottonmouths (water moccasins), and coral snakes. Individuals, zoos, or laboratories may own other poisonous species, however. Rattlesnakes account for most snakebites and nearly all fatalities from snakebites. Most snakebites occur near the home, as opposed to in the wild. Because it is often difficult to identify a snake, any unidentified snake should be considered poisonous. General signs and symptoms of a bite from a poisonous snake include puncture marks on the skin, pain and swelling at the puncture site, rapid pulse, nausea, vomiting, unconsciousness, and convulsions.

Emergency Care for Snakebites

1. Wash the bite area gently with soap and water.
2. Immobilize the injured part, and position it below the level of the heart.
3. Call emergency personnel. Do not apply ice to a snakebite. Do not apply a tourniquet, and do not cut or suction the wound.
4. If the snake is dead, inform emergency personnel of its location so that it can be transported to the hospital for identification.

Animal Bites

Bites and other injuries from animals range in severity from minor to serious and fatal. Most people who are bitten by animals do not report the bite to a physician. Because of this factor, the incidence of animal bites in the United States each year is unknown but has been estimated at approximately 1 to 2 million for dog bites and 400,000 for cat bites.

The most serious type of bite is one from an animal with rabies. Rabies is a viral infection transmitted through the saliva of an infected animal. If the condition is not treated, rabies is generally fatal. Certain animals tend to have a higher incidence of rabies than others. These include skunks, bats, raccoons, cats, dogs, cattle, and foxes. Hamsters, gerbils, guinea pigs, chipmunks, rats, mice, gophers, and rabbits are rarely infected with the rabies virus.

An individual who has been bitten by an animal that has rabies or is suspected of having rabies must obtain medical care. To prevent rabies, a rabies vaccine, which produces antibodies to fight the rabies virus, is administered to the individual.

Emergency Care for Animal Bites

Minor Animal Bites. Wash the wound with soap and water. Apply an antibiotic ointment and a dry sterile dressing. Transport the individual to a physician so that medical care can be provided to prevent infection and to ensure that the patient's tetanus toxoid immunization is up-to-date.

Serious Bites. If the wound is bleeding heavily, first control the bleeding with direct pressure. Do not clean the wound because this may result in more bleeding. Transport the patient to a physician, or if the bite is serious enough, call the local EMS.

All Animal Bites. If you suspect that the animal has rabies, relay this information to the appropriate authorities, such as medical personnel, the police, or animal control personnel. If possible, try to remember what the animal looked like and the area in which you last saw it.

Heat and Cold Exposure

Exposure to excessive environmental heat or cold can result in injury to the body ranging in severity from minor to life-threatening. Heat-related injuries are most apt to occur on very hot days that are accompanied by high humidity with little or no air movement. The three conditions caused by overexposure to heat are heat cramps, heat exhaustion, and heatstroke.

The two major types of cold-related injury are frostbite and hypothermia. Although cold-related injuries are most apt to occur in the winter months, they can occur at other times of the year, such as when an individual is exposed to cold water in a near-drowning incident.

Certain individuals are at higher risk for developing heat-related and cold-related injuries, as follows:
- Elderly individuals
- Young children, particularly infants
- Individuals who work or exercise outdoors
- Individuals with medical conditions that cause poor blood circulation, such as diabetes mellitus and cardiovascular disease
- Individuals who have had heat-related or cold-related injuries in the past
- Individuals under the influence of drugs or alcohol

Heat Cramps

Heat cramps are the least serious of the three types of heat-related injury. Heat cramps are most apt to occur when an individual is exercising or working in a hot environment and fails to replace lost fluids and electrolytes. Lost electrolytes can be replaced with a commercial sports drink (e.g., Gatorade).

Signs and symptoms of heat cramps include painful muscle spasms, particularly of the legs, calves, and abdomen; hot, sweaty skin; weakness; and a rapid pulse. These symptoms are a warning that an individual is having a problem with the heat. If the problem is ignored, heat cramps may progress to a more serious condition, such as heat exhaustion or heatstroke.

Treatment of heat cramps consists of removal of the patient to a cool environment, rest, and replacement of fluids and electrolytes. If the patient's condition does not improve, he or she should be transported to an emergency care facility for further treatment.

Heat Exhaustion

Heat exhaustion is the most common heat-related injury. It occurs most often in individuals involved in vigorous physical activity on a hot and humid day, such as athletes and construction workers. It also can occur in people who are wearing too much clothing on a hot and humid day. Signs and symptoms of heat exhaustion are similar to those of influenza: cold and clammy skin that is pale or gray, profuse sweating, headache, nausea, dizziness, weakness, and diarrhea.

Treatment of heat exhaustion consists of removal of the patient to a cool environment, replacement of fluids and electrolytes, application of a cold compress to the forehead, and rest (Figure 21-15). Tight clothing should be loosened, and excessive layers of clothing should be removed. In most cases, these measures improve the patient's condition in approximately 30 minutes. If the patient's condition does not improve, however, he or she should be transported to an emergency care facility.

Heatstroke

Heatstroke is the least common, but most serious, of the three heat-related injuries. Heatstroke is most apt to occur in elderly people during a heat wave and in athletes who overexert in a hot and humid environment. Heatstroke can occur in a very short time, as when a child has been left to wait in a closed car on a hot day.

During heatstroke, the body becomes so overheated that the heat-regulating mechanism breaks down and is unable to cool the body. The body temperature increases to a dangerous level, causing destruction of tissues. Signs and symptoms of heatstroke include a body temperature of 105° F (40° C) or greater; red, hot, dry skin; a rapid, weak pulse; dizziness and weakness; rapid, shallow breathing; decreased levels of consciousness; and seizures.

Heatstroke is a life-threatening emergency that requires immediate transport of the patient to an emergency care

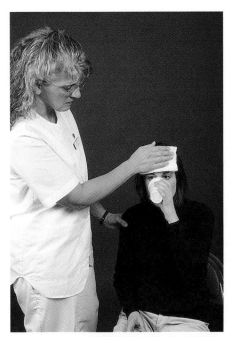

Figure 21-15. Treatment of heat exhaustion consists of moving the patient to a cool environment, replacing fluids and electrolytes, and applying a cold compress to the forehead; the patient should then rest.

What Would You Do? What Would You *Not* Do?

Case Study 3
David Brently has come to the medical office. He is a member of Kiwanis, and this year it was his turn to deliver Easter candy and flowers to patients at the local hospital and nursing home while wearing a bunny costume. It is a very warm day, and David says that he got really hot and sweaty in his costume and then started feeling dizzy and nauseous. He got a little worried and decided to drive himself to the medical office. David says he cannot get his costume off because the zipper is stuck. He does not want to cut it off because that would ruin it and Kiwanis would not be able to use it next year. He is hoping the physician can fix him up well enough so that he can drive home. David says he is sure his wife can get the costume off without damaging it. ■

---

facility by the fastest way possible. If not treated, heatstroke is always fatal. During transport, every attempt should be made to lower the body temperature, such as setting the air conditioner to its maximal capacity; covering the victim with cool, wet sheets; and fanning the victim.

Frostbite

Frostbite is the localized freezing of body tissue as a result of exposure to cold. The severity of frostbite depends on the environmental temperature, the duration of exposure, and the wind-chill factor. Frostbite most commonly affects the hands, fingers, feet, toes, ears, nose, and cheeks. Although frostbite is not life-threatening, it can cause severe tissue damage that may require amputation of the affected body

part. Signs and symptoms of frostbite include loss of feeling in the affected area; cold and waxy skin; and white, yellow, or blue discoloration of the skin.

Treatment of frostbite requires rewarming of the affected body part to prevent permanent damage. This is best accomplished in an emergency care facility because improper rewarming can result in further tissue damage. To transport the patient, loosely wrap warm clothing or blankets around the affected body part. The frozen area also can be placed in contact with another body part that is warm. It is important to handle the affected area gently. Do not rub or massage the affected area because this can damage frozen tissue further.

Hypothermia

Hypothermia is a life-threatening emergency in which the temperature of the entire body falls to a dangerously low level. Hypothermia can occur rapidly, such as when an individual falls through the ice on a frozen lake. It also can occur slowly when an individual is exposed to a cold environment for a long time, such as when a hiker is lost in the woods.

When the core body temperature decreases too much, the body loses its ability to regulate its temperature and to generate body heat. Signs and symptoms of hypothermia include shivering, numbness, drowsiness, apathy, a glassy stare, and decreased levels of consciousness.

Treatment of hypothermia should focus on preventing further heat loss. Remove the patient from the cold, or, if this is impossible, wrap him or her in blankets. Do not attempt to rewarm the patient such as through immersion in warm water. Rapid rewarming can result in serious respiratory and cardiac problems. The patient should be transported immediately to an emergency care facility.

Diabetic Emergencies

Glucose is the end product of carbohydrate metabolism. It serves as the chief source of energy to perform normal body functions and to assist in maintaining body temperature. The body maintains a constant blood glucose level to ensure a continuous source of energy for the body. Glucose that is not needed for energy can be stored in the form of glycogen in muscle and liver tissue for later use. When no more tissue storage is possible, excess glucose is converted to fat and stored as adipose tissue.

Insulin, a hormone secreted by the beta cells of the pancreas, is required for normal use of glucose in the body. Insulin enables glucose to enter the body's cells and be converted to energy. Insulin also is needed for proper storage of glycogen in liver and muscle cells.

Diabetes mellitus is a disease in which the body is unable to use glucose for energy because of a lack of insulin in the body. There are two types of diabetes—a severe form, usually appearing in childhood, known as *type 1 diabetes,* and a mild form, usually appearing in adulthood, known as *type 2 diabetes.* Most individuals with diabetes (90%) have type 2 diabetes. No cure for diabetes mellitus is known, but significant advances have been made in controlling the disease through a combination of drug therapy, diet therapy, and activity. The goal for the diabetic patient is to balance food intake and level of activity with the body's insulin.

A diabetic patient can experience two types of emergency: *hypoglycemia,* commonly referred to as "insulin shock," and *diabetic ketoacidosis,* commonly known as "diabetic coma." Insulin shock (hypoglycemia) occurs when there is too much insulin in the body and not enough glucose. Insulin shock can be caused by administration of too much insulin, skipping meals, and unexpected or unusual exercise. Symptoms of insulin shock include normal or rapid respirations; pale, cold, and clammy skin; sweating; dizziness and headache; full, rapid pulse; normal or high blood pressure; extreme hunger; aggressive or unusual behavior; fainting; and seizure or coma. The onset of insulin shock occurs rapidly, usually over 5 to 20 minutes, after the blood glucose level begins to decrease. Because the brain requires a constant supply of glucose for proper functioning, permanent brain damage or death can result from severe hypoglycemia.

Diabetic coma (diabetic ketoacidosis) occurs when there is not enough insulin in the body. This causes the blood glucose level to increase, resulting in hyperglycemia. When glucose cannot be used for energy, fat is broken down. This results in a buildup of acid waste products in the blood, known as *ketoacidosis.* The combined effect of the hyperglycemia and the ketoacidosis causes the following symptoms: polyuria; excessive thirst and hunger; vomiting; abdominal pain; dry, warm skin; rapid, deep sighing respirations; a sweet or fruity (acetone) odor to the breath; and a rapid, weak pulse.

If the condition is not treated, diabetic coma can progress to dehydration, hypotension, coma, and death. In contrast to insulin shock, however, the onset of diabetic coma is gradual, usually developing over 12 to 48 hours. Diabetic coma can be caused by illness and infection, over-

eating, forgetting to administer an insulin injection, or administering an insufficient amount of insulin.

Most individuals with diabetes have a thorough knowledge of their disease and manage it effectively. Because of this, diabetic emergencies are most apt to occur when there is an unusual upset in the insulin/glucose balance in the body, such as might be caused by illness or infection. An emergency situation also may arise in an individual who has diabetes but in whom the condition has not yet been diagnosed.

It may be difficult to tell the difference between insulin shock and diabetic coma because the symptoms are similar. Often a patient with either of these conditions seems to be intoxicated. If he or she is conscious, the diabetic patient usually knows what the trouble is; you should listen carefully to the patient to determine what may have caused the problem (e.g., not eating, forgetting to administer an insulin injection). If the patient is unconscious and unable to communicate, you should observe the patient's respirations. A patient in insulin shock has normal or rapid respirations, whereas a patient in diabetic coma has deep, labored respirations. Most diabetic patients carry an emergency medical identification, such as a medical alert bracelet or necklace and a wallet card (Figure 21-16), to alert others to their condition when they cannot.

Emergency Care in Diabetes

Insulin Shock (Hypoglycemia)

A patient in insulin shock needs sugar immediately. For a conscious patient, glucose should be administered by mouth in the form of fruit juice (e.g., orange juice), nondiet soft drinks, candy, honey, or table sugar dissolved in water (Figure 21-17). Improvement is usually rapid after the glucose has been consumed. If the patient is unconscious, do not give anything by mouth because it may be aspirated into the lungs. Instead, provide the fastest possible transportation of the patient to an emergency care facility.

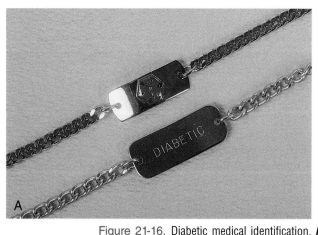

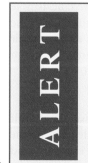

I HAVE TYPE I DIABETES

If I appear to be intoxicated or am unconscious, I may be having a reaction to diabetes or its treatment.

EMERGENCY TREATMENT

If I am able to swallow, please give me a beverage that contains sugar, such as orange juice, cola or even sugar in water. Then please send me to the nearest hospital **IMMEDIATELY.**

Figure 21-16. Diabetic medical identification. **A,** Diabetic medical alert bracelet. **B,** Diabetic wallet card.

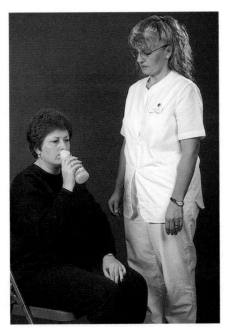

Figure 21-17. Orange juice is administered to a diabetic patient showing signs and symptoms of insulin shock.

Diabetic Coma (Diabetic Ketoacidosis)
A patient in diabetic coma needs insulin and must be transported as soon as possible to an emergency care facility.

Doubtful Situations

If you are ever in doubt as to whether a patient is developing insulin shock or diabetic coma, give sugar, even though the final diagnosis may be diabetic coma. This is because insulin shock develops much more rapidly than diabetic coma and can quickly cause permanent brain damage or death. If you give sugar to a patient in diabetic coma, there is little risk of making the condition worse because a patient can withstand a high blood glucose level longer than he or she can tolerate a low blood glucose level.

 evolve *Check out the Evolve site to access additional interactive activities.*

MEDICAL PRACTICE *and the* LAW

Emergency medicine is one of the most litigious (lawsuit-prone) areas of health care. Owing to the nature of emergencies, there is little time to plan your actions, and one misstep could cause damage. Keep in mind that your actions would be compared in court with those of a "reasonably prudent medical assistant with similar education and experience." Do not perform procedures you are not comfortable performing.

Whenever possible, obtain written consent for all procedures. In a life-or-death situation, this usually is not possible. In this case, you are held accountable to try to save the life of the patient, even without consent.

Patients or families often become hysterical during emergencies. As a health care professional, you are expected to keep a cool head and calm the patient and family while attending to the emergency situation.

If you are out of the office and encounter an emergency situation, many states have a "Good Samaritan" law that protects you from legal action if you perform only procedures with which you are familiar, such as emergency first aid or CPR. ∎

What Would You Do? What Would You *Not* Do? RESPONSES

Case Study 1
Page 813

What Did Judy Do?
❑ Gave Beth the National Poison Control hotline number (1-800-222-1222) and told her to call it immediately. Explained that was the fastest way to obtain information on what to do.
❑ Told Beth not to give the syrup of ipecac to Olivia unless she was told to do so by the poison control center.
❑ Told Beth to have the vitamin bottle in her hand when she calls. Told her that the poison control center would want to know information from the label and would especially want to know whether the vitamins contained iron.
❑ Told Beth to call the office back if she needs any more help after talking with the poison control center.

What Did Judy Not *Do?*
❑ Did not tell Beth she should give Olivia syrup of ipecac, because some poisons can cause additional problems if they are brought back up.

What Would You Do?/What Would You *Not* Do? Review Judy's response and place a checkmark next to the information you included in your response. List additional information you included in your response.

_____

_____

_____

_____

Continued

Case Study 2
Page 814

What Did Judy Do?
❑ Told Anita that Garon needs to get to the hospital as soon as possible. Explained that he is having a very serious allergic reaction that could be life-threatening.
❑ Told her to stay calm and call 911 immediately.
❑ Notified the physician of the situation.

What Did Judy Not *Do?*
❑ Did not tell her to bring Garon to the office because he may need special life-support equipment available at the hospital.

What Would You Do?/What Would You *Not* Do? Review Judy's response and place a checkmark next to the information you included in your response. List additional information you included in your response.

_____
_____
_____
_____

Case Study 3
Page 817

What Did Judy Do?
❑ Took David to an examining room that was cool and gave him a glass of water.
❑ Told David she needed to get his costume off as soon as possible. Explained that if his condition gets worse, it could become life-threatening.
❑ Helped David out of the costume and gave him another glass of water.

What Did Judy Not *Do?*
❑ Did not let David keep the costume on.

What Would You Do?/What Would You *Not* Do? Review Judy's response and place a checkmark next to the information you included in your response. List additional information you included in your response.

_____
_____
_____
_____

CERTIFICATION REVIEW

❑ **First aid** is the immediate care that is administered before complete medical care can be provided to an individual who is injured or suddenly becomes ill. The emergency medical services (EMS) system is a network of community resources, equipment, and medical personnel that provides emergency care to victims of injury or sudden illness.

❑ **Respiratory distress** indicates that the patient is breathing but is having great difficulty in doing so. Asthma is a condition characterized by wheezing, coughing, and dyspnea. Emphysema is a progressive lung disorder in which the terminal bronchioles that lead into the alveoli become plugged with mucus. Hyperventilation is a manner of breathing in which the respirations become rapid and deep, causing an individual to exhale too much carbon dioxide.

❑ **A heart attack,** also known as a *myocardial infarction* (MI), is caused by partial or complete obstruction of one or both of the coronary arteries or their branches. The principal symptom of a heart attack is chest pain or discomfort. The pain usually is felt behind the sternum and may radiate to the neck, throat, jaw, both shoulders, and arms.

❑ **A stroke** results when an artery to the brain is blocked or ruptures, interrupting the blood flow to the brain. Signs and symptoms of a stroke include sudden weakness or numbness of the face, arm, or leg on one side of the body; difficulty in speaking; dimmed vision or loss of vision in one eye; double vision; dizziness; confusion; severe headache; and loss of consciousness.

❑ **Shock** is the failure of the cardiovascular system to deliver enough blood to all of the body's vital organs. Shock accompanies many types of emergency—hemorrhaging, MI, and severe allergic reaction. The five major types of shock are hypovolemic, cardiogenic, neurogenic, anaphylactic, and psychogenic. General signs and symptoms of shock include weakness, restlessness, anxiety, disorientation, pallor, cold and clammy skin, rapid breathing, and rapid pulse.

❑ **Hypovolemic shock** is caused by a loss of blood or other body fluids. Cardiogenic shock is caused by failure of the heart to pump blood adequately to all of the vital organs of the body. Neurogenic shock occurs when the nervous system is unable to control the diameter of the blood vessels. Anaphylactic shock is a life-threatening reaction of the body to an allergen. Psychogenic shock is caused by an unpleasant experience or emotional stimulus, such as pain, fright, or the sight of blood.

❑ **Bleeding or hemorrhaging** is the escape of blood from a severed blood vessel. External bleeding is bleeding that can be seen coming from a wound. The most effective way to control bleeding is through the application of direct pressure to the bleeding site. If bleeding cannot be controlled with direct pressure, a pressure point can be used. A pressure point is a site on the body where an artery lies close to the surface of the skin and can be compressed against an underlying bone. Internal bleeding is bleeding that flows into a body cavity or an organ, or between tissues.

❑ **A wound** is a break in the continuity of an external or internal surface caused by physical means. An open wound is a break in the skin surface or mucous membrane that exposes the underlying tissues; examples include incisions, lacerations, punctures, and abrasions.

❑ **An incision** is a clean, smooth cut caused by a sharp cutting instrument, such as a knife, a razor, or a piece of glass. A laceration is a wound in which the tissues are torn apart, rather than cut, leaving ragged and irregular edges. A puncture is a wound made by a sharp, pointed object piercing the skin layers and sometimes the underlying structures. An abrasion is a wound in which the outer layers of the skin are scraped or rubbed off.

❑ **A closed wound** involves an injury to the underlying tissues of the body without a break in the skin or mucous membrane; an example is a contusion or bruise.

❑ **A fracture** is any break of a bone. A closed fracture occurs when there is a broken bone, but no break in the skin over the fracture site. An open fracture involves a break in the bone along with penetration of the overlying skin surface. Signs and symptoms of a fracture include pain and tenderness, deformity, swelling and discoloration, loss of function of the body part, and numbness or tingling.

❑ **A dislocation** is an injury in which one end of a bone making up a joint is separated or displaced from its normal position. A sprain is a tearing of ligaments at a joint. A strain is a stretching and tearing of muscles or tendons. A splint is any item that immobilizes a body part.

❑ **A burn** is an injury to the tissues caused by exposure to thermal, chemical, electrical, or radioactive agents. A superficial (first-degree) burn involves only the epidermis; an example is sunburn. A partial-thickness (second-degree) burn involves the epidermis and extends into the dermis. A full-thickness (third-degree) burn completely destroys the epidermis and the dermis and extends into the underlying tissues, such as fat, muscle, bone, and nerves.

❑ **A seizure** is a sudden episode of involuntary muscle contractions and relaxation often accompanied by a change in sensation, behavior, and level of consciousness. Seizures are classified as partial or generalized. In a partial seizure, the abnormal electrical activity is localized into specific areas of the brain; only the brain functions in those areas are affected. With a generalized seizure, the abnormal electrical activity spreads through the entire brain.

❑ **A poison** is any substance that causes illness, injury, or death if it enters the body. Poisons that are ingested enter the body by being swallowed. A poison that is inhaled is breathed into the body in the form of gas, vapor, or spray. A poison that is absorbed enters the body through the skin. An injected poison enters the body through bites, through stings, or by a needle.

❑ **Heat cramps** are most apt to occur when an individual is exercising or working in a hot environment and fails to replace lost fluids and electrolytes. Symptoms include painful muscle spasms, particularly of the legs, calves, and abdomen; hot, sweaty skin; weakness; and a rapid pulse.

❑ **Heat exhaustion** occurs most often in individuals involved in vigorous physical activity on a hot and humid day. Symptoms of heat exhaustion include cold and clammy skin, profuse sweating, headache, nausea, dizziness, weakness, and diarrhea.

❑ **Heatstroke** is the most serious heat-related injury and is most apt to occur in elderly individuals during a heat wave and in athletes who overexert in a hot and humid environment. Symptoms of heatstroke include a body temperature of 105° F or greater; red, hot, dry skin; a rapid, weak pulse; dizziness and weakness; rapid, shallow breathing; decreased level of consciousness; and seizures.

❑ **Frostbite** is the localized freezing of body tissue as a result of exposure to cold. Frostbite commonly affects the hands, fingers, feet, toes, ears, nose, and cheeks. Hypothermia is a life-threatening emergency in which the temperature of the entire body falls to a dangerously low level.

❑ **Diabetes mellitus** is a disease in which the body is unable to use glucose for energy because the body lacks enough insulin. Insulin shock (hypoglycemia) occurs when there is too much insulin in the body and not enough glucose. Diabetic coma occurs when there is not enough insulin in the body. This causes the blood glucose level to increase in the body, resulting in hyperglycemia.

⟲ TERMINOLOGY REVIEW

Medical Term	Word Parts	Definition
Burn		An injury to the tissues caused by exposure to thermal, chemical, electrical, or radioactive agents.
Crash cart		A specially equipped cart for holding and transporting medications, equipment, and supplies needed for life-saving procedures in an emergency.
Crepitus		A grating sensation caused by fractured bone fragments rubbing against each other.
Dislocation	*dis-:* to undo, free from	An injury in which one end of a bone making up a joint is separated or displaced from its normal anatomic position.
Emergency medical services (EMS) system		A network of community resources, equipment, and personnel that provides care to victims of injury or sudden illness.
First aid		The immediate care administered before complete medical care can be provided to an individual who is injured or suddenly becomes ill.
Fracture		Any break in a bone.
Hypothermia	*hypo-:* below, deficient *therm/o:* heat *-ia:* condition of diseased or abnormal state	A life-threatening condition in which the temperature of the entire body falls to a dangerously low level.
Poison		Any substance that causes illness, injury, or death if it enters the body.
Pressure point		A site on the body where an artery lies close to the surface of the skin and can be compressed against an underlying bone to control bleeding.
Seizure		A sudden episode of involuntary muscular contractions and relaxation, often accompanied by changes in sensation, behavior, and level of consciousness.
Shock		The failure of the cardiovascular system to deliver enough blood to all of the vital organs of the body.
Splint		Any device that immobilizes a body part.
Sprain		Trauma to a joint that causes tearing of ligaments.
Strain		A stretching or tearing of muscles or tendons caused by trauma.
Wound		A break in the continuity of an external or internal surface, caused by physical means.

🖰 ON THE WEB

For Information on Emergency Medicine:

American Red Cross: www.redcross.org

Federal Emergency Management Agency: www.fema.gov

Medical Abbreviations

a̅a̅	of each
AA	affected area; Alcoholics Anonymous
AAA	abdominal aortic aneurysm
AAL	anterior axillary line
AAMA	American Association of Medical Assistants
Ab	abortion; antibody
ABC	airway, breathing, circulation
abd	abdomen
ABE	acute bacterial endocarditis
ABG	arterial blood gases
ABN	abnormal
ABO	a blood group system
ABP	arterial blood pressure
Abs	absent
ac	before meals (Latin: *ante cibum*)
ACLS	advanced cardiac life support
ACOA	adult child of an alcoholic
ACTH	adrenocorticotropic hormone
AD	right ear (Latin: *auris dextra*)
ADA	American Diabetic Association; American Dental Association
ADH	antidiuretic hormone
ADL	activities of daily living
ad lib	as desired
adm	admission, admit
admin	administer
AFB	acid-fast bacillus
A Fib	atrial fibrillation
AFL	atrial flutter
AFP	alpha-fetoprotein
A/G	albumin-to-globulin ratio
AGA	appropriate for gestational age
AGN	acute glomerular nephritis
AHA	American Heart Association
AI	aortic insufficiency
AICD	automatic implantable cardioverter-defibrillator
AIDS	acquired immunodeficiency syndrome
AJ	ankle jerk
AKA	above the knee amputation
AL	acute leukemia
alb	albumin
ALL	acute lymphoblastic leukemia
ALP	alkaline phosphatase
ALS	amyotrophic lateral sclerosis
ALT	alanine aminotransferase
AM or a.m.	before noon, morning (Latin: *ante meridiem*)
AMA	against medical advice; American Medical Association
amb	ambulatory
AMI	acute myocardial infarction
amnio	amniocentesis
amt	amount
anes	anesthesia, anesthetist
ant	anterior
A/O	alert and oriented
AOM	acute otitis media
AP	apical pulse; angina pectoris
APC	atrial premature complex
approx	approximately
appt	appointment
aq	water
ARC	American Red Cross; AIDS-related complex
ARD	acute respiratory distress
ARDS	acute respiratory distress syndrome
AS	left ear (Latin: *auris sinistra*)
ASA	acetylsalicylic acid (aspirin)
ASAP	as soon as possible
ASCVD	arteriosclerotic cardiovascular disease
ASD	atrial septal defect
ASHD	arteriosclerotic heart disease
ASO	antistreptolysin-O; arteriosclerosis obliterans
AST	aspartate aminotransferase
ATR	Achilles tendon reflex
AU	both ears (Latin: *aurus unitas*); in each ear (Latin: *auris uterque*)
aud	auditory
AVR	aortic valve replacement
A & W	alive and well
ax	axillary
BA	backache
Ba	barium
Bab	Babinski (reflex)
bas	basophil
BBB	bundle branch block; blood-brain barrier
BBT	basal body temperature

b/c	because		CFS	chronic fatigue syndrome
BC	birth control; bone conduction		CGL	chronic granulocytic leukemia
BCP	birth control pills		CH	crown-heel (length of baby)
BE	barium enema		CHB	complete heart block
BEA	below elbow amputation		CHD	congenital heart disease; coronary heart disease
BG	blood glucose		chemo	chemotherapy
bid	twice a day (Latin: *bis in die*)		CHF	congestive heart failure
bili	bilirubin		CHL	conductive hearing loss
BJ	biceps jerk		Chol	cholesterol
BJM	bones, joints, and muscles		CIS	carcinoma in situ
BK	below knee		CK	creatine kinase
BKA	below knee amputation		cl	chloride, chlorine
BLS	basic life support		CLD	chronic lung disease
BM	bowel movement		cldy	cloudy
BMR	basal metabolic rate		cm	centimeter
BOM	bilateral otitis media		cm^3	cubic centimeter
BP	blood pressure		CMA	Certified Medical Assistant
BPAD	bipolar affective disorder		CMV	cytomegalovirus
BPH	benign prostatic hyperplasia		CNS	central nervous system
BPM	beats per minute		CO	cardiac output
BR	bathroom		c/o	complains of
BRB	bright red blood		CO_2	carbon dioxide
BrBx	breast biopsy		COPD	chronic obstructive pulmonary disease
BS	blood sugar; breath sounds		CP	cerebral palsy
BSA	body surface area		CPK	creatine phosphokinase
BSE	breast self-examination		CPN	chronic pyelonephritis
BSN	bowel sounds normal		CPR	cardiopulmonary resuscitation
BTL	bilateral tubal ligation		CR	crown-rump (length of baby)
BUN	blood urea nitrogen		CRC	colorectal cancer
BW	birth weight		CRD	chronic respiratory disease
Bx	biopsy		CS	cesarean section
c̄	with		C & S	culture and sensitivity
C	Celsius		CSF	cerebrospinal fluid
C1	first cervical vertebra		CST	contraction stress test
C2	second cervical vertebra		CT	computed tomography
Ca	calcium		CTS	carpal tunnel syndrome
CA	cancer; cardiac arrest		CV	cardiovascular
CAD	coronary artery disease		CVA	cerebrovascular accident
CAHD	coronary atherosclerotic heart disease		CVP	central venous pressure
cal	calorie(s)		CVS	chorionic villous sampling; cardiovascular system
CAPD	continuous ambulatory peritoneal dialysis			
caps	capsules		Cx	cervix
CAT	computed axial tomography		CXR	chest x-ray
cath	catheter, catheterize		Cysto	cystoscopy
CB	cesarean birth		d	day
CBC	complete blood count		/day	per day
CBD	common bile duct		db	decibel
CBF	cerebral blood flow		DBE	deep breathing exercise
CBR	complete bedrest		DBM	diabetic management
CC	chief complaint		DBP	diastolic blood pressure
cc	cubic centimeter		d/c	discontinue
CCU	coronary care unit; critical care unit		D & C	dilation and curettage
CD	chemical dependence		DD	discharge diagnosis
C & D	cystoscopy and dilation		DDD	degenerative disc disease
CDC	Centers for Disease Control and Prevention		D/DW	dextrose, distilled water
cerv	cervical, cervix		DDx	differential diagnosis
CF	cystic fibrosis			

D & E	dilation and evacuation
DEA	Drug Enforcement Administration
del	delivery
DES	diethylstilbestrol
DI	diabetes insipidus
D & I	dry and intact
diab	diabetic
diff	differential white blood cell count
dil	dilute
disch	discharge
disp	dispense
DIU	death in utero
DJD	degenerative joint disease
DKA	diabetic ketoacidosis
dL	deciliter
DM	diabetes mellitus
DNA	deoxyribonucleic acid
DNKA	did not keep appointment
DNR	do not resuscitate
d/o	disorder
DOA	dead on arrival
DOB	date of birth
DOE	dyspnea on exertion
DOI	date of injury
DP	diastolic pressure
DPT	diphtheria, pertussis, and tetanus (vaccine)
DR	delivery room
dr	dram
DRE	digital rectal exam
DRG	diagnosis-related group
drsg	dressing
DS	double strength
D/S	discharge summary
DSD	dry sterile dressing
DT	diphtheria and tetanus toxoid
DTaP	diphtheria and tetanus toxoids and acellular pertussis vaccine
DTR	deep tendon reflex
DU	duodenal ulcer
DUB	dysfunctional uterine bleeding
DUI	driving under the influence (of alcohol)
D & V	diarrhea and vomiting
DVA	distance visual acuity
DVT	deep venous thrombosis
DW	distilled water
D/W	dextrose in water
Dx	diagnosis
Dz	disease
ea	each
EAB	elective abortion
EAC	external auditory canal
EAM	external auditory meatus
EBL	estimated blood loss
EBV	Epstein-Barr virus
EC	enteric-coated
ECD	esophagogastroduodenoscopy
ECF	extended care facility

ECG	electrocardiogram
Echo	echocardiogram
E. coli	*Escherichia coli*
ECT	electroconvulsive therapy
ED	emergency department
EDD	expected date of delivery
EEG	electroencephalogram
EENT	eye, ear, nose, and throat
EGA	estimated gestational age
elect stim	electrical stimulation
ELISA	enzyme-linked immunosorbent assay
elix	elixir
EmBx	endometrial biopsy
EMG	electromyogram
EMS	emergency medical services
ENT	ear, nose, and throat
EOM	extraocular movement
eos	eosinophil
ER	emergency room
ESR	erythrocyte sedimentation rate
est	estimated
ESWL	extracorporeal shock-wave lithotripsy
ETT	endotracheal tube
EVAL	evaluation
ex	exercise
ext	extract
Ez	eczema
F	Fahrenheit
FA	fluorescent antibody
FB	foreign body
FBP	femoral blood pressure
FBS	fasting blood sugar
FD	fully dilated
FDA	Food and Drug Administration
Fe	iron
Fe def	iron deficiency
FEF	forced expiratory flow
FEKG	fetal electrocardiogram
FEV	forced expiratory volume
FFP	fresh frozen plasma
FH	family history
FHR	fetal heart rate
FHT	fetal heart tones
fl	fluid
flex sig	flexible sigmoidoscopy
FMP	first menstrual period
FOB	fetal occult blood
FOBT	fecal occult blood test
FP	family practice
freq	frequent
FS	finger-stick
FSH	follicle-stimulating hormone
ft	foot
FT	full term
FTND	full-term normal delivery
FTT	failure to thrive
F/U	follow-up

FUO	fever of undetermined origin	H & P	history and physical
FVC	forced vital capacity	hpf	high-power field
FWB	full weight bearing	HPI	history of present illness
Fx	fracture	*H. pylori*	*Helicobacter pylori*
g	gram	hr	hour
G	gravida	HR	heart rate
GA	general anesthesia; gestational age	HRT	hormone replacement therapy
GB	gallbladder	hs	at bedtime (Latin: *hora somni*)
GC	gonorrhea; gas chromatography	HSV	herpes simplex virus
GCT	glucose challenge test	ht	height
GDM	gestational diabetes mellitus	HTN	hypertension
gen	general	HVD	hypertensive vascular disease
GFR	glomerular filtration rate	Hx	history
GH	growth hormone	Hz	hertz
GI	gastrointestinal	IA	intraarterial
glu	glucose	IABP	intraaortic balloon pump
GM	gross motor	IBS	irritable bowel syndrome
Gm−	gram negative	IBW	ideal body weight
Gm+	gram positive	ICCU	intensive coronary care unit
GP	general practitioner	ICD	International Classification of Diseases (of the World Health Organization)
gr	grain		
GSW	gunshot wound	ICDA	International Classification of Diseases, Adapted
gtt(s)	drop (drops)		
GTT	glucose tolerance test	ICF	intracellular fluid
GU	genitourinary	ICP	intracranial pressure
G/W	glucose in water	ICS	intercostal space
GYN	gynecology	ICU	intensive care unit
H/A	headache	ID	intradermal
HAL	hyperalimentation	I & D	incision and drainage
HAV	hepatitis A virus	IDDM	insulin-dependent diabetes mellitus
HBIG	hepatitis B immunoglobulin	IM	intramuscular
HBP	high blood pressure	Immuniz	immunizations
HBsAg	hepatitis B surface antigen	imp	impression
HBV	hepatitis B virus	in	inch
HC	head circumference	IN	inhalation
HCG	human chorionic gonadotropin	I & O	intake and output
HCl	hydrochloric acid	IOP	intraocular pressure
Hct	hematocrit	IPPB	intermittent positive-pressure breathing
HCVD	hypertensive cardiovascular disease	IPV	inactivated polio vaccine
HD	Hodgkin's disease	IQ	intelligence quotient
HDL	high-density lipoprotein	IU	international unit
HDN	hemolytic disease of the newborn	IUD	intrauterine device
HEENT	head, eye, ear, nose, and throat	IUFD	intrauterine fetal death
Hep	heparin	IUGR	intrauterine growth rate
Hep B	hepatitis B vaccine	IV	intravenous
Hg	mercury	IVP	intravenous pyelogram
Hgb	hemoglobin	*JAMA*	*Journal of the American Medical Association*
HGM	home glucose monitoring	jaund	jaundice
HH	home health	JODM	juvenile-onset diabetes mellitus
H & H	hemoglobin and hematocrit	JP	Jackson Pratt (drain)
Hib	*Haemophilus influenzae* type b conjugate vaccine	JRA	juvenile rheumatoid arthritis
		JVD	jugular venous distention
HIV	human immunodeficiency virus	JVP	jugular venous pressure
H & L	heart and lungs	K	potassium
HMO	health maintenance organization	KCl	potassium chloride
H/O	history of	kg	kilogram
H_2O	water	KOH	potassium hydroxide

KUB	kidney, ureter, and bladder		med(s)	medication(s)
L	liter		mEq/L	milliequivalents per liter
l	length		mg	milligram
LA	left atrium		MG	myasthenia gravis
lab	laboratory		MGF	maternal grandfather
lac	laceration		MGM	maternal grandmother
lap	laparotomy		MH	marital history
lat	lateral		MHx	medical history
LAVH	laparoscopic-assisted vaginal hysterectomy		MI	myocardial infarction
lax	laxative		min	minute
LB	lower back		ml	milliliter
lb	pound		mm	millimeter
LBBB	left bundle branch block		mm^3	cubic millimeter
LBP	low back pain		mm Hg	millimeters of mercury
LBW	low birth weight		mmol	millimole
LD	lactate dehydrogenase		MMR	measles, mumps, and rubella (vaccine)
L & D	labor and delivery		MO	month old
LDL	low-density lipoprotein		mod	moderate
LE	lupus erythematosus		MODM	mature-onset diabetes mellitus
LFD	low forceps delivery		mono	mononucleosis
LFT	liver function test		MP	menstrual period
lg	large		MR	mitral regurgitation; mental retardation
LGA	large for gestational age		MRI	magnetic resonance imaging
LH	luteinizing hormone		MRM	modified radical mastectomy
liq	liquid		MS	multiple sclerosis
LLC	long leg cast		MSL	midsternal line
LLE	left lower extremity		MSU	midstream urine specimen
LLL	left lower leg		MT	medical technologist
LLQ	left lower quadrant		multip	multipara
LMP	last menstrual period		MV	mitral valve
LNMP	last normal menstrual period		MVA	motor vehicle accident
LOC	loss of consciousness		MVP	mitral valve prolapse
LOM	loss of motion		MVR	mitral valve replacement
LP	lumbar puncture		Na	sodium
lpf	low-power field		N/A	not applicable
LR	labor room		NaCl	sodium chloride
LRQ	lower right quadrant		NAD	nothing abnormal detected; no appreciable disease
LS	lumbosacral			
lt	left		narc	narcotic
LTC	long-term care		NB	newborn
LTM	long-term memory		NBS	normal bowel sounds; normal breath sounds
LUE	left upper extremity			
LUQ	left upper quadrant		NBW	normal birth weight
LV	left ventricle		NC	no change
L & W	living and well		N/C	no complaints
lymphs	lymphocytes		NED	no evidence of disease
m	meter		neg	negative
mcg	microgram		NG	nasogastric
MCH	mean corpuscular hemoglobin		NGT	nasogastric tube
MCHC	mean corpuscular hemoglobin concentration		NGU	nongonococcal urethritis
			NH	nursing home
MCL	midclavicular line		NHL	non-Hodgkin's lymphoma
MCV	mean corpuscular volume		NI	not improved
MD	muscular dystrophy; medical doctor		NICU	newborn intensive care unit
MDE	major depressive episode		NIDDM	non–insulin-dependent diabetes mellitus
MDI	metered-dose inhaler		NKA	no known allergies
MDR	minimum daily requirement		NKDA	no known drug allergies

NL	normal limits		PAC	premature atrial contraction
NMP	normal menstrual period		Pap	Pap test
NMR	nuclear magnetic resonance		PAT	paroxysmal atrial tachycardia
noct	nocturnal		path	pathology
non rep	do not repeat		Pb	lead
nor	normal		PBI	protein-bound iodine
NPO	nothing by mouth (Latin: *nil per os*)		pc	after meals (Latin: *post cibum*)
NR	no refill		PC	platelet count
N/R	not responsible		PCC	Poison Control Center
NS	normal saline		PCV	packed cell volume
NSAID	nonsteroidal anti-inflammatory drug		PD	Parkinson's disease
NSR	normal sinus rhythm		*PDR*	*Physician's Desk Reference*
NSS	normal saline solution		PE	physical examination
NST	nonstress test		peds	pediatrics
NSU	nonspecific urethritis		PEG	pneumoencephalogram; pneumoencephalography
NSVD	normal spontaneous vaginal delivery			
NT	nontender		PEN	penicillin; pharmacy equivalent name
N & T	nose and throat		per	by, through
nullip	nullipara (never gave birth)		peri	perineal
N & V	nausea and vomiting		PERRLA	pupils equal, round, regular, react to light, and accommodation (normal)
NVA	near visual acuity			
NVD	nausea, vomiting, and diarrhea		PET	positron emission tomography
N & W	normal and well		PFS	pulmonary function studies
NWB	non–weight-bearing		PFT	pulmonary function test
NYD	not yet diagnosed		PGF	paternal grandfather
O	oral		PGH	pituitary growth hormone
O₂	oxygen		PGM	paternal grandmother
OA	osteoarthritis		pH	hydrogen ion concentration
OB	obstetrics		PH	past history
OB/GYN	obstetrics and gynecology		pharm	pharmacy
obs	observed		PI	present illness
occ	occasionally		PID	pelvic inflammatory disease
OCD	obsessive-compulsive disorder		PIH	pregnancy-induced hypertension
OCT	oxytocin challenge test		PKU	phenylketonuria
OD	right eye		PM or p.m.	afternoon, evening (Latin: *post meridiem*)
O & E	observation and examination		PMB	postmenopausal bleeding
O/E	on examination		PMH	past medical history
OH	occupational history		PMN	polymorphonuclear neutrophils
oint	ointment		PMP	past menstrual period
OM	otitis media		PMS	premenstrual syndrome
OOB	out of bed		PMT	premenstrual tension
op	operation		PN	progress notes
OP	outpatient		PND	paroxysmal nocturnal dyspnea
O & P	ova and parasites		PNX	pneumothorax
OPV	oral polio vaccine		po	by mouth (Latin: *per os*)
OR	operating room		PO	by mouth (Latin: *per os*)
ortho	orthopedics		POL	physician's office laboratory
OS	left eye		POR	problem-oriented medical record
OT	occupational therapy		pos	positive
OTC	over the counter (nonprescription medication)		postop	postoperative (after surgery)
			PP	postpartum
OU	in each eye (Latin: *oculus uterque*); both eyes		PPB	positive-pressure breathing
			PPBS	postprandial blood sugar
OV	office visit		PPD	purified protein derivative
oz	ounce		PPH	postpartum hemorrhage
P	pulse		PPT	partial prothrombin time
PA	posteroanterior; physician assistant		preop	preoperative (before surgery)

prep	preparation	RHF	right heart failure
primip	woman bearing first child	RI	respiratory illness
prn	as the occasion arises, as necessary (Latin: *pro re nata*)	RLQ	right lower quadrant
		RMA	Registered Medical Assistant
procto	proctoscopy	RMSF	Rocky Mountain spotted fever
prog	prognosis	RNA	ribonucleic acid
PROM	premature rupture of membranes	R/O	rule out
prox	proximal	ROM	rupture of membranes; range of motion
PSA	prostate-specific antigen	ROS	review of systems
pt	patient; pint	RP	retrograde pyelogram
Pt	patient	RQ	respiratory quotient
PT	physical therapy; prothrombin time	RRR	regular rate and rhythm
PTA	prior to admission	RSV	respiratory syncytial virus
PTB	prior to birth	rt	right
PTD	prior to discharge	RT	room temperature; radiation therapy
PTH	parathyroid hormone	R/T	related to
PTT	partial thromboplastin time	RTW	return to work
PUD	peptic ulcer disease	RUE	right upper extremity
PVC	premature ventricular contraction	RUQ	right upper quadrant
PVD	peripheral vascular disease	RV	right ventricle
PWB	partial weight bearing	RVH	right ventricular hypertrophy
Px	physical examination	Rx	prescription
q	each; every (Latin: *quaque*)	$\bar{s}$	without
q AM	every morning	SA	sinoatrial
qd	every day (Latin: *quaque die*)	SAB	spontaneous abortion
qh	every hour (Latin: *quaque hora*)	SARS	severe acute respiratory syndrome
q2h (q3h, q4h)	every 2 (3, 4) hours	SB	stillborn; sinus bradycardia
		SBE	subacute bacterial endocarditis
qid	4 times a day (Latin: *quater in die*)	SBO	small-bowel obstruction
qn	every night (Latin: *quaque nocturnus*)	SBP	systolic blood pressure
QNS	quantity not sufficient	SC	subcutaneous
qod	every other day (Latin: *quater in die*)	SCD	sudden cardiac death
QS	quantity sufficient	schiz	schizophrenia
qt	quart	SCI	spinal cord injury
quad	quadriplegic	SD	spontaneous delivery; standard deviation
R	respiration	SDH	subdural hematoma
RA	rheumatoid arthritis	S/E	side effects
RAF	rheumatoid arthritis factor	sec	second
RAST	radioallergosorbent test	sed rate	sedimentation rate
RBC/hpf	red blood cells per high-power field	segs	segmented neutrophils
RBC	red blood cell; red blood (cell) count	seq	sequela
RBCV	red blood cell volume	SF	scarlet fever; spinal fluid
RBS	random blood sugar	SG	specific gravity
RCV	red cell volume	SGA	small for gestational age
RD	respiratory distress	SH	social history; serum hepatitis
RDA	recommended daily allowance	sid	once a day (Latin: *semel in die*)
RDS	respiratory distress syndrome	SIDS	sudden infant death syndrome
RE	rectal examination	sig	write on label
reg	regular	sigmoid	sigmoidoscopy
rehab	rehabilitation	sl	slight
REM	rapid eye movement	SLC	short leg cast
REP	retrograde pyelogram	SLE	systemic lupus erythematosus
resp	respiration	SM	simple mastectomy
RF	rheumatic fever	sm	small
RG	random glucose	SNF	skilled nursing facility
Rh	rhesus blood factor	SOAP	subjective data, objective data, assessment, and plan
RHD	rheumatic heart disease		

SOB	shortness of breath	TPM	temporary pacemaker
sol	solution	TPN	total parenteral nutrition
SOM	serous otitis media	TPR	temperature, pulse, and respiration
sp gr	specific gravity	Tq	tourniquet
SP	systolic pressure	tr	trace
SPA	suprapubic aspiration	trig	triglycerides
spec	specimen	TRUS	transrectal ultrasound
spont ab	spontaneous abortion	TSE	testicular self-examination
SQ	subcutaneous	TSH	thyroid-stimulating hormone
SR	sustained release	tsp	teaspoon
SROM	spontaneous rupture of membranes	TSP	total serum protein
ss	one half	TSS	toxic shock syndrome
Staph	*Staphylococcus*	TVH	total vaginal hysterectomy
STAT	immediately	Tx	treatment
STD	sexually transmitted disease	U	unit
std	standard	UA	urinalysis
STM	short-term memory	UC	ulcerative colitis
Strep	*Streptococcus*	U/C	urine culture
subcut	subcutaneous	UCG	urinary chorionic gonadotropin
sup	superior	UCHD	usual childhood diseases
supp	suppository	UE	upper extremity
surg	surgery	UGI	upper gastrointestinal
SV	stroke volume	ULQ	upper left quadrant
Sx	symptoms	UOQ	upper outer quadrant
Sz	seizure	UR	upper respiratory
T	temperature	URI	upper respiratory infection
T_3	triiodothyronine	Urol	urology
T_4	thyroxine	URQ	upper right quadrant
T & A	tonsils and adenoids	US	ultrasound
tab(s)	tablet(s)	USI	urinary stress incontinence
TAB	therapeutic abortion	*USP*	*United States Pharmacopoeia*
TAH	total abdominal hysterectomy	UT	urinary tract
TB	tuberculosis	UTI	urinary tract infection
TBF	total body fat	UV	ultraviolet
TBLC	term birth, living child	VA	visual acuity
tbsp	tablespoon	VAD	vascular access device
TBW	total body water	vag	vagina; vaginal
TC	total capacity	VAP	vascular access port
T & C	type and cross-match	VC	vital capacity
temp	temperature	VD	venereal disease
TENS	transcutaneous electrical nerve stimulation	VDRL	Venereal Disease Research Laboratory (test)
TF	tube feeding; transfer factor	VE	vaginal examination
ther	therapy	VFib	ventricular fibrillation
THR	total hip replacement	VH	vaginal hysterectomy
TIA	transient ischemic attack	VHD	valvular heart disease
tid	3 times a day (Latin: *ter in die*)	VHDL	very high density lipoprotein
tinct	tincture	vit	vitamin
TKR	total knee replacement	VLDL	very low density lipoprotein
TLC	total lung capacity; tender loving care	VO	verbal order
TM	tympanic membrane	VP	venipuncture
TMJ	temporomandibular joint	VS	vital signs
TND	term normal delivery	VSD	ventricular septal defect
TO	telephone order	VSS	vital signs stable
tol	tolerate, tolerated	VT	ventricular tachycardia
TOP	termination of pregnancy	VV	varicose veins
TOPV	trivalent oral poliovirus vaccine	WB	weight bearing
TP	total protein	WBAT	weight bearing as tolerated

WBC	white blood cell; white blood (cell) count	w/o	without
WC	white cell	WR	weakly reactive
W/C	wheelchair	wt	weight
WDWN	well developed, well nourished	W/U	workup
wk	week	X	magnification
WN	well nourished	XM	cross-match
WNF	well-nourished female	XR	x-ray
WNL	within normal limits	yd	yard(s)
WNM	well-nourished male	YOB	year of birth
WO	written order	yr	year(s)

Glossary

Abortion The termination of a pregnancy before the fetus has reached the stage of viability (20 wefis).

Abrasion A wound in which the outer layers of the skin are damaged; a scrape.

Abscess A collection of pus in a cavity surrounded by inflamed tissue.

Absorbable suture Suture material that is gradually digested by tissue enzymes and absorbed by the body.

Adnexal Adjacent.

Adolescent An individual from 12 to 18 years old.

Adventitious sounds Abnormal breath sounds.

Adverse reaction An unintended and undesirable effect produced by a drug.

Aerobe A microorganism that needs oxygen to live and grow.

Afebrile Without fever; the body temperature is normal.

Agglutination (As it pertains to blood) Clumping of blood cells.

Allergen A substance that is capable of causing an allergic reaction.

Allergy An abnormal hypersensitivity of the body to substances that are ordinarily harmless.

Alveolus (*pl.* alveoli) A thin-walled air sac of the lungs in which the exchange of oxygen and carbon dioxide takes place.

Ambulation Walking or moving from one place to another.

Ambulatory Able to walk, as opposed to being confined to bed or a wheelchair.

Ameboid movement Movement used by leukocytes that permits them to propel themselves from the capillaries into the tissues.

Amenorrhea The absence or cessation of the menstrual period. Amenorrhea occurs normally before puberty, during pregnancy, and after menopause.

Amplitude Refers to amount, extent, size, abundance, or fullness.

Ampule A small sealed glass container that holds a single dose of medication.

Anaerobe A microorganism that grows best in the absence of oxygen.

Analyte A substance that is being identified or measured in a laboratory test.

Anaphylactic reaction A serious allergic reaction that requires immediate treatment.

Anemia A condition in which there is a decrease in the number of erythrocytes or in the amount of hemoglobin in the blood.

Anisocytosis A variation in the size of red blood cells.

Antecubital space The surface of the arm in front of the elbow.

Antibody A substance capable of combining with an antigen, resulting in an antigen-antibody reaction.

Anticoagulant A substance that inhibits blood clotting.

Antigen A substance capable of stimulating the formation of antibodies.

Antipyretic An agent that reduces fever.

Antiseptic An agent that kills disease-producing microorganisms but not their spores. An antiseptic is usually applied to living tissue.

Antiserum (*pl.* antisera) A serum that contains antibodies.

Anuria Failure of the kidneys to produce urine.

Aorta The major trunk of the arterial system of the body. The aorta arises from the upper surface of the left ventricle.

Apnea The temporary cessation of breathing.

Approximation The process of bringing two parts, such as tissue, together, through the use of sutures or other means.

Artifact Additional electrical activity picked up by the electrocardiograph that interferes with the normal appearance of the ECG cycles.

Asepsis Free from infection or pathogens; the actions practiced to make and maintain an object free from infection or pathogens.

Astigmatism A refractive error that causes distorted and blurred vision for both near and far objects due to a cornea that is oval-shaped.

Atherosclerosis Buildup of fibrous plaques of fatty deposits and cholesterol on the inner walls of an artery that causes narrowing, obstruction, and hardening of the artery.

Attending physician The physician responsible for the care of a hospitalized patient.

Atypical Deviation from the normal.

Audiometer An instrument used to measure hearing acuity quantitatively for the various frequencies of sound waves.

Auscultation The process of listening to the sounds produced within the body to detect signs of disease.

Autoclave An apparatus for the sterilization of materials, using steam under pressure.

Autoimmune disease A condition in which the body's immune system produces antibodies that attack the body's own cells. The cause is unknown.

Axilla The armpit.

Bacilli (*sing.* bacillus) Bacteria that have a rod shape.

Bandage A strip of woven material used to wrap or cover a part of the body.

Bariatrics The branch of medicine that deals with the treatment and control of obesity and diseases associated with obesity.

Baseline The flat horizontal line that separates the various waves of the ECG cycle.

Bilirubin An orange bile pigment produced by the breakdown of heme from the hemoglobin molecule.

Bilirubinuria The presence of bilirubin in the urine.

Biopsy The surgical removal and examination of tissue from the living body. Biopsies are generally performed to determine whether a tumor is benign or malignant.

Bladder catheterization The passing of a sterile catheter through the urethra and into the bladder to remove urine.

Blood antibody A protein in blood plasma that is capable of combining with its corresponding blood antigen to produce an antigen-antibody reaction.

Blood antigen A protein present on the surface of red blood cells that determines a person's blood type.

Body mechanics Utilization of the correct muscles to maintain proper balance, posture, and body alignment to accomplish a task safely and efficiently without undue strain on any muscle or joint.

Bounding pulse A pulse with an increased volume that feels very strong and full.

Brace An orthopedic device used to support and hold a part of the body in the correct position to allow functioning and healing.

Bradycardia An abnormally slow heart rate (fewer than 60 beats per minute).

Bradypnea An abnormal decrease in the respiratory rate of fewer than 10 respirations per minute.

Braxton Hicks contractions Intermittent and irregular painless uterine contractions that occur throughout pregnancy. They occur more frequently toward the end of pregnancy and are sometimes mistaken for true labor pains.

Buffy coat A thin, light-colored layer of white blood cells and platelets that lays between a top layer of plasma and a bottom layer of red blood cells when an anticoagulant has been added to a blood specimen.

Burn An injury to the tissues caused by exposure to thermal, chemical, electrical, or radioactive agents.

Calibration A mechanism to check the precision and accuracy of a test system, such as an automated analyzer, to determine if the system is providing accurate results. Calibration is typically performed using a calibration device called a *standard.*

Canthus The junction of the eyelids at either corner of the eye.

Capillary action The action that causes liquid to rise along a wick, a tube, or a gauze dressing.

Cardiac arrest A condition in which the heart has stopped beating or beats too irregularly to circulate blood effectively through the body.

Cardiac cycle One complete heartbeat.

Celsius scale A temperature scale on which the freezing point of water is 0° and the boiling point of water is 100°; also called the centigrade scale.

Cerumen Earwax.

Cervix The lower narrow end of the uterus that opens into the vagina.

Charting The process of making written entries about a patient in the medical record.

Chemotherapy The use of chemicals to treat disease. Chemotherapy is most often used to refer to the treatment of cancer using antineoplastic medications.

Cilia Slender, hairlike projections that constantly beat toward the outside to remove microorganisms from the body.

Clinical diagnosis A tentative diagnosis of a patient's condition obtained through evaluation of the health history and the physical examination, without the benefit of laboratory or diagnostic tests.

Cocci (*sing.* coccus) Bacteria that have a round shape.

Colonoscope An endoscope that is specially designed for passage through the anus to permit visualization of the rectum and the entire length of the colon.

Colonoscopy The visualization of the rectum and the entire colon using a colonoscope.

Colony A mass of bacteria growing in a solid culture medium that have arisen from the multiplication of a single bacterium.

Colposcope A lighted instrument with a binocular magnifying lens used to examine the vagina and cervix.

Colposcopy Examination of the vagina and cervix using a colposcope.

Compress A soft, moist, absorbent cloth that is folded in several layers and applied to a part of the body in the local application of heat or cold.

Conduction The transfer of energy, such as heat, from one object to another by direct contact.

Consultation report A narrative report of an opinion about a patient's condition by a practitioner other than the attending physician.

Contagious Capable of being transmitted directly or indirectly from one person to another.

Contaminate To soil or to make impure.

Contrast medium A substance that is used to make a particular structure visible on a radiograph.

Control A solution that is used to monitor a test system to ensure the reliability and accuracy of test results.

Controlled drug A drug that has restrictions placed on it by the federal government because of its potential for abuse.

Contusion An injury to the tissues under the skin causing blood vessels to rupture, allowing blood to seep into the tissues; a bruise.

Convection The transfer of energy, such as heat, through air currents.

Conversion Changing from one system of measurement to another.

Crash cart A specially equipped cart for holding and transporting medications, equipment, and supplies needed for performing lifesaving procedures in an emergency.

Crepitus A grating sensation caused by fractured bone fragments rubbing against each other.

Crisis (pertaining to fever) A sudden falling of an elevated body temperature to normal.

Critical item An item that comes in contact with sterile tissue or the vascular system.

Cryosurgery The therapeutic use of freezing temperatures to destroy abnormal tissue.

Cubic centimeter The amount of space occupied by 1 milliliter (1 ml = 1 cc).

Culture The propagation of a mass of microorganisms in a laboratory culture medium.

Culture medium A mixture of nutrients in which microorganisms are grown in the laboratory.

Cyanosis A bluish discoloration of the skin and mucous membranes.

Cytology The science that deals with the study of cells, including their origin, structure, function, and pathology.

DEA number A registration number assigned to physicians by the Drug Enforcement Administration for prescribing or dispensing controlled drugs.

Decontamination The use of physical or chemical means to remove, inactivate, or destroy bloodborne pathogens on a surface or item to the point where they are no longer capable of transmitting infectious particles and the surface or item is rendered safe for handling, use, or disposal.

Detergent An agent that cleanses by emulsifying dirt and oil.

Diagnosis The scientific method of determining and identifying a patient's condition.

Diagnostic procedure A procedure performed to assist in the diagnosis, management, and treatment of a patient's condition.

Diapedesis The ameboid movement of blood cells (especially leukocytes) through the wall of a capillary and out into the tissues.

Diastole The phase in the cardiac cycle in which the heart relaxes between contractions.

Diastolic pressure The point of lesser pressure on the arterial wall, which is recorded during diastole.

Differential diagnosis A determination of which of two or more diseases with similar symptoms is producing the patient's symptoms.

Dilation (of the cervix) The stretching of the external os from an opening a few millimeters wide to an opening large enough to allow the passage of an infant (approximately 10 cm).

Discharge summary report A brief statement of the significant events of a patient's hospitalization.

Disinfectant An agent used to destroy pathogenic microorganisms but not necessarily their spores. Disinfectants are usually applied to inanimate objects.

Dislocation An injury in which one end of a bone making up a joint is separated or displaced from its normal anatomic position.

Diuresis Secretion and passage of large amounts of urine.

Donor One who furnishes something such as blood, tissue, or organs to be used in another person.

Dose The quantity of a drug to be administered at one time.

Drug A chemical used for the treatment, prevention, or diagnosis of disease.

Dysmenorrhea Pain associated with the menstrual period.

Dyspareunia Pain in the vagina or pelvis experienced by a woman during sexual intercourse.

Dysplasia The growth of abnormal cells. Dysplasia is a precancerous condition that may or may not develop into cancer.

Dyspnea Shortness of breath or difficulty in breathing.

Dysrhythmia An irregular heart rhythm; also termed arrhythmia.

Dysuria Difficult or painful urination.

ECG cycle The graphic representation of a heartbeat.

Echocardiogram An ultrasound examination of the heart.

Ectocervix The part of the cervix that projects into the vagina and is lined with stratified squamous epithelium.

EDD Expected date of delivery, or due date.

Edema The retention of fluid in the tissues, resulting in swelling.

Effacement The thinning and shortening of the cervical canal from its normal length of 1 to 2 cm to a structure with paper-thin edges in which there is no canal at all. Effacement occurs late in pregnancy or during labor, or both. The purpose of effacement along with dilation is to permit passage of the infant into the birth canal.

Electrocardiogram (ECG) The graphic representation of the electrical activity of the heart.

Electrocardiograph The instrument used to record the electrical activity of the heart.

Electrode A conductor of electricity which is used to promote contact between the body and the electrocardiograph.

Electrolyte A chemical substance that promotes conduction of an electrical current.

Electronic medical record (EMR) A medical record that is stored on a computer.

Embryo The child in utero from the time of conception to the beginning of the first trimester.

Emergency medical services (EMS) system A network of community resources, equipment, and personnel that provides care to victims of injury or sudden illness.

Endocervix The mucous membrane lining the cervical canal.

Endoscope An instrument that consists of a tube and an optical system that is used for direct visual inspection of organs or cavities.

Enema An injection of fluid into the rectum to aid in the elimination of feces from the colon.

Engagement The entrance of the fetal head or the presenting part into the pelvic inlet.

Enteral nutrition The delivery of nutrients through a tube inserted into the gastrointestinal tract.

Erythema Reddening of the skin caused by dilation of superficial blood vessels in the skin.

Eupnea Normal respiration. The rate is 16 to 20 respirations per minute, the rhythm is even and regular, and the depth is normal.

Evacuated tube A closed glass or plastic tube that contains a premeasured vacuum.

Exhalation The act of breathing out.

External os The opening of the cervical canal of the uterus into the vagina.

Exudate A discharge produced by the body's tissues.

Fahrenheit scale A temperature scale on which the freezing point of water is 32° and the boiling point of water is 212°.

False-negative A test result indicating that a condition is absent when, in actuality, it is present.

False-positive A test result indicating that a condition is present when, in actuality, it is absent.

Familial Occurring in or affecting members of a family more frequently than would be expected by chance.

Fastidious Extremely delicate, difficult to culture, therefore involving specialized growth requirements.

Fasting Abstaining from food or fluids (except water) for a specified amount of time before the collection of a specimen.

Febrile Pertaining to fever.

Fetal heart rate The number of times per minute the fetal heart beats.

Fetal heart tones The sounds of the heartbeat of the fetus heard through the mother's abdominal wall.

Fetus The child in utero, from the third month after conception to birth; during the first 2 months of development, it is called an embryo.

Fever A body temperature that is above normal. Synonym for pyrexia.

Fibroblast An immature cell from which connective tissue can develop.

First aid The immediate care that is administered to an individual who is injured or suddenly becomes ill before complete medical care can be provided.

Flow rate The number of liters of oxygen per minute that comes out of an oxygen delivery system.

Fluoroscope An instrument used to view internal organs and structures directly.

Fluoroscopy Examination of a patient with a fluoroscope.

Forceps A two-pronged instrument for grasping and squeezing.

Fracture Any break in a bone.

Frenulum linguae The midline fold that connects the undersurface of the tongue with the floor of the mouth.

Frequency The condition of having to urinate often.

Fundus The dome-shaped upper portion of the uterus between the fallopian tubes.

Furuncle A localized staphylococcal infection that originates deep within a hair follicle; also known as a boil.

Gauge The diameter of the lumen of a needle used to administer medication.

Gene A unit of heredity.

Gestation The period of intrauterine development from conception to birth; the period of pregnancy. The average pregnancy lasts about 280 days, or 40 wefis, from the date of conception to childbirth.

Gestational age The age of the fetus between conception and birth.

Glycogen The form in which carbohydrate is stored in the body.

Glycosuria The presence of sugar in the urine.

Glycosylation The process of glucose attaching to hemoglobin.

Gravidity The total number of pregnancies a woman has had regardless of duration, including a current pregnancy.

Gynecology The branch of medicine that deals with diseases of the reproductive organs of women.

Hand hygiene The process of cleansing or sanitizing the hands.

Hazardous chemical Any chemical that presents a threat to the health and safety of an individual coming into contact with it.

HDL cholesterol A lipoprotein consisting of protein and cholesterol that removes excess cholesterol from the cells.

Health history report A collection of subjective data about a patient.

Hematology The study of blood and blood-forming tissues.

Hematoma A swelling or mass of coagulated blood caused by a break in a blood vessel.

Hematuria Blood present in the urine.

Hemoconcentration An increase in the concentration of nonfilterable blood components such as red blood cells, enzymes, iron, and calcium as a result of a decrease in the fluid content of the blood.

Hemoglobin The iron-containing pigment of erythrocytes that transports oxygen in the body.

Hemoglobin A$_{1c}$ Compound formed when glucose attaches or glycosylates to the protein in hemoglobin.

Hemolysis The breakdown of erythrocytes with the release of hemoglobin into the plasma; the breakdown of blood cells.

Hemophilia An inherited bleeding disorder caused by a deficiency of a clotting factor needed for proper coagulation of the blood.

Hemostasis The arrest of bleeding by natural or artificial means.

Home health care The provision of medical and nonmedical care in a patient's home or place of residence.

Homeostasis The state in which body systems are functioning normally and the internal environment of the body is in equilibrium; the body is in a healthy state.

Hyperglycemia An abnormally high level of glucose in the blood.

Hyperopia Farsightedness.

Hyperpnea An abnormal increase in the rate and depth of respiration.

Hyperpyrexia An extremely high fever.

Hypertension High blood pressure.

Hyperventilation An abnormally fast and deep type of breathing usually associated with acute anxiety conditions.

Hypochromic A red blood cell with a decreased concentration of hemoglobin.

Hypoglycemia An abnormally low level of glucose in the blood.

Hypopnea An abnormal decrease in the rate and depth of respiration.

Hypotension Low blood pressure.

Hypothermia A body temperature that is below normal.

Hypoxemia A decrease in the oxygen saturation of the blood. Hypoxemia may lead to hypoxia.

Hypoxia A reduction in the oxygen supply to the tissues of the body.

Immune globulins A blood product consisting of pooled human plasma containing antibodies.

Immunity The resistance of the body to the effects of a harmful agent such as a pathogenic microorganism or its toxins.

Immunization (active, artificial) The process of becoming immune or of rendering an individual immune through the use of a vaccine or toxoid.

Impacted Wedged firmly together so as to be immovable.

Incision A clean cut caused by a cutting instrument.

Incubate To provide proper conditions for growth and development. In microbiology, the act of placing a culture in a chamber (incubator), that meets optimal growth requirements for multiplication of the organisms, such as the proper temperature, humidity, and darkness.

Incubation period The interval of time between invasion by a pathogenic microorganism and the appearance of first symptoms of the disease.

Induration An abnormally raised hardened area of the skin with clearly defined margins.

Infant A child from birth to 12 months of age.

Infection The condition in which the body, or part of it, is invaded by a pathogen.

Infectious disease A disease caused by a pathogen that produces harmful effects on its host.

Infiltration The process by which a substance passes into and is deposited within the substance of a cell, tissue, or organ.

Inflammation A protective response of the body to trauma and the entrance of foreign matter. The purpose of inflammation is to destroy invading microorganisms and to remove damaged tissue debris from the area so that proper healing can occur. Symptoms at the site of inflammation include pain, swelling, redness, and warmth.

Informed consent Consent given by a patient for a medical procedure after being informed of the nature of his or her condition, the purpose of the procedure, and has been given an explanation of risks involved with the procedure, alternative treatments or procedures available, the likely outcome of the procedure, and the risks involved with declining or delaying the procedure.

Infusion The administration of fluids, medications, or nutrients into a vein.

Inhalation The act of breathing in.

Inhalation administration The administration of medication by way of air or other vapor being drawn into the lungs.

Inoculate To introduce microorganisms into a culture medium for growth and multiplication.

Inpatient A patient who has been admitted to a hospital for at least one overnight stay.

Inscription The part of a prescription that indicates the name of the drug and the drug dosage.

Inspection The process of observing a patient to detect signs of disease.

Instillation The dropping of a liquid into a body cavity.

Insufflate To blow a powder, vapor, or gas (such as air) into a body cavity.

Intercostal Between the ribs.

Internal os The internal opening of the cervical canal into the uterus.

Interval The length of a wave or the length of a wave with a segment.

Intradermal injection The introduction of medication into the dermal layer of the skin.

Intramuscular injection The introduction of medication into the muscular layer of the body.

Intravenous therapy The administration of a liquid agent directly into a patient's vein, where it is distributed throughout the body by way of the circulatory system.

In vitro Occurring in glass. Refers to tests performed under artificial conditions, as in the laboratory.

In vivo Occurring in the living body or organism.

Irrigation The washing of a body canal with a flowing solution.

Ischemia Deficiency of blood in a body part.

Ketonuria The presence of ketone bodies in the urine.

Ketosis An accumulation of large amounts of ketone bodies in the tissues and body fluids.

Korotkoff sounds Sounds heard during the measurement of blood pressure that are used to determine the systolic and diastolic blood pressure readings.

Laboratory test The clinical analysis and study of materials, fluids, or tissues obtained from patients to assist in diagnosing and treatment of disease.

Laceration A wound in which the tissues are torn apart, leaving ragged and irregular edges.

LDL cholesterol A lipoprotein, consisting of protein and cholesterol, that picks up cholesterol and delivers it to the cells.

Length (recumbent) The measurement from the vertex of the head to the heel of the foot in a supine position.

Leukocytosis An abnormally high number of white blood cells (greater than 11,000 per cubic millimeter of blood).

Leukopenia An abnormal decrease in the number of white blood cells (less than 4500 per cubic millimeter of blood).

Ligate To tie off and close a structure such as a severed blood vessel.

Lipoprotein A complex molecule consisting of protein and a lipid fraction such as cholesterol. Lipoproteins function in transporting lipids in the blood.

Load Articles that are being sterilized.

Local anesthetic A drug that produces a loss of feeling and an inability to perceive pain in only a specific part of the body.

Lochia A discharge from the uterus after delivery, that consists of blood, tissue, white blood cells, and some bacteria.

Long arm cast A cast that extends from the axilla to the fingers, usually with a bend in the elbow.

Long leg cast A cast that extends from the midthigh to the toes.

Maceration The softening and breaking down of the skin as a result of prolonged exposure to moisture.

Macrocytic An abnormally large red blood cell.

Malaise A vague sense of body discomfort, weakness, and fatigue that often marks the onset of a disease and continues through the course of the illness.

Manometer An instrument for measuring pressure.

Material safety data sheet (MSDS) A sheet that provides information regarding a chemical, its hazards, and measures to take to prevent injury and illness when handling the chemical.

Mayo tray A broad, flat metal tray placed on a stand and used to hold sterile instruments and supplies once it has been covered with a sterile towel.

Medical asepsis Practices that are employed to reduce the number and hinder the transmission of pathogens.

Medical impressions Conclusions drawn by the physician from an interpretation of data. Other terms for impressions include *provisional diagnosis* and *tentative diagnosis*.

Medical record A written record of important information regarding a patient, including the care of that individual and the progress of the patient's condition.

Medical record format The way a medical record is organized. The two main types of medical record format are the source-oriented record and the problem-oriented record.

Melena The darkening of the stool caused by the presence of blood in an amount of 50 ml or greater.

Meniscus The curved surface on a column of liquid in a tube.

Menopause The permanent cessation of menstruation, which usually occurs between the ages of 45 and 55.

Menorrhagia Excessive bleeding during a menstrual period, in the number of days or the amount of blood or both; also called dysfunctional uterine bleeding (DUB).

Mensuration The process of measuring the patient.

Metrorrhagia Bleeding between menstrual periods.

Microbiology The scientific study of microorganisms and their activities.

Microcytic An abnormally small red blood cell.

Microorganism A microscopic plant or animal.

Micturition The act of voiding urine.

Mucous membrane A membrane lining body passages or cavities that open to the outside.

Multigravida A woman who has been pregnant more than once.

Multipara A woman who has completed two or more pregnancies to the age of fetal viability regardless of whether they ended in live infants or stillbirths.

Myopia Nearsightedness.

Needle biopsy A type of biopsy in which tissue from deep within the body is obtained by the insertion of a biopsy needle through the skin.

Nephron The functional unit of the kidney.

Nocturia Excessive (voluntary) urination during the night.

Nocturnal enuresis Inability of an individual to control urination at night during sleep (bedwetting).

Nonabsorbable suture Suture material that is not absorbed by the body and either remains permanently in the body tissue and becomes encapsulated by fibrous tissue or is removed.

Noncritical item An item that comes into contact with intact skin but not mucous membranes.

Nonintact skin Skin that has a break in the surface. This includes, but is not limited to, abrasions, cuts, hangnails, paper cuts, and burns.

Nonpathogen A microorganism that does not normally produce disease.

Nonwaived test A complex laboratory test that does not meet the CLIA criteria for waiver and is subject to the CLIA regulations.

Normal flora Harmless, nonpathogenic microorganisms that normally reside in many parts of the body but do not cause disease.

Normal sinus rhythm Refers to an ECG that is within normal limits.

Normochromic A red blood cell with a normal concentration of hemoglobin.

Normocytic A normal-sized red blood cell.

Nullipara A woman who has not carried a pregnancy to the point of fetal viability (20 wefis of gestation).

Objective symptom A symptom that can be observed by an examiner.

Obstetrics The branch of medicine concerned with the care of the woman during pregnancy, childbirth, and the postpartum period.

Occult blood Blood in such a small amount that it is not detectable by the unaided eye.

Oliguria Decreased or scanty output of urine.

Ophthalmoscope An instrument for examining the interior of the eye.

Opportunistic infection An infection that results from a defective immune system that cannot defend the body from pathogens normally found in the environment.

Optimum growth temperature The temperature at which an organism grows best.

Oral administration Administration of medication by mouth.

Orthopedist A physician who specializes in the diagnosis and treatment of disorders of the musculoskeletal system, which includes the bones, joints, ligaments, tendons, muscles, and nerves.

Orthopnea The condition in which breathing is easier when an individual is in a standing or sitting position.

Osteochondritis Inflammation of bone and cartilage.

Osteomyelitis Inflammation of the bone or bone marrow due to bacterial infection.

Otoscope An instrument for examining the external ear canal and tympanic membrane.

Oxygen therapy The administration of supplemental oxygen in concentrations greater than room air to treat or prevent hypoxemia.

Oxyhemoglobin Hemoglobin that has combined with oxygen.

Palpation The process of feeling with the hands to detect signs of disease.

Paper-based patient record (PPR) A medical record in paper form.

Parenteral Taken into the body through piercing of the skin barrier or mucous membranes, such as through needlesticks, human bites, cuts, and abrasions. Administration of medication by injection.

Parity The condition of having borne offspring regardless of the outcome.

Pathogen A disease-producing microorganism.

Patient An individual receiving medical care.

Peak flow rate The maximum volume of air that can be exhaled when the patient blows into a peak flow meter as forcefully and as rapidly as possible.

Pediatrician A medical doctor who specializes in the care and development of children and the diagnosis and treatment of children's diseases.

Pediatrics The branch of medicine that deals with the care and development of children and the diagnosis and treatment of children's diseases.

Percussion The process of tapping the body to detect signs of disease.

Percussion hammer An instrument with a rubber head, used for testing reflexes.

Perimenopause Before the onset of menopause, the phase during which the woman with regular periods changes to irregular cycles and increased periods of amenorrhea.

Perinatal Relating to the period shortly before and after birth.

Perineum The external region between the vaginal orifice and the anus in a female and between the scrotum and the anus in a male.

Peroxidase (as it pertains to the guaiac slide test) A substance that is able to transfer oxygen from hydrogen peroxide to oxidize guaiac, causing the guaiac to turn blue.

pH The unit that describes the acidity or alkalinity of a solution.

Phagocytosis The engulfing and destruction of foreign particles, such as bacteria, by special cells called phagocytes.

Pharmacology The study of drugs.

Phlebotomist A health professional trained in the collection of blood specimens.

Phlebotomy Incision of a vein for the removal or withdrawal of blood; the collection of blood.

Physical examination An assessment of each part of the patient's body to obtain objective data about the patient that assists the physician in determining the patient's state of health.

Physical examination report A report of the objective findings from the physician's assessment of each body system.

Plasma The liquid part of the blood, consisting of a clear, straw-colored fluid that makes up approximately 55% of the total blood volume.

Poison Any substance that causes illness, injury, or death if it enters the body.

Polycythemia A disorder in which there is an increase in the red cell mass.

Polyuria Increased output of urine.

Position The relation of the presenting part of the fetus to the maternal pelvis.

Postexposure prophylaxis (PEP) Treatment administered to an individual after exposure to an infectious disease to prevent the disease.

Postoperative After a surgical operation.

Postpartum Occurring after childbirth.

Preeclampsia A major complication of pregnancy, the cause of which is unknown, characterized by increasing hypertension, albuminuria, and edema. If this condition is neglected or is not treated properly, it may develop into eclampsia, which could cause maternal convulsions and coma. Preeclampsia generally occurs between the twentieth wefi of pregnancy and the end of the first wefi postpartum.

Prenatal Before birth.

Preoperative Preceding a surgical operation.

Presbyopia A decrease in the elasticity of the lens that occurs with aging, resulting in a decreased ability to focus on close objects.

Preschool child A child from 3 to 6 years old.

Prescription A physician's order authorizing the dispensing of a drug by a pharmacist.

Presentation Indication of the part of the fetus that is closest to the cervix and will be delivered first. A cephalic presentation is a delivery in which the fetal head is presenting against the cervix. A breech presentation is a delivery in which the buttocks or feet are presented instead of the head.

Pressure point A site on the body where an artery lies close to the surface of the skin and can be compressed against an underlying bone to control bleeding.

Preterm birth Delivery occurring at between 20 and 37 wefis regardless of whether the child was born alive or stillborn.

Primigravida A woman who is pregnant for the first time.

Primipara A woman who has carried a pregnancy to viability (20 wefis of gestation) for the first time, regardless of whether the infant was stillborn or alive at birth.

Product insert A printed document supplied by the manufacturer with a laboratory test product that contains information on the proper storage and use of the product.

Problem Any condition that requires further observation, diagnosis, management, or patient education.

Profile An array of laboratory tests for identifying a disease state or evaluating a particular organ or organ system.

Prognosis The probable course and outcome of a patient's condition and the patient's prospects for recovery.

Proteinuria The presence of protein in the urine.

Puerperium The period of time, usually 4 to 6 wefis after delivery, in which the uterus and the body systems are returning to normal.

Pulse oximeter A computerized device consisting of a probe and a monitor used to measure the oxygen saturation of arterial blood.

Pulse oximetry The use of a pulse oximeter to measure the oxygen saturation of arterial blood.

Pulse pressure The difference between the systolic and diastolic pressures.

Pulse rhythm The time interval between heartbeats.

Pulse volume The strength of the heartbeat.

Puncture A wound made by a sharp pointed object piercing the skin.

Pyuria The presence of pus in the urine.

Qualitative test A test that indicates whether or not a substance is present in the specimen being tested and also provides an approximate indication of the amount of the substance present.

Quality control The application of methods to ensure that test results are reliable and valid, and that errors are detected and eliminated.

Quantitative test A test that indicates the exact amount of a chemical substance that is present in the body with the results being reported in measurable units.

Quickening The first movements of the fetus in utero as felt by the mother, which usually occurs between the sixteenth and twentieth wefis of gestation, and are felt consistently thereafter.

Radiation The transfer of energy, such as heat, in the form of waves.

Radiograph A permanent record of a picture of an internal body organ or structure produced on radiographic film.

Radiography The taking of permanent records (radiographs) of internal body organs and structures by passing x-rays through the body to act on a specially sensitized film.

Radiologist A physician who specializes in the diagnosis and treatment of disease using radiation and other imaging techniques (such as ultrasound, CT scans, MRIs, and nuclear medicine).

Radiology The branch of medicine that deals with the use of radiation and other imaging techniques in the diagnosis and treatment of disease.

Radiolucent Describing a structure that permits the passage of x-rays.

Radiopaque Describing a structure that obstructs the passage of x-rays.

Reagent A substance that produces a reaction with a patient specimen that allows detection or measurement of the substance by the test system.

Recipient One who receives something, such as a blood transfusion, from a donor.

Reference range (for laboratory tests) A certain established and acceptable parameter or reference range within which the laboratory test results of a healthy individual are expected to fall. (Also known as reference value and reference interval).

Refraction The deflection or bending of light rays by a lens.

Regulated medical waste Medical waste that poses a threat to health and safety.

Renal threshold The concentration at which a substance in the blood that is not normally excreted by the kidneys begins to appear in the urine.

Reservoir host The organism that becomes infected by a pathogen and also serves as a source of transfer of the pathogen to others.

Resident flora Harmless, nonpathogenic microorganisms that normally reside on the skin and usually do not cause disease; also known as normal flora.

Resistance The natural ability of an organism to remain unaffected by harmful substances in its environment.

Retention The inability to empty the bladder. The urine is being produced normally but is not being voided.

Reverse chronological order Arranging documents with the most recent document on top or in the front, which means that the oldest document is on the bottom or at the back of a section or file.

Risk factor Anything that increases an individual's chance of developing a disease. Some risk factors (e.g., smoking) can be avoided, but others (e.g., age, family history) cannot.

Routine test Laboratory test performed routinely on apparently healthy patients to assist in the early detection of disease.

Sanitization A process to remove organic matter from an article and to lower the number of microorganisms to a safe level as determined by public health requirements.

SaO$_2$ (saturation of arterial oxygen) Abbreviation for the percentage of hemoglobin that is saturated with oxygen in arterial blood.

Scalpel A surgical knife used to divide tissues.

School-age child A child from 6 to 12 years of age.

Scissors A cutting instrument.

Sebaceous cyst A thin, closed sac or capsule that contains fatty secretions from a sebaceous gland.

Segment The portion of the ECG between two waves.

Seizure A sudden episode of involuntary muscular contractions and relaxation, often accompanied by a change in sensation, b›avior, and level of consciousness.

Semicritical item An item that comes into contact with nonintact skin and intact mucous membranes.

Sequela (*pl.* sequelae) A morbid (secondary) condition occurring as a result of a less serious primary infection.

Serum The clear, straw-colored part of the blood (plasma) that remains after the solid elements and the clotting factor fibrinogen have been removed.

Shock The failure of the cardiovascular system to deliver enough blood to all the vital organs of the body.

Short arm cast A cast that extends from below the elbow to the fingers.

Short leg cast A cast that begins just below the knee and extends to the toes.

Sigmoidoscope An endoscope that is specially designed for passage through the anus to permit visualization of the rectum and sigmoid colon.

Sigmoidoscopy The visual examination of the rectum and sigmoid colon using a sigmoidoscope.

Signatura The part of a prescription that indicates the information to print on the medication label.

Smear Material spread on a slide for microscope examination.

Soak The direct immersion of a body part in water or a medicated solution.

SOAP format A method of organization for recording progress notes. The SOAP format includes the following categories: subjective data, objective data, assessment, and plan.

Sonogram The record obtained with ultrasonography.

Specific gravity The weight of a substance compared with the weight of an equal volume of a substance known as the standard. In urinalysis, the specific gravity refers to the measurement of the amount of dissolved substance in the urine, compared with the same amount of distilled water.

Specimen A small sample of something taken to show the nature of the whole.

Speculum An instrument for opening a body orifice or cavity for viewing.

Sphygmomanometer An instrument for measuring arterial blood pressure.

Spirilla (*sing.* spirillum) Bacteria that have a spiral or curved shape.

Spirometer An instrument for measuring air taken into and expelled from the lungs.

Spirometry Measurement of an individual's breathing capacity by means of a spirometer.

Splint An orthopedic device used to immobilize, restrain, or support a part of the body.

SpO₂ (saturation of peripheral oxygen) Abbreviation for the percentage of hemoglobin that is saturated with oxygen in arterial blood as measured by a pulse oximeter.

Sponge A porous, absorbent pad, such as a 4-inch gauze pad or cotton surrounded by gauze, used to absorb fluids, to apply medication, or to cleanse an area.

Spore A hard, thick-walled capsule formed by some bacteria that contains only the essential parts of the protoplasm of the bacterial cell.

Sprain Trauma to a joint that causes injury to the ligaments.

Sterile Free of all living microorganisms and bacterial spores.

Sterilization The process of destroying all forms of microbial life, including bacterial spores.

Stethoscope An instrument for amplifying and hearing sounds produced by the body.

Strain An overstretching of a muscle caused by trauma.

Streaking In microbiology, the process of inoculating a culture to provide for the growth of colonies on the surface of a solid medium. Streaking is accomplished by skimming a wire inoculating loop that contains the specimen across the surface of the medium, using a back-and-forth motion.

Streptolysin An exotoxin produced by beta-hemolytic streptococci, which completely hemolyzes red blood cells.

Subcutaneous injection Introduction of medication beneath the skin, into the subcutaneous or fatty layer of the body.

Subjective symptom A symptom that is felt by the patient but is not observable by an examiner.

Sublingual administration Administration of medication by placing it under the tongue, where it dissolves and is absorbed through the mucous membrane.

Subscription The part of the prescription that gives directions to the pharmacist and usually designates the number of doses to be dispensed.

Supernatant The clear liquid that remains at the top after a precipitate settles.

Superscription The part of a prescription consisting of the symbol Rx (from the Latin word *recipe*, meaning "take").

Suppuration The process of pus formation.

Suprapubic aspiration The passing of a sterile needle through the abdominal wall into the bladder to remove urine.

Surgery The branch of medicine that deals with operative and manual procedures for correction of deformities, repair of injuries, and diagnosis and treatment of certain diseases.

Surgical asepsis Practices that keep objects and areas sterile or free from microorganisms.

Susceptible Easily affected; lacking resistance.

Sutures Material used to approximate tissues with surgical stitches.

Swaged needle A needle with suturing material permanently attached to its end.

Symptom Any change in the body or its functioning that indicates the presence of disease.

Systole The phase in the cardiac cycle in which the ventricles contract, sending blood out of the heart and into the aorta and pulmonary aorta.

Systolic pressure The point of maximum pressure on the arterial walls, which is recorded during systole.

Tachycardia An abnormally fast heart rate (more than 100 beats per minute).

Tachypnea An abnormal increase in the respiratory rate of more than 20 respirations per minute.

Term birth Delivery occurring after 37 wefis, regardless of whether the child was born alive or stillborn.

Test system A setup that includes all of the test components required to perform a laboratory test such as testing devices, controls, and testing reagents.

Thermolabile Easily affected or changed by heat.

Thready pulse A pulse with a decreased volume that feels weak and thin.

Toddler A child from 1 to 3 years old.

Topical administration Application of a drug to a particular spot, usually for a local action.

Toxemia A pathologic condition occurring in pregnant women that includes preeclampsia and eclampsia. If preeclampsia goes undiagnosed or is not satisfactorily controlled, it could develop into eclampsia, characterized by convulsions and coma.

Toxoid A toxin (poisonous substance produced by a bacterium) that has been treated by heat or chemicals to destroy its harmful properties. It is administered to an individual to prevent an infectious disease by stimulating the production of antibodies in that individual.

Transfusion The administration of whole blood or blood products through the intravenous route.

Transient flora Microorganisms that reside on the superficial skin layers and are picked up in the course of daily activities. They are often pathogenic but can be removed easily from the skin by sanitizing the hands.

Trimester Three months, or one third, of the gestational period of pregnancy.

Tympanic membrane A thin, semitransparent membrane located between the external ear canal and the middle ear that receives and transmits sound waves; also known as the eardrum.

Ultrasonography The use of high-frequency sound waves (ultrasound) to produce an image of an organ or tissue.

Urgency The immediate need to urinate.

Urinalysis The physical, chemical, and microscopic analysis of urine.

Urinary incontinence The inability to retain urine.

Vaccine A suspension of attenuated (weakened) or killed microorganisms administered to an individual to prevent an infectious disease by stimulating the production of antibodies in that individual.

Venipuncture Puncturing of a vein.

Venous reflux The backflow of blood (from an evacuated tube) into the patient's vein.

Venous stasis The temporary cessation or slowing of the venous blood flow.

Vertex The top of the head.

Vial A closed glass container with a rubber stopper that holds medication.

Void To empty the bladder.

Vulva The region of the external female genital organs.

Waived test A laboratory test that meets the CLIA criteria for being a simple procedure that is easy to perform and has a low risk of erroneous test results. Waived tests include tests that have been FDA-approved for use by patients at home.

Wheal A tense, pale raised area of the skin.

Wheezing A continuous high-pitched whistling musical sound heard particularly during exhalation and sometimes during inhalation.

Wound A break in the continuity of an external or internal surface caused by physical means.

Index